BRITISH
NATIONAL
FORMULARY
1988

BRITISH NATIONAL FORMULARY

Number 16 (1988)

British Medical Association
and
Royal Pharmaceutical Society of Great Britain

Copies may be obtained through any bookseller or, in any case of difficulty, direct from the publishers:

British Medical Association
Tavistock Square
London WC1H 9JP, England

The Pharmaceutical Press
1 Lambeth High Street
London SE1 7JN, England

ISBN: 0 85369 196 7. ISSN: 0260–535X

Typeset in Great Britain by Page Bros (Norwich) Ltd, Norwich, Norfolk NR6 6SA and printed and bound by The Bath Press, Bath, Avon BA2 3BL.

Joint Formulary Committee
1988–89

Chairman

C. F. George, BSc, MD, FRCP

Deputy Chairman

J. P. Kerr, FRPharmS

Committee Members

M. Goodman, MRCS, LRCP, FRCGP, DObstRCOG

C. R. Hitchings, BPharm, MSc, FRPharmS, MCPP

G. Jones, BA, PhD, FRCP

F. P. Marsh, MA, MB, BChir, FRCP

G. M. Mitchell, KStJ, MB, ChB, FRPharmS

R. H. Smith, MB, BS

B. A. Wills, BPharm, PhD, FRPharmS, CChem, FRSC

N. L. Wood, BPharm, MRPharmS

Joint Secretaries

Vivienne H. Nathanson, MB, BS

A. Wade, BPharm, MPhil, FRPharmS

Executive Editor

Anne B. Prasad, FRPharmS

Assistant Editor

Sheenagh M. Townsend-Smith, BSc, DipLib

Editorial Staff

K. B. K. Davis, MRPharmS

Brenda M. Ecclestone, MRPharmS, ALA

D. K. Mehta, BPharm, MSc, MRPharmS

Executive Secretary

Susan M. Thomas, BSc(Econ), MA

Contents

APPENDIXES AND INDEXES

Arrangement of Information

Guidance on prescribing
This chapter includes information on prescription writing, prescribing for children and elderly patients, prescribing in terminal care, and prescribing for patients with liver disease or renal impairment, and in pregnancy or lactation. Information is also given on adverse reactions, controlled drugs, and dependence.

Emergency treatment of poisoning
The main intention of this chapter is to provide information on the management of acute poisoning when first seen in the home, although certain aspects of hospital-based treatment are mentioned.

Classified notes on drugs and preparations
The main text consists of classified notes on drugs and preparations used in the treatment of diseases and conditions. These notes are split into 15 chapters, each of which is related to a particular system of the human body or to another main subject. Each chapter is divided into sections which begin with appropriate *notes for prescribers*. These notes are intended to provide information to doctors, pharmacists, nurses etc. to facilitate the selection of suitable treatment. The notes are followed by details of relevant drugs and preparations.

DRUGS appear under pharmacopoeial or other non-proprietary titles. When there is an *appropriate current monograph* (Medicines Act 1968, Section 65) preference is given to a name at the head of that monograph; otherwise a British Approved Name, if available, is used. If there is an acknowledged reference drug, information on it is usually given first; otherwise the drugs are arranged alphabetically.

PREPARATIONS usually follow immediately after the drug which is their main ingredient. They are printed in text-sized type but those considered by the Committee to be less suitable for prescribing are described in smaller type. Small type is also used for the entries describing foods for special diets, preparations for stoma care, and wound management products. Preparations are included under a non-proprietary title only if
  (a) they are marketed under such a title,
  (b) they are not otherwise prescribable under the NHS, or
  (c) they may be prepared extemporaneously.
  If proprietary preparations are of a distinctive colour this is stated, but flavour is not usually mentioned.
  In the case of compound preparations the indications, cautions, contra-indications, side-effects, and drug interactions of all constituents should be taken into account in prescribing; usually the ingredients should be looked up separately. Compound preparations may contain ingredients not suggested by the name or title; e.g. Sandocal® contains potassium.

PREPARATIONS NOT AVAILABLE FOR NHS PRESCRIPTION. The symbol NHS has been placed against those preparations included in the BNF that are not prescribable under the NHS. Those prescribable only for specific disorders have a foot-note specifying the condition(s) for which the preparation remains available. Prescribers are reminded that although some preparations are not *prescribable* by brand name under the NHS the brand in question may nevertheless be *dispensed* if no non-proprietary preparation is marketed.

PRESCRIPTION-ONLY MEDICINES. The symbol PoM has been placed against those preparations that are available only on medical or dental prescription. For more detailed information see *Medicines and Poisons Guide*, 4th edition, London, Pharmaceutical Press, 1984. The symbol CD indicates that the preparation is subject to the prescription requirements of the Misuse of Drugs Act. For regulations governing prescriptions for such preparations see pages 7–9.

PRICES (see p. 1) have been calculated whenever possible from the basic cost used in pricing NHS prescriptions dispensed in February 1988; these prices are based on the largest pack size of the preparation in use in pharmacies or, in the case of an extemporaneous preparation, on the net cost of the ingredients used to make it.

DILUENTS indicated in the entries for certain creams, ointments, elixirs, and mixtures are intended to be used when lower strengths or doses are ordered, as indicated under 'General Guidance'.

Appendixes and indexes
The appendixes include information on drug interactions, intravenous additives, borderline substances, and cautionary and advisory labels for dispensed medicines. Where relevant they are designed for use in association with the main body of the text.
  The Formulary (for extemporaneous preparations) and the Dental Practitioners' List are also included in this section. The indexes consist of the Index of Manufacturers and the Main Index.

Preface

A new type of British National Formulary was introduced in February 1981, and the scope of the book was considerably increased although it still remained a pocket book for those concerned with the prescribing, dispensing and administration of medicines. Earlier editions of the BNF included only those products that had the confidence of the Joint Formulary Committee, and consequently only a limited selection of the many drugs and preparations available were described in the book. From 1981, the basis of selection has been changed and information is included on most products available to prescribers in the United Kingdom. The entries, coupled with the relevant notes for prescribers, are intended to help in the choice of appropriate treatment of each patient.

Most of the preparations now follow immediately after the notes for prescribers with which they are associated. It is considered that this arrangement will help in the selection process. A small formulary section has been retained for convenience in dispensing those formulated preparations that are commonly prepared extemporaneously.

In preparing the sixteenth edition an attempt has been made to clarify some portions of the guidance on controlled drugs and drug dependence. In chapter 1 the presentation of section 1.7 (preparations for haemorrhoids) has been extensively reorganised. In chapter 2 the presentation of sections 2.3 (anti-arrhythmics) and 2.12 (lipid-lowering drugs) have been revised and reorganised. In chapter 5 significant amendments have been made to section 5.4.1 (anti-malarials). In chapter 9 extensive revision has been carried out on the presentation of doses of iron salts (section 9.1.1); section 9.2.1.2 (oral rehydration) has been rewritten, and revised guidelines on fluoride supplementation have been introduced into section 9.5.3. Significant amendments have been made to some of the vaccines in chapter 14 to reflect the new DHSS guidelines. For ease of reference the list of dental preparations in the Dental Practitioners' Formulary has been reorganised into alphabetical order.

This is the first BNF to include a section on intra-uterine contraceptive devices (section 7.3.4); in section 7.3.1 combined oral contraceptives have been grouped according to their oestrogen content.

The 1988 BP has now been published and will become official from 1st December 1988; significant changes affecting preparations in the BNF have been noted in this edition, particularly in the formulary section.

The BNF continues to include details of prices. Basic net prices have been introduced to provide better indications of relative cost and enable prescribers to take into account the need to make the best use of available resources. Good prescribing requires careful consideration of the needs of the patient and the condition being treated; these factors may result in a limitation of choice. However, where there is a choice of a number of suitable preparations to treat a particular disease or condition the relative net prices may be used in making a selection on a basis of cost. It should be emphasised that cost-effective prescribing must take into account other factors such as dose frequency and duration of treatment that affect the total cost. The use of more expensive drugs is also justified if it will result in better treatment of the patient or a reduction of the length of an illness or the time spent in hospital.

The BNF is revised twice yearly and numerous changes are made between issues. All copies of BNF Number 15 (1988) should therefore be withdrawn and replaced by BNF Number 16 (1988). Changes made after the preparation of the main text are included on p. xii. Dose and classification changes are also there.

The BNF is intended to be a pocket book for rapid reference and so cannot contain all the information necessary for prescribing and dispensing. It should be supplemented as necessary from specialised publications. Manufacturers' data sheets prepared in accordance with the Medicines (Data Sheet) Regulations 1972 are available for most proprietary medicines and these should also be consulted. Less detail is given in the chapters on malignant disease and immunosuppression, and anaesthesia, as it is expected that those undertaking treatment will have specialised knowledge and will consult specialist literature. Supplementary information may be available from local drug information services.

The Joint Formulary Committee acknowledges the help of individuals and organisations that provided information or advised on specific matters. The principal contributors for this edition were J. M. Aitken, S. P. Allison, D. G. Arkell, R. S. Atkinson, C. G. Barnes, L. Beeley, D. R. Bell, D. J. Bradley, D. A. Chamberlain, W. A. M. Cutting, J. F. Davidson, S. I. Davidson, R. Dinwiddie, J. A. Dudgeon, A. J. Duxbury, H. M. Elliston, A. M. Geddes, A. H. Ghodse, J. Guillebaud, C. H. Hawkes, P. Hobson, A. V. Hoffbrand, M. J. S. Langman, R. Marks, M. W. McNicol, G. M. Mead, D. J. Oliver, P. Phillips-Howard, A. T. Proudfoot, L. E. Ramsay, R. S. Sawers, M. C. Sheppard, S. D. Shorvon, C. W. Smith, E. R. Tallett, A. Tattersfield, G. R. Thompson, V. R. Tindall, T. D. Turner, D. A. Warrell, P. Watkins. The Committee also wishes to express its thanks to correspondents in the pharmaceutical industry who provided information and made numerous comments on points of detail, to colleagues who have advised members of the committee and the editorial staff on specific matters, to D. M. Salisbury for advice on the DHSS vaccine guidelines, to C. Loewe for supplementary checks, to H. Johns for legal advice, and to T. M. Roberts for clerical assistance. Finally, the Committee would like to thank those doctors, pharmacists, nurses, and others who sent comments and suggestions.

Comments and constructive criticism will be welcome, and should be sent to the Executive Editor, British National Formulary, 1 Lambeth High Street, London SE1 7JN.

Product liability
The Consumer Protection Act 1987 came into force on 1 March 1988.
Guidance is provided in:
British Medical Journal, 27 February 1988, *296*, 635.
The Pharmaceutical Journal, 2 January 1988, *240*, 25.

New Preparations

Preparations included in appropriate sections of BNF No. 16

Adalat IC	Bricanyl Turbohaler	Froben SR	Paritane
Almodan	Britiazim	Mercilon	Pred Forte
Anexate	Carbo Cort (r)	Minims Metipranolol	Sinemet LS
Bactroban Nasal	Dalacin T	Minulet	Slow Sodium (r)
Balneum with Tar	Elantan LA50	Monocor	Trosyl
Baltar	Emcor	Nimotop	Ventodisks
Becodisks	Erwinase	Oramorph	

(r) indicates discontinued preparation reintroduced by manufacturer
Note. NHS Paxalgesic Tablets remain available

Preparations too late for inclusion in appropriate sections of BNF No. 16

Alphosyl® (Stafford-Miller)

Shampoo, allantoin 0.2%, refined coal tar extract 5%. Net price 125 ml = £1.30. ACBS: for psoriasis and other scaly disorders of the scalp

PoM **Becotide**® (A&H)

Rotacaps®, dark brown/clear, beclomethasone dipropionate 400 micrograms. Net price 100 = £27.27. Label: 8, counselling advised, dose (see p. 122)

Calcichew® (Shire)

Tablets (chewable), calcium carbonate 1.26 g (500 mg calcium or 12.6 mmol Ca^{2+}). Net price 100 = £9.78. Label: 24

Dose: calcium supplement, 1 to be chewed 3 times a day

▼ PoM **Carace**® (Morson)

Tablets, lisinopril 2.5 mg (blue), net price 50 = £15.30; 5 mg (scored), 28-tab pack = £10.14; 10 mg (yellow, scored), 28-tab pack = £12.13; 20 mg (orange, scored), 28-tab pack = £20.30

Dose: hypertension, initially 2.5 mg daily; usual maintenance dose 10–20 mg daily; max. 40 mg daily; diuretic should be stopped for few days before starting lisinopril
Heart failure, see manufacturer's literature
Cautions: see ACE inhibitors (section 2.5.5)

▼ PoM **Corwin**® (Stuart)

Tablets, yellow, f/c, xamoterol (as fumarate) 200 mg. Net price 56-tab pack = £26.60

Dose: chronic heart failure (in patients who have symptoms on exertion) 1 tablet twice daily

▼ PoM **Cymevene**® (Syntex)

Intravenous infusion, powder for reconstitution, ganciclovir (as sodium salt). Net price 500-mg vial = £17.15
For life-threatening or sight-threatening cytomegalovirus infection in immunocompromised patients

PoM **Dimotane**® **Plus LA** (Robins)

Tablets, s/r, f/c, brompheniramine maleate 12 mg, pseudoephedrine hydrochloride 120 mg. Net price 14-tab pack = 91p. Label: 2, 25

Dose: adults, 1 tablet twice daily

▼ PoM **Epilim**® Intravenous (Labaz)

Injection, powder for reconstitution, sodium valproate. Net price 400-mg vial (with 4-ml amp water for injections) = £9.00

Dose: continuation of treatment when oral valproate not possible, *by intravenous infusion*, at same dosage as by mouth; other patients, *by intravenous injection* over 3–5 minutes, 400–800 mg (up to 10 mg/kg) followed by intravenous infusion up to max. of 2.5 g daily

PoM **Franol**® (Winthrop) [New formulation]

Tablets, ephedrine hydrochloride 11 mg, theophylline 120 mg. Net price 100-tab pack = £5.11. Label: 21

Plus tablets, ephedrine sulphate 15 mg, theophylline 120 mg. Net price 50-tab pack = £4.15. Label: 21

Note. New formulations are not subject to Controlled Drug Regulations

Hydromol® (Quinoderm Ltd)

Cream, arachis oil 10%, isopropyl myristate 5%, liquid paraffin 10%, sodium pyrrolidone carboxylate 2.5%, sodium lactate 1%. Net price 50 g = £1.82; 100 g = £2.97; 500 g = £9.49. *Additives:* fragrance

NHS **Kaltocarb**® (BritCair)

Dressing, 3 layers: wound-facing layer of calcium alginate fibre; absorbent middle layer of activated charcoal cloth; backing layer of bonded polyester and viscose non-woven material. Net price 7.5 cm × 12 cm, each = £1.50
Uses: treatment of discharging infected malodorous wounds and ulcers

Manevac® (Galen) [formerly Agiolax®]

Granules, coated, senna fruit 12.4%, ispaghula 54.2%. Net price 250 g = £2.48. Label: 14, 25, 27

Dose: 1–2 level 5-ml spoonfuls with water or warm drink after supper and, if necessary, before breakfast or every 6 hours in resistant cases for 1–3 days; CHILD 5–12 years 1 level 5-ml spoonful daily

PoM **Mantadine**® (Du Pont)

Capsules, red, amantadine hydrochloride 100 mg. Net price 14-cap pack = £2.05; 100 = £14.70

Milupa PKU 2® (Milupa)

Granules, containing essential and non-essential amino acids except phenylalanine; with vitamins, minerals, trace elements, 7.1% sucrose. Flavour: vanilla. Net price 500 g = £36.00. For phenylketonuria, not recommended for child under 1 year

▼ PoM **Nalorex**® (Du Pont)

Tablets, orange, scored, naltrexone hydrochloride 50 mg. Net price 50-tab pack = £79.49
For adjunctive therapy of detoxified, formerly opioid-dependent, patients

▼ PoM **Nizoral**® (Janssen)

Shampoo, ketoconazole 2%. Net price 100 ml = £7.95.
For seborrhoeic dermatitis and dandruff, apply twice weekly for 2–4 weeks; pityriasis versicolor, once daily for max. 5 days. *Additives:* fragrance

Nutrizym® **GR** (Merck)

Capsules, green/orange, enclosing e/c pellets of pancreatin, providing minimum of: protease 650 units, lipase 10000 units, amylase 10000 units. Net price 100 = £12.52. Counselling advised, see dose

Dose: 1–2 capsules with meals swallowed whole or contents sprinkled on soft food (then swallowed immediately without chewing); may be increased in severe cases

P.K.U. Drink® (GF Supplies)

Liquid, whey, butterfat, providing protein 1 g (phenylalanine 30 mg), lactose 9.4 g, fat 4 g, energy 300kJ/200 ml. Net price 200 ml = 26p. For phenylketonuria

Platet® (Nicholas)

Tablets, effervescent, aspirin 100 mg. Net price 30-tab pack = 90p. Label: 13

Dose: antiplatelet following bypass surgery, 1 tablet daily at the same time of day

▼ PoM **Primaxin**® (MSD)

Intravenous infusion, powder for reconstitution, imipenem (as monohydrate) 250 mg with cilastatin (as sodium salt) 250 mg. Net price 60-ml vial = £9.00

Intravenous infusion, powder for reconstitution, imipenem (as monohydrate) 500 mg with cilastatin (as sodium salt) 500 mg. Net price 120-ml vial = £15.00

NHS PoM **Regaine**® (Upjohn)

Topical solution, minoxidil 2% in an aqueous alcoholic

basis. Net price 60-ml bottle = £20.00. For pattern baldness in males. *Additives:* propylene glycol
Cautions: flammable; wash hands after application
▼ PoM **Sandimmun**® (Sandoz)
Capsules, both pink, cyclosporin 25 mg, net price 30-cap pack = £20.46; 100 mg, 30-cap pack = £76.01
▼ PoM **Stiemycin**® (Stiefel)
Solution, erythromycin 2% in an alcoholic basis. Net price 2 × 25-ml applicator bottles = £9.00. Acne vulgaris, apply twice daily. *Additives:* propylene glycol

Uniphyllin Continus® (Napp)
Tablets, s/r, scored, theophylline 300 mg. Net price 56-tab pack = £5.50. Label: 25
▼ PoM **Zestril**® (ICI)
Tablets, lisinopril (as dihydrate) 2.5 mg, net price 28-tab pack = £7.84; 5 mg (pink, scored), 28-tab pack = £9.83; 10 mg (pink), 28-tab pack = £12.13; 20 mg (red), 28-tab pack = £20.96
Dose and *Cautions:* see Carace®, p. xii

Discontinued Preparations

Preparations discontinued during the compilation of BNF No. 16

Actonorm
Alavac-P
Alavac-S
Amoxidin
Ampilar
Ancoloxin
Antasil
Betnovate
  Compound
  Suppositories
Bronchodil Elixir
Ce-Cobalin Syrup
Centrax
Chenocedon
Cosylan
Dalivit Syrup
Defencin
Dettol Lotion

Dia-tuss
Duvadilan Retard
Duvadilan Tablets
Feospan Z
Gondafon
Hibitane Lozenges
Hypurin Soluble
Ibumetin
Iliadin Mini
Ilotycin
Klyx
Lejguar
Levius
Libraxin
Librium Injection
Locan
Mestinon Injection
Migen

Monophane
Mucolex
Mycifradin
Neoplatin
Norflex Tablets
Norgesic
Nutrizym [replaced
  by Nutrizym GR]
Omnopon Tablets
Opilon Injection
Opobyl
Ototbyl
Panasorb
Pernivit
Pharmidone
Pollinex

Prempak
  [Prempak-C still
  available]
Quicksol
SDV
Selora
Solpadeine Forte
Synandone
Syntocinon Nasal Spray
Synuretic
Tempulin
Tenormin CCU
Theograd
Tridesilon Ointment
Ureaphil
Wyeth Standard
  Enteral Feed
Xylodase

Dose Changes

Drugs and preparations affected by changes in dose statements introduced into BNF No. 16:

Betamethasone Valerate, p.123
Clomiphene, p. 255
Corticosteroids, Compound
  (rectal), pp.68–9 [more detail]
Desmopressin, p. 257

Diazoxide, p.91
Diflunisal, p. 325
Doxapram Hydrochloride, p.130
Fluorides [age], p. 314
Hormonin, p. 250

Methohexitone sodium, p. 418
Promethazine, p.127, p.167
Terfenadine, p.127
Trimeprazine Tartrate, p.127
Xylocaine Viscous, p. 431

Classification Changes

Amendments have been made in the following sections:
1.2   Atropine tablets now in 15.1.3
1.4.3   Other Antidiarrhoeal Preparations deleted
1.6.5   Rectally Administered Laxatives deleted
1.7   now called Preparations for Haemorrhoids
1.7.2   Rectal Corticosteroids (preparations now in 1.5)
1.7.3   now 1.7.2
1.7.4   now 1.7.3 (now called Rectal Sclerosants)
2.3.1   now called Management of Arrhythmias
2.3.2   now called Drugs for Arrhythmias (atropine injection now in 15.1.3)
2.3.3   section incorporated into 2.3.2
2.12   now called Lipid-lowering Drugs
3.1.1.2 Adrenaline now in 3.4.3
3.8   now called Aromatic Inhalations
3.9.2   Pavacol-D now in 3.9.1
5.4.1   Hydroxychloroquine now in 10.1.3 only
6.1.2   now called Oral Antidiabetic Drugs
6.5.2   now called Posterior Pituitary Hormones and Antagonists
6.5.3   section incorporated into 6.5.2
7.3.4   new: Intra-uterine Contraceptive Devices
8.1.6   deleted, mesna now in 8.1.1
9.1.2   Folinic acid now in 8.1.3
9.4   now called Oral Nutrition
9.4.2   now called Enteral Nutrition

New Name

The following approved name has been adopted:
Co-amilozide, compounded preparations of amiloride hydrochloride and hydrochlorothiazide in the proportions of 1 part to 10 parts respectively.
Tablets containing amiloride hydrochloride 5 mg and hydrochlorothiazide 50 mg respectively may be described as co-amilozide 5/50 (available as: Amilco®, Hypertane 50®, Moduretic®, and Normetic®)
Tablets containing amiloride hydrochloride 2.5 mg and hydrochlorothiazide 25 mg respectively may be described as co-amilozide 2.5/25 (available as: Moduret 25®).

For further reference to significant changes made for BNF No. 16 see Preface, p. x.

Drug Information Services

Information on any aspect of drug therapy can be obtained, free of charge, from Regional and District Drug Information Services. Details regarding the *local* services provided within your Region can be obtained by telephoning the following numbers.

England

Birmingham	021-378 2211	Extn 3565
Bristol	0272 250256	Direct Line
Guildford	0483 504312	Direct Line
Ipswich	0473 712233	Extn 4322/4323
or	0473 718687	Direct Line
Leeds	0532 430715	Direct Line
Leicester	0533 555779	Direct Line
Liverpool	051-236 4620	Extn 2126/2127/2128
London (Guy's Hospital)	01-407 7600	Extn 2548
London (London Hospital)	01-377 7487	Direct Line
or	01-377 7488	Direct Line
London (Northwick Park)	01-423 4535	Direct Line
Manchester	061-225 2063	Direct Line
or	061-276 6270	Direct Line
Newcastle	091-232 1525	Direct Line
Oxford	0865 742424	Direct Line
Southampton	0703 780323	Direct Line

Northern Ireland

Belfast	0232 248095	Direct Line
Londonderry	0504 45171	Extn 3262

Scotland

Aberdeen	0224 681818	Extn 52316
Dundee	0382 60111	Extn 2351
Edinburgh	031-229 2477	Extn 2234/2936
Glasgow	041-552 4726	Direct Line
Inverness	0463 234151	Extn 288
or	0463 220157	Direct Line

Wales

Cardiff	0222 759541	Direct Line

POISONS INFORMATION CENTRES

See p. 37

Guidance on Prescribing

Prices in the BNF

Basic **net prices** have been introduced into the BNF in order to provide better indications of relative cost. Whenever possible they have been calculated from the basic cost used in pricing NHS prescriptions dispensed in February 1988; these prices are based on the largest pack size of the preparation in use in community pharmacies or, in the case of an extemporaneous preparation, on the net cost of the ingredients used to make it.

The unit of 20 is still used as a basis for comparison, but where suitable original packs are available (e.g. calendar packs) these are priced instead.

Gross prices vary as follows:
1. Costs to the NHS are greater than the net prices quoted and include professional fees and overhead allowances;
2. Private prescription charges are calculated on a separate basis;
3. Over-the-counter sales are at retail price, as opposed to basic net price, and include VAT.

BNF prices are NOT, therefore, suitable for quoting to patients seeking private prescriptions or contemplating over-the-counter purchases.
A fuller explanation of costs to the NHS may be obtained from the Drug Tariff.

General Guidance

Medicines should be prescribed only when they are essential, and in all cases the benefit of administering the medicine should be considered in relation to the risk involved. This is particularly important during pregnancy where the risk to both mother and fetus must be considered (for further details see Prescribing in Pregnancy, see p. 27).

ABBREVIATION OF TITLES. In general, titles of drugs and preparations should be written *in full*. Unofficial abbreviations should not be used as they may be misinterpreted; obsolete titles, such as Mist. Expect. and Mist. Tussis should not be used.

NON-PROPRIETARY TITLES. Where non-proprietary ('generic') titles are given, they should be used in prescribing. This will enable any suitable product to be dispensed, thereby saving delay to the patient and sometimes expense to the health service. The only exception is where bio-availability problems are so important that the patient should always receive the same brand; in such cases, the brand name or the manufacturer should be stated.

Titles used as headings for monographs may be used freely in Great Britain and Northern Ireland but in other countries may be subject to restriction.

Many of the non-proprietary titles used in this book are titles of monographs in the European Pharmacopoeia, British Pharmacopoeia 1980[1] or British Pharmaceutical Codex 1973. In such cases the preparations must comply with the standard (if any) in the appropriate publication, as required by the Medicines Act (section 65).

PROPRIETARY TITLES. Names followed by the symbol® are or have been used as proprietary names in the United Kingdom. These names may in general be applied only to products supplied by the owners of the trade marks.

DOSES. The doses stated in the BNF are intended for general guidance and represent, unless otherwise stated, the usual range of doses that are generally regarded as being suitable for adults; unless otherwise indicated the quantities are those generally suitable for administration on one occasion.

DILUTIONS. When fractional doses are prescribed *liquid preparations for oral use* will be diluted with a suitable vehicle to dose-volumes of 5 ml or a multiple thereof, unless otherwise directed in the text. Dilution should be effected at the time of dispensing and such diluted preparations may be less stable than the original undiluted preparations. Where a complete recipe is given in the formulary section the diluent is the specified vehicle, otherwise the diluent specified in the text should be used.

In the case of *creams, ointments etc.*, where a complete recipe is available the diluent is the

specified vehicle, otherwise only diluents specified in the text should be used.

STRENGTHS AND QUANTITIES. The strength or quantity to be contained in capsules, lozenges, tablets, etc. should be stated by the prescriber.

If a pharmacist receives an incomplete prescription for a systemically administered preparation other than a prescription for a controlled drug and considers it would not be appropriate for the patient to return to the doctor, the following procedures will apply:
(a) an attempt must always be made to contact the prescriber to ascertain the intention;
(b) if the attempt is successful the pharmacist must, where practicable, subsequently arrange for details of quantity, strength where applicable, and dosage to be inserted by the prescriber on the incomplete form;
(c) where, although the prescriber has been contacted, it has not proved possible to obtain the written intention regarding an incomplete prescription, the pharmacist may endorse the form 'p.c.' (prescriber contacted) and add details of the quantity and strength where applicable of the preparation supplied, and of the dose indicated. The endorsement should be initialled and dated by the pharmacist;
(d) where the prescriber cannot be contacted and the pharmacist has sufficient information to make a professional judgment a sufficient quantity of the preparation may be dispensed to complete up to 5 days' treatment; except that where a combination pack (i.e., a proprietary pack containing more than one medicinal product) or oral contraceptive is prescribed by name only, the smallest pack shall be dispensed. In all cases the prescription must be endorsed 'p.n.c.' (prescriber not contacted) the quantity, the dose, and the strength (where applicable) of the preparation supplied must be indicated, and the endorsement must be initialled and dated;
(e) if the pharmacist has any doubt about exercising discretion, an incomplete prescription must be referred back to the prescriber.

CONTROLLED DRUGS. A prescription for a controlled drug other than those in schedules 4 and 5 to the Misuse of Drugs Regulations 1985 may not be dispensed by a pharmacist unless the requirements of Regulation 15 of the Misuse of Drugs Regulations are met. The pharmacist may not add to the prescription or otherwise exercise discretion on the quantity, dosage, or strength of the drug which is to be dispensed. All incomplete prescriptions must therefore be referred back to the prescriber.

APPLIANCES AND CHEMICAL REAGENTS. A limited selection of appliances (including dressings, elastic hosiery, and trusses) and chemical reagents is available for prescribing by general medical practitioners in the NHS; dressings are included

---

1. BP 1988 will be effective from 1st December 1988.

in BNF section 13.13 (Wound Management Products). For full details the appropriate edition of the Drug Tariff should be consulted.

DRUGS AND DRIVING. Prescribers should advise patients if treatment is likely to affect their ability to drive motor vehicles. This applies particularly to drugs with sedative effects and patients should be warned that these effects are increased by alcohol. See also Appendix 4.

NOTICE CONCERNING PATENTS. In the BNF certain drugs have been included notwithstanding the existence of actual or potential patent rights. In so far as such substances are protected by Letters Patent, their inclusion in this Formulary neither conveys, nor implies, licence to manufacture.

HEALTH AND SAFETY. When handling chemical or biological materials particular attention should be given to the possibility of allergy, fire, explosion, radiation, or poisoning. Some substances, including corticosteroids, antibiotics, phenothiazines, and many cytotoxics, are irritant or very potent and should be handled with caution. Contact with the skin and inhalation of dust should be avoided.

SAFETY IN THE HOME. Patients must be warned to keep all medicines out of the reach of children, in a safe locked place. As an additional precaution certain medicines may be supplied in child-resistant containers or strip packaging. Arthritic or infirm patients should be advised to ask the pharmacist to replace child-resistant closures by suitable ordinary closures. All patients should be advised to dispose of unwanted medicines by flushing them down a WC or returning them to the supplier for destruction.

LABELLING OF CONTAINERS WITH THE NAME OF THE PREPARATION. The Councils of the British Medical Association and the Royal Pharmaceutical Society have agreed that the name of the preparation should appear on the label unless the prescriber indicates otherwise.

1. Subject to the conditions of paragraphs 4 and 6 below, the name of the prescribed preparation is stated on the label of dispensed medicines unless the prescriber deletes the letters 'NP' which appear on National Health Service prescription forms.

2. The strength is also stated on the label in the case of tablets, capsules, and similar preparations that are available in different strengths.

3. If it is the wish of the prescriber that a description of the preparation such as 'The Sedative Tablets' should appear on the label, the prescriber should write the desired description on the prescription form.

4. The arrangement will extend to approved names, proprietary names or titles given in the BP, BPC, BNF, or DPF. The arrangement does not apply when a prescription is written so that several ingredients are given.

5. The name written on the label is that used by the prescriber on the prescription.

6. If more than one item is prescribed on one form and the prescriber does not delete the letters 'NP', each dispensed medicine is named on the label, subject to the conditions given above in paragraph 4. If the prescriber wants only selected items on such a prescription to be so labelled this should be indicated by deleting the letters 'NP' on the form and writing 'NP' alongside the medicines to be labelled.

7. When a prescription is written other than on a National Health Service prescription form the name of the prescribed preparation will be stated on the label of the dispensed medicine unless the prescriber indicates otherwise.

8. The Council of the Royal Pharmaceutical Society advises that the labels of dispensed medicines should indicate the total quantity of the product dispensed in the container to which the label refers. This requirement applies equally to solid, liquid, internal, and external preparations. If a product is dispensed in more than one container, the reference should be to the amount in each container.

SCOPE OF THE BNF. The BNF is intended for the guidance of medical practitioners, pharmacists, dentists, nurses, and other workers who have the necessary training and experience to interpret the information it provides. It is intended as a reference book for the pocket, and should be supplemented by a study of more detailed publications when required.

Security and validity of prescriptions

The Councils of the British Medical Association and the Royal Pharmaceutical Society have issued a joint statement on the security and validity of prescriptions.

In particular, prescription forms should:
(i) not be left unattended at reception desks;
(ii) not be left in a car where they may be visible; and
(iii) when not in use, be kept in a locked drawer within the surgery and at home.

Where there is any doubt about the authenticity of a prescription, the pharmacist should contact the prescriber. If this is done by telephone, the number should be obtained from the directory rather than relying on the prescription form information, which may be false.

Prescription Writing

The following recommendations are acceptable for prescription-only medicines (PoM). For items marked **CD** see Controlled Drugs and Drug Dependence. It should be noted that internationally recognised units and symbols are used in the BNF wherever possible.

Prescriptions should be written legibly in ink or typewritten, should be dated, and the full name and address of the individual patient added, and should be signed by the prescriber. The age of the patient should preferably be stated, and is a legal requirement in the case of prescription-only medicines for children under 12 years of age. In general practice the following should be noted:

(a) For solids, quantities of 1 gram or more should be written as 1 g etc.

Quantities less than 1 gram should be written in milligrams, e.g. 500 mg, not 0.5 g.

Quantities less than 1 mg should be written in micrograms, e.g. 100 micrograms, not 0.1 mg.

When decimals are unavoidable a zero should be written in front of the decimal point where there is no other figure, e.g. 0.5 ml, not .5 ml.

Use of the decimal point is acceptable to express a range, e.g. 0.5 to 1 g.

(b) 'Micrograms' and 'nanograms' should **not** be abbreviated. Similarly 'units' should **not** be abbreviated.

(c) The term 'millilitre' (ml) is used in medicine and pharmacy, and cubic centimetre, c.c., or cm^3 should not be used.

(d) Dose and dose frequency should be stated.

For oral liquid preparations of the linctus or elixir type and for preparations for children, doses should preferably be stated in terms of 5-ml spoonfuls.

For mixtures for adults, doses should preferably be stated in 10-ml quantities; unless the prescription states otherwise, the patient will be directed to take the dose with water.

When doses other than 5 or 10 ml are prescribed the dose-volume will be diluted to 5 or 10 ml or a multiple thereof (except for preparations intended to be measured with a pipette).

The volume of liquid preparations should normally be 50, 100, 150, 200, 300, or 500 ml. Suitable quantities of liquid preparations:

Elixirs, Linctuses, and Paediatric
  Mixtures (5-ml dose), 50, 100, or 150 ml
Adult Mixtures (10-ml dose), 200 or 300 ml
Ear Drops, Eye-drops, and Nasal Drops,
  10 ml (or the manufacturer's pack)
Eye Lotions, Gargles, and Mouth-washes, 200 ml
Liniments, 100 ml

(e) Quantities of solids prescribed should normally be 15, 25, 50, 100, 200, 300, or 500 grams (or the manufacturer's appropriate pack).

For suitable quantities of dermatological preparations, see section 13.1.

(f) The names of drugs and preparations should be written clearly and **not** abbreviated.

(g) The symbol 'NP' on NHS forms should be deleted if it is required that the name of the preparation should not appear on the label. For full details see under General Guidance.

(h) The quantity to be supplied may be stated by indicating the number of days of treatment required in the box provided on NHS forms. In most cases the exact amount will be supplied. This does not apply to items directed to be used as required; if the dose and frequency are not given the quantity to be supplied should be stated.

When several items are ordered on one form the box can be marked with the number of days of treatment providing the quantity is added for any item for which the amount cannot be calculated.

(i) Directions should preferably be in English without abbreviation, e.g. one at night, not i.o.n.

(j) A prescription for a preparation that has been withdrawn or needs to be specially imported for a named patient should be handwritten. The name of the preparation should be endorsed with the prescriber's signature and the letters 'WD' (withdrawn or specially-imported drug); this will be a valuable indication to the pharmacist of the prescriber's intentions. There may be considerable delay in obtaining a withdrawn medicine.

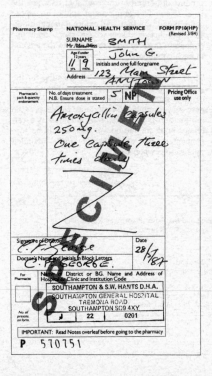

Hospital Prescriptions

In hospitals the following should also be noted:

1. There should be a prescription sheet on which prescriptions and a record of dispensing and administration *only* are written.

2. Not more than one prescription sheet should be in use at any one time for any one patient.

3. Frequency of administration of 'as required' medicines should be indicated by clear and definitely stated intervals.

4. The route of administration should be clearly shown.

5. The prescription sheet should show signed and dated cancellations of any prescriptions no longer current.

Arrangements should be made for doses to be given at special times when intervals are critical.

Computer-issued Prescriptions

For computer-issued prescriptions the following should also be noted:

1. The computer must print out the date, the patient's surname, one forename, other initials, and address, and may also print out the patient's title. The age of children under 12 years must be printed in the box available; a facility may exist to print out the age of older children and adults as well.

2. The doctor's name[1] must be printed at the bottom of the prescription form; this will be the name of the doctor responsible for the prescription (who will normally sign it). The doctor's surgery address, reference number, and Family Practitioner Committee[2] are also necessary. In addition, the surgery telephone number should be printed.

3. When prescriptions are to be signed by trainees, assistants, locums, or deputising doctors, the name of the doctor printed at the bottom of the form must still be that of the responsible principal. To avoid difficulties for the pharmacist checking the prescription, the name of the signing doctor may be printed in the signature box, to be signed over on prescribing.

4. Names of medicines must come from a dictionary held in the computer memory, to provide a check on the spelling and ensure that the name is written in full. The computer can be programmed to recognise both the non-proprietary and the proprietary name of a particular drug and to print out the preferred choice, but must not print out both names. For medicines not in the dictionary, separate checking mechanisms are required—the user must be warned that no check was possible and the entire prescription must be entered in the lexicon.

5. The dictionary may contain information on the usual doses, formulations, and (where relevant) pack sizes to produce standard predetermined prescriptions for common preparations, and to provide a check on the validity of an individual prescription on entry.

6. The prescription must be printed in English without abbreviation, see (i) above; information may be entered or stored in abbreviated form. The dose must be in numbers, the frequency in words, and the quantity in numbers (in brackets), thus:

40 mg four times daily (112)

It must also be possible to prescribe by indicating the length of treatment required, see (h) above.

7. The BNF recommendations should be followed as in (a), (b), (c), (d), and (e) above.

8. Checks may be incorporated to ensure that all the information required for dispensing a particular drug has been filled in. Instructions such as 'as directed' should be avoided. For the instruction 'when required' the maximum daily dose should normally be specified.

9. Numbers and codes used in the system for organising and retrieving data must never appear on the form.

10. Supplementary warnings or advice should be written in full, should not interfere with the clarity of the prescription itself, and should be in line with any warnings or advice in the BNF; numerical codes should not be used.

11. A mechanism (such as printing a series of non-specific characters) may be incorporated to cancel out unused space, or wording such as 'no more items on this prescription' may be added after the last item. Otherwise the doctor should delete the space manually.

12. To avoid forgery the computer may print on the form the number of items to be dispensed (somewhere separate from the box for the pharmacist). The number of items per form need be limited only by the ability of the printer to produce clear and well-demarcated instructions with sufficient space for each item and a spacer line before each fresh item.

13. Handwritten alterations should only be made in exceptional circumstances—it is preferable to print out a new prescription. Any alterations that are made must be written in the doctor's own handwriting and countersigned.

14. Prescriptions for controlled drugs cannot be produced by a printer (except in the case of phenobarbitone, see Controlled Drugs and Drug Dependence). If there is a record of such a prescription in the computer, it must not be printed. Instead the computer may print out a blank form with the doctor's name[1] and other details printed at the bottom.

15. The strip of paper on the side of the FP10[3](Comp) may be used for various purposes but care should be taken to avoid including confidential information. It may be advisable for the patient's name to appear at the top, but this should be preceded by 'confidential'.

16. In rural dispensing practices prescription requests (or details of medicines dispensed) will normally be entered in one surgery. The prescriptions (or dispensed medicines) may then need to be delivered to another surgery or location; if possible the computer should hold up to 10 alternatives.

---

1. Except in Scotland where it does not appear.
2. Health Board in Scotland.
3. GP10 in Scotland.

Emergency Supply of PoM at Patient's Request[1]

The Medicines (Products Other Than Veterinary Drugs) (Prescription Only) Order 1983, as amended, allows exemptions from the Prescription Only requirements for emergency supply to be made by a person lawfully conducting a retail pharmacy business provided:

(a) that the pharmacist has interviewed the person requesting the prescription-only medicine and is satisfied: (i) that there is immediate need for the prescription-only medicine and that it is impracticable in the circumstances to obtain a prescription without undue delay; (ii) that the treatment with the prescription-only medicine has on a previous occasion been prescribed by a doctor for the person requesting it; and (iii) as to the dose which it would be appropriate for the person to take;

(b) that no greater quantity shall be supplied than will provide five days' treatment except when the prescription-only medicine is: (i) an ointment, cream, or preparation for the relief of asthma in an aerosol dispenser when the smallest pack can be supplied; (ii) an oral contraceptive when a full cycle may be supplied; or (iii) an antibiotic in liquid form for oral adminstration when the smallest quantity that will provide a full course of treatment can be supplied;

(c) that an entry shall be made in the prescription book stating: (i) the date of supply; (ii) the name, quantity and, where appropriate, the pharmaceutical form and strength; (iii) the name and address of the patient; and (iv) the nature of the emergency;

(d) that the container or package must be labelled to show: (i) the date of supply; (ii) the name, quantity and, where appropriate, the pharmaceutical form and strength; (iii) the name of the patient; (iv) the name and address of the pharmacy; and (v) the words "Emergency supply".

(e) that the prescription-only medicine is not a substance specifically excluded from the emergency supply provision, and does not contain a Controlled Drug specified in schedules 1, 2, or 3 to the Misuse of Drugs Regulations 1985 except for phenobarbitone or phenobarbitone sodium for the treatment of epilepsy: for details see *Medicines and Poisons Guide*, 4th Edition, London, Pharmaceutical Press, 1984.

ROYAL PHARMACEUTICAL SOCIETY'S GUIDELINES
(1) The pharmacist should consider the medical consequences, if any, of **not** supplying.
(2) The pharmacist should identify the patient by means of documentary evidence and/or personal knowledge.
(3) The doctor who prescribed on a previous occasion should be identified and contacted, if possible.
(4) The patient should be asked whether the doctor has stopped the treatment.
(5) The patient should be asked whether any other medicine is being taken at the same time to check drug interactions.
(6) An emergency supply should not be made if the item requested was prescribed previously more than six months prior to the request. Variations may be made in the case of illnesses which occur infrequently, e.g. hay fever, asthma attack, or migraine.
(7) Consideration should be given to providing less than five days' supply if this is justified.
(8) Labelling should be clear and legible and there should be some suitable identification of emergency supply entries in the prescription book.

1. For emergency supply at the request of a doctor see *Medicines and Poisons Guide*, 4th Edition, London, Pharmaceutical Press, 1984.

Plasma concentrations in the BNF are expressed in mass units per litre (e.g. mg/litre). The approximate equivalent in terms of amount of substance units (e.g. micromol/litre) is given in brackets.

Approximate Conversions and Units

lb	kg	stones	kg	ml	fl. oz
1	0.45	1	6.35	50	1.8
2	0.91	2	12.70	100	3.5
3	1.36	3	19.05	150	5.3
4	1.81	4	25.40	200	7.0
5	2.27	5	31.75	500	17.6
6	2.72	6	38.10	1000	35.2
7	3.18	7	44.45		
8	3.63	8	50.80		
9	4.08	9	57.15		
10	4.54	10	63.50		
11	4.99	11	69.85		
12	5.44	12	76.20		
13	5.90	13	82.55		
14	6.35	14	88.90		
		15	95.25		

Mass
1 kilogram (kg)	= 1000 grams (g)
1 gram (g)	= 1000 milligrams (mg)
1 milligram (mg)	= 1000 micrograms
1 microgram	= 1000 nanograms
1 nanogram	= 1000 picograms

Volume
1 litre	= 1000 millilitres (ml)
1 millilitre	= 1000 microlitres
1 pint	≈ 568 ml

Other units
1 kilocalorie (kcal)	= 4186.8 joules (J)
1000 kilocalories (kcal)	= 4.1868 megajoules (MJ)
1 megajoule (MJ)	= 238.8 kilocalories (kcal)
1 millimetre of mercury (mmHg)	= 133.3 pascals (Pa)
1 kilopascal (kPa)	= 7.5 mmHg (pressure)

Controlled Drugs and Drug Dependence

PRESCRIPTIONS. Preparations which are subject to the prescription requirements of the Misuse of Drugs Regulations 1985, i.e. preparations specified in schedules 2 and 3, are distinguished throughout the BNF by the symbol **CD** (Controlled Drugs). The principal legal requirements relating to medical prescriptions are listed below.

Prescriptions ordering Controlled Drugs subject to prescription requirements must be *signed* and *dated*[1] by the prescriber and specify the prescriber's *address*. The prescription must always state *in the prescriber's own handwriting*[2] in ink or otherwise so as to be indelible:

1. The name and address of the patient;
2. In the case of a preparation, the form[3] and where appropriate the strength of the preparation;
3. The total quantity of the preparation, or the number of dose units, *in both words and figures;*
4. The dose.

A prescription may order a Controlled Drug to be dispensed by instalments; the amount of the instalments and the intervals to be observed must be specified.[4] 'Repeat' prescriptions are **not** permitted.

It is an offence for a doctor to issue an incomplete prescription and a pharmacist is **not** allowed to dispense a Controlled Drug unless all the information required by law is given on the prescription. Failure to comply with the regulations concerning the writing of prescriptions will result in inconvenience to patients and delay in supplying the necessary medicine.

DEPENDENCE AND MISUSE. The prevalence of drug dependence and misuse in Great Britain, particularly amongst young people, continues to give cause for concern to teachers, social workers, and the police, as well as doctors.

The most serious drugs of addiction are **diamorphine** (heroin), **morphine**, and the **synthetic opioids.** The likelihood that the dose will be increased is considerable, psychic dependence is common, and the withdrawal syndrome may be severe.

Although a campaign by doctors led to marked reduction in the prescribing of **amphetamines** there is still concern that they are widely used illicitly.

The principal **barbiturates** are now Controlled Drugs (class B of the Act and schedule 3 of the Regulations), but phenobarbitone and phenobarbitone sodium or a preparation containing either of these are exempt from the handwriting requirement; moreover, for the treatment of epilepsy phenobarbitone and phenobarbitone sodium are available under the emergency supply regulations (p. 6).

Cannabis (Indian hemp) has no approved medicinal use and cannot be prescribed by doctors (except under licence from the Home Secretary). Its use is illegal but has become widespread in certain sections of society. Cannabis is a mild hallucinogen seldom accompanied by a desire to increase the dose; withdrawal symptoms are unusual. **Lysergide** (lysergic acid diethylamide, LSD) is a much more potent hallucinogen; its use can lead to severe psychotic states in which life may be at risk.

---

1. A prescription is valid for 13 weeks from the date stated thereon
2. Unless the prescriber has been specifically exempted from this requirement or unless the prescription contains no controlled drug other than phenobarbitone or phenobarbitone sodium or a preparation containing either of these.
3. The dosage form (e.g. tablets) must be included on a Controlled Drugs prescription irrespective of whether it is implicit in the proprietary name (e.g. Tenuate Dospan®) or of whether only one form is available.
4. A special form, FP10HP(ad), in Scotland HBP(A), is available to certain doctors in the NHS for prescribing cocaine, dextromoramide, diamorphine, dipipanone, methadone, morphine, or pethidine by instalments. Forms FP10 and FP10HP, in Scotland GP10 and HBP, are not suitable for this purpose but a new form FP10(MDA) is now available for general practitioners to prescribe by instalments (**important:** a special licence is still necessary, however, to prescribe cocaine, diamorphine, or dipipanone).

PRESCRIBING DRUGS LIKELY TO CAUSE DEPEN-
DENCE OR MISUSE. The prescriber has three main
responsibilities:

1. To avoid creating dependence by introducing
drugs to patients without sufficient reason. In this
context, the proper use of the morphine-like drugs
is well understood. The dangers of other controlled drugs are less clear because recognition of
dependence is not easy and its effects, and those
of withdrawal, are less obvious. Consequently,
divergent views are held. Perhaps the most
notable result of uninhibited prescribing is that a
very large number of patients in the country take
tablets which do them neither much good nor
much harm, but are committed to them indefinitely because they cannot readily be stopped.

2. To see that the patient does not gradually
increase the dose of a drug, given for good medical
reasons, to the point where dependence becomes
more likely. This tendency is seen especially with
the barbiturates and also with other hypnotics and
tranquillisers, including the benzodiazepines. The
prescriber should keep a close eye on the amount
prescribed to prevent patients from accumulating
stocks that would enable them to arrange their
own dosage or even that of their families and
friends. A minimal amount should be prescribed
in the first instance, or when seeing a new patient
for the first time.

3. To avoid being used as an unwitting source
of supply for addicts. This manoeuvre is often
attempted by addicts to opioid analgesics and they
may be very skilled, plausible, and persistent in
attaining their ends. Methods include visiting
more than one doctor, fabricating stories to sub-
stantiate demands, and forging prescriptions. A
doctor should therefore be wary of prescribing for
strangers and may be able to get information
about suspected opiate addicts from the Drugs
Branch of the Home Office or in Northern Ireland
from the Drugs Branch, Department of Health
and Social Services (see p. 9).

Patients under temporary care should be given
only small supplies of drugs unless they present
an unequivocal letter from their own doctors.
Doctors should also remember that their own
patients may be doing a collecting round with
other doctors, especially in hospitals. It is sensible
to decrease dosages steadily or to issue weekly or
even daily prescriptions for small amounts if it is
apparent that dependence is occurring.

The stealing and misuse of prescription forms
could be minimised by the following precautions:

(a) do not leave unattended if called away from
the consulting room or at reception desks; do
not leave in a car where they may be visible;
when not in use, keep in a locked drawer
within the surgery and at home;

(b) draw a diagonal line across the blank part of
the form under the prescription;

(c) write the quantity in words and figures when
prescribing drugs prone to abuse; this is
obligatory for controlled drugs (see Prescriptions, above);

(d) alterations are best avoided but if any are
made they should be clear and unambiguous;
add initials against altered items;

(e) if prescriptions are left for collection they
should be left in a safe place in a sealed
envelope.

TRAVELLING ABROAD. Prescribed drugs listed in
schedules 4 and 5 to the Misuse of Drugs Regulations 1985 are not subject to import or export
licensing but doctors are advised that patients
travelling abroad may only carry 15 days' supply
of any schedule 2 or 3 prescribed controlled drug
without a licence. If especially high doses are
prescribed, however, or if prescriptions are for a
longer period, an import or export licence may
be required. Licences are issued by the Home
Secretary, Home Office, Drugs Branch, Queen
Anne's Gate, London SW1H 9AT, telephone 01-
273 3806.

There is no standard application form but applications must be supported by a letter from a
doctor giving details of:

the patient's name and current address;
the quantities of drugs to be carried;
the strength and form in which the drugs will be
dispensed;
the dates of travel to and from the United Kingdom.

Ten days should be allowed for processing the
application.

Individual doctors who wish to take Controlled
Drugs abroad while accompanying patients, may
similarly be issued with licences. Licences are
not normally issued to doctors who wish to take
Controlled Drugs abroad solely in case a family
emergency should arise.

These import/export licences for named individuals do not have any legal status outside the
UK and are only issued to comply with the Misuse
of Drugs Act and facilitate passage through UK
Customs control. For clearance in the country to
be visited it would be necessary to approach that
country's embassy in the UK.

The Misuse of Drugs Act, 1971

This Act was passed in 1971 to provide more
flexible and more comprehensive control over the
misuse of drugs of all kinds than was possible
under the earlier Dangerous Drugs Act. The Act
as amended prohibits certain activities in relation
to 'Controlled Drugs', in particular their manufacture, supply, and possession. The penalties
applicable to offences involving the different
drugs are graded broadly according to the *harm-
fulness attributable to a drug when it is misused*
and for this purpose the drugs are defined in the
following three classes:

Class A includes: alfentanil, cocaine, dextromoramide,
diamorphine (heroin), dipipanone, lysergide (LSD)
methadone, morphine, opium, pethidine, phencycli-
dine, and class B substances when prepared for injection

Class B includes: oral amphetamines, barbiturates, cannabis, cannabis resin, codeine, ethylmorphine, glutethimide, pentazocine, phenmetrazine, and
pholcodine

Class C includes: certain drugs related to the amphet
amines such as benzphetamine and chlorphentermine
diethylpropion, mazindol, meprobamate, methypry
lone, pipradrol, and most benzodiazepines

The Misuse of Drugs Regulations 1985 define
the classes of person who are authorised to supply
and possess controlled drugs while acting in their
professional capacities and lay down the con

ditions under which these activities may be carried out. In the regulations drugs are divided into five schedules each specifying the requirements governing such activities as import, export, production, supply, possession, prescribing, and record keeping which apply to them.

Schedule 1 includes drugs such as cannabis and lysergide which are not used medicinally. Possession and supply are prohibited except in accordance with Home Office authority.

Schedule 2 includes drugs such as diamorphine (heroin), morphine, pethidine, quinalbarbitone, glutethimide, amphetamine, and cocaine and are subject to the full controlled drug requirements relating to prescriptions, safe custody, the need to keep registers, etc. (unless exempted in schedule 5).

Schedule 3 includes the barbiturates (except quinalbarbitone, now schedule 2), diethylpropion, mazindol, meprobamate, methyprylone, pentazocine, and phentermine. They are subject to the special prescription requirements but not to the safe custody requirements (except for diethylpropion) nor to the need to keep registers (although there are requirements for the retention of invoices for 2 years).

Schedule 4 includes 33 benzodiazepines which are subject to minimal control. In particular, controlled drug prescription requirements do not apply and they are not subject to safe custody.

Schedule 5 includes those preparations which, because of their strength, are exempt from virtually all Controlled Drug requirements other than retention of invoices for two years.

Notification of Addicts

The Misuse of Drugs (Notification of and Supply to Addicts) Regulations 1973 require that any doctor who attends a person who the doctor considers or has reasonable grounds to suspect, is addicted to any drug shall, within seven days of the attendance, furnish in writing particulars of that person to:

Chief Medical Officer,
Home Office, Drugs Branch,
Queen Anne's Gate, London SW1H 9AT.

The drugs commonly in use to which the Regulations apply are:

Cocaine	Methadone
Dextromoramide	Morphine
Diamorphine	Opium
Dipipanone	Oxycodone
Hydrocodone	Pethidine
Hydromorphone	Phenazocine
Levorphanol	Piritramide

Note. Dipipanone is only legally available as Diconal® Tablets. These have been much misused by opiate addicts in recent years; only medical practitioners with a special licence may now prescribe them for addicts to treat addiction. Doctors and others should be suspicious of young people who ask for them, especially as temporary residents.

Particulars[1] to be notified to the Chief Medical Officer are:

Name and address
Sex
Date of birth
National Health Service number
Date of attendance
Name of drug or drugs concerned[2]

Notification must be confirmed annually in writing if the patient is still being treated by the practitioner. Notified information is incorporated in an Index of Addicts which is maintained in the Home Office and information from this is available on a confidential basis to doctors; in fact, it is good medical practice to check all new cases of addiction or suspected addiction with the Index before prescribing or supplying controlled drugs since this is a safeguard against addicts obtaining supplies simultaneously from two or more doctors. Enquiries can be made either in writing to the Chief Medical Officer or, preferably, by telephoning 01-273 2213. To keep notified information confidential, such enquiries are normally answered by means of a return telephone call. The reply will come from lay staff who are not qualified to give guidance on the clinical handling of cases.

The preceding paragraph applies only to medical practitioners in England, Scotland, and Wales. In Northern Ireland notification should be sent to the Chief Medical Officer, Department of Health and Social Services, Dundonald House, Belfast BT4 3SF, and any enquiries about the Northern Ireland Regulations or addicts should be made to that Department, also at Dundonald House, telephone number 0232 63939 extension 2874.

Prescribing of diamorphine (heroin), dipipanone, and cocaine for addicts

The Misuse of Drugs (Notification of and Supply to Addicts) Regulations 1973 also provide that only medical practitioners who hold a special licence issued by the Home Secretary may prescribe diamorphine, dipipanone (Diconal®), or cocaine for addicts; other practitioners must refer any addict who requires these drugs to a treatment centre. General practitioners and other doctors may still prescribe diamorphine, dipipanone, and cocaine for patients (including addicts) for relief of pain due to organic disease or injury without a special licence. Whenever possible the addict will be introduced to a member of staff from the treatment centre to a pharmacist whose agreement has been obtained and whose pharmacy is conveniently sited for the patient. Prescriptions for weekly supplies will be sent to the pharmacy by post and will be dispensed on a daily basis as indicated by the doctor. If any alterations of the arrangements are requested by the addict, the portion of the prescription affected must be represcribed and not merely altered.

---

1. Only the particulars of which the doctor has knowledge need be notified immediately; the remainder may be notified at a later date; forms for notification may be obtained from the Chief Medical Officer, Home Office, Drugs Branch, Queen Anne's Gate, London SW1H 9AT.
2. The Home Office has also requested that notification be made of any drug prescribed or of whether the doctor declined to prescribe.

PREPARATIONS FOR DRUG DEPENDENCE

CD Methadone Mixture 1 mg/ml, methadone hydrochloride 1 mg/ml (see Formulary). Net price 100 ml = 72p. Label: 2. Used in replacement and maintenance treatment

Note. This preparation is 2½ times the strength of methadone linctus.

Adverse Reactions to Drugs

Any drug may produce unwanted or unexpected adverse reactions. The detection and recording of these reactions is of vital importance.

Doctors are urged to help by reporting adverse reactions to:

CSM
Freepost
London SW8 5BR
(01-720 2188)

Yellow prepaid lettercards for reporting are available from the above address or by dialling 100 and asking for 'CSM Freefone'; also, forms are bound in this book (inside back cover).

A 24-hour Freefone service is now available to all parts of the United Kingdom, for doctors seeking advice and information on adverse reactions. The service may be obtained by dialling 100 and asking for 'CSM Freefone'. Outside office hours a telephone-answering machine will take messages. When, on rare occasions, it is considered essential to report particularly serious and unexpected adverse reactions immediately, a doctor may use the Freefone service. Written confirmation will be requested, however, and this method does not supersede the normal system.

The following regional centres also collect data:

CSM Wales
Freepost
Cardiff CF4 1ZZ
(0222 759541 Direct Line).

CSM West Midlands
Freepost
Birmingham B15 1BR
(021-472 1311 Extn 4516)

CSM Northern
Freepost 1085
Newcastle upon Tyne NE1 1BR
(0632 321525 Direct Line)

Suspected adverse reactions to *any* therapeutic agent should be reported, including drugs, blood products, vaccines, X-ray contrast media, dental or surgical materials, intra-uterine contraceptive devices, absorbable sutures, and contact lens fluids.

Newer drugs

These are indicated by the sign ▼ in the BNF, MIMS, and ABPI Data Sheet Compendium. Doctors are asked to report any adverse or any unexpected event, however minor, which could conceivably be attributed to the drug. Reports should be made despite uncertainty in the doctor's mind about a causal relationship, irrespective of whether the reaction is well recognized, and even if other drugs have been given concurrently.

'Red alert' scheme. This is a trial of a new drug monitoring scheme aimed at encouraging doctors to report serious adverse reactions to new drugs. The scheme will cover every new drug marketed over the trial period; inclusion of a drug does not imply any special concern about its safety. General practitioners in England who prescribe drugs included in the scheme will be sent yellow cards marked with red triangles, printed with the name of the patient and of the drug; they should only be used to report serious or life-threatening reactions or death of the patient. Other reactions should be reported to the CSM on an ordinary yellow card.

Established drugs

Doctors are asked to report *all* serious suspected reactions, including those that are fatal, life-threatening, disabling, incapacitating, or which result in or prolong hospitalisation; they should be reported even though the toxic effect is well recognised.

Examples include anaphylaxis, blood disorders, endocrine disturbances, effects on fertility, haemorrhage from any site, renal impairment, jaundice, ophthalmic disorders, severe CNS effects, severe skin reactions, reactions in pregnant women, and any drug interactions. Reports of serious adverse reactions are required to enable risk/benefit ratios to be compared with other drugs of a similar class. For established drugs doctors are asked not to report well-known, relatively minor side-effects, such as dry mouth with tricyclic antidepressants, constipation with opiates, or nausea with digoxin.

Special problems

Delayed drug effects. Doctors are reminded that some reactions (e.g. the development of cancers, chloroquine retinopathy, and retroperitoneal fibrosis) may become manifest months or years after drug exposure. Any suspicion of such an association should be reported.

Drugs in the elderly. Doctors are asked to be particularly alert to the possibility of adverse reactions when drugs are given to the elderly.

Congenital abnormalities. When an infant is born with a congenital abnormality or there is a malformed aborted fetus doctors are asked to consider the possibility that this might be an adverse reaction to a drug and to report all drugs (including self-medication) taken by the mother during pregnancy.

Vaccines. Doctors are asked to report all suspected reactions to both new and established vaccines. The balance between risks and benefits from vaccines is liable to change and needs to be kept under continuous review.

Prevention of adverse reactions

Adverse reactions may be prevented as follows:

1. Never use any drug unless there is a good indication. If the patient is pregnant do not use a drug unless the need for it is imperative.

2. It is very important to recognise allergy and idiosyncrasy as causes of adverse drug reactions. Ask if the patient had previous reactions.

3. Ask if the patient is already taking other drugs *including self-medication* and remember that drug interactions may occur.

4. Remember that age, hepatic disease, or renal disease may alter the metabolism or excretion of drugs, so that they may need to be prescribed in much smaller doses than usual. Pharmacogenetic factors may also be responsible for variations in the rate of metabolism of drugs, notably isoniazid and the tricyclic antidepressants. Appropriate dose adjustments may be necessary to compensate for these variations.

5. Prescribe as few drugs as possible and give very clear instructions to the elderly or any patient likely to misunderstand complicated instructions.

6. When possible use a drug with which you are familiar. If you use a new drug be particularly alert for adverse reactions or unexpected events.

7. If serious adverse reactions are liable to occur warn the patient.

Prescribing for Children

All children, and particularly neonates, differ from adults in their response to drugs. Special care is needed in the neonatal period (first 30 days of life) and doses should always be calculated according to weight. At this age, the risk of toxicity is increased by inefficient renal filtration, relative enzyme deficiencies, differing target organ sensitivity, and inadequate detoxifying systems causing delayed excretion. In childhood dosage should be adjusted for weight until 50 kg or puberty is reached.

Prescriptions should be written according to the guidelines in Prescription Writing (p. 4). Inclusion of age is a legal requirement in the case of prescription-only medicines for children under 12 years of age, but it is preferable to state the age for **all** prescriptions.

It is particularly important to state the strengths of capsules or tablets. Although liquid preparations are particularly suitable for children, many contain sucrose which encourages dental decay. When taken over a long period, sugar-free tablets, liquid medicines, and diluents should be used when possible.

When a prescription for a liquid oral preparation is written and the dose ordered is smaller than 5 ml, the preparation will normally be diluted so that the required dose is contained in 5 ml. Parents must be instructed to use the standard 5-ml spoon to measure the dose and not to heap up a viscous preparation. They should also be advised not to add any medicines to the contents of the infant's feeding bottle, since the drug may interact with the milk or other liquid in it; moreover the ingested dosage may be reduced, if the child does not drink all the contents.

See also General Guidance, Safety in the home, p. 3.

Dosage in Children

Doses for children are stated in the individual drug entries as far as possible, except where paediatric use is not recommended, as with tetracyclines, or where there are special hazards.

Doses are generally based on body-weight (in kilograms) or the following age ranges:

first month (neonate)
up to 1 year (infant)
1–5 years
6–12 years

Where a single dose is quoted for a given range, it applies to the middle of the age range and some extrapolation may be necessary to obtain doses for ages at the lower and upper limits of the stated range.

DOSE CALCULATION. If no dose is stated in the BNF, children's doses may be calculated from adult doses by using age, body-weight, or body-surface area, or by a combination of these factors.

The most reliable methods are those based on body-surface area.

Body-weight may be used to calculate doses expressed in mg/kg, and some children's doses in the BNF are stated in this way. Young children may require a higher dose per kilogram body-weight than adults because of their higher metabolic rates. Other problems need to be considered. For example, calculation by body-weight in the obese child would result in much higher doses being administered than necessary. In such cases, dose should be calculated from an ideal weight, related to height and age. Where new or potentially toxic drugs are used, the manufacturers' recommended doses should be carefully followed.

Body-surface estimates are more accurate for calculation of paediatric doses than body-weight since many physical phenomena are more closely related to body-surface area. The average body-surface area of a 70-kilogram human is about $1.8\,m^2$. Thus, to calculate the dose for a child the following formula may be used:

Approximate dose for patient =

$$\frac{\text{surface area of patient (m}^2)}{1.8} \times \text{adult dose}$$

The percentage method using the table below may be conveniently used to calculate children's doses of commonly prescribed drugs with a wide margin between the therapeutic and the toxic dose.

Age	Ideal body-weight kg	lb	Height mm	in	Body-surface m^2	Percentage of adult dose
Newborn*	3.4	7.5	500	20	0.23	12.5
1 month*	4.2	9	550	22	0.26	14.5
3 months*	5.6	12	590	23	0.32	18
6 months	7.7	17	670	26	0.40	22
1 year	10	22	760	30	0.47	25
3 years	14	31	940	37	0.62	33
5 years	18	40	1080	42	0.73	40
7 years	23	51	1200	47	0.88	50
12 years	37	81	1480	58	1.25	75
Adult						
Male	68	150	1727	68	1.8	100
Female	56	123	1626	64	1.6	100

* The figures relate to full term and not preterm infants who may need reduced dosage according to their clinical condition.

More precise body-surface values may be calculated from height and weight by means of a table (e.g. *Martindale: The Extra Pharmacopoeia*, 28th Edition, London, Pharmaceutical Press, 1982) or a nomogram (e.g. J. Insley and B. Wood, *A Paediatric Vademecum*, 11th Edition, London, Lloyd Luke, 1986).

Prescribing for the Elderly

Old people, especially the very old, require special care and consideration from prescribers.

Elderly patients are apt to receive multiple drugs for their multiple diseases. This greatly increases the risk of drug interactions as well as other adverse reactions. Moreover, symptoms such as headache, sleeplessness, and lightheadedness which may be associated with social stress, as in widowhood, loneliness, and family dispersal can lead to further prescribing, especially of psychotropics. The use of drugs in such cases can at best be a poor substitute for effective social measures and at worst pose a serious threat from adverse reactions.

In very old subjects, manifestations of normal ageing may be mistaken for disease and lead to inappropriate prescribing. For example, drugs such as prochlorperazine are commonly misprescribed for giddiness due to age-related loss of postural stability. Not only is such treatment ineffective but the patient may experience serious side-effects such as drug-induced parkinsonism, postural hypotension, and mental confusion.

Self-medication with over-the-counter products or with drugs prescribed for a previous illness (or even for another person) may be an added complication. Discussion with relatives and a home visit may be needed to establish exactly what is being taken.

The ageing nervous system shows increased *susceptibility* to many commonly used drugs, such as opioid analgesics, benzodiazepines, and antiparkinsonian drugs, all of which must be used with caution.

PHARMACOKINETICS. While drug distribution and metabolism may be significantly altered, the most important effect of age is reduction in renal clearance, frequently aggravated by the effects of prostatism, nephrosclerosis, or chronic urinary tract infection. Many aged patients thus possess only limited reserves of renal function, excrete drugs slowly, and are highly susceptible to nephrotoxic drugs. Acute illness may lead to rapid reduction in renal clearance, especially if accompanied by dehydration. Hence, a patient stabilised on digoxin may rapidly develop adverse effects in the aftermath of a myocardial infarction or a respiratory tract infection.

The net result of pharmacokinetic changes is that tissue concentrations are commonly increased by over 50%, and aged and debilitated patients may show even larger changes.

COMMON ADVERSE REACTIONS. Adverse reactions often present in the elderly in a vague and nonspecific fashion. *Mental confusion* is often the presenting symptom (caused by almost any of the commonly used drugs). Other common manifestations are *constipation* (as with anticholinergics and many tranquillisers) and postural *hypotension* and *falls* (as with diuretics and many psychotropics).

Many hypnotics with long half-lives have serious hangover effects of drowsiness, unsteady gait, and even slurred speech and confusion. Those with short half-lives should be used but they too can present problems (see section 4.1.1). Short courses of hypnotics are occasionally useful for helping a patient through an acute illness or some other crisis but every effort must be made to avoid dependence.

Diuretics are overprescribed in old age and should not be used to treat simple gravitational oedema which will usually respond to increased movement, raising the legs, and support stockings. A few days of diuretic treatment may speed the clearing of the oedema but it should rarely need continued drug therapy.

Other drugs which commonly cause adverse reactions are antiparkinsonian drugs, antihypertensives, psychotropics, and digoxin; the usual maintenance dose of digoxin in very old patients should be 125 micrograms daily (toxicity is common in those given 250 micrograms).

Drug-induced blood disorders are much more common in the elderly. Therefore drugs with a tendency to cause bone marrow depression (e.g. co-trimoxazole) should be avoided whenever possible.

GUIDELINES. First one must always pose the question of whether a drug is indicated at all.

It is a sensible policy to prescribe from a limited range of drugs and to be thoroughly familiar with their effects in the elderly.

Dosage should generally be substantially lower than for younger patients and it is common to start with about 50% of the adult dose. Some drugs (e.g. chlorpropamide) should be avoided altogether.

Review repeat prescriptions regularly. It may be possible to stop the drug (e.g. digoxin can often be withdrawn) or it may be necessary to reduce the dose to match diminishing renal function.

Simplify regimens. Elderly patients cannot normally cope with more than three different drugs and, ideally, these should not be given more than twice daily. In particular, regimens which call for a confusing array of dosage intervals should be avoided.

Write full instructions on every prescription (*including* repeat prescriptions) so that containers can be properly labelled with full directions. Avoid imprecisions like 'as directed'. Child-resistant containers may be unsuitable.

If these guidelines are followed most elderly people will cope adequately with their own medicines. If not then it is essential to enrol the help of a third party, usually a relative but sometimes a home help, neighbour, or a sheltered-housing warden.

Prescribing in Terminal Care

In recent years there has been increased interest in providing better treatment and support for patients with terminal illness. The aim is to keep them as comfortable, alert, and free of pain as possible. If patients are to end their days in serenity it may also be necessary to direct attention to emotional, financial, social, or family problems. The patient's minister or the hospital chaplain may give invaluable help.

DOMICILIARY TREATMENT. Whenever possible patients should end their days in their own homes with their families. Although families may at first be resistant to, or frightened of, caring for the patient at home, they will usually do so if extra support from district nursing services and social services is provided. Families may be reassured if an assurance is given that the patient will be admitted to hospital if they are unable to cope.

HOSPITAL TREATMENT. The most important lesson to be drawn from the experience of hospices is that both doctors and nurses must give time to listen to the patient. This gives great support and comfort to a patient who may otherwise suffer intolerable loneliness. Often problems come to light that can easily be dealt with—adjusting a blind in the late afternoon, an irritating noise to be avoided, drinks to be placed in easier reach, someone to read the newspaper, or the TV to be replaced by radio. The staff should not exclude the family from contributing to the patient's care; if prevented they may be resentful or subsequently suffer a feeling of guilt.

DRUG TREATMENT. The number of drugs should be as few as possible, for even the taking of medicine may be an effort.

PAIN. Analgesics are always more effective in preventing the development of pain than in the relief of established pain. The non-opioid analgesics **aspirin** or **paracetamol** given regularly will often make the use of opioids unnecessary.

Anti-inflammatory analgesics may control the pain of *bone secondaries* if aspirin is inadequate. Naproxen, flurbiprofen, and indomethacin are valuable and if necessary can be given rectally. Corticosteroids or radiotherapy are often useful for pain due to bone metastasis.

Morphine is the most useful opioid analgesic (see section 4.7.2). It is given by mouth regularly every 4 hours as a simple solution in chloroform water. The dose should be the lowest which prevents pain; a dose of 5–20 mg every 4 hours is usually effective but there need be no hesitation in increasing it to 30–60 mg or occasionally to 90–150 mg if necessary. Sustained-release preparations of morphine are available for oral administration which need only be given twice daily.

For patients unable to swallow, morphine (or sometimes oxycodone, see section 4.7.2.) may be given as suppositories. **Diamorphine** is preferred for injection (and for subcutaneous infusion via syringe driver[1]) since it is more soluble and can be given in a smaller volume; diamorphine hydrochloride 1 mg by intramuscular injection is generally considered to be as effective as morphine hydrochloride (or sulphate) 3 or 4 mg by mouth.

Nausea and vomiting may occur in the initial stages of morphine therapy and can be prevented by giving an anti-emetic such as prochlorperazine (usually only necessary for the first 4 or 5 days).

MISCELLANEOUS CONDITIONS. *Headache due to raised intracranial pressure* often responds to a high dose of a corticosteroid, e.g. dexamethasone 16 mg daily for 4 to 5 days, subsequently reduced to 4 to 6 mg daily if possible. *Intractable cough* may be relieved by inhalations or may require diamorphine linctus; oral morphine hydrochloride solution in an initial dose of 5 mg every 4 hours may be preferable; methadone linctus has a long duration of action and tends to accumulate. *Dyspnoea* may be relieved by regular oral morphine hydrochloride solution in carefully titrated doses, starting at 5 mg every 4 hours; diazepam 2 mg every 8 hours and a corticosteroid, such as dexamethasone 4 to 8 mg daily, may also be helpful. *Excessive respiratory secretion* (death rattle) may be reduced by subcutaneous injection of hyoscine hydrobromide 400 to 600 micrograms every 4 to 8 hours. *Restlessness and confusion* may require treatment with chlorpromazine hydrochloride 50 to 100 mg by mouth initially, followed by 25 to 50 mg every 8 hours, or haloperidol 1 to 3 mg by mouth every 8 hours; methotrimeprazine is used occasionally for restlessness in terminal illness. *Hiccup* may be treated with chlorpromazine 10 to 25 mg every 6 to 8 hours or metoclopramide 10 mg every 6 to 8 hours by mouth or by intramuscular injection. *Anorexia* may be helped by prednisolone 15 to 30 mg daily or dexamethasone 2 to 4 mg daily. *Constipation* is a very common cause of distress and should be prevented if possible by the regular administration of laxatives; a faecal softener with a peristaltic stimulant (e.g. lactulose solution with a senna preparation) should be used. *Fungating growth* may be treated by cleansing with a mixture of 1 part of 4% povidone-iodine skin cleanser solution and 4 parts of liquid paraffin. *Capillary bleeding* may be reduced by applying gauze soaked in adrenaline solution (1 in 1000). *Dry mouth* may be due to candidiasis which can be treated by nystatin mixture 100 000 units or amphotericin lozenges after food. *Pruritus*, even when associated with obstructive jaundice, often responds to simple measures such as emollients; further measures include administration of cholestyramine or an anabolic steroid.

---

1. Health Equipment Information No. 175, October 1987 contains an evaluation of infusion pumps and controllers. Doctors working for the NHS can obtain the report free from Regional or District Administrators; others can obtain it for £5 from DHSS (Leaflets), PO Box 21, Stanmore, Middx HA7 1AY.

Prescribing in Liver Disease

Liver disease may alter the response to drugs in several ways as indicated below, and drug prescribing should be kept to a minimum in all patients with severe liver disease. The main problems occur in patients with jaundice, ascites, or evidence of encephalopathy.

IMPAIRED DRUG METABOLISM. Metabolism by the liver is the main route of elimination for many drugs, but the hepatic reserve appears to be large and liver disease has to be severe before important changes in drug metabolism occur. Routine liver-function tests are a poor guide to the capacity of the liver to metabolise drugs, and in the individual patient it is not possible to predict the extent to which the metabolism of a particular drug may be impaired.

A few drugs, e.g. rifampicin and fusidic acid, are excreted in the bile unchanged and may accumulate in patients with intrahepatic or extrahepatic obstructive jaundice.

HYPOPROTEINAEMIA. The hypoalbuminaemia in severe liver disease is associated with reduced protein binding and increased toxicity of some highly protein-bound drugs such as phenytoin and prednisolone.

REDUCED CLOTTING. Reduced hepatic synthesis of blood-clotting factors, indicated by a prolonged prothrombin time, increases the sensitivity to oral anticoagulants such as warfarin and phenindione.

HEPATIC ENCEPHALOPATHY. In severe liver disease many drugs can further impair cerebral function and may precipitate hepatic encephalopathy. These include all sedative drugs, narcotic analgesics, those diuretics that produce hypokalaemia, and drugs that cause constipation.

FLUID OVERLOAD. Oedema and ascites in chronic liver disease may be exacerbated by drugs that give rise to fluid retention, e.g. NSAIDs, corticosteroids, and carbenoxolone.

HEPATOTOXIC DRUGS. Hepatotoxicity is either dose-related or unpredictable (idiosyncratic). Drugs causing dose-related toxicity may do so at lower doses than in patients with normal liver function, and some drugs producing reactions of the idiosyncratic kind do so more frequently in patients with liver disease. These drugs should be avoided.

Table of drugs to be avoided or used with caution in liver disease

The list of drugs given below is not comprehensive and is based on current information concerning the use of these drugs in therapeutic dosage.

Drugs	Comment	Drugs	Comment
Alfentanil see Opioid Analgesics		Anxiolytics and Hypnotics	All can precipitate coma; small dose of lorazepam or oxazepam probably safest; reduce oral dose of chlormethiazole
Alprazolam see Anxiolytics and Hypnotics			
Aminophylline see Theophylline			
Amitriptyline see Antidepressants			
Analgesics see NSAIDs and Opioid Analgesics			
Androgens and Anabolic Steroids	Avoid—dose-related toxicity	Aspirin	Avoid—increased risk of gastro-intestinal bleeding
Antacids	In patients with fluid retention, avoid those containing large amounts of sodium, e.g. magnesium trisilicate mixture, *Gaviscon®*. Avoid those causing constipation—can precipitate coma	Astemizole see Antihistamines	
		Auranofin see Gold	
		Aurothiomalate see Gold	
		Azapropazone see NSAIDs	
		Azatadine see Antihistamines	
		Bendrofluazide see Thiazides	
		Benorylate [aspirin-paracetamol ester] see Aspirin	
		Benperidol see Antipsychotics	
		Benzodiazepines see Anxiolytics and Hypnotics	
		Beta-blockers see individual drugs	
Anticoagulants, Oral	Avoid, especially if prothrombin time is already prolonged	Bezafibrate	Avoid in severe liver disease
		Bromazepam see Anxiolytics and Hypnotics	
Antidepressants	Tricyclics preferable to MAOIs but sedative effects increased. Iprindole and MAOIs may cause idiosyncratic hepatotoxicity	Brompheniramine see Antihistamines	
		Bumetanide see Loop Diuretics	
		Buprenorphine see Opioid Analgesics	
		Butriptyline see Antidepressants	
Antihistamines	Avoid—may precipitate coma	Carbenoxolone	Produces fluid retention and hypokalaemia
Anti-inflammatory Analgesics (NSAIDs)	Increased risk of gastro-intestinal bleeding and can cause fluid retention	Chenodeoxycholic acid	Avoid in chronic liver disease; patients with non-functioning gall-bladder do not respond
Antipsychotics	All can precipitate coma; phenothiazines are hepatotoxic	Chloral hydrate see Anxiolytics and Hypnotics	

Table of drugs to be avoided or used with caution in liver disease (*continued*)

Drugs	Comment	Drugs	Comment
Chloramphenicol	Avoid—increased risk of bone-marrow depression	Ergotamine	Avoid in severe liver disease—risk of toxicity increased
Chlordiazepoxide *see* Anxiolytics and Hypnotics		Erythromycin	May cause idiosyncratic hepatotoxicity
Chlormethiazole	Reduce oral dose; *see* Anxiolytics and Hypnotics	Ethacrynic acid *see* Loop Diuretics	
Chlormezanone *see* Anxiolytics and Hypnotics		Etodolac *see* NSAIDs	
Chlorothiazide *see* Thiazides		Etretinate	Avoid—further impairment of liver function may occur
Chlorpheniramine *see* Antihistamines		Fenbufen *see* NSAIDs	
Chlorpromazine	*see* Antipsychotics	Fenoprofen *see* NSAIDs	
Chlorpropamide	Avoid—increased risk of hypoglycaemia and can produce jaundice	Flecainide	Avoid (or reduce dose) in severe liver disease
Chlorprothixene *see* Antipsychotics		Flunitrazepam *see* Anxiolytics and Hypnotics	
Chlorthalidone *see* Thiazides		Flupenthixol *see* Antipsychotics	
Cholestyramine	Interferes with absorption of fat-soluble vitamins and may aggravate malabsorption in primary biliary cirrhosis	Fluphenazine *see* Antipsychotics	
		Flurazepam *see* Anxiolytics and Hypnotics	
		Flurbiprofen *see* NSAIDs	
Choline magnesium trisalicylate *see* Aspirin		Fluspirilene *see* Antipsychotics	
Choline theophyllinate *see* Theophylline		Frusemide *see* Loop diuretics	
Cimetidine	Increased risk of confusion; reduce dose	Fusidic acid	Impaired biliary excretion; may be increased risk of hepatotoxicity; avoid or reduce dose
Cinnarizine *see* Antihistamines			
Clemastine *see* Antihistamines			
Clindamycin	Reduce dose	Gemfibrozil	Avoid in severe liver disease
Clobazam *see* Anxiolytics and Hypnotics		Gold (auranofin, aurothiomalate)	Avoid in severe liver disease—hepatotoxicity may occur
Clofibrate	Avoid in severe liver disease		
Clomiphene	Avoid in severe liver disease		
Clomipramine *see* Antidepressants		Haloperidol *see* Antipsychotics	
Clopamide *see* Thiazides		Hydrochlorothiazide *see* Thiazides	
Clorazepate *see* Anxiolytics and Hypnotics		Hydroflumethiazide *see* Thiazides	
Codeine *see* Opioid Analgesics		Hydroxyzine *see* Antihistamines	
Contraceptives, oral	Avoid in cholestatic liver disease and in patients with a history of pruritus or cholestasis during pregnancy	Hypnotics *see* Anxiolytics and Hypnotics	
		Ibuprofen *see* NSAIDs	
		Imipramine *see* Antidepressants	
		Indapamide *see* Thiazides	
Cyclizine *see* Antihistamines		Indomethacin *see* NSAIDs	
Cyclofenil	Avoid in severe liver disease	Iprindole	May cause idiosyncratic hepatotoxicity; *see* Antidepressants
Cyclopenthiazide *see* Thiazides			
Cyproheptadine *see* Antihistamines			
Cyproterone	Avoid—dose-related toxicity	Isocarboxazid *see* Antidepressants	
Dantrolene	Avoid—may cause severe liver damage	Isoniazid	Avoid—idiosyncratic hepatotoxicity more common
Dehydrocholic acid	Avoid in intra-hepatic cholestasis or complete biliary obstruction	Ketazolam *see* Anxiolytics and Hypnotics	
		Ketoconazole	Induces hepatitis-like reaction; may accumulate in severe liver disease; contra-indicated unless no alternative
Desipramine *see* Antidepressants			
Dextromethorphan *see* Opioid Analgesics			
Dextromoramide *see* Opioid Analgesics			
Dextropropoxyphene *see* Opioid Analgesics		Ketoprofen *see* NSAIDs	
Diamorphine *see* Opioid Analgesics		Ketotifen *see* Antihistamines	
Diazepam *see* Anxiolytics and Hypnotics		Labetalol	Reduce oral dose
Dichloralphenazone *see* Anxiolytics and Hypnotics		Levorphanol *see* Opioid Analgesics	
Diclofenac *see* NSAIDs		Lignocaine	Avoid (or reduce dose) in severe liver disease
Diflunisal *see* NSAIDs			
Dihydrocodeine *see* Opioid Analgesics		Lincomycin	Avoid if possible
Dimenhydrinate *see* Antihistamines		Lofepramine *see* Antidepressants	
Dimethindene *see* Antihistamines		Loop diuretics	Hypokalaemia may precipitate coma; potassium-sparing diuretic should be used to prevent this; increased risk of hypomagnesaemia in alcoholic cirrhosis
Diphenoxylate *see* Opioid Analgesics			
Diphenylpyraline *see* Antihistamines			
Dipipanone *see* Opioid Analgesics			
Dothiepin *see* Antidepressants			
Doxepin *see* Antidepressants			
Doxorubicin	Reduce dose according to bilirubin concentration		
		Loprazolam *see* Anxiolytics and Hypnotics	
Droperidol *see* Antipsychotics		Lorazepam *see* Anxiolytics and Hypnotics	
Epirubicin	Reduce dose according to bilirubin concentration	Lormetazepam *see* Anxiolytics and Hypnotics	

Table of drugs to be avoided or used with caution in liver disease (*continued*)

Drugs	Comment
Magnesium sulphate	Avoid in hepatic coma if risk of renal failure
MAOIs *see* Antidepressants	
Maprotiline *see* Antidepressants	
Mebhydrolin *see* Antihistamines	
Medazepam *see* Anxiolytics and Hypnotics	
Mefenamic acid *see* NSAIDs	
Mefruside *see* Thiazides	
Meprobamate *see* Anxiolytics and Hypnotics	
Meptazinol *see* Opioid Analgesics	
Mequitazine *see* Antihistamines	
Metformin	Avoid—increased risk of lactic acidosis
Methadone *see* Opioid Analgesics	
Methotrexate	Dose-related toxicity—avoid in non-malignant conditions (e.g. psoriasis)
Methotrimeprazine *see* Antipsychotics	
Methyclothiazide *see* Thiazides	
Methyldopa	Avoid—increased risk of hepatotoxicity
Methyltestosterone *see* Androgens and Anabolic Steroids	
Metoprolol	Reduce oral dose
Metronidazole	Reduce dose in severe liver disease
Mexiletine	Avoid—or reduce dose in severe liver disease
Mianserin *see* Antidepressants	
Monoamine-oxidase inhibitors (MAOIs)	May cause idiosyncratic hepatotoxicity; *see* Antidepressants
Morphine *see* Opioid Analgesics	
Nabumetone *see* NSAIDs	
Nalbuphine *see* Opioid Analgesics	
Nandrolone *see* Androgens and Anabolic Steroids	
Naproxen *see* NSAIDs	
Narcotic Analgesics *see* Opioid Analgesics	
Nicardipine	Reduce dose
Nifedipine	Reduce dose
Niridazole	Increased CNS toxicity in patients with cirrhosis or portal-systemic shunts
Nitrazepam *see* Anxiolytics and Hypnotics	
Nitroprusside	Avoid in severe liver disease
Nortriptyline *see* Antidepressants	
NSAIDs	Increased risk of gastro-intestinal bleeding and can cause fluid retention
Oestrogens	Avoid; *see also* Contraceptives, oral
Opioid Analgesics	Avoid—may precipitate coma
Oxatomide *see* Antihistamines	
Oxazepam *see* Anxiolytics and Hypnotics	
Oxprenolol	Reduce oral dose
Oxymetholone *see* Androgens and Anabolic Steroids	
Oxypertine *see* Antipsychotics	
Papaveretum *see* Opioid Analgesics	
Paracetamol	Dose-related toxicity—avoid large doses
Pentazocine *see* Opioid Analgesics	
Pericyazine *see* Antipsychotics	
Perphenazine *see* Antipsychotics	
Pethidine *see* Opioid Analgesics	
Phenazocine *see* Opioid Analgesics	
Phenelzine *see* Antidepressants	
Phenindamine *see* Antihistamines	
Pheniramine *see* Antihistamines	
Phenobarbitone	May precipitate coma
Phenoperidine *see* Opioid Analgesics	
Phenothiazines *see* Antipsychotics	
Phenylbutazone *see* NSAIDs	
Phenytoin	Reduce dose to avoid toxicity
Pholcodine *see* Opioid Analgesics	
Pimozide *see* Antipsychotics	
Pipothiazine *see* Antipsychotics	
Piretanide *see* Loop Diuretics	
Piroxicam *see* NSAIDs	
Polythiazide *see* Thiazides	
Prazepam *see* Anxiolytics and Hypnotics	
Prednisolone	Side-effects more common; prednisolone preferable to prednisone (needs conversion to prednisolone by liver before active)
Prednisone	Prednisolone is preferable
Primidone	May precipitate coma
Prochlorperazine *see* Antipsychotics	
Progestogens	Avoid; *see also* Contraceptives, oral
Promazine *see* Antipsychotics	
Promethazine *see* Antihistamines	
Propranolol	Reduce oral dose
Protriptyline *see* Antidepressants	
Pyrazinamide	Avoid—idiosyncratic hepatotoxicity more common
Ranitidine	Increased risk of confusion; reduce dose
Rifampicin	Impaired elimination; may be increased risk of hepatotoxicity; avoid or reduce dose
Salsalate *see* Aspirin	
Sodium aurothiomalate *see* Gold	
Sodium salicylate *see* Aspirin	
Sodium nitroprusside *see* Nitroprusside	
Sodium valproate *see* Valproate	
Stanozolol *see* Androgens and Anabolic Steroids	
Sulindac *see* NSAIDs	
Suxamethonium	Prolonged apnoea may occur in severe liver disease due to reduced hepatic synthesis of pseudocholinesterase
Temazepam *see* Anxiolytics and Hypnotics	
Terfenadine *see* Antihistamines	
Testosterone *see* Androgens and Anabolic Steroids	
Tetracyclines	Avoid—dose-related toxicity by i/v route
Theophylline	Reduce dose
Thiazides	Hypokalaemia may precipitate coma (potassium-sparing diuretic can prevent); increased risk of hypomagnesaemia in alcoholic cirrhosis
Thiethylperazine *see* Antipsychotics	
Thiopentone	Reduce dose for induction in severe liver disease
Thioridazine *see* Antipsychotics	
Tiaprofenic acid *see* NSAIDs	
Tocainide	Avoid—or reduce dose in severe liver disease

Table of drugs to be avoided or used with caution in liver disease (*continued*)

Drugs	Comment	Drugs	Comment
Tolbutamide	Avoid—increased risk of hypoglycaemia; can produce jaundice	Triprolidine *see* Antihistamines	
Tolmetin *see* NSAIDs		Ursodeoxycholic acid	Avoid in chronic liver disease; patients with non-functioning gall-bladder do not respond
Tranylcypromine *see* Antidepressants			
Trazodone *see* Antidepressants		Valproate	Avoid if possible—hepatotoxicity and liver failure may occasionally occur (usually in first 6 months)
Triazolam *see* Anxiolytics and Hypnotics			
Triclofos *see* Anxiolytics and Hypnotics			
Trifluoperazine *see* Antipsychotics			
Trifluperidol *see* Antipsychotics		Verapamil	Reduce dose
Trimeprazine *see* Antihistamines			
Trimipramine *see* Antidepressants			

Prescribing in Renal Impairment

The use of drugs in patients with reduced renal function can give rise to problems for several reasons:

> failure to excrete a drug or its metabolites may produce toxicity;
> sensitivity to some drugs is increased even if elimination is unimpaired;
> many side-effects are tolerated poorly by patients in renal failure;
> some drugs cease to be effective when renal function is reduced.

Many of these problems can be avoided by reducing the dose or by using alternative drugs.

Principles of dose adjustment in renal impairment

The level of renal function below which the dose of a drug must be reduced depends on whether the drug is eliminated entirely by renal excretion or is partly metabolised, and on how toxic it is.

For many drugs with only minor or no dose-related side-effects very precise modification of the dose regimen is unnecessary and a simple scheme for dose reduction is sufficient.

For more toxic drugs with a small safety margin dose regimens based on glomerular filtration rate should be used. For those where both efficacy and toxicity are closely related to plasma concentrations recommended regimens should be seen only as a guide to initial treatment; subsequent treatment must be adjusted according to clinical response and plasma concentration.

The total daily maintenance dose of a drug can be reduced either by reducing the size of the individual doses or by increasing the interval between doses. For some drugs, if the size of the maintenance dose is reduced it will be important to give a loading dose if an immediate effect is required. This is because when a patient is given a regular dose of any drug it takes more than five times the half-life to achieve steady-state plasma concentrations. As the plasma half-life of drugs excreted by the kidney is prolonged in renal failure it may take many days for the reduced dosage to achieve a therapeutic plasma concentration.

The loading dose should usually be the same size as the initial dose for a patient with normal renal function.

Nephrotoxic drugs should, if possible, be avoided in patients with renal disease because the consequences of nephrotoxicity are likely to be more serious when the renal reserve is already reduced.

Use of dosage table

Dose recommendations are based on the severity of renal impairment. This is expressed in terms of glomerular filtration rate (GFR), usually measured by the **creatinine clearance**. The serum-creatinine concentration can be used instead as a measure of renal function but is only a rough guide unless corrected for age, weight, and sex. Nomograms are available for making the correction and should be used where accuracy is important.

Renal impairment is arbitrarily divided into 3 grades:

Grade	GFR	Serum creatinine (approx.)
Mild	20–50 ml/min	150–300 µmol/litre
Moderate	10–20 ml/min	300–700 µmol/litre
Severe	< 10 ml/min	> 700 µmol/litre

Renal function declines with age; many elderly patients have a glomerular filtration rate below 50 ml/minute which, because of reduced muscle mass, may not be indicated by a raised serum creatinine. It is wise to assume at least mild impairment of renal function when prescribing for the elderly.

The following table may be used as a guide to drugs which are known to require a reduction in dose in renal impairment, and to those which are potentially harmful or are ineffective. Drug prescribing should be kept to the minimum in all patients with severe renal disease.

Renal function should be checked before prescribing **any** drug which requires dose modification in the presence of mild renal impairment.

Table of drugs to be avoided or used with caution in renal impairment

Drugs	GFR ml/minute	Dosage recommendations	Comments
Acebutolol	<10	Start with small dose	Active metabolite accumulates
Acetazolamide	<10	Avoid	Metabolic acidosis
Acetohexamide	<50	Avoid	Tolbutamide and gliquidone suitable alternatives
Acyclovir	<50	Reduce dose	Possible transient increase in plasma urea
Alcuronium	<20	Reduce dose	Prolonged paralysis with large or repeated doses

Alfentanil see Opioid Analgesics

Table of drugs to be avoided or used with caution in renal impairment (*continued*)

Drugs	GFR ml/minute	Dosage recommendations	Comments
Allopurinol	10–20 <10	Max. 200 mg daily Max. 100 mg daily	Increased toxicity; rashes
Alprazolam *see* Anxiolytics and Hypnotics			
Amantadine	<50	Avoid	Excreted by kidney
Amikacin *see* Aminoglycosides			
Amiloride *see* Potassium-sparing diuretics			
Aminoglycosides	<50	Reduce dose. Monitor plasma concentrations	Ototoxic; nephrotoxic
Amoxycillin	<10	Reduce dose	Rashes more common
Amphotericin	<50	Use only if no alternative	Nephrotoxic
Ampicillin	<10	Reduce dose	Rashes more common
Amylobarbitone	<10	Reduce dose	Active metabolite accumulates
Analgesics *see* Opioid Analgesics and NSAIDs			
Anti-inflammatory analgesics (NSAIDs)	<50	Avoid if possible	Fluid retention and deterioration in renal function
Antipsychotics	<10	Start with small doses	Increased cerebral sensitivity
Anxiolytics and Hypnotics	<10	Start with small doses	Increased cerebral sensitivity
Aspirin	<10	Avoid	Fluid retention; deterioration in renal function; increased risk of gastro-intestinal bleeding
Atenolol	<20	Reduce dose	Excreted unchanged
Augmentin®	<20	Reduce dose	
Auranofin *see* Gold			
Aurothiomalate, sodium *see* Gold			
Azapropazone	<20	Avoid	Excreted by kidney; *see also* NSAIDs
Azathioprine	<10	Reduce dose	
Azlocillin	<20	Reduce dose	
Aztreonam	<20	Reduce dose	
Bacampicillin	<10	Avoid	Potentially toxic products of hydrolysis of ester may accumulate
Baclofen	<50	Use smaller doses	Excreted by kidney
Bendrofluazide *see* Thiazides			
Benorylate [aspirin-paracetamol ester] *see* Aspirin			
Benperidol *see* Antipsychotics			
Benzodiazepines *see* Anxiolytics and Hypnotics			
Benzylpenicillin	<10	Max. 6 g daily	Neurotoxicity—high doses may cause convulsions
Beta-blockers	<10	Start with small dose	
Betaxolol *see* Beta-blockers			
Bethanidine	<20	Avoid	Increased postural hypotension; decrease in renal blood flow
Bezafibrate	10–50 <10	Reduce dose Avoid	Further deterioration in renal function
Bicarbonate *see* Sodium bicarbonate			
Bisoprolol *see* Beta-blockers			
Bleomycin	<20	Reduce dose	

Table of drugs to be avoided or used with caution in renal impairment (*continued*)

Drugs	GFR ml/minute	Dosage recommendations	Comments
Bromazepam *see* Anxiolytics and Hypnotics			
Bumetanide	<20	May need high doses	
Buprenorphine *see* Opioid Analgesics			
Capreomycin	<50	Reduce dose	Neurotoxic; ototoxic
Captopril	<50	Reduce dose and monitor response; avoid if possible	Excreted by kidney; hyperkalaemia and other side-effects more common
Carbenicillin	<20	Reduce dose	Neurotoxic; may produce bleeding diathesis; 1 g contains 5.4 mmol sodium
Carbenoxolone	<10	Avoid	Fluid retention
Cefadroxil	<20	Reduce dose	
Cefotaxime	<5	Use half dose	
Cefoxitin	<50	Reduce dose	
Cefsulodin	<20	Reduce dose	
Ceftazidime	<50	Reduce dose	
Ceftizoxime	<50	Reduce dose	
Cefuroxime	<50	Reduce dose	
Cephalexin	<10	Max. 500 mg daily	
Cephalothin	<50	Avoid	Nephrotoxic
Cephamandole	<50	Reduce dose	
Cephazolin	<50	Reduce dose	
Cephradine	<50	Reduce dose	
Chloral hydrate *see* Anxiolytics and Hypnotics			
Chloramphenicol	<10	Avoid unless no alternative	Dose-related depression of haemopoiesis
Chlordiazepoxide *see* Anxiolytics and Hypnotics			
Chlormethiazole *see* Anxiolytics and Hypnotics			
Chlormezanone *see* Anxiolytics and Hypnotics			
Chloroquine	20–50	Max. 75 mg daily	Only on prolonged use
	10–20	Max. 50 mg daily	
	<10	Avoid	
Chlorothiazide *see* Thiazides			
Chlorpropamide	<50	Avoid	Tolbutamide and gliquidone suitable alternatives
Chlorpromazine *see* Antipsychotics			
Chlorprothixene *see* Antipsychotics			
Chlorthalidone *see* Thiazides			
Choline magnesium trisalicylate *see* Aspirin			
Ciclacillin	<50	Reduce dose	
Cimetidine	10–20	400–600 mg daily	Occasional risk of confusion
	<10	400 mg daily	
Cinoxacin	<20	Avoid	Nausea, rashes
Ciprofloxacin	<20	Use half dose	
Cisplatin	<50	Avoid if possible	Nephrotoxic
Clavulanic acid [ingredient] *see Augmentin®, Timentin®*			
Clobazam *see* Anxiolytics and Hypnotics			
Clofibrate	10–50	Reduce dose	Further deterioration in renal function; myopathy
	<10	Avoid	
Clopamide *see* Thiazides			
Clorazepate *see* Anxiolytics and Hypnotics			

Table of drugs to be avoided or used with caution in renal impairment (*continued*)

Drugs	GFR ml/minute	Dosage recommendations	Comments
Codeine	<20	Avoid	Increased and prolonged effect; *see also* Opioid Analgesics
Colchicine	<10	Avoid or reduce dose if no alternative	
Colistin sulphomethate sodium	<50	Reduce dose	Nephrotoxic; neurotoxic
Colven®	<10	Avoid	High sodium content
Co-trimoxazole	<10	Max. 960 mg daily	Rashes and blood disorders; may cause further deterioration in renal function
Cyclopenthiazide *see* Thiazides			
Cyclophosphamide	<20	Reduce dose	
Cycloserine	<50	Avoid	
Debrisoquine	<20	Avoid	Increased postural hypotension; decrease in renal blood flow
De-Nol®, De-Noltab®	<10	Avoid	
Dextromethorphan *see* Opioid Analgesics			
Dextromoramide *see* Opioid Analgesics			
Dextropropoxyphene	<10	Avoid	Increased CNS toxicity
Diamorphine *see* Opioid Analgesics			
Diazepam *see* Anxiolytics and Hypnotics			
Diazoxide	<10	75–150 mg i/v	Increased sensitivity to hypotensive effect
Dichloralphenazone *see* Anxiolytics and Hypnotics			
Diclofenac *see* NSAIDs			
Diflunisal	<10	Avoid	Excreted by kidney; *see also* NSAIDs
Digitoxin	<10	Max. 100 micrograms daily	As digoxin
Digoxin	20–50	250 micrograms daily	Toxicity increased by electrolyte disturbances in severe impairment
	10–20	125–250 micrograms daily	
	<10	Up to 125 micrograms daily	
Dihydrocodeine	<20	Avoid	Increased and prolonged effect; *see also* Opioid Analgesics
Diphenoxylate *see* Opioid Analgesics			
Dipipanone *see* Opioid Analgesics			
Disodium etidronate	20–50	Max. 5 mg/kg daily	Excreted by kidney
	<20	Avoid	
Disopyramide	20–50	100 mg every 8 hours *or* 150 mg every 12 hours	
	10–20	100 mg every 12 hours	
	<10	150 mg every 24 hours	
Droperidol *see* Antipsychotics			
Domperidone	<10	Reduce dose by 30–50%	
Enalapril	<50	Initial daily dose 2.5 mg	As for Captopril
Ergotamine	<20	Avoid	Nausea and vomiting; risk of renal vasoconstriction
Ethacrynic acid	<10	Avoid	Ototoxic
Ethambutol	<50	Avoid	Optic nerve damage
Etodolac *see* NSAIDs			
Famotidine	<20	Reduce dose	
Fenbufen *see* NSAIDs			

Table of drugs to be avoided or used with caution in renal impairment (*continued*)

Drugs	GFR ml/minute	Dosage recommendations	Comments
Fenoprofen *see* NSAIDs			
Fentanyl *see* Opioid Analgesics			
Flecainide	<50	Reduce dose	
Flucytosine	<50	Reduce dose	
Flunitrazepam *see* Anxiolytics and Hypnotics			
Flupenthixol *see* Antipsychotics			
Fluphenazine *see* Antipsychotics			
Flurazepam *see* Anxiolytics and Hypnotics			
Flurbiprofen *see* NSAIDs			
Fluspirilene *see* Antipsychotics			
Frusemide	<20	May need high doses	Deafness may follow rapid i/v injection
Gallamine	<20	Avoid	Prolonged paralysis
Gaviscon®	<10	Avoid	High sodium content
Gemfibrozil	<10	Start with 900 mg daily	
Gentamicin *see* Aminoglycosides			
Glibenclamide	<10	Avoid	Increased risk of prolonged hypoglycaemia
Gliclazide	<10	Start with small dose	Increased risk of hypoglycaemia
Glipizide	<10	Start with small dose	Increased risk of hypoglycaemia
Gliquidone	<10	May need dose reduction	Increased risk of hypoglycaemia
Glymidine	<10	Avoid	Increased risk of hypoglycaemia
Gold (auranofin, aurothiomalate)	<50	Avoid	Nephrotoxic
Guanethidine	<20	Avoid	Increased postural hypotension and decrease in renal blood flow
Haloperidol *see* Antipsychotics			
Hexamine	<50	Avoid	Ineffective
Hydralazine	<10	Start with small dose	Increased hypotensive effect
Hydrochlorothiazide *see* Thiazides			
Hydroflumethiazide *see* Thiazides			
Hydroxychloroquine	20–50 10–20 <10	Max. 75 mg daily Max. 50 mg daily Avoid	Only on prolonged use
Hypnotics *see* Anxiolytics and Hypnotics			
Ibuprofen *see* NSAIDs			
Ifosfamide	<20	Reduce dose	
Indapamide *see* Thiazides			
Indomethacin *see* NSAIDs			
Inosine pranobex	<50	Avoid	Metabolised to uric acid
Insulin	<10	May need dose reduction	Insulin requirements fall; compensatory response to hypoglycaemia is impaired
Isoniazid	<10	Max. 200 mg daily	Peripheral neuropathy
Kanamycin *see* Aminoglycosides			
Ketazolam *see* Anxiolytics and Hypnotics			
Ketoprofen *see* NSAIDs			
Latamoxef	<50	Reduce dose	
Levorphanol *see* Opioid Analgesics			
Lincomycin	<20	Use clindamycin instead	

Table of drugs to be avoided or used with caution in renal impairment (*continued*)

Drugs	GFR ml/minute	Dosage recommendations	Comments
Lithium	20–50	Avoid if possible or reduce dose and monitor plasma concentration carefully	
	<20	Avoid	
Loprazolam *see* Anxiolytics and Hypnotics			
Lorazepam *see* Anxiolytics and Hypnotics			
Lormetazepam *see* Anxiolytics and Hypnotics			
Magnesium salts	<20	Avoid or reduce dose	Increased risk of toxicity; magnesium carbonate mixture and magnesium trisilicate mixture also have high sodium content
Medazepam *see* Anxiolytics and Hypnotics			
Mefenamic acid *see* NSAIDs			
Mefruside *see* Thiazides			
Melphalan	<20	Reduce dose	
Meprobamate *see* Anxiolytics and Hypnotics			
Meptazinol *see* Opioid Analgesics			
Mercaptopurine	<20	Reduce dose	
Mesalazine	<50	Avoid	Manufacturer recommends avoidance as metabolite excreted by kidney
Metformin	<50	Avoid	Increased risk of lactic acidosis
Methadone *see* Opioid Analgesics			
Methocarbamol	<50	Avoid	Increased plasma urea and acidosis
Methotrexate	20–50	Reduce dose	Accumulates; nephrotoxic
	<20	Avoid	
Methotrimeprazine *see* Antipsychotics			
Methyclothiazide *see* Thiazides			
Methyldopa	<10	Start with small dose	Increased sensitivity to hypotensive and sedative effect
Metoclopramide	<10	Avoid or use small dose	Increased risk of extrapyramidal reactions
Metolazone *see* Thiazides			
Metoprolol	<10	Start with small dose	Higher plasma concentrations after oral administration; may reduce renal blood flow and adversely affect renal function in severe impairment
Mezlocillin	<10	Reduce dose	
Morphine	<20	Avoid	Increased and prolonged effect; *see also* Opioid Analgesics
Nabumetone *see* NSAIDs			
Nadolol	<20	Reduce dose	Excreted unchanged
Nalbuphine *see* Opioid Analgesics			
Nalidixic acid	<20	Avoid	Increased risk of nausea, vomiting, rashes, photosensitivity
Naproxen *see* NSAIDs			
Narcotic Analgesics *see* Opioid Analgesics			

Table of drugs to be avoided or used with caution in renal impairment (*continued*)

Drugs	GFR ml/minute	Dosage recommendations	Comments
Neomycin	<50	Avoid	Ototoxic; nephrotoxic
Netilmicin *see* Aminoglycosides			
Nicardipine	<20	Start with small dose	
Nifedipine	<20	Start with small dose	Reversible deterioration in renal function has been reported
Nitrazepam *see* Anxiolytics and Hypnotics			
Nitrofurantoin	<50	Avoid	Peripheral neuropathy
Nitroprusside	<20	Avoid prolonged use	
Nizatidine	20–50	150 mg daily	
	<20	150 mg on alternate days	
NSAIDs	<50	Avoid if possible	Fluid retention and deterioration in renal function.
Opioid Analgesics	<20	Use small doses—avoid codeine, dihydrocodeine, morphine	Increased cerebral sensitivity; *see also* individual entries
	<10	Avoid dextroproproxyphene, pethidine	
Oxazepam *see* Anxiolytics and Hypnotics			
Oxprenolol *see* Beta-blockers			
Oxypertine *see* Antipsychotics			
Pancuronium	<20	Reduce dose	Prolonged paralysis with large or repeated doses
Papaveretum *see* Opioid Analgesics			
Penbutolol *see* Beta-blockers			
Penicillamine	<50	Avoid if possible or reduce dose	Nephrotoxic
Pentazocine *see* Opioid Analgesics			
Pericyazine *see* Antipsychotics			
Perphenazine *see* Antipsychotics			
Pethidine	<10	Avoid	Increased CNS toxicity; *see also* Opioid Analgesics
Phenazocine *see* Opioid Analgesics			
Phenobarbitone	<10	Avoid large doses	
Phenoperidine *see* Opioid Analgesics			
Phenothiazines *see* Antipsychotics			
Phenylbutazone *see* NSAIDs			
Pholcodine *see* Opioid Analgesics			
Pimozide *see* Antipsychotics			
Pindolol	<20	Reduce dose	Excreted unchanged
Piperacillin	<20	Reduce dose	
Piperazine	<10	Reduce dose	Neurotoxic
Pipothiazine *see* Antipsychotics			
Piroxicam *see* NSAIDs			
Pivampicillin	<10	Avoid	Potentially toxic products of hydrolysis of ester may accumulate
Polythiazide *see* Thiazides			
Potassium salts	<20	Avoid routine use	High risk of hyperkalaemia
Potassium-sparing diuretics	20–50	Monitor plasma K$^+$	High risk of hyperkalaemia in renal impairment
	<20	Avoid	

Table of drugs to be avoided or used with caution in renal impairment (*continued*)

Drugs	GFR ml/minute	Dosage recommendations	Comments
Prazosin	<10	Start with small dose	Increased sensitivity to hypotensive effect and possible CNS toxicity
Primidone	<10	Avoid large doses	
Probenecid	<20	Avoid	Ineffective and toxicity increased
Procainamide	<50	Avoid or reduce dose	
Procarbazine	<20	Reduce dose	
Prochlorperazine *see* Antipsychotics			
Proguanil	<10	Avoid or reduce dose	Increased risk of haematological toxicity
Promazine *see* Antipsychotics			
Propranolol	<10	Start with small dose	Higher plasma concentrations after oral administration; may reduce renal blood flow and adversely affect renal function in severe impairment
Propylthiouracil	<50	Reduce dose	
Ranitidine	<10	Use half normal dose	
Salsalate *see* Aspirin			
Salt substitutes	<20	Avoid routine use	High risk of hyperkalaemia
Sandocal®	<10	Avoid	High potassium content
Sodium aurothiomalate *see* Gold			
Sodium bicarbonate	<10	Avoid	
Sodium nitroprusside *see* Nitroprusside			
Sodium salicylate *see* Aspirin			
Solpadeine®	<10	Avoid	High sodium content
Sotalol	<20	Reduce dose	Excreted unchanged
Spironolactone *see* Potassium-sparing diuretics			
Streptomycin *see* Aminoglycosides			
Sulfametopyrazine *see* Sulphonamides			
Sulindac	<20	Avoid	Excreted by kidney; *see also* NSAIDs
Sulphadiazine	<10	Avoid	High risk of crystalluria
Sulphadimidine *see* Sulphonamides			
Sulphasalazine	<10	Ensure high fluid intake	Rashes and blood disorders; crystalluria a risk
Sulphaurea *see* Sulphonamides			
Sulphinpyrazone	<20	Avoid	Ineffective as uricosuric
Sulphonamides	<10	Ensure high fluid intake	Rashes and blood disorders; crystalluria a risk
Sulphonylureas *see* under individual drugs			
Sulpiride	<20	Avoid if possible, or reduce dose	
Talampicillin	<10	Avoid	Potentially toxic products of hydrolysis of ester may accumulate
Temazepam *see* Anxiolytics and Hypnotics			
Tetracyclines (except doxycycline and minocycline)	<50	Avoid—use doxycycline or minocycline if necessary	Anti-anabolic effect, increased plasma urea, further deterioration in renal function

Table of drugs to be avoided or used with caution in renal impairment (*continued*)

Drugs	GFR ml/minute	Dosage recommendations	Comments
Thiazides and related diuretics (except metolazone)	<20	Avoid	Ineffective (metolazone remains effective but risk of excessive diuresis)
Thiethylperazine *see* Antipsychotics			
Thioguanine	<20	Reduce dose	
Thioridazine *see* Antipsychotics			
Tiaprofenic acid *see* NSAIDs			
Ticarcillin	<20	Reduce dose	1 g contains 5.3 mmol sodium
Timentin®	<20	Reduce dose	
Timolol *see* Beta-blockers			
Tobramycin *see* Aminoglycosides			
Tocainide	<50	Reduce dose	
Tolazamide	<10	May need dose reduction	Increased risk of hypoglycaemia
Tolbutamide	<10	May need dose reduction	Increased risk of hypoglycaemia
Tolmetin	<50	*See* NSAIDs	
	<10	Avoid	
Triamterene *see* Potassium-sparing diuretics			
Triazolam *see* Anxiolytics and Hypnotics			
Triclofos *see* Anxiolytics and Hypnotics			
Trifluoperazine *see* Antipsychotics			
Trifluperidol *see* Antipsychotics			
Trimethoprim	<10	Reduce dose	Possible deterioration in renal function
Tubocurarine	<20	Reduce dose	Prolonged paralysis with large or repeated doses
Vancomycin	<50	Avoid parenteral use if possible	Ototoxic; nephrotoxic
Xipamide *see* Thiazides			
Zuclopenthixol *see* Antipsychotics			

Prescribing in Pregnancy

Drugs can have harmful effects on the fetus at any time during pregnancy. Experience with many drugs in pregnancy is limited.

During the *first trimester* they may produce congenital malformations (teratogenesis), and the period of greatest risk is from the third to the eleventh week of pregnancy.

During the *second* and *third trimesters* drugs may affect the growth and functional development of the fetus or have toxic effects on fetal tissues; and drugs given shortly before term or during labour may have adverse effects on the neonate after delivery.

The following table lists drugs which may have harmful effects in pregnancy and indicates the trimester of risk.

The table is based on human data but information on *animal* studies has been included for some newer drugs when its omission might be misleading.

> Drugs should be prescribed in pregnancy only if the expected benefit to the mother is thought to be greater than the risk to the fetus, and all drugs should be avoided if possible during the first trimester. Drugs which have been extensively used in pregnancy and appear to be usually safe should be prescribed in preference to new or untried drugs; and the smallest effective dose should be used.
>
> Few drugs have been shown conclusively to be teratogenic in man but no drug is safe beyond all doubt in early pregnancy.
>
> Absence of a drug from the list does not imply safety.

Table of drugs to be avoided or used with caution in pregnancy

Drug (Trimester of risk)	Comments	Drug (Trimester of risk)	Comments
Acebutolol *see* Beta-blockers		Anticoagulants, Oral (*cont.*)	haemorrhage; subcutaneous heparin should be substituted in the last few weeks of pregnancy in patients with prosthetic heart valve and can be substituted throughout for deep-vein thrombosis; *see also* section 2.8
Acetazolamide *see* Diuretics			
Acetohexamide *see* Sulphonylureas			
Alclometasone *see* Corticosteroids			
Alcohol			
(1, 2)	Regular daily drinking is teratogenic and may cause growth retardation; occasional single drinks are probably safe		
(3)	Withdrawal syndrome may occur in babies of alcoholic mothers	Antidepressants, Tricyclic (and related) (3)	Tachycardia, irritability, muscle spasms, and convulsions in neonate reported occasionally
Alfentanil *see* Opioid Analgesics		Antiepileptics	Benefit of treatment outweighs risk to the fetus; *see also* section 4.8
Allyloestrenol *see* Progestogens			
Alprazolam *see* Anxiolytics and Hypnotics		Anti-inflammatory Analgesics *see* NSAIDs	
Amikacin *see* Aminoglycosides		Antimalarials (1, 3)	Benefit of prophylaxis and treatment in malaria outweighs risk
Amiloride *see* Diuretics			
Aminoglycosides (2, 3)	Auditory or vestibular nerve damage; risk greatest with streptomycin and kanamycin; probably small with gentamicin and tobramycin	Antipsychotics (3)	Extrapyramidal effects in neonate occasionally reported
Aminophylline *see* Theophylline		Anxiolytics and Hypnotics (3)	Depress neonatal respiration. Benzodiazepines cause neonatal drowsiness, hypotonia, and withdrawal symptoms; avoid large doses and regular use; short-acting benzodiazepines preferable to long-acting
Amiodarone (2, 3)	Releases iodine with possible risk of neonatal goitre; use only if no alternative		
Amitriptyline *see* Antidepressants, Tricyclic			
Amodiaquine *see* Antimalarials			
Amylobarbitone *see* Barbiturates			
Anabolic Steroids (1, 2, 3)	Virilisation of female fetus		
Analgesics *see* Opioid Analgesics and NSAIDs		Aspirin (3)	Impaired platelet function and risk of haemorrhage; delayed onset and increased duration of labour with increased blood loss; avoid if possible in last week; with high doses, closure of fetal ductus arteriosus *in utero* and possibly persistent pulmonary hypertension of newborn; kernicterus in jaundiced neonates
Androgens (1, 2, 3)	Virilisation of female fetus		
Anaesthetics, General (3)	Depress neonatal respiration		
Anaesthetics, Local (3)	With large doses, neonatal respiratory depression, hypotonia, and bradycardia after paracervical or epidural block		
Anticoagulants, Oral (1, 2, 3)	Congenital malformations; fetal and neonatal	Astemizole	Manufacturer advises toxicity in *animal* studies

Table of drugs to be avoided or used with caution in pregnancy (*continued*)

Drug (Trimester of risk)	Comments
Atenolol *see* Beta-blockers	
Auranofin *see* Gold	
Aurothiomalate *see* Gold	
Azapropazone *see* NSAIDs	
Azathioprine (1)	Risk of teratogenicity appears to be small
Barbiturates (3)	Withdrawal effects in neonate
Beclomethasone *see* Corticosteroids	
Bendrofluazide *see* Diuretics	
Benorylate [aspirin-paracetamol ester] *see* Aspirin	
Benperidol *see* Antipsychotics	
Benzodiazepines *see* Anxiolytics and Hypnotics	
Beta-blockers (3)	Neonatal hypoglycaemia and bradycardia; risk greater in severe hypertension
Betamethasone *see* Corticosteroids	
Betaxolol *see* Beta-blockers	
Bethanidine *see* Guanethidine	
Bezafibrate *see* Clofibrate	
Bisoprolol *see* Beta-blockers	
Bromazepam *see* Anxiolytics and Hypnotics	
Bumetanide *see* Diuretics	
Buprenorphine *see* Opioid Analgesics	
Bupivacaine *see* Anaesthetics, local	
Butriptyline *see* Antidepressants, Tricyclic	
Captopril (1, 2, 3)	Avoid; may adversely affect fetal and neonatal blood pressure control and renal function and manufacturers advise toxicity in *animal* studies
Carbamazepine *see* Antiepileptics	
Carbimazole (2, 3)	Has been associated with aplasia cutis of the neonate
Chenodeoxycholic acid (1, 2, 3)	Theoretical risk of effects on fetal metabolism
Chloral hydrate *see* Anxiolytics and Hypnotics	
Chloramphenicol (3)	Neonatal 'grey syndrome'
Chlordiazepoxide *see* Anxiolytics and Hypnotics	
Chlormethiazole *see* Anxiolytics and Hypnotics	
Chlormezanone *see* Anxiolytics and Hypnotics	
Chloroquine *see* Antimalarials	
Chlorothiazide *see* Diuretics	
Chlorpromazine *see* Antipsychotics	
Chlorpropamide *see* Sulphonylureas	
Chlorprothixene *see* Antipsychotics	
Chlorthalidone *see* Diuretics	
Choline magnesium trisalicylate *see* Aspirin	
Ciprofloxacin (1, 2, 3)	Arthropathy in *animal* studies
Clobazam *see* Anxiolytics and Hypnotics	
Clobetasol *see* Corticosteroids	
Clobetasone *see* Corticosteroids	
Clofibrate (1, 2, 3)	Avoid—theoretical possibility of interference with embryonic growth and development due to anticholesterol effect
Clomipramine *see* Antidepressants, Tricyclic	
Clonazepam *see* Antiepileptics	
Clorazepate *see* Anxiolytics and Hypnotics	
Codeine *see* Opioid Analgesics	
Contraceptives, Oral (1)	May possibly be a small risk of congenital malformations

Drug (Trimester of risk)	Comments
Corticosteroids (2, 3)	High doses (>10 mg prednisolone daily) may produce fetal and neonatal adrenal suppression; corticosteroid cover required by mother during labour
Cortisone acetate *see* Corticosteroids	
Co-trimoxazole (1)	Possible teratogenic risk (trimethoprim a folate antagonist)
(3)	Neonatal haemolysis and methaemoglobinaemia; increased risk of kernicterus in jaundiced neonates (due to sulphamethoxazole)
Cyclopenthiazide *see* Diuretics	
Cyclopropane *see* Anaesthetics, General	
Cyproterone [ingredient] *see* Dianette®	
Danazol (1, 2, 3)	Has weak androgenic effects and virilisation of female fetus reported
Dapsone (3)	Neonatal haemolysis and methaemoglobinaemia; folate supplements should be given to mother
Debrisoquine *see* Guanethidine	
Desipramine *see* Antidepressants, Tricyclic	
Desonide *see* Corticosteroids	
Desoxymethasone *see* Corticosteroids	
Dexamethasone *see* Corticosteroids	
Dextromethorphan *see* Opioid Analgesics	
Dextromoramide *see* Opioid Analgesics	
Dextropropoxyphene *see* Opioid Analgesics	
Diamorphine *see* Opioid Analgesics	
Dianette® (1, 2, 3)	Feminisation of male fetus (due to cyproterone)
Diazepam *see* Anxiolytics and Hypnotics	
Diazoxide (2, 3)	Prolonged use may produce alopecia and impaired glucose tolerance in neonate; inhibits uterine activity during labour
Dichloralphenazone *see* Anxiolytics and Hypnotics	
Diclofenac *see* NSAIDs	
Diflucortolone *see* Corticosteroids	
Diflunisal *see* NSAIDs	
Dihydrocodeine *see* Opioid Analgesics	
Diltiazem	May inhibit labour and manufacturers advise toxicity in *animal* studies
Diphenoxylate *see* Opioid Analgesics	
Dipipanone *see* Opioid Analgesics	
Distigmine	Manufacturer advises avoid (may stimulate uterine contractions)
Disulfiram (1)	High concentrations of acetaldehyde which occur in presence of alcohol may be teratogenic
Diuretics (3)	Reduce plasma volume and placental perfusion and should not be used to treat hypertension in pregnancy; thiazides may cause neonatal thrombocytopenia
Dothiepin *see* Antidepressants, Tricyclic	

Table of drugs to be avoided or used with caution in pregnancy (*continued*)

Drug (Trimester of risk)	Comments	Drug (Trimester of risk)	Comments
Doxepin *see* Antidepressants, Tricyclic		Guanethidine (*cont.*)	perfusion; should not be used to treat hypertension in pregnancy
Droperidol *see* Antipsychotics			
Dydrogesterone *see* Progestogens		Halcinonide *see* Corticosteroids	
Enalapril (1, 2, 3)	Avoid; may adversely affect fetal and neonatal blood pressure control and renal function and manufacturers advise toxicity in *animal* studies	Haloperidol *see* Antipsychotics	
		Halothane *see* Anaesthetics, general	
		Heparin (1, 2, 3)	Osteoporosis has been reported after prolonged use
		Hydrochlorothiazide *see* Diuretics	
Enflurane *see* Anaesthetics, General		Hydrocortisone *see* Corticosteroids	
Ergotamine (1, 2, 3)	Oxytocic effects on the pregnant uterus	Hydroflumethiazide *see* Diuretics	
		Hydroxychloroquine *see* Antimalarials	
Ethacrynic acid *see* Diuretics		Hydroxyprogesterone *see* Progestogens	
Ether *see* Anaesthetics, general		Hypnotics *see* Anxiolytics and Hypnotics	
Ethosuximide (1)	May possibly be teratogenic; *see* Antiepileptics	Imipramine *see* Antidepressants, Tricyclic	
Etomidate *see* Anaesthetics, general		Indapamide *see* Diuretics	
Etretinate (1, 2, 3)	Teratogenic; effective contraception must be continued for one year after stopping treatment	Indomethacin *see* NSAIDs	
		Iodine and Iodides (2, 3)	Neonatal goitre and hypothyroidism
		Radioactive iodine (1, 2, 3).	Permanent hypothyroidism— avoid
Fansidar® (1)	Possible teratogenic risk (pyrimethamine a folate antagonist)	Iprindole *see* Antidepressants, Tricyclic (and related)	
		Isoflurane *see* Anaesthetics, general	
(3)	Neonatal haemolysis and methaemoglobinaemia; increased risk of kernicterus in jaundiced neonates (due to sulfadoxine) *See* Antimalarials	Isotretinoin (1, 2, 3)	Teratogenic; causes serious CNS malformations; effective contraception must be continued for at least 4 weeks after stopping
		Kanamycin *see* Aminoglycosides	
		Ketamine *see* Anaesthetics, General	
Fenoprofen *see* NSAIDs		Ketazolam *see* Anxiolytics and Hypnotics	
Fentanyl *see* Opioid Analgesics		Ketoconazole	Manufacturer advises teratogenicity in *animal* studies
Flecainide	Manufacturer advises toxicity in *animal* studies		
Fluclorolone *see* Corticosteroids		Ketoprofen *see* NSAIDs	
Flucytosine (1)	Possible teratogenic risk	Labetalol *see* Beta-blockers	
		Levorphanol *see* Opioid Analgesics	
Flunitrazepam *see* Anxiolytics and Hypnotics		Lidoflazine	May inhibit labour and manufacturers advise toxicity in *animal* studies
Fluocinolone *see* Corticosteroids			
Fluocinonide *see* Corticosteroids		Lignocaine *see* Anaesthetics, Local	
Fluocortolone *see* Corticosteroids		Lithium (1, 2, 3)	Congenital malformations; neonatal goitre has been reported; lithium toxicity (hypotonia and cyanosis) in neonate if maternal therapy poorly controlled; maternal dose requirement increased in pregnancy
Flupenthixol *see* Antipsychotics			
Fluphenazine *see* Antipsychotics			
Flurandrenolone *see* Corticosteroids			
Flurazepam *see* Anxiolytics and Hypnotics			
Fluspirilene *see* Antipsychotics			
Frusemide *see* Diuretics			
Gemfibrozil *see* Clofibrate		Lofepramine *see* Antidepressants, Tricyclic	
Gentamicin *see* Aminoglycosides		Loprazolam *see* Anxiolytics and Hypnotics	
Glibenclamide *see* Sulphonylureas		Lorazepam *see* Anxiolytics and Hypnotics	
Gliclazide *see* Sulphonylureas		Lormetazepam *see* Anxiolytics and Hypnotics	
Glipizide *see* Sulphonylureas		*Maloprim*®	
Gliquidone *see* Sulphonylureas		(1)	Possible teratogenic risk (pyrimethamine a folate antagonist)
Glymidine *see* Sulphonylureas			
Gold		(3)	Neonatal haemolysis and methaemoglobinaemia (due to dapsone); folate supplements should be given to mother *see* Antimalarials
Auranofin	Manufacturer advises teratogenicity in *animal* studies		
Aurothiomalate (1, 2, 3)	No good evidence of harm but avoid if possible		
Griseofulvin	CRM advises avoid (fetotoxicity and teratogenicity in *animals*)		
Guanethidine (3)	Postural hypotension and reduced uteroplacental	Maprotiline *see* Antidepressants, Tricyclic	

Table of drugs to be avoided or used with caution in pregnancy (*continued*)

Drug (Trimester of risk)	Comments
Mebendazole	Manufacturer advises toxicity in *animal* studies
Medazepam *see* Anxiolytics and Hypnotics	
Mefenamic acid *see* NSAIDs	
Mefruside *see* Diuretics	
Menadiol sodium diphosphate (3)	Neonatal haemolysis; increased risk of kernicterus in jaundiced neonates
Meprobamate *see* Anxiolytics and Hypnotics	
Meptazinol *see* Opioid Analgesics	
Mesterolone *see* Androgens	
Metaraminol (1, 2, 3)	Avoid—may reduce placental perfusion
Metformin (1, 2, 3)	Avoid
Methadone *see* Opioid Analgesics	
Methohexitone *see* Anaesthetics, General	
Methotrimeprazine *see* Antipsychotics	
Methylclothiazide *see* Diuretics	
Methylphenobarbitone *see* Antiepileptics	
Methylprednisolone *see* Corticosteroids	
Methyltestosterone *see* Androgens	
Metolazone *see* Diuretics	
Metoprolol *see* Beta-blockers	
Metronidazole	Manufacturer advises avoidance of high-dose regimens
Metyrapone	Avoid (may impair biosynthesis of fetal-placental steroids)
Mianserin *see* Antidepressants, Tricyclic (and related)	
Morphine *see* Opioid Analgesics	
Nabumetone *see* NSAIDs	
Nadolol *see* Beta-blockers	
Nalbuphine *see* Opioid Analgesics	
Nalidixic acid (1, 2, 3)	Arthropathy in *animal* studies
Nandrolone *see* Anabolic Steroids	
Naproxen *see* NSAIDs	
Narcotic Analgesics *see* Opioid Analgesics	
Neomycin *see* Aminoglycosides	
Neostigmine (3)	Neonatal myasthenia with large doses
Netilmicin *see* Aminoglycosides	
Nicoumalone *see* Anticoagulants, Oral	
Nifedipine	May inhibit labour and manufacturers advise toxicity in *animal* studies
Nitrazepam *see* Anxiolytics and Hypnotics	
Nitrous oxide *see* Anaesthetics, general	
Noradrenaline (1, 2, 3)	Avoid—may reduce placental perfusion
Nortriptyline *see* Antidepressants, Tricyclic	
NSAIDs (3)	With regular use closure of fetal ductus arteriosus *in utero* and possibly persistent pulmonary hypertension of the newborn. Delayed onset and increased duration of labour
Opioid Analgesics (3)	Depress neonatal respiration; withdrawal effects in neonates of dependent mothers; gastric stasis and risk of inhalation

Drug (Trimester of risk)	Comments
Opioid Analgesics (*cont.*)	pneumonia in mother during labour
Oxazepam *see* Anxiolytics and Hypnotics	
Oxprenolol *see* Beta-blockers	
Oxypertine *see* Antipsychotics	
Papaveretum *see* Opioid Analgesics	
Penbutolol *see* Beta-blockers	
Penicillamine (1, 2, 3)	Fetal abnormalities reported rarely; avoid if possible
Pentazocine *see* Opioid Analgesics	
Pericyazine *see* Antipsychotics	
Perphenazine *see* Antipsychotics	
Pethidine *see* Opioid Analgesics	
Phenindione *see* Anticoagulants, Oral	
Phenobarbitone (1, 3)	Congenital malformations. Neonatal bleeding tendency—prophylactic vitamin K_1 should be given; *see* Antiepileptics
Phenoperidine *see* Opioid Analgesics	
Phenothiazines *see* Antipsychotics	
Pholcodine *see* Opioid Analgesics	
Phenytoin (1, 3)	Congenital malformations. Neonatal bleeding tendency—prophylactic vitamin K_1 should be given. Caution in interpreting plasma concentrations—bound may be reduced but free (i.e. effective) unchanged *See* Antiepileptics
Pimozide *see* Antipsychotics	
Pindolol *see* Beta-blockers	
Piperazine	Packs sold to the general public carry a warning to avoid in pregnancy except on medical advice
Pipothiazine *see* Antipsychotics	
Piroxicam *see* NSAIDs	
Podophyllum resin (1, 2, 3)	Avoid—neonatal death and teratogenesis have been reported
Polythiazide *see* Diuretics	
Povidone-iodine (2, 3)	Sufficient iodine may be absorbed to affect the fetal thyroid
Prednisolone *see* Corticosteroids	
Prednisone *see* Corticosteroids	
Prilocaine (3)	Neonatal methaemo-globinaemia *See* Anaesthetics, Local
Primaquine (3)	Neonatal haemolysis and methaemoglobinaemia *See* Antimalarials
Primidone *see* Antiepileptics	
Probucol *see* Clofibrate	
Prochlorperazine *see* Antipsychotics	
Procaine (3)	Neonatal methaemoglobinaemia *See* Anaesthetics, Local
Progestogens (used to prevent abortion) (1)	May possibly be teratogenic
Proguanil *see* Antimalarials	
Promazine *see* Antipsychotics	

Table of drugs to be avoided or used with caution in pregnancy (*continued*)

Drug (Trimester of risk)	Comments
Promethazine theoclate	Packs sold to the general public carry a warning to avoid in pregnancy
Propofol *see* Anaesthetics, General	
Propranolol *see* Beta-blockers	
Propylthiouracil (2, 3)	Neonatal goitre and hypothyroidism
Protriptyline *see* Antidepressants, Tricyclic	
Pyridostigmine (3)	Neonatal myasthenia with large doses
Pyrimethamine (1)	Possible teratogenic risk (folate antagonist); *See also* Antimalarials
Quinine (1)	High doses are teratogenic; but in malaria benefit of treatment outweighs risk
Reserpine (3)	Neonatal bradycardia, drowsiness, and nasal stuffiness
Rifampicin (3)	Risk of neonatal bleeding may be increased
Salbutamol (3)	Large parenteral doses given at term for asthma could delay onset of labour
Salsalate *see* Aspirin	
Sodium aurothiomalate *see* Gold	
Sodium valproate *see* Valproate	
Sotalol *see* Beta-blockers	
Spironolactone	Potential human metabolic products carcinogenic in *rodents*
Stanozolol *see* Anabolic Steroids	
Stilboestrol (1)	High doses associated with vaginal carcinoma in female offspring
Streptokinase (1, 2, 3)	Possibility of premature separation of placenta in first 18 weeks; theoretical possibility of fetal haemorrhage throughout pregnancy; avoid postpartum use—maternal haemorrhage
Streptomycin *see* Aminoglycosides	
Sulfadoxine *see* Sulphonamides	
Sulfametopyrazine *see* Sulphonamides	
Sulindac *see* NSAIDs	
Sulphadiazine *see* Sulphonamides	
Sulphadimidine *see* Sulphonamides	
Sulphasalazine (3)	Theoretical risk of neonatal haemolysis; folate supplements should be given to mother
Sulphaurea *see* Sulphonamides	
Sulphonamides (3)	Neonatal haemolysis and methaemoglobinaemia; increased risk of kernicterus in jaundiced neonates
Sulphonylureas (3)	Neonatal hypoglycaemia; insulin is normally substituted in all diabetics; if oral drugs are used therapy should be stopped at least 2 days before delivery
Sulpiride *see* Antipsychotics	
Temazepam *see* Anxiolytics and Hypnotics	

Drug (Trimester of risk)	Comments
Terbutaline (3)	Large parenteral doses given at term for asthma could delay onset of labour
Testosterone *see* Androgens	
Tetracyclines (2, 3)	Dental discoloration; maternal hepatotoxicity with large parenteral doses
Theophylline (3)	Neonatal irritability and apnoea have been reported
Thiazides (3)	May cause neonatal thrombocytopenia; *See also* Diuretics
Thiethylperazine *see* Antipsychotics	
Thiopentone *see* Anaesthetics, General	
Thioridazine *see* Antipsychotics	
Tiaprofenic acid *see* NSAIDs	
Timolol *see* Beta-blockers	
Tobramycin *see* Aminoglycosides	
Tocainide	Manufacturer advises toxicity in *animal* studies
Tolbutamide *see* Sulphonylureas	
Tolmetin *see* NSAIDs	
Trazodone *see* Antidepressants, Tricyclic (and related)	
Triamcinolone *see* Corticosteroids	
Triamterene *see* Diuretics	
Triazolam *see* Anxiolytics and Hypnotics	
Trichloroethylene *see* Anaesthetics, General	
Triclofos *see* Anxiolytics and Hypnotics	
Trifluoperazine *see* Antipsychotics	
Trifluperidol *see* Antipsychotics	
Trilostane (1, 2, 3)	Interferes with placental sex hormone production
Trimethoprim (1)	Possible teratogenic risk (folate antagonist)
Trimipramine *see* Antidepressants, Tricyclic	
Urokinase (1, 2, 3)	Possibility of premature separation of placenta in first 18 weeks; theoretical possibility of fetal haemorrhage throughout pregnancy; avoid postpartum use—maternal haemorrhage
Vaccines (live) (1)	Theoretical risk of congenital malformations
Valproate (1, 3)	Increased risk of neural tube defects reported; neonatal bleeding and hepatotoxicity also reported
Verapamil (3)	May inhibit labour
Vidarabine	Manufacturer advises teratogenic in *animal* studies
Viloxazine *see* Antidepressants, Tricyclic (and related)	
Vitamin A (1)	Excessive doses may be teratogenic
Warfarin *see* Anticoagulants, Oral	
Xipamide *see* Diuretics	
Zuclopenthixol *see* Antipsychotics	

Prescribing during Breast-feeding

Administration of some drugs to nursing mothers may cause toxicity in the infant (e.g. ergotamine), whereas administration of others (e.g. digoxin), has little effect on the neonate. Some drugs inhibit lactation (e.g. bromocriptine).

Toxicity to the infant can occur if the drug enters the milk in pharmacologically significant quantities. Milk concentrations of some drugs (e.g. iodides), may exceed those in the maternal plasma so that therapeutic doses in the mother may cause toxicity to the infant. Some drugs inhibit the infant's sucking reflex (e.g. phenobarbitone). Drugs in breast milk may, at least theoretically, cause hypersensitivity in the infant even when concentrations are too low for a pharmacological effect.

The following table lists drugs:

which should be used with caution or which are contra-indicated in breast-feeding for the reasons given above;

which, on present evidence, may be given to the mother during breast-feeding, because they are excreted in milk in amounts which are too small to be harmful to the infant;

which are not known to be harmful to the infant although they are present in milk in significant amounts.

For many drugs there is insufficient evidence available to provide guidance and it is advisable only to administer essential drugs to a mother during breast-feeding. Because of the inadequacy of currently available information on drugs in breast milk the following table should be used only as a guide; absence from the table does not imply safety.

Table of drugs excreted in breast milk

Drug	Comments
Acebutolol *see* Beta-blockers	
Acetazolamide	Amount too small to be harmful
Acetohexamide *see* Sulphonylureas	
Alcohol	Large amounts may affect infant
Alfacalcidol *see* Vitamin D	
Alprazolam *see* Benzodiazepines	
Aminophylline *see* Theophylline	
Amiodarone	Avoid; present in milk in significant amounts; theoretical risk from release of iodine; *see also* Iodine
Amitriptyline *see* Antidepressants, Tricyclic	
Amylobarbitone *see* Barbiturates	
Androgens	Avoid; may cause masculinisation in the female infant or precocious development in the male infant; high doses suppress lactation
Anthraquinones	Avoid; large doses may cause increased gastric motility and diarrhoea (particularly cascara and danthron)
Anticoagulants, Oral	Risk of haemorrhage; increased by vitamin-K deficiency; warfarin appears safe but phenindione should be avoided
Antidepressants, Tricyclic (and related)	Amount of tricyclic antidepressants (including related drugs such as mianserin and trazodone) too small to be harmful
Antihistamines	Significant amount but not known to be harmful
Antipsychotics	Amount excreted in milk probably too small to be harmful; drowsiness in infant reported with chlorpromazine
Aspirin	Avoid—possible risk of Reye's syndrome; regular

Drug	Comments
Aspirin *(cont.)*	use of high doses could impair platelet function and produce hypoprothrombinaemia in infant if neonatal vitamin K stores low
Astemizole *see* Antihistamines	
Atenolol *see* Beta-blockers	
Atropine	May possibly have anticholinergic effects in infants
Auranofin *see* Gold	
Aurothiomalate *see* Gold	
Azatadine *see* Antihistamines	
Azathioprine	Amount too small to be harmful
Baclofen	Amount too small to be harmful
Barbiturates	Avoid if possible (*see also* phenobarbitone); large doses may produce drowsiness
Bendrofluazide *see* Thiazides	
Benperidol *see* Antipsychotics	
Benzodiazepines	Avoid repeated doses; lethargy and weight loss may occur in infant
Beta-blockers and Labetalol	Monitor infant; possible toxicity due to beta-blockade but amount of most beta-blockers excreted in milk too small to affect infant; acebutolol, nadolol, and sotalol are present in greater amounts than other beta-blockers
Betamethasone *see* Corticosteroids	
Betaxolol *see* Beta-blockers	
Bisoprolol *see* Beta-blockers	
Bromazepam *see* Benzodiazepines	
Bromide salts	Avoid; sedation and rash in infant
Bromocriptine	Suppresses lactation
Brompheniramine *see* Antihistamines	
Butobarbitone *see* Barbiturates	
Butriptyline *see* Antidepressants, Tricyclic	

Table of drugs excreted in breast milk (*continued*)

Drug	Comments
Calciferol *see* Vitamin D	
Calcitriol *see* Vitamin D	
Carbamazepine	Amount too small to be harmful
Carbimazole	Amounts in milk may be sufficient to affect neonatal thyroid function
Carisoprodol	Concentrated in milk; no adverse effects reported but best avoided
Cascara *see* Anthraquinones	
Chloral hydrate	Sedation in infant
Chloramphenicol	Stop breast-feeding; may cause bone-marrow toxicity in infant; concentration in milk usually insufficient to cause 'grey syndrome'
Chlordiazepoxide *see* Benzodiazepines	
Chlormethiazole	Amount too small to be harmful
Chloroquine	Amount too small to be harmful
Chlorothiazide *see* Thiazides	
Chlorpheniramine *see* Antihistamines	
Chlorpromazine	Drowsiness in infant reported; *see* Antipsychotics
Chlorpropamide *see* Sulphonylureas	
Chlortetracycline *see* Tetracyclines	
Chlorthalidone *see* Thiazides	
Cholecalciferol *see* Vitamin D	
Cimetidine	Significant amount but not known to be harmful
Clavulanic acid (in *Augmentin®*, *Timentin®*)	Amount too small to be harmful
Clemastine	Drowsiness in infant reported
Clobazam *see* Benzodiazepines	
Clomipramine *see* Antidepressants, Tricyclic	
Clomocycline *see* Tetracyclines	
Clorazepate *see* Benzodiazepines	
Codeine	Amount too small to be harmful
Colchicine	Caution because of its cytotoxicity
Contraceptives, Oral	Oestrogen/progestogen contraceptives usually have little effect on milk flow; in some women, usually when lactation not well established, suppression may occur; one report of neonatal folate deficiency; progestogen-only contraceptives do not appear to adversely affect established milk flow
Corticosteroids	Continuous therapy with high doses (>10 mg prednisolone daily) could possibly affect infant's adrenal function—monitor carefully
Corticotrophin	Amount too small to be harmful
Cortisone acetate *see* Corticosteroids	
Co-trimoxazole	Small risk of kernicterus in jaundiced infants and of haemolysis in G6PD-deficient infants (due to sulphamethoxazole)
Cough mixtures containing iodides	Use alternative cough mixtures; *see* Iodine
Cyclobarbitone *see* Barbiturates	
Cyclopenthiazide *see* Thiazides	
Cycloserine	Amount too small to be harmful
Cyclosporin	Caution—excreted in milk
Cyproheptadine *see* Antihistamines	
Cyproterone	Caution; possibility of anti-androgen effects in neonate
Cytotoxics	Discontinue breast-feeding
Danazol	No data available but avoid because of possible androgenic effects in infant
Danthron *see* Anthraquinones	
Dapsone	Haemolytic anaemia; risk to infant very small
Demeclocycline *see* Tetracyclines	
Desipramine *see* Antidepressants, Tricyclic	
Dextropropoxyphene	Amount too small to be harmful
Dexamethasone *see* Corticosteroids	
Diamorphine	Therapeutic doses unlikely to affect infant; withdrawal symptoms in infants of dependent mothers; breast-feeding no longer considered best method of treating dependence in offspring of dependent mothers and should be stopped
Diazepam *see* Benzodiazepines	
Dichloralphenazone	Sedation in infant
Diclofenac	Amount too small to be harmful
Digoxin	Amount too small to be harmful
Dihydrotachysterol *see* Vitamin D	
Diltiazem	Significant amount but not known to be harmful
Dimethindene *see* Antihistamines	
Diphenylpyraline *see* Antihistamines	
Disopyramide	Amount too small to be harmful
Domperidone	Amount too small to be harmful
Dothiepin *see* Antidepressants, Tricyclic	
Doxepin *see* Antidepressants, Tricyclic	
Doxycycline *see* Tetracyclines	
Droperidol *see* Antipsychotics	
Ephedrine	Irritability and disturbed sleep reported
Ergocalciferol *see* Vitamin D	
Ergotamine	Avoid where possible; ergotism may occur in infant; repeated doses may inhibit lactation
Erythromycin	Significant amount but not known to be harmful
Ethambutol	Amount too small to be harmful
Ethamsylate	Significant amount but not known to be harmful

Table of drugs excreted in breast milk (*continued*)

Drug	Comments	Drug	Comments
Ethosuximide	Significant amount but not known to be harmful	Isoniazid	Monitor infant for possible toxicity; theoretical risk of convulsions and neuropathy; prophylactic pyridoxine advisable in mother and infant
Fansidar®	Small risk of kernicterus in jaundiced infants and of haemolysis in G6PD-deficient infants (due to sulfadoxine)		
		Ketazolam *see* Benzodiazepines	
Fenbufen	Amount too small to be harmful	Ketoprofen	Amount too small to be harmful
Fenoprofen	Amount too small to be harmful	Ketotifen *see* Antihistamines	
		Labetalol *see* Beta-blockers	
Flunitrazepam *see* Benzodiazepines		Liothyronine	May interfere with neonatal screening for hypothyroidism
Flupenthixol	Amount too small to be harmful	Lithium salts	Monitor infant for possible intoxication; low incidence of adverse effects but increased by continuous ingestion; good control of maternal plasma concentrations minimises the risk
Fluphenazine *see* Antipsychotics			
Flurazepam *see* Benzodiazepines			
Flurbiprofen	Amount too small to be harmful		
Frusemide	Amount too small to be harmful		
Glibenclamide *see* Sulphonylureas			
Gliclazide *see* Sulphonylureas		Lofepramine *see* Antidepressants, Tricyclic	
Glipizide *see* Sulphonylureas		Loprazolam	Amount too small to be harmful
Gliquidone *see* Sulphonylureas			
Glymidine *see* Sulphonylureas		Lorazepam *see* Benzodiazepines	
		Lormetazepam *see* Benzodiazepines	
		Lymecycline *see* Tetracyclines	
Gold (auranofin, aurothiomalate)	Caution—excreted in milk; theoretical possibility of rashes and idiosyncratic reactions	*Maloprim*®	Haemolytic anaemia (due to dapsone); risk to infant very small
		Maprotiline *see* Antidepressants, Tricyclic	
Haloperidol	Amount excreted in milk probably too small to be harmful	Mebeverine	Amount too small to be harmful
		Mebhydrolin *see* Antihistamines	
Heparin	Amount too small to be harmful	Medazepam *see* Benzodiazepines	
		Mefenamic acid	Amount too small to be harmful
Hydrochlorothiazide *see* Thiazides			
Hydrocortisone *see* Corticosteroids		Mefruside *see* Thiazides	
Hydroflumethiazide *see* Thiazides		Meprobamate	Concentration in milk may exceed maternal plasma concentrations fourfold and may cause drowsiness in infant
Hydroxychloroquine	Amount too small to be harmful		
Hydroxyzine *see* Antihistamines			
Hyoscine	Amount too small to be harmful	Mequitazine *see* Antihistamines	
		Metformin	Caution; theoretical possibility of hypoglycaemia in infant
Ibuprofen	Amount too small to be harmful		
Idoxuridine	May possibly make milk taste unpleasant	Methadone	Withdrawal symptoms in infant; breast-feeding permissible during maintenance dosage
Imipramine *see* Antidepressants, Tricyclic			
Indapamide *see* Thiazides			
Indomethacin	Significant amounts are present in milk; convulsions reported in one infant	Methotrimeprazine *see* Antipsychotics	
		Methyclothiazide *see* Thiazides	
Insulin	Amount too small to be harmful	Methyldopa	Amount too small to be harmful
		Methylprednisolone *see* Corticosteroids	
Iodine	Stop breast-feeding; danger of neonatal hypothyroidism or goitre; appears to be concentrated in milk	Metoclopramide	Amount too small to be harmful
		Metolazone *see* Thiazides	
		Metoprolol *see* Beta-blockers	
Radioactive iodine	Breast-feeding contra-indicated after therapeutic doses. With diagnostic doses withhold breast-feeding for at least 24 hours	Metronidazole	May give a bitter taste to the milk, also manufacturer advises avoidance of high-dose regimens
Iprindole *see* Antidepressants, Tricyclic (and related)			
		Mexiletine	Amount too small to be harmful
		Mianserin	Amount too small to be harmful

Table of drugs excreted in breast milk (*continued*)

Drug	Comments	Drug	Comments
Minocycline *see* Tetracyclines		Prednisone *see* Corticosteroids	
Minoxidil	Significant amount but not known to be harmful	Prochlorperazine *see* Antipsychotics	
Morphine	Therapeutic doses unlikely to affect infant; withdrawal symptoms in infants of dependent mothers; breast-feeding not best method of treating dependence in offspring and should be stopped	Progestogens	High doses suppress lactation but *see also* Contraceptives, Oral
		Promazine *see* Antipsychotics	
		Promethazine *see* Antihistamines	
		Propranolol *see* Beta-blockers	
		Propylthiouracil	Monitor infant's thyroid status but amounts in milk probably too small to affect infant; high doses might affect neonatal thyroid function
Nadolol *see* Beta-blockers			
Nalidixic acid	Risk to infant very small but one case of haemolytic anaemia reported	Protriptyline *see* Antidepressants, Tricyclic	
		Pseudoephedrine	Amount too small to be harmful
Naproxen	Amount too small to be harmful	Pyrazinamide	Amount too small to be harmful
Nefopam	Amount too small to be harmful	Pyridostigmine	Amount too small to be harmful
Nicoumalone *see* Anticoagulants, Oral		Pyrimethamine	Significant amount but not known to be harmful
Nitrazepam *see* Benzodiazepines			
Nitrofurantoin	Only small amounts in milk but could be enough to produce haemolysis in G6PD-deficient infants	Quinalbarbitone *see* Barbiturates	
		Quinidine	Significant amount but not known to be harmful
		Ranitidine	Significant amount but not known to be harmful
Nortriptyline *see* Antidepressants, Tricyclic		Rifampicin	Amount too small to be harmful
NSAIDs *see* individual entries			
		Senna *see* Anthraquinones	
Oestrogens	High doses suppress lactation but *see also* Contraceptives, Oral	Sex hormones *see* Contraceptives Oral *and* Androgens, Oestrogens, and Progestogens	
		Sodium valproate *see* Valproate	
Oxatomide *see* Antihistamines		Sotalol *see* Beta-blockers	
Oxazepam *see* Benzodiazepines		Spironolactone	Avoid; significant amounts and potential human metabolic products carcinogenic in *rodents*
Oxypertine *see* Antipsychotics			
Oxprenolol *see* Beta-blockers			
Oxytetracycline *see* Tetracyclines			
Paracetamol	Significant amount but not known to be harmful	Sulfametopyrazine *see* Sulphonamides	
		Sulphadiazine *see* Sulphonamides	
Penbutolol *see* Beta-blockers		Sulphadimidine *see* Sulphonamides	
Pericyazine *see* Antipsychotics		Sulphasalazine	Theoretical risk of neonatal haemolysis especially in G6PD-deficient infants
Perphenazine *see* Antipsychotics			
Phenindamine *see* Antihistamines		Sulphaurea *see* Sulphonamides	
Phenindione *see* Anticoagulants, Oral		Sulphonamides	Small risk of kernicterus in jaundiced infants particularly with long-acting sulphonamides, and of haemolysis in G6PD-deficient infants
Pheniramine *see* Antihistamines			
Phenobarbitone	Avoid when possible; drowsiness may occur but risk probably small; one report of methaemoglobinaemia with phenobarbitone and phenytoin		
		Sulphonylureas	Caution; theoretical possibility of hypoglycaemia in infant
		Sulpiride	Best avoided; significant amounts in milk
Phenolphthalein	Avoid; increased gastric motility, diarrhoea, and possibly rash	Temazepam *see* Benzodiazepines	
		Terbutaline	Amount too small to be harmful
Phenytoin	Amount too small to be harmful	Terfenadine *see* Antihistamines	
Pimozide *see* Antipsychotics		Tetracyclines	Some authorities recommend avoidance but absorption and therefore discoloration of teeth in infant probably prevented by chelation with calcium in milk
Pindolol *see* Beta-blockers			
Pirenzepine	Amount too small to be harmful		
Piroxicam	Amount too small to be harmful		
Polythiazide *see* Diuretics			
Povidone-iodine	Avoid; iodine absorbed from vaginal preparations is concentrated in milk		
Primidone *see* Phenobarbitone			
Prednisolone *see* Corticosteroids			

Table of drugs excreted in breast milk (*continued*)

Drug	Comments	Drug	Comments
Theophylline	Irritability in infant reported; sustained-release preparations probably safe	Triazolam *see* Benzodiazepines	
		Trifluoperazine *see* Antipsychotics	
		Trifluperidol *see* Antipsychotics	
Thiamine	Severely thiamine-deficient mothers should avoid breast-feeding as toxic methylglyoxal excreted in milk	Trimeprazine *see* Antihistamines	
		Trimethoprim	Significant amount but not known to be harmful
		Trimipramine *see* Antidepressants, Tricyclic	
		Triprolidine *see* Antihistamines	
Thiazides	Amount too small to be harmful	Valproate	Amount too small to be harmful
Thiethylperazine *see* Antipsychotics		Verapamil	Amount too small to be harmful
Thioridazine *see* Antipsychotics			
Thyroxine	May interfere with neonatal screening for hypothyroidism	Viloxazine *see* Antidepressants, Tricyclic (and related)	
Tiaprofenic acid	Amount too small to be harmful	Vitamin A	Theoretical risk of toxicity in infants of mothers taking large doses
Timolol *see* Beta-blockers			
Tolazamide *see* Sulphonylureas		Vitamin D (and related compounds)	Caution with high doses; may cause hypercalcaemia in infant
Tolbutamide *see* Sulphonylureas			
Tolmetin	Amount too small to be harmful	Warfarin *see* Anticoagulants, Oral	
		Xipamide *see* Thiazides	
Trazodone	Amount too small to be harmful	Zuclopenthixol *see* Antipsychotics	
Triamcinolone *see* Corticosteroids			

Emergency Treatment of Poisoning

Poisons Information Services

Belfast	0232 240503
Birmingham	021-554 3801
Cardiff	0222 709901
Dublin	0001 379964
	or 0001 379966
Edinburgh	031-229 2477
	031-228 2441
	(Viewdata)
Leeds	0532 430715
	or 0532 432799
London	01-635 9191
	or 01-407 7600
Newcastle	091-232 5131

Note. Some of these centres also advise on laboratory analytical services which may be of help in the diagnosis and management of a small number of cases.

**CONSULT POISONS
INFORMATION CENTRES
DAY AND NIGHT**

Emergency Treatment of Poisoning

These notes deal with the initial management of acute poisoning in the home; brief mention only is given of hospital-based treatment. The notes are only guidelines and it is strongly recommended that **poisons information services** (see previous page) be consulted in cases where there is doubt about the degree of risk or about appropriate management.

HOSPITAL ADMISSION. All patients who show features of poisoning should generally be admitted to hospital. Patients who have taken poisons with delayed actions should also be admitted, even if they appear well; delayed-action poisons include aspirin, iron, paracetamol, tricyclic antidepressants, diphenoxylate with atropine (Lomotil®), and paraquat, also sustained-release capsules or tablets. A note should be sent of what is known and what treatment has been given.

It is often impossible to establish with certainty the identity of the poison and the size of the dose. Fortunately this is not usually important because only a few poisons (such as opioids, paracetamol, and iron) have specific antidotes and few patients require active removal of the poison. Most patients must be treated symptomatically. Nevertheless, knowledge of the type of poisoning does help in anticipating the course of events. Patients' reports may be of little help, as they may be confused or may only be able to say that they have taken an undefined amount, possibly of mixed drugs. Parents may think a child has taken something which could be poisonous and may exaggerate or underplay the risks out of anxiety or guilt. Sometimes symptoms are due to an illness such as appendicitis. Accidents can arise from a number of domestic and industrial products (the contents of which are not generally known).

The **poisons information services** (see previous page) will provide advice on all aspects of poisoning.

General care

Respiration

Respiration is often impaired in unconscious patients. An obstructed airway requires immediate attention. Pull the tongue forward, remove dentures and oral secretions, hold the jaw forward, insert an oropharyngeal airway if one is available, and turn the patient semiprone. The risk of inhaling vomit is minimised with the patient positioned semiprone and head down.

Most poisons that impair consciousness also depress respiration. Assisted ventilation by mouth-to-mouth or Ambu bag inflation may be needed. Oxygen is not a substitute for adequate ventilation, though it should be given in the highest concentration possible in poisoning with carbon monoxide and irritant gases.

Respiratory stimulants do not help and are **potentially dangerous**.

Blood pressure

Hypotension is common in severe poisoning with central nervous system depressants. A systolic blood pressure of less than 70 mmHg may lead to irreversible brain damage or renal tubular necrosis. The patient should be carried head downwards on a stretcher and nursed in this position in the ambulance. Oxygen should be given to correct hypoxia and an intravenous infusion should be set up if at all practicable. Vasopressor drugs should **not** be used.

Fluid depletion without hypotension is common after prolonged coma and after aspirin poisoning due to vomiting, sweating, and hyperpnoea.

Heart

Cardiac conduction defects and arrhythmias may occur in acute poisoning, notably with tricyclic antidepressants. Arrhythmias often respond to correction of underlying hypoxia or acidosis. Ventricular arrhythmias that have been confirmed by emergency electrocardiography and which are causing serious hypotension may require treatment with lignocaine 50–100 mg by slow intravenous injection. Supraventricular arrhythmias are seldom life-threatening and drug treatment is best withheld until the patient reaches hospital.

Body temperature

Hypothermia may develop in patients of any age who have been deeply unconscious for some hours particularly following overdose with barbiturates or phenothiazines. It may be missed unless temperature is measured rectally using a low-reading rectal thermometer. It is best treated by wrapping the patient in blankets to conserve body heat. Hot-water bottles are of little value and may cause burns.

Convulsions

Single short-lived convulsions do not require treatment. Diazepam, up to 10 mg by slow intravenous injection, preferably in emulsion form, should be given if convulsions are protracted or recur frequently; it should not be given intramuscularly.

Removal and elimination

Removal from the stomach

The dangers of attempting to empty the stomach have to be balanced against the toxicity of the ingested poison, as assessed by the quantity ingested, the inherent toxicity of the poison, and the time since ingestion. Gastric emptying is clearly unnecessary if the risk of toxicity is small or if the patient presents too late.

Emptying the stomach by **gastric lavage** or **emesis** is of doubtful value if attempted more than 4 hours after ingestion. However, a worthwhile recovery of salicylates can be achieved up to 24 hours after ingestion and of tricyclic antidepressants (which delay gastric emptying) up to 8 hours after ingestion. The chief danger of gastric aspiration and lavage is inhalation of stomach contents, and it should **not** be attempted in drowsy or comatose patients unless there is a good enough cough reflex or the airway can be protected by a cuffed endotracheal tube. Stomach tubes should **not** be passed after corrosive poisoning.

Petroleum products are more dangerous in the lungs than in the stomach and therefore removal from the stomach is **not** advised because of the risk of inhalation.

On balance gastric lavage is seldom practicable or desirable before the patient reaches hospital.

Emesis induced by using **ipecacuanha** (Paediatric Ipecacuanha Emetic Mixture BP[1]) is favoured in children and is also effective in adults. It may be given safely in the home providing that the patient is fully conscious and that the poison ingested is neither a corrosive nor a petroleum distillate.

Salt solutions, copper sulphate, apomorphine, and mustard are dangerous and should **not** be used.

Ipecacuanha Emetic Mixture, Paediatric[1], total alkaloids (as emetine) 14 mg/10 ml (see Formulary). Net price 100 ml = 11p
Dose: ADULT 30 ml; CHILD 6–18 months 10 ml, older children 15 ml; the dose is followed by a tumblerful of water and repeated after 20 minutes if necessary

Adsorbents

Given by mouth, activated charcoal can bind many poisons in the stomach, thereby *reducing their absorption*, but it is only effective if given within 1–2 hours of ingestion. It is safe and is particularly useful for the prevention of absorption of poisons which are toxic in small amounts, e.g. antidepressants.

For the use of adsorbents in active elimination techniques, see below.

CHARCOAL, ACTIVATED
Indications; Dose: see notes above

Carbomix® (Penn)
Powder, activated charcoal. Net price 50-g bottle = £7.80
Medicoal® (Lundbeck)
Granules, effervescent, activated charcoal 5 g/sachet. Net price 10 sachets = £4.66.
Dose: 5–10 g in 100–200 ml water repeated every 15–20 min; max. 50 g, but see notes above

Active elimination techniques

Repeated doses of activated charcoal by mouth *enhance the elimination* of some drugs after they have been absorbed; repeated doses are given after overdosage with aspirin, carbamazepine, digoxin, phenobarbitone and other barbiturates, phenytoin, quinine, and theophylline. The usual

adult dose is 50 g every 4 hours or 25 g every 2 hours.

Other techniques intended to enhance the elimination of poisons after absorption are only practicable in hospital and are only suitable for a small number of severely poisoned patients. Moreover, they only apply to a limited number of poisons. Examples include:

Forced alkaline diuresis for salicylates and phenobarbitone
Haemodialysis for salicylates, phenobarbitone, methyl alcohol (methanol), ethylene glycol, and lithium
Charcoal haemoperfusion for medium- and short-acting barbiturates, chloral hydrate, and meprobamate.

Specific drugs

> CONSULT POISONS INFORMATION CENTRES
> DAY AND NIGHT—see p. 37

Alcohol

Acute intoxication with alcohol (ethanol) is common in adults but also occurs in children. The features include ataxia, dysarthria, nystagmus, and drowsiness, which may progress to coma, with hypotension and acidosis. Aspiration of vomit is a special hazard and hypoglycaemia may occur in children and some adults. Patients are managed supportively with particular attention to maintaining a clear airway and measures to reduce the risk of aspiration of gastric contents. The blood glucose is measured and glucose given if indicated.

Analgesics

ASPIRIN

Absorption of aspirin and other salicylates may be delayed, especially if enteric-coated tablets have been taken; blood concentrations taken within the first 6 hours may therefore be misleadingly low.

The chief features of poisoning are hyperventilation, tinnitus, deafness, vasodilatation, and sweating. Coma is uncommon but indicates very severe poisoning. The associated acid-base disturbances are complex.

Gastric emptying is carried out in all cases; a worthwhile recovery of salicylates can be achieved up to 24 hours after ingestion.

Treatment must be in hospital where plasma salicylate, pH, and electrolytes can be measured. Fluid losses are replaced and forced alkaline diuresis is considered when the plasma-salicylate concentration is greater than
500 mg/litre (3.6 mmol/litre) in adults *or*
300 mg/litre (2.2 mmol/litre) in children.

NON-STEROIDAL ANTI-INFLAMMATORY DRUGS (NSAIDs)

Mefenamic acid is the most significant member of this group encountered in overdosage. Con-

---

[1] Paediatric Ipecacuanha Emetic Mixture BP is equivalent in strength to Ipecac Syrup USP

vulsions are the only important feature of toxicity and are treated with diazepam.

Ibuprofen may cause nausea, vomiting, and tinnitus, but more serious toxicity is very uncommon. Gastric emptying is indicated if more than 10 tablets have been ingested within the preceding 4 hours, followed by symptomatic measures.

PARACETAMOL

As little as 10–15 g (20–30 tablets) of paracetamol may cause severe hepatocellular necrosis and, less frequently, renal tubular necrosis. Nausea and vomiting, the only early features of poisoning, usually settle within 24 hours. Persistence beyond this time, often associated with the onset of right subcostal pain and tenderness, usually indicates development of hepatic necrosis. Liver damage is maximal 3–4 days after ingestion and may lead to encephalopathy, haemorrhage, hypoglycaemia, cerebral oedema, and death.

Therefore, despite a lack of significant early symptoms, patients who have taken an overdose of paracetamol should be transferred to hospital urgently.

Gastric emptying is carried out if the overdose was taken within 4 hours of admission.

Antidotes such as **acetylcysteine** and **methionine** protect the liver if given within 10–12 hours of ingestion; this may also apply to periods up to and beyond 15 hours but expert advice is **essential**.

Patients at risk of liver damage and therefore requiring treatment can be identified from a single measurement of the plasma-paracetamol concentration, related to the time from ingestion, provided this time interval is not less than 4 hours; earlier samples may be misleading. The concentration is compared against a reference line joining plots of 200 mg/litre (1.32 mmol/litre) at 4 hours and 30 mg/litre (0.2 mmol/litre) at 15 hours, on a semi-logarithmic graph. Those whose concentrations are above that line are treated either with acetylcysteine intravenously or with methionine by mouth.

In remote areas, emesis should be induced if the patient presents within 4 hours of the overdose. Methionine (2.5 g) should be given by mouth once vomiting has occurred; it is seldom practicable to give acetylcysteine outside hospital. Once the patient reaches hospital the need to continue treatment with the antidote will be assessed from the plasma-paracetamol concentration (related to the time from ingestion).

See also Co-proxamol, under Opioids.

ACETYLCYSTEINE

Indications: paracetamol overdosage (above)
Cautions: asthma
Side-effects: bronchoconstriction, rashes
Dose: by intravenous infusion, in glucose intravenous infusion 5%, initially 150 mg/kg in 200 ml over 15 minutes, followed by 50 mg/kg in 500 ml over 4 hours, then 100 mg/kg in 1000 ml over 16 hours

PoM **Parvolex®** (DF)
Injection, acetylcysteine 200 mg/ml. Net price course of 12 amps of 10 ml = £31.75

METHIONINE

Indications: paracetamol overdosage, see notes above
Dose: by mouth, 2.5 g initially, followed by 3 further doses of 2.5 g every 4 hours

Methionine Tablets (Evans), DL-methionine 250 mg. Net price course of 40 tabs = £3.16

OPIOIDS

Opioids (narcotic analgesics) cause varying degrees of coma, respiratory depression, and pinpoint pupils. The specific antidote **naloxone** is indicated if there is coma or bradypnoea. Since naloxone is short-acting repeated injections are necessary according to the respiratory rate and depth of coma. Alternatively, it may be given by continuous intravenous infusion, the rate of administration being adjusted according to response.

CO-PROXAMOL. Combinations of dextropropoxyphene and paracetamol (now called co-proxamol) (in Distalgesic® etc.) are frequently taken in overdosage. The initial features are those of acute opioid overdosage with coma, respiratory depression, and pinpoint pupils. Patients may die of acute cardiovascular collapse before reaching hospital (particularly if alcohol has also been consumed) unless adequately resuscitated or given **naloxone** as antidote to the dextropropoxyphene. Paracetamol hepatotoxicity may develop later and should be anticipated and treated as indicated above.

NALOXONE HYDROCHLORIDE

Indications: overdosage with opioids; for postoperative respiratory depression, see section 15.1.7
Cautions: physical dependence on opioids; naloxone is short-acting, see notes above
Dose: by intravenous injection, 0.8–2 mg repeated at intervals of 2–3 minutes to a max. of 10 mg if respiratory function does not improve (then question diagnosis); CHILD 10 micrograms/kg; subsequent dose of 100 micrograms/kg if no response
By subcutaneous or intramuscular injection, as intravenous injection but only if intravenous route not feasible (onset of action slower)
By continuous intravenous infusion, 2 mg diluted in 500 ml intravenous infusion solution at a rate adjusted according to the response

PoM **Naloxone Hydrochloride** (Non-proprietary)
Injection, naloxone hydrochloride 400 micrograms/ml. Net price 1-ml amp = £4.92
PoM **Min-I-Jet Naloxone Hydrochloride®** (IMS)
Injection, naloxone hydrochloride 400 micrograms/ml. Net price 1-ml disposable syringe = £6.45; 2-ml disposable syringe = £10.97
PoM **Narcan®** (Du Pont)
Injection, naloxone hydrochloride 400 micrograms/ml. Net price 1-ml amp = £4.92; 10-ml vial = £44.25
Neonatal preparations —see section 15.1.7

Antidepressants

Tricyclic and related antidepressants cause dry mouth, coma of varying degree, hypotension, hypothermia, hyperreflexia, extensor plantar responses, convulsions, respiratory failure, cardiac conduction defects, and arrhythmias. Dilated pupils and urinary retention also occur. Metabolic acidosis may complicate severe poisoning; delirium with confusion, agitation, and visual and auditory hallucinations, is common during recovery.

Symptomatic treatment and activated charcoal by mouth may reasonably be given in the home before transfer but hospital admission is strongly advised, and supportive measures to ensure a patent airway and adequate ventilation during transfer are mandatory. Intravenous diazepam may be required for control of convulsions (preferably in emulsion form). Although arrhythmias are worrying, the use of anti-arrhythmic drugs is best avoided. Diazepam given by mouth is usually adequate to sedate delirious patients but large doses may be required.

Hypnotics and anxiolytics

BARBITURATES

These cause drowsiness, coma, respiratory depression, hypotension, and hypothermia. The duration and depth of cerebral depression vary greatly with the drug, the dose, and the tolerance of the patient. The severity of poisoning is often greater with a large dose of barbiturate hypnotics than with the longer-acting phenobarbitone. The majority of patients survive with supportive measures alone. Forced alkaline diuresis may be considered in severe phenobarbitone poisoning. Charcoal haemoperfusion is the treatment of choice for the small minority of patients with very severe barbiturate poisoning who fail to improve, or who deteriorate despite good supportive care.

BENZODIAZEPINES

Benzodiazepines taken alone cause drowsiness, ataxia, dysarthria, and occasionally minor and short-lived depression of consciousness. They potentiate the effects of other central nervous system depressants taken concomitantly.

Iron salts

Iron poisoning is commonest in childhood and is usually accidental. The symptoms are nausea, vomiting, abdominal pain, diarrhoea, haematemesis, and rectal bleeding. Hypotension, coma, and hepatocellular necrosis occur later. Mortality is reduced with intensive and specific therapy with **desferrioxamine**, which chelates iron. The stomach should be emptied at once, preferably by inducing vomiting as this is quickest. Gastric lavage in hospital should follow as soon as possible, leaving a solution of 10 g of desferrioxamine mesylate in 50 ml water in the stomach. The serum-iron concentration is measured as an emergency and parenteral desferrioxamine given to chelate absorbed iron in excess of the expected iron binding capacity.

DESFERRIOXAMINE MESYLATE

Indications: removal of iron from the body in poisoning; for use in chronic iron overload, see section 9.1.3

Side-effects: pain at site of intramuscular injection, anaphylactic reactions, and hypotension when given too rapidly by intravenous injection

Dose: by mouth after gastric lavage, 5–10 g in 50–100 ml of liquid

By intramuscular injection, 1–2 g in 10–20 ml of water for injections every 3–12 hours

By continuous intravenous infusion, up to 15 mg/kg/hour; max. in 24 hours 80 mg/kg

PoM **Desferal**® (Ciba)

Injection, powder for reconstitution, desferrioxamine mesylate. Net price 500-mg vial = £1.94

Lithium salts

Most cases of lithium intoxication occur as a complication of long-term therapy and are caused by reduced excretion of the drug due to a variety of factors including deterioration of renal function, infections, dehydration, and co-adminstration of diuretics. Acute deliberate overdoses may also occur with delayed onset of symptoms (12 hours or more) due to slow entry of lithium into the tissues and continuing absorption from sustained-release formulations.

The early clinical features are non-specific and may include apathy and restlessness which could be confused with mental changes due to the patient's depressive illness. Vomiting, diarrhoea, ataxia, weakness, dysarthria, muscle twitching, and tremor may follow. Severe poisoning is associated with convulsions, coma, renal failure, electrolyte imbalance, and hypotension.

Therapeutic lithium concentrations are within the range of 0.6–1.2 mmol/litre; concentrations in excess of 2.0 mmol/litre are usually associated with serious toxicity and such cases may need treatment with forced diuresis or dialysis (if there is renal failure). In acute overdosage much higher serum concentrations may be present without features of toxicity and measures to increase urine production are usually all that are necessary. Otherwise treatment is supportive with special regard to electrolyte balance, renal function, and control of convulsions.

Phenothiazines and related drugs

Phenothiazines cause less depression of consciousness and respiration than other sedatives. Hypotension, hypothermia, sinus tachycardia, and arrhythmias (particularly with thioridazine) may complicate poisoning. Dystonic reactions can occur with therapeutic doses, (particularly with prochlorperazine and trifluoperazine) and convulsions may occur in severe cases. Drugs to control arrhythmias and convulsions may be needed. Dystonic reactions are rapidly abolished by injection of drugs such as orphenadrine or procyclidine (see section 4.9.2).

Stimulants

AMPHETAMINES

These cause wakefulness, excessive activity, paranoia, hallucinations, and hypertension followed by exhaustion, convulsions, hyperthermia, and coma. The early stages can be controlled by chlorpromazine and, if necessary, beta-blockers. Later, tepid sponging, anticonvulsants, and artificial respiration may be needed. Amphetamine excretion can be increased by forced acid diuresis but this is seldom necessary.

COCAINE

Cocaine can be smoked, sniffed, or injected. It stimulates the central nervous system causing agitation, dilated pupils, tachycardia, hypertension, hallucinations, hypertonia, and hyperreflexia. Convulsions, coma and metabolic acidosis may develop in the worst cases. Sedation, with intravenous diazepam, may be all that is necessary but intravenous propranolol may be indicated for severe intoxication.

Theophylline

Theophylline and related drugs are often prescribed as sustained-release formulations and toxicity may therefore be delayed. They cause vomiting (which may be severe and intractable), agitation, restlessness, dilated pupils, and sinus tachycardia. More serious effects are haematemesis, convulsions, and supraventricular and ventricular arrhythmias. Profound hypokalaemia may develop rapidly.

The stomach should be emptied as early as possible. Elimination of theophylline may be enhanced by repeated doses of activated charcoal by mouth (see also under Active Elimination Techniques). Hypokalaemia is corrected by intravenous infusion of potassium chloride and may be so severe as to require 60 mmol/hour (high doses under ECG monitoring). Convulsions should be controlled by intravenous administration of diazepam (emulsion preferred). Sedation with chlorpromazine or diazepam may be necessary in agitated patients. In non-asthmatic patients extreme tachycardia, hypokalaemia, and hyperglycaemia may be reversed by intravenous administration of propranolol (see section 2.4).

Other poisons

CONSULT POISONS INFORMATION CENTRES
DAY AND NIGHT—see p. 37

Cyanides

Cyanide antidotes include dicobalt edetate, given alone, and sodium nitrite, followed by sodium thiosulphate. These antidotes are held for emergency use in hospitals as well as in centres where cyanide poisoning is a risk such as factories and laboratories.

DICOBALT EDETATE

Indications: acute poisoning with cyanides
Cautions: toxic in absence of cyanides
Side-effects: transient hypotension, tachycardia, and vomiting
Dose: by intravenous injection, 300 mg (20 ml) over 1 minute, followed by 50 ml of glucose intravenous infusion 50%, both repeated once or twice if necessary

PoM **Kelocyanor**® (Lipha)
Injection, dicobalt edetate 300 mg/20 ml. Net price 20-ml amp = £2.66

SODIUM NITRITE

Indications: poisoning with cyanides in conjunction with sodium thiosulphate
Side-effects: flushing and headache due to vasodilatation

PoM **Sodium Nitrite Injection**
Injection, sodium nitrite 3% (30 mg/ml) in water for injections
Dose: 10 ml by intravenous injection over 3 minutes, followed by 25 ml of sodium thiosulphate injection 50%, by intravenous injection over 10 minutes
Available from Macarthys, Penn, etc. (special order)

SODIUM THIOSULPHATE

Indications: poisoning with cyanides in conjunction with sodium nitrite

PoM **Sodium Thiosulphate Injection**
Injection, sodium thiosulphate 50% (500 mg/ml) in water for injections
Dose: see above under Sodium Nitrite Injection
Available from Macarthys, Penn, etc. (special order)

Heavy metals

Heavy metal antidotes include dimercaprol, penicillamine, and sodium calciumedetate.

DIMERCAPROL
(BAL)
Indications: poisoning by antimony, arsenic, bismuth, gold, mercury, thallium; adjunct (with sodium calciumedetate) in lead poisoning.
Cautions: hypertension
Contra-indications: not indicated for iron or cadmium poisoning; severe hepatic impairment
Side-effects: hypertension, tachycardia, malaise, nausea, vomiting, lachrymation, sweating, burning sensation (mouth and eyes), constriction of throat and chest, headache, muscle spasm, abdominal pain, tingling of extremities; pyrexia in children; pain on injection
Dose: by intramuscular injection, 2.5–3 mg/kg every 4 hours for 2 days, 2–4 times on the 3rd day, then 1–2 times daily for 10 days or until recovery

PoM **Dimercaprol Injection** (Boots), dimercaprol 50 mg/ml. Net price 2-ml amp = 55p

PENICILLAMINE

Indications: poisoning by certain toxic metal ions, particularly by copper and lead

Cautions; Contra-indications; Side-effects: see section 10.1.3

Dose: 1–2 g daily in divided doses before food until urinary lead is stabilised at less than 500 micrograms/day; CHILD 20 mg/kg daily

Preparations

See section 10.1.3

SODIUM CALCIUMEDETATE

Indications: poisoning by heavy metals, especially lead

Cautions: renal impairment

Side-effects: nausea, cramp; in overdosage renal damage

Dose: by intravenous infusion, adults and children, up to 40 mg/kg twice daily in sodium chloride intravenous infusion 0.9% or glucose intravenous infusion 5% for up to 5 days, repeated if necessary after 48 hours

PoM **Ledclair®** (Sinclair)

Injection, sodium calciumedetate 200 mg/ml. Net price 5-ml amp = £2.38

Noxious gases

CARBON MONOXIDE

Carbon monoxide poisoning is now usually due to inhalation of smoke, car exhaust, or fumes caused by blocked flues or incomplete combustion of fuel gases in confined spaces. Its toxic effects are entirely due to hypoxia.

Immediate treatment is essential. The person should be removed into the fresh air, the airway cleared, and **oxygen** 100% administered as soon as available. Artificial respiration should be given as necessary and continued until adequate spontaneous breathing starts, or stopped only after persistent and efficient treatment of cardiac arrest has failed. Admission to hospital is desirable because complications may arise after a delay of hours or days. Cerebral oedema should be anticipated in severe poisoning and is treated with an intravenous infusion of mannitol (see section 2.2.5). Referral for hyperbaric oxygen treatment should be discussed with the poisons information services if the victim is or has been unconscious or has a blood carboxyhaemoglobin concentration of more than 40%.

SULPHUR DIOXIDE, CHLORINE, PHOSGENE, AMMONIA

The immediate effect of all except phosgene is coughing and choking. Pulmonary oedema, with severe breathlessness and cyanosis may develop suddenly up to 36 hours after exposure. Death may occur. Patients are kept under observation and those who develop pulmonary oedema are given corticosteroids and oxygen. Assisted ventilation may be necessary in the most serious cases.

Pesticides

PARAQUAT

Concentrated liquid paraquat preparations (e.g. Gramoxone®), available to farmers and horticulturists, contain 10–20% paraquat and are extremely toxic. Granular preparations, for garden use, contain only 2.5% paraquat and have caused few deaths.

Paraquat has local and systemic effects. Splashes in the eyes irritate and ulcerate the cornea and conjunctiva. Copious washing of the eye and instillation of antibacterial eye-drops, should aid healing but it may be a slow process. Skin irritation, blistering, and ulceration can occur from prolonged contact both with the concentrated and dilute forms. Inhalation of spray, mist, or dust containing paraquat may cause nose bleeding and sore throat but not systemic toxicity.

Ingestion of concentrated paraquat solutions is followed by nausea, vomiting, and diarrhoea. Painful ulceration of the tongue, lips, and fauces may appear after 36 to 48 hours together with renal failure. Some days later there may be dyspnoea with pulmonary fibrosis due to proliferative alveolitis and bronchiolitis.

Treatment should be started immediately. The single most useful measure is oral administration of either **Fuller's earth** or **bentonite** to adsorb paraquat and reduce absorption. The stomach is then emptied by careful gastric lavage and 300 ml of a suspension containing 30 g of Fuller's earth and 15 g of magnesium sulphate should be left in the stomach. Further quantities of 300 ml of a 30% Fuller's earth suspension are given after 2 and after 4 hours; magnesium sulphate or mannitol is given as required to produce diarrhoea and empty the gut. Some authorities prefer regimens employing 15% Fuller's earth suspensions. Intravenous fluids and analgesics are given as necessary. Oxygen therapy should be avoided if possible since this may exacerbate damage to the lungs. Measures to enhance elimination of absorbed paraquat are probably valueless but should be discussed with the poisons information services who will also give guidance on predicting the likely outcome from plasma concentrations. Paraquat absorption can be confirmed by a simple qualitative urine test.

ORGANOPHOSPHORUS INSECTICIDES

Organophosphorus insecticides are usually supplied as powders or dissolved in organic solvents. All are absorbed through the bronchi and intact skin as well as through the gut and inhibit cholinesterase activity thereby prolonging and intensifying the effects of acetylcholine. Toxicity between different organophosphorus compounds varies considerably, and onset may be delayed after skin exposure.

Anxiety, restlessness, dizziness, headache, miosis, nausea, hypersalivation, vomiting, abdominal colic, diarrhoea, bradycardia, and sweating are common. Muscle weakness and fasciculation may develop and progress to generalised flaccid paralysis including the ocular and respiratory muscles. Convulsions, coma, pulmonary oedema with copious bronchial secretions, hypoxia, and arrhythmias occur in severe cases. Hyperglycaemia and glycosuria without ketonuria may also be present.

Further absorption should be prevented by emptying the stomach, removing the patient to fresh air, or removing soiled clothing and washing contaminated skin as appropriate. In severe poisoning it is vital to ensure a clear airway, frequent removal of bronchial secretions, and adequate ventilation and oxygenation. **Atropine** will reverse the muscarinic effects of acetylcholine and is given in a dose of 2 mg as atropine sulphate injection (intramuscularly or intravenously according to the severity of poisoning) every 20 to 30 minutes until the skin becomes flushed and dry, the pupils dilate, and tachycardia develops.

Pralidoxime mesylate (P2S), a cholinesterase reactivator, is indicated, as an adjunct to atropine, in moderate or severe poisoning but is only effective if given within 24 hours. It may be obtained from designated centres, the names of which are held by the poisons information services (see p. 37). A dose of 1 g by intramuscular injection or, diluted with 10–15 ml water for injections, by slow intravenous injection should produce improvement in muscle power within 30 minutes but repeated doses or, in severe cases, an intravenous infusion of up to 500 mg/hour may be required.

PRALIDOXIME MESYLATE

Indications: adjunct to atropine in the treatment of organophosphorus poisoning

Cautions: renal impairment, myasthenia gravis

Contra-indications: poisoning due to carbamates and to organophosphorus compounds without anticholinesterase activity

Side-effects: drowsiness, dizziness, disturbances of vision, nausea, tachycardia, headache, hyperventilation, and muscular weakness

Dose: by intramuscular injection, 1 g initially followed by 1–2 further doses if necessary; in very severe poisoning the initial dose can be doubled; usual max. 12 g in 24 hours

By slow intravenous injection (diluted to 10–15 ml with water for injections and given over 5–10 minutes), 1 g initially followed by 1–2 further doses if necessary; in very severe poisoning the initial dose can be doubled; usual max. 12 g in 24 hours

CHILD 20–60 mg/kg as required depending on severity of poisoning and response

PoM **Pralidoxime Mesylate Injection,** pralidoxime mesylate 200 mg/ml. Available as 5-ml amps (from designated centres)

Snake and Insect Bites

SNAKE BITE. Acute poisoning due to venomous snakes is extremely rare in the United Kingdom and the only indigenous venomous snake is the adder. The bite may cause local and systemic effects. The local effects include pain and swelling. Systemic effects include agitation, restlessness, abdominal colic, diarrhoea, and vomiting. Death is unlikely except in the case of a very weak debilitated person who receives a large amount of venom.

Only patients with persistent or recurrent hypotension, polymorphonuclear leucocytosis, electrocardiographic abnormalities, or extensive limb swelling within 4 hours of the bite should be given antivenom. Two ampoules of **Zagreb antivenom** (Regent) diluted with 2–3 volumes of sodium chloride intravenous infusion 0.9% are given intravenously and repeated in 1–2 hours if there is no clinical improvement (the dose is the same for adults and children). Adrenaline injection should be immediately to hand for treatment of serum hypersensitivity reactions (for full details see section 3.4.3).

For slight or moderate poisoning (local pain and swelling, possibly vomiting and diarrhoea), symptomatic treatment only is required. The site should be cleaned, covered with a dry dressing, and immobilised. Antibiotics and antitetanus immunoglobulin are of no value; an antihistamine may be given by injection.

Antivenom is available for certain foreign snakes. Information on supply, telephone:

London (also identification and management)   01-635 9191

Liverpool (Walton Hospital Pharmacy) (supply only)   051-525 3611

INSECT BITES. Stings from ants, wasps, bees, and hornets cause local pain and swelling but seldom cause severe toxicity. If the bite is in the mouth or on the tongue marked swelling may cause respiratory distress. The stings from these insects are usually treated by cleansing the area, applying a cooling lotion (such as a calamine preparation), and giving an antihistamine by mouth. Bee stings should be removed by scraping them off with a finger nail or knife before cleansing the area. Anaphylactic reactions require treatment with **adrenaline**. Inhalation of adrenaline (Medihaler-epi®, see section 3.4.3) is sufficient for mild attacks and is convenient for patients at risk to carry. A dose of 0.5–1 ml of adrenaline injection 1 in 1000 (1 mg/ml) should be given intramuscularly in more severe cases (for full details see section 3.4.3).

Classified Notes on Drugs and Preparations

1: Drugs acting on the
GASTRO-INTESTINAL SYSTEM

The drugs and preparations in this chapter are described under the following sections:
1.1 Antacids
1.2 Antispasmodics and other drugs altering gut motility
1.3 Ulcer-healing drugs
1.4 Antidiarrhoeal drugs
1.5 Treatment of chronic diarrhoeas
1.6 Laxatives
1.7 Preparations for haemorrhoids
1.8 Stoma care
1.9 Drugs affecting intestinal secretions

For antibacterial prophylaxis in abdominal surgery see section 5.1, Table 2.

1.1   Antacids

1.1.1 Aluminium- and magnesium-containing antacids
1.1.2 Sodium bicarbonate
1.1.3 Calcium- and bismuth-containing antacids

Antacids are still useful for treating gastro-intestinal disease; they can often relieve symptoms in both ulcer and non-ulcer dyspepsia, and in reflux oesophagitis. They are best given when symptoms occur or are expected, usually between meals and at bedtime, four or more times daily; additional doses may be required up to once an hour. High doses of magnesium- or aluminium-containing antacids, such as 200 to 300 ml of aluminium hydroxide mixture daily, to give a neutralising capacity of about 150 to 1000 mmol daily, will promote duodenal ulcer healing, but possibly less well than antisecretory agents (section 1.3); proof of a relationship between healing and neutralising capacity is lacking. Liquid preparations are more effective than solids.

Antacids should not be taken at the same time as other drugs as they may impair their absorption. Antacids may also damage enteric coatings designed to prevent dissolution in the stomach. Drug interactions: see Appendix 1 (sections *1*, *2.3*, *4.2*, *4.7*, *5.1*, *5.2*, *5.4*, *10*).

For the use of aluminium- and calcium-containing antacids as phosphate-binding agents in the management of renal failure, see section 9.5.2.2.

1.1.1   Aluminium- and magnesium-containing antacids

Magnesium- and aluminium-containing antacids, such as magnesium carbonate, hydroxide and trisilicate, and aluminium glycinate and hydroxide, being relatively insoluble in water, are long-acting if retained in the stomach. They are suitable for most antacid purposes. Magnesium-containing antacids tend to be laxative whereas aluminium-containing antacids may be constipating.

Compound preparations have no clear advantages over simpler preparations: neutralising capacity may be the same.

Complexes, such as alexitol sodium, almasilate, and hydrotalcite, confer no special advantage.

ALUMINIUM HYDROXIDE
Indications: dyspepsia
Cautions: see notes above

Aluminium-only preparations
Aluminium Hydroxide (Non-proprietary)
Tablets, dried aluminium hydroxide 500 mg. Net price 20 = 28p
Dose: 1–2 tablets chewed 4 times daily and at bedtime or as required
Mixture (gel), about 4% w/w Al_2O_3 in water. Diluent water for preparations, life of diluted mixture 14 days. Net price 200 ml = 36p
Dose: antacid, 5–10 ml 4 times daily between meals and at bedtime or as required
Note. The brand name ℕℍS Aludrox® (Wyeth) relates to aluminium hydroxide mixture; net price 200 ml = 49p. For ℕℍS Aludrox® tablets see preparations, with magnesium, below.

Alu-Cap® (Riker)
Capsules, green/red, dried aluminium hydroxide 475 mg (low Na^+). Net price 20 = 64p
Dose: dyspepsia, 1 capsule 4 times daily and at bedtime

With magnesium
ℕℍS Aludrox® (Wyeth)
Tablets, aluminium hydroxide-magnesium carbonate co-dried gel 282 mg, magnesium hydroxide 85 mg. Net price 20 = 37p
Dose: 1 or 2 tablets chewed 4 times daily between meals and at bedtime when required
ℕℍS Dijex® (Crookes)
Tablets, pink, aluminium hydroxide-magnesium carbonate co-dried gel 400 mg (low Na^+). Net price 30 = 42p
Dose: 1–2 tablets chewed every 2–4 hours when required
Liquid, aluminium hydroxide mixture 98%, magnesium hydroxide 1.7%. Net price 200 ml = 86p
Dose: 5–10 ml every 2–4 hours when required
ℕℍS Gastrils® (Jackson)
Pastilles, green (mint-flavoured) or yellow (fruit-flavoured), s/c, aluminium hydroxide-magnesium carbonate co-dried gel 500 mg. Net price 22 = 51p
Dose: 1–2 pastilles sucked when required; CHILD 1 pastille 3 times daily
ℕℍS Gelusil® (W-L)
Tablets, dried aluminium hydroxide 250 mg, magnesium trisilicate 500 mg (low Na^+). Net price 20 = 56p
Dose: 1–2 tablets chewed or sucked after meals or when required; CHILD half adult dose

Maalox® (Rorer)
Tablets, dried aluminium hydroxide 400 mg, magnesium hydroxide 400 mg (low Na⁺). Net price 20 = 25p
Dose: 1–2 tablets chewed after meals and at bedtime or when required
Suspension, sugar-free, dried aluminium hydroxide 220 mg, magnesium hydroxide 195 mg/5 ml (low Na⁺). Net price 100 ml = 38p; 20 × 10-ml sachets = 76p
Dose: 10–20 ml after meals and at bedtime or when required

¹**Maalox TC®** (Rorer)
Tablets, dried aluminium hydroxide 600 mg, magnesium hydroxide 300 mg (low Na⁺). Net price 100 = £3.60
Suspension, sugar-free, dried aluminium hydroxide 600 mg, magnesium hydroxide 300 mg/5 ml (low Na⁺). Net price 500 ml = £3.60
Dose: prevention of recurrence of duodenal ulcer, 3 tablets or 15 ml suspension twice daily (in the morning after food and at bedtime)
¹formerly Maalox Concentrate

Mucogel® (Pharmax)
Tablets, dried aluminium hydroxide 400 mg, magnesium hydroxide 400 mg (low Na⁺). Net price 100 = £1.36
Dose: 1–2 tablets to be chewed after meals and at bedtime or as required
Suspension, sugar-free, dried aluminium hydroxide 220 mg, magnesium hydroxide 195 mg/5 ml (low Na⁺). Net price 100 ml = 41p
Dose: 10–20 ml 3 times daily, preferably between meals, and at bedtime or when required

Polyalk Revised Formula® (Galen)
Suspension, dried aluminium hydroxide 440 mg, light magnesium oxide 70 mg/5 ml (low Na⁺). Net price 100 ml = 38p
Dose: 10–20 ml after meals and at bedtime or when required

N̶H̶S̶ **Prodexin®** (Bencard)
Tablets, aluminium glycinate 900 mg, magnesium carbonate 100 mg (low Na⁺). Net price 30 = 91p
Dose: 1 or more tablets chewed or sucked when required

ALEXITOL SODIUM

Sodium poly(hydroxyaluminium) carbonate-hexitol complex
Indications: dyspepsia
Cautions: see notes above

Alexitol Sodium (Non-proprietary)
Tablets, alexitol sodium 360 mg. Net price 20 = 20p
Dose: 1–2 tablets chewed or sucked when required
Note. The brand name N̶H̶S̶ Actal® (Winthrop) relates to alexitol sodium.

With magnesium

N̶H̶S̶ **Droxalin®** (Sterling Health)
Tablets, alexitol sodium 200 mg, magnesium trisilicate 162 mg (low Na⁺). Net price 20 = 33p
Dose: 1–2 tablets chewed when required

MAGNESIUM CARBONATE

Indications: dyspepsia
Cautions: renal impairment; see also notes above. Drug interactions: see Appendix 1 (sections *9*, *15*)
Side-effects: diarrhoea; belching due to liberated carbon dioxide

Magnesium Carbonate Mixture (see Formulary). Contains about 9 mmol Na⁺/10 ml. Net price 200 ml = 33p
Dose: 10 ml 3 times daily in water

Magnesium Carbonate Mixture, Aromatic, (see Formulary). Contains about 6 mmol Na⁺/10 ml. Net price 200 ml = 28p
Dose: 10 ml 3 times daily in water

For compound preparations with aluminium, see under Aluminium Hydroxide (above)

MAGNESIUM TRISILICATE

Indications: dyspepsia
Cautions: renal impairment; see also notes above. Drug interactions: see Appendix 1 (sections *9*, *15*)
Side-effects: diarrhoea

Magnesium Trisilicate Tablets, Compound, magnesium trisilicate 250 mg, dried aluminium hydroxide 120 mg. Net price 20 = 19p
Dose: 1–2 tablets chewed when required

Magnesium Trisilicate Mixture (see Formulary). Contains about 6 mmol Na⁺/10 ml. Net price 200 ml = 22p
Dose: 10 ml 3 times daily in water

Magnesium Trisilicate (powder). (Low Na⁺). Net price 20 g = 11p. Label: 13
Dose: 0.5–2 g in liquid when required

Magnesium Trisilicate Oral Powder, Compound, magnesium trisilicate 250 mg, chalk 250 mg, heavy magnesium carbonate 250 mg, sodium bicarbonate 250 mg/g. Contains about 3 mmol Na⁺/g. Net price 20 g = 16p. Label: 13
Dose: 1–5 g in liquid when required

For compound preparations with aluminium, see under Aluminium Hydroxide (above)

ALUMINIUM-MAGNESIUM COMPLEXES

ALMASILATE

Aluminium magnesium silicate hydrate (artificial)
Indications: dyspepsia
Cautions: see notes above

Almasilate (Non-proprietary)
N̶H̶S̶ *Tablets*, almasilate 500 mg. Net price 12 = 52p
Dose: 2 tablets chewed with meals and at bedtime or when required

---

Suspension, almasilate 500 mg/5 ml. Net price 200 ml = 76p

Dose: 10 ml with meals and at bedtime or when required

Note. The brand name NHS Malinal® (Robins) relates to almasilate tablets and suspension.

HYDROTALCITE

Aluminium magnesium carbonate hydroxide hydrate

Indications: dyspepsia
Cautions: see notes above

Hydrotalcite (Non-proprietary)
Tablets, hydrotalcite 500 mg. Net price 20 = 25p

Dose: 2 tablets chewed between meals and at bedtime; CHILD 6–12 years 1 tablet

Suspension, hydrotalcite 500 mg/5 ml. Net price 100 ml = 35p

Dose: 10 ml between meals and at bedtime; CHILD 6–12 years 5 ml

Note. Both tablets and suspension were formerly marketed as NHS Altacite® (Roussel); see section 1.1.1.1 for Altacite Plus® preparations.

MAGALDRATE

A synthetic combination of aluminium and magnesium hydroxides and sulphuric acid

Indications: dyspepsia
Cautions: see notes above

Magaldrate (Non-proprietary)
Suspension, magaldrate 800 mg/5 ml. Net price 100 ml = 38p

Dose: 5–10 ml after meals and at bedtime; CHILD 6–12 years 2.5–5 ml

Note. The brand name NHS Dynese® (Galen) relates to magaldrate suspension.

1.1.1.1   Aluminium- and magnesium-containing antacids with additional ingredients

Activated dimethicone (simethicone USP) either given alone or added to antacids as an antifoaming agent, to relieve flatulence, is of uncertain value. Alginates added as protectants against reflux oesophagitis in Gastrocote®, Gaviscon® and Topal® may be useful, but the antacid content of all three is relatively low; Gastrocote® and Gaviscon® both contain sodium as the bicarbonate. Surface anaesthetics (oxethazaine in Mucaine®) may be included in antacids to relieve the discomfort in oesophagitis but they are of doubtful efficacy.

NHS **Actonorm**® (Wallace Mfg)
Gel, dried aluminium hydroxide 220 mg, activated dimethicone 25 mg, magnesium hydroxide 200 mg/5 ml (low Na⁺). Net price 200 ml = £1.34

Dose: 5–20 ml when required

Algicon® (Rorer)
Tablets, aluminium hydroxide-magnesium carbonate co-dried gel 360 mg, magnesium alginate 500 mg, magnesium carbonate 320 mg,

potassium bicarbonate 100 mg, sucrose 1.5 g (low Na⁺). Net price 60 = £2.61

Dose: 1–2 tablets chewed after meals and at bedtime

Suspension, yellow, aluminium hydroxide-magnesium carbonate co-dried gel 140 mg, magnesium alginate 250 mg, magnesium carbonate 175 mg, potassium bicarbonate 50 mg/5 ml (low Na⁺). Net price 500 ml = £2.88

Dose: 10–20 ml after meals and at bedtime

Altacite Plus® (Roussel)
NHS *Tablets*, activated dimethicone 250 mg, hydrotalcite 500 mg (low Na⁺). Net price 20 = 99p

Dose: 2 tablets chewed between meals and at bedtime when required; CHILD 8–12 years 1 tablet

Suspension, sugar-free, activated dimethicone 125 mg, hydrotalcite 500 mg/5 ml (low Na⁺). Do not dilute. Net price 100 ml = 37p

Dose: 10 ml between meals and at bedtime when required; CHILD 8–12 years 5 ml

NHS **Andursil**® (Ciba Consumer)
Tablets, aluminium hydroxide-magnesium carbonate co-dried gel 750 mg, activated dimethicone 250 mg. Contains about 1 mmol Na⁺/tablet. Net price 20 = 76p

Dose: 1–2 tablets 3 or 4 times daily and at bedtime when required

Suspension, sugar-free, Al₂O₃ 200 mg (as aluminium hydroxide mixture), magnesium hydroxide 200 mg, aluminium hydroxide-magnesium carbonate co-dried gel 200 mg, activated dimethicone 150 mg/5 ml (low Na⁺). Do not dilute. Net price 100 ml = 65p

Dose: 5–10 ml 3 or 4 times daily and at bedtime when required

Asilone® (Rorer)
NHS *Tablets*, dried aluminium hydroxide 500 mg, activated dimethicone 270 mg (low Na⁺). Net price 20 = 77p

Dose: 1–2 tablets chewed or sucked before meals and at bedtime

Gel and suspension, sugar-free, dried aluminium hydroxide 420 mg, activated dimethicone 135 mg, light magnesium oxide 70 mg/5 ml (low Na⁺). Diluent purified water, freshly boiled and cooled, life of diluted gel or suspension 14 days. Net price 100 ml (both) = 38p

Dose: 5–10 ml before meals and at bedtime

Asilone for Infants® (Rorer)
Paediatric suspension, sugar-free, dried aluminium hydroxide 84 mg, activated dimethicone 27 mg, light magnesium oxide 14 mg/5 ml (low Na⁺). Diluent as above. Net price 100 ml = £1.00

Dose: CHILD 1–3 months 2.5 ml, over 3 months 5 ml, 3 or 4 times daily before or with feeds

Diovol® (Pharmax)
Suspension, sugar-free, white (mint-flavoured) or yellow (fruit-flavoured), aluminium hydroxide 200 mg, dimethicone 25 mg, magnesium hydroxide 200 mg/5 ml (low Na⁺). Net price 300 ml (both) = £1.16

Dose: 10–20 ml when required; CHILD 6–12 years 5–10 ml

Gastrocote® (MCP)

Tablets, alginic acid 200 mg, dried aluminium hydroxide 80 mg, magnesium trisilicate 40 mg, sodium bicarbonate 70 mg. Contains about 1 mmol Na⁺/tablet. Net price 100 = £3.76
Dose: 1–2 tablets chewed 4 times daily, after meals and at bedtime. Not recommended for children under 6 years

Liquid, peach-coloured, dried aluminium hydroxide 80 mg, magnesium trisilicate 40 mg, sodium alginate 220 mg, sodium bicarbonate 70 mg/5 ml. Contains 1.8 mmol Na⁺/5 ml. Net price 500 ml = £2.86
Dose: 5–15 ml 4 times daily, after meals and at bedtime. Not recommended for children under 6 years

Gastron® (Winthrop)

Tablets, alginic acid 600 mg, dried aluminium hydroxide 240 mg, magnesium trisilicate 60 mg, sodium bicarbonate 210 mg. Contains about 2.5 mmol Na⁺/tablet. Net price 20 = 78p
Dose: 1–2 tablets chewed 3 times daily after meals and 2 tablets at bedtime

Gaviscon® (R&C)

Tablets, alginic acid 500 mg, dried aluminium hydroxide 100 mg, magnesium trisilicate 25 mg, sodium bicarbonate 170 mg, with glucose and sucrose. Contains 2 mmol Na⁺/tablet. Net price 60 = £2.25
Dose: 1–2 tablets chewed after meals and at bedtime, followed by liquid; CHILD 1 tablet

Liquid, pink, sodium alginate 250 mg, sodium bicarbonate 133.5 mg, calcium carbonate 80 mg/5 ml. Contains about 3 mmol Na⁺/5 ml. Net price 100 ml = 58p
Dose: 10–20 ml after meals and at bedtime; CHILD 5–10 ml

Infant Gaviscon® (R&C)

Oral powder, sugar-free, alginic acid 924 mg, dried aluminium hydroxide 200 mg, magnesium trisilicate 50 mg, sodium bicarbonate 340 mg, with mannitol and colloidal silica/2-g sachet. Contains 4 mmol Na⁺/sachet. Net price 10 sachets = £1.64
Dose: INFANT ½–1 sachet mixed with feeds when required; up to 2 months, not more than ½ sachet; CHILD 1 sachet after food

Infacol® (Pharmax)

Liquid, sugar-free, activated dimethicone 40 mg/ml (low Na⁺). Net price 50 ml = £1.38. Counselling advised, use of dropper
Dose: INFANT 0.5–1 ml before feeds

Maalox Plus® (Rorer)

NHS *Tablets*, white/yellow, dried aluminium hydroxide 200 mg, activated dimethicone 25 mg, magnesium hydroxide 200 mg (low Na⁺). Net price 50 = £1.41
Dose: 1–2 tablets chewed 4 times daily after meals and at bedtime or when required

Suspension, sugar-free, dried aluminium hydroxide 220 mg, activated dimethicone 25 mg, magnesium hydroxide 195 mg/5 ml (low Na⁺). Net price 500 ml = £1.90
Dose: 5–10 ml 4 times daily after meals and at bedtime or when required

PoM **Mucaine**® (Wyeth)

Suspension, sugar-free, aluminium hydroxide mixture 4.75 ml, magnesium hydroxide 100 mg, oxethazaine 10 mg/5 ml. Diluent water for preparations, life of diluted suspension 14 days. Net price 500 ml = £1.20
Dose: 5–10 ml (without fluid) 3–4 times daily 15 minutes before meals and at bedtime or when required

Phazyme® (Stafford-Miller)

Tablets, pink, s/c, activated dimethicone 20 mg outer layer, 40 mg core (low Na⁺). Net price 20 = 74p
Dose: 1–2 tablets with meals and at bedtime or when required

Polycrol® (Nicholas)

Tablets, green/white, aluminium hydroxide-magnesium carbonate co-dried gel 275 mg, activated dimethicone 25 mg, magnesium hydroxide 100 mg (low Na⁺). Net price 20-tab pack = 46p; 200-tab pack = £2.71
Dose: 1–2 tablets chewed between meals and at bedtime or when required; CHILD 5–12 years 1 tablet 2–3 times daily

Gel, sugar-free, aluminium hydroxide mixture 4.75 ml, activated dimethicone 25 mg, magnesium hydroxide 100 mg/5 ml (low Na⁺). Net price 300 ml = £1.16
Dose: 5–10 ml between meals and at bedtime or when required; CHILD 5–12 years 5 ml up to six times daily

Polycrol Forte® (Nicholas)

Tablets, aluminium hydroxide-magnesium carbonate co-dried gel 275 mg, activated dimethicone 250 mg, magnesium hydroxide 100 mg (low Na⁺). Net price 12-tab pack = 46p; 120-tab = £1.63
Dose: 1–2 tablets chewed between meals and at bedtime or when required

Gel, sugar-free, aluminium hydroxide mixture 4.75 ml, activated dimethicone 125 mg, magnesium hydroxide 100 mg/5 ml (low Na⁺). Net price 300 ml = £1.16
Dose: 5–10 ml between meals and at bedtime or when required; CHILD 5–12 years 5 ml, up to six times daily

NHS **Siloxyl**® (Martindale)

Tablets, dried aluminium hydroxide 500 mg, activated dimethicone 250 mg (low Na⁺). Net price 20 = 53p
Dose: 1–2 tablets chewed or sucked when required

Suspension, dried aluminium hydroxide 420 mg, activated dimethicone 125 mg, light magnesium oxide 70 mg/5 ml (low Na⁺). Net price 300 ml = £1.62
Dose: 5–10 ml when required; CHILD 7–12 years 5 ml

NHS **Simeco**® (Wyeth)

Tablets, pink/white, aluminium hydroxide–magnesium carbonate co-dried gel 282 mg, activated dimethicone 25 mg, magnesium hydroxide 85 mg. Net price 60 = £3.15
Dose: 2 tablets to be chewed after or between meals and at bedtime

Suspension, aluminium hydroxide 215 mg, activated dimethicone 25 mg, magnesium hydroxide 80 mg/5 ml. Net price 200 ml = £1.35

Dose: 10 ml after or between meals and at bedtime

Topal® (ICI)

Tablets, alginic acid 200 mg, dried aluminium hydroxide 30 mg, light magnesium carbonate 40 mg with lactose 220 mg, sucrose 880 mg (low Na⁺). Net price 42 = £1.67

Dose: 1–3 tablets chewed 4 times daily after meals and at bedtime

NHS **Unigest®** (Unigreg)

Tablets, dried aluminium hydroxide 450 mg, dimethicone 400 mg (low Na⁺). Net price 12 = 89p

Dose: 1–2 tablets chewed or sucked after meals and at bedtime or when required

1.1.2   Sodium bicarbonate

Sodium bicarbonate, being soluble in water, is rapid-acting, but absorbed bicarbonate can cause alkalosis in excessive doses. Like other carbonate-containing antacids it liberates carbon dioxide which causes belching. Sodium bicarbonate and antacid preparations with a high sodium content, such as magnesium trisilicate mixture, should be avoided in patients on salt-restricted diets (in heart failure, hepatic and renal impairment, and during pregnancy).

SODIUM BICARBONATE

Indications: rapid relief of dyspepsia

Cautions: renal impairment; patients on a sodium-restricted diet; avoid prolonged use. Drug interactions: see Appendix 1 (section *4.2*)

Side-effects: belching due to liberated carbon dioxide and, with prolonged use, alkalosis

Dose: 1–5 g in water when required

Sodium Bicarbonate (powder). Net price 50 g = 5p. Label: 13

Sodium Bicarbonate Mixture, Paediatric (see Formulary). Net price 100 ml = 14p

Dose: CHILD up to 1 year 5 ml, 1–5 years 10 ml

Sodium Bicarbonate Tablets, Compound (Soda Mint Tablets), sodium bicarbonate 300 mg. Contains about 4 mmol Na⁺/tab. Net price 20 = 6p

Dose: 2–6 tablets sucked when required

1.1.3   Calcium- and bismuth-containing antacids

Bismuth-containing antacids are best avoided because absorbed bismuth can be neurotoxic, causing encephalopathy; they tend to be constipating. Calcium-containing antacids can induce rebound acid secretion: with modest doses the clinical significance is doubtful, but prolonged high doses also cause hypercalcaemia and alkalosis, and can precipitate the milk alkali syndrome.

Calcium Carbonate Mixture, Compound, Paediatric (see Formulary). Net price 100 ml = 5p

Dose: CHILD up to 1 year 5 ml, 1–5 years 10 ml

Calcium Carbonate Powder, Compound, calcium carbonate 375 mg, light kaolin 125 mg, heavy magnesium carbonate 125 mg, sodium bicarbonate 375 mg/g. Net price 100 g = 26p. Label: 13

Dose: 1–5 g in liquid when required

Magnesium Carbonate Tablets, Compound, heavy magnesium carbonate 200 mg, light kaolin 60 mg, sodium bicarbonate 120 mg, calcium carbonate 200 mg. Net price 20 = 20p

Dose: 1–2 tablets chewed when required

Magnesium Carbonate Powder, Compound, heavy magnesium carbonate 333 mg, light kaolin 83 mg, sodium bicarbonate 250 mg, calcium carbonate 333 mg. Net price 100 g = 26p. Label: 13

Dose: 1–5 g in liquid when required

NHS **Nulacin®** (Bencard)

Tablets, calcium carbonate 130 mg, heavy magnesium carbonate 30 mg, heavy magnesium oxide 130 mg, magnesium trisilicate 230 mg, with milk solids, dextrins and maltose (low Na⁺). Net price 25 = 67p

Note. Contains gluten

Dose: 1–2 tablets chewed or sucked when required

NHS **Roter®** (Roterpharma)

Tablets, pink, bismuth subnitrate 300 mg, frangula 25 mg, magnesium carbonate 400 mg, sodium bicarbonate 200 mg. Net price 20 = 48p

Dose: 1–2 tablets dispersed in warm water 3 times daily after meals

---

1.2   Antispasmodics and other drugs altering gut motility

The smooth muscle relaxant properties of anti-cholinergic and other antispasmodic drugs may be useful as adjunctive treatment in non-ulcer dyspepsia, in the irritable bowel syndrome, and in diverticular disease. The gastric antisecretory effects of conventional anticholinergic drugs are of little practical importance since dosage is limited by atropine-like side-effects. Moreover, they have been superseded by more powerful and specific antisecretory drugs, including the histamine H₂-receptor antagonists and the selective anticholinergic pirenzepine.

The dopamine-receptor antagonists metoclopramide and domperidone have different properties, tending to stimulate transit in the gut.

ANTICHOLINERGICS

The anticholinergics (more correctly termed 'antimuscarinics') can be divided into atropine and its related alkaloids (including the belladonna alkaloids), and synthetic anticholinergics. The synthetic anticholinergics can, in turn, be divided into **tertiary amines** (dicyclomine hydrochloride and piperidolate hydrochloride) and **quaternary ammonium compounds** (ambutonium bromide, glycopyrronium bromide, mepenzolate bromide, pipenzolate bromide, poldine methylsulphate, and propantheline bromide). The tertiary amine dicyclomine hydrochloride has a much less marked anticholinergic action than atropine and may also have some direct action on smooth muscle.

Quaternary ammonium compounds are less lipid soluble than atropine and so may be less likely to cross the blood–brain barrier; they are also less well absorbed. Although central atropine-like side-effects, such as confusion, are thereby reduced, peripheral atropine-like side-effects remain common with dry mouth, difficult visual accommodation, hesitant micturition, and constipation at doses which act as gut neuromuscular relaxants or inhibitors of acid secretion. The elderly are particularly susceptible; glaucoma and urinary retention may occur.

Anticholinergics tend to relax the oesophageal sphincter and should be avoided in patients with symptomatic reflux; all antispasmodics should be avoided in paralytic ileus. Despite these side-effects anticholinergics are nevertheless useful in some dyspeptics, in the irritable bowel syndrome, and in diverticular disease. A dose at night will delay gastric emptying and prolong the gastric retention of antacids, thus helping to reduce nocturnal acidity; side-effects are also better tolerated then.

The quaternary ammonium compound, **hyoscine butylbromide** is advocated as a gastro-intestinal antispasmodic, but it is poorly absorbed and its action is brief; the injection is a useful antispasmodic in endoscopy and radiology.

ATROPINE SULPHATE

Indications: see notes above; see also section 15.1.3

Cautions: in the elderly, urinary retention, prostatic enlargement, tachycardia, cardiac insufficiency, paralytic ileus, ulcerative colitis, and pyloric stenosis; may aggravate gastro-oesophageal reflux; breast-feeding. Drug interactions of anticholinergic drugs: see Appendix 1 (sections *2.3, 2.6, 4.6, 4.9, 5.2*)

Contra-indications: glaucoma

Side-effects: dry mouth with difficulty in swallowing and thirst, dilatation of the pupils with loss of accommodation and sensitivity to light, increased intra-ocular pressure, flushing, dry skin, bradycardia followed by tachycardia, palpitations and arrhythmias, difficulty with micturition, and constipation; rarely fever, confusional states and rashes

Dose and **Preparations**
See section 15.1.3

AMBUTONIUM BROMIDE

Indications: adjunct in gastro-intestinal disorders characterised by smooth muscle spasm

Cautions; Contra-indications; Side-effects: see under Atropine Sulphate and notes above

NHS PoM Aludrox SA® (Wyeth)
Suspension, sugar-free, green, ambutonium bromide 2.5 mg, aluminium hydroxide mixture 4.75 ml, magnesium hydroxide 100 mg/5 ml. Diluent water for preparations, life of diluted suspension 14 days. Net price 100 ml = 24p
Dose: 5–10 ml 3–4 times daily between meals and at bedtime

BELLADONNA ALKALOIDS

Indications: adjunct in gastro-intestinal disorders characterised by smooth muscle spasm

Cautions; Contra-indications; Side-effects: see under Atropine Sulphate

Aluminium Hydroxide and Belladonna Mixture, belladonna alkaloids 300 micrograms/10 ml (see Formulary). Net price 100 ml = 23p
Dose: 5 ml between meals

Belladonna Mixture, Paediatric, belladonna alkaloids 45 micrograms/5 ml (see Formulary). Net price 100 ml = 12p
Dose: CHILD up to 1 year 5 ml, 1–5 years 10 ml half an hour before meals

Magnesium Trisilicate and Belladonna Mixture, belladonna alkaloids 150 micrograms/10 ml (see Formulary). Contains about 6 mmol Na+/10 ml. Net price 200 ml = 26p
Dose: 10–20 ml between meals when necessary

NHS Alka-Donna® (Carlton)
Tablets, belladonna alkaloids 80 micrograms (calc. as hyoscyamine), dried aluminium hydroxide 250 mg, magnesium trisilicate 500 mg. Net price 20 = 7p
Dose: 1–2 tablets, sucked 3 times daily before meals

Suspension, belladonna alkaloids 60 micrograms (calc. as hyoscyamine), aluminium hydroxide mixture 2.15 ml, magnesium trisilicate 342.5 mg/5 ml. Net price 100 ml = 13p
Dose: 5–10 ml 3 times daily between meals

NHS Aluhyde® (Sinclair)
Tablets, scored, belladonna liquid extract 7.8 mg, dried aluminium hydroxide 245 mg, magnesium trisilicate 245 mg. Net price 50 = £2.94
Dose: 2 tablets 3 times daily

NHS Bellocarb® (Sinclair)
Tablets, beige, scored, belladonna dry extract 10 mg (equivalent to 100 micrograms of hyoscyamine), magnesium carbonate 300 mg, magnesium trisilicate 300 mg. Net price 50 = £2.51
Dose: 1–2 tablets 4 times daily

NHS Carbellon® (Torbet)
Tablets, black, belladonna dry extract 6 mg (equivalent to 60 micrograms hyoscyamine), charcoal 100 mg, magnesium hydroxide 100 mg, peppermint oil 0.003 ml. Net price 20 = 25p
Dose: flatulence and abdominal distension, 2–4 tablets 3 times daily

PoM Peptard® (Riker)
Tablets, s/r, hyoscyamine sulphate 200 micrograms. Net price 100 = £5.05. Label: 25
Dose: 2–3 tablets twice daily; CHILD over 10 years 1–2 tablets

DICYCLOMINE HYDROCHLORIDE

Indications: adjunct in gastro-intestinal disorders characterised by smooth muscle spasm

Cautions; Contra-indications; Side-effects: see under Atropine Sulphate. Contra-indicated in infants under 6 months

Dose: 10–20 mg 3 times daily; CHILD 6–24 months 5–10 mg up to 3–4 times daily, 15 minutes before feeds, 2–12 years 10 mg 3 times daily

PoM **Merbentyl**® (Merrell)

Tablets, dicyclomine hydrochloride 10 mg. Net price 20 = 58p

Syrup, dicyclomine hydrochloride 10 mg/5 ml. Diluent syrup, life of diluted preparation 14 days. Net price 100 ml = 88p

PoM **Merbentyl 20**® (Merrell)

Tablets, dicyclomine hydrochloride 20 mg. Net price 84 = £4.89

Compound preparations
Kolanticon® (Merrell)

Gel, sugar-free, dicyclomine hydrochloride 2.5 mg, dried aluminium hydroxide 200 mg, light magnesium oxide 100 mg, activated dimethicone (simethicone USP) 20 mg/5 ml. Diluent purified water, freshly boiled and cooled, life of diluted gel 14 days. Net price 200 ml = £1.15; 500 ml = £1·90

Dose: 10–20 ml every 4 hours when required

NHS **Kolantyl**® (Merrell)

Gel, sugar-free, dicyclomine hydrochloride 2.5 mg, dried aluminium hydroxide 200 mg, light magnesium oxide 100 mg/5 ml. Diluent purified water, freshly boiled and cooled, life of diluted gel 14 days. Net price 500 ml = £1.38

Dose: 10–20 ml every 4 hours when required

GLYCOPYRRONIUM BROMIDE

Indications: adjunct in gastro-intestinal disorders characterised by smooth muscle spasm

Cautions; Contra-indications; Side-effects: see under Atropine Sulphate and notes above

Dose: 1–4 mg 2–3 times daily

PoM **Robinul**® (Robins)

Tablets, pink, scored, glycopyrronium bromide 2 mg. Net price 20 = £1.88

HYOSCINE BUTYLBROMIDE

Indications: adjunct in gastro-intestinal disorders characterised by smooth muscle spasm

Cautions; Contra-indications; Side-effects: see under Atropine Sulphate and notes above

Dose: by mouth, 20 mg 4 times daily; CHILD 6–12 years, 10 mg 3 times daily

By intramuscular or intravenous injection (acute spasm), 20 mg, repeated after 30 minutes if necessary

PoM **Buscopan**® (Boehringer Ingelheim)

Tablets, s/c, hyoscine butylbromide 10 mg. Net price 20 = 68p

Injection, hyoscine butylbromide 20 mg/ml. Net price 1-ml amp = 19p

MEPENZOLATE BROMIDE

Indications: adjunct in gastro-intestinal disorders characterised by smooth muscle spasm

Cautions; Contra-indications; Side-effects: see under Atropine Sulphate and notes above

Dose: 25–50 mg 3–4 times daily; CHILD 6–12 years 12.5 mg

PoM **Cantil**® (MCP)

Tablets, yellow, scored, mepenzolate bromide 25 mg. Net price 20 = 96p

Elixir, red, mepenzolate bromide 12.5 mg/5 ml. Diluent water for preparations, life of diluted elixir 7 days. Net price 100 ml = £1.76

PIPENZOLATE BROMIDE

Indications: adjunct in gastro-intestinal disorders characterised by smooth muscle spasm

Cautions; Contra-indications; Side-effects: see under Atropine Sulphate and notes above

Dose: 5 mg 3 times daily and 5–10 mg at night

PoM **Piptal**® (MCP)

Tablets, peach, pipenzolate bromide 5 mg. Net price 50 = £1.14

Compound preparations
PoM **Piptalin**® (MCP)

Suspension, orange, sugar-free, pipenzolate bromide 4 mg, activated dimethicone 40 mg/5 ml. Diluent syrup or water for preparations, life of diluted suspension 14 days. Net price 100 ml = £1.03

Dose: 10 ml 3–4 times daily before meals; CHILD up to 10 kg 2.5 ml, 10–20 kg 2.5–5 ml, 20–40 kg 5 ml, 3–4 times daily 15 minutes before meals (or feeds)

PIPERIDOLATE HYDROCHLORIDE

Indications: adjunct in gastro-intestinal disorders characterised by smooth muscle spasm

Cautions; Contra-indications; Side-effects: see under Atropine Sulphate

Dose: 50 mg 4 times daily

PoM **Dactil**® (MCP)

Tablets, piperidolate hydrochloride 50 mg. Net price 50 = £2.00

POLDINE METHYLSULPHATE

Indications: adjunct in gastro-intestinal disorders characterised by smooth muscle spasm

Cautions; Contra-indications; Side-effects: see under Atropine Sulphate and notes above

Dose: 2–4 mg 3 times daily and at bedtime

PoM **Nacton**® (Bencard)

Tablets, scored, poldine methylsulphate 2 mg. Net price 112-tab pack = £1.89

Tablets forte, orange, scored, poldine methylsulphate 4 mg. Net price 112-tab pack = £3.61

PROPANTHELINE BROMIDE

Indications: adjunct in gastro-intestinal disorders characterised by smooth muscle spasm; for use with retention enemas see section 1.5; for use in enuresis see section 7.4.2

Cautions; Contra-indications; Side-effects: see under Atropine Sulphate and notes above

Dose: 15 mg 3 times daily 1 hour before meals and 30 mg at night, max. 120 mg daily

PoM **Pro-Banthine**® (Gold Cross)
Tablets, pink, s/c, propantheline bromide 15 mg.
Net price 100 = £2.34. Label: 22

OTHER ANTISPASMODICS

Alverine citrate (Spasmonal®), mebeverine
hydrochloride (Colofac®), and peppermint oil
(Colpermin®) are believed to be direct relaxants
of intestinal smooth muscle and may relieve pain
in the irritable bowel syndrome and diverticular
disease. They have no serious adverse effects but,
like all antispasmodics, should be avoided in paralytic ileus. Peppermint oil occasionally causes
heartburn.

ALVERINE CITRATE
Indications: irritable bowel syndrome
Cautions: paralytic ileus
Dose: 60–120 mg 1–3 times daily

Spasmonal® (Norgine)
Capsules, blue/grey, alverine citrate 60 mg. Net
price 20 = £1.99

Compound preparations
NHS **Normacol Antispasmodic**® (Norgine)
Granules, orange, coated, sterculia 62%, alver-
ine citrate 0.5%. Net price 500 g = £11.00.
Label: 25, 27, see dose below
Dose: 1–2 heaped 5-ml spoonfuls swallowed
without chewing with water once or twice daily
after meals; CHILD 6–12 years, half adult dose

MEBEVERINE HYDROCHLORIDE
Indications: irritable bowel syndrome
Cautions: paralytic ileus

PoM **Colofac**® (Duphar)
Tablets, s/c, mebeverine hydrochloride 135 mg.
Net price 20 = £1.67. Label: 22
Dose: 1 tablet 3 times daily preferably 20 minutes before meals
Liquid, yellow, sugar-free, mebeverine hydrochloride 50 mg (as embonate)/5 ml. Diluent
water for preparations, life of diluted liquid 14
days. Net price 300 ml = £3.50. Label: 22
Dose: adults and children over 10 years, 15 ml
3 times daily, preferably 20 minutes before food

Compound preparations
▼ PoM **Colven**® (R&C)
Granules, yellowish-brown, effervescent,
ispaghula husk 3.5 g, mebeverine
hydrochloride 135 mg/sachet. Contains
6.1 mmol Na+/sachet; caution in renal impairment. Net price 60 sachets = £15.00. Label: 13,
22
Dose: irritable bowel syndrome, 1 sachet in
water twice daily 30 minutes before meals

PEPPERMINT OIL
Indications: relief of abdominal colic and
distension, particularly in irritable bowel
syndrome

Cautions: ulcerative colitis, paralytic ileus, rarely
sensitivity to menthol
Side-effects: heartburn, local irritation

Colpermin® (Tillotts)
Capsules, e/c, light blue/dark blue, green band,
peppermint oil 0.2 ml. Net price 20 = £2.12.
Label: 5, 22, 25
Dose: 1–2 capsules, swallowed whole with
water, 3 times daily before meals for up to 2–3
months if necessary
Mintec® (Bridge)
Capsules, e/c, green/ivory, peppermint oil
0.2 ml. Net price 20 = £2.33. Label: 5, 22, 25
Dose: 1–2 capsules, swallowed whole with
water, 3 times daily before meals for up to 2–3
months if necessary

DOPAMINE ANTAGONIST MOTILITY STIMULANTS

Metoclopramide hydrochloride (Maxolon® etc.)
and domperidone (Motilium® etc.) stimulate gastric emptying and small intestinal transit, and
enhance the strength of oesophageal sphincter
contraction. Metoclopramide is used in some
patients with non-ulcer dyspepsia, for speeding
the transit of barium during intestinal follow-
through examination and as accessory treatment
for oesophageal reflux. Both metoclopramide and
domperidone are useful in nonspecific or cyto-
toxic-induced nausea and vomiting (see section
4.6).

Metoclopramide and, occasionally, domperidone induce extrapyramidal reactions with facial
and skeletal muscle spasms and oculogyric crises.
These are more common in the young (especially
girls and young women) and the very old, usually
occur shortly after starting treatment, and subside
within 24 hours of stopping the drug. Injection of
an anti-parkinsonian agent such as procyclidine
(see section 4.9.2) will abort attacks. Other side-
effects are rare, but gynaecomastia and galactorrhoea can occur. Dosage of both drugs should
be reduced in renal impairment and both drugs
should be avoided in the period immediately after
abdominal surgery.

DOMPERIDONE
Indications: see notes above; for use in nausea
and vomiting, see section 4.6
Cautions; Side-effects; Dose: see notes above and
section 4.6

Preparations: see section 4.6

METOCLOPRAMIDE HYDROCHLORIDE
Indications: see notes above; for use in nausea
and vomiting, see section 4.6
Cautions; Side-effects; Dose: see notes above and
section 4.6

Preparations: see section 4.6

1.2.1 Compound antispasmodic preparations

These preparations should be **avoided**, especially where they contain barbiturates. Sedatives should only be used in gastro-intestinal disease on their own individual merits.

NHS **CD Alka-Donna-P**® (Carlton)
Tablets, belladonna dry extract 8 mg, phenobarbitone 8 mg, dried aluminium hydroxide 250 mg, magnesium trisilicate 500 mg. Net price 20 = 7p
Dose: 1–2 tablets sucked before meals when required

NHS PoM **APP Stomach Tablets**® (Consolidated)
Tablets, homatropine methylbromide 1.5 mg, papaverine hydrochloride 3 mg, aluminium hydroxide mixture 15 mg, bismuth carbonate 12.5 mg, calcium carbonate 180.5 mg, magnesium carbonate 195 mg, magnesium trisilicate 92.5 mg. Net price 20 = 24p
Dose: 1–2 tablets 3–4 times daily after meals

NHS PoM **APP Stomach Powder**® (Consolidated)
Powder, homatropine methylbromide 1 mg, papaverine hydrochloride 1 mg, aluminium hydroxide mixture 30 mg, bismuth carbonate 20 mg, calcium carbonate 378 mg, magnesium carbonate 375 mg, magnesium trisilicate 195 mg/g. Net price 100 g = 84p. Label: 13
Dose: 5-ml spoonful in liquid 3–4 times daily

Emetrol® (Fisons)
Oral solution, yellow, fructose 1.87 g, glucose 1.87 g, phosphoric acid 21.5 mg/5 ml. Net price 100 ml = 72p
Dose: nausea, 15–30 ml every 15 minutes; prevention of morning sickness 15–30 ml every 3 hours; avoid fluids within 15 minutes; CHILD, nausea, 5–10 ml every 15 minutes or, to prevent regurgitation, 15 minutes before feeds

1.3 Ulcer-healing drugs

Peptic ulceration is a common condition involving the stomach, duodenum, oesophagus, and, after gastric surgery, the gastro-enterostomy stoma. Duodenal ulcers occur about four times more commonly than gastric ulcers and each type of ulcer has a distinct pathogenesis with differing complications and management problems.

Ulcer healing may be accelerated by simple measures such as bedrest and the avoidance of smoking whilst regular meals and antacids may provide symptomatic relief. Antacids are effective in healing duodenal ulcers but probably less so than antisecretory and other drugs. Originally carbenoxolone and tripotassium dicitratobismuthate were introduced and were later followed by cimetidine and ranitidine and, more recently, sucralfate and pirenzepine. The main problem with all drugs is the high rate of relapse after treatment is discontinued (slightly slower following bismuth chelate); surgery may be necessary when relapse is frequent.

H₂-RECEPTOR BLOCKING DRUGS

Cimetidine (Tagamet®) and **ranitidine** (Zantac®) heal peptic ulcers, by reducing gastric acid output, as a result of H_2-receptor blockade.

They may also relieve heartburn in peptic oesophagitis, in high doses reduce gastric acid output in the Zollinger-Ellison syndrome, and inhibit acid peptic breakdown of pancreatic enzyme supplements. Given prophylactically they reduce the frequency of bleeding from gastroduodenal erosions in patients with fulminating hepatic coma and possibly in others undergoing intensive care. Clear proof that they prevent rebleeding in haematemesis and melaena is lacking. Use of these drugs in undiagnosed dyspepsia may be justified in younger patients but is undesirable in older uninvestigated patients because the diagnosis of gastric cancer may be delayed.

Both drugs are well tolerated and symptomatic side-effects are rare. Cimetidine binds to androgen receptors, occasionally causes gynaecomastia and may, rarely, cause impotence. Cimetidine also retards the oxidative phase of hepatic drug metabolism by binding to microsomal cytochrome P450. Clinical effects due to the potentiation of drugs such as benzodiazepines and some beta-blockers are unlikely to be noticed but may be important where other drugs, such as phenytoin, warfarin, and theophylline are in use where the margin between toxic and therapeutic concentrations is small. Tubular excretion of drugs such as procainamide is retarded. Confusion which rapidly reverses on stopping treatment is also described, particularly in elderly and severely ill patients. Acute pancreatitis, thrombocytopenia and interstitial nephritis occur rarely.

Ranitidine does not have anti-androgenic effects, does not inhibit the metabolism of phenytoin, warfarin, theophyllines, or, materially, that of other drugs. Ranitidine, like cimetidine, may cause reversible confusion. Headache, constipation, and nausea have been reported occasionally. Hepatitis, anaphylactoid reactions, thrombocytopenia, and leucopenia occur rarely; agranulocytosis or pancytopenia has also rarely been reported, sometimes with marrow hypoplasia; male breast tenderness has been described.

Reports of diarrhoea, rash, and photosensitivity with either drug are of doubtful significance. Evidence that hypochlorhydria induced by H_2-receptor blockade allows nitrosamine formation in the stomach and so could predispose to gastric cancer has been contested, and no coherent evidence exists to show that any clinical hazard arises.

Maintenance treatment with 400 mg of cimetidine or 150 mg of ranitidine at night will prevent ulcer relapse, but does not seem to modify natural history once treatment has stopped.

Treatment is probably best given in courses of 4–8 weeks, with further short courses if symptoms recur. Maintenance treatment is likely to be particularly appropriate where recurrences are severe and frequent and where, because of age or concomitant disease, surgery is likely to be hazardous.

Famotidine (Pepcid PM®) and **nizatidine** (Axid®) are two newly introduced H_2-receptor blocking drugs with properties broadly the same as those of ranitidine.

CIMETIDINE

Indications: benign gastric and duodenal ulceration, stomal ulcer, reflux oesophagitis, Zollinger-Ellison syndrome, other conditions where gastric acid reduction is beneficial (see notes above and section 1.9.4)

Cautions: see notes above; renal and hepatic impairment (reduce dose). Avoid intravenous injection in high dosage (may rarely cause arrhythmias) and in cardiovascular impairment. Drug interactions: see Appendix 1 (sections 1, 2.3, 2.4, 2.6, 2.8B, 3, 4.1, 4.3, 4.7, 4.8, 5.1, 5.2, 5.4, 6.1, 8)

Side-effects: see notes above

Dose: by mouth, 400 mg twice daily (with breakfast and at night) *or* 800 mg as a single daily dose at night (benign gastric and duodenal ulceration). Doses should be taken for at least 4 weeks (6 weeks in gastric ulceration); when necessary the dose may be increased to 400 mg 4 times daily or rarely (e.g. as in stress ulceration) to a max. of 2.4 g daily in divided doses; CHILD 20–30 mg/kg daily in divided doses

Maintenance, 400 mg at night *or* 400 mg morning and night

Reflux oesophagitis, 400 mg 4 times daily for 4–8 weeks, Zollinger-Ellison syndrome, 400 mg 4 times daily or more

Gastric acid reduction (prophylaxis of acid aspiration; do not use syrup), obstetrics 400 mg at start of labour, then up to 400 mg every 4 hours if required (max. of 2.4 g daily); surgical procedures 400 mg 90–120 minutes before induction of general anaesthesia

Short-bowel syndrome, 400 mg twice daily (with breakfast and at bedtime) adjusted according to response

To reduce degradation of pancreatic enzyme supplements, 0.8–1.6 g daily in 4 divided doses according to response 1–1½ hours before meals

By intramuscular injection, 200 mg every 4–6 hours; max. 2.4 g daily

By slow intravenous injection, 200 mg given over at least 2 minutes; may be repeated every 4–6 hours; if a larger dose is needed or there is cardiovascular impairment, the dose should be diluted and given over at least 10 minutes (infusion is preferable); max. 2.4 g daily

By intravenous infusion, 400 mg in 100 ml of sodium chloride 0.9% intravenous infusion infused over ½–1 hour (may be repeated every 4–6 hours) *or* by continuous infusion at an average rate of 50–100 mg/hour over 24 hours, max. 2.4 g daily; CHILD, *by intramuscular injection or slow intravenous injection or infusion*, 20–30 mg/kg daily in divided doses

PoM **Dyspamet**® (Bridge)
Chewtab® (chewable tablets), cimetidine 200 mg. Net price 120-tab pack = £16.73. Counselling advised, chew thoroughly before swallowing
Suspension, cimetidine 200 mg/5 ml. Contains sorbitol 2.79 g/5 ml. Net price 600 ml = £21.89

PoM **Tagamet**® (SK&F)
Tablets, all green, f/c, cimetidine 200 mg, net price 120 = £17.80; 400 mg, 60-tab pack = £17.80; 800 mg, 30-tab pack = £16.91
Syrup, orange, cimetidine 200 mg/5 ml. Diluent syrup, life of diluted syrup 28 days. Net price 600 ml = £23.04
Injection, cimetidine 100 mg/ml. Net price 2-ml amp = 30p
Intravenous infusion, cimetidine 4 mg/ml in sodium chloride intravenous infusion 0.9%. Net price 100-ml infusion bag = £1.86

FAMOTIDINE

Indications: see under Dose

Cautions: see notes above; renal impairment (reduce dose)

Side-effects: rarely headache, dizziness, constipation, and diarrhoea; also reported dry mouth, nausea, vomiting, abdominal discomfort, anorexia, rash, and fatigue

Dose: benign gastric and duodenal ulceration, treatment, 40 mg at night for 4–8 weeks; maintenance, 20 mg at night
Zollinger–Ellison syndrome, 20 mg every 6 hours (higher dose in those who have previously been receiving another H_2-antagonist)

▼ PoM **Pepcid PM**® (Morson)
Tablets, famotidine 20 mg (beige), net price 28-tab pack = £14.00; 40 mg (brown), 28-tab pack = £26.60

NIZATIDINE

Indications: see under Dose

Cautions: see notes above; renal and hepatic impairment (reduce dose)

Side-effects: reported, headache, asthenia, chest pain, myalgia, abnormal dreams, somnolence, rhinitis, pharyngitis, cough, pruritus, and sweating; reversible increases in liver enzymes also reported

Dose: benign gastric and duodenal ulceration, treatment, 300 mg at night *or* 150 mg twice daily for 4–8 weeks; maintenance, 150 mg at night for up to 1 year

▼ PoM **Axid**® (Lilly)
Capsules, nizatidine 150 mg (pale yellow/dark yellow), net price 28-tab pack = £11.52; 300 mg (pale yellow/brown), 28-tab pack = £23.04

RANITIDINE

Indications: benign gastric and duodenal ulceration, stomal ulcer, reflux oesophagitis, Zollinger–Ellison syndrome, other conditions where reduction of gastric acidity is beneficial (see notes above and section 1.9.4)

Cautions: see notes above; hepatic and renal impairment (reduce dose). Drug interactions: see Appendix 1 (sections *1*, 5.2)

Side-effects: see notes above

Dose: by mouth, 150 mg twice daily (morning and night), or for patients with gastric and duodenal ulceration 300 mg as a single daily dose at night, for 4 to 8 weeks, and up to 8 weeks in reflux oesophagitis; Zollinger–Ellison syndrome,

150 mg 3 times daily increased if necessary to
6 g daily in divided doses
Maintenance, 150 mg at night
CHILD 8–18 years up to 150 mg twice daily
Gastric acid reduction (prophylaxis of acid
aspiration) in obstetrics, *by mouth*, 150 mg at
onset of labour, then every 6 hours; surgical
procedures, *by intramuscular or slow intravenous injection*, 50 mg 45–60 minutes before
induction (intravenous injection diluted to
20 ml and given over at least 2 minutes), or *by
mouth*, 150 mg 2 hours before induction, and
also, when possible on the preceding evening
By intramuscular injection, 50 mg every 6–8
hours
By slow intravenous injection, 50 mg diluted to
20 ml and given over at least 2 minutes; may be
repeated every 6–8 hours
By intravenous infusion, 25 mg/hour for 2 hours;
may be repeated every 6–8 hours

▼ PoM **Zantac**® (Glaxo)
Tablets, f/c, ranitidine 150 mg (as
hydrochloride). Net price 60-tab pack = £29.76
Dispersible tablets, f/c, scored, ranitidine 150 mg
(as hydrochloride). Net price 60-tab pack =
£31.25. Label: 13
Tablets, f/c, ranitidine 300 mg (as
hydrochloride). Net price 30-tab pack = £27.43
Syrup, sugar-free, ranitidine (as hydrochloride)
75 mg/5 ml. Net price 300 ml = £22.32
Injection, ranitidine 25 mg (as hydrochloride)/
ml. Net price 2-ml amp = 64p

SELECTIVE ANTICHOLINERGICS

Pirenzepine (Gastrozepin®) is a selective anticholinergic drug. It specifically inhibits gastric acid
and pepsin secretion and has fewer peripheral
side-effects than the drugs in section 1.2; as it
does not cross the blood-brain barrier it is unlikely
to have central effects. It is as effective as cimetidine in healing gastric and duodenal ulcers and
may also be useful in maintenance treatment.
It has also been used in conjunction with H_2
antagonists in resistant cases.

PIRENZEPINE
Indications: gastric and duodenal ulceration
Side-effects: occasionally dry mouth and visual
disturbances; agranulocytosis and thrombocytopenia have been reported
Dose: 50 mg twice daily, increased if necessary
to a max. of 150 mg daily in 3 divided doses,
for 4–6 weeks, or in resistant cases for up to 3
months. Doses should preferably be taken 30
minutes before meals

▼ PoM **Gastrozepin**® (Boots)
Tablets, scored, pirenzepine 50 mg (as hydrochloride). Net price 60 = £20.50. Label: 22

CHELATES AND COMPLEXES

Tripotassium dicitratobismuthate (De-Nol®) is

a bismuth chelate which promotes healing of gastric and duodenal ulcers. Healing may be longer
lasting but relapse still occurs. Encephalopathy
has followed the use of older bismuth preparations
and therefore, although it has not been demonstrated with this preparation, its use should be
restricted to short courses. It may act by coating
the ulcer or by stimulating bicarbonate secretion.
As the elixir, which has a pungent ammoniacal
odour, is likely to adhere to food rather than to
the surface of the ulcer, patients should be advised
to avoid food, antacids, and large quantities of
milk when taking doses. Tablets (De-Noltab®)
are as effective as the elixir and more palatable.

Sucralfate (Antepsin®) is another effective
treatment for gastric and duodenal ulcers and may
act by protecting the mucosa from acid-pepsin
attack. It is a complex of aluminium hydroxide
and sulphated sucrose but has minimal antacid
properties. Long-term use needs further assessment because some aluminium may be absorbed.

BISMUTH CHELATE
Indications: peptic ulceration
Cautions: avoid in severe renal impairment; see
also notes above
Side-effects: may darken tongue and blacken
faeces

De-Nol® (Brocades)
Liquid, red, tripotassium dicitratobismuthate
120 mg/5 ml. Net price 560 ml = £14.65. Counselling advised, see below
Dose: adults, 10 ml twice daily *or* 5 ml 4 times
daily; taken for 28 days, followed by further 28
days if necessary; maintenance not indicated
but course may be repeated after interval of 1
month; CHILDREN, no longer recommended
COUNSELLING. Each dose to be diluted with 15 ml of
water; twice daily dosage to be taken 30 minutes before
breakfast and main evening meal; four times daily
dosage to be taken as follows: one dose 30 minutes
before breakfast, midday meal and main evening meal,
and one dose 2 hours after main evening meal; milk
should not be drunk by itself during treatment but small
quantities may be taken in tea or coffee or on cereal;
antacids should not be taken half an hour before or
after a dose
De-Noltab® (Brocades)
Tablets, pink, tripotassium dicitratobismuthate
120 mg. Net price 112-tab pack = £20.98. Counselling advised, see below
Dose: adults 2 tablets twice daily *or* 1 tablet 4
times daily; taken for 28 days followed by
further 28 days if necessary; maintenance not
indicated but course may be repeated after
interval of 1 month; CHILDREN, no longer
recommended
COUNSELLING. Each dose to be swallowed with a tumblerful of water then as above under De-Nol

SUCRALFATE
Indications: gastric and duodenal ulceration;
chronic gastritis
Cautions: renal disease. Drug interactions: see
Appendix 1 (sections 1, *4.8*, *5.1*)

Side-effects: constipation; gastric discomfort reported

Dose: 2 g twice daily (on rising and at bedtime) *or* 1 g 4 times daily 1 hour before meals and at bedtime, taken for up to 6 weeks or in resistant cases 12 weeks; max. 8 g daily

COUNSELLING. Tablets may be dispersed in 10–15 ml of water; antacids should not be taken half an hour before or after a dose

▼ PoM **Antepsin**® (Wyeth)
Tablets, scored, sucralfate 1 g. Net price 20 = £2.50. Label: 5, counselling advised, see dose above

OTHER ULCER-HEALING DRUGS

Carbenoxolone (Biogastrone®, Duogastrone®), a synthetic derivative of glycyrrhizinic acid (a constituent of liquorice) is effective in gastric ulcer; it is also effective in duodenal ulcer if released at the site of the lesion. It is better suited to younger patients rather than older patients because of the nature of its side-effects, which include sodium retention and hypokalaemia and which may aggravate conditions such as oedema, hypertension, cardiac failure, and muscle weakness. For these reasons regular monitoring of weight, blood pressure, and electrolytes is advisable during treatment. Carbenoxolone may act by protecting the mucosal barrier from acid–pepsin attack and increasing mucosal mucin production. **Deglycyrrhizinised liquorice** is free from these side-effects but is of doubtful efficacy.

CARBENOXOLONE SODIUM

Indications: gastric and duodenal ulceration in young and middle-aged patients
Cautions: elderly patients, cardiac disease, hypertension, impaired hepatic and renal function. See also notes above. Potassium supplements and thiazide diuretics may be necessary. Drug interactions: see Appendix 1 (sections 1, *2.1, 2.2, 2.5, 6.3*)
Contra-indications: avoid use with spironolactone and amiloride
Side-effects: sodium and water retention leading to oedema, alkalosis, hypertension, hypokalaemia

PoM **Biogastrone**® (Winthrop)
Tablets, scored, carbenoxolone sodium 50 mg. Net price 20 = £3.96. Label: 21
Dose: for gastric ulceration, 2 tablets 3 times daily after meals for 1 week, then 1 tablet 3 times daily until the ulcer is healed (4–6 weeks)
PoM **Duogastrone**® (Winthrop)
Capsules (for duodenal release), carbenoxolone sodium 50 mg. Net price 28 = £11.13. Label: 22, 25

Dose: for duodenal ulceration, 1 capsule with liquid 4 times daily 15–30 minutes before meals for 6–12 weeks

Compound preparation
PoM **Pyrogastrone**® (Winthrop)
Tablets, chewable, carbenoxolone sodium 20 mg, alginic acid 600 mg, dried aluminium hydroxide 240 mg, magnesium trisilicate 60 mg, sodium bicarbonate 210 mg (Na^+ 2.6 mmol/tablet). Net price 20 = £4.64. Label: 21, 24
Dose: for oesophageal inflammation and ulceration, 1 tablet, chewed, 3 times daily immediately after meals, and 2 at night, for 6–12 weeks
Liquid, carbenoxolone sodium 10 mg, dried aluminium hydroxide 150 mg (Na^+ 0.85 mmol, K^+ 1.5 mmol)/5 ml when reconstituted with water for preparations. Net price 500 ml = £11.55. Label: 21
Dose: 10 ml 3 times daily after meals and 20 ml at night, for 6–12 weeks

LIQUORICE, DEGLYCYRRHIZINISED
Indications: peptic ulceration

Caved-S® (Tillotts)
Tablets, brown, deglycyrrhizinised liquorice 380 mg, aluminium hydroxide mixture 100 mg, magnesium carbonate 200 mg, sodium bicarbonate 100 mg. Net price 20 = 80p. Label: 24
Dose: 1–2 tablets chewed 3–6 times daily; CHILD over 10 years half adult dose
Rabro® (Sinclair)
Tablets, brown, deglycyrrhizinised liquorice 400 mg, calcium carbonate 500 mg, frangula 25 mg, magnesium oxide 100 mg. Net price 20 = £1.10. Label: 21, 24
Dose: 1–2 tablets chewed and swallowed with liquid 3 times daily after meals for 1–2 months

1.4 Antidiarrhoeal drugs

1.4.1 Antidiarrhoeal adsorbent mixtures
1.4.2 Antidiarrhoeal drugs which reduce motility
1.4.3 Other antidiarrhoeal preparations

The **first line** of treatment in acute diarrhoea, as in gastro-enteritis, is prevention or treatment of fluid and electrolyte depletion. This is particularly important in infants and in frail and elderly patients. Clinical signs of severe dehydration require immediate admission to hospital and urgent replacement of fluid, sodium, potassium, and chloride deficits. For details of *oral rehydration therapy* and of preparations available, see section 9.2.1.2.

Antidiarrhoeal drugs are of secondary value in the treatment of diarrhoea, may have undesirable side-effects, and may distract from giving fluids.

Antispasmodics (section 1.2) are occasionally of value in treating abdominal cramp associated with diarrhoea but they should not be used for primary treatment. Antispasmodics and anti-emetics should generally be **avoided** in young children with gastro-enteritis as they are rarely effective and have troublesome side-effects.

Antibiotics and sulphonamides are generally unnecessary in simple gastro-enteritis, even when a bacterial cause is suspected, because the complaint will usually resolve quickly without such treatment, and most infective diarrhoeas in this country are caused by viral infections. Systemic bacterial infection does, however, need appropriate systemic treatment. **Erythromycin** (see section 5.1.5) is the drug of choice for treating enteritis caused by *Campylobacter* spp. **Co-trimoxazole** (see section 5.1.8) is used to treat shigella infections with severe systemic involvement and salmonella gastro-enteritis with suspected or confirmed septicaemia and is effective in both these conditions. The general use of sulphonamides in treating diarrhoea of travellers is inadvisable because of the risks of rash and agranulocytosis.

Poorly-absorbed drugs such as dihydrostreptomycin, neomycin, and sulphaguanidine should be **avoided** altogether in gastro-intestinal infection. They prolong rather than shorten the time taken to control diarrhoea by causing masked bacterial diarrhoea, carrier states, or pseudomembranous colitis. Clioquinol should be avoided as it is neurotoxic and of doubtful efficacy and the lactobacillus preparations are probably valueless.

For treatment of diarrhoea associated with chronic disease see section 1.5; for antibacterial treatment in gastro-intestinal infections see Table 1, section 5.1; for amoebicides see section 5.4.2; for anthelmintic treatment see section 5.5.

1.4.1   Antidiarrhoeal adsorbent mixtures

Mixtures of **chalk** and **kaolin** may be effective particularly in mild chronic diarrhoea but fluid replacement is of prime importance in acute disease, especially in children (see section 9.2.1.2). **Methylcellulose** is used in diarrhoea and is also useful in controlling faecal consistency in ileostomy and colostomy.

KAOLIN, LIGHT

Indications: diarrhoea but see notes above
Cautions: drug interactions: see Appendix 1 (section *5.1*)

Kaolin Mixture (see Formulary). Net price 200 ml = 31p
Dose: 10–20 ml every 4 hours
Kaolin Mixture, Paediatric (see Formulary). Net price 100 ml = 27p
Dose: CHILD up to 1 year 5 ml, 1–5 years 10 ml every 4 hours
Kaopectate® (Upjohn)
Mixture, sugar-free, kaolin 1.03 g/5 ml. Diluent water for preparations, life of diluted mixture 14 days. Net price 100 ml = 86p

Dose: 10–30 ml every 4 hours; CHILD up to 1 year 5 ml, 1–5 years 10 ml every 4 hours but see notes above
KLN® (Ashe)
Mixture, kaolin 1.15 g, pectin 57.5 mg, sodium citrate 17.25 mg/5 ml. Net price 100 ml = 78p
Dose: CHILD 6 months–1 year 5 ml, 1–3 years 10 ml, 3–10 years 20 ml every 4 hours

CERATONIA
Indications: diarrhoea

Arobon® (Nestlé)
Powder, sugar-free, ceratonia 80%, starch 15%, cocoa 5%. Net price 150 g (with measure) = £1.49
Dose: adults and children 20–40 g, in liquid, daily; infants 2–10%, premature infants 1%, added to feeds

CHALK
Indications: diarrhoea but see notes above

Chalk Mixture, Paediatric (see Formulary). Net price 100 ml = 8p
Dose: CHILD up to 1 year 5 ml, 1–5 years 10 ml, every 4 hours (but see notes above)
Chalk Powder, Aromatic, chalk 250 mg, cardamom seed 30 mg, clove 40 mg, nutmeg 80 mg, cinnamon 100 mg, sucrose 500 mg/g. Net price 100 g = 91p. Label: 13
Dose: 0.5–5 g in water, every 4 hours

ISPAGHULA HUSK
Indications: diarrhoea (also constipation, section 1.6.1)
Side-effects: flatulence, abdominal distension
Note. For diarrhoea the dose given in section 1.6.1 should be taken with a minimum of water.

Preparations: section 1.6.1

METHYLCELLULOSE
Indications: diarrhoea (also ileostomy, colostomy control, and constipation, section 1.6.1)
Note. For diarrhoea the dose given in section 1.6.1 should be taken with a minimum of water.

Preparations: section 1.6.1

STERCULIA
Indications: diarrhoea (also ileostomy and colostomy control and constipation, section 1.6.1)
Note. For diarrhoea the dose given in section 1.6.1 should be taken with a minimum of water.

Preparations: section 1.6.1

1.4.2   Antidiarrhoeal drugs which reduce motility

Codeine, diphenoxylate (Lomotil®), **loperamide** (Imodium®), **morphine** (Kaolin and Morphine Mixture), and **opium** (Aromatic Chalk with Opium Mixture) are useful symptomatic treatment for chronic diarrhoeas, but in acute diarrhoeas fluid and electrolyte replacement are the prime requirements, especially in children (see section 1.4). In chronic diarrhoeas (section 1.5) loperamide may be preferable to the centrally acting opioids (morphine, codeine, and diphenoxylate) as it is unlikely to cause dependence.

There are few side-effects associated with these drugs but, except in the case of loperamide, excessive sedation may occur in children and in patients with chronic liver disease. They should be used with caution in colitic attacks as they may possibly increase the risk of toxic megacolon. Prolonged use could possibly aggravate irritable bowel syndrome. Drug interactions: see Appendix 1 (sections *1, 2.3, 4.1, 4.3*).

They should be used with caution in the elderly as they may induce faecal impaction, producing incontinence, spurious diarrhoea, abdominal pain, and rarely colonic obstruction. In acute gastro-enteritis, fluid and electrolyte replacement are the vital measures (see section 9.2.1.2).

CODEINE PHOSPHATE
Indications: see notes above
Cautions; Contra-indications; Side-effects: see notes above and section 4.7.2; use with caution in children (respiratory depression); tolerance and dependence may occur with prolonged use
Dose: 10–60 mg every 4–6 hours; CHILD over 4 years 1–3 mg/kg daily in divided doses

PoM **Codeine Phosphate Tablets,** codeine phosphate 15 mg, net price 20 = 38p; 30 mg, 20 = 39p; 60 mg, 20 = £1.22. Label: 2
Note. Travellers needing to take codeine phosphate tablets abroad may require a doctor's letter explaining why they are necessary.
PoM **Diarrest**® (Galen)
Liquid, yellow, codeine phosphate 5 mg, dicyclomine hydrochloride 2.5 mg, potassium chloride 40 mg, sodium chloride 50 mg, sodium citrate 50 mg/5 ml. For diarrhoea, vomiting, and cramp. Net price 100 ml = £1.67
Dose: 20 ml; CHILD 4–5 years 5 ml, 6–9 years 10 ml, 10–13 years 15 ml. Doses should be taken with water 4 times daily
Kaodene® (Boots)
Mixture, codeine phosphate 10 mg, light kaolin 3 g/10 ml. Net price 250 ml = 89p
Dose: 20 ml 3–4 times daily; CHILD over 5 years 10 ml

DIPHENOXYLATE HYDROCHLORIDE
Indications: adjunct to rehydration in acute diarrhoea (but see notes above); chronic mild ulcerative colitis
Cautions; Contra-indications; Side-effects: see notes above and under Codeine Phosphate; young children are particularly susceptible to overdosage and symptoms may be delayed so that observation is needed for at least 48 hours after ingestion; in addition the presence of subclinical doses of atropine may give rise to the side-effects of atropine in susceptible individuals or in overdosage

Dose: initially 10 mg, followed by 5 mg every 6 hours until diarrhoea is controlled; CHILD 4–8 years 2.5 mg 3 times daily, 9–12 years 2.5 mg 4 times daily, 13–16 years 5 mg 3 times daily but see notes above

PoM **Lomotil**® (Gold Cross)
Tablets, diphenoxylate hydrochloride 2.5 mg, atropine sulphate 25 micrograms. Net price 20 = £1.96
Liquid, red, sugar-free, diphenoxylate hydrochloride 2.5 mg, atropine sulphate 25 micrograms/5 ml. Diluent glycerol, life of diluted preparation 14 days. Net price 100 ml = £3.73

LOPERAMIDE HYDROCHLORIDE
Indications: acute diarrhoea in adults and children over 4 years (but see notes above); chronic diarrhoea in adults only
Side-effects: occasional rashes
Dose: acute diarrhoea, 4 mg initially followed by 2 mg after each loose stool for up to 5 days; usual dose 6–8 mg daily; max. 16 mg daily; CHILD 4–8 years 1 mg 4 times daily for up to *3 days only*, 9–12 years 2 mg 4 times daily for up to 5 days
Chronic diarrhoea in adults, initially, 4–8 mg daily in divided doses, subsequently adjusted according to response and given in 2 divided doses for maintenance

PoM[1] **Loperamide**(Non-proprietary)
Capsules, loperamide hydrochloride 2 mg. Net price 30 = £3.35
PoM[1] **Imodium**® (Janssen)
Capsules, green/grey, loperamide hydrochloride 2 mg. Net price 30 = £3.36
Syrup, red, sugar-free, loperamide hydrochloride 1 mg/5 ml. Diluent water for preparations, life of diluted preparation 14 days. Net price 100 ml = £1.90
[1]*Note.* Loperamide capsules can be sold to the public provided they are licensed and labelled for the treatment of acute diarrhoea; a proprietary brand (Arret® capsules and adult syrup) is also on sale to the public

OPIUM AND MORPHINE
Indications: see notes above
Cautions; Contra-indications; Side-effects: see notes above and under Codeine Phosphate, sedation and the risk of dependence are greater

PoM **Aromatic Chalk with Opium Mixture,** morphine 5 mg/10 ml (see Formulary). Net price 200 ml = 62p
Dose: 10–20 ml every 4 hours
Kaolin and Morphine Mixture, morphine hydrochloride 916 micrograms/10 ml (see Formulary). Net price 200 ml = 27p
Dose: 10 ml every 4 hours

1.5   Treatment of chronic diarrhoeas

Once tumours are ruled out individual complaints need specific treatment including dietary manipulation as well as drug treatment and the maintenance of a liberal fluid intake (see section 9.2). See also section 9.4.1 Foods for special diets.

IRRITABLE BOWEL SYNDROME. This can present with pain, constipation, or diarrhoea, all of which may benefit from a high-fibre diet with bran or other agents which increase stool bulk (section 1.6.1) if necessary. In some patients there may be important psychological aggravating factors which respond to reassurance. Antidiarrhoeal drugs such as **loperamide** may sometimes be necessary but prolonged use may aggravate the condition (section 1.4.2). Antispasmodics (section 1.2), may relieve the pain.

MALABSORPTION SYNDROMES. Individual conditions need specific treatment and also general nutritional consideration. Thus coeliac disease (gluten enteropathy) usually needs a gluten-free diet (section 9.4.1) and pancreatic insufficiency needs pancreatin supplements (section 1.9.4).

ULCERATIVE COLITIS. For localised rectal disease, topical treatment with **corticosteroids** such as prednisolone enemas or suppositories will induce remission; foam preparations may be a useful alternative for patients with difficulty in retaining enemas. More extensive disease is treated with corticosteroids by mouth or, if mild, with **sulphasalazine** (Salazopyrin®). Severe extensive or fulminating disease requires hospital admission and intravenous administration of a corticosteroid (usually prednisolone), with full supportive therapy. Once remission is obtained maintenance with sulphasalazine reduces relapse frequency, and in resistant cases **azathioprine** (Imuran®), in a dose of 2 mg/kg, given under close supervision may be helpful. **Mesalazine** (Asacol®) can be substituted for sulphasalazine in those sensitive to sulphonamides.

Laxatives are required to facilitate bowel movement when proctitis is present but a high-fibre diet and bulk-forming drugs such as **methylcellulose** are more useful in adjusting faecal consistency (section 1.6.1).

Symptoms of mild ulcerative colitis may be relieved with antidiarrhoeal drugs such as **codeine** or **loperamide** but they should be used with caution in severe cases as paralytic ileus and toxic megacolon may be precipitated. For similar reasons antispasmodics should **not** be used in ulcerative colitis.

CROHN'S DISEASE. Treatment particularly of colonic disease is similar to that for ulcerative colitis. In small bowel disease **sulphasalazine** is of doubtful value. **Oral corticosteroids** (e.g. prednisolone) suppress inflammation, and **metronidazole** may be beneficial possibly through antibacterial activity. Other antibacterials should be given if specifically indicated and for managing bacterial overgrowth in the small bowel.

In both colitis and Crohn's disease general nutritional care and appropriate supplements are essential.

Cholestyramine (Questran®) and **aluminium hydroxide mixture** (section 1.1.1), bind unabsorbed bile salts and provide symptomatic relief of diarrhoea following ileal disease or resection, in bacterial colonisation of the small bowel, and in post-vagotomy diarrhoea.

PSEUDOMEMBRANOUS COLITIS. This is due to colonisation of the colon with *Clostridium difficile* which may develop after antibiotic therapy. It is usually of acute onset, but may run a chronic course. Ampicillin, clindamycin, and lincomycin have been implicated most frequently but few antibiotics are free of this side-effect. Oral **vancomycin** (see section 5.1.7) or **metronidazole** (see section 5.1.11) have been advocated as specific treatment.

DIVERTICULAR DISEASE. This is treated with a high-fibre diet, **bran supplements**, and **bulk-forming laxatives**. **Antispasmodics** may provide symptomatic relief when colic is a problem (section 1.2). **Antibiotics** should be used only when the diverticula in the intestinal wall become infected. **Antidiarrhoeal** drugs which slow intestinal motility, for example codeine, diphenoxylate, and loperamide could possibly exacerbate the symptoms of diverticular disease and are therefore **contra-indicated**.

AZATHIOPRINE

Indications: maintenance of remission in resistant cases of ulcerative colitis and Crohn's disease
Cautions; Side-effects: see section 8.2.1
Dose: see notes above

Preparations
See section 8.2.1

CHOLESTYRAMINE

Indications: diarrhoea associated with Crohn's disease, ileal resection, vagotomy, diabetic vagal neuropathy, and radiation; pruritus in liver disease
Cautions; Contra-indications; Side-effects: see section 2.12
Dose: diarrhoea, 12–24 g daily mixed with water, in single or divided doses, subsequently adjusted as required; max. 36 g daily
Pruritus, 4–8 g daily mixed with water
Cholesterol reduction, as for diarrhoea, see also section 2.12
COUNSELLING. Other drugs should be taken at least 1 hour before or 4–6 hours after cholestyramine to reduce possible interference with absorption

PoM **Questran®** (Bristol-Myers)
Powder, peach, cholestyramine (anhydrous) 4 g/ sachet. Net price 10 sachets = £4.18. Label: 13, counselling advised, avoid other drugs at same time (see above)

HYDROCORTISONE

Indications: inflammation associated with colitis, proctitis

Cautions; Contra-indications; Side-effects: systemic absorption may occur, see section 6.3.3; prolonged use should be avoided; avoid use of enemas and rectal foams in obstruction, bowel perforation, and extensive fistulas; contra-indicated in untreated infection

Dose: rectal, see under Preparations

ADMINISTRATION OF RETENTION ENEMAS. They are best administered by laying patient on left side with knees drawn up and buttock elevated on small pillow; tip of applicator (if necessary lubricated with soft paraffin) is inserted into rectum; contents slowly expressed, then applicator removed, and patient instructed to roll over face downwards for 3–5 minutes; patient then sleeps in most comfortable position, retaining enema for as long as possible; in patients who have difficulty in retaining enemas, oral administration of an anticholinergic (such as propantheline bromide 30 mg) half an hour beforehand may help

PoM **Hydrocortisone Suppositories,** hydrocortisone or hydrocortisone acetate 25 mg in theobroma oil or other suitable basis. Net price 6 = £2.15

Dose: proctitis, 1 suppository inserted night and morning after a bowel movement

PoM **Colifoam**® (Stafford-Miller)

Foam in aerosol pack, hydrocortisone acetate 10%. Net price 25 g (= 14 applications) with applicator = £7.25

Dose: initially 1 metered application (125 mg hydrocortisone acetate) inserted into the rectum once or twice daily for 2–3 weeks, then once on alternate days

PoM **Cortenema**® (Bengué)

Retention enema, hydrocortisone 100 mg/60 ml in viscous suspension, in single-dose disposable packs with nozzle. Net price 7 = £4.73

Dose: initially 1 enema at bedtime for 2–3 weeks; then alternate days

PoM **Proctofoam HC**® (Stafford-Miller)

Foam in aerosol pack, hydrocortisone acetate 1%, pramoxine hydrochloride 1%. Net price 24-g pack (approx. 40 applications) with applicator = £4.83

Dose: haemorrhoids and proctitis, 1 applicatorful (4–6 mg hydrocortisone acetate, 4–6 mg pramoxine hydrochloride) by rectum 2–3 times daily and after a bowel movement

MESALAZINE

Indications: maintenance of remission in ulcerative colitis for patients intolerant of sulphasalazine

Cautions: renal impairment

Contra-indications: salicylate hypersensitivity; avoid administration with lactulose

Side-effects: nausea, diarrhoea, and abdominal pain; headache; rarely exacerbation of symptoms of colitis

Dose: 400–800 mg 3 times daily

▼ PoM **Asacol**® (SK&F)

Tablets, red, coated with an acrylic-based resin, mesalazine 400 mg. Net price 20 = £4.37. Label: 25

PREDNISOLONE

Indications: induction and maintenance of remission in ulcerative colitis, and Crohn's disease

Cautions; Contra-indications; Side-effects: see under Hydrocortisone and section 6.3.3

Dose: by mouth, initial dose 40 mg daily, in single or divided doses, until remission occurs, followed by reducing doses

By intravenous injection, for emergency treatment (under hospital supervision only), the equivalent of 20 mg of prednisolone (as prednisolone sodium phosphate) every 8 hours

By rectum, see under Preparations

Oral and parenteral preparations, see section 6.3.4

Rectal preparations

PoM **Predenema**® (Pharmax)

Retention enema, prednisolone 20 mg (as sodium metasulphobenzoate) in 100-ml single-dose disposable pack. Net price 10 (standard tube) = £7.72, 7 (long tube) = £9.26

Dose: initially 1 enema at bedtime for 2–4 weeks, extending course if good response obtained

ADMINISTRATION. See under Hydrocortisone

PoM **Predfoam**® (Pharmax)

Foam in aerosol pack, prednisolone 20 mg (as metasulphobenzoate sodium)/metered application. Net price 25 g (14 applications) with disposable applicators = £7.00

Dose: 1 metered application (20 mg prednisolone) inserted into the rectum once or twice daily for 2 weeks, continued for further 2 weeks if good response

PoM **Predsol**® (Glaxo)

Retention enema, prednisolone 20 mg (as sodium phosphate) in 100-ml single-dose disposable packs fitted with a nozzle. Net price 7 = £5.24

Dose: initially 1 enema at bedtime for 2–4 weeks, extending course if good response obtained

ADMINISTRATION. See under Hydrocortisone

Suppositories, prednisolone 5 mg (as sodium phosphate). Net price 10 = £1.00

Dose: proctitis and rectal complications of Crohn's disease, 1 suppository inserted night and morning after a bowel movement

---

SODIUM CROMOGLYCATE

Indications: food allergy (in conjunction with dietary restriction)

Side-effects: occasional nausea, rashes, and joint pain

Dose: 200 mg 4 times daily before meals; CHILD 2–14 years 100 mg; capsules may be swallowed whole or the contents dissolved in hot water and diluted with cold water before taking. May be increased if necessary after 2–3 weeks to a max. of 40 mg/kg daily and then reduced according to the response

PoM **Nalcrom**® (Fisons)
Capsules, sodium cromoglycate 100 mg. Net price 100 = £13.72. Label: 22, counselling advised, see dose above

SULPHASALAZINE

Indications: induction and maintenance of remission in ulcerative colitis and colonic Crohn's disease (for use in rheumatoid arthritis see section 10.1.3)

Cautions: maintain adequate fluid intake to prevent crystalluria; pregnancy; hepatic and renal disease; G6PD deficiency (including breast-feeding of affected infants); slow acetylator status; withdraw treatment if blood disorders or hypersensitivity reactions develop; side-effects become common with doses over 4 g daily

Contra-indications: salicylate and sulphonamide hypersensitivity; porphyria

Side-effects: nausea, vomiting, epigastric discomfort, headache, rashes; *occasionally:* fever, minor haematological abnormalities such as Heinz-body anaemia, reversible neutropenia, folate deficiency; reversible azoospermia; *rarely:* pancreatitis, hepatitis, exacerbation of colitis, thrombocytopenia, agranulocytosis, Stevens–Johnson syndrome, neurotoxicity, photosensitisation, lupus erythematosus-like syndrome, and pneumonitis; urine may be coloured orange; contact lenses may be stained

Dose: by mouth, acute attack 1–2 g 4 times daily (but see **cautions**) until remission occurs (if necessary corticosteroids may also be given), reducing to a maintenance dose of 500 mg 4 times daily; CHILD over 2 years, acute attack 40–60 mg/kg daily, maintenance dose 20–30 mg/kg daily

By rectum, in suppositories, alone or in conjunction with oral treatment 0.5–1 g morning and night after a bowel movement. As an enema, 3 g at night, retained for at least 1 hour

PoM **Salazopyrin**® (Pharmacia)
Tablets, orange-brown, scored, sulphasalazine 500 mg. Net price 20 = £1.34. Label: 14
EN-tablets® (= tablets e/c), yellow, f/c, sulphasalazine 500 mg. Net price pack of 125 = £11.94. Label: 5, 14, 25

Suspension, yellow, sulphasalazine 250 mg/5 ml. Net price 473 ml = £15.95. Label: 14
Suppositories, brown, sulphasalazine 500 mg. Net price 10 = £2.67
Retention enema, sulphasalazine 3 g in 100-ml single-dose disposable packs fitted with a nozzle. Net price 7 × 100 ml = £12.14

1.6 Laxatives

1.6.1 Bulk-forming drugs
1.6.2 Stimulant laxatives
1.6.3 Faecal softeners
1.6.4 Osmotic laxatives

Misconceptions about bowel habits have led to excessive laxative use. Abuse may lead to hypokalaemia and an atonic non-functioning colon. Simple constipation is usually relieved by increasing the intake of dietary fibre. The use of laxatives in children is undesirable and the introduction of fruit purée into the diet may be sufficient to regulate bowel action. In infants constipation is often remedied by adjustment of the diet.

Laxatives should generally be **avoided** except where straining will exacerbate a condition (such as angina) or increase the risk of rectal bleeding as in haemorrhoids. Laxatives are also of value in drug-induced constipation, for the expulsion of parasites after anthelmintic treatment, and to clear the alimentary tract before surgery and radiological procedures.

The laxatives that follow have been divided into 4 main groups (sections 1.6.1–1.6.4). This simple classification disguises the fact that some laxatives have a complex action.

1.6.1 Bulk-forming drugs

These relieve constipation by increasing faecal mass which stimulates peristalsis, but patients should be told that the full effect may take some days to develop. They are useful in the management of patients with colostomy, ileostomy, haemorrhoids, anal fissure, chronic diarrhoea associated with diverticular disease, irritable bowel syndrome, and ulcerative colitis (section 1.5). Adequate fluid intake must be maintained to avoid intestinal obstruction. Unprocessed wheat bran, taken with food or fruit juice, is a most effective bulk-forming preparation. Finely ground bran, though more palatable, has poorer water-retaining properties, but can be taken as bran bread or biscuits in appropriately increased quantities. Oat bran is also used.

Methylcellulose, **ispaghula**, and **sterculia** are useful in patients who cannot tolerate bran. Methylcellulose also acts as a faecal softener.

BRAN

Indications: see notes above

Cautions; Contra-indications; Side-effects: see under Ispaghula Husk. Calcium and iron absorption may be impaired. Avoid in gluten enteropathies and coeliac disease

Dose: 8–24 g or more daily in divided doses

NHS **Fybranta**® (Norgine)
Tablets, brown, bran 2 g. Net price 20 = 46p.
Label: 24, 27
Dose: 1–3 tablets chewed and swallowed with
water 3–4 times daily, preferably with meals

NHS **Lejfibre**® (Britannia)
Biscuits, bran (oat) 40%. Net price 25 × 10 g =
£1.95. Label: 24, 27
Dose: 2 biscuits with fluid

NHS **Proctofibe**® (Roussel)
Tablets, beige, f/c, fibrous grain extract 375 mg,
fibrous citrus extract 94 mg. Net price 20 = 56p.
Counselling advised, see dose below
Dose: adults and children over 3 years 4–12
tablets daily in divided doses chewed,
swallowed, or dispersed in water

ISPAGHULA HUSK

Indications: see notes above
Cautions: adequate fluid intake should be maintained to avoid intestinal obstruction; ulcerative
colitis
Contra-indications: intestinal obstruction,
colonic atony, faecal impaction
Side-effects: flatulence, abdominal distension
COUNSELLING. Preparations that swell in contact with
liquid should always be carefully swallowed with water
and should not be taken immediately before going to
bed

Fybogel® (R&C)
Granules, buff or orange, effervescent, sugar-
and gluten-free, ispaghula husk 3.5 g/sachet.
Net price 60 sachets (plain or orange
flavoured) = £4.24. Label: 13
Dose: 1 sachet in water twice daily preferably
after meals; CHILD ½–1 level 5-ml spoonful

Isogel® (A&H)
Granules, pink, sugar-free, ispaghula husk 90%.
Net price 200 g = 97p. Label: 13
Dose: constipation, 2 teaspoonfuls in water
once or twice daily, preferably at mealtimes;
CHILD 1 teaspoonful
Diarrhoea (section 1.4.1), 1 teaspoonful 3 times
daily

Metamucil® (Searle)
Powder, buff, ispaghula husk 49%, gluten-free.
Net price 200 g = 96p. Label: 13
Dose: one 5-ml spoonful 1–3 times daily in
150 ml water; CHILD 6–12 years 2.5–5 ml

Regulan® (Gold Cross)
Powder, beige, effervescent, ispaghula husk
3.6 g/6.4-g sachet (gluten-free). Net price 10
sachets = 71p. Label: 13
Dose: 1 sachet in 150 ml water 1–3 times daily;
CHILD 6–12 years 2.5–5 ml

METHYLCELLULOSE

Indications: see notes above
Cautions; Contra-indications; Side-effects: see
under Ispaghula Husk

Methylcellulose Granules, pink, methylcellulose '450', '2500', or '4500' 64%. Net price
100 g = £1.19. Label: see dose below
Dose: 1.5–6 g (2.5–10 ml) with water

Methylcellulose Mixture, methylcellulose '450'
900 mg/10 ml. Diluent water for preparations,
life of diluted mixture 14 days. Net price
100 ml = 57p. Label: see dose below
Dose: 5–15 ml taken with a tumblerful of water preferably after meals 3 times
daily initially, reducing to a maintenance dose of
5–15 ml daily

Celevac® (Boehringer Ingelheim)
Tablets, pink, methylcellulose '450' 500 mg. Net
price 20 = 17p. Label: see dose below
NHS *Granules*, pink, methylcellulose '450' 64%.
Net price 100 g = £1.19. Label: see dose below
Dose: 3–6 tablets (5–10 ml granules) twice
daily. In constipation the dose should be taken
with at least 300 ml of water. In diarrhoea,
ileostomy, and colostomy control, minimise
liquid intake for 30 minutes before and after
the dose. Liquid and intragastric feeding, 5 ml
granules per litre

Cellucon® (Medo)
Tablets, brown, methylcellulose '2500' 500 mg.
Net price 20 = 16p. Label: see dose below
Dose: constipation, 1–4 tablets, chewed 3 times
daily; CHILD 1–2 tablets 3–4 times daily. Doses
should be followed by a tumblerful of liquid.
Colostomy control 3 tablets chewed 2–3 times
daily, adjusted according to response; minimise
liquid intake for 30 minutes before and after
the dose

NHS **Cologel**® (Lilly)
Mixture, sugar-free, methylcellulose '450'
900 mg/10 ml. Diluent water for preparations,
life of diluted mixture 14 days. Net price
100 ml = 57p. Label: see dose below
Dose: constipation, 5–15 ml taken with a tumblerful of water preferably after meals 3 times
daily initially, reducing to a maintenance dose
of 5–15 ml daily

STERCULIA

Indications: see notes above
Cautions; Contra-indications; Side-effects: see
under Ispaghula Husk

[1]**Normacol**® (Norgine)
Granules, coated, sterculia 62%. Net price
100 g = 96p; 60 × 7-g sachets = £4.98. Label:
25, 27, see dose below
Dose: 1–2 heaped 5-ml spoonfuls, or the contents of 1–2 sachets, washed down without
chewing with plenty of liquid once or twice daily
after meals; CHILD 6–12 years half adult dose
[1]formerly Normacol Special®

Compound preparation
[2]**Normacol Plus**® (Norgine)
Granules, brown, coated, sterculia 62%, frangula (standardised) 8%. Net price 100 g = 96p;
60 × 7-g sachets = £4.98. Label: 25, 27, see
dose below

Dose: constipation and after haemorrhoidec-
tomy, 1–2 heaped 5-ml spoonfuls or the contents of 1–2 sachets washed down without
chewing with plenty of liquid once or twice daily
after meals
[2]formerly Normacol Standard

1.6.2   Stimulant laxatives

The recognised stimulant laxatives include bisacodyl and members of the anthraquinone group, e.g. senna. Docusate sodium probably acts both as a stimulant and as a softening agent. Danthron is mutagenic and should be reserved for managing opioid-induced constipation in patients with terminal illness. Powerful stimulants such as cascara and castor oil are seldom needed at all.

Stimulant laxatives increase intestinal motility and often cause abdominal cramp. They should not be used in intestinal obstruction, and prolonged use can precipitate the onset of an atonic non-functioning colon and hypokalaemia. They should preferably be avoided in children.

Glycerol suppositories act as a rectal stimulant by virtue of the mildly irritant action of glycerol.

Soft soap is a more severe irritant; the use of soft soap enema should be **avoided**, expecially in pregnancy, as it may inflame the colonic mucosa.

The **parasympathomimetics** bethanechol, distigmine, neostigmine, and pyridostigmine (see sections 7.4.1 and 10.2.1) enhance parasympathetic activity in the gut and increase intestinal motility. They are rarely used for their gastrointestinal effects but may be needed in cases of paralytic ileus, for example postoperatively. Organic obstruction of the gut must first be excluded and they should be used with caution in bowel anastomosis.

Oxyphenisatin is indicated for diagnostic procedures or surgery only, since it causes hepatitis in chronic use.

BISACODYL

Indications: see under Dose. Tablets act within 10–12 hours; suppositories act within 20 minutes to an hour

Cautions; Contra-indications; Side-effects: see general notes on stimulant laxatives; tablets may cause griping; suppositories may cause local irritation

Dose: by mouth for constipation, 10 mg at night; occasionally necessary to increase to 15–20 mg; CHILD 5 mg

By rectum in suppositories for constipation, 10 mg in the morning; CHILD 5 mg

Before radiological procedures and surgery, 10 mg by mouth at bedtime for 2 days before examination and, if necessary, a 10-mg suppository 1 hour before examination.

Oral preparations
Bisacodyl Tablets, e/c, s/c, bisacodyl 5 mg. Net price 20 = 26p. Label: 5, 25
Dulcolax® (Boehringer Ingelheim)
NHS *Tablets*, yellow, e/c, s/c, bisacodyl 5 mg. Net price 20 = 38p. Label: 5, 25

Rectal preparations
Bisacodyl Suppositories, bisacodyl 10 mg, net price 12 = 90p; 5 mg (paediatric), 12 = 63p
Dulcolax® (Boehringer Ingelheim)
NHS *Suppositories*, bisacodyl 10 mg. Net price 12 = £1.10
Paediatric suppositories, bisacodyl 5 mg. Net price 12 = 96p

CASCARA

Indications: constipation. Acts within 6–8 hours
Cautions; Contra-indications; Side-effects: see notes on stimulant laxatives, urine may be coloured red; avoid in breast-feeding

NHS **Cascara Tablets,** s/c unless otherwise indicated, 20 mg total hydroxyanthracene derivatives of which not less than 40% consists of cascarosides. Net price 20 (s/c) = 18p. Label: 14
Dose: 1–2 tablets, usually at bedtime

CASTOR OIL

Indications: constipation; bowel evacuation before radiological procedures, endoscopy, surgery. Acts within 2–8 hours
Cautions: menstruation, pregnancy. See also notes on stimulant laxatives
Contra-indications: intestinal obstruction
Side-effects: nausea, vomiting
Dose: 5–20 ml when required (best given in milk or fruit juice)
Net price 100 ml = 68p

DANTHRON

Indications: see notes above and under preparations. Acts within 6–12 hours
Cautions; Contra-indications; Side-effects: see notes on stimulant laxatives; urine may be coloured red; avoid prolonged contact with skin (as in incontinent patients) since irritation and excoriation may occur; avoid in breast-feeding; *rodent* studies indicate potential carcinogenic risk
Dose: see below

Co-danthramer preparations. These are no longer available, as the proprietary brand, Dorbanex®, has been withdrawn by the manufacturer and there is no nonproprietary version marketed.

Co-danthrusate Capsules (Danthron and Docusate Sodium Capsules). When co-danthrusate capsules are prescribed and no strength is stated capsules containing danthron 50 mg and docusate sodium 60 mg should be dispensed
NHS **Normax®** (Bencard)
Capsules, brown, danthron 50 mg, docusate sodium 60 mg. Net price 20 = 48p. Label: 14
Dose: 1–3 capsules, usually at bedtime; CHILD 6–12 years 1 capsule

Note. Indicated only for: constipation in geriatric practice; analgesic-induced constipation in terminally ill patients of all ages; constipation in cardiac failure and coronary thrombosis (conditions in which defaecation must be free of strain)

DOCUSATE SODIUM

(Dioctyl Sodium Sulphosuccinate)

Indications: constipation (acts within 1–2 days); adjunct in abdominal radiological procedures

Cautions; Contra-indications; Side-effects: see notes on stimulant laxatives

Dose: by mouth, constipation, up to 500 mg daily in divided doses; initial doses should be large and gradually reduced; CHILD 12.5–25 mg 3 times daily

With barium meal, 400 mg

By rectum, see under preparations

Dioctyl® (Medo)

Tablets, yellow, s/c, docusate sodium 100 mg. Net price 20 = 51p

Paediatric syrup, yellow, docusate sodium 12.5 mg/5 ml. Diluent syrup, life of diluted syrup 14 days. Net price 125 ml = 73p

Syrup, docusate sodium 50 mg/5 ml. Diluent as above. Net price 100 ml = 75p

Note. The paediatric syrup may be used as an enema in the following *dose*:

By rectum, ADULT 15–40 ml; CHILD up to 1 year 5–10 ml, over 1 year 7.5–15 ml. One-quarter the amount of adult syrup diluted with 3 parts of water may also be used as an enema

Fletchers' Enemette® (Pharmax)

Enema, docusate sodium 90 mg, glycerol 3.78 g, macrogol 2.25 g, sorbic acid 5 mg/5 ml. Net price 5-ml unit = 30p

Dose: adults and children over 3 years, 5 ml when required

Klyx® (Ferring)

Product discontinued

FIG

Indications: constipation

NHS **Figs Elixir, Compound** (figs syrup, compound), fig 3.2 g, cascara elixir 0.5 ml, compound rhubarb tincture 0.5 ml, senna liquid extract 1 ml/10 ml

Dose: 2.5–10 ml when required

GLYCEROL

Indications: constipation

Dose: see below

Glycerol Suppositories, gelatin 140 mg, glycerol 700 mg, purified water to 1 g. Net price 12 = 42p (infant), 47p (child), 55p (adult)

Dose: 1 suppository moistened with water before use. The usual sizes are for *infants* small (1-g mould), *children* medium (2-g mould), *adults* large (4-g mould)

OXYPHENISATIN

Indications: see under Dose

Cautions; Contra-indications; Side-effects: see notes on stimulant laxatives; avoid repeated use owing to liver toxicity

Veripaque® (Sterling Research)

Enema, powder for reconstitution, oxyphenisatin 50 mg in 3 g. Net price 1 vial = £1.65

Dose: before diagnostic procedures or surgery, oxyphenisatin 50 mg dissolved in 2 litres of water given over 5–8 minutes

Adjuvant to barium enema, oxyphenisatin 50 mg mixed thoroughly with 2 litres of barium sulphate enema

SENNA

Indications: constipation; bowel evacuation before abdominal radiological procedures, endoscopy, and surgery. Acts in 8–12 hours

Cautions; Contra-indications; Side-effects: see notes on stimulant laxatives; urine may be coloured red

Senna Tablets, ≡ total sennosides 7.5 mg. Net price 20 = 9p. Label: 14

Dose: 2–4 tablets, usually at night; initial dose should be low then gradually increased; CHILD over 6 years, half adult dose

Senokot® (R&C)

NHS *Tablets*, brown, ≡ total sennosides (calculated as sennoside B) 7.5 mg. Net price 20 = 10p. Label: 14

Dose: 2–4 tablets, usually at bedtime; initial dose should be low then gradually increased; CHILD over 6 years, half adult dose

Note. For Senokot tablets on general sale to the public the maximum recommended dose is 2 tablets.

Granules, brown, total sennosides (calculated as sennoside B) 15 mg/5 ml or 5.5 mg/g (one 5-ml spoonful = 2.7 g). Net price 100 g = 46p. Label: 14

Dose: 5–10 ml, usually at bedtime; CHILD over 6 years 2.5–5 ml

Syrup, brown, ≡ total sennosides (calculated as sennoside B) 7.5 mg/5 ml. Diluent syrup, life of diluted syrup 14 days. Net price 100 ml = 36p. Label: 14

Dose: 10–20 ml, usually at bedtime; CHILD 2–6 years 2.5–5 ml, over 6 years 5–10 ml

X-Prep® (Napp)

Liquid, brown, total sennosides 72 mg/72 ml (for bowel evacuation before radiological procedures). Net price 72-ml bottle = 47p

Dose: patients weighing 72 kg or more, 72 ml on day before procedure (in 2 divided doses between 2 and 4 p.m. with 1 hour between doses); each dose followed by 2 tumblerfuls of water and a further 2 tumberfuls drunk every hour throughout afternoon and evening; lighter patients, 1 ml/kg

Acts within 6–8 hours

SODIUM PICOSULPHATE

Indications: constipation, bowel evacuation before abdominal radiological procedures, endoscopy, and surgery
Cautions; Contra-indications; Side-effects: see notes on stimulant laxatives
Dose: see below

Sodium Picosulphate Elixir, sodium picosulphate 5 mg/5 ml. Diluent purified water, freshly boiled and cooled, life of diluted elixir 14 days. Acts within 10–14 hours. Net price 100 ml = £1.16
Dose: 5–15 ml at night; CHILD 2–5 years 2.5 ml, 5–10 years 2.5–5 ml
Note. The brand name NHS Laxoberal® (Windsor) relates to sodium picosulphate elixir 5 mg/5 ml

Picolax® (Nordic)
Oral powder, sugar-free, sodium picosulphate 10 mg/sachet, with magnesium citrate (for bowel evacuation before radiological procedures, endoscopy, and surgery). Net price 2 sachets = 59p. Label: 13, counselling advised, see below
Dose: adults and children over 9 years, 1 sachet in water in morning and a second in afternoon of day preceding procedures; CHILD 1–2 years ¼ sachet morning and afternoon, 2–4 years ½ sachet morning and afternoon, 4–9 years 1 sachet morning and ½ sachet afternoon
Acts within 3 hours of first dose
COUNSELLING. Patients should be warned that heat is generated on addition to water; for this reason the powder should be added initially to 30 ml (2 tablespoonfuls) of water; after 5 minutes (when reaction complete) the solution should be further diluted to 150 ml (about a tumblerful)

OTHER STIMULANT LAXATIVES

Unstandardised preparations of cascara, frangula, rhubarb, and senna should be **avoided** as their laxative action is unpredictable.

Aloes, colocynth, and jalap should be **avoided** as they have a drastic purgative action.

Phenolphthalein should be **avoided** as it may cause rashes. Its laxative effects may continue for several days because of enterohepatic recycling; alkaline urine may be coloured pink.

NHS **Liquid Paraffin and Phenolphthalein Mixture,** phenolphthalein 30 mg/10 ml in liquid paraffin mixture. Net price 100 ml = 22p. Label: 14
Dose: 5–20 ml, usually at bedtime

NHS **Phenolphthalein Tablets,** phenolphthalein 125 mg. Net price 20 = 60p. Label: 14
Dose: 125 mg, usually at bedtime

NHS **Rhubarb Mixture, Compound** (see Formulary). Net price 100 ml = 16p
Dose: 10–20 ml, usually at bedtime

NHS **Rhubarb and Soda Mixture, Ammoniated** (see Formulary). Net price 100 ml = 12p
Dose: 10–20 ml, usually at bedtime

NHS **Agarol®** (W-L)
Mixture, sugar-free, phenolphthalein 66 mg, liquid paraffin 1.6 ml, agar 10 mg/5 ml. Diluent water for preparations, life of diluted mixture 28 days. Net price 100 ml = 46p. Label: 14
Dose: 5–15 ml, usually at bedtime

NHS **Alophen®** (W-L)
Pills, brown, f/c, aloin 15 mg, belladonna dry extract 5 mg, ipecacuanha 4 mg, phenolphthalein 30 mg. Net price 50 pills = 99p. Label: 14
Dose: 1–3 pills, usually at bedtime

NHS **Kest®** (Berk)
Tablets, magnesium sulphate 300 mg, phenolphthalein 50 mg. Net price 50 = 46p. Label: 14
Dose: 1 tablet with water at bedtime and 2 tablets in the morning

1.6.3   Faecal softeners

Liquid paraffin, the classical lubricating agent, has disadvantages (see below). Bulk laxatives (section 1.6.1), non-ionic surfactant 'wetting' agents e.g. docusate sodium, and glycerol suppositories (both section 1.6.2) also have softening properties. Such drugs are useful in the management of haemorrhoids and anal fissure.

Enemas containing **arachis oil** lubricate and soften impacted faeces and promote a bowel movement.

ARACHIS OIL

Indications: see notes above
Dose: see below

Fletchers' Arachis Oil Retention Enema® (Pharmax)
Enema, arachis oil in 130-ml single-dose disposable packs. Net price 130 ml = £1.01
Dose: to soften impacted faeces, 130 ml; the enema should be warmed before use

LIQUID PARAFFIN

Indications: constipation
Cautions: avoid prolonged use
Side-effects: anal seepage of paraffin and consequent anal irritation after prolonged use, granulomatous reactions caused by absorption of small quantities of liquid paraffin (especially from the emulsion), lipoid pneumonia, and interference with the absorption of fat-soluble vitamins
Dose: 10–30 ml when required

Liquid Paraffin Mixture, liquid paraffin 5 ml/10 ml. Net price 100 ml = 18p
Dose: 10–30 ml when required

NHS ***Petrolagar®** (Wyeth)
Emulsion, sugar-free, liquid paraffin 7%, light liquid paraffin 18%. Net price 100 ml = 30p
Dose: 10 ml morning and night or after meals
*formerly Petrolagar No. 1®

1.6.4   Osmotic laxatives

These act by maintaining a volume of fluid in the bowel by osmosis.

Saline purgatives are commonly abused but are satisfactory for occasional use. Adequate fluid intake should be maintained. **Magnesium sulphate** is useful where rapid bowel evacuation is required; a dose taken before breakfast or on an empty stomach and followed by a tumblerful of warm fluid usually causes evacuation within 2 hours. Sodium salts should be avoided as they may give rise to sodium and water retention in

---

susceptible individuals. **Phosphate enemas** are useful in bowel clearance before radiological procedures, endoscopy, and surgery.

Lactulose is a semi-synthetic disaccharide which is not absorbed from the gastro-intestinal tract. It produces an osmotic diarrhoea of low faecal pH, and discourages the proliferation of ammonia-producing organisms. It is therefore useful in the treatment of hepatic encephalopathy.

LACTULOSE

Indications: constipation (may take up to 48 hours to act), hepatic encephalopathy
Contra-indications: galactosaemia, intestinal obstruction
Side-effects: occasional nausea and vomiting
Dose: expressed in terms of the elixir containing lactulose 3.35 g/5 ml
Constipation, initially 15 ml twice daily, gradually reduced according to patient's needs; CHILD under 1 year 2.5 ml, 1–5 years 5 ml, 6–12 years 10 ml twice daily, gradually reduced
Hepatic encephalopathy, 30–50 ml 3 times daily, subsequently adjusted to produce 2–3 soft stools daily

Lactulose Solution, lactulose 3.35 g/5 ml with other ketoses. Net price 100 ml = 77p
NHS **Duphalac**® (Duphar)
Syrup, pale yellow, lactulose 3.35 g/5 ml with other ketoses. Net price 100 ml = 77p

MAGNESIUM HYDROXIDE

Indications: mild constipation (acts within 2–4 hours)
Cautions: use only occasionally; the elderly, in renal impairment. Drug interactions: see Appendix 1 (section *15*)
Contra-indications: intestinal obstruction
Dose: see below

Liquid Paraffin and Magnesium Hydroxide Mixture, magnesium hydroxide mixture 7.35 ml, liquid paraffin 2.5 ml, chloroform spirit 0.15 ml/10 ml. Net price 100 ml = 20p
Dose: 5–20 ml when required
Magnesium Hydroxide Mixture, magnesium oxide (hydrated) about 550 mg/10 ml. Do not store in a cold place. Net price 100 ml = 17p
Dose: 25–50 ml when required

MAGNESIUM SULPHATE

Indications: rapid bowel evacuation (acts within 2–4 hours when given by mouth)
Cautions; Contra-indications: see under Magnesium Hydroxide; hepatic impairment (see Table)
Side-effects: colic
Dose: see below

Magnesium Sulphate (Epsom salts). Net price 20 g = 2p. Label: 13, 23
Dose: 5–10 g in a tumblerful of water preferably before breakfast

Magnesium Sulphate Mixture, magnesium sulphate 4 g/10 ml (see Formulary). Net price 200 ml = 17p. Label: 23
Dose: 10–20 ml, followed by a tumblerful of water, preferably before breakfast
Fletchers' Magnesium Sulphate Retention Enema® (Pharmax)
Enema, magnesium sulphate 50%, in 130-ml single-dose disposable packs. Net price 130 ml = 54p (Hosp. only)
Dose: 130 ml, as an adjunct in neurosurgery to lower cerebrospinal fluid pressure

---

PHOSPHATES (RECTAL)

Indications: rectal use in constipation; bowel evacuation before abdominal radiological procedures, endoscopy, and surgery
Cautions: see notes above
Contra-indications: acute gastro-intestinal conditions
Dose: see below

¹**Carbalax**® (Pharmax)
Suppositories, sodium acid phosphate 1.72 g in an effervescent basis. Net price 12 = £2.30
Dose: 1 suppository, inserted 30 minutes before evacuation is required; moisten with water before use; CHILD, not recommended
¹ formerly Beogex
Fletchers' Phosphate Enema® (Pharmax)
Enema, sodium acid phosphate 12.8 g, sodium phosphate 10.24 g, purified water, freshly boiled and cooled, to 128 ml (corresponds to Phosphates Enema Formula B). Net price 128 ml with standard tube = 43p, with long rectal tube = 60p
Dose: 128 ml; CHILD according to age

SODIUM CITRATE

Indications: rectal use in constipation
Cautions: see notes above
Contra-indications: acute gastro-intestinal conditions
Dose: see below

Micolette Micro-enema® (Wyeth)
Enema, sodium citrate 450 mg, sodium lauryl sulphoacetate 45 mg, glycerol 625 mg, together with citric acid, potassium sorbate, and sorbitol in a viscous solution, in 5-ml single-dose disposable packs with nozzle. Net price 5 ml = 18p
Dose: adults and children over 3 years, 5–10 ml
Micralax Micro-enema® (SK&F)
Enema, sodium citrate 450 mg, sodium alkyl-sulphoacetate 45 mg, sorbic acid 5 mg, together with glycerol and sorbitol in a viscous solution in 5-ml single-dose disposable packs with nozzle. Net price 5 ml = 30p
Dose: adults and children over 3 years, 5 ml
Relaxit Micro-enema® (Pharmacia)
Enema, sodium citrate 450 mg, sodium lauryl sulphate 75 mg, sorbic acid 5 mg, together with glycerol and sorbitol in a viscous solution in 5-

---

ml single-dose disposable packs with nozzle. Net price 5 ml = 30p

Dose: adults and children over 3 years, 5 ml

1.7   Preparations for haemorrhoids

1.7.1 Soothing preparations
1.7.2 Compound preparations with corticosteroids
1.7.3 Rectal sclerosants

Anal and perianal pruritus, soreness, and excoriation are best treated by application of bland ointments, suppositories, and dusting-powders (section 1.7.1). These conditions occur commonly in patients suffering from haemorrhoids, fistulas, and proctitis. Careful local toilet as well as adjustment of the diet to avoid hard stools, and bulk-forming materials such as bran (section 1.6.1) and a high residue diet are also helpful. In proctitis these measures may supplement treatment with corticosteroids or sulphasalazine.

When necessary topical preparations containing **local anaesthetics** (section 1.7.1) or **corticosteroids** (section 1.7.2) are used provided perianal thrush has been excluded. Perianal thrush is best treated with **nystatin** by mouth and by local application (see sections 5.2, 7.2.2, and 13.10.2).

See also sections 13.2.1 and 13.10.5 for preparations used in napkin rash.

1.7.1   Soothing preparations

Bland soothing preparations containing mild astringents such as bismuth subgallate, zinc oxide, and hamamelis may give symptomatic relief in haemorrhoids. Many proprietary preparations also contain lubricants, vasoconstrictors, or mild antiseptics.

Prolonged application of preparations containing **resorcinol** should be **avoided** because it may interfere with thyroid function. Heparinoids are claimed to promote the resorption of local oedema and extravasated blood.

Local anaesthetics are used to relieve pain associated with haemorrhoids, anal fissure, and pruritus ani but good evidence is lacking. Lignocaine gel and ointment (see section 15.2) are best applied on a plastic dilator which ensures contact with the base of the fissure. Alternative local anaesthetics include amethocaine, cinchocaine, and pramoxine, but they are more irritant.

Local anaesthetics should be used for short periods only (no longer than 2 weeks) since they may cause sensitisation of the anal skin.

ADMINISTRATION. Unless otherwise indicated a suppository is usually inserted into the rectum night and morning and after a bowel movement. Rectal ointments and creams are applied night and morning and after a bowel movement, externally or by rectum using a rectal nozzle.

Note. Local anaesthetic ointments can be absorbed through the rectal mucosa therefore excessive application should be avoided, particularly in infants and children.

Bismuth Subgallate Suppositories, Compound, bismuth subgallate 200 mg, castor oil 60 mg, resorcinol 60 mg, zinc oxide 120 mg, in theobroma oil or other suitable basis. Net price 12 = £1.35

Hamamelis Suppositories, hamamelis dry extract, usual strength 200 mg in theobroma oil or other suitable basis. Net price 12 = £1.87

Hamamelis and Zinc Oxide Suppositories. Usual strength hamamelis dry extract 200 mg, zinc oxide 600 mg. Net price 12 = £2.35

Alcos-Anal® (Norgine)
Ointment, sodium oleate 10%, laureth '9' 2%, chlorothymol 0.1%. Net price 20 g (with applicator) = £2.20
Suppositories, sodium oleate 200 mg, laureth '9' 20 mg, chlorothymol 700 micrograms. Net price 10 = £2.20

Anodesyn® (Crookes)
Ointment, ephedrine hydrochloride 0.25%, lignocaine hydrochloride 0.5%, allantoin 0.5%. Net price 25 g = 73p
Suppositories, ephedrine hydrochloride 5.1 mg, lignocaine hydrochloride 10.25 mg, allantoin 10.25 mg, bronopol 4.1 mg. Net price 12 = 87p

Anusol® (W-L)
Cream, bismuth oxide 2.14%, Peru balsam 1.8%, zinc oxide 10.75%. Net price 23 g (with rectal nozzle) = 98p
Ointment, bismuth oxide 0.875%, bismuth subgallate 2.25%, zinc oxide 10.75%, Peru balsam 1.875%. Net price 25 g (with rectal nozzle) = 94p
Suppositories, bismuth oxide 24 mg, bismuth subgallate 59 mg, Peru balsam 49 mg, zinc oxide 296 mg. Net price 12 = 90p

Bismodyne® (Loveridge)
Suppositories, bismuth subgallate 150 mg, hexachlorophane 2.5 mg, lignocaine 10 mg, zinc oxide 120 mg. Net price 12 = 98p

Lasonil® (Bayer)
Ointment, hyaluronidase 150 units, heparinoid 50 units/g. Net price 14 g = 38p; 40 g = £1.08 (both with applicator)

1.7.2   Compound preparations with corticosteroids

Corticosteroids are often combined with antibiotics, local anaesthetics, and soothing agents.

Antibiotics may do little more than encourage the growth of resistant bacteria and should be avoided. See section 1.7.1 for comment on local anaesthetics.

PoM **Anacal**® (Panpharma)
Rectal ointment, hexachlorophane 0.5%, laureth '9' 5%, heparinoid 0.2%, prednisolone 0.15%. Net price 30 g (with rectal nozzle) = £3.04
Apply 1-4 times daily
Suppositories, hexachlorophane 5 mg, laureth '9' 50 mg, a heparinoid 4 mg, prednisolone 1 mg. Net price 10 = £1.70
Insert 1 suppository once or twice daily

PoM **Anugesic-HC**® (P-D)

Cream, benzyl benzoate 1.2%, bismuth oxide 0.875%, hydrocortisone acetate 0.5%, Peru balsam 1.85%, pramoxine hydrochloride 1%, resorcinol 0.875%, zinc oxide 12.35%. Net price 25 g (with rectal nozzle) = £4.87

Apply night and morning and after a bowel movement

PoM **Anugesic-HC**® (P-D)

Suppositories, benzyl benzoate 33 mg, bismuth oxide 24 mg, bismuth subgallate 59 mg, hydrocortisone acetate 5 mg, Peru balsam 49 mg, pramoxine hydrochloride 27 mg, zinc oxide 296 mg. Net price 12 = £2.49

Insert 1 suppository night and morning and after a bowel movement

PoM **Anusol-HC**® (P-D)

Ointment, benzyl benzoate 1.25%, bismuth oxide 0.875%, bismuth subgallate 2.25%, hydrocortisone acetate 0.25%, Peru balsam 1.875%, resorcinol 0.875%, zinc oxide 10.75%. Net price 15 g (with rectal nozzle) = £2.74

Apply night and morning and after a bowel movement

Suppositories, benzyl benzoate 33 mg, bismuth oxide 24 mg, bismuth subgallate 59 mg, hydrocortisone acetate 10 mg, Peru balsam 49 mg, resorcinol 24 mg, zinc oxide 296 mg. Net price 12 = £2.49

Insert 1 suppository night and morning and after a bowel movement

PoM **Betnovate**® (Glaxo)

Rectal ointment, betamethasone valerate 0.05%, lignocaine hydrochloride 2.5%, phenylephrine hydrochloride 0.1%. Net price 25 g (with applicator) = 85p

Apply 2–3 times daily until inflammation subsides then once daily, externally or by rectum; do not use for longer than 7 days

PoM **Proctosedyl**® (Roussel)

Ointment, aesculin 1%, cinchocaine hydrochloride 0.5%, framycetin sulphate 1%, hydrocortisone 0.5%. Net price 30 g = £6.33 (with cannula)

Apply morning and night and after a bowel movement, externally or by rectum

Suppositories, aesculin 10 mg, cinchocaine hydrochloride 5 mg, framycetin sulphate 10 mg, hydrocortisone 5 mg. Net price 12 = £2.86

Insert 1 suppository night and morning and after a bowel movement

PoM **Scheriproct**® (Schering)

Ointment, cinchocaine hydrochloride 0.5%, clemizole undecenoate 1%, prednisolone hexanoate 0.19%. Net price 30 g = £4.41

Apply twice daily for 5–7 days (3–4 times daily on 1st day if necessary), then once daily for few days after symptoms have cleared

Suppositories, cinchocaine hydrochloride 1 mg, clemizole undecenoate 5 mg, prednisolone hexanoate 1.3 mg. Net price 12 = £2.08

Insert 1 suppository daily after a bowel movement, for 5–7 days (in severe cases initially 2–3 times daily)

PoM **Ultraproct**® (Schering)

Ointment, cinchocaine hydrochloride 0.5%, clemizole undecenoate 1%, fluocortolone hexanoate 0.095%, fluocortolone pivalate 0.092%. Net price 30 g (with rectal nozzle) = £4.57

Apply twice daily for 5–7 days (3–4 times daily on 1st day if necessary), then once daily for few days after symptoms have cleared

Suppositories, cinchocaine hydrochloride 1 mg, clemizole undecenoate 5 mg, fluocortolone hexanoate 630 micrograms, fluocortolone pivalate 610 micrograms. Net price 12 = £2.15

Insert 1 suppository daily after a bowel movement, for 5–7 days (in severe cases initially 2–3 times daily) then 1 suppository every other day for 1 week

PoM **Uniroid**® (Unigreg)

Ointment, cinchocaine hydrochloride 0.5%, hydrocortisone 0.5%, neomycin sulphate 3400 units, polymyxin B sulphate 6250 units/g. Net price 15 g (with applicator) = £2.52

Apply 3 times daily, preferably after a bowel movement, externally or by rectum

Suppositories, cinchocaine hydrochloride 5 mg, hydrocortisone 5 mg, neomycin sulphate 6800 units, polymyxin B sulphate 12 500 units. Net price 10 = £1.90

Insert 1 suppository 3 times daily, preferably after a bowel movement

PoM **Xyloproct**® (Astra)

Ointment (water-miscible), aluminium acetate 3.5%, hydrocortisone acetate 0.275%, lignocaine 5%, zinc oxide 18%. Net price 30 g (with applicator) = £3.48

Apply several times daily

Suppositories, aluminium acetate 50 mg, hydrocortisone acetate 5 mg, lignocaine 60 mg, zinc oxide 400 mg. Net price 10 = £1.63

Insert 1 suppository at night and after a bowel movement

1.7.3 Rectal sclerosants

Oily phenol injection is used to inject haemorrhoids particularly when unprolapsed.

PHENOL

Indications: injection of haemorrhoidal veins

Side-effects: irritation, tissue necrosis

Dose: 2–3 ml of oily phenol injection into the submucosal layer at the base of the pile; several injections may be given at different sites, max. total injected 10 ml at any one time

Oily Phenol Injection, phenol 5% in almond oil or other suitable oil. Net price 2-ml amp = 41p; 5-ml amp = 94p; 25-ml vial = £2.11

1.8 Stoma care

1.8.1 Local care of stoma
1.8.2 Prescribing for patients with stoma

1.8.1 Local care of stoma

Patients are usually given advice about the use of cleansing agents, protective creams, lotions, deodorants, or sealants whilst in hospital, either by the surgeon or by the health authority stoma care nurses. Voluntary organisations offer help and support to patients with stoma.

Items in the following list are prescribable as drugs or as accessories to stoma appliances (see Drug Tariff).

Adhesives
Aquadry® (Thackraycare)
Medical adhesive. Net price 20 ml (with brush) = £2.55

Dow Corning DC 355® (Dow Corning)
Medical adhesive brushable. Net price 20-ml bottle (with brush) = £2.55
Dow Corning Medical Adhesive B Spray® (Dow Corning)
Spray adhesive. Net price 206-g aerosol spray = £8.42
Hollister® (Abbott)
Medical adhesive spray (with silicones). Net price 170-g aerosol spray = £14.21
Latex adhesive solution (Salt)
Net price per tube = £1.25
Caution: flammable

Adhesive removers
Dow Corning Remover® (Dow Corning)
Adhesive remover spray. For removal of Medical Adhesive B Spray. Net price 227-g aerosol spray = £6.63
Hollister® (Abbott)
Adhesive remover spray. Net price 170-g aerosol spray = £14.21
Salts 'SPR' Plaster Remover® (Salt)
Adhesive remover spray. Net price 150-g aerosol spray = £1.85
Caution: flammable

Deodorants
Atmocol® is used as a deodorising spray when emptying the appliance. The other deodorants listed are placed in the appliance.

Atmocol® (Thackraycare)
Aerosol deodorant. Net price 1 unit (400 sprays) = £1.70
Chironair Odour Control Liquid® (Simcare)
Deodorant solution. Net price 113 g = £3.73
Colostomy Plus® (Shannon)
Deodorant. Net price 1 unit = £2.17
Dor® (Simpla)
Deodorant solution. Net price 7 ml = £1.16
Forest Breeze® (Shaw)
Deodorant. Net price 1 unit = £2.10
Nilodor® (Loxley)
Deodorant solution. Net price (with dropper) 7.5 ml = £1.40; 15 ml = £2.55
Ostobon® (Coloplast)
Deodorant powder. Net price 22 g = £2.31
Saltair No-Roma® (Salt)
Deodorant solution. Net price 30 ml = £1.50; 300 ml = £4.90
Stomogel® (Raymed)
Deodorant gel. Net price 50 g = £2.30
Sween® (Francol)
Deodorant. Net price 15 ml = £2.59
Translet Plus One® (Franklin)
Deodorant solution for men. Net price 7 ml = £2.07
Translet Plus Two® (Franklin)
Deodorant solution for women. Net price 7 ml = £2.07

Skin protectives, fillers, and cleansers
Bullen Karaya Gum Powder® (Bullen)
Powder. Net price 70 g = £3.28
Chiron® (Simcare)
Barrier cream (with antiseptic). Net price 52 g = £3.20
Comfeel® (Coloplast)
Barrier cream. Net price 60 g = £2.54
Downs Karaya Gel® (Simcare)
Gel. Net price 35 g = £3.94
Downs Karaya Gum Powder® (Simcare)
Powder. Net price 100 g = £4.53
Downs Ostomy Seal Protective Paste® (Simcare)
Paste. Net price 52 g = £4.47
Hollister® (Abbott)
Karaya paste. Net price 128 g = £4.44
Do not apply to severely excoriated skin

Karaya powder. Net price 71 g = £5.28
Skin gel. Net price 28 g = £3.86
Caution: flammable
Do not apply to severely excoriated skin
Orabase® (Squibb)
Paste, see section 12.3.1
Orahesive® (Squibb)
Powder (with adherent properties), see section 12.3.1
Saltair® (Salt)
Karaya gum powder. Net price per puffer pack = £3.00
Lotion. Net price 110 g = £1.50. For sore or excoriated skin
Ostomy cleansing soap (soap spirit). Net price 110-ml = £1.75
'Protect' Friar's Balsam Spray (compound benzoin tincture). Net price 150 g aerosol spray = £2.50
Simpla Sassco® (Simpla)
Gel. Net price 95 g = £4.10
Stomahesive® (Squibb)
Paste. Net price 60 g = £4.55. For filling and sealing skin creases
Stomobar® (Thackraycare)
Barrier cream. Net price 20 g = £1.60
Stomosol® (Thackraycare)
Antiseptic liquid. Dilute before use. Net price 200 ml = £3.70
Translet® (Franklin)
Barrier cream. Net price 51 g = £1.80

1.8.2   Prescribing for patients with stoma

Enteric-coated and *sustained-release* preparations are **unsuitable**, particularly in patients with ileostomies, as there may not be sufficient release of the active ingredient.

Laxatives. Enemas and washouts should **not** be prescribed for patients with ileostomies as they may cause rapid and severe dehydration.

Colostomy patients may suffer from constipation and whenever possible should be treated by increasing fluid intake or dietary fibre. **Bulk-forming laxatives** (section 1.6.1) should be tried. If they are insufficient, as small a dose as possible of senna (section 1.6.2) should be used. Preparations such as X-Prep® should be avoided when preparing patients for radiological procedures as they may cause severe dehydration with nausea, vomiting, and griping.

Antidiarrhoeals. Intestinal sedatives such as **loperamide, codeine phosphate**, or **diphenoxylate** (with atropine) are effective. Bulk-forming drugs (section 1.6.1) may be tried but it is often difficult to adjust the dose appropriately.

Antibiotics should **not** be given for an episode of acute diarrhoea.

Antacids. The tendency to diarrhoea from magnesium salts or constipation from aluminium salts may be increased in these patients.

Diuretics should be used with caution in patients with ileostomies as they may become excessively dehydrated and potassium depletion may easily occur. It is usually advisable to use a **potassium-sparing** diuretic (see section 2.2.3).

Digoxin. Patients with a stoma are particularly susceptible to hypokalaemia if on digoxin therapy and potassium supplements or a potassium-sparing diuretic may be advisable (for comment see section 9.2.1.1).

Potassium supplements. Liquid formulations are preferred to sustained-release formulations (see above).

Analgesics. Opioid analgesics (see section 4.7.2) may cause troublesome constipation in colostomy patients. When a non-opioid analgesic is required **paracetamol** is usually suitable but anti-inflammatory analgesics may cause gastric irritation and bleeding.

Iron preparations may cause loose stools and sore skin in these patients. If this is troublesome and if iron is definitely indicated one of the intramuscular iron preparations (see section 9.1.1.2) should be used. Sustained-release preparations should be **avoided** for the reasons given above.

1.9   Drugs affecting intestinal secretions

1.9.1 Drugs acting on the gall bladder
1.9.2 Drugs which increase gastric acidity
1.9.3 Aprotinin
1.9.4 Pancreatin supplements

1.9.1   Drugs acting on the gall bladder

The bile acids **chenodeoxycholic** or **ursodeoxycholic acid** are used in selected patients to dissolve cholesterol gallstones as an alternative to surgery. They are only suitable for patients who have mild symptoms, unimpaired gall bladder function, and small or medium sized radiolucent stones; they are not suitable for radio-opaque stones, which are unlikely to be dissolved. Patients should preferably be supervised in hospital because radiological monitoring is required. Long-term prophylaxis may be needed after complete dissolution of the gallstones has been confirmed (preferably with cholecystograms and ultrasound on two separate occasions) as gallstones may recur in up to 25% of patients within one year of stopping treatment.

Dehydrocholic acid is used to improve biliary drainage by stimulating the secretion of thin watery bile. It is given after surgery of the biliary tract to flush the common duct and drainage tube and wash away small calculi obstructing flow through the common bile duct but its value has not been established.

A **terpene** mixture (Rowachol®) also raises biliary cholesterol solubility. It is less effective than the bile acids but may be a useful adjunct.

CHENODEOXYCHOLIC ACID

Indications: dissolution of cholesterol gallstones (see notes above)
Cautions: see notes above
Contra-indications: do not use when stones are radio-opaque, in pregnancy, in non-functioning gall bladders, in chronic liver disease, and inflammatory diseases of the small intestine and colon
Side-effects: diarrhoea particularly initially with high dosage (reduce dose for few days), pruritus, minor hepatic abnormalities and transient rise in serum transaminases
Dose: 10–15 mg/kg daily as a single dose at bedtime *or* in divided doses for 3–24 months, depending on size of stone; treatment is continued for 3 months after stones dissolve

PoM **Chendol**® (CP)
Capsules, orange/white, chenodeoxycholic acid 125 mg. Net price 20 = £3.36
Tablets, orange, f/c, scored, chenodeoxycholic acid 250 mg. Net price 20 = £7.41
PoM **Chenofalk**® (Thames)
Capsules, chenodeoxycholic acid 250 mg. Net price 60 = £16.00

DEHYDROCHOLIC ACID

Indications: see notes above
Contra-indications: complete mechanical biliary obstruction and occlusive hepatitis, chronic liver disease
Dose: 250–750 mg, 3 times daily
Cholecystography, 500–750 mg every 4 hours for 12 hours before and after the examination

Dehydrocholic Acid (Non-proprietary)
Tablets, dehydrocholic acid 250 mg. Net price 20 = £4.16

URSODEOXYCHOLIC ACID

Indications; Cautions; Contra-indications: see under Chenodeoxycholic Acid
Side-effects: see under Chenodeoxycholic Acid; diarrhoea occurs rarely; liver changes have not been reported
Dose: 8–12 mg/kg (obese patients up to 15 mg/kg) daily as a single dose at bedtime or in divided doses, for up to 2 years; treatment is continued for 3–4 months after stones dissolve

PoM **Destolit**® (Merrell)
Tablets, scored, ursodeoxycholic acid 150 mg. Net price 60 = £19.40. Label: 21
▼ PoM **Ursofalk**® (Thames)
Capsules, ursodeoxycholic acid 250 mg. Net price 60 = £28.00. Label: 21

OTHER PREPARATIONS FOR BILIARY DISORDERS

Rowachol® (Tillotts)
PoM *Capsules,* green, e/c, borneol 5 mg, camphene 5 mg, cineole 2 mg, menthol 32 mg, menthone 6 mg, pinene 17 mg in olive oil. Net price 20 = £2.18. Label: 22
Dose: 1–2 capsules 3 times daily before food
Liquid, yellow, borneol 50 mg, camphene 50 mg, cineole 20 mg, menthol 320 mg, menthone 60 mg, pinene 170 mg/g in olive oil. Net price 10-ml dropper bottle = £5.70. Label: 22
Dose: 3–5 drops 4–5 times daily before food
Drug interactions: see Appendix 1 (section *2.8C*)

1.9.2   Drugs which increase gastric acidity

Muripsin® is used in achlorhydria and hypochlorhydria but is of uncertain value; it replaced dilute hydrochloric acid.

Muripsin® (Norgine)
Tablets, orange, f/c, glutamic acid hydrochloride 500 mg, pepsin 35 mg: 1 tablet ≈ 1 ml dilute hydrochloric acid. Net price 50 = £3.04. Label: 21
Dose: 1–2 tablets with meals

1.9.3   Aprotinin

Aprotinin is a proteolytic enzyme inhibitor used in the treatment of acute pancreatitis. Its value has not been substantiated.

APROTININ

Indications: prevention of pancreatitis after abdominal surgery; acute pancreatitis; disseminated intravascular coagulation
Side-effects: occasional hypersensitivity reactions
Dose: therapeutic, *by slow intravenous injection*, 500 000 kallidinogenase (kallikrein) inactivator units, then 200 000 units *by intravenous infusion* every 4 hours. In disseminated intravascular coagulation dosage may be increased to 1 000 000 units
Prophylactic, *by slow intravenous injection*, 200 000 kallidinogenase (kallikrein) inactivator units pre-operatively, repeated postoperatively every 4 hours by slow intravenous injection or continuous infusion for 2 days

PoM **Trasylol**® (Bayer)
Injection, aprotinin 20 000 kallidinogenase (kallikrein) inactivator units/ml. Net price 5-ml amp = £3.42; 10-ml amp = £6.50

1.9.4   Pancreatin

Supplements of pancreatin are given by mouth to compensate for reduced or absent exocrine secretion in cystic fibrosis, and following pancreatectomy, total gastrectomy, or chronic pancreatitis. They assist the digestion of starch, fat, and protein.

Pancreatin is inactivated by gastric acid therefore pancreatin preparations are best taken with food (or immediately before or after food). Gastric acid secretion may be reduced by giving cimetidine or ranitidine an hour beforehand (section 1.3). Concurrent use of antacids also reduces gastric acidity but may dissolve enteric coatings.

Since pancreatin is also inactivated by heat, excessive heat should be avoided if preparations are mixed with liquids or food; the resulting mixtures should not be kept for more than one hour.

Dosage is adjusted according to size, number, and consistency of stools, so that the patient thrives; extra allowance may be needed if snacks are taken between meals.

Pancreatin may irritate the skin around mouth and anus, particularly if preparations are retained in the mouth or dosage is excessive. Hypersensitivity reactions occur occasionally and may affect those handling the powder.

For reference to acetylcysteine in cystic fibrosis, see Acetylcysteine Granules (section 3.7).

PANCREATIN

Indications; Cautions; Side-effects: see above
Dose: see below

Pancreatin, BP (Non-proprietary)
Powder, pancreatin, providing minimum of: protease 1400 units, lipase 20000 units, amylase 24000 units/g

Cotazym® (Organon)
Capsules, green, pancreatin, providing minimum of: protease 450 units, lipase 13000 units, amylase 9000 units. Net price 100 = £3.33. Counselling advised, see dose
Dose: 6 capsules daily in divided doses; contents sprinkled on food

Creon® (Duphar)
Capsules, brown/yellow, enclosing buff-coloured e/c granules of pancreatin, providing: protease 210 units, lipase 8000 units, amylase 9000 units. Net price 100 = £13.33. Counselling advised, see dose
Dose: 5–15 capsules daily in divided doses with meals either taken whole or contents mixed with fluid or soft food (then swallowed immediately without chewing)

Nutrizym® (Merck)
Replaced by **Nutrizym GR** (see p. xii)

Pancrease® (Ortho-Cilag)
Capsules, enclosing e/c beads of pancreatin, providing minimum of: protease 330 units, lipase 5000 units, amylase 2900 units. Net price 100 = £15.98. Counselling advised, see dose
Dose: 1–2 (occasionally 3) capsules during each meal and 1 capsule with snacks swallowed whole or contents sprinkled on liquid or soft food (then swallowed immediately without chewing)

Pancrex® (Paines & Byrne)
Granules, pancreatin, providing minimum of: protease 300 units, lipase 5000 units, amylase 4000 units/g. Net price 100 g = £4.79, 500 g = £19.16. Label: 25, counselling advised, see dose
Dose: 5–10 g 4 times daily with meals washed down or mixed with liquid

Pancrex V® (Paines & Byrne)
Capsules, pancreatin, providing minimum of: protease 430 units, lipase 8000 units, amylase 9000 units. Net price 100 = £3.71. Counselling advised, see dose
Dose: up to 1 year 1–2 capsules mixed with feeds; adults and children over 1 year 2–6 capsules 4 times daily with meals, swallowed whole or sprinkled on food

Capsules '125', pancreatin, providing minimum of: protease 160 units, lipase 2950 units, amylase 3000 units. Net price 50 = £1.10. Counselling advised, see dose
Dose: NEONATE 1–2 capsules with feeds

Tablets, e/c, s/c, pancreatin, providing minimum of: protease 110 units, lipase 1900 units, amylase 1700 units. Net price 100 = £1.79. Label: 5, 25, counselling advised, see dose
Dose: 5–15 tablets 4 times daily before meals

Tablets forte, e/c, s/c, pancreatin, providing minimum of: protease 330 units, lipase 5600 units, amylase 5000 units. Net price 100 = £3.23. Label: 5, 25, counselling advised, see dose
Dose: 6–10 tablets 4 times daily before meals

Powder, pancreatin, providing minimum of: protease 1400 units, lipase 25000 units, amylase 30000 units/g. Net price 100 g = £6.53, 250 g = £13.90. Counselling advised, see dose
Dose: 0.5–2 g 4 times daily washed down or mixed with liquid

2: Drugs used in the treatment of diseases of the
CARDIOVASCULAR SYSTEM

In this chapter, drug treatment is discussed under the following headings:

2.1   Cardiac glycosides

Cardiac glycosides are most useful in the treatment of *supraventricular tachycardias*, especially for controlling ventricular response in atrial fibrillation. *Heart failure* may also be improved, even in patients in sinus rhythm, because of changes in the availability of intracellular calcium; this action is relatively unimportant, however, compared with effects that can be achieved with diuretics and vasodilators. Except when needed to maintain satisfactory rhythm, cardiac glycosides can often be withdrawn from patients with heart failure that is well controlled, without clinical deterioration. Their use for heart failure alone is therefore best avoided in the elderly who are particularly susceptible to digitalis toxicity.

Loss of appetite, nausea, and vomiting are common toxic effects. Sinus bradycardia, atrioventricular block, ventricular extrasystoles, and sometimes ventricular tachycardia or atrial tachycardia with block also occur—especially in the presence of underlying conducting system defects or myocardial disease. These unwanted effects depend both on the plasma concentrations of the drugs and on the sensitivity of the conducting system or myocardium, which is often increased in patients with heart disease. Thus, no one plasma concentration can indicate toxicity reliably but the likelihood increases progressively through the range 1.5 to 3 micrograms/litre. Higher steady-state concentrations must certainly be avoided. Measurements of plasma concentration are not necessary, however, unless problems occur during maintenance treatment. Hypokalaemia predisposes to toxicity.

Renal function is the most important determinant of digoxin dosage, whereas elimination of digitoxin depends on metabolism by the liver. Manifestations of toxicity can often be managed by discontinuing therapy and correcting hypokalaemia if appropriate. Serious manifestations require urgent specialist management. Digoxin-specific antibody fragments are now available for the reversal of life-threatening overdosage (see overleaf).

Digoxin (Lanoxin® etc.) is the glycoside most commonly used. In patients with mild failure a loading dose is not required, and a satisfactory plasma concentration can be achieved over a period of about a week, using a dose of 125 to 250 micrograms twice a day which may then be reduced having special regard to renal function. For management of atrial fibrillation, the most common indication, the maintenance dose can usually be governed by ventricular response which should not be allowed to fall below 60 beats per minute except in special and recognised circumstances e.g. with the concomitant administration of beta-blockers.

When very rapid control is needed, digoxin may be given intravenously in a digitalising dose of 0.75 to 1 mg, preferably as an infusion (suggested volume 50 ml) over two or more hours, followed by normal maintenance therapy. The intramuscular route is not recommended, except when other methods of administration are not available.

Lanatoside C (Cedilanid®) is less well absorbed than digoxin. Most is converted to digoxin after ingestion. The maintenance dose is about twice that of digoxin, and depends in part on renal function.

Digitoxin has a long half-life and consequently maintenance doses need only be given once daily.

CHILDREN. The dose is based on body-weight; they require a relatively larger dose of digoxin than adults.

DIGOXIN

Indications: heart failure, supraventricular arrhythmias (particularly atrial fibrillation)

Cautions: recent infarction, hypothyroidism; reduce dose in the elderly and in renal impairment; avoid hypokalaemia. Drug interactions: see Appendix 1 (sections 2.1, *15*)

Contra-indications: supraventricular arrhythmias caused by Wolff-Parkinson-White syndrome

Side-effects: anorexia, nausea, vomiting, visual disturbances, arrhythmias, heart block

Dose: by mouth, rapid digitalisation, 1–1.5 mg in divided doses over 24 hours; less urgent digitalisation and maintenance, 125–250 micrograms twice daily; elderly 125 micrograms daily

For intravenous doses, see notes above

PoM **Digoxin** (Non-proprietary)
Tablets, digoxin 62.5 micrograms, net price 20 = 8p; 125 micrograms, 20 = 6p; 250 micrograms, 20 = 8p

PoM **Digoxin Injection, Paediatric** (Boots)
Paediatric injection, digoxin 100 micrograms/ml. (Hosp. only)

PoM **Lanoxin**® (Wellcome)
Tablets, digoxin 125 micrograms, net price 20 = 22p; 250 micrograms, 20 = 20p
Injection, digoxin 250 micrograms/ml. Net price 2-ml amp = 45p

PoM **Lanoxin-PG**® (Wellcome)
Tablets, blue, digoxin 62.5 micrograms. Net price 20 = 22p
Elixir, yellow, digoxin 50 micrograms/ml. Do not dilute, measure with pipette. Net price 60 ml = £3.62. Counselling advised, use of pipette

DIGITOXIN

Indications: heart failure, supraventricular arrhythmias (particularly atrial fibrillation)
Cautions; Side-effects: see under Digoxin
Dose: 50–200 micrograms daily

PoM **Digitoxin** (Non-proprietary)
Tablets, digitoxin 100 micrograms, net price 20 = 28p

LANATOSIDE C

Indications: heart failure, supraventricular arrhythmias (particularly atrial fibrillation)
Cautions; Side-effects: see under Digoxin
Dose: slow digitalisation 1.5–2 mg daily for 3–5 days; maintenance 0.25–1 mg daily

PoM **Cedilanid**® (Sandoz)
Tablets, scored, lanatoside C 250 micrograms. Net price 20 = 30p

DIGOXIN-SPECIFIC ANTIBODY

▼ PoM **Digibind**® (Wellcome)
Injection, powder for preparation of an infusion, digoxin-specific antibody fragments (F(ab)) 40 mg. Net price per vial = £87.44
For reversal of life-threatening manifestations of intoxication by digoxin; although designed specifically to treat digoxin overdose has successfully reversed digitoxin overdose

2.2   Diuretics

2.2.1 Thiazides and related diuretics
2.2.2 Loop diuretics
2.2.3 Potassium-sparing diuretics
2.2.4 Potassium-sparing diuretics with other diuretics
2.2.5 Osmotic diuretics
2.2.6 Mercurial diuretics
2.2.7 Carbonic anhydrase inhibitors
2.2.8 Diuretics with potassium

Thiazides (section 2.2.1) are used to relieve oedema due to heart failure, a condition characterised by reduced glomerular filtration, increased reabsorption of sodium from the renal tubules, and an increased production of aldosterone contributing to fluid retention. They are also used in lower doses to reduce blood pressure.

The more potent **'loop' diuretics** such as frusemide or bumetanide (section 2.2.2) are used in patients with pulmonary oedema due to left ventricular failure and in patients with long-standing heart failure who no longer respond to the thiazides.

Diuretics are usually administered early in the day so that the diuresis does not interfere with sleep.

In patients with oedema resistant to treatment with one diuretic, combination treatment may be effective. For example, a loop diuretic may be combined with a potassium-sparing diuretic (section 2.2.3).

POTASSIUM LOSS. Hypokalaemia may occur with both thiazide and loop diuretics. Often the use of potassium-sparing diuretics (section 2.2.3) avoids the need to take potassium supplements. Intermittent diuretic therapy is less likely to induce hypokalaemia than daily treatment.

The combination of a thiazide with spironolactone is of value in less severe heart failure when hypokalaemia is difficult to counter or when any degree of hypokalaemia should be avoided, as in patients with a continuing tendency to life-threatening ventricular arrhythmias.

In hepatic failure hypokalaemia caused by diuretics can precipitate encephalopathy. Diuretics may also increase the risk of hypomagnesaemia in alcoholic cirrhosis.

Potassium supplements (see section 9.2.1.1) are seldom necessary when thiazides are used in routine treatment of hypertension (section 2.5). For further comment see section 9.2.1.1.

2.2.1   Thiazides and related diuretics

Thiazides and related compounds act at the beginning of the distal convoluted tubule and are moderately potent diuretics. Side-effects include impotence, hypokalaemia, hypochloraemic alkalosis, hyperuricaemia, hyperglycaemia, and increases in plasma cholesterol concentration. Hypokalaemia is dangerous in severe coronary artery disease and in patients being treated with cardiac glycosides. Less common side-effects include rashes and thrombocytopenia, and when given in late pregnancy thiazides have been reported to cause neonatal thrombocytopenia.

All thiazides are active by mouth with an onset of action within 1 to 2 hours and duration of 12 to 24 hours.

Small doses of thiazides are used long-term to control hypertension (section 2.5)—alone in mild hypertension, and with other drugs in more severe hypertension. They act in part by reducing peripheral vascular resistance. Increasing the dose has little additional antihypertensive effect, yet augments the long-term effects on glucose tolerance and plasma lipids, which are cause for concern. Optimum doses for the control of heart failure may be larger, and long-term effects are of less importance.

Bendrofluazide is an appropriate drug for mild or moderate cardiac failure when the patient is not desperately ill and severe pulmonary oedema is not present. This drug is also effective either alone in the treatment of mild hypertension or with other drugs in more severe hypertension.

Chlorthalidone (Hygroton®), a thiazide-related compound, has a longer duration of action than the thiazides and may be given on alternate days to control hypertension. It is also useful if acute retention may be precipitated by a more rapid diuresis or if patients dislike the altered pattern of micturition promoted by diuretics.

Other thiazides do not offer any significant advantage over those mentioned.

NEWER COMPOUNDS. **Xipamide** (Diurexan®) resembles chlorthalidone structurally, and is more potent than the other thiazides. **Indapamide** (Natrilix®) is chemically related to chlorthalidone. It is claimed to lower blood pressure with less metabolic disturbance, particularly less aggravation of diabetes mellitus. The advantages of these newer agents over longer-established thiazides need further evaluation.

BENDROFLUAZIDE

Indications: oedema, hypertension
Cautions: may cause hypokalaemia, aggravates diabetes and gout; pregnancy; renal and hepatic impairment; see also notes above. Drug interactions: see Appendix 1 (sections *2.1, 2.2, 2.2, 2.3, 2.4, 2.5, 2.6, 4.2, 4.7, 6.1, 6.3, 9*)
Contra-indications: hypercalcaemia, renal failure, Addison's disease
Side-effects: gout, rashes and photosensitivity, thrombocytopenia; impotence (reversible on withdrawal of treatment); see also notes above
Dose: oedema, initially 5–10 mg in the morning daily *or* on alternate days; maintenance 2.5–10 mg 1–3 times weekly
Hypertension, 2.5–5 mg in the morning

PoM **Bendrofluazide** (Non-proprietary)
Tablets, bendrofluazide 2.5 mg, net price 20 = 10p; 5 mg, 20 = 5p
PoM **Aprinox**® (Boots)
Tablets, bendrofluazide 2.5 mg, net price 20 = 8p; 5 mg, 20 = 13p
PoM **Berkozide**® (Berk)
Tablets, bendrofluazide 2.5 mg, net price 20 = 8p; 5 mg (scored), 20 = 11p
PoM **Centyl**® (Leo)
Tablets, bendrofluazide 2.5 mg, net price 20 = 39p; 5 mg (scored), 20 = 57p
PoM **Neo-NaClex**® (DF)
Tablets, scored, bendrofluazide 5 mg, net price 20 = 20p

CHLOROTHIAZIDE

Indications: oedema, hypertension
Cautions; Contra-indications; Side-effects: see under Bendrofluazide
Dose: oedema, initially 0.5–1 g 1–2 times daily; maintenance 0.5–1 g daily, on alternate days, or less frequently
Hypertension, 0.5–1 g daily in single or divided doses

PoM **Saluric**® (MSD)
Tablets, scored, chlorothiazide 500 mg. Net price 20 = 38p

CHLORTHALIDONE

Indications: oedema, hypertension, diabetes insipidus (see section 6.5.2)
Cautions; Contra-indications; Side-effects: see under Bendrofluazide
Dose: oedema, initially 50 mg in the morning *or* 100–200 mg on alternate days, reduced for maintenance if possible
Hypertension, 25 mg, increased to 50 mg if necessary, in the morning

PoM **Hygroton**® (Geigy)
Tablets, both scored, chlorthalidone 50 mg (yellow), net price 20 = 68p; 100 mg, 20 = £1.32

CLOPAMIDE

Cautions; Contra-indications; Side-effects: see under Bendrofluazide

Preparation
Ingredient of Viskaldix® (section 2.4)

CYCLOPENTHIAZIDE

Indications: oedema, hypertension
Cautions; Contra-indications; Side-effects: see under Bendrofluazide
Dose: oedema, initially 0.5–1 mg in the morning; maintenance 500 micrograms on alternate days
Hypertension, 250–500 micrograms in the morning
Max. 1.5 mg daily

PoM **Navidrex**® (Ciba)
Tablets, scored, cyclopenthiazide 500 micrograms. Net price 20 = 35p

HYDROCHLOROTHIAZIDE

Indications: oedema, hypertension
Cautions; Contra-indications; Side-effects: see under Bendrofluazide
Dose: oedema, initially 50–100 mg daily; maintenance 25–50 mg on alternate days
Hypertension, 25 mg daily, can be increased to 50–100 mg daily if necessary

PoM **Esidrex**® (Ciba)
Tablets, both scored, hydrochlorothiazide 25 mg, net price 20 = 57p; 50 mg, 20 = £1.05
PoM **HydroSaluric**® (MSD)
Tablets, both scored, hydrochlorothiazide 25 mg, net price 20 = 29p; 50 mg, 20 = 54p

HYDROFLUMETHIAZIDE

Indications: oedema, hypertension
Cautions; Contra-indications; Side-effects: see under Bendrofluazide
Dose: oedema, initially 50–200 mg in the morning; maintenance 25–50 mg on alternate days
Hypertension, 25–50 mg daily

PoM **Hydrenox**® (Boots)
Tablets, hydroflumethiazide 50 mg. Net price
20 = 32p

INDAPAMIDE
Indications: hypertension
Cautions: severe hepatic or renal impairment.
Drug interactions: see Appendix 1 (section 2.2)
Side-effects: nausea, headache, slight weight loss;
diuresis with doses above 2.5 mg daily
Dose: 2.5 mg in the morning

PoM **Natrilix**® (Servier)
Tablets, pink, s/c, indapamide 2.5 mg. Net price
60 = £11.72

MEFRUSIDE
Indications: oedema, hypertension
Cautions; Contra-indications; Side-effects: see
under Bendrofluazide
Dose: initially 25–50 mg in the morning,
increased to 75–100 mg for oedema; maintenance 25 mg daily *or* on alternate days

PoM **Baycaron**® (Bayer)
Tablets, scored, mefruside 25 mg. Net price 20 =
£1.41

METHYCLOTHIAZIDE
Indications: oedema, hypertension
Cautions; Contra-indications; Side-effects: see
under Bendrofluazide
Dose: 2.5–5 mg in the morning, increased to
10 mg daily if required

PoM **Enduron**® (Abbott)
Tablets, pink, scored, methyclothiazide 5 mg.
Net price 20 = 41p

METOLAZONE
Indications: oedema, hypertension
Cautions; Contra-indications; Side-effects: see
under Bendrofluazide; also profound diuresis
on concomitant administration with frusemide
(monitor patient carefully)
Dose: oedema, 5–10 mg in the morning,
increased if necessary; max. 80 mg daily
Hypertension, initially 5 mg in the morning;
maintenance 5 mg on alternate days

PoM **Metenix 5**® (Hoechst)
Tablets, blue, metolazone 5 mg. Net price 20 =
£1.75

POLYTHIAZIDE
Indications: oedema, hypertension
Cautions; Contra-indications; Side-effects: see
under Bendrofluazide
Dose: usually 1–4 mg daily; in hypertension 500
micrograms daily may be adequate

PoM **Nephril**® (Pfizer)
Tablets, scored, polythiazide 1 mg. Net price
20 = 55p

XIPAMIDE
Indications: oedema, hypertension
Cautions; Contra-indications: see under Bendrofluazide. Drug interactions: see Appendix 1
(section 2.2)
Side-effects: slight gastro-intestinal disturbances;
mild dizziness
Dose: oedema, initially 40 mg in the morning,
increased to 80 mg in resistant cases; maintenance 20 mg in the morning
Hypertension, usual dose 20 mg in the morning
(may be increased to 40 mg if necessary, but not
if other antihypertensive therapy being given)

PoM **Diurexan**® (Degussa)
Tablets, scored, xipamide 20 mg. Net price 20 =
£1.95

2.2.2   Loop diuretics
These drugs inhibit resorption from the ascending
loop of Henle in the renal tubule and are powerful
diuretics. Hypokalaemia frequently develops, and
care is needed to avoid hypotension. If there is
an enlarged prostate, urinary retention may
occur; this is less likely if small doses and less
potent diuretics are used initially.

Frusemide and **bumetanide** have similar
activity. Oral administration is effective within 1
hour and diuresis is complete within 6 hours, so
that the drugs can be given twice daily without
interfering with sleep. Given intravenously they
act rapidly, the peak effect occurring within 30
minutes. The diuresis is related to the size of dose,
and in patients with impaired renal function very
large doses may occasionally have to be given. In
such doses both drugs can cause deafness and
bumetanide can cause myalgia.

Ethacrynic acid has a similar onset and duration
of action. Gastro-intestinal side-effects are more
severe and deafness may occur in patients with
renal failure, especially when it is given
intravenously.

Piretanide is the newest member of this group;
it has properties similar to those of frusemide and
bumetanide, but is promoted for the treatment of
hypertension.

FRUSEMIDE
Indications: oedema, oliguria due to renal failure
Cautions: pregnancy; may cause hypokalaemia
and hyponatraemia; aggravates diabetes and
gout; liver failure, prostatism. Drug
interactions: see Appendix 1 (sections *2.1, 2.2,
2.2, 2.3, 2.4, 2.5, 2.6, 4.2, 4.7, 5.1, 6.1, 6.3*)
Contra-indications: precomatose states associated with liver cirrhosis
Side-effects: rashes; tinnitus and deafness in
impaired renal function
Dose: by mouth, oedema, initially 40 mg in the
morning; maintenance 20 mg daily *or* 40 mg on
alternate days, increased in resistant oedema to
80 mg daily; CHILD 1–3 mg/kg daily
Oliguria, initially 250 mg daily; if necessary
larger doses, increasing in steps of 250 mg, may

---

be given every 4–6 hours to a max. of a single dose of 2 g

By intramuscular or slow intravenous injection, initially 20–50 mg; CHILD 0.5–1.5 mg/kg

By intravenous infusion, in oliguria, 0.25–1 g at a rate not exceeding 4 mg/minute

PoM **Frusemide** (Non-proprietary)

Tablets, frusemide 20 mg, net price 20 = 16p; 40 mg, 20 = 8p; 500 mg, 20 = £6.00

Injection: frusemide 10 mg/ml, net price 2-ml amp = 17p; 5-ml amp = 45p

PoM **Aluzine**® (Steinhard)

Tablets, all scored, frusemide 20 mg, net price 20 = 58p; 40 mg, 20 = 90p; 500 mg (yellow), 20 = £9.51

PoM **Diuresal**® (Lagap)

Injection, frusemide 10 mg/ml. Net price 2-ml amp = 21p; 5-ml amp = 49p

PoM **Dryptal**® (Berk)

Tablets, scored, frusemide 40 mg, net price 20 = 37p; 500 mg (yellow), 20 = £9.74

Injection, frusemide 10 mg/ml. Net price 2-ml amp = 23p; 5-ml amp = 45p; 25-ml amp = £2.25 (Hosp. only)

PoM **Frusetic**® (Unimed)

Tablets, scored, frusemide 40 mg. Net price 20 = 51p

PoM **Frusid**® (DDSA)

Tablets, scored, frusemide 40 mg. Net price 20 = 35p

PoM **Lasix**® (Hoechst)

Tablets, all scored, frusemide 20 mg, net price 28-tab pack = 99p; 40 mg, 20 = 93p; 500 mg (yellow), 20 = £11.74

Paediatric liquid, sugar-free, frusemide 1 mg/ml when reconstituted with purified water, freshly boiled and cooled, net price 150 ml = £1.13

Injection, frusemide 10 mg/ml, net price 2-ml amp = 26p; 5-ml amp = 54p; 25-ml amp = £2.27

BUMETANIDE

Indications: oedema, oliguria due to renal failure

Cautions; Contra-indications: see under Frusemide. Drug interactions: see Appendix 1 (sections *2.1, 2.2, 2.2, 2.3, 2.4, 2.5, 2.6, 4.2, 4.7, 6.1, 6.3*)

Side-effects: see under Frusemide; also myalgia

Dose: by mouth, 1 mg in the morning, repeated after 6–8 hours if necessary; severe cases, increased up to 5 mg or more daily

By intramuscular or intravenous injection, 1–2 mg, repeated after 20 minutes

By intravenous infusion, 2–5 mg over 30–60 minutes

PoM **Burinex**® (Leo)

Tablets, scored, bumetanide 1 mg. Net price 20 = £1.14

Tablets, scored, bumetanide 5 mg. Net price 20 = £5.72

Liquid, green, sugar-free, bumetanide 1 mg/5 ml. Net price 150 ml = £3.25

Injection, bumetanide 500 micrograms/ml. Net price 2-ml amp = 41p; 4-ml amp = 71p; 10-ml amp = £1.49

ETHACRYNIC ACID

Indications: oedema, oliguria due to renal failure

Cautions; Contra-indications; Side-effects: see under Frusemide and notes above; also pain on injection. Drug interactions: see Appendix 1 (sections *2.1, 2.2, 2.2, 2.3, 2.4, 2.5, 2.6, 4.2, 4.7, 5.1, 6.1, 6.3*)

Dose: by mouth, initially 50 mg daily after food, maintenance 50–150 mg daily or on alternate days; max. 400 mg daily

By slow intravenous injection or infusion, 50 mg, increased to 100 mg if necessary

PoM **Edecrin**® (MSD)

Tablets, scored, ethacrynic acid 50 mg. Net price 20 = 75p. Label: 21

Injection, powder for reconstitution, ethacrynic acid (as sodium salt). Net price 50-mg vial = £1.05

PIRETANIDE

Indications: hypertension

Cautions: causes hypokalaemia, monitor plasma electrolytes in hepatic and renal impairment; prostatism. Drug interactions: see Appendix 1 (sections *2.1, 2.2, 2.2, 2.3, 2.4, 2.5, 2.6, 4.2, 4.7, 5.1, 6.3*)

Contra-indications: severe electrolyte imbalance, hypovolaemia

Side-effects: rarely nausea, vomiting, diarrhoea, rashes; myalgia after high doses

Dose: 6–12 mg in the morning with food

PoM **Arelix**® (Hoechst)

Capsules, s/r, green/orange, enclosing yellow pellets, piretanide 6 mg. Net price 28 = £3.37. Label: 21

2.2.3 Potassium-sparing diuretics

Amiloride (Midamor®) and **triamterene** (Dytac®) on their own are weak diuretics. They cause retention of potassium and are therefore used as an alternative to giving potassium supplements with thiazide or loop diuretics. (See section 2.2.4 for compound preparations with thiazides or loop diuretics.)

Spironolactone (Aldactone® etc.) is also a potassium-sparing diuretic, and potentiates thiazide or loop diuretics by antagonising aldosterone. It is of value in the treatment of the oedema of cirrhosis of the liver and occasionally may help in oedema of cardiac failure that is resistant to therapy, particularly when congestion has caused hepatic engorgement.

Spironolactone is also used in primary hyperaldosteronism (Conn's syndrome).

Potassium canrenoate (Spiroctan-M®) has similar uses to spironolactone, but can be given parenterally. It is metabolised to canrenone, which is also a metabolite of spironolactone.

Potassium supplements must **not** be given with potassium-sparing diuretics.

AMILORIDE HYDROCHLORIDE

Indications: oedema, potassium conservation with thiazide and loop diuretics
Cautions: pregnancy; diabetes mellitus. Drug interactions: see Appendix 1 (sections *1*, 2.2, *2.5*, *4.2*, *4.7*, *8*)
Contra-indications: hyperkalaemia, renal failure
Side-effects: rashes, mental confusion
Dose: alone, initially 10 mg daily *or* 5 mg twice daily, adjusted according to response; max. 20 mg daily
With other diuretics, congestive heart failure and hypertension, initially 5–10 mg daily
Cirrhosis with ascites, initially 5 mg daily

PoM **Amiloride** (Non-proprietary)
Tablets, amiloride hydrochloride 5 mg, net price 20 = £1.35
PoM **Midamor**® (Morson)
Tablets, yellow, amiloride hydrochloride 5 mg. Net price 20 = £1.46

POTASSIUM CANRENOATE

Indications: oedema associated with secondary aldosteronism, liver failure, chronic decompensated heart disease
Cautions; Contra-indications: see under Spironolactone; also contra-indicated in hyponatraemia
Side-effects: nausea and vomiting, particularly after high doses; pain and irritation at injection site
Dose: by slow intravenous injection or intravenous infusion, 200–400 mg daily (exceptionally 800 mg)

▼ PoM **Spiroctan-M**® (MCP)
Injection, potassium canrenoate 20 mg/ml. Net price 10-ml amp = 72p

SPIRONOLACTONE

Indications: oedema in cirrhosis of the liver, nephrotic syndrome, congestive heart failure, primary aldosteronism
Cautions: potential human metabolic products carcinogenic in *rodents*. Drug interactions: see Appendix 1 (sections *1*, *2.1*, 2.2, *2.5*, *4.7*, *8*)
Contra-indications: hyperkalaemia, renal failure; pregnancy and breast-feeding; Addison's disease
Side-effects: gastro-intestinal disturbances, gynaecomastia
Dose: 100–200 mg daily, increased to 400 mg if required; CHILD 3 mg/kg daily in divided doses

PoM **Spironolactone** (Non-proprietary)
Tablets, spironolactone 25 mg, net price 20 = 54p; 50 mg, 20 = £2.40; 100 mg, 20 = £2.40
PoM **Aldactone**® (Searle)
Tablets, all f/c, spironolactone 25 mg (buff), net price 20 = £1.80; 50 mg (off-white), 20 = £3.59; 100 mg (buff), 20 = £7.18

PoM **Diatensec**® (Gold Cross)
Tablets, off-white, f/c, spironolactone 50 mg. Net price 20 = £3.59
PoM **Laractone**® (Lagap)
Tablets, both f/c, spironolactone 25 mg, net price 20 = 54p; 50 mg, 20 = £2.40; 100 mg, 20 = £2.20
PoM **Spiretic**® (DDSA)
Tablets, yellow, spironolactone 25 mg, net price 20 = £1.19; 100 mg, 20 = £4.92
PoM **Spiroctan**® (MCP)
Tablets, both s/c, spironolactone 25 mg (blue), net price 20 = £1.44; 50 mg (green), 20 = £2.84
Capsules, green, spironolactone 100 mg. Net price 28-tab pack = £7.75
PoM **Spirolone**® (Berk)
Tablets, all s/c, spironolactone 25 mg, net price 20 = £1.25; 50 mg, 20 = £2.48; 100 mg, 20 = £5.02

TRIAMTERENE

Indications: oedema, potassium conservation with thiazide and loop diuretics
Cautions; Contra-indications: see under Amiloride Hydrochloride; monitor plasma urea and potassium, particularly in the elderly and in renal impairment; also may cause blue fluorescence of urine. Drug interactions: see Appendix 1 (sections 2.2, *2.5*, *4.7*, *8*)
Side-effects: gastro-intestinal disturbances, dry mouth, rashes; triamterene found in kidney stones
Dose: initially 150–250 mg daily, reducing to alternate days after 1 week; taken in divided doses after breakfast and lunch; lower initial dose when given with other diuretics
COUNSELLING. Urine may look slightly blue in some lights

PoM **Dytac**® (Bridge)
Capsules, maroon, triamterene 50 mg. Net price 20 = £1.24. Label: 21, counselling, see above

2.2.4 Potassium-sparing diuretics with other diuretics

Although it is preferable to prescribe thiazides and potassium-sparing diuretics separately, the use of fixed combinations may be justified if compliance is a problem. There is an increased risk of hyponatraemia if these are given with chlorpropamide (see Appendix 1, section 2.2).

PoM **Aldactide 25**® (Gold Cross)
Tablets, buff, spironolactone 25 mg, hydroflumethiazide 25 mg. Net price 20 = £3.07
Dose: congestive heart failure, initially 4 tablets daily; range 1–8 daily
PoM **Aldactide 50**® (Gold Cross)
Tablets, buff, f/c, spironolactone 50 mg, hydroflumethiazide 50 mg. Net price 20 = £5.79
Dose: congestive heart failure, initially 2 tablets daily; range 1–4 daily

PoM **Amilco**® (Norton)
Tablets, peach, scored, amiloride hydrochloride 5 mg, hydrochlorothiazide 50 mg. Net price 20 = £1.58
Dose: 1–2 tablets, increased if necessary to a max. of 4, daily

PoM **Dyazide**® (Bridge)
Tablets, peach, scored, triamterene 50 mg, hydrochlorothiazide 25 mg. Net price 30-tab pack = £1.95. Label: 21, counselling, see under triamterene, above
Dose: hypertension, 1 tablet daily after breakfast
Oedema, 2 tablets daily (1 after breakfast and 1 after lunch) increased to 3 daily if necessary (2 after breakfast and 1 after lunch); usual maintenance, 1 daily or 2 on alternate days; max. 4 daily

PoM **Dytide**® (Bridge)
Capsules, clear/maroon, triamterene 50 mg, benzthiazide 25 mg. Net price 20 = £1.35. Label: 21, counselling, see under triamterene, above
Dose: oedema, initially 3 capsules daily (2 after breakfast and 1 after lunch) for 1 week then 1 or 2 on alternate days

▼ PoM **Frumil**® (Rorer)
Tablets, orange, scored, amiloride hydrochloride 5 mg, frusemide 40 mg. Net price 28-tab pack = £3.97; 56-tab pack = £7.77
Dose: 1–2 tablets in the morning

PoM **Frusene**® (Fisons)
Tablets, yellow, scored, triamterene 50 mg, frusemide 40 mg. Net price 20 = £1.75. Label: 21, counselling, see under triamterene, above
Dose: 1–2 tablets daily

PoM **Hypertane 50**® (Schwarz)
Tablets, scored, amiloride hydrochloride 5 mg, hydrochlorothiazide 50 mg. Net price 28 = £2.11
Dose: 1–2 tablets, increased if necessary to a max. of 4, daily

▼ PoM **Kalspare**® (Armour)
Tablets, orange, f/c, scored, triamterene 50 mg, chlorthalidone 50 mg. Net price 28-tab pack = £1.93. Label: 21, counselling, see under triamterene, above
Dose: 1–2 tablets in the morning

▼ PoM **Lasilactone**® (Hoechst)
Capsules, blue/white, spironolactone 50 mg, frusemide 20 mg. Net price 28-tab pack = £5.04
Dose: resistant oedema, 1–4 capsules daily

▼ PoM **Lasoride**® (Hoechst)
Tablets, yellow, amiloride hydrochloride 5 mg, frusemide 40 mg. Net price 28-tab pack = £3.86
Dose: 1–2 tablets in the morning

PoM **Moduret 25**® (Morson)
Tablets, off-white, amiloride hydrochloride 2.5 mg, hydrochlorothiazide 25 mg. Net price 28-tab pack = £2.08
Dose: 1–4 tablets, increased if necessary to a max. of 8, daily

PoM **Moduretic**® (MSD)
Tablets, peach, scored, amiloride hydrochloride 5 mg, hydrochlorothiazide 50 mg. Net price 20 = £1.80
Dose: 1–2 tablets, increased if necessary to a max. of 4, daily
Oral solution, amiloride hydrochloride 5 mg, hydrochlorothiazide 50 mg/5 ml. Do not dilute. Net price 200 ml = £4.95
Dose: as for tablets above (5 ml = 1 tablet)

PoM **Normetic**® (Abbott)
Tablets, peach, scored, amiloride hydrochloride (anhydrous) 5 mg, hydrochlorothiazide 50 mg. Net price 20 = £1.32
Dose: 1–2 tablets, increased if necessary to a max. of 4, daily

PoM **Triamco**® (Norton)
Tablets, peach, scored, triamterene 50 mg, hydrochlorothiazide 25 mg. Net price 20 = £1.19. Label: 21, counselling, see under triamterene, above
Dose: 1–2 tablets daily; max. 4 daily

2.2.5 Osmotic diuretics

Osmotic diuretics are rarely used in heart failure as they may acutely expand the blood volume. **Mannitol** is the most commonly used—in forced diuresis in cases of drug overdose, and in cerebral oedema.

MANNITOL
Indications: cerebral oedema, forced diuresis
Cautions: extravasation causes inflammation and thrombophlebitis
Contra-indications: congestive cardiac failure, pulmonary oedema
Side-effects: chills, fever
Dose: by intravenous infusion, 50–200 g over 24 hours, preceded by a test dose of 200 mg/kg by slow intravenous injection

PoM **Mannitol** (Non-proprietary)
Intravenous infusion, mannitol 10%, 15%, 20%, and 25%
Different strengths and volumes available from different manufacturers

2.2.6 Mercurial diuretics

They are effective diuretics but are now little used because of their nephrotoxicity. Mersalyl **must** be given by intramuscular injection; intravenous use may cause severe hypotension and sudden death.

MERSALYL
Indications: oedema unresponsive to other diuretics
Cautions: recent myocardial infarction, treatment with cardiac glycosides, frequent extrasystoles; pregnancy
Contra-indications: renal impairment
Side-effects: gastro-intestinal disturbances, allergic reactions

PoM **Mersalyl Injection**, mersalyl sodium 100 mg, theophylline 50 mg/ml
Dose: by deep intramuscular injection, 0.5–2 ml

2.2.7   Carbonic anhydrase inhibitors

Acetazolamide and dichlorphenamide are weak diuretics, and are little used for their diuretic effect. They inhibit the formation of aqueous fluid, and are used in glaucoma (see section 11.6). Although acetazolamide is used as a prophylactic measure for mountain sickness it is not a substitute for acclimatisation.

2.2.8   Diuretics with potassium

Many patients on diuretics do not need potassium supplements (see section 9.2.1.1). For many of those who do, the amount of potassium ion in combined preparations may not be enough, and for this reason their use is to be discouraged.

Diuretics with potassium and potassium-sparing diuretics should **not** usually be given together.

COUNSELLING. Sustained-release potassium tablets should be swallowed whole with plenty of fluid during meals while sitting or standing

PoM **Burinex K**® (Leo)
Tablets, bumetanide 500 micrograms, potassium 7.7 mmol for sustained release. Net price 20 = 85p.
Label: 25, 27, counselling, see above

PoM **Centyl K**® (Leo)
Tablets, green, bendrofluazide 2.5 mg, potassium 7.7 mmol for sustained release. Net price 20 = 58p.
Label: 25, 27, counselling, see above

PoM **Diumide-K Continus**® (Degussa)
Tablets, white/orange, frusemide 40 mg, potassium 8 mmol for sustained release. Net price 20 = £1.34.
Label: 25, 27, counselling, see above

PoM **Esidrex-K**® (Ciba)
Tablets, s/c, hydrochlorothiazide 12.5 mg, potassium 8.1 mmol for sustained release. Net price 20 = 32p.
Label: 25, 27, counselling, see above

PoM **Hygroton-K**® (Geigy)
Tablets, red, s/c, chlorthalidone 25 mg, potassium 6.7 mmol for sustained release. Net price 20 = 40p.
Label: 25, 27, counselling, see above

PoM **Lasikal**® (Hoechst)
Tablets, white/yellow, f/c, frusemide 20 mg, potassium 10 mmol for sustained release. Net price 20 = £1.04.
Label: 25, 27, counselling, see above

PoM **Lasix + K**® (Hoechst)
Calendar pack, 30 white scored tablets, frusemide 40 mg; 60 s/r yellow tablets, potassium chloride (potassium 10 mmol). Net price = £3.05. Label: 25, 27, counselling, see above

PoM **Navidrex-K**® (Ciba)
Tablets, yellow, s/c, cyclopenthiazide 250 micrograms, potassium 8.1 mmol for sustained release. Net price 20 = 23p. Label: 25, 27, counselling, see above

PoM **Neo-NaClex-K**® (DF)
Tablets, pink/white, f/c, bendrofluazide 2.5 mg, potassium 8.4 mmol for sustained release. Net price 20 = 27p. Label: 25, 27, counselling, see above

2.3   Anti-arrhythmic drugs

2.3.1 Management of arrhythmias
2.3.2 Drugs for arrhythmias

2.3.1   Management of arrhythmias

Management of an arrhythmia, apart from the treatment of associated heart failure, requires precise diagnosis of the type of arrhythmia, and electrocardiography is essential.

Ectopic beats. If spontaneous with a normal heart, these rarely require treatment beyond reassurance. If they are particularly troublesome, beta-blockers are sometimes effective and may be safer than other suppressant drugs.

Atrial fibrillation. The ventricular rate can be controlled by digoxin (section 2.1).

Atrial flutter. The ventricular rate can often be controlled with digoxin. Reversion to sinus rhythm (if indicated) is best achieved by appropriately synchronised d.c. shock, rather than by drug therapy. If the arrhythmia is long-standing a period of treatment with anticoagulants should be considered before cardioversion to avoid the complication of emboli.

Paroxysmal supraventricular tachycardia. In most patients this remits spontaneously or can be returned to sinus rhythm by reflex vagal stimulation with respiratory manoeuvres, prompt squatting, or pressure over one carotid sinus (**important:** pressure over carotid sinus should be restricted to monitored patients, it can be dangerous in recent ischaemia, digitalis toxicity, or the elderly).

If vagal stimulation fails, digitalisation or intravenous administration of a beta-blocker may be effective. Intravenous adminstration of verapamil is useful for patients without myocardial or valvular disease (**important:** never in patients recently treated with beta-blockers, see section 2.3.2). For arrhythmias that are poorly tolerated, synchronised d.c. shock usually provides rapid relief.

In cases of paroxysmal atrial tachycardia with block, digitalis toxicity should be suspected. In addition to stopping administration of the cardiac glycoside and giving potassium supplements, intravenous administration of a beta-blocker or phenytoin may be useful. Specific digoxin antibody is available if the toxicity is considered life-threatening (see section 2.1).

Acute arrhythmias after myocardial infarction. It is best to do nothing in patients with a paroxysmal tachycardia or rapid irregularity of the pulse until an ECG record is obtainable. If the condition of the patient is such that death due to the arrhythmia seems possible 100 mg of lignocaine should be given intravenously. Bradycardia, particularly if complicated by hypotension, should be treated with atropine sulphate (section 15.1.3) in an initial dose of 300 micrograms, increasing to 1 mg if necessary.

Ventricular tachycardia. Drug treatment is used both for the treatment of ventricular tachycardia and for prophylaxis of recurrent attacks that merit suppression. Ventricular tachycardia requires treatment most commonly in the acute stage of myocardial infarction, but the likelihood of this and other life-threatening arrhythmias diminishes sharply over the first 24 hours after the attack, especially in patients without heart failure or shock. Lignocaine is the preferred drug for emergency use. Other drugs are best administered under specialist supervision. Very rapid ventricular tachycardia causes profound circulatory collapse and should be treated urgently with d.c. shock.

2.3.2   Drugs for arrhythmias

Anti-arrhythmic drugs can be classified clinically into those that act on supraventricular arrhythmias (e.g. verapamil), those that act on both supraventricular and ventricular arrhythmias (e.g. quinidine), and those that act on ventricular arrhythmias (e.g. lignocaine).

They can also be classified according to their effects on the electrical behaviour of myocardial cells during activity (termed 'action potential'), but this has less clinical relevance.

CAUTIONS. The negative inotropic effects of anti-arrhythmic drugs tend to be additive therefore special care should be taken if two or more are used, especially in patients with impaired myocardial function. Most or all drugs that are effective in countering arrhythmias can also provoke them in some circumstances; moreover, hypokalaemia enhances the pro-arrhythmic effect of many drugs.

DRUGS FOR SUPRAVENTRICULAR ARRHYTHMIAS

Oral administration of a **cardiac glycoside** (such as digoxin, section 2.1) is the treatment of choice in slowing ventricular response in cases of atrial fibrillation and atrial flutter. Intravenous digoxin, preferably infused slowly, is occasionally required if the ventricular rate needs rapid control. Ouabain acts more quickly but may be difficult to obtain since it is not on the UK market.

Verapamil (section 2.6.2) is usually effective for supraventricular tachycardias, including those associated with the Wolff-Parkinson-White syndrome; an initial intravenous dose may be followed by oral treatment. Hypotension may occur with larger doses (see below). It should not be used in children with arrhythmias without specialist advice; some supraventricular arrhythmias in childhood can be accelerated by verapamil with dangerous consequences.

Verapamil and beta-blockers. Verapamil should not be injected into patients recently treated with beta-blockers because of the risk of hypotension and asystole. It has been suggested that when verapamil injection has been given first, an interval of 30 minutes before giving a beta-blocker is sufficient but this too is open to doubt.

CARDIAC GLYCOSIDES
Section 2.1

VERAPAMIL
Section 2.6.2.

DRUGS FOR SUPRAVENTRICULAR AND VENTRICULAR ARRHYTHMIAS

Amiodarone (Cordarone X®) is used in the treatment of the Wolff-Parkinson-White syndrome. It may only be used for the treatment of other arrhythmias when other drugs are ineffective or contra-indicated. These include supraventricular and ventricular tachycardias, atrial fibrillation and flutter, and recurrent ventricular fibrillation. Since amiodarone has a very long half-life it only needs to be given once daily (but larger doses may cause nausea unless divided). It may be given by intravenous infusion as well as by mouth, and has the advantage of causing little or no myocardial depression. Unlike oral amiodarone, intravenous amiodarone may act relatively rapidly.

Most patients taking amiodarone develop corneal microdeposits; these rarely interfere with vision and are reversible on withdrawal of treatment. Because of the possibility of phototoxic reactions, patients should be advised to shield the skin from light and to use a wide-spectrum sunscreen such as RoC Total Sunblock (section 13.8.1) to protect against both long ultraviolet and visible light.

Amiodarone contains iodine and can cause disorders of thyroid function; both hypothyroidism and hyperthyroidism may occur. Thyroid function tests which rely on plasma concentrations of thyroxine alone, rather than on both thyroxine and triiodothyronine, may be spuriously elevated, but where doubt exists amiodarone should be withdrawn.

Beta-blockers (section 2.4) act as an anti-arrhythmic drugs principally by attenuating the effects of the sympathetic system on automaticity and conductivity within the heart. Some have additional anti-arrhythmic effects. They may be used in conjunction with digoxin to control the ventricular response in atrial fibrillation, especially in patients with thyrotoxicosis. Beta-blockers are also useful in the management of supraventricular tachycardias.

Evidence is now available that at least some **beta-blockers** (such as metoprolol) can reduce the incidence of life-threatening arrhythmias in the acute stage of myocardial infarction (see also section 2.4).

Disopyramide may be given by intravenous injection to control arrhythmias after myocardial infarction including those not responding to lignocaine, but it impairs cardiac contractility. Oral administration of disopyramide is useful but it has an anticholinergic effect which limits its use in patients with glaucoma or prostatic hypertrophy.

Flecainide is a newer agent in the same general class as lignocaine; it is of value in ventricular and supraventricular arrhythmias.

Procainamide can be given by intramuscular or intravenous injection to control ventricular and supraventricular arrhythmias, but prolonged oral use can cause a syndrome resembling systemic lupus erythematosus.

Cautionary label wordings, see inside back cover   Prices are **net**, see p. 1

Quinidine may be effective in suppressing supraventricular and ventricular arrhythmias. The drug itself may precipitate rhythm disorders, and is best used on specialist advice; it can cause hypersensitivity reactions and gastro-intestinal upsets.

AMIODARONE HYDROCHLORIDE

Indications: see notes above.

Cautions: liver-function and thyroid-function tests required in long-term therapy; interferes with tests of thyroid function. Drug interactions: see Appendix 1 (sections *2.1*, 2.3, *2.3*, *2.8B*, *4.8*)

Contra-indications: sinus bradycardia, atrioventricular block, thyroid dysfunction; pregnancy and breast-feeding; iodine sensitivity

Side-effects: corneal microdeposits, peripheral neuropathy, phototoxicity and rarely persistent slate-grey skin discoloration (see also notes above); hypothyroidism, hyperthyroidism, diffuse pulmonary alveolitis, hepatitis; rarely nausea, vomiting, metallic taste, tremor, nightmares, vertigo, headache, sleeplessness, fatigue; epididymitis with higher doses; blood disorders and increased prothrombin time reported

Dose: by mouth, 200 mg 3 times daily for 1 week reduced to 200 mg twice daily for a further week; maintenance, usually 200 mg daily or the minimum required to control the arrhythmia

By intravenous infusion via caval catheter, up to 5 mg/kg over 20–120 minutes with ECG monitoring; max. 1.2 g in 24 hours

▼ PoM **Cordarone X**® (Labaz)
Tablets, scored, amiodarone hydrochloride 100 mg. Net price 30 = £5.50. Label: 11
Tablets, scored, amiodarone hydrochloride 200 mg. Net price 30 = £9.00. Label: 11
Injection, amiodarone hydrochloride 50 mg/ml. Net price 3-ml amp = £1.54

DISOPYRAMIDE

Indications: ventricular arrhythmias, especially after myocardial infarction; supraventricular arrhythmias

Cautions: glaucoma; heart failure or diminished cardiac output; prostatic enlargement; reduce dose in renal impairment. Drug interactions: see Appendix 1 (sections 2.3, *2.6*, *4.9*)

Side-effects: myocardial depression, hypotension, atrioventricular block; anticholinergic effects include dry mouth, blurred vision, urinary retention

Dose: by mouth, 300–800 mg daily in divided doses

By slow intravenous injection, 2 mg/kg over at least 5 minutes to a max. of 150 mg, with ECG monitoring, followed immediately *either* by 200 mg *by mouth*, then 200 mg every 8 hours for 24 hours *or* 400 micrograms/kg/hour *by intravenous infusion*; max. 300 mg in first hour and 800 mg daily

PoM **Disopyramide** (Non-proprietary)
Capsules, disopyramide 100 mg, net price 20 = £1.60; 150 mg, 20 = £2.68
PoM **Dirythmin SA**® (Astra)
Durules® (= tablets, s/r), f/c, disopyramide 150 mg (as phosphate). Net price 20 = £2.53. Label: 25
Dose: 300 mg every 12 hours; max. 900 mg daily
PoM **Rythmodan**® (Roussel)
Capsules, disopyramide 100 mg (green/beige), net price 20 = £1.79; 150 mg, 20 = £2.68
Injection, disopyramide 10 mg (as phosphate)/ml, net price 5-ml amp = 70p
PoM **Rythmodan Retard**® (Roussel)
Tablets, s/r, scored, f/c, disopyramide 250 mg (as phosphate). Net price 20 = £5.14. Label: 25
Dose: 250–375 mg every 12 hours

FLECAINIDE ACETATE

Indications: ventricular and supraventricular arrhythmias

Cautions: patients with pacemakers; reduce dose in hepatic and renal impairment; pregnancy (toxicity in *animal* studies). Drug interactions: see Appendix 1 (section 2.3)

Contra-indications: heart failure, sino-atrial disorders, atrioventricular block

Side-effects: dizziness, visual disturbances; rarely nausea and vomiting

Dose: by mouth, 100–200 mg twice daily; max. 400 mg daily, reduced after 3–5 days if possible; elderly patients 100 mg twice daily, reduced after 1 week if possible

By slow intravenous injection, 2 mg/kg over 10–30 minutes, max. 150 mg; followed if required by *infusion* at a rate of 1.5 mg/kg/hour for 1 hour, then 250 micrograms/kg/hour; transfer to *oral* treatment, 100-mg tablet, then withdraw infusion over 4 hours by hourly decrements of 20%, and continue oral treatment as above

▼ PoM **Tambocor**® (Riker)
Tablets, scored, flecainide acetate 100 mg. Net price 20 = £5.64
Injection, flecainide acetate 10 mg/ml. Net price 15-ml amp = £3.60

PROCAINAMIDE HYDROCHLORIDE

Indications: ventricular arrhythmias, especially after myocardial infarction; supraventricular arrhythmias

Cautions: renal impairment, asthma, myasthenia gravis. Drug interactions: see Appendix 1 (section 2.3)

Contra-indications: heart block, heart failure, hypotension

Side-effects: nausea, diarrhoea, rashes, fever, myocardial depression, heart failure, lupus erythematosus-like syndrome, agranulocytosis after prolonged treatment

Dose: by mouth, 250 mg every 4–6 hours, preferably controlled by measurement of plasma concentration

By *slow intravenous injection*, 25–50 mg/minute with ECG monitoring, until arrhythmia is controlled; max. 1 g

Maintenance, *by mouth* as above or *by intramuscular injection*, 100–250 mg every 4–6 hours, preferably controlled by measurement of plasma concentration

PoM **Procainamide Durules®** (Astra)
Tablets, s/r, yellow, procainamide hydrochloride 500 mg. Net price 20 = £1.46. Label: 25
  Dose: 1–1.5 g every 8 hours

PoM **Pronestyl®** (Squibb)
Tablets, scored, procainamide hydrochloride 250 mg. Net price 20 = 94p
Injection, procainamide hydrochloride 100 mg/ml. Net price 10-ml vial = £1.90

QUINIDINE

Indications: prevention of supraventricular tachycardias, ventricular arrhythmias

Cautions: 200-mg test dose to detect hypersensitivity reactions. Drug interactions: see Appendix 1 (sections *2.1*, 2.3, *2.8C*, *10*, *15*)

Contra-indications: heart block

Side-effects: see under Procainamide Hydrochloride; also ventricular arrhythmias, thrombocytopenia, haemolytic anaemia; rarely granulomatous hepatitis; also cinchonism (see Quinine, section 5.4.1) with tinnitus, visual disturbances, headache, hot and flushed skin, confusion, vertigo, vomiting, and abdominal pain

Dose: by mouth, quinidine sulphate 200–400 mg 3–4 times daily

Note: quinidine sulphate 200 mg ≡ quinidine bisulphate 250 mg

PoM **Quinidine Sulphate** (Non-proprietary)
Tablets, quinidine sulphate 200 mg, net price 20 = £1.30; 300 mg, 20 = £1.76

PoM **Kiditard®** (Delandale)
Capsules, s/r, blue, quinidine bisulphate 250 mg. Net price 20 = £2.43. Label: 25
  Dose: 500 mg every 12 hours, adjusted as required

PoM **Kinidin Durules®** (Astra)
Tablets, s/r, f/c, quinidine bisulphate 250 mg. Net price 20 = £2.15. Label: 25
  Dose: 500 mg every 12 hours, adjusted as required

DRUGS FOR VENTRICULAR ARRHYTHMIAS

Bretylium is only used as an anti-arrhythmic drug in resuscitation. It is given both intramuscularly and intravenously but can cause severe hypotension, particularly after intravenous administration; nausea and vomiting can occur with either route. The intravenous route should only be used in emergency when there is doubt about absorption because of inadequate circulation.

Lignocaine is relatively safe when used by slow intravenous injection and should be considered

first for emergency use. Though effective in suppressing ventricular tachycardia and reducing the risk of ventricular fibrillation following myocardial infarction, it has not been shown convincingly to reduce mortality when used prophylactically in this condition. In patients with cardiac or hepatic failure doses may need to be reduced to avoid convulsions, depression of the central nervous system, or depression of the cardiovascular system.

Mexiletine may be given as a slow intravenous injection if lignocaine is ineffective; it has a similar action. Adverse cardiovascular and central nervous system effects may limit the dose tolerated; nausea and vomiting may prevent an effective dose being given by mouth.

Phenytoin by slow intravenous injection is sometimes useful in ventricular arrhythmias particularly those caused by cardiac glycosides.

Tocainide is an analogue of lignocaine; because of a high incidence of blood disorders its use is limited to treatment of life-threatening symptomatic ventricular tachyarrhythmias associated with severely compromised left ventricular function in patients who do not respond to other therapy or for whom other therapy is contra-indicated.

BRETYLIUM TOSYLATE

Indications: ventricular arrhythmias resistant to other treatment

Cautions: do not give noradrenaline or other sympathomimetic amines

Side-effects: hypotension, nausea and vomiting

Dose: by *Intramuscular injection*, 5 mg/kg repeated after 6–8 hours if necessary

By *slow intravenous injection*, 5–10 mg/kg over 8–10 minutes; may be repeated after 1–2 hours to a total dosage of 30 mg/kg (initial dose being diluted to 10 mg/ml in glucose 5% or sodium chloride intravenous infusion)

Maintenance 5–10 mg/kg *by intramuscular injection* every 6–8 hours *or* 1–2 mg/minute *by intravenous infusion*

PoM **Bretylate®** (Wellcome)
Injection, bretylium tosylate 50 mg/ml. Net price 2-ml amp = £2.74

LIGNOCAINE HYDROCHLORIDE

Indications: ventricular arrhythmias, especially after myocardial infarction

Cautions: lower doses in congestive cardiac failure, in hepatic failure, and following cardiac surgery. Drug interactions: see Appendix 1 (section 2.3, *2.4*)

Contra-indications: sino-atrial disorders, all grades of atrioventricular block, severe myocardial depression

Side-effects: confusion, convulsions

Dose: by *intravenous injection*, in patients without gross circulatory impairment, 100 mg as a bolus over a few minutes, followed by *infusion* of 4 mg/minute for 30 minutes, 2 mg/minute for 2 hours, then 1 mg/minute

PoM **Lignocaine in Glucose Injection,** lignocaine hydrochloride 0.1% (1 mg/ml) and 0.2% (2 mg/ml) in glucose intravenous infusion 5%. 500-ml and 1-litre containers

PoM **Min-I-Jet   Lignocaine   Hydrochloride®** (IMS)
Injection, lignocaine hydrochloride 1% (10 mg/ml), net price 10-ml disposable syringe = £2.65; 2% (20 mg/ml), 5-ml disposable syringe = £2.39

PoM **Select-A-Jet   Lignocaine   Hydrochloride®** (IMS)
Injection, lignocaine hydrochloride 20% (200 mg/ml). To be diluted before use. Net price 5-ml vial = £3.55

PoM **Xylocard®** (Astra)
Injection 100 mg, lignocaine hydrochloride (anhydrous) 20 mg/ml. Net price 5-ml syringe = £1.65
Intravenous infusion, lignocaine hydrochloride (anhydrous) 200 mg/ml. To be diluted before use. Net price 5-ml syringe (1 g) = £2.01; 10-ml syringe (2 g) = £2.35

MEXILETINE HYDROCHLORIDE

Indications: ventricular arrhythmias, especially after myocardial infarction
Cautions: hepatic impairment. Drug interactions: see Appendix 1 (section 2.3)
Contra-indications: bradycardia, heart block
Side-effects: bradycardia, hypotension, confusion, convulsions, psychiatric disorders, dysarthria, nystagmus, tremor; jaundice, hepatitis, and blood disorders reported
Dose: by mouth, initial dose 400 mg, followed after 2 hours by 200–250 mg 3–4 times daily
By intravenous injection, 100–250 mg at a rate of 25 mg/minute followed by *infusion* of 250 mg as a 0.1% solution over 1 hour, 125 mg/hour for 2 hours, then 500 micrograms/minute

PoM **Mexitil®** (Boehringer Ingelheim)
Capsules, purple/red, mexiletine hydrochloride 50 mg. Net price 20 = 91p
Capsules, red, mexiletine hydrochloride 200 mg. Net price 20 = £2.18
Injection, mexiletine hydrochloride 25 mg/ml. Net price 10-ml amp = £1.36

PoM **Mexitil PL®** (Boehringer Ingelheim)
Perlongets® (= capsules, s/r, each enclosing 5 miniature tablets), turquoise/scarlet, mexiletine hydrochloride 360 mg. Net price 60 = £11.76. Label: 25
Dose: 1 capsule twice daily

PHENYTOIN SODIUM

Indications: supraventricular and ventricular arrhythmias, especially those caused by cardiac glycosides (for use in epilepsy, see section 4.8.1)
Cautions: do not give with lignocaine
Contra-indications: supraventricular tachycardias (except those induced by digitalis), heart block

Side-effects: bradycardia, hypotension, asystole, confusion
Dose: by intravenous injection via caval catheter, 3.5–5 mg/kg at a rate not exceeding 50 mg/minute. Repeat after 10 minutes if necessary

PoM **Epanutin Ready Mixed Parenteral®** (P-D)
Injection, phenytoin sodium 50 mg/ml. Net price 5-ml amp = £3.65

TOCAINIDE HYDROCHLORIDE

Indications: ventricular arrhythmias (restricted use—see notes above)
Cautions: weekly blood counts essential for first 12 weeks, then monthly; severe hepatic or renal impairment, uncompensated heart failure, pregnancy (toxicity in *animal* studies). Drug interactions: see Appendix 1 (section 2.3)
Contra-indications: see under Lignocaine Hydrochloride
Side-effects: CNS effects including tremor, dizziness, convulsions, paraesthesia; gastro-intestinal effects including nausea and vomiting; bradycardia and hypotension after injection; rash and fever; lupus erythematosus-like syndrome, fibrosing alveolitis, agranulocytosis, aplastic anaemia, and thrombocytopenia—see also notes above; psychiatric disorders reported
Dose: chronic arrhythmias, *by mouth*, 1.2 g daily in 2–3 divided doses; max. 2.4 g daily
Acute treatment, *by slow intravenous injection or infusion*, 500–750 mg over 15–30 minutes, followed immediately by 600–800 mg by mouth
Maintenance, *by mouth*, 1.2 g daily, in 2–3 divided doses

▼ PoM **Tonocard®** (Astra)
Tablets, yellow, f/c, tocainide hydrochloride 400 mg. Net price 20 = £3.35
Tablets, yellow, f/c, tocainide hydrochloride 600 mg. Net price 20 = £4.50
Injection, tocainide hydrochloride 50 mg/ml. Net price 15-ml vial = £5.80

2.4   Beta-adrenoceptor blocking drugs

This group of drugs blocks the beta-adreno-receptors in the heart, peripheral vasculature, bronchi, pancreas, and liver.

Many beta-blockers are now available and in general they are all equally effective. There are, however, differences between them which may affect choice in treating particular diseases or individual patients.

Intrinsic sympathomimetic activity (ISA, partial agonist activity) represents the capacity of beta-blockers to stimulate as well as to block adrenergic receptors. Oxprenolol, pindolol, and acebutolol have ISA; they tend to cause less bradycardia than the other beta-blockers and may also cause less coldness of the extremities.

Some beta-blockers are lipid soluble and some are water soluble. Atenolol, nadolol, and sotalol are the most water-soluble; they are less likely to enter the brain, and may therefore cause less sleep disturbance and nightmares. Water-soluble beta-blockers are excreted by the kidneys; they accumulate in renal impairment and dosage reduction is therefore often necessary.

Some beta-blockers have a relatively short duration of action and have to be given twice or three times daily. Many of these are, however, available in slow-release formulations so that in general it is not necessary to give beta-blockers more often than once daily for hypertension (for angina twice-daily treatment may sometimes be needed even with a slow-release formulation).

All beta-blockers slow the heart and may induce myocardial depression and precipitate heart failure. They should not therefore be given to patients who have incipient cardiac failure or those with second- or third-degree heart block. Sotalol may prolong the QT interval, and has occasionally caused life-threatening ventricular arrhythmias. Particular care should be taken to avoid hypokalaemia in patients taking sotalol.

Beta-blockers may precipitate asthma and this effect can be dangerous. Some, such as acebutolol, atenolol, betaxolol, and metoprolol, have less effect on the beta$_2$ (bronchial) receptors and are, therefore, relatively cardioselective, but they are not cardiospecific. They have a lesser effect on airways resistance but are not free of this side-effect. Patients who have a tendency towards obstructive airways disease must be treated with great caution and may require to take increased doses of their beta$_2$-stimulants (e.g. salbutamol) to overcome the effect of blockade of the bronchial adrenoceptors.

CSM advice. Beta-blockers, even those with apparent cardioselectivity, should not be used in patients with asthma or a history of obstructive airways disease, unless no alternative treatment is available. In such cases the risk of inducing bronchospasm should be appreciated and appropriate precautions taken.

Beta-blockers may occasionally aggravate intermittent claudication.

Beta-blockers can lead to a small deterioration of glucose tolerance in diabetics; they also interfere with metabolic and autonomic responses to hypoglycaemia. Their use is not contra-indicated in diabetics, but cardioselective beta-blockers may be preferable and they should be avoided altogether in those with frequent episodes of hypoglycaemia.

Practolol is restricted to use by injection for the treatment of arrhythmias.

Labetalol (Trandate®) combines alpha- and beta-receptor blocking activity. Alpha-blocking activity in the peripheral vessels lowers peripheral resistance. There is no evidence that labetalol has an important advantage over other beta-blockers as regards reduction of blood pressure. The alpha-blocking properties tend to offset the lack of cardioselectivity of the beta blockade, with the net effect that labetalol and atenolol have roughly similar effects on airways resistance.

HYPERTENSION

Beta-blockers are effective antihypertensive drugs but their mode of action is not understood; they reduce cardiac output, alter baroceptor reflex sensitivity, and block peripheral adrenoceptors. Some beta-blockers depress plasma renin secretion. It is possible that a central effect may also explain their mode of action. Despite the many contra-indications blood pressure can usually be controlled with relatively few side-effects. In general the dose of beta-blocker does not have to be as high as originally thought. The maximum dose of oxprenolol and propranolol necessary is probably 320 mg daily. Atenolol can usually be given in a dose of 50 mg daily and it is only rarely necessary to increase to 100 mg.

Combined thiazide/beta-blocker preparations are now available (for details see under Compound Preparations at end of section). These may help compliance with treatment regimens but combined preparations should only be used when blood pressure is uncontrolled by thiazide or beta-blocker alone. Beta-blockers reduce, but do not abolish, the tendency for diuretics to cause hypokalaemia.

Beta-blockers can be used to control the pulse rate in patients with *phaeochromocytoma*. However, they should never be used alone as beta-blockade without concurrent alpha-blockade may lead to a hypertensive crisis. For this reason phenoxybenzamine should always be used together with the beta-blocker.

ANGINA

Beta-blockers improve exercise tolerance and relieve symptoms in patients with angina; this effect is caused by their reduction of cardiac work. As with hypertension there is no good evidence of the superiority of any one drug, although occasionally a patient will respond better to one beta-blocker than to another. There is some evidence that sudden withdrawal may cause an exacerbation of angina therefore gradual reduction of dose is preferable when beta-blockers are to be stopped. There is a risk of precipitating heart failure when beta-blockers and verapamil are used together in patients with established ischaemic heart disease (**important:** see section 2.3.2).

MYOCARDIAL INFARCTION

Several studies have now shown that some beta-blockers can cause a reduction in the recurrence rate of myocardial infarction. However, pre-existing heart failure, hypotension, bradyarrhythmias, and obstructive airways disease render this group of drugs unsuitable in some patients who have recovered from a myocardial infarction.

Atenolol and metoprolol may reduce early mortality after intravenous and subsequent oral administration in the acute phase, while timolol and propranolol have protective value when started in the early convalescent phase. The evidence relating to other beta-blockers is less convincing; some have not been tested in trials of secondary protection. It is also not known whether the protective effect of beta-blockers continues after two years; it is possible that sudden cessation may cause a rebound worsening of myocardial ischaemia.

ARRHYTHMIAS

Beta-blockers are used to control supraventricular tachycardia following myocardial infarction, see above.

THYROTOXICOSIS

Beta-blockers are used in pre-operative preparation for thyroidectomy. Administration of propranolol can reverse clinical features of thyrotoxicosis within 4 days. Routine tests of increased thyroid function remain unaltered. The thyroid gland is rendered less vascular thus making surgery easier (see section 6.2.2).

OTHER USES

Beta-blockers have been used to alleviate some symptoms of anxiety; probably patients with palpitations, tremor, and tachycardia respond best. (See also sections 4.1.2 and 4.9.3.) Beta-blockers are also used in the prophylaxis of migraine (see section 4.7.4.2.) Beta-blockers are used topically in the management of glaucoma (see section 11.6).

PROPRANOLOL HYDROCHLORIDE

Indications: see under Dose
Cautions: late pregnancy; breast-feeding; avoid abrupt withdrawal in angina; reduce oral dose of propranolol in liver disease; reduce initial dose in renal impairment. See also notes above. Drug interactions: see Appendix 1 (sections 2.3, 2.4, 2.5, 2.7, 3, 4.2, 6.1, 10, 15)
Contra-indications: asthma, heart failure, second or third degree heart block, cardiogenic shock
Side-effects: bradycardia, heart failure, bronchospasm, peripheral vasoconstriction, gastrointestinal disturbances
Dose: by mouth, hypertension, initially 80 mg twice daily, increased at weekly intervals as required; maintenance 160–320 mg daily
Angina, initially 40 mg 2–3 times daily; maintenance 120–240 mg daily
Arrhythmias, hypertrophic obstructive cardiomyopathy, anxiety tachycardia, and thyrotoxicosis, 10–40 mg 3–4 times daily
Prophylaxis after infarction, 40 mg 4 times daily for 2–3 days, then 80 mg twice daily, beginning 5 to 21 days after infarction

Migraine prophylaxis and essential tremor, initially 40 mg 2–3 times daily; maintenance 80–160 mg daily
By intravenous injection, arrhythmias and thyrotoxic crisis, 1 mg over 1 minute; if necessary repeat at 2-minute intervals; max. 10 mg (5 mg in anaesthesia)
Note. Excessive bradycardia can be countered with intravenous injection of atropine 0.6–2.4 mg in divided doses of 600 micrograms

PoM **Propranolol** (Non-proprietary)
Tablets, propranolol hydrochloride 10 mg, net price 20 = 5p; 40 mg, 20 = 8p; 80 mg, 20 = 15p; 160 mg, 20 = 26p. Label: 8
PoM **Angilol**® (DDSA)
Tablets, all pink, f/c, propranolol hydrochloride 10 mg, net price 20 = 21p; 40 mg, 20 = 50p; 80 mg, 20 = 76p; 160 mg, 20 = £1.51. Label: 8
PoM **Apsolol**® (APS)
Tablets, all pink, f/c, scored, propranolol hydrochloride 10 mg, net price 20 = 6p; 40 mg, 20 = 10p; 80 mg, 20 = 17p; 160 mg, 20 = 46p. Label: 8
PoM **Berkolol**® (Berk)
Tablets, all pink, f/c, scored, propranolol hydrochloride 10 mg, net price 20 = 23p; 40 mg, 20 = 54p; 80 mg, 20 = 82p; 160 mg, 20 = £1.64. Label: 8
PoM **Half-Inderal LA**® (ICI)
Capsules, s/r, lavender/pink, propranolol hydrochloride 80 mg. Net price 28 = £4.48. Label: 8, 25
PoM **Inderal**® (ICI)
Tablets, all pink, f/c, propranolol hydrochloride 10 mg, net price 20 = 20p; 40 mg, 20 = 54p; 80 mg, 20 = 88p; 160 mg, 20 = £1.56. Label: 8
Injection, propranolol hydrochloride 1 mg/ml, net price 1-ml amp = 24p
PoM **Inderal-LA**® (ICI)
Capsules, s/r, lavender/pink, propranolol hydrochloride 160 mg. Net price 28 = £6.66. Label: 8, 25
PoM **Sloprolol**® (CP)
Capsules, s/r, green/clear enclosing off-white pellets, propranolol hydrochloride 160 mg. Net price 20 = £3.64. Label: 8, 25

ACEBUTOLOL

Indications: see under Dose
Cautions; Contra-indications; Side-effects: see under Propranolol Hydrochloride
Dose: hypertension, initially 400 mg once daily or 200 mg twice daily, increased after 2 weeks to 400 mg twice daily
Angina, initially 400 mg once daily or 200 mg twice daily; 300 mg 3 times daily in severe angina; maintenance up to 1.2 g daily
Arrhythmias, 0.4–1.2 g daily in 2–3 divided doses

PoM **Sectral**® (M&B)
Capsules, buff/white, acebutolol 100 mg (as hydrochloride). Net price 20 = £1.59. Label: 8

Capsules, buff/pink, acebutolol 200 mg (as hydrochloride). Net price 20 = £3.06. Label: 8
Tablets, f/c, acebutolol 400 mg (as hydrochloride). Net price 28 = £8.30. Label: 8

ATENOLOL

Indications: see under Dose
Cautions; Contra-indications; Side-effects: see under Propranolol Hydrochloride; reduce dose in renal impairment
Dose: by mouth, hypertension, 50–100 mg daily
Angina, 100 mg daily in 1 or 2 doses
Arrhythmias, 50–100 mg daily
By intravenous injection, 2.5 mg at a rate of 1 mg/minute, repeated at 5-minute intervals to a max. of 10 mg

Note. Excessive bradycardia can be countered with intravenous injection of atropine 0.6–2.4 mg in divided doses of 600 micrograms

By intravenous infusion, 150 micrograms/kg over 20 minutes, repeated every 12 hours if required
Early intervention within 12 hours of infarction, 5–10 mg *by slow intravenous injection*, then *by mouth* 50 mg after 15 minutes, 50 mg after 12 hours, then 100 mg daily

PoM **Atenolol** (Non-proprietary)
Tablets, atenolol 50 mg, net price 28-tab pack = £4.67; 100 mg, 28-tab pack = £6.60. Label: 8
PoM **Tenormin**® (Stuart)
Tablets, orange, f/c, atenolol 100 mg. Net price 28 = £6.98. Label: 8
Syrup, sugar-free, atenolol 25 mg/5 ml. Diluent purified water freshly boiled and cooled, life of diluted syrup diluted not more than 50% 14 days. Net price 300 ml = £8.35. Label: 8
Injection, atenolol 500 micrograms/ml. Net price 10-ml amp = 90p (Hosp. only)
PoM **Tenormin LS**® (Stuart)
Tablets, orange, f/c, scored, atenolol 50 mg. Net price 28 = £4.88. Label: 8
▼ PoM **Tenormin CCU Pack**® (Stuart)
Product discontinued

BETAXOLOL HYDROCHLORIDE

Indications: hypertension
Cautions; Contra-indications; Side-effects: see under Propranolol Hydrochloride; reduce dose in renal impairment
Dose: 20 mg daily (elderly patients 10 mg), increased to 40 mg if required

▼ PoM **Kerlone**® (Lorex)
Tablets, f/c, scored, betaxolol hydrochloride 20 mg. Net price 28 = £7.70. Label: 8

BISOPROLOL FUMARATE

Indications: hypertension, angina
Cautions; Contra-indications; Side-effects: see under Propranolol Hydrochloride; reduce dose in hepatic and renal impairment

Dose: usual dose 10 mg daily (5 mg may be adequate in some patients); max. recommended dose 20 mg daily

▼ PoM **Emcor**® (Merck)
LS Tablets, yellow, f/c, scored, bisoprolol fumarate 5 mg. Net price 28-tab pack = £7.98. Label: 8
Tablets, orange, f/c, scored, bisoprolol fumarate 10 mg. Net price 28-tab pack = £8.96. Label: 8
▼ PoM **Monocor**® (Cyanamid)
Tablets, both f/c, bisoprolol fumarate 5 mg, (pink), net price 28-tab pack = £7.98; 10 mg, 28-tab pack = £8.96. Label: 8

LABETALOL HYDROCHLORIDE

Indications: hypertension (including hypertension in pregnancy, hypertension with angina, and hypertension following acute myocardial infarction); hypertensive crisis; controlled hypotension in surgery
Cautions: late pregnancy, breast-feeding; avoid abrupt withdrawal; reduce oral dose in liver disease; interferes with laboratory tests for catecholamines. Drug interactions: see Appendix 1 (see under Propranolol Hydrochloride)
Contra-indications: as for Propranolol Hydrochloride
Side-effects: postural hypotension, tiredness, weakness, headache, rashes, scalp tingling, difficulty in micturition, epigastric pain, nausea, vomiting; rarely lichenoid rash
Dose: by mouth, initially 100–200 mg (elderly patients 50 mg) twice daily with food, increased at 14-day intervals; max. 2.4 g daily
By intravenous injection, 50 mg over 1 minute, repeated after 5 minutes if necessary; max. 200 mg

Note. Excessive bradycardia can be countered with intravenous injection of atropine 0.6–2.4 mg in divided doses of 600 micrograms

By intravenous infusion, 2 mg/minute to a max. of 200 mg
Hypertension of pregnancy, 20 mg/hour, doubled every 30 minutes; max. 160 mg/hour
Hypertension following infarction, 15 mg/hour, gradually increased to max. 120 mg/hour

PoM **Labetalol Hydrochloride** (Non-proprietary)
Tablets, all f/c, labetalol hydrochloride 100 mg, net price 20 = £1.52; 200 mg, 20 = £2.40; 400 mg, 20 = £3.87. Label: 8, 21
PoM **Labrocol**® (Lagap)
Tablets, all orange, f/c, labetalol hydrochloride 100 mg, net price 20 = £1.32; 200 mg, 20 = £2.09; 400 mg, 20 = £3.54. Label: 8, 21
PoM **Trandate**® (DF)
Tablets, all orange, f/c, labetalol hydrochloride 50 mg, net price 56-tab pack = £5.05; 100 mg, 56-tab pack = £5.56; 200 mg, 56-tab pack = £9.02; 400 mg, 20 = £4.48. Label: 8, 21
Injection, labetalol hydrochloride 5 mg/ml. Net price 20-ml amp = £2.83

METOPROLOL TARTRATE

Indications: see under Dose

Cautions; Contra-indications; Side-effects: see under Propranolol Hydrochloride. Reduce initial dose in renal impairment

Dose: by mouth, hypertension, initially 100 mg daily, maintenance 100–400 mg daily in 1–2 doses

Angina, 50–100 mg 2–3 times daily

Arrhythmias, usually 50 mg 2–3 times daily, up to 300 mg daily in divided doses if necessary

Migraine prophylaxis, 100–200 mg in divided doses

Thyrotoxicosis, 50 mg 4 times daily

By intravenous injection, up to 5 mg at rate 1–2 mg/minute, repeated after 5 minutes if necessary, total dose 10–15 mg

Note. Excessive bradycardia can be countered with intravenous injection of atropine 0.6–2.4 mg in divided doses of 600 micrograms

In surgery, 2–4 mg *by slow intravenous injection* at induction or to control arrhythmias developing during anaesthesia; 2-mg doses may be repeated to a max. of 10 mg

Early intervention within 12 hours of infarction, 5 mg *by intravenous injection* every 2 minutes to a max. of 15 mg, then 50 mg *by mouth* every 6 hours for 48 hours; maintenance 200 mg daily

PoM **Metoprolol Tartrate** (Non-proprietary)

Tablets, metoprolol tartrate 50 mg, net price 20 = 94p; 100 mg, 20 = £1.74. Label: 8

PoM **Betaloc**® (Astra)

Tablets, both scored, metoprolol tartrate 50 mg, net price 20 = 92p; 56-tab pack = £2.90; 100 mg, 20 = £1.71. Label: 8

Injection, metoprolol tartrate 1 mg/ml. Net price 5-ml amp = 45p

PoM **Betaloc-SA**® (Astra)

Durules® (= tablets, s/r), metoprolol tartrate 200 mg. Net price 28-tab pack = £6.51. Label: 8, 25

Dose: 200–400 mg daily

PoM **Lopresor**® (Geigy)

Tablets, both f/c, scored, metoprolol tartrate 50 mg (pink), net price 20 = 94p; 100 mg (blue), 14-tab   pack = £1.23,   56-tab   pack = £4.90. Label: 8

Injection, metoprolol tartrate 1 mg/ml. 5-ml amp (Hosp. only)

PoM **Lopresor SR**® (Geigy)

Tablets, s/r, yellow, f/c, metoprolol tartrate 200 mg. Net price 28 = £7.20. Label: 8, 25

Dose: 200–400 mg daily

NADOLOL

Indications: see under Dose

Cautions; Contra-indications; Side-effects: see under Propranolol Hydrochloride; reduce dose in renal impairment

Dose: hypertension, 80 mg daily, increased at weekly intervals if required; max. 240 mg daily

Angina, 40 mg daily, increasing at weekly intervals if required; max. usually 160 mg daily

Arrhythmias, 80 mg daily, increased to 160 mg if required; reduce to 40 mg if bradycardia occurs

Migraine prophylaxis, 80 mg daily, increased by 40 mg at weekly intervals; usual maintenance dose 80–160 mg daily

Thyrotoxicosis, 80–160 mg daily

PoM **Corgard**® (Squibb)

Tablets, blue, nadolol 40 mg. Net price 28 = £5.22. Label: 8

Tablets, blue, scored, nadolol 80 mg. Net price 28 = £7.55. Label: 8

OXPRENOLOL HYDROCHLORIDE

Indications: see under Dose

Cautions; Contra-indications; Side-effects: see under Propranolol Hydrochloride

Dose: hypertension, initially 80 mg twice daily, increased as required at weekly intervals; max. 480 mg daily

Angina, 40–160 mg 3 times daily

Arrhythmias, initially 20–40 mg 3 times daily, increased as necessary

Anxiety symptoms, 160 mg daily in divided doses

PoM **Oxprenolol** (Non-proprietary)

Tablets, all f/c, oxprenolol hydrochloride 20 mg, net price 20 = 30p; 40 mg, 20 = 43p; 80 mg, 20 = 71p; 160 mg, 20 = £1.38. Label: 8

PoM **Apsolox**® (APS)

Tablets, all f/c, oxprenolol hydrochloride 20 mg, net price 20 = 37p; 40 mg, 20 = 52p; 80 mg (yellow),   20 = 86p;   160 mg   (orange),   20 = £1.56. Label: 8

PoM **Paritane**® (Berck)

Tablets, oxprenolol hydrochloride 20 mg, net price,   20 = 40p;   40 mg,   20 = 66p;   80 mg (yellow),   20 = £1.01;   160 mg (orange),   20 = £1.81. Label: 8

PoM **Slow-Pren**® (Norton)

Tablets, s/r, f/c, oxprenolol hydrochloride 160 mg. Net price 28 = £6.10. Label: 8, 25

Dose: 160–480 mg daily

PoM **Slow-Trasicor**® (Ciba)

Tablets, s/r, f/c, oxprenolol hydrochloride 160 mg. Net price 28 = £6.84. Label: 8, 25

Dose: 160–480 mg daily

PoM **Trasicor**® (Ciba)

Tablets, all f/c, oxprenolol hydrochloride 20 mg, net price 20 = 58p; 40 mg, 20 = 96p; 80 mg (beige), 20 = £1.46; 160 mg (orange), 20 = £2.64. Label: 8

PENBUTOLOL SULPHATE

Indications: hypertension

Cautions; Contra-indications; Side-effects: see under Propranolol Hydrochloride

Dose: 40 mg daily, increased to twice daily if required

Preparations

See under Compound Preparations

PINDOLOL

Indications: see under Dose
Cautions; Contra-indications; Side-effects: see under Propranolol Hydrochloride; reduce dose in renal impairment
Dose: hypertension, initially 5 mg 2–3 times daily *or* 15 mg once daily, increased as required at weekly intervals; max. 45 mg daily
Angina, 2.5–5 mg up to 3 times daily

PoM **Betadren**® (Lagap)
Tablets, pindolol 5 mg, net price 20 = £1.81; 15 mg, 30-tab pack = £8.15. Label: 8
PoM **Visken**® (Sandoz)
Tablets, both scored, pindolol 5 mg, net price 20 = £2.13; 15 mg, 30 = £9.59. Label: 8

PRACTOLOL

Indications: supraventricular tachycardias; ventricular tachycardias, especially after myocardial infarction
Cautions: chronic obstructive airways disease; for cautions with verapamil see notes (section 2.3.2). Drug interactions: see Appendix 1 (sections *2.3*, 2.4, *2.5*, *2.7*, *6.1*, *15*)
Side-effects: bradycardia, hypotension, heart failure, bronchospasm
Dose: by slow intravenous injection, 5 mg, repeated if required

PoM **Eraldin**® (ICI)
Injection, practolol 2 mg/ml. Net price 5-ml amp = 90p (Hosp. only)

SOTALOL HYDROCHLORIDE

Indications: see under Dose
Cautions; Contra-indications; Side-effects: see under Propranolol Hydrochloride; reduce dose in renal impairment; occasionally causes atypical ventricular arrhythmias (torsade de pointes)—special need to avoid hypokalaemia (stop if severe or persistent diarrhoea etc.)
Dose: by mouth, hypertension and angina, initially 80 mg twice daily *or* 160 mg once daily; maintenance 160 mg daily, increased to 400–600 mg daily if necessary
Arrhythmias, 120–240 mg daily in single or divided doses
Thyrotoxicosis, 120–240 mg daily in single or divided doses
Prophylaxis after infarction, 320 mg daily, starting 5–14 days after infarction
By slow intravenous injection, 20–60 mg over 2–3 minutes with ECG monitoring, repeated if necessary with 10-minute intervals between injections; up to 100 mg over 3 minutes or longer
Note. Excessive bradycardia can be countered with intravenous injection of atropine 0.6–2.4 mg in divided doses of 600 micrograms

PoM **Beta-Cardone**® (DF)
Tablets, green, scored, sotalol hydrochloride 40 mg. Net price 20 = 79p. Label: 8
Tablets, pink, scored, sotalol hydrochloride 80 mg. Net price 20 = £1.17. Label: 8

Tablets, scored, sotalol hydrochloride 200 mg. Net price 30 = £4.15. Label: 8
PoM **Sotacor**® (Bristol-Myers)
Tablets, pink, sotalol hydrochloride 80 mg. Net price 28-tab pack = £2.05. Label: 8
Tablets, blue, sotalol hydrochloride 160 mg. Net price 28-tab pack = £4.05. Label: 8
Injection, sotalol hydrochloride 2 mg/ml. Net price 5-ml amp = 44p
Injection, sotalol hydrochloride 10 mg/ml. 10-ml amp (available on special order)

TIMOLOL MALEATE

Indications: see under Dose
Cautions; Contra-indications; Side-effects: see under Propranolol Hydrochloride
Dose: hypertension, initially 5 mg twice daily *or* 10 mg once daily; max. 60 mg daily
Angina, initially 5 mg 2–3 times daily, maintenance 15–45 mg daily
Prophylaxis after infarction, initially 5 mg twice daily, increased after 2 days to 10 mg twice daily, starting 7 to 28 days after infarction
Migraine prophylaxis, 10–20 mg daily

PoM **Betim**® (Leo)
Tablets, scored, timolol maleate 10 mg. Net price 20 = £1.75. Label: 8
PoM **Blocadren**® (MSD)
Tablets, blue, scored, timolol maleate 10 mg. Net price 20 = £2.12. Label: 8

COMPOUND PREPARATIONS

PoM **Co-Betaloc**® (Astra)
Tablets, scored, metoprolol tartrate 100 mg, hydrochlorothiazide 12.5 mg. Net price 28-tab pack = £6.65. Label: 8
PoM **Co-Betaloc SA**® (Astra)
Tablets, yellow, f/c, metoprolol tartrate 200 mg (sustained release), hydrochlorothiazide 25 mg. Net price 28-tab pack = £8.20. Label: 8, 25
▼ PoM **Corgaretic 40**® (Squibb)
Tablets, scored, nadolol 40 mg, bendrofluazide 5 mg. Net price 28-tab pack = £6.07. Label: 8
▼ PoM **Corgaretic 80**® (Squibb)
Tablets, scored, nadolol 80 mg, bendrofluazide 5 mg. Net price 28-tab pack = £8.69. Label: 8
PoM **Inderetic**® (ICI)
Capsules, propranolol hydrochloride 80 mg, bendrofluazide 2.5 mg. Net price 20 = £2.19. Label: 8
PoM **Inderex**® (ICI)
Capsules, pink/grey, propranolol hydrochloride 160 mg (sustained release), bendrofluazide 5 mg. Net price 28-tab pack = £7.44. Label: 8, 25
▼ PoM **Kalten**® (Stuart)
Capsules, red/ivory, atenolol 50 mg, amiloride hydrochloride (anhydrous) 2.5 mg, hydrochlorothiazide 25 mg. Net price 28-tab pack = £6.70. Label: 8

▼ PoM **Lasipressin**® (Hoechst)

Tablets, yellow-white, f/c, scored, penbutolol sulphate 40 mg, frusemide 20 mg. Net price 30-tab pack = £8.49. Label: 8

PoM **Lopresoretic**® (Geigy)

Tablets, f/c, scored, metoprolol tartrate 100 mg, chlorthalidone 12.5 mg. Net price 56 = £7.25. Label: 8

PoM **Moducren**® (Morson)

Tablets, blue, scored, timolol maleate 10 mg, amiloride hydrochloride 2.5 mg, hydrochlorothiazide 25 mg. Net price 28-tab pack = £8.00. Label: 8

PoM **Prestim**® (Leo)

Tablets, scored, timolol maleate 10 mg, bendrofluazide 2.5 mg. Net price 20 = £2.79. Label: 8

PoM **Prestim Forte**® (Leo)

Tablets, scored, timolol maleate 20 mg, bendrofluazide 5 mg. Net price 20 = £5.88. Label: 8

PoM **Secadrex**® (M&B)

Tablets, f/c, acebutolol 200 mg (as hydrochloride), hydrochlorothiazide 12.5 mg. Net price 28-tab pack = £7.84. Label: 8

PoM **Sotazide**® (Bristol-Myers)

Tablets, blue, sotalol hydrochloride 160 mg, hydrochlorothiazide 25 mg. Net price 28-tab pack = £7.12. Label: 8

PoM **Tenoret 50**® (Stuart)

Tablets, brown, f/c, atenolol 50 mg, chlorthalidone 12.5 mg. Net price 28-tab pack = £5.20. Label: 8

PoM **Tenoretic**® (Stuart)

Tablets, brown, f/c, atenolol 100 mg, chlorthalidone 25 mg. Net price 28-tab pack = £7.44. Label: 8

▼ PoM **Tolerzide**® (Bristol-Myers)

Tablets, lilac, sotalol hydrochloride 80 mg, hydrochlorothiazide 12.5 mg. Net price 28-tab pack = £4.05. Label: 8

PoM **Trasidrex**® (Ciba)

Tablets, red, s/c, oxprenolol hydrochloride 160 mg (for sustained release), cyclopenthiazide 250 micrograms. Net price 28-tab pack = £7.92. Label: 8

PoM **Viskaldix**® (Sandoz)

Tablets, scored, pindolol 10 mg, clopamide 5 mg. Net price 28-tab pack = £8.17. Label: 8

2.5   Antihypertensive therapy

2.5.1 Vasodilator antihypertensive drugs
2.5.2 Centrally acting antihypertensive drugs
2.5.3 Adrenergic neurone blocking drugs
2.5.4 Alpha-adrenoceptor blocking drugs
2.5.5 Angiotensin-converting enzyme inhibitors
2.5.6 Ganglion blocking drugs
2.5.7 Tyrosine hydroxylase inhibitors

Antihypertensive therapy has improved the outlook for patients with high blood pressure by decreasing the frequency of stroke, heart failure, and renal failure. In general, patients whose average diastolic pressure exceeds 100 mmHg should

receive antihypertensive therapy. Below that level the benefits of therapy are unproven. The usual aim should be to reduce the diastolic blood pressure preferably to below 90 mmHg and certainly below 100 mmHg. The quality of control of blood pressure at follow-up is an important predictor of outcome, and efficient long-term care is necessary.

Malignant (or accelerated) hypertension or very severe hypertension (diastolic blood pressure >140 mmHg) is not an indication for parenteral antihypertensive therapy. Normally treatment should be by mouth with a beta-blocker (atenolol or labetalol), a calcium-channel blocker (nifedipine), or a vasodilator (hydralazine). Within the first 24 hours the diastolic blood pressure should not be reduced to below 110 mmHg. Over the next two or three days blood pressure should be normalised by using beta-blockers, calcium-channel blockers, diuretics, vasodilators, or angiotensin-converting enzyme inhibitors. Very rapid falls in blood pressure can cause reduced cerebral perfusion leading to cerebral infarction, a reduction in renal perfusion causing a deterioration in renal function, and myocardial ischaemia. Parenteral antihypertensive drugs are, therefore, hardly ever necessary.

Sodium nitroprusside by infusion is the parenteral antihypertensive drug of choice. Small doses of diazoxide by slow intravenous injection, labetalol by infusion, or hydralazine by slow intravenous injection may also be used, but again precipitate falls in blood pressure should be carefully avoided.

The strategy for reducing blood pressure is probably best as follows:

1. *Non-drug treatment*—high salt intake, obesity, and high alcohol intake may elevate blood pressure and these should be corrected.

2. *Diuretic therapy*—any thiazide diuretic will be effective, e.g. bendrofluazide 2.5 mg/day (section 2.2.1). The optimum dose of a thiazide used to treat hypertension is the lowest possible dose; higher doses do not have a major additional antihypertensive effect, but do cause more metabolic side-effects. Potassium supplements are seldom necessary but plasma potassium concentration should be checked 3 to 4 weeks after starting treatment. Potassium-sparing diuretics (amiloride or triamterene) are usually not necessary in the routine treatment of hypertension, unless hypokalaemia develops.

3. *Beta-adrenoceptor blocking drugs* (section 2.4) should be used in combination with a thiazide where they are not effective alone.

4. *Calcium-channel blockers*—nifedipine, nicardipine, and verapamil (section 2.6.2) have antihypertensive efficacy broadly similar to that of thiazides or beta-blockers. Minor side-effects are more common, and their safety during long-term treatment is less well established; they should therefore be considered for hypertension only when thiazides and beta-blockers are contra-indicated, are not tolerated, or fail to control blood pressure.

There are important differences between verapamil and the dihydropyridine calcium-channel blockers, nifedipine and nicardipine. Nifedipine and nicardipine act primarily as arteriolar vasodilators and frequently cause flushing, headache, palpitation, and oedema (which does not respond to diuretics); they can be combined with beta-blockers. Verapamil reduces cardiac output, slows the heart rate, and may impair atrioventricular conduction. It is contra-indicated in heart failure or second- or third-degree heart block, and should **not** be combined with beta-blockers; constipation is the most common side-effect.

5. *ACE inhibitors*—Captopril (section 2.5.5) is a potent vasodilator; proteinuria, rashes, and leucopenia were described at the high doses used previously but few side-effects are encountered with doses below 100 mg daily. Enalapril (section 2.5.5) is newer and longer acting. Both captopril and enalapril may cause a precipitate drop in blood pressure in patients with renal impairment and/or receiving diuretic therapy; they should be given in low initial doses and where possible diuretic therapy should be omitted for a few days before starting.

6. *Vasodilator therapy*—patients are usually maintained on a thiazide with a beta-blocker and a vasodilator is added to this regimen. Hydralazine (section 2.5.1) 25 to 50 mg may be given twice daily; higher doses can cause a lupus erythematosus-like syndrome.

Diazoxide and minoxidil (section 2.5.1) are extremely potent vasodilator antihypertensive drugs, with many side-effects. They should only be used where other vasodilators have failed.

7. *Other drugs*—The addition of either methyldopa or prazosin to beta-blocker/thiazide/hydralazine therapy is sometimes effective.

SYSTOLIC HYPERTENSION. High systolic blood pressure carries a poor prognosis. This may be because the height of the systolic blood pressure reflects evidence of end-organ damage caused by the hypertension itself. The quality of control of systolic blood pressure may have some importance in determining the outcome in patients with antihypertensive treatment.

HYPERTENSION IN PREGNANCY. It is important to control blood pressure in pregnancy. High blood pressure may be due to pre-existing essential hypertension or to pre-eclampsia. Oral methyldopa or atenolol or labetalol are safe in pregnancy. Thiazides and other diuretics are best avoided as they may reduce placental blood flow. Hydralazine by mouth is useful as second-line therapy, and by intravenous injection can be used to control hypertensive crises associated with eclampsia.

HYPERTENSION IN THE ELDERLY. There is evidence that treating hypertension in patients up to the age of 80 years is worthwhile provided treatment is carefully supervised. Little or no benefit has been shown in those over 80.

DRUG INTERACTIONS. The effects of antihypertensive drugs are modified by a number of other drugs. See Appendix 1 (sections 2.5 and *15*), and also under individual entries.

2.5.1 Vasodilator antihypertensive drugs

These are potent drugs, especially when used in combination with a beta-blocker and a thiazide.

Diazoxide is diabetogenic and is not used by mouth, except in very severe hypertension; it can be used by intravenous injection in hypertensive emergencies.

Hydralazine given by mouth is a useful adjunct to other treatment, but when used alone causes tachycardia and fluid retention. Side-effects can be few if the dose is kept below 100 mg daily.

Sodium nitroprusside is given by intravenous infusion to control severe hypertensive crises.

Minoxidil should be reserved for the treatment of severe hypertension resistant to other drugs. Vasodilatation is accompanied by increased cardiac output and tachycardia and the patients develop fluid retention. For this reason a beta-blocker and a diuretic (usually frusemide) are mandatory. Hypertrichosis is troublesome and renders this drug unsuitable for women.

Prazosin and **terazosin** (section 2.5.4) have alpha-blocking and vasodilator properties.

DIAZOXIDE

Indications: hypertensive crisis (for use in hypoglycaemia, see section 6.1.4)

Cautions: ischaemic heart disease, pregnancy, labour, impaired renal function. Drug interactions: see Appendix 1 (section *6.1*)

Side-effects: tachycardia, hyperglycaemia, fluid retention

Dose: by rapid intravenous injection (less than 30 seconds), 1–3 mg/kg to max. single dose of 150 mg (see below); may be repeated after 5–15 minutes if required

Note. Single doses of 300 mg have been associated with angina and with myocardial and cerebral infarction

PoM **Eudemine®** (A&H)
Injection, diazoxide 15 mg/ml. Net price 20-ml amp = £2.70

HYDRALAZINE HYDROCHLORIDE

Indications: moderate to severe hypertension, with beta-blocker and thiazide; hypertensive crisis

Cautions: reduce initial dose in renal impairment; over-rapid blood pressure reduction is occasionally encountered even with low parenteral doses

Side-effects: tachycardia, fluid retention, nausea, and vomiting; systemic lupus erythematosus-like syndrome after long-term therapy with over 100 mg daily (or less in women)

Dose: by mouth, 25 mg twice daily, increased to a max. of 50 mg twice daily (see notes above)

By slow intravenous injection, 5–20 mg over 20 minutes; may be repeated after 20–30 minutes (see Cautions)

By intravenous infusion, 20 mg, repeated if necessary

PoM **Hydralazine** (Non-proprietary)
Tablets, hydralazine hydrochloride 25 mg, net price 20 = 27p; 50 mg, 20 = 55p
PoM **Apresoline**® (Ciba)
Tablets, both s/c, hydralazine hydrochloride 25 mg (yellow), net price 20 = 36p; 50 mg (violet), 20 = 70p
Injection, powder for reconstitution, hydralazine hydrochloride. Net price 20-mg amp = 32p

MINOXIDIL

Indications: severe hypertension, in addition to a diuretic and a beta-blocker

Cautions: avoid oedema, may aggravate heart failure and angina, lower doses in dialysis patients

Contra-indications: phaeochromocytoma

Side-effects: gastro-intestinal disturbances, weight gain, peripheral oedema, tachycardia, hypertrichosis, breast tenderness

Dose: initially 5 mg daily, in 1–2 doses, increased by 5–10 mg every 3 or more days; max. usually 50 mg daily

PoM **Loniten**® (Upjohn)
Tablets, all scored, minoxidil 2.5 mg, net price 20 = £2.38; 5 mg, 20 = £4.25; 10 mg, 20 = £8.24

SODIUM NITROPRUSSIDE

Indications: hypertensive crisis (but see notes in section 2.5); controlled hypotension in surgery; acute or chronic heart failure

Cautions: hypothyroidism, severe renal impairment, impaired cerebral circulation, elderly patients; monitor plasma-cyanide concentration

Contra-indications: severe hepatic impairment; vitamin B_{12} deficiency; Leber's optic atrophy; compensatory hypertension

Side-effects: headache, dizziness, nausea, retching, abdominal pain, perspiration, palpitations, apprehension, retrosternal discomfort—reduce infusion rate

Dose: hypertensive crisis, in patients not already receiving antihypertensives, *by intravenous infusion*, 0.3–1 micrograms/kg/minute initially, then adjusted; usual range 0.5–6 micrograms/kg/minute (usual range 20–400 micrograms/minute; max. 8 micrograms/kg/minute); lower doses for patients already being treated with antihypertensives

Lower doses should also be employed for con-trolled hypotension in surgery (max. 1.5 micrograms/kg/minute)

Heart failure, *by intravenous infusion*, initially 10–15 micrograms/minute, increased every 5–10 minutes as necessary; usual range 10–200 micrograms/minute; max. 400 micrograms/minute (6 micrograms/kg/minute)

PoM **Sodium Nitroprusside** (Non-proprietary)
Intravenous solution, sodium nitroprusside 10 mg/ml. For dilution and use as an infusion. Net price 5-ml vial = £1.77
PoM **Nipride**® (Roche)
Infusion, sodium nitroprusside 50-mg amp (with solvent for reconstitution). Net price = £4.00

2.5.2   Centrally acting antihypertensive drugs

This group includes methyldopa and clonidine and is largely falling from use.

Methyldopa, however, has the advantage of being safe in asthmatics, in heart failure, and in pregnancy. Side-effects are minimised if the daily dose is kept below 1 g.

Clonidine has the disadvantage that sudden withdrawal may cause a hypertensive crisis. Reserpine and rauwolfia are not used much in Britain but if their dose is kept low and they are taken at night, blood pressure control can be achieved with few side-effects in mild hypertension.

CLONIDINE HYDROCHLORIDE

Indications: hypertension (for use in migraine, see section 4.7.4.2)

Cautions: must be withdrawn gradually to avoid hypertensive crisis. Drug interactions: see Appendix 1 (section 2.5)

Contra-indications: history of depression

Side-effects: dry mouth, sedation, depression, fluid retention, bradycardia, Raynaud's phenomenon

Dose: by mouth, 50–100 micrograms 3 times daily, increased every second or third day; max. daily dose usually 1.2 mg

By slow intravenous injection, 150–300 micrograms; max. 750 micrograms in 24 hours

PoM **Catapres**® (Boehringer Ingelheim)
Tablets, both scored, clonidine hydrochloride 100 micrograms, net price 20 = £1.21; 300 micrograms, 20 = £2.99. Label: 3, 8
Perlongets® (= capsules s/r), red/yellow, clonidine hydrochloride 250 micrograms. Net price 56-tab pack = £12.74. Label: 3, 8, 25
Dose: initially 250 micrograms in the evening; maintenance usually 250–750 micrograms daily in divided doses
Injection, clonidine hydrochloride 150 micrograms/ml. Net price 1-ml amp = 27p
Dixarit (migraine), see section 4.7.4.2

METHYLDOPA

Indications: hypertension, in conjunction with diuretic; hypertensive crisis

---

Cautions: positive direct Coombs' test in 20% of patients (may affect blood cross-matching); interference with laboratory tests; reduce initial dose in renal impairment; blood counts and liver-function tests advised. Drug interactions: see Appendix 1 (sections *4.2, 4.9*)

Contra-indications: history of depression, active liver disease, phaeochromocytoma

Side-effects: dry mouth, sedation, depression, drowsiness, diarrhoea, fluid retention, failure of ejaculation, liver damage, haemolytic anaemia, systemic lupus erythematosus-like syndrome

Dose: by mouth, 250 mg 2–3 times daily, gradually increased; max. daily dose 3 g

By intravenous infusion, methyldopa hydrochloride 250–500 mg, repeated after 6 hours if required

PoM **Methyldopa** (Non-proprietary)
Tablets, f/c, methyldopa (anhydrous) 125 mg, net price 20 = 52p; 250 mg, 20 = 68p; 500 mg, 20 = £1.38. Label: 3, 8

PoM **Aldomet**® (MSD)
Tablets, all yellow, f/c, methyldopa (anhydrous) 125 mg, net price 20 = 77p; 250 mg, 20 = £1.19; 500 mg, 20 = £2.34. Label: 3, 8
Suspension, methyldopa 250 mg/5 ml. Do not dilute. Net price 200 ml = £3.96. Label: 3, 8
Injection, methyldopa hydrochloride 50 mg/ml. Net price 5-ml amp = £2.31

PoM **Dopamet**® (Berk)
Tablets, all yellow, f/c, methyldopa (anhydrous) 125 mg, net price 20 = 43p; 250 mg, 20 = 73p; 500 mg, 20 = £1.46. Label: 3, 8

PoM **Medomet**® (DDSA)
Capsules, yellow, methyldopa (anhydrous) 250 mg, net price 20 = 52p. Label: 3, 8
Tablets, yellow, f/c, methyldopa (anhydrous) 250 mg, net price 20 = 53p; 500 mg, 20 = £1.14. Label: 3, 8

Compound preparations
PoM **Hydromet**® (MSD)
Tablets, pink, f/c, methyldopa (anhydrous) 250 mg, hydrochlorothiazide 15 mg. Net price 20 = £1.52. Label: 3, 8

RESERPINE AND RAUWOLFIA ALKALOIDS

Indications: hypertension
Cautions: late pregnancy, breast-feeding. Drug interactions: see Appendix 1 (sections 2.5, *4.3, 4.9*)
Contra-indications: history of depression, phaeochromocytoma, peptic ulcer, Parkinson's disease
Side-effects: dry mouth, nasal congestion, sedation, depression, postural hypotension, bradycardia, fluid retention

PoM **Reserpine** (Non-proprietary)
Tablets, reserpine 100 micrograms, net price 20 = 9p; 250 micrograms, 20 = 18p. Label: 3

PoM **Decaserpyl**® (Roussel)
Tablets, scored, methoserpidine 5 mg, net price 20 = £1.71; 10 mg (pink), 20 = £3.13. Label: 3

PoM **Hypercal**® (Carlton)
Tablets, rauwolfia alkaloids 2 mg. Net price 20 = 10p. Label: 3

PoM **Serpasil**® (Ciba)
Tablets, blue, reserpine 100 micrograms, net price 20 = 9p; 250 micrograms (scored), 20 = 19p. Label: 3

Compound preparations
PoM **Decaserpyl Plus**® (Roussel)
Tablets, scored, methoserpidine 10 mg, benzthiazide 20 mg. Net price 20 = £3.34. Label: 3

PoM **Serpasil-Esidrex**® (Ciba)
Tablets, scored, reserpine 150 micrograms, hydrochlorothiazide 10 mg. Net price 20 = 38p. Label: 3

With barbiturate
Note. There is no justification for the use of barbiturates in the treatment of hypertension

CD **Hypercal-B**® (Carlton)
Tablets, rauwolfia alkaloids 2 mg, amylobarbitone 15 mg. Net price 20 = 10p. Label: 2

2.5.3 Adrenergic neurone blocking drugs

These drugs prevent the release of noradrenaline from postganglionic adrenergic neurones. Guanethidine also depletes the nerve endings of noradrenaline. These drugs do not control supine blood pressure and may cause postural hypotension. For this reason they have largely fallen from use, but they may be necessary in combination with other therapy in resistant hypertension.

BETHANIDINE SULPHATE

Indications: hypertension, in conjunction with diuretic or beta-blocker
Cautions; Contra-indications; Side-effects: see under Guanethidine Monosulphate (except diarrhoea)
Dose: 10 mg 3 times daily after food, increased by 5 mg at intervals; max. daily dose 200 mg

PoM **Bethanidine** (Non-proprietary)
Tablets, bethanidine sulphate 10 mg, net price 20 = 95p; 50 mg, 20 = £4.20. Label: 21

PoM **Bendogen**® (Lagap)
Tablets, scored, bethanidine sulphate 10 mg, net price 20 = 95p; 50 mg, 20 = £4.20. Label: 21

PoM **Esbatal**® (Calmic)
Tablets, peach, scored, bethanidine sulphate 10 mg, net price 20 = £1.64; 50 mg, 20 = £7.38. Label: 21

DEBRISOQUINE

Indications: hypertension, in conjunction with a diuretic or beta-blocker
Cautions; Contra-indications; Side-effects: see under Guanethidine Monosulphate (except diarrhoea)
Dose: 10 mg 1–2 times daily, increased by 10 mg every 3 days; max. daily dose usually 120 mg

PoM **Declinax**® (Roche)
Tablets, both scored, debrisoquine (as sulphate) 10 mg, net price 20 = 77p; 20 mg (blue), 20 = £1.12

GUANETHIDINE MONOSULPHATE

Indications: hypertension, in conjunction with diuretic or beta-blocker

Cautions: postural hypotension may cause falls in elderly patients; pregnancy. Drug interactions: see Appendix 1 (section 2.5)

Contra-indications: phaeochromocytoma, renal failure

Side-effects: postural hypotension, failure of ejaculation, fluid retention, nasal congestion, diarrhoea

Dose: by mouth, 20 mg daily, increased by 10 mg at weekly intervals; max. daily dose usually 100 mg

By intramuscular injection, 10–20 mg, repeated after 3 hours if required

PoM **Ismelin**® (Ciba)
Tablets, guanethidine monosulphate 10 mg, net price 20 = 46p; 25 mg (pink), 20 = £1.03
Injection, guanethidine monosulphate 10 mg/ml. Net price 1-ml amp = 23p

2.5.4 Alpha-adrenoceptor blocking drugs

Prazosin has post-synaptic alpha-blocking and vasodilator properties and rarely causes tachycardia. It may, however, cause a rapid reduction in blood pressure after the first dose and should be introduced with caution. **Terazosin** has properties similar to those of prazosin.

Phenoxybenzamine and **indoramin** are alpha-blockers which are effective agents, but have many side-effects. They can be used in conjunction with beta-blockers and/or diuretics. Phenoxybenzamine is used with a beta-blocker in the short-term management of severe hypertensive episodes associated with phaeochromocytoma.

Phentolamine is used rarely as a suppression test for phaeochromocytoma.

INDORAMIN

Indications: hypertension, usually in conjunction with thiazide or beta-blocker

Cautions: patient's ability to drive or operate machinery may be impaired; avoid alcohol (enhances rate and extent of absorption); control incipient heart failure with diuretics and digoxin; hepatic or renal impairment; elderly patients; Parkinson's disease; epilepsy (convulsions in *animal* studies); history of depression

Contra-indications: established heart failure; patients receiving MAOIs

Side-effects: sedation; also dizziness, depression, failure of ejaculation, dry mouth, nasal congestion, extrapyramidal effects

Dose: initially 25 mg twice daily, increased by 25–50 mg daily at intervals of 2 weeks; max. daily dose 200 mg in 2–3 divided doses

▼ PoM **Baratol**® (Wyeth)
Tablets, both f/c, indoramin (as hydrochloride) 25 mg (blue), net price 20 = £2.86; 50 mg (green), scored, 20 = £5.07. Label: 2

PHENOXYBENZAMINE HYDROCHLORIDE

Indications: phaeochromocytoma only (see notes above)

Cautions: elderly patients; congestive heart failure; ischaemic heart disease, marked arteriosclerosis; renal impairment; carcinogenic in *animals*

Side-effects: postural hypotension with dizziness and marked tachycardia, lassitude, nasal congestion, miosis, retrograde ejaculation; rarely gastro-intestinal disturbances

Dose: by mouth, phaeochromocytoma, 10 mg daily, increased by 10 mg daily; usual dose 1–2 mg/kg daily in 2 divided doses

PoM **Dibenyline**® (SK&F)
Capsules, red/white, phenoxybenzamine hydrochloride 10 mg. Net price 20 = £2.13
Injection, phenoxybenzamine hydrochloride 50 mg/ml. To be diluted before use. 2-ml amp (Hosp. only)

PHENTOLAMINE MESYLATE

Indications: hypertensive crises due to phaeochromocytoma or interaction of foods with MAOIs, clonidine withdrawal; acute left ventricular failure

Side-effects: hypotension, tachycardia, dizziness; nausea, diarrhoea, nasal congestion after high doses

Dose: by intravenous injection, 5–10 mg repeated as necessary

By intravenous infusion, 5–60 mg over 10–30 minutes at a rate of 0.1–2 mg/minute

PoM **Rogitine**® (Ciba)
Injection, phentolamine mesylate 10 mg/ml. Net price 1-ml amp = 27p; 5-ml amp = £1.32

PRAZOSIN HYDROCHLORIDE

Indications: see under Dose

Cautions: first dose may cause collapse due to hypotension (therefore should be taken on retiring to bed); reduce initial dose in renal failure. Drug interactions: see Appendix 1 (section 2.5)

Side-effects: postural hypotension, drowsiness, weakness

Dose: hypertension, 500 micrograms 2–3 times daily, the initial dose on retiring to bed at night (to avoid collapse, see Cautions); increased to a max. of 20 mg daily

Congestive heart failure, 500 micrograms initially (at bedtime, see above); then 1 mg 3–4 times daily; maintenance 4–20 mg daily

Raynaud's syndrome, initially 500 micrograms twice daily (initial dose at bedtime, see above); maintenance 1–2 mg twice daily

Benign prostatic hypertrophy, initially 500 micrograms twice daily for 3–7 days (initial dose at bedtime, see above), dose subsequently adjusted according to response; usual maintenance (and max.) 2 mg twice daily

PoM **Hypovase**® (Pfizer)
Tablets, prazosin hydrochloride 500 micrograms, net price 20 = 86p; 1 mg (orange, scored), 20 = £1.11; 2 mg (scored), 20 = £1.50; 5 mg (scored), 20 = £3.24. Label: 3, counselling advised, see dose above

B.d. starter pack, 8 tablets, prazosin hydrochloride 500 micrograms; 32 orange tablets, prazosin hydrochloride 1 mg. Net price = £2.90. Label: 3, counselling advised, see dose above

TERAZOSIN

Indications: mild to moderate hypertension
Cautions: first dose may cause collapse due to hypotension (within 30–90 minutes, therefore should be taken on retiring to bed) (may also occur with rapid dose increase). Drug interactions: see Appendix 1 (section 2.5)
Side-effects: dizziness, lack of energy, peripheral oedema
Dose: 1 mg at bedtime (compliance with bedtime dose important to avoid collapse, see Cautions); dose doubled after 7 days if necessary; usual maintenance dose 2–10 mg daily; more than 20 mg daily rarely improves efficacy

▼ PoM **Hytrin**® (Abbott)
Tablets, terazosin (as hydrochloride) 2 mg (yellow), net price 28 = £12.32; 5 mg (tan), 28 = £16.63; 10 mg (blue), 28 = £23.41. Label: 3, counselling advised, see dose above
Starter pack, 7 white tablets terazosin (as hydrochloride) 1 mg; 7 yellow tablets terazosin (as hydrochloride) 2 mg. Net price per pack = £6.79. Label: 3, counselling advised, see dose above

2.5.5 Angiotensin-converting enzyme inhibitors

(ACE inhibitors)

Captopril (Capoten®, Acepril®) and **enalapril** (Innovace®) inhibit the conversion of angiotensin I to angiotensin II. They are effective and generally well tolerated, but experience is limited as regards long-term use.

They should therefore be considered for *hypertension* only when thiazides and beta-blockers are contra-indicated, not tolerated, or fail to control blood pressure. Both may cause very rapid falls of blood pressure in some patients. Therefore where possible diuretic therapy should be stopped for a few days before initiating therapy and the first dose should preferably be given at bedtime.

Captopril and enalapril are also used in the treatment of *heart failure*, as adjuncts to digitalis and diuretics. Since it may not be possible to

suspend diuretics in heart failure treatment should be initiated under direct supervision in hospital.

CAPTOPRIL

Indications: mild to moderate hypertension as an adjunct to thiazide therapy; severe hypertension resistant to other treatment; adjunctive treatment in severe congestive heart failure
Cautions: where possible stop any diuretic a few days before initiating; first doses may cause hypotension especially in patients taking diuretics, on a low-sodium diet, on dialysis, or dehydrated; monitor renal function; reduce dose or avoid in renal impairment (white cell counts and urinary protein estimations needed). Drug interactions: see Appendix 1 (sections 2.2, 2.5, 4.2, 4.7, 8)
Contra-indications: pregnancy (toxicity in *animal* studies)
Side-effects: persistent dry cough; loss of taste, stomatosis, abdominal pain, rash, angioedema, hypotension (see Cautions); proteinuria, agranulocytosis, neutropenia, hyperkalaemia (all more common in renal impairment)
Dose: hypertension, used alone, initially 12.5 mg twice daily; used in addition to a diuretic, in elderly, or in renal impairment, initially 6.25 mg twice daily (first dose at bedtime); usual maintenance dose 25 mg twice daily; max. 50 mg twice daily (rarely 3 times daily in severe hypertension)
Heart failure, with a diuretic, initially 6.25–12.5 mg under close hospital supervision; usual maintenance dose 25 mg 3 times daily

▼ PoM **Acepril**® (DF)
Tablets, captopril 12.5 mg (scored), net price 100 = £16.40; 25 mg, 56-tab pack = £13.37, 100 = £23.88; 50 mg (scored), 56-tab pack = £20.50, 100 = £36.61
▼ PoM **Capoten**® (Squibb)
Tablets, captopril 12.5 mg (scored), net price 100 = £16.40; 25 mg, 56-tab pack = £13.37, 100 = £23.88; 50 mg (scored), 56-tab pack = £20.50, 100 = £36.61

With diuretic
▼ PoM **Acezide**® (DF)
Tablets, scored, captopril 50 mg, hydrochlorothiazide 25 mg. Net price 28-tab pack = £16.07
▼ PoM **Capozide**® (Squibb)
Tablets, scored, captopril 50 mg, hydrochlorothiazide 25 mg. Net price 28-tab pack = £16.07

ENALAPRIL MALEATE

Indications: all grades of essential hypertension and renovascular hypertension (where standard therapy is ineffective or inappropriate); congestive heart failure (adjunct)
Cautions; Contra-indications: see under Captopril

Side-effects: persistent dry cough; dizziness, headache, fatigue, weakness, hypotension (see Cautions), change of taste, nausea, diarrhoea, muscle cramps, rash, and angioedema

Dose: hypertension, used alone, initially 5 mg daily; used in addition to a diuretic, in elderly patients, or in renal impairment, initially 2.5 mg daily; usual maintenance dose 10–20 mg daily; max. 40 mg daily

Heart failure, with a diuretic, initially 2.5 mg daily under close hospital supervision

▼ PoM **Innovace**® (MSD)
Tablets, enalapril maleate 2.5 mg, net price 50 = £10.00; 5 mg (scored), 28-tab pack = £7.86, 50 = £14.03; 10 mg (red), 28-tab pack = £11.03, 50 = £19.69; 20 mg (peach), 28-tab pack = £13.10, 50 = £23.40

2.5.6   Ganglion-blocking drugs

Trimetaphan is used to provide hypotension in surgery.

TRIMETAPHAN CAMSYLATE
Indications: see notes above
Cautions: hepatic or renal impairment, diabetes mellitus, Addison's disease, CNS degenerative disease
Contra-indications: severe arteriosclerosis or cardiac disease
Side-effects: tachycardia and respiratory depression (particularly with muscle relaxants); pupillary dilatation
Dose: by intravenous infusion, 3–4 mg/minute initially, then adjusted according to response

PoM **Arfonad**® (Roche)
Injection, trimetaphan camsylate 50 mg/ml. Net price 5-ml amp = £3.12

2.5.7   Tyrosine hydroxylase inhibitors

Metirosine inhibits the enzyme tyrosine hydroxylase, and hence the synthesis of catecholamines. It is used in the pre-operative management of phaeochromocytoma, and long term in patients unsuitable for surgery; an alpha-adrenoceptor blocking drug (e.g. phenoxybenzamine) may also be required. Metirosine should **not** be used to treat essential hypertension.

METIROSINE
Indications: see notes above
Cautions: maintain high fluid intake and adequate blood volume; may impair ability to drive or operate machinery. Drug interactions: see Appendix 1 (sections 2.5, 4.9)
Side-effects: sedation; extrapyramidal symptoms; diarrhoea (may be severe); hypersensitivity reactions
Dose: initially 250 mg 4 times daily, increased to max. of 4 g daily in divided doses; doses of 2–3 g daily should be given for 5–7 days before surgery

PoM **Demser**® (MSD)
Capsules, blue, metirosine 250 mg (Hosp. only). Label: 2

2.6   Nitrates and other vasodilators, and calcium-channel blockers

2.6.1 Nitrates
2.6.2 Calcium-channel blockers
2.6.3 Peripheral vasodilators
2.6.4 Cerebral vasodilators

Most patients with *angina pectoris* are treated with beta-blockers (section 2.4) or calcium-channel blockers (section 2.6.2). However, short-acting nitrates (section 2.6.1) retain an important role both for prophylactic use before exertion and for chest pain occurring at rest. Nitrates are sometimes used as sole therapy, especially in elderly patients with infrequent symptoms.

Vasodilators act in *heart failure* either by:
arteriolar dilatation which reduces both peripheral vascular resistance and left ventricular pressure at systole and results in improved cardiac output, *or*
venous dilatation which results in a dilatation of capacitance vessels, an increase of venous pooling, and diminution of venous return to the heart thus decreasing left ventricular end-diastolic pressure.

Three groups of drugs should be considered—nitrates (section 2.6.1) which act predominantly by venous dilatation; captopril and enalapril (section 2.5.5) and hydralazine (section 2.5.1) which act predominantly by arteriolar dilatation; and phentolamine and prazosin (section 2.5.4) and sodium nitroprusside (section 2.5.1) which produce both arteriolar and venous dilatation. Combinations of drugs with different effects can be tried. Abrupt withdrawal of treatment may be hazardous.

2.6.1   Nitrates

Sublingual **glyceryl trinitrate** is one of the most effective drugs for providing rapid symptomatic relief, but its effect lasts only for 20 to 30 minutes. Though a potent coronary vasodilator, its principal benefit follows from a reduction in venous return which reduces left ventricular work. Unwanted effects such as flushing, headache, and postural hypotension may limit therapy, especially when angina is severe or when patients are unusually sensitive to the effects of nitrates. The 300-microgram tablet is often appropriate when glyceryl trinitrate is first used and tolerance to the unwanted effects has not developed. Duration of action may be prolonged by slow-release preparations. The aerosol spray provides an alternative method of rapid relief of symptoms for those who find difficulty in dissolving sublingual preparations. The percutaneous preparations may be useful in the prophylaxis of angina for patients who suffer attacks at rest, especially at night.

Isosorbide dinitrate is active sublingually and is a more stable preparation for those who only require nitrates infrequently. It is also effective by mouth for prophylaxis; although the effect is slower in onset, it may persist for several hours. Duration of action of up to 12 hours is claimed for sustained-release preparations. The activity of isosorbide dinitrate may depend on the production of active metabolites, the most important of which is isosorbide mononitrate. **Isosorbide mononitrate** itself is also available for angina prophylaxis, though the advantages over isosorbide dinitrate have not yet been firmly established.

Glyceryl trinitrate injection or isosorbide dinitrate injection may be tried when the sublingual form is ineffective in patients with chest pain due to myocardial infarction or severe ischaemia. The intravenous preparations are also useful in the treatment of acute left ventricular failure.

GLYCERYL TRINITRATE

Indications: prophylaxis and treatment of angina; left ventricular failure
Cautions: hypotensive conditions. Drug interactions: see Appendix 1 (section 2.5, 2.6)
Side-effects: throbbing headache, flushing, dizziness, postural hypotension, tachycardia
Dose: sublingually, 0.3–1 mg, repeated as required
By mouth, 2.6–6.4 mg as sustained-release tablets, 2–3 times daily
By intravenous infusion, 10–200 micrograms/minute

Short-acting tablets and sprays
Glyceryl Trinitrate (Non-proprietary)
Tablets, glyceryl trinitrate 300 micrograms, net price 100 = £1.06; 500 micrograms, 100 = 44p; 600 micrograms, 100 = 58p. Label: 16
Note. Glyceryl trinitrate tablets should be supplied in glass containers of not more than 100 tablets, closed with a foil-lined cap, and containing no cotton wool wadding; they should be discarded after 8 weeks in use
▼ **Coro-Nitro Spray®** (MCP)
Aerosol spray, glyceryl trinitrate 400 micrograms/metered dose. Net price 200-dose unit = £3.36
Dose: treatment or prophylaxis of angina, 1–2 metered doses sprayed on the oral mucosa (preferably on or under the tongue) and the mouth then closed
Caution: flammable
GTN 300 mcg (Martindale)
Tablets, glyceryl trinitrate 300 micrograms. Net price 100 = 80p. Label: 16
▼ **Nitrolingual Spray®** (Lipha)
Aerosol spray, glyceryl trinitrate 400 micrograms/metered dose. Net price 200-dose unit = £4.36
Dose: treatment or prophylaxis of angina, spray 1–2 doses on the oral mucosa (preferably on or under tongue) and then close mouth
Note. No need to shake canister; caution flammable

Sustained-release tablets
Nitrocontin Continus® (Degussa)
Tablets, s/r, pink, glyceryl trinitrate 2.6 mg. Net price 20 = 67p. Label: 25
Tablets, s/r, pink, glyceryl trinitrate 6.4 mg. Net price 20 = 88p. Label: 25
Suscard Buccal® (Pharmax)
Tablets, s/r, glyceryl trinitrate 1 mg. Net price 20 = £1.93. Counselling advised, see administration below
Tablets, s/r, glyceryl trinitrate 2 mg. Net price 20 = £2.87. Counselling advised, see administration below
Tablets, s/r, glyceryl trinitrate 3 mg. Net price 20 = £4.02. Counselling advised, see administration below
Tablets, s/r, glyceryl trinitrate 5 mg. Net price 20 = £5.63. Counselling advised, see administration below
Dose: treatment of angina, 1–2 mg as required; prophylaxis 1–2 mg 3 times daily; 5 mg in severe angina
Congestive heart failure, 5 mg 3 times daily, increased to 10 mg 3 times daily in severe cases
Administration. Tablets are placed between upper lip and gum, and left to dissolve
Sustac® (Pharmax)
Tablets, s/r, pink, glyceryl trinitrate 2.6 mg. Net price 20 = £1.19. Label: 25
Tablets, s/r, pink, glyceryl trinitrate 6.4 mg. Net price 20 = £1.72. Label: 25
Tablets, s/r, pink, glyceryl trinitrate 10 mg. Net price 20 = £2.39. Label: 25
Dose: severe angina, 10 mg 3 times daily

Parenteral preparations
▼ PoM **Glyceryl Trinitrate** (Non-proprietary)
Injection, glyceryl trinitrate 5 mg/ml. To be diluted before use. Net price 5-ml amp = £8.50; 10-ml amp = £17.00
Note. Glass or polyethylene apparatus is preferable; loss of potency will occur if PVC is used
▼ PoM **Nitrocine®** (Schwarz)
Injection, glyceryl trinitrate 1 mg/ml. To be diluted before use or given undiluted with syringe pump. Net price 10-ml amp = £9.45; 50-ml bottle = £22.15
Note. Glass or polyethylene apparatus is preferable; loss of potency will occur if PVC is used
▼ PoM **Nitronal®** (Lipha)
Injection, glyceryl trinitrate 1 mg/ml. To be diluted before use or given undiluted with syringe pump. Net price 5-ml vial = £2.20; 25-ml vial = £7.50; 50-ml vial = £18.00
Note. Glass or polyethylene apparatus is preferable; loss of potency will occur if PVC is used
▼ PoM **Tridil®** (Du Pont)
Injection, glyceryl trinitrate 500 micrograms/ml. To be diluted before use. Net price 10-ml amp = £4.50
Injection, glyceryl trinitrate 5 mg/ml. To be diluted before use. Net price 10-ml amp = £21.88; 10-ml amp with polyethylene giving set = £24.98
Note. Glass or polyethylene apparatus is preferable; loss of potency will occur if PVC is used

---

Transdermal preparations

▼ Deponit® (Schwarz)

'5' dressing, self-adhesive, peach-coloured, releasing glyceryl trinitrate approx. 5 mg/24 hours when in contact with skin. Net price 30 = £19.25. Counselling advised, see administration below

'10' dressing, self-adhesive, peach-coloured, releasing glyceryl trinitrate approx. 10 mg/24 hours when in contact with skin. Net price 30 = £21.19. Counselling advised, see administration below

Administration: prophylaxis of angina, apply 1 dressing to lateral chest wall; replace every 24 hours, siting replacement dressing on different area

▼ Percutol® (Rorer)

Ointment, glyceryl trinitrate 2%. Net price 30 g = £3.97. Counselling advised, see administration below

Administration: prophylaxis of angina, ½–2 inches of ointment measured on to Applirule, which is applied to body (usually chest, arm, or thigh) without rubbing in, and secured with a dressing; repeat every 3–4 hours or as required *Note.* 1 inch of ointment contains glyceryl trinitrate 16.64 mg

▼ Transiderm-Nitro® (Geigy)

'5' dressing, self-adhesive, pink, releasing glyceryl trinitrate approx. 5 mg/24 hours when in contact with skin. Net price 30 = £19.33. Counselling advised, see administration below

'10' dressing, self-adhesive, pink, releasing glyceryl trinitrate approx. 10 mg/24 hours when in contact with skin. Net price 30 = £21.26. Counselling advised, see administration below

Administration: prophylaxis of angina, apply 1 dressing to lateral chest wall; replace every 24 hours, siting replacement dressing on different area

---

ISOSORBIDE DINITRATE

Indications: prophylaxis and treatment of angina; left ventricular failure

Cautions; Side-effects: see under Glyceryl Trinitrate

Dose: sublingually, 5–10 mg

By mouth, daily in divided doses, angina 30–120 mg, left ventricular failure 40–160 mg, up to 240 mg if required

By intravenous infusion, 2–10 mg/hour

Short-acting tablets

Cedocard-5® (Tillotts)

Tablets (sublingual), scored, isosorbide dinitrate 5 mg. Net price 20 = 44p

Cedocard-10® (Tillotts)

Tablets, pink, scored, isosorbide dinitrate 10 mg. Net price 20 = 31p

PoM **Cedocard-20®** (Tillotts)

Tablets, blue, scored, isosorbide dinitrate 20 mg. Net price 20 = 58p

Cedocard-40® (Tillotts)

Tablets, green, scored, isosorbide dinitrate 40 mg. Net price 20 = £1.37

Isoket 5® (Schwarz)

Tablets, scored, isosorbide dinitrate 5 mg. Net price 20 = 24p (Hosp.)

Isoket 10® (Schwarz)

Tablets, scored, isosorbide dinitrate 10 mg. Net price 20 = 30p (Hosp.)

Isoket 20® (Schwarz)

Tablets, scored, isosorbide dinitrate 20 mg. Net price 20 = 48p (Hosp.)

Isordil® (Wyeth)

Tablets (sublingual), pink, isosorbide dinitrate 5 mg. Net price 20 = 27p. Label: 26

Tablets, scored, isosorbide dinitrate 10 mg. Net price 20 = 27p

Tablets, scored, isosorbide dinitrate 30 mg. Net price 20 = 64p

Sorbichew® (Stuart)

Tablets (chewable), green, scored, isosorbide dinitrate 5 mg. Net price 20 = 29p. Label: 24

Sorbitrate® (Stuart)

Tablets, yellow, scored, isosorbide dinitrate 10 mg. Net price 20 = 29p

Tablets, blue, scored, isosorbide dinitrate 20 mg. Net price 20 = 43p

Vascardin® (Nicholas)

Tablets, scored, isosorbide dinitrate 10 mg (as diluted isosorbide dinitrate). Net price 20 = 28p

Tablets, scored, isosorbide dinitrate 30 mg (as diluted isosorbide dinitrate). Net price 20 = 54p

Sustained-release tablets

Cedocard Retard-20® (Tillotts)

Tablets, s/r, yellow, scored, isosorbide dinitrate 20 mg. Net price 20 = £1.39. Label: 25

Dose: prophylaxis of angina, 1 tablet every 12 hours

Cedocard Retard-40® (Tillotts)

Tablets, s/r, orange-red, scored, isosorbide dinitrate 40 mg. Net price 20 = £3.22. Label: 25

Dose: prophylaxis of angina, 1–2 tablets every 12 hours

Isoket Retard-20® (Schwarz)

Tablets, s/r, yellow, scored, isosorbide dinitrate 20 mg. Net price 50-tab pack = £3.24. Label: 25

Dose: prophylaxis of angina, 20–40 mg every 12 hours

Isoket Retard-40® (Schwarz)

Tablets, s/r, orange, scored, isosorbide dinitrate 40 mg. Net price 50-tab pack = £7.99. Label: 25

Dose: prophylaxis of angina, 20–40 mg every 12 hours

Isordil Tembids® (Wyeth)

Capsules, s/r, blue/clear, isosorbide dinitrate 40 mg. Net price 20 = £1.50. Label: 25

Dose: prophylaxis of angina, 1 capsule 2–3 times daily

Soni-Slo® (Lipha)

Capsules, s/r, pink/clear, enclosing off-white pellets, isosorbide dinitrate 20 mg. Net price 20 = £1.19. Label: 25

Capsules, s/r, red/clear, enclosing off-white pellets, isosorbide dinitrate 40 mg. Net price 20 = £1.40. Label: 25

Dose: prophylaxis of angina, 40–80 mg daily in divided doses

Sorbid-20 SA® (Stuart)
Capsules, s/r, red/yellow, isosorbide dinitrate 20 mg. Net price 56-tab pack = £7.83. Label: 25
Dose: prophylaxis of angina, 1–2 capsules twice daily

Sorbid-40 SA® (Stuart)
Capsules, s/r, red/clear, isosorbide dinitrate 40 mg. Net price 56-tab pack = £9.00. Label: 25
Dose: prophylaxis of angina, 1–2 capsules twice daily

Parenteral preparations

PoM **Cedocard IV®** (Tillotts)
Injection, isosorbide dinitrate 1 mg/ml. To be diluted before use or given undiluted with syringe pump. Net price 10-ml amp = £3.94; 50-ml infusion bottle = £19.47; 100-ml infusion bottle = £26.85
Note. Glass or polyethylene infusion apparatus is preferable; loss of potency if PVC used

PoM **Isoket 0.1%®** (Schwarz)
Injection, isosorbide dinitrate 1 mg/ml. To be diluted before use. Net price 10-ml amp = £4.33; 50-ml infusion bottle = £21.50; 100-ml bottle = £29.69
Note. Glass or polyethylene infusion apparatus is preferable; loss of potency if PVC used

ISOSORBIDE MONONITRATE

Indications: prophylaxis and treatment of angina; adjunct in congestive heart failure
Cautions; Side-effects: see under Glyceryl Trinitrate
Dose: initially 20 mg 2–3 times daily (10 mg twice daily in those who have not previously received nitrates); up to 120 mg daily in divided doses if required

▼ PoM **Elantan 20®** (Schwarz)
Tablets, scored, isosorbide mononitrate 20 mg. Net price 20 = £1.64. Label: 25

▼ PoM **Elantan 40®** (Schwarz)
Tablets, scored, isosorbide mononitrate 40 mg. Net price 20 = £2.83. Label: 25

▼ **Elantan LA50®** (Schwarz)
Capsules s/r, pink/dark pink, enclosing white micropellets, isosorbide mononitrate 50 mg. Net price 30-cap pack = £12.19. Label: 25
Dose: prophylaxis of angina, 1 capsule daily in the morning

▼ PoM **Imdur®** (Astra)
Durules® (= tablets s/r), yellow, f/c, scored, isosorbide mononitrate 60 mg. Net price 28-tab pack = £11.43. Label: 25
Dose: prophylaxis of angina, 1 tablet in the morning, increased to 2 tablets if required

▼ PoM **Ismo®** (MCP)
Ismo 10 tablets, isosorbide mononitrate 10 mg. Net price 20 = £1.16. Label: 25
Ismo 20 tablets, isosorbide mononitrate 20 mg. Net price 20 = £1.60. Label: 25
Starter pack, 8 tablets, isosorbide mononitrate 10 mg; 60 tablets, scored, isosorbide mononitrate 20 mg. Net price = £5.52. Label: 25
Ismo 40 tablets, isosorbide mononitrate 40 mg. Net price 20 = £2.79. Label: 25

▼ PoM **Monit®** (Stuart)
Tablets, scored, isosorbide mononitrate 20 mg. Net price 28 = £2.39. Label: 25

▼ **Monit LS®** (Stuart)
Tablets, isosorbide mononitrate 10 mg. Net price 56-tab calendar pack = £3.32. Label: 25

▼ PoM **Mono-Cedocard 20®** (Tillotts)
Tablets, scored, isosorbide mononitrate 20 mg. Net price 20 = £1.75. Label: 25

▼ **Mono-Cedocard 40®** (Tillotts)
Tablets, scored, isosorbide mononitrate 40 mg. Net price 20 = £2.97. Label: 25

PENTAERYTHRITOL TETRANITRATE

Indications: prophylaxis of angina
Cautions; Side-effects: see under Glyceryl Trinitrate
Dose: see below

Cardiacap® (Consolidated)
Capsules, s/r, blue/yellow, pentaerythritol tetranitrate 30 mg. Net price 20 = 66p. Label: 22, 25
Dose: prophylaxis of angina, 30 mg every 12 hours

Mycardol® (Winthrop)
Tablets, scored, pentaerythritol tetranitrate 30 mg. Net price 20 = 78p. Label: 22
Dose: 2 tablets 3–4 times daily

2.6.2 Calcium-channel blockers

Calcium-channel blockers interfere with the inward displacement of calcium ions through the slow channels of active cell membranes. They influence the myocardial cells, the cells within the specialised conducting system of the heart, and the cells of vascular smooth muscle. Thus, myocardial contractility may be reduced, the formation and propagation of electrical impulses within the heart may be depressed, and coronary or systemic vascular tone may be diminished.

Calcium-channel blockers differ in their predelection for the various possible sites of action therefore their therapeutic effects are disparate, with much greater variation than those of beta-blockers. The indications, unwanted effects, and contra-indications of each calcium-channel blocker differ to a lesser or greater degree from the others; they cannot be considered as equivalents.

Verapamil is used for the treatment of angina, hypertension, and arrhythmias (section 2.3.2). It decreases myocardial contractility and influences the sinus node and particularly the atrioventricular node. It may precipitate heart failure, exacerbate conduction disorders, and cause hypotension at high doses and should be used with caution with beta-blockers.

Nifedipine relaxes vascular smooth muscle and dilates coronary and peripheral arteries. It has more influence on vessels and less on the myocardium than does verapamil, and unlike verapamil has no anti-arrhythmic activity. It rarely precipitates heart failure because any negative inotropic effect is offset by a reduction in left ventricular work. **Nicardipine** has similar effects;

Prices are **net**, see p. 1

it does not reduce myocardial contractility. Both drugs are valuable in forms of angina associated with unusual coronary constriction; they are useful as adjuncts to beta-blockers for patients with severe symptoms, and as alternative treatment for those who are intolerant of beta-blockers. Minor side-effects associated with vasodilatation such as flushing and headache (which become less obtrusive after a few days), and ankle swelling are common.

Nifedipine in a dose of 20 mg as a sustained-release preparation twice daily, increasing to 40 mg twice daily, is very useful in managing hypertensive patients, especially in conjunction with beta-blockers.

Diltiazem is effective in most forms of angina. It may be used in patients for whom beta-blockers are contra-indicated or ineffective, but because of the risk of bradycardia, should be used with caution with beta-blockers. Significant myocardial depression occurs rarely.

Lidoflazine is a long-acting coronary vaso-dilator. Increased exercise tolerance develops gradually over several weeks.

Prenylamine can cause an unusual form of ventricular tachycardia (torsade de pointes) especially in the presence of hypokalaemia, and usually associated with syncope. It should not, therefore, be regarded as a first-line drug. It is available on a named-patient basis only (as *Synadrin®*, Hoechst).

WITHDRAWAL. There is some evidence that sudden withdrawal of calcium-channel blockers may be associated with an exacerbation of angina.

DILTIAZEM HYDROCHLORIDE

Indications: prophylaxis and treatment of angina
Cautions: reduce dose in hepatic and renal impairment. Drug interactions: see Appendix 1 (section *2.1*, *2.3*, *2.4*, *2.6*, *4.2*, *4.8*, *8*)
Contra-indications: bradycardia, second- or third-degree heart block, sick sinus syndrome; pregnancy (toxicity in *animal* studies)
Side-effects: bradycardia, hypotension, ankle oedema; rarely headache, nausea, rashes
Dose: initially 60 mg 3 times daily (elderly patients twice daily); max. 360 mg daily

▼ PoM **Britiazim®** (Thames)
Tablets, diltiazem hydrochloride 60 mg. Net price 100 = £16.49
▼ PoM **Calcicard®** (Riker)
Tablets, off-white, diltiazem hydrochloride 60 mg. Net price 100 = £16.67
▼ PoM **Tildiem®** (Lorex)
Tablets, off-white, diltiazem hydrochloride 60 mg. Net price 100 = £16.67

LIDOFLAZINE

Indications: prophylaxis of angina
Cautions: may precipitate ventricular tachycardia; avoid in pregnancy. Drug interactions: see Appendix 1 (section 2.6)

Side-effects: gastro-intestinal upsets, dizziness, tinnitus, headaches; rarely bad dreams
Dose: 1st week, 120 mg once daily with or after food; 2nd week, 120 mg twice daily; 3rd and subsequent weeks, 120 mg 3 times daily

PoM **Clinium®** (Janssen)
Tablets, lidoflazine 120 mg. Net price 20 = £2.31.
Label: 21

NICARDIPINE HYDROCHLORIDE

Indications: prophylaxis and treatment of angina; mild to moderate hypertension
Cautions: withdraw if ischaemic pain occurs or existing pain worsens within 30 minutes of initiating treatment or increasing dose; hepatic or renal impairment. Drug interactions: see Appendix 1 (sections *2.1*, 2.6, *8*)
Contra-indications: advanced aortic stenosis
Side-effects: dizziness, headache, peripheral oedema, flushing, palpitations, nausea; also gastro-intestinal disturbances, drowsiness, hypotension, rashes, salivation, frequency of micturition
Dose: initially 20 mg 3 times daily, increased to 30 mg 3 times daily (usual range 60–120 mg daily); patients with hypertension controlled on 20–30 mg 3 times daily can be given 30–40 mg twice daily

▼ PoM **Cardene®** (Syntex)
Capsules, blue/white, nicardipine hydrochloride 20 mg. Net price 20 = £2.73
Capsules, blue/pale blue, nicardipine hydrochloride 30 mg. Net price 20 = £3.27

NIFEDIPINE

Indications: prophylaxis and treatment of angina; hypertension; Raynaud's phenomenon
Cautions: withdraw if ischaemic pain worsens shortly after initiating treatment; may inhibit labour. Drug interactions: see Appendix 1 (sections *2.1*, *2.4*, *2.5*, 2.6, *6.1*)
Contra-indications: cardiogenic shock
Side-effects: headache, flushing, lethargy; also peripheral oedema and gum hyperplasia
Dose: by mouth, angina, *capsules*, initially 10 mg 3 times daily with or after food, increased to 20 mg 3 times daily if necessary; in elderly patients, initially 5 mg 3 times daily; for immediate effect bite into capsule and retain liquid in mouth
Raynaud's phenomenon, *capsules*, 10 mg 3 times daily; max. 20 mg 3 times daily
Hypertension and angina prophylaxis, *tablets*, 20 mg twice daily after food (initial titration 10 mg twice daily), increased to 40 mg twice daily if necessary
By intracoronary injection, see preparation below

PoM **Nifedipine** (Non-proprietary)
Capsules, nifedipine 5 mg, net price 100 = £7.75; 10 mg, 100 = £12.20. Label: 21, counselling advised, see dose

---

PoM **Adalat**® (Bayer)
Capsules, both orange, nifedipine 5 mg, net price 20 = £1.63; 10 mg, 20 = £2.44. Label: 21, counselling advised, see dose

PoM **Adalat**® **Retard** (Bayer)
Tablets, pink, nifedipine 20 mg. Net price 20 = £3.86. Label: 21, 25

PoM **Adalat**® **Retard 10** (Bayer)
Tablets, pink, nifedipine 10 mg. Net price 56-tab pack = £8.94. Label: 21, 25

PoM **Adalat**® **IC** (Bayer)
Coronary injection, nifedipine 100 micrograms/ml. Net price 2-ml pre-filled syringe = 74p
Note. Use polyethylene catheters only
Dose: for treatment of coronary spasm during coronary angiography and balloon angioplasty, 100–200 micrograms via coronary catheter over 90–120 seconds; lasts 15 minutes; do not exceed total of six 200-microgram injections in 3 hours

NIMODIPINE

Indications: treatment of ischaemic neurological deficits caused by arterial spasm following subarachnoid haemorrhage
Cautions: cerebral oedema or severely raised intracranial pressure; avoid concomitant administration of other calcium-channel blockers (monitor carefully if unavoidable); impaired renal function or nephrotoxic drugs
Side-effects: hypotension, variation in heart-rate, flushing, headache, gastro-intestinal disorders, nausea, and feeling of warmth; transient increase in liver enzymes after intravenous administration
Dose: by intravenous infusion via central catheter, 1 mg/hour initially, increased after 2 hours to 2 mg/hour, providing no severe decrease in blood pressure; patients with unstable blood pressure or weighing less than 70 kg, 500 micrograms/hour initially or less if necessary; treatment should start as soon as possible and should continue for 5 days; in the event of surgical intervention during treatment continue for at least 5 days after

▼ PoM **Nimotop**® (Bayer)
Intravenous infusion, nimodipine 200 micrograms/ml; also contains ethanol 20% and macrogol '400' 17%. Net price 50-ml vial (with polyethylene infusion catheter) = £13.24
Note. Glass, polyethylene, or polypropylene apparatus should be used; PVC should be avoided

VERAPAMIL HYDROCHLORIDE

Indications: supraventricular arrhythmias, angina, hypertension
Cautions: first-degree heart block; intravenous route in patients taking beta-blockers (**important:** see section 2.3.2), only give by mouth with beta-blockers if myocardial function is well preserved; reduce dose in hepatic impairment. Drug interactions: see Appendix 1 (sections *2.1, 2.3, 2.5, 2.6, 4.2, 4.8, 8, 15*)
Contra-indications: bradycardia, second- and third-degree heart block, sick sinus syndrome,

heart failure; atrial flutter or fibrillation complicating Wolff-Parkinson-White syndrome
Side-effects: nausea, vomiting, constipation, headache; rarely reversible impairment of liver function; after intravenous administration, hypotension, bradycardia, heart block, and asystole
Dose: by mouth, arrhythmias, 40–120 mg 3 times daily; angina, 80–120 mg 3 times daily; hypertension, 240–480 mg daily in 2–3 divided doses
By slow intravenous injection, 5–10 mg (preferably with ECG monitoring); in paroxysmal tachyarrhythmias a further 5 mg after 5–10 minutes if required

PoM **Verapamil** (Non-proprietary)
Tablets, verapamil hydrochloride 40 mg, net price 20 = 89p; 80 mg, 20 = £1.78; 120 mg, 20 = £2.72; 160 mg, 20 = £3.27

PoM **Berkatens**® (Berk)
Tablets, all yellow, f/c, verapamil hydrochloride 40 mg, net price 20 = 90p; 80 mg, 20 = £1.80; 120 mg, 20 = £2.59; 160 mg, 20 = £3.27

PoM **Cordilox**® (Abbott)
Tablets, all yellow, f/c, verapamil hydrochloride 40 mg, net price 20 = £1.28; 80 mg, 20 = £2.55; 120 mg, 20 = £3.60; 160 mg, 56-tab pack = £13.10
Injection, verapamil hydrochloride 2.5 mg/ml, net price 2-ml amp = £1.11

PoM **Securon**® (Knoll)
Tablets, f/c, verapamil hydrochloride 40 mg, net price 100 = £4.69; 80 mg, 100 = £9.38; 120 mg, 56-tab pack = £7.87, 100 = £14.05; 160 mg, 56-tab pack = £10.49, 100 = £18.73

▼ PoM **Securon SR**® (Knoll)
Tablets, s/r, pale green, f/c, verapamil hydrochloride 240 mg. Net price 28-tab pack = £10.92. Label: 25
Dose: hypertension, 1 tablet daily, increased to twice daily if necessary (new patients, initial dose ½ tablet)

▼ PoM **Univer**® (Rorer)
Capsules, all s/r, verapamil hydrochloride 120 mg (yellow/dark blue), net price 28-cap pack = £7.00; 180 mg (yellow), 56-cap pack = £16.92; 240 mg (yellow/dark blue), 28-cap pack = £11.42. Label: 25
Dose: hypertension, 240 mg daily, increased to a max. of 480 mg daily if necessary (new patients, initial dose 120 mg)

2.6.3 Peripheral vasodilators and related drugs

Most serious peripheral disorders are now known to be due to occlusion of vessels, either by spasm or sclerotic plaques; use of vasodilators may increase blood flow at rest, but no controlled studies have shown any improvement in walking distance or sustained increase in muscle blood flow during exercise. Rest pain is rarely affected.

CHILBLAINS. Vasodilator therapy is not recommended for chilblains (see section 13.14).

CINNARIZINE

Indications: peripheral vascular disease, Raynaud's syndrome

Cautions; Side-effects: see under Cyclizine (section 4.6); also hypersensitivity reactions, caution in hypotension; rarely, extrapyramidal symptoms in elderly on prolonged therapy

Dose: initially, 75 mg 3 times daily; maintenance, 75 mg 2–3 times daily

Stugeron Forte® (Janssen)
Capsules, orange/ivory, cinnarizine 75 mg. Net price 20 = £1.61. Label: 2
Stugeron: see section 4.6

NICOTINIC ACID DERIVATIVES

Indications: peripheral vascular disease (for the use of nicotinic acid and nicofuranose in hyperlipidaemia, see section 2.12)

Side-effects: flushing, dizziness, nausea, vomiting, hypotension (more frequent with nicotinic acid than derivatives); occasional diabetogenic effect reported with nicotinic acid

Bradilan® (Napp)
Tablets, e/c and s/c, nicofuranose 250 mg. Net price 20 = £1.41. Label: 5, 25
Dose: 500 mg 3 times daily, increased if required
Hexopal® (Winthrop)
Tablets, scored, inositol nicotinate 500 mg. Net price 20 = £3.71
Dose: 0.5–1 g 3 times daily, increased to 4 g daily if required
Tablets forte, scored, inositol nicotinate 750 mg. Net price 112-tab pack = £30.99
Dose: 1.5–3 g daily
Suspension, sugar-free, inositol nicotinate 1 g/5 ml. Diluent syrup, life of diluted suspension 14 days. Net price 300 ml = £19.00
Dose: as for tablets (above)
N̶H̶S **Pernivit**® (DF)
Tablets, pink, s/c, nicotinic acid 25 mg, acetomenaphthone 7 mg. Net price 20 = 17p
Ronicol® (Roche)
Tablets, scored, nicotinyl alcohol 25 mg (as tartrate). Net price 20 = 37p
Dose: 25–50 mg 4 times daily
Timespan® (= tablets s/r), red, s/c, nicotinyl alcohol 150 mg (as tartrate). Net price 20 = £1.58. Label: 25
Dose: 150–300 mg twice daily

OXPENTIFYLLINE

Indications: peripheral vascular disease
Cautions: hypotension
Side-effects: nausea, dizziness, flushing
Dose: 400 mg 2–3 times daily

PoM **Trental**® (Hoechst)
Tablets, s/r, pink, s/c, oxpentifylline 400 mg. Net price 20 = £3.28. Label: 21, 25

THYMOXAMINE

Indications: Raynaud's syndrome, peripheral vascular disease, vascular spasm
Cautions: coronary artery disease, diabetes mellitus

Side-effects: nausea, diarrhoea, flushing, headache, dizziness
Dose: 40 mg 4 times daily

PoM **Opilon**® (P-D)
Tablets, yellow, scored, thymoxamine 40 mg (as hydrochloride). Net price 20 = £3.77. Label: 21

OTHER PREPARATION USED IN PERIPHERAL VASCULAR DISEASE

Rutosides (oxerutins, Paroven®) are not vasodilators and are not generally regarded as effective preparations as capillary sealants or for the treatment of cramps.

Paroven® (Zyma)
Capsules, yellow, oxerutins 250 mg. Net price 20 = £2.17
Label: 21

2.6.4   Cerebral vasodilators

These drugs are claimed to improve mental function. Some improvements in performance of psychological tests have been reported but the drugs have not been shown clinically to be of much benefit in senile dementia.

CO-DERGOCRINE MESYLATE

A mixture in equal proportions of dihydroergocornine mesylate, dihydroergocristine mesylate, and (in the ratio 2:1) α- and β-dihydroergocryptine mesylate

Indications: adjunct in senile dementia
Cautions: severe bradycardia
Side-effects: nausea, vomiting, flushing, headache, rash, nasal congestion, postural hypotension in hypertensive patients
Dose: 1.5 mg 3 times daily *or* 4.5 mg once daily

PoM **Hydergine**® (Sandoz)
Tablets, co-dergocrine mesylate 1.5 mg (scored), net price 20 = £3.16; 4.5 mg, 28 = £15.80. Label: 22

CYCLANDELATE

Indications: peripheral vascular disease; adjunct in the management of senile dementia
Contra-indications: acute phase of cerebrovascular accident
Side-effects: nausea, flushing, dizziness with high doses
Dose: 1.2–1.6 g daily in 2–4 divided doses

Cyclobral® (Norgine)
Capsules, pink/brown, cyclandelate 400 mg. Net price 20 = £1.93
Cyclospasmol® (Brocades)
Capsules, pink/grey, cyclandelate 400 mg. Net price 20 = £2.40
Tablets, pink, s/c, cyclandelate 400 mg. Net price 112 = £15.91
Suspension, cyclandelate 400 mg/5 ml when reconstituted with freshly boiled and cooled purified water. Diluent syrup, life of diluted suspension 14 days. Net price 450-ml pack = £11.87

ISOXSUPRINE HYDROCHLORIDE

Indications: cerebral and peripheral vascular disease

Contra-indications: recent arterial haemorrhage

Side-effects: flushing, tachycardia, palpitations, nausea, vomiting

Defencin CP® (Bristol-Myers)
Product discontinued
Duvadilan® (Duphar)
Tablets—discontinued
PoM *Injection* (obstetrics)—see section 7.1.2
Duvadilan Retard® (Duphar)
Product discontinued

NAFTIDROFURYL OXALATE

Indications: cerebral and peripheral vascular disease

Contra-indications: parenteral administration in atrioventricular block

Side-effects: nausea, epigastric pain

Dose: see below

PoM **Praxilene®** (Lipha)
Capsules, pink, naftidrofuryl oxalate 100 mg. Net price 20 = £1.99
  Dose: peripheral vascular disease, 100–200 mg 3 times daily; cerebral vascular disease, 100 mg 3 times daily
Injection forte, naftidrofuryl oxalate 20 mg/ml. Net price 10-ml amp = £1.10
  Dose: peripheral vascular disease only, by intravenous or intra-arterial infusion, 200 mg over at least 90 minutes, twice daily

2.7 Sympathomimetics

2.7.1 Sympathomimetics with inotropic activity
2.7.2 Sympathomimetics causing vasoconstriction

The properties of sympathomimetics vary according to whether they act on alpha or on beta receptors. Adrenaline acts on both alpha and beta receptors and increases both heart rate and contractility; it can cause peripheral vasodilation (a beta effect) or vasoconstriction (an alpha effect). Adrenaline injection 1 in 1000 is used in the emergency treatment of acute allergic and anaphylactic reactions (see section 3.4.3).

In *cardiac arrest* adrenaline 1 in 10000 is recommended in a dose of 10 ml by central intravenous injection. In ventricular fibrillation, adrenaline injection should be reserved for patients who have not responded to d.c. shocks at 200 and 400 J, and should precede further shocks only after lignocaine has been tried. For asystole, adrenaline is usually tried after atropine; the intracardiac route is not recommended except as a last resort. Sodium bicarbonate (see section 9.2.2) should be given only when arrest is prolonged and when ventilation is adequate. Calcium should only be used as a last resort for electromechanical dissociation.

ADRENALINE

Indications: cardiac arrest—see notes above

Cautions: ischaemic heart disease, diabetes mellitus, hyperthyroidism, hypertension; increased risk of arrhythmias with antidepressants, digoxin, or quinidine

Side-effects: anxiety, tremor, tachycardia, headache, cold extremities; in overdosage arrhythmias, cerebral haemorrhage, pulmonary oedema

Dose: by subcutaneous or intramuscular injection, 500 micrograms (0.5 ml of 1 in 1000 injection), repeated if required
By central intravenous injection, 0.5–1 mg (5–10 ml of 1 in 10000 injection)
By intracardiac injection, 100–200 micrograms (1–2 ml of 1 in 10000 injection)

PoM **Adrenaline Injection,** adrenaline 1 in 1000 (adrenaline 1 mg/ml as acid tartrate). Net price 0.5-ml amp = 27p; 1-ml amp = 28p
PoM **Min-I-Jet Adrenaline®** (IMS)
Injection, adrenaline 1 in 1000 (1 mg/ml as hydrochloride). Net price 0.5-ml = £2.45; 1-ml = £2.32; disposable syringe (both)
Intracardiac injection, adrenaline 1 in 10000 (100 micrograms/ml as hydrochloride). Net price 10-ml disposable syringe = £2.45 and £3.10 (longer needle)

2.7.1 Sympathomimetics with inotropic activity

The cardiac stimulants **dobutamine** (Dobutrex®) and **dopamine** (Intropin®) act on sympathetic receptors in cardiac muscle, and increase contractility with little effect on rate; they are used in cardiogenic shock. Dosage of dopamine is critical since although low doses induce vasodilatation and increase renal perfusion, higher doses (more than 5 micrograms per kg per minute) lead to vasoconstriction and may exacerbate heart failure.

Isoprenaline also acts on sympathetic receptors and increases both heart rate and contractility; it may prevent Stokes-Adams attacks, but insertion of a pacemaker is preferable.

DOBUTAMINE HYDROCHLORIDE

Indications: inotropic support in infarction, cardiac surgery, cardiomyopathies, septic shock, and cardiogenic shock

Cautions: severe hypotension complicating cardiogenic shock

Side-effects: tachycardia and marked increase in systolic blood pressure indicate overdosage

Dose: by intravenous infusion, 2.5–10 micrograms/kg/minute, adjusted according to response

PoM **Dobutrex**® (Lilly)

Injection, powder for preparation of an infusion, dobutamine (as hydrochloride). Net price 250-mg vial = £11.77

Intravenous solution, dobutamine (as hydrochloride) 12.5 mg/ml. For dilution and use as an infusion. Net price 20-ml vial = £12.95

DOPAMINE HYDROCHLORIDE

Indications: cardiogenic shock in infarction or cardiac surgery

Cautions: correct hypovolaemia; low dose in shock due to acute myocardial infarction—see notes above

Contra-indications: tachyarrhythmia, phaeochromocytoma

Side-effects: nausea and vomiting, peripheral vasoconstriction, hypotension, hypertension, tachycardia

Dose: by intravenous infusion, 2–5 micrograms/kg/minute initially (see notes above)

PoM **Dopamine Hydrochloride** (Non-proprietary)

Injection, dopamine hydrochloride 40 mg/ml, net price 5-ml amp = £4.30; 160 mg/ml, 5-ml amp = £17.25. For dilution and use as an infusion

PoM **Dopamine Hydrochloride in Dextrose (Glucose) Injection** (Abbott)

Intravenous infusions (in glucose 5% intravenous infusion), dopamine hydrochloride 800 micrograms/ml, 1.6 mg/ml, and 3.2 mg/ml. 250-ml containers (all hosp. only)

PoM **Intropin**® (Du Pont)

Injection, dopamine hydrochloride 40 mg/ml. For dilution and use as an infusion. Net price 5-ml amp or syringe = £4.80

Injection, dopamine hydrochloride 160 mg/ml. For dilution and use as an infusion. Net price 5-ml amp = £19.20

PoM **Select-A-Jet Dopamine**® (IMS)

Injection, dopamine hydrochloride 40 mg/ml. For dilution and use as an infusion. Net price 5-ml vial = £4.90; 10-ml vial = £9.03; 20-ml vial = £15.48

ISOPRENALINE HYDROCHLORIDE

Indications: heart block, severe bradycardia

Cautions: ischaemic heart disease, diabetes mellitus, hyperthyroidism. Drug interactions: see Appendix 1 (section *15*)

Side-effects: tachycardia, arrhythmias, hypotension, sweating, tremor, headache

Dose: by mouth, 30 mg every 8 hours, then increased; max. daily dose usually 840 mg

By intravenous infusion, 0.5–10 micrograms/minute

PoM **Isuprel**® (Winthrop)

Injection, isoprenaline hydrochloride 200 micrograms/ml. Net price 1-ml amp = £4.42; 5-ml amp = £15.94

PoM **Min-I-Jet Isoprenaline**® (IMS)

Injection, isoprenaline hydrochloride 20 micro-grams/ml. Net price 10-ml disposable syringe = £2.58 and £3.10 (longer needle)

PoM **Saventrine**® (Pharmax)

Tablets, isoprenaline hydrochloride 30 mg. Net price 20 = £1.72

PoM **Saventrine IV**® (Pharmax)

Injection, isoprenaline hydrochloride 1 mg/ml. For dilution and use as an infusion. Net price 2-ml amp = 45p

2.7.2 Sympathomimetics causing vasoconstriction

Vasoconstrictors raise blood pressure transiently by constricting peripheral vessels. They are sometimes used as an emergency method of elevating blood pressure while preparations are being made for more effective therapy such as transfusion. They may also be used in general and spinal anaesthesia to control blood pressure.

The danger of vasoconstrictors is that although they raise blood pressure they do so at the expense of perfusion of vital organs such as the kidney. Further, in many patients with shock the peripheral resistance is already high, and to raise it further is unhelpful. Thus the use of vasoconstrictors in the treatment of shock is to be generally **deprecated**. The use of volume expanders such as blood or plasma, or the inotropic agents dopamine, dobutamine, or isoprenaline is more appropriate (section 2.7.1). Treatment of the underlying condition, e.g. with antibiotics, in septic shock, is obviously important.

METARAMINOL

Indications: acute hypotension

Cautions; Contra-indications: see under Noradrenaline Acid Tartrate

Side-effects: tachycardia, arrhythmias, reduced renal blood flow

Dose: by subcutaneous or intramuscular injection, 2–10 mg

By intravenous infusion, 15–100 mg in 500 ml, adjusted according to response

PoM **Aramine**® (MSD)

Injection, metaraminol 10 mg (as tartrate)/ml. Net price 1-ml amp = 48p

METHOXAMINE HYDROCHLORIDE

Indications: hypotension in anaesthesia

Cautions: hyperthyroidism; pregnancy. Drug interactions: see Appendix 1 (section 2.7)

Contra-indications: severe coronary or cardiovascular disease

Side-effects: headache, hypertension, bradycardia

Dose: by intramuscular injection, 5–20 mg

By slow intravenous injection, 5–10 mg (rate 1 mg/minute)

PoM **Vasoxine**® (Calmic)

Injection, methoxamine hydrochloride 20 mg/ml. Net price 1-ml amp = 36p

NORADRENALINE ACID TARTRATE

Indications: acute hypotension, cardiac arrest
Cautions: extravasation at injection site may cause necrosis. Drug interactions: see Appendix 1 (section 2.7)
Contra-indications: myocardial   infarction, pregnancy
Side-effects: headache, palpitations, bradycardia
Dose: by intravenous infusion, of a solution containing noradrenaline acid tartrate 8 micrograms/ml (equivalent to noradrenaline base 4 micrograms/ml) at an initial rate of 2 to 3 ml/minute, adjusted according to response
By rapid intravenous or intracardiac injection, 0.5 to 0.75 ml of a solution containing noradrenaline acid tartrate 200 micrograms/ml (equivalent to noradrenaline base 100 micrograms/ml)

PoM **Levophed**® (Winthrop)
Injection, noradrenaline acid tartrate 2 mg/ml. For dilution and use as an infusion. Net price 2-ml amp = 75p; 4-ml amp = £1.10
Special injection, noradrenaline acid tartrate 200 micrograms/ml. Net price 2-ml amp = 73p

PHENYLEPHRINE HYDROCHLORIDE

Indications: acute hypotension
Cautions; Contra-indications: see under Noradrenaline Acid Tartrate; also contra-indicated in severe hypertension and hyperthyroidism
Side-effects: hypertension with headache, palpitations, vomiting; tachycardia or reflex bradycardia; tingling and coolness of skin
Dose: by subcutaneous or intramuscular injection, 5 mg
By slow intravenous injection, 100–500 micrograms
By intravenous infusion, 5–20 mg in 500 ml, adjusted according to response

PoM **Phenylephrine Injection 1%** (Boots)
Injection, phenylephrine hydrochloride 10 mg/ml. Net price 1-ml amp = 49p

2.8   Anticoagulants and Protamine

2.8.1   Parenteral anticoagulants
2.8.2   Oral anticoagulants
2.8.3   Protamine sulphate

The main use of anticoagulants is to prevent thrombus formation or the extension of an existing thrombus in the slower-moving venous side of the circulation, where the thrombus consists of a fibrin web enmeshed with platelets and red cells. Anticoagulants are therefore widely used in the prevention and treatment of deep-vein thrombosis in the legs.

Anticoagulants are of less use in preventing thrombus formation in arteries, for in faster-flowing vessels thrombi are composed mainly of platelets with little fibrin. Anticoagulants are used to prevent thrombi forming on prosthetic heart valves.

2.8.1   Parenteral anticoagulants

Heparin is given to initiate anticoagulation and is rapidly effective. As its effects are short-lived it is best given by continuous infusion; if given by intermittent intravenous injection, the interval between doses must not exceed 6 hours. Oral anticoagulants are started at the same time, and the heparin infusion withdrawn after 3 days.

If oral anticoagulants cannot be given and heparin is continued, its dose is adjusted after determination of the activated partial thromboplastin time.

If haemorrhage occurs it is usually sufficient to withdraw heparin, but if rapid reversal of the effects of heparin is required, protamine sulphate is a specific antidote (section 2.8.3).

For the prophylaxis of thrombosis in patients undergoing heart surgery or renal dialysis full therapeutic doses of heparin are given for the duration of the procedure. Low-dose heparin by subcutaneous injection is widely advocated to prevent postoperative deep-vein thrombosis and pulmonary embolism in 'high risk' patients, i.e. those with obesity, malignant disease, or previous history of thrombosis. Laboratory monitoring is not required with this regimen.

Epoprostenol (prostacyclin) can be given to inhibit platelet aggregation during renal dialysis either alone or with heparin. Since its half-life is only about 3 minutes it must be given by continuous intravenous infusion. It is a potent vasodilator and therefore its side-effects include flushing, headache, and hypotension.

Ancrod (Arvin®), an enzymatic principle derived from Malaysian pit-viper venom, reduces plasma fibrinogen by cleavage of fibrin. It has been shown to be as effective as heparin in the resolution of deep-vein thromboses, but some patients develop resistance. The initial infusion must be given slowly, as there is a risk of massive intravascular formation of unstable fibrin. Response can be monitored by observing clot size after the blood has been allowed to stand for about 2 hours, the aim being to predict a dose that produces a 2–3 mm clot. Alternatively, plasma-fibrinogen concentrations can be measured directly.

The major complication of ancrod is haemorrhage, and since it takes 12 to 24 hours for haemostatic fibrinogen concentrations to be restored after stopping administration it may be necessary to give ancrod antivenom as an antidote (0.2-ml test dose subcutaneously followed by 0.8 ml intramuscularly, and 30 minutes later 1 ml intravenously). Since the antivenom may cause anaphylaxis adrenaline, chlorpheniramine, and hydrocortisone should be available. (For details see Allergic Emergencies, section 3.4.3.) As an alternative to the antivenom reconstituted freeze-dried fibrinogen may be given, or if this is not available one litre of fresh frozen plasma.

Ancrod has been used subcutaneously for prophylaxis in patients likely to develop deep-vein thrombosis, but is not in common use.

HEPARIN

Indications: deep-vein thrombosis, disseminated intravascular coagulation, prevention of post-operative thrombosis

Cautions: pregnancy. Drug interactions: see Appendix 1 (section 2.8)

Contra-indications: haemophilia and other haemorrhagic disorders, peptic ulcer, cerebral aneurysm, severe hypertension, severe liver disease, recent surgery of eye or nervous system, hypersensitivity to heparin

Side-effects: haemorrhage, thrombocytopenia, hypersensitivity reactions; osteoporosis after prolonged use, alopecia

Dose: by intravenous injection, loading dose of 12 500 units followed by continuous *infusion* of 20 000–40 000 units over 24 hours *or* 5000–10 000 units by *intravenous injection* every 4 hours

By subcutaneous injection, prophylaxis of deep-vein thrombosis, 5000 units 2 hours before surgery, then every 8–12 hours until patient is ambulant; in pregnancy, 10 000 units every 12 hours

Treatment of deep-vein thrombosis, initially 10 000–20 000 units every 12 hours *or* 2500 units/10 kg every 12 hours, adjusted daily by laboratory monitoring

Intravenous preparations

PoM **Heparin Injection** (heparin sodium)
1000 units/ml, net price 1-ml amp = 20p; 5-ml amp = 57p; 5-ml vial = 52p
5000 units/ml, net price 1-ml amp = 31p; 5-ml amp = 98p; 5-ml vial = £1.43
10 000 units/ml, net price 1-ml amp = 45p
25 000 units/ml, net price 1-ml amp = 81p; 5-ml vial = £6.24

PoM **Monoparin**® (CP)
Injection, heparin sodium (mucous) 1000 units/ml, net price 1-ml amp = 17p; 5-ml amp = 46p; 10-ml amp = 66p; 5000 units/ml, 1-ml amp = 32p; 5-ml amp = 98p; 25 000 units/ml, 1-ml amp = £1.27

PoM **Multiparin**® (CP)
Injection, heparin sodium (mucous) 1000 units/ml, net price 5-ml vial = 45p; 5000 units/ml, 5-ml vial = £1.32; 25 000 units/ml, 5-ml vial = £5.41

PoM **Pump-Hep**® (Leo)
Intravenous infusion, heparin sodium (mucous) 1000 units/ml. Net price 5-ml amp = 40p; 10-ml amp = 66p; 20-ml amp = £1.06
Dose: by continuous infusion pump, 20 000–40 000 units daily

PoM **Unihep**® (Leo)
Injection, heparin sodium (mucous) 1000 units/ml, net price 1-ml amp = 14p; 5000 units/ml, 1-ml amp = 27p; 10 000 units/ml, 1-ml amp = 45p; 25 000 units/ml, 1-ml amp = £1.07

Subcutaneous preparations

PoM **Heparin Injection** (heparin sodium or heparin calcium)
25 000 units/ml (subcutaneous). Net price 0.2-ml amp = 53p; syringe = 70p

PoM **Calciparine**® (Labaz)
Injection (subcutaneous), heparin calcium 25 000 units/ml. Net price 0.2-ml syringe = 70p; 0.5-ml amp = £1.50; 0.8-ml amp = £1.80

PoM **Minihep**® (Leo)
Darts (= subcutaneous injection), heparin sodium 10 000 units/ml. Net price 0.5-ml injector system = 51p
Injection (subcutaneous), heparin sodium 25 000 units/ml. Net price 0.2-ml amp = 42p

PoM **Minihep Calcium**® (Leo)
Darts (= subcutaneous injection), heparin calcium 10 000 units/ml. Net price 0.5-ml injector system = 55p
Injection (subcutaneous), heparin calcium 25 000 units/ml. Net price 0.2-ml amp = 45p

PoM **Monoparin**® (CP)
Injection (subcutaneous), heparin sodium (mucous) 25 000 units/ml. Net price 0.2-ml amp = 41p

PoM **Monoparin Calcium**® (CP)
Injection (subcutaneous), heparin calcium 25 000 units/ml. Net price 0.2 ml amp = 52p

PoM **Uniparin**® (CP)
Injection (subcutaneous), heparin sodium 25 000 units/ml. Net price 0.2-ml syringe = 72p

PoM **Uniparin Calcium**® (CP)
Injection (subcutaneous), heparin calcium 25 000 units/ml. Net price 0.2-ml syringe = 72p

PoM **Uniparin Forte**® (CP)
Injection (subcutaneous), heparin sodium 25 000 units/ml. Net price 0.4-ml syringe = £1.30

HEPARIN FLUSHES

PoM **Heparinised Saline**® (Paines & Byrne)
Solution, heparin sodium (mucous) 10 units/ml. Net price 5-ml amp = 32p
To maintain patency of catheters, cannulas, etc., 50 units flushed through every 4 hours or as required. Not for therapeutic use

PoM **Hep-Flush**® (Leo)
Solution, heparin sodium 100 units/ml. Net price 2-ml amp = 33p
To maintain patency of catheters, cannulas, etc., 200 units flushed through every 4–8 hours. Not for therapeutic use

PoM **Heplok**® (Leo)
Solution, heparin sodium 10 units/ml. Net price 5-ml amp = 30p
To maintain patency of catheters, cannulas, etc., 10–50 units flushed through every 4 hours. Not for therapeutic use

PoM **Hepsal**® (CP)
Solution, heparin sodium 10 units/ml. Net price 5-ml amp = 30p
To maintain patency of catheters, cannulas, etc., 50 units flushed through every 4 hours or as required. Not for therapeutic use

ANCROD

Indications: deep-vein thrombosis, prevention of postoperative thrombosis

Cautions; Contra-indications; Side-effects: see under Heparin; resistance may develop; avoid administration with dextrans

Dose: by intravenous infusion, 2–3 units/kg over 4–12 hours (usually 6–8 hours), then *by infusion or slow intravenous injection,* 2 units/kg every 12 hours

By subcutaneous injection, prophylaxis of deep-vein thrombosis, 280 units immediately after surgery, then 70 units daily for 4 days (fractured femur) or 8 days (hip replacement)

PoM **Arvin**® (Armour)
Injection, ancrod 70 units/ml. Net price 1-ml amp = £9.25 (Hosp. only)
Note. Arvin Antidote is available from Armour

EPOPROSTENOL

Indications: see notes above

Cautions: anticoagulant monitoring required when given with heparin

Side-effects: see notes above; also bradycardia, pallor, sweating with higher doses

Dose: see manufacturer's literature

▼ PoM **Flolan**® (Wellcome)
Infusion, powder for reconstitution, epoprostenol (as sodium salt). Net price 500-microgram vial (with diluent) = £103.86

2.8.2   Oral anticoagulants

Oral anticoagulants antagonise the effects of vitamin K, and take at least 36 to 48 hours for the anticoagulant effect to develop; if an immediate effect is required, heparin must be given concomitantly.

The main indication for oral anticoagulant therapy is deep-vein thrombosis. Patients with poorly controlled atrial fibrillation who are at risk of embolisation should also be treated, as should patients with heart valve prostheses, to prevent emboli developing on the valves; antiplatelet drugs may also be useful in these patients.

Oral anticoagulants should not be used in cerebral thrombosis or peripheral arterial occlusion, but may be of value in patients with transient brain ischaemic attacks whether due to carotid or vertebrobasilar arterial disease; if these patients also have severe hypertension anticoagulants are contra-indicated, and antiplatelet drugs are an alternative (section 2.9).

Warfarin and other coumarins are the drugs of choice, as they are less likely to cause sensitivity reactions than phenindione.

Whenever possible, the base-line prothrombin time should be determined before the initial dose is given. A typical induction dose is 10 mg daily for 3 days but this should be reduced if the base-

line prothrombin time is prolonged, the liver-function tests are abnormal, or the patient is in cardiac failure, is on parenteral feeding, is less than average weight, or is over 80 years of age. The subsequent maintenance dose must depend upon the prothrombin time reported by the laboratory as the International Normalised Ratio (INR) which has now replaced the British Ratio (BR). The currently recommended therapeutic ranges are 2–2.5 for prophylactic therapy of deep-vein thrombosis including high-risk surgery; 2–3 for prophylactic therapy in hip surgery and fractured femur operations, for treatment of deep-vein thrombosis, pulmonary embolism, and transient ischaemic attacks; 3–4.5 for recurrent deep-vein thrombosis and pulmonary embolism, arterial disease including myocardial infarction, arterial grafts, and prosthetic heart valves and grafts.

It is essential that the INR be determined on the second and third days of treatment, then on alternate days with longer intervals once stability of dosage has been achieved. The daily maintenance dose is usually 3 to 9 mg and should be taken at the same time each day.

Change in the patient's clinical condition, particularly associated with liver disease or drug administration, necessitates more frequent testing. Patients taking a fixed dose of warfarin and a microsomal enzyme-inducing agent such as phenobarbitone or phenytoin are at risk of haemorrhage if the agent is withdrawn and the anticoagulant dose maintained. There is an increased risk of haemorrhage if patients on warfarin are prescribed drugs such as aspirin or clofibrate. For further interactions with warfarin, see Appendix 1 (section 2.8). Major changes in diet may also affect warfarin control.

The main adverse effect of all oral anti-coagulants is haemorrhage. Omission of dosage with checking of the INR is essential. The following recommendations of the British Society for Haematology are based on the result of the INR and the clinical state:

INR 4.5–7 without haemorrhage—withhold warfarin for 1 or more days, according to INR

INR > 7 without haemorrhage—withhold warfarin and consider giving phytomenadione (vitamin K_1) 5–10 mg by mouth

INR < 4.5 with haemorrhage—give fresh frozen plasma and investigate cause

INR > 2 with life-threatening haemorrhage—phytomenadione 2.5–10 mg by slow intravenous injection with factors II, IX, and X (or fresh frozen plasma) and investigate cause.

Phytomenadione will take up to 12 hours to act and will prevent oral anticoagulants from acting for several days or even weeks (see section 9.6.6.).

PREGNANCY. Oral anticoagulants are weakly teratogenic and should not be given in the first trimester of pregnancy. Women at risk of pregnancy should be warned of this danger. Also, oral anticoagulants cross the placenta with risk of placental or fetal haemorrhage; they should therefore not be given during the last few weeks of pregnancy.

Anticoagulant treatment cards must be carried by patients, and are available from:

DHSS Store   SHHD (Div IIID)
No. 2 Site   Room 9
Manchester Rd   St. Andrew's House
Heywood   Edinburgh EH1 3DE
Lancs OL10 2PZ

Cards giving advice for patients on anticoagulant treatment may be given to patients at the discretion of the doctor or pharmacist.

WARFARIN SODIUM

Indications: deep-vein thrombosis, transient brain ischaemic attacks, prophylaxis with prosthetic heart valves
Cautions: hepatic or renal disease, recent surgery. Drug interactions: see Appendix 1 (section 2.8)
Contra-indications: pregnancy, peptic ulcer, severe hypertension, bacterial endocarditis
Side-effects: haemorrhage
Dose: see notes above

PoM **Marevan**® (DF)
Tablets, brown, scored, warfarin sodium 1 mg. Net price 20 = 9p. Label: 10 anticoagulant card
Tablets, blue, scored, warfarin sodium 3 mg. Net price 20 = 10p. Label: 10 anticoagulant card
Tablets, pink, scored, warfarin sodium 5 mg. Net price 20 = 16p. Label: 10 anticoagulant card
PoM **Warfarin WBP** (Boehringer Ingelheim)
Tablets, brown, scored, warfarin sodium 1 mg. Net price 20 = 9p. Label: 10 anticoagulant card
Tablets, blue, scored, warfarin sodium 3 mg. Net price 20 = 10p. Label: 10 anticoagulant card
Tablets, pink, scored, warfarin sodium 5 mg. Net price 20 = 16p. Label: 10 anticoagulant card

NICOUMALONE

Indications: deep-vein thrombosis, transient brain ischaemic attacks, prophylaxis with prosthetic heart valves
Cautions; Contra-indications; Side-effects: see under Warfarin Sodium; avoid breast-feeding
Dose: 8–12 mg on 1st day; 4–8 mg on 2nd day; maintenance dose usually 1–8 mg daily

PoM **Sinthrome**® (Geigy)
Tablets, pink, nicoumalone 1 mg. Net price 20 = 15p. Label: 10 anticoagulant card
Tablets, scored, nicoumalone 4 mg. Net price 20 = 31p. Label: 10 anticoagulant card

PHENINDIONE

Indications: deep-vein thrombosis
Cautions; Contra-indications; Side-effects: see under Warfarin Sodium; also hypersensitivity reactions including rashes, fever, leucopenia, agranulocytosis, diarrhoea, renal and hepatic damage; urine coloured pink; avoid breast-feeding. Drug interactions: see Appendix 1 (section 2.8)
Dose: 200 mg on 1st day; 100 mg on 2nd day; maintenance dose usually 50–150 mg daily

PoM **Dindevan**® (DF)
Tablets, phenindione 10 mg; net price 20 = 26p; 25 mg (green), 20 = 36p; 50 mg, 20 = 46p. Label: 10 anticoagulant card, 14

2.8.3   Protamine sulphate

Although protamine sulphate is used to counteract overdosage with heparin, if used in excess it has an anticoagulant effect.

PROTAMINE SULPHATE

Indications; Cautions: see above
Side-effects: flushing, hypotension, bradycardia
Dose: *by slow intravenous injection*, 1 mg neutralises 100 units heparin (mucous) or 80 units heparin (lung) when given within 15 minutes; if longer time, less protamine required as heparin rapidly excreted; max. 50 mg

PoM **Protamine Sulphate Injection,** protamine sulphate 10 mg/ml. Net price 5- and 10-ml amp (both) = 84p

2.9   Antiplatelet drugs

By decreasing platelet adhesiveness, these drugs may inhibit thrombus formation on the arterial side of the circulation, where thrombi are formed by platelet aggregation and anticoagulants have little effect. Antiplatelet drugs have little effect in venous thromboembolism. **Dipyridamole** is used with anticoagulants to prevent thrombus formation on prosthetic valves.

Encouraging results have been obtained using **aspirin** 300 mg for the *secondary* prevention of cerebrovascular or cardiovascular disease; studies are still needed to determine whether lower doses (such as 75 mg daily or 300 mg on alternate days) might not be equally (or more) effective. Physicians in the USA have demonstrated that 325 mg on alternate days can have a *primary* preventive action for myocardial infarction but further analysis is awaited before aspirin can be recommended for routine use in primary prevention.

For use of epoprostenol, see section 2.8.1.

DIPYRIDAMOLE

Indications: modification of platelet function
Cautions: rapidly worsening angina, aortic stenosis, recent myocardial infarction; may exacerbate migraine, hypotension. Drug interactions: see Appendix 1 (sections *2.8, 2.8E*)
Side-effects: nausea, diarrhoea, throbbing headache, hypotension
Dose: *by mouth*, 300–600 mg daily in 3–4 divided doses before food
By intravenous injection, diagnostic only, see manufacturer's literature

PoM **Dipyridamole** (Non-proprietary)
Tablets, dipyridamole 25 mg, net price 20 = 74p; 100 mg, 20 = £2.06. Label: 22

PoM **Persantin**® (Boehringer Ingelheim)
Tablets, both s/c, dipyridamole 25 mg (orange), net price 20 = 68p; 100 mg, 20 = £1.89. Label: 22
Injection, dipyridamole 5 mg/ml. Net price 2-ml amp = 10p

2.10 Fibrinolytic drugs

These activate plasminogen to form plasmin, which degrades fibrin and so breaks up thrombi. **Streptokinase** is used in the treatment of life-threatening venous thrombosis, and in pulmonary embolism. Treatment must be started rapidly, within an hour of the event, and be controlled by measurement of the thrombin clotting time. Adrenaline, chlorpheniramine, and hydrocortisone should be available to control allergic reactions. (For details see Allergic Emergencies, section 3.4.3.)

Urokinase is currently used for thrombolysis in the eye and in arteriovenous shunts. It has the advantage of being non-immunogenic.

Stanozolol (see section 6.4.3) in a dosage of 10 mg daily produces some fibrinolytic enhancement, and is used in the treatment of Raynaud's syndrome associated with systemic sclerosis and lipodermatosclerosis.

STREPTOKINASE

Indications: deep-vein thrombosis, pulmonary embolism, acute arterial thromboembolism, thrombosed arteriovenous shunts; myocardial infarction (see specialist literature)
Cautions: atrial fibrillation, recovery from streptococcal infection; concurrent anticoagulant and antiplatelet therapy
Contra-indications: recent haemorrhage, coagulation defects, severe hypertension, streptococcal infections, surgery or needle biopsy in previous 72 hours, menstruation, pregnancy
Side-effects: allergic reactions, fever, rashes, haemorrhage (if due to overdose, can give tranexamic acid)
Dose: by intravenous infusion, 250 000–600 000 units over 30–60 minutes, then 100 000 units every hour for up to 48–72 hours

PoM **Kabikinase**® (KabiVitrum)
Injection, powder for reconstitution, streptokinase; net price 100 000-unit vial = £9.60; 250 000-unit vial = £17.00; 600 000-unit vial = £36.00
PoM **Streptase**® (Hoechst)
Injection, powder for reconstitution, streptokinase 100 000, 250 000, and 750 000 units per vial

UROKINASE

Indications: thrombosed arteriovenous shunts; thrombolysis in the eye
Contra-indications: recent haemorrhage, surgery or needle biopsy in previous 72 hours, pregnancy

Side-effects: haemorrhage (if due to overdose, give tranexamic acid), fever
Dose: by instillation into arteriovenous shunt, 5000–37 500 International units in 2–3 ml sodium chloride intravenous infusion 0.9%
Intra-ocular administration, 5000–37 500 International units in 2 ml sodium chloride intravenous infusion 0.9%
Note. 1.5 International units ≈ 1 Ploug unit

PoM **Ukidan**® (Serono)
Injection, powder for reconstitution, urokinase; net price 5000 International unit vial = £6.71; 25 000 International unit vial = £23.58
PoM **Urokinase** (Leo)
Injection, powder for reconstitution, urokinase; net price 7500 International unit (5000 Ploug unit) amp = £9.75; 37 500 International unit (25 000 Ploug unit) amp = £27.79

2.11 Antifibrinolytic drugs and haemostatics

Fibrin dissolution can be impaired by the administration of **tranexamic acid** (Cyklokapron®), which inhibits plasminogen activation and fibrinolysis. It may be useful when haemorrhage cannot be staunched, e.g. in prostatectomy, dental extraction in haemophiliacs, or menorrhagia; it may also be used in streptokinase overdose.

Aprotinin (see section 1.9.3) is a proteolytic enzyme inhibitor acting on plasmin and kallidinogenase (kallikrein). Its value in the treatment of disseminated intravascular coagulation has not been substantiated.

Ethamsylate (Dicynene®) reduces capillary bleeding in the presence of a normal number of platelets. It does not act by fibrin stabilisation, but probably by correcting abnormal platelet adhesion.

ETHAMSYLATE

Indications: haemorrhage from small blood vessels; menorrhagia
Side-effects: nausea, headache, rashes
Dose: by mouth, 500 mg 4 times daily
By intramuscular or intravenous injection, 1 g; maintenance 500 mg every 4–6 hours

PoM **Dicynene**® (Delandale)
Tablets, ethamsylate 250 mg. Net price 20 = £2.03
Tablets, ethamsylate 500 mg. Net price 20 = £4.02
Injection, ethamsylate 125 mg/ml. Net price 2-ml amp = 74p
Injection, ethamsylate 500 mg/ml. Net price 2-ml amp = £1.25

TRANEXAMIC ACID

Indications: see notes above
Cautions: reduce dose in renal impairment; massive haematuria (ureteric obstruction); regular eye examinations and liver function tests in long-term treatment of hereditary angioedema

Contra-indications: thromboembolic disease
Side-effects: nausea, vomiting, diarrhoea (reduce dose); giddiness on rapid intravenous injection
Dose: by mouth, 1–1.5 g 2–4 times daily
By slow intravenous injection, 1 g 3 times daily

PoM **Cyklokapron®** (KabiVitrum)
Tablets, f/c, scored, tranexamic acid 500 mg. Net price 50 = £10.80
Syrup, tranexamic acid 500 mg/5 ml. Diluent syrup, life of diluted syrup 14 days. Net price 300 ml = £15.60
Injection, tranexamic acid 100 mg/ml. Net price 5-ml amp = £1.35

2.12   Lipid-lowering drugs

There are a number of common conditions, some familial, in which there are very high plasma concentrations of cholesterol, or triglycerides, or both. There is evidence that therapy which lowers low density lipoprotein (LDL) cholesterol and raises high density lipoprotein (HDL) cholesterol reduces the progression of coronary atherosclerosis and may even induce regression. Lipid-lowering drugs should be reserved for patients in whom severe hyperlipidaemia is inadequately controlled by a modified fat diet. Any drug therapy must be combined with strict adherence to diet, maintenance of near-ideal body weight and, if appropriate, reduction of blood pressure and cessation of smoking.

ANION-EXCHANGE RESINS

Cholestyramine and **colestipol** are anion-exchange resins used in the management of hypercholesterolaemia. They act by binding bile acids, preventing their reabsorption; this promotes hepatic conversion of cholesterol into bile acids; the resultant increased LDL-receptor activity of liver cells increases the breakdown of LDL-cholesterol, thus both compounds effectively reduce LDL-cholesterol but can aggravate hypertriglyceridaemia.

COUNSELLING. Other drugs should be taken at least 1 hour before or 4–6 hours after cholestyramine or colestipol to reduce possible interference with absorption

---

CHOLESTYRAMINE

Indications: see notes above
Cautions: supplements of fat-soluble vitamins and of folic acid may be required with high doses, particularly in children. Drug interactions: see Appendix 1 (sections *2.1, 2.2, 2.8, 2.8C, 4.7, 5.1, 6.2, 10*)
Contra-indications: complete biliary obstruction, pregnancy
Side-effects: nausea, constipation or diarrhoea, heartburn, flatulence, abdominal discomfort, rashes; rarely steatorrhoea (with large doses)
Dose: usually 12–24 g daily in liquid in single or divided doses; up to 36 g daily in resistant cases

PoM **Questran®** (Bristol-Myers)
Powder, peach, cholestyramine (anhydrous) 4 g/sachet. Net price 10 sachets = £4.18. Label: 13, counselling advised, avoid other drugs at same time (see notes above)

COLESTIPOL HYDROCHLORIDE

Indications: see notes above
Cautions; Contra-indications; Side-effects: see under Cholestyramine. Drug interactions: see Appendix 1 (section *2.1*)
Dose: 5–10 g 2–3 times daily in liquid

PoM **Colestid®** (Upjohn)
Granules, yellow, colestipol hydrochloride. Net price 30 × 5-g sachets = £17.07. Label: 13, counselling advised, avoid other drugs at same time (see notes above)

CLOFIBRATE GROUP

Clofibrate, bezafibrate, and **gemfibrozil** can be regarded as broad-spectrum lipid-modulating agents in that although their main action is to decrease serum triglycerides they also tend to reduce LDL-cholesterol and to raise HDL-cholesterol.

All three can cause a myositis-like syndrome, especially in patients with impaired renal function. In addition, clofibrate predisposes to gallstones by increasing biliary cholesterol excretion; it is therefore only indicated in patients who have had a cholecystectomy.

BEZAFIBRATE

Indications: see notes above
Cautions: reduce dose in moderate renal impairment. Drug interactions: see Appendix 1 (sections *2.8, 2.8B, 6.1*)
Contra-indications: severe renal or hepatic impairment, hypoalbuminaemia, primary biliary cirrhosis, gall bladder disease, nephrotic syndrome, pregnancy
Side-effects: nausea, abdominal discomfort; rarely myositis-like syndrome, pruritus, urticaria, impotence
Dose: 200 mg 3 times daily with or after food; may be reduced to 200 mg twice daily in hypertriglyceridaemia

▼ PoM **Bezalip®** (MCP)
Tablets, f/c, bezafibrate 200 mg. Net price 20 = £2.05. Label: 21
▼ PoM **Bezalip-Mono®** (MCP)
Tablets, f/c, bezafibrate 400 mg. Net price 28 = £8.72. Label: 21, 25
Dose: 1 tablet daily in the evening

CLOFIBRATE

Indications: see notes above
Cautions; Contra-indications: see under Bezafibrate. Drug interactions: see Appendix 1 (sections *2.8, 2.8B, 6.1*)

Side-effects: see under Bezafibrate; also cholesterol cholelithiasis
Dose: 500 mg 2–3 times daily after meals

PoM **Atromid-S**® (ICI)
Capsules, red, clofibrate 500 mg. Net price 20 = 65p. Label: 21

GEMFIBROZIL

Indications: hyperlipidaemia (see also notes above)
Cautions: lipid profile, blood counts, and liver-function tests before initiating long-term treatment; renal impairment; annual eye examinations. Drug interactions: see Appendix 1 (sections *2.8*, *2.8B*)
Contra-indications: alcoholism, hepatic impairment, gallstones; pregnancy
Side-effects: gastro-intestinal disturbances; pruritus, rash, headache, dizziness, blurred vision, painful extremities; rarely myalgia
Dose: 1.2 g daily, usually in 2 divided doses; range 0.9–1.5 g daily

▼ PoM **Lopid**® (P-D)
Capsules, white/maroon, gemfibrozil 300 mg. Net price 20 = £4.80

NICOTINIC ACID GROUP

The value of nicotinic acid and nicofuranose is limited by their side-effects, especially vasodilatation. In doses of 1.5 to 3 g daily they lower both cholesterol and triglyceride concentrations by inhibiting synthesis; they also increase HDL-cholesterol.

ACIPIMOX

Indications: hyperlipidaemia
Contra-indications: peptic ulcer
Side-effects: vasodilatation, flushing, itching, rashes, erythema; occasionally, heartburn, epigastric pain, nausea, diarrhoea, headache, malaise
Dose: usually 500–750 mg daily in divided doses

▼ PoM **Olbetam**® (Farmitalia Carlo Erba)
Capsules, brown/pink, acipimox 250 mg. Net price 100-cap pack = £40.00. Label: 21

NICOFURANOSE

Indications: see notes above (for use in peripheral vascular disease, see section 2.6.3)
Cautions; Side-effects: see under Nicotinic Acid, but prostaglandin-mediated symptoms less severe
Dose: 0.5–1 g 3 times daily

Bradilan® (Napp)
Tablets, e/c and s/c, nicofuranose 250 mg. Net price 20 = £1.41. Label: 5, 25

NICOTINIC ACID

Indications: see notes above
Cautions: diabetes mellitus, gout, liver disease, peptic ulcer
Contra-indications: pregnancy, breast-feeding
Side-effects: flushing, dizziness, palpitations, pruritus (prostaglandin-mediated symptoms can be reduced by low initial doses taken with meals, or by taking aspirin 300 mg 30 minutes before the dose—needed in only a very small proportion of patients); nausea, vomiting; rarely impaired liver function and rashes
Dose: initially 100–200 mg 3 times daily (see above), gradually increased over 2–4 weeks to 1–2 g 3 times daily

Nicotinic Acid Tablets, nicotinic acid 25 mg, net price 20 = 9p; 50 mg, 20 = 12p; 100 mg, 20 = 20p. Label: 21

FISH OILS

A fish-oil preparation (Maxepa®), rich in omega-3 marine triglycerides, is useful in the treatment of severe hypertriglyceridaemia.

OMEGA-3 MARINE TRIGLYCERIDES

Indications: reduction of plasma triglycerides in patients with severe hypertriglyceridaemia judged to be at special risk of ischaemic heart disease and/or pancreatitis, in conjunction with dietary and other methods (see notes above)
Side-effects: occasional nausea and belching
Dose: see under preparations below

▼ **Maxepa**® (DF)
Capsules, 1 g (approx. 1.1 ml) concentrated fish oils of composition below. Net price 200 = £28.57. Label: 21
Dose: 5 capsules twice daily with food
Liquid, golden-coloured, concentrated fish oils containing, as percentage of total fatty acid composition, eicosapentaenoic acid 18% w/w, docosahexaenoic acid 12% w/w. Vitamin A content less than 100 units/g, vitamin D content less than 10 units/g. Net price 150 ml = £21.43. Label: 21
Dose: 5 ml twice daily with food

OTHER DRUGS

Probucol decreases both LDL- and HDL-cholesterol; despite the latter effect it appears to promote resolution of xanthomata.
Dextrothyroxine (Choloxin®) is no longer recommended as a lipid-lowering drug. It lowers the plasma cholesterol concentration but may cause tachycardia and, in patients with ischaemic heart disease, angina.

DEXTROTHYROXINE SODIUM

Indications: see notes above
Cautions: drug interactions: see Appendix 1 (section *2.8B*)

Contra-indications: severe kidney or liver disease; ischaemic heart disease

Side-effects: tachycardia, angina in patients with pre-existing subclinical coronary artery disease

Dose: 1–2 mg daily, increased by 1–2 mg at monthly intervals; max. dose 8 mg daily

PoM **Choloxin**® (Baxter)
Tablets, yellow, scored, dextrothyroxine sodium 2 mg. Net price 20 = £4.00

PROBUCOL

Indications: see notes above

Cautions: avoid pregnancy during and for 6 months after stopping treatment

Contra-indications: breast-feeding

Side-effects: nausea, vomiting, flatulence, diarrhoea, abdominal pain; rarely angioedema, hypersensitivity reactions

Dose: 500 mg twice daily with food

PoM **Lurselle**® (Merrell)
Tablets, probucol 250 mg. Net price 20 = £2.23. Label: 21

2.13   Local sclerosants

Ethanolamine oleate and sodium tetradecyl sulphate are used in sclerotherapy of varicose veins, and phenol is used in thrombosed haemorrhoids (see section 1.7.3).

ETHANOLAMINE OLEATE

Indications: sclerotherapy of varicose veins

Cautions: extravasation may cause necrosis of tissues

Contra-indications: inability to walk, acute phlebitis, oral contraceptive use, obese legs

Side-effects: allergic reactions

PoM **Ethanolamine Oleate Injection**, ethanolamine oleate 5%. Net price 2-ml amp = 49p; 5-ml amp = 59p
Dose: by intravenous injection, 2–5 ml divided between 3–4 sites; repeated at weekly intervals

SODIUM TETRADECYL SULPHATE

Indications: sclerotherapy of varicose veins

Cautions; Contra-indications; Side-effects: see under Ethanolamine Oleate

PoM **STD**® (STD Pharmaceutical)
Injection, sodium tetradecyl sulphate 3%. Net price 1-ml amp = 45p; 30-ml vial = £8.75
Dose: by intravenous injection, 0.5–1 ml at up to 4 sites

3: Drugs used in the treatment of diseases of the
RESPIRATORY SYSTEM

In this chapter, drug treatment is described under the following headings:

3.1 Bronchodilators
3.2 Corticosteroids
3.3 Prophylaxis of asthma
3.4 Allergic disorders
3.5 Respiratory stimulants
3.6 Oxygen
3.7 Mucolytics
3.8 Aromatic inhalations
3.9 Antitussives
3.10 Systemic nasal decongestants

The initial treatment of exacerbations of chronic bronchitis and bacterial pneumonia is indicated in section 5.1 (Table 1) and the treatment of tuberculosis is discussed in section 5.1.9.

3.1 Bronchodilators

3.1.1 Adrenoceptor stimulants
3.1.2 Anticholinergic bronchodilators
3.1.3 Theophylline
3.1.4 Compound bronchodilator preparations

3.1.1 Adrenoceptor stimulants
(sympathomimetics)

3.1.1.1 Selective beta$_2$-adrenoceptor stimulants
3.1.1.2 Other adrenoceptor stimulants

Most mild to moderate attacks of asthma respond rapidly to aerosol administration of a selective beta$_2$-adrenoceptor stimulant such as salbutamol or terbutaline (section 3.1.1.1). In frequently occurring moderate asthma the introduction of a corticosteroid inhalation (section 3.2), sodium cromoglycate (section 3.3), or oral theophylline (section 3.1.3) may stabilise the asthma and avoid the use of oral corticosteroids. However in more severe attacks a short course of an oral corticosteroid may be necessary to bring the asthma under control (section 3.2).

Treatment of patients with severe acute asthma or airways obstruction (see also below) is safer in hospital where oxygen and resuscitation facilities are immediately available.

Patients with chronic bronchitis and emphysema are often described as having irreversible airways obstruction, but they usually respond partially to the beta$_2$-adrenoceptor stimulant drugs or to the anticholinergic drug ipratropium (section 3.1.2).

CHOICE OF DRUG. The **selective beta$_2$-adrenoceptor stimulants** (section 3.1.1.1) such as salbutamol or terbutaline (preferably given by aerosol inhalation) are the safest and most effective preparations. The drugs described in section 3.1.1.2 should be avoided whenever possible.

There is little difference between the various selective beta$_2$-adrenoceptor stimulant drugs. **Sal-** **butamol** and **terbutaline** are available in the widest range of formulations. **Rimiterol** has a shorter duration of action than salbutamol, terbutaline and fenoterol. **Pirbuterol**, which has recently been introduced, is similar to the others. The dose or frequency of administration of beta$_2$-adrenoceptor stimulants can often be reduced by concurrent treatment with prophylactic drugs such as corticosteroid inhalations (section 3.2) or sodium cromoglycate (section 3.3).

CHOICE OF FORMULATION. The *pressurised aerosol inhaler* is an effective and convenient method of administration for mild to moderate airways obstruction. Aerosol inhalers usually act for about 3 to 5 hours (rimiterol less than the others) but this depends to some extent on the severity of the asthma and on the dose administered. Aerosol inhalation is preferred because it provides relief more rapidly and causes fewer side-effects (such as tremor and nervous tension) than tablets; the drug is delivered directly to the bronchi and is therefore effective in smaller doses.

Patients should be given careful instruction on the use of their pressurised aerosol inhalers and it is important to check that they continue to use them correctly as inadequate technique may be mistaken for drug failure. In particular, it should be emphasised that they must inhale slowly and hold their breath for 10 seconds after inhalation. Most patients can be successfully taught to use pressurised aerosol inhalers but some patients, particularly the elderly, the arthritic, and small children are unable to use them; some patients are unable to synchronise their breathing with the administration of aerosol.

The dose should be stated explicitly in terms of the number of inhalations at one time, the frequency, and the maximum number of inhalations allowed in 24 hours. Very high doses of beta$_2$-stimulants can be dangerous in some patients, but excessive use is usually an indication of inadequately treated asthma. Patients should be advised to seek medical advice when they fail to obtain their usual degree of symptomatic relief as this usually indicates a worsening of the asthma and may require alternative medication. When patients with asthma are not adequately controlled with 6 to 8 puffs daily, addition of a prophylactic drug such as a corticosteroid inhalation should be considered; this is more convenient for the patient than higher doses of beta$_2$-stimulants and usually provides better overall control.

Dry powder inhalers (e.g. Ventolin Rotacaps®) are actuated by the patient's inspiration and hence are of particular value in subjects who cannot use pressurised aerosol inhalers correctly. Children as young as 2 years can inhale the drug once the capsule has been placed in the inhaler. Bioavailability of the drug appears to be lower, so the

---

recommended doses are twice those in a metered inhaler. The dry powder occasionally causes coughing.

A variety of spacing devices are now available for use with metered dose inhalers. By providing a space between inhaler and mouth, they reduce the velocity of the aerosol and subsequent impaction on the oropharynx; in addition they allow more time for evaporation of the propellent so that a larger proportion of the particles can be inhaled and deposited in the lungs; also co-ordination of inspiration with actuation of the aerosol is less important. They range from the Bricanyl Spacer® (for terbutaline), a collapsible extended mouthpiece, to larger cone-shaped spacing devices with a one-way valve (Nebuhaler®, Volumatic®). Spacing devices are particularly useful for patients with poor inhalation technique, for children, for patients requiring higher doses, for nocturnal asthma, and for patients prone to develop candidiasis with inhaled corticosteroids.

Aqueous aerosols (respirator solutions) of salbutamol and terbutaline, and more recently fenoterol and reproterol, are increasingly used for the treatment of acute asthma both in hospital and in general practice. Aqueous aerosols are usually administered over a period of about 15 minutes from a nebuliser, usually driven from an oxygen cylinder in hospital. An electrical compressor is most suitable for domiciliary use but these are costly and not currently prescribable under the NHS. Patients with a severe attack of asthma should have oxygen during nebulisation since beta-adrenoceptor stimulants can cause an increase in arterial hypoxaemia. For patients with chronic bronchitis and hypercapnoea, however, oxygen can be dangerous, and the nebuliser should be driven by air. The dose prescribed by nebuliser is substantially higher than that prescribed by metered dose inhaler. For example, a 2.5-ml Ventolin Nebule® contains 2.5 mg of salbutamol, which is equivalent to 25 puffs from the aerosol inhaler. Patients should therefore be warned that it is dangerous to exceed the stated dose and that if they fail to respond to the usual dose of beta₂-adrenoceptor stimulant they should call for help.

Oral preparations are available for patients who cannot manage the inhaled route. They are sometimes used for children, though the inhaled route is better and most children can use one or other of the inhalation devices available. They have a slower onset but slightly more prolonged action than the aerosol inhalers. The *sustained-release* preparations (Ventolin Spandets®; Bricanyl SA®) may be of value in patients with nocturnal asthma as an alternative to the sustained-release theophylline preparations (section 3.1.3).

Intravenous, and occasionally *subcutaneous*, injections of salbutamol and terbutaline are given for severe acute asthma.

EMERGENCY TREATMENT OF SEVERE ACUTE ASTHMA. Severe asthma can be fatal and **must** be treated promptly and energetically. It is characterised by persistent dyspnoea poorly relieved by broncho-dilators, restlessness, exhaustion, a high pulse rate (usually over 110/minute), often pulsus paradoxus of over 10 mmHg, and a very low peak expiratory flow. The respiration is so shallow that wheezing may be absent. Such patients should be given a large dose of a **corticosteroid** (see section 6.3.4)—for adults hydrocortisone 200 mg (as sodium phosphate or succinate) intravenously or prednisolone 40 mg by mouth, children half these doses. They should also be given a beta₂-selective adrenoceptor stimulant such as **salbutamol** or **terbutaline** by nebuliser. If there is little response the following additional treatment should be considered: **ipratropium** by nebuliser (section 3.1.2), **aminophylline** by slow intravenous injection, if the patient has not already been receiving theophylline (section 3.1.3), or change of administration of the beta₂-selective adrenoceptor stimulant to the intravenous route.

Further treatment of these patients is safer in hospital where oxygen therapy and resuscitation facilities are immediately available. Treatment should **never** be delayed for investigations, patients should **never** be sedated, and the possibility of a pneumothorax should also be remembered.

If the patient deteriorates despite appropriate pharmacological treatment, intermittent positive pressure ventilation may be needed temporarily.

3.1.1.1 SELECTIVE BETA₂-ADRENOCEPTOR STIMULANTS

SALBUTAMOL

Indications: reversible airways obstruction, severe acute asthma

Cautions: hyperthyroidism, ischaemic heart disease, hypertension, pregnancy, elderly patients; intravenous administration to diabetics (monitor blood glucose). See also notes above

Side-effects: fine tremor (usually hands), nervous tension, headache, peripheral vasodilatation, tachycardia (seldom troublesome when given by aerosol inhalation); hypokalaemia after high doses; slight pain on intramuscular injection

Dose: by mouth, 4 mg (elderly and sensitive patients initially 2 mg) 3–4 times daily; max. 8 mg (but unlikely to be tolerated); CHILD 2–6 years 1–2 mg 3–4 times daily, 6–12 years 2 mg

By subcutaneous or intramuscular injection, 500 micrograms, repeated every 4 hours if necessary

By slow intravenous injection, 250 micrograms, repeated if necessary

By intravenous infusion, initially 5 micrograms/ minute, adjusted according to response usually in range 3–20 micrograms/minute, or more if necessary

By aerosol inhalation, acute and intermittent episodes of wheezing and asthma, 100–200 micrograms (1–2 puffs); CHILD 100 micrograms (1 puff)

Prophylaxis in exercise-induced bronchospasm,

200 micrograms (2 puffs); CHILD 100 micrograms (1 puff)
Chronic maintenance therapy, 200 micrograms (2 puffs) 3–4 times daily; CHILD 100 micrograms (1 puff) 3–4 times daily, increased to 200 micrograms (2 puffs) if necessary
By inhalation of a powder (Rotacaps®, Ventodisks®), acute and intermittent episodes of wheezing and asthma, 200–400 micrograms; CHILD 200 micrograms
Prophylaxis in exercise-induced bronchospasm, 400 micrograms; CHILD 200 micrograms
Chronic maintenance therapy, 400 micrograms 3–4 times daily; CHILD 200 micrograms 3–4 times daily
By inhalation of nebulised solution, chronic bronchospasm unresponsive to conventional therapy and severe acute asthma, 2.5 mg, repeated up to 4 times daily, increased to 5 mg if necessary; in refractory patients with severe acute asthma 10 mg can be used if side-effects permit; CHILD 2.5 mg, increased to 5 mg if required

Oral preparations
PoM **Asmaven®** (APS)
Tablets, both pink, salbutamol (as sulphate), 2 mg, net price 20 = 23p; 4 mg, 20 = 42p
PoM **Cobutolin®** (Cox Pharmaceuticals)
Tablets, both pink, salbutamol (as sulphate), 2 mg, net price 20 = 18p; 4 mg, 20 = 35p
PoM **Salbulin®** (Riker)
Tablets, salbutamol (as sulphate), 2 mg, net price 20 = 18p; 4 mg, 20 = 35p
PoM **Ventolin®** (A&H)
Tablets, both pink, scored, salbutamol (as sulphate), 2 mg, net price 20 = 22p; 4 mg, 20 = 43p
Spandets® (= tablets s/r), pink/white, salbutamol 8 mg (as sulphate). Net price 50 = £2.25. Label: 25
Dose: 8 mg twice daily, increased if necessary to a max. of 32 mg daily; CHILD over 12 years 8 mg twice daily
Syrup, sugar-free, salbutamol 2 mg (as sulphate)/5 ml. Diluent purified water, freshly boiled and cooled, life of diluted syrup 28 days. Net price 100 ml = 45p
PoM **Volmax®** (DF)
Tablets, s/r, salbutamol (as sulphate) 4 mg, net price 56-tab pack = £10.00; 8 mg, 56-tab pack = £12.00. Label: 25
Dose: 8 mg twice daily; CHILD 3–12 years 4 mg twice daily

Parenteral preparations
PoM **Ventolin®** (A&H)
Injection, salbutamol 50 micrograms (as sulphate)/ml. Net price 5-ml amp = 57p
Injection, salbutamol 500 micrograms (as sulphate)/ml. Net price 1-ml amp = 43p
Solution for intravenous infusion, salbutamol 1 mg (as sulphate)/ml. Dilute before use. Net price 5-ml amp = £3.08

Inhalation preparations
PoM **Aerolin 400®** (Riker)
Aerosol inhalation, salbutamol 100 micrograms (as sulphate)/metered inhalation. Net price 400-dose unit = £4.98
COUNSELLING. Advise patients not to exceed prescribed dose and to follow manufacturer's directions
PoM **Aerolin Auto®** (Riker)
Aerosol inhalation, salbutamol 100 micrograms (as sulphate)/metered inhalation. Net price 400-dose breath-actuated unit = £11.50; refill = £4.98
COUNSELLING. Advise patients as above
PoM **Asmaven®** (APS)
Aerosol inhalation, salbutamol 100 micrograms/metered inhalation. Net price 200-dose unit = £2.18
COUNSELLING. Advise patients not to exceed prescribed dose and to follow manufacturer's directions
PoM **Cobutolin®** (Cox Pharmaceuticals)
Aerosol inhalation, salbutamol 100 micrograms/metered inhalation. Net price 200-dose unit = £2.08
COUNSELLING. Advise patients not to exceed prescribed dose and to follow manufacturer's directions
PoM **Salbulin®** (Riker)
Aerosol inhalation, salbutamol 100 micrograms/metered inhalation. Net price 200-dose unit = £2.08
COUNSELLING. Advise patients not to exceed prescribed dose and to follow manufacturer's directions
PoM **Ventodisks®** (A&H)
Powder for inhalation, disks containing 8 blisters of salbutamol (as sulphate) 200 micrograms/blister, net price pack of 14 × 8 = £7.11; 400 micrograms/blister, pack of 14 × 8 = £12.02 (both with Diskhaler®)
PoM **Ventolin®** (A&H)
Aerosol inhalation, salbutamol 100 micrograms/metered inhalation. Net price 200-dose unit = £2.62
COUNSELLING. Advise patients not to exceed prescribed dose and to follow manufacturer's directions
Nebules® (= single-dose ampoules for nebulisation), salbutamol 0.1% (1 mg/ml, as sulphate), net price 2.5-ml amp (2.5 mg) = 19p; 0.2% (2 mg/ml), 2.5-ml amp (5 mg) = 39p. May be diluted with physiological saline
Rotacaps®, light blue/clear, salbutamol 200 micrograms (as sulphate). Net price 20 = £1.06
Rotacaps®, dark blue/clear, salbutamol 400 micrograms (as sulphate). Net price 20 = £1.43
Respirator solution (for use with a nebuliser or ventilator), salbutamol 0.5% (5 mg/ml, as sulphate). Net price 20 ml = £2.71. Before use dilute with physiological saline

Devices
Rotahaler® (A&H)
Breath actuated inhaler for use with Rotacaps. Net price = 78p
Volumatic® (A&H)
Inhaler, large-volume spacer device. For use with Ventolin, Becotide, Becloforte, and Ventide inhalers. Net price = £2.75

TERBUTALINE SULPHATE

Indications; Cautions; Side-effects: see under Salbutamol

Dose: by mouth, 5 mg 2–3 times daily; CHILD 3–7 years 0.75–1.5 mg 3 times daily, 7–15 years 2.5 mg 2–3 times daily

By subcutaneous, intramuscular, or slow intravenous injection, 250–500 micrograms up to 4 times daily; CHILD 2–15 years 10 micrograms/ kg to a max. of 300 micrograms

By continuous intravenous infusion as a solution containing 3–5 micrograms/ml, 1.5–5 micrograms/minute for 8–10 hours; reduce dose for children

By aerosol inhalation, prophylaxis, adults and children 250–500 micrograms (1–2 puffs) repeated after 4 hours if necessary; not more than 8 inhalations should be necessary in any 24 hours

By inhalation of powder (Turbohaler®), 500 micrograms (1 inhalation) as required; not more than 4 inhalations in any 24 hours

By inhalation of nebulised solution, 5–10 mg 2–4 times daily; additional doses may be necessary in acute severe asthma; CHILD, up to 3 years 2 mg, 3–6 years 3 mg; 6–8 years 4 mg, over 8 years 5 mg, 2–4 times daily

PoM **Bricanyl**® (Astra)

Tablets, scored, terbutaline sulphate 5 mg. Net price 20 = 71p

Syrup, sugar-free, terbutaline sulphate 1.5 mg/ 5 ml. Diluent water for preparations, life of diluted syrup 14 days. Net price 100 ml = 75p

Injection, terbutaline sulphate 500 micrograms/ ml. Net price 1-ml amp = 28p

Aerosol inhalation, terbutaline sulphate 250 micrograms/metered inhalation. Net price 400-dose unit = £5.31; 400-dose unit with Spacer inhaler (collapsible extended mouthpiece) = £7.21; 400-dose refill cannister for use with Nebuhaler or Spacer inhaler = £5.21

COUNSELLING. Advise patients not to exceed prescribed dose and to follow manufacturer's directions

Turbohaler® (= breath-actuated dry powder inhaler), terbutaline sulphate 500 micrograms/ metered inhalation. Net price 200-dose unit = £17.88

COUNSELLING. Advise patients not to exceed prescribed dose and to follow manufacturer's directions

Respules® (= single-dose units for nebulisation), terbutaline sulphate 2.5 mg/ml. Net price 20 × 2-ml units = £3.76

Respirator solution (for use with a nebuliser or ventilator), terbutaline sulphate 10 mg/ml. Net price 10 ml = £1.35. Before use dilute with sterile physiological saline

PoM **Bricanyl SA**® (Astra)

Tablets, s/r, terbutaline sulphate 7.5 mg. Net price 20 = £1.59. Label: 25

Dose: 7.5 mg twice daily

PoM **Monovent**® (Lagap)

Tablets, scored, terbutaline sulphate 5 mg. Net price 20 = 64p

Syrup, terbutaline sulphate 1.5 mg/5 ml. Diluent

PoM **Monovent SA**® (Lagap)

Tablets, s/r, terbutaline sulphate 7.5 mg. Net price 20 = £1.43. Label: 25

Dose: 7.5 mg twice daily

Nebuhaler® (Astra)

Inhaler, fitted with plastic cone and one-way valve. For use with Bricanyl and Pulmicort refill canisters. Net price £4.75

FENOTEROL HYDROBROMIDE

Indications; Cautions; Side-effects: see under Salbutamol

Dose: by aerosol inhalation, chronic maintenance therapy, 180–360 micrograms (1–2 puffs) 3 times daily, if necessary increased to every 4 hours; CHILD 6–12 years 180 micrograms (1 puff)

By inhalation of nebulised solution, 0.5–2.5 mg (increased in severe cases to a max. of 5 mg) up to 4 times daily, dilution adjusted to equipment and length of administration; CHILD 6–14 years, up to 1 mg up to 3 times daily

PoM **Berotec**® (Boehringer Ingelheim)

Aerosol inhalation, fenoterol hydrobromide 180 micrograms/metered inhalation. Net price 200-dose unit = £2.78 (extension tube also available)

COUNSELLING. Advise patients not to exceed prescribed dose and to follow manufacturer's directions

Nebuliser solution, fenoterol hydrobromide 0.5% (5 mg/ml, 20 drops ≈1 ml). Net price 20 ml (with dropper) = £1.76. For use with nebuliser or ventilator; if dilution is necessary, use only sterile sodium chloride 0.9% solution.

PIRBUTEROL

Indications: reversible airways obstruction

Cautions; Side-effects: see under Salbutamol

Dose: by mouth, 10–15 mg 3–4 times daily; CHILD 6–12 years 7.5 mg up to 4 times daily

By aerosol inhalation, intermittent episodes, prophylaxis in exercise-induced bronchospasm, 200–400 micrograms (1–2 puffs) repeated after 4 hours if necessary; max. 2.4 mg (12 puffs) daily

Chronic maintenance therapy, 400 micrograms (2 puffs) 3–4 times daily or in severe bronchospasm every 4 hours; max. 2.4 mg (12 puffs) daily

▼ PoM **Exirel**® (Pfizer)

Capsules, turquoise/olive, pirbuterol 10 mg (as hydrochloride). Net price 20 = 48p

Capsules, turquoise/beige, pirbuterol 15 mg (as hydrochloride). Net price 20 = 71p

Syrup, pirbuterol 7.5 mg (as hydrochloride)/ 5 ml. Net price 150 ml = £1.71

Aerosol inhalation, pirbuterol 200 micrograms (as acetate)/metered inhalation. Net price 200-dose unit = £2.86

COUNSELLING. Advise patients not to exceed prescribed dose and to follow manufacturer's directions

REPROTEROL HYDROCHLORIDE

Indications: reversible airways obstruction

Cautions; Side-effects: see under Salbutamol

Dose: by mouth, 10–20 mg 3 times daily; CHILD 6–12 years 10 mg 3 times daily

By aerosol inhalation, intermittent episodes and prophylaxis in exercise-induced bronchospasm, 0.5–1 mg (1–2 puffs) repeated after 3–6 hours if necessary; CHILD 6–12 years 500 micrograms (1 puff)

Chronic maintenance therapy, 1 mg (2 puffs) 3 times daily or in severe bronchospasm every 3–6 hours; CHILD 6–12 years 500 micrograms (1 puff) 3 times daily

By inhalation of nebulised solution (respirator solution), 10–20 ml diluted to 3 ml with sterile physiological saline, over 10 minutes, when required. Dilution may be adjusted to equipment and length of administration

▼ PoM **Bronchodil**® (Degussa)

Tablets, scored, reproterol hydrochloride 20 mg. Net price 20 = 68p.

Aerosol inhalation, reproterol hydrochloride 500 micrograms/metered inhalation. Net price 400-dose unit = £6.84

COUNSELLING. Advise patients not to exceed prescribed dose and to follow manufacturer's directions

Respirator solution, reproterol hydrochloride 10 mg/ml. Net price 50 ml = £4.70

RIMITEROL HYDROBROMIDE

Indications: reversible airways obstruction (particularly when short action required)

Cautions; Side-effects: see under Salbutamol

Dose: by aerosol inhalation, adults and children 200–600 micrograms (1–3 puffs); should not be repeated in less than 30 minutes; max. 8 doses daily

PoM **Pulmadil**® (Riker)

Aerosol inhalation, rimiterol hydrobromide 200 micrograms/metered inhalation. Net price 300-dose unit = £6.32

COUNSELLING. Advise patients not to exceed prescribed dose and to follow manufacturer's directions

PoM **Pulmadil Auto**® (Riker)

Aerosol inhalation, rimiterol hydrobromide 200 micrograms/metered inhalation. Net price 300-dose cartridge in breath-actuated unit = £7.93; replacement cartridge = £6.32

COUNSELLING. Advise patients as above

3.1.1.2 OTHER ADRENOCEPTOR STIMULANTS

These preparations (including the partially selective orciprenaline) are now regarded as less suitable and less safe for use as bronchodilators than the selective beta$_2$-adrenoceptor stimulants, as they are more likely to cause arrhythmias and other side-effects. They should be avoided whenever possible. For use as nasal decongestants see section 3.10.

Adrenaline injection (1 in 1000) is used in the emergency treatment of acute allergic and anaphylactic reactions (section 3.4.3).

EPHEDRINE HYDROCHLORIDE

Indications: reversible airways obstruction

Cautions; Side-effects: see under Adrenaline, (section 3.4.3); incidence of tachycardia lower; anxiety, restlessness, and insomnia common; may cause acute retention in prostatic hypertrophy; interaction with MAOIs a disadvantage. Drug interactions: see Appendix 1 (section *4.3*)

Dose: 3 times daily, 15–60 mg; CHILD 3 times daily, up to 1 year 7.5 mg, 1–5 years 15 mg, 6–12 years 30 mg

PoM **Ephedrine Hydrochloride Tablets,** ephedrine hydrochloride 15 mg, net price 20 = 6p; 30 mg, 20 = 7p; 60 mg, 20 = 15p

PoM **Ephedrine Elixir,** ephedrine hydrochloride 15 mg/ 5 ml. Net price 100 ml = 42p

ISOETHARINE HYDROCHLORIDE

Indications: reversible airways obstruction

Cautions; Side-effects: see under Salbutamol (section 3.1.1.1)

PoM **Numotac**® (Riker)

Tablets, s/r, isoetharine hydrochloride 10 mg. Net price 20 = 55p. Label: 25

Dose: 10–20 mg 3–4 times daily

ISOPRENALINE SULPHATE

Indications: reversible airways obstruction

Cautions; Side-effects: see under Salbutamol (section 3.1.1.1) and notes above. Drug interactions: see Appendix 1 (section *15*)

Dose: sublingually, 10–20 mg 1–3 times daily; CHILD 5–10 mg 1–3 times daily

By aerosol inhalation, see below.

By inhalation of a nebulised solution containing 1%, not recommended

PoM **Iso-Autohaler**® (Riker)

Aerosol inhalation, isoprenaline sulphate 80 micrograms/metered inhalation. Net price 400-dose vial in breath-actuated unit = £4.34; refill vial = £2.73.

Dose: by aerosol inhalation, 80–240 micrograms (1–3 puffs); do not repeat within 30 minutes and not more than 8 times in 24 hours

COUNSELLING. Advise patients not to exceed prescribed dose and to follow manufacturer's directions

PoM **Medihaler-iso**® (Riker)

Aerosol inhalation, isoprenaline sulphate 80 micrograms/ metered inhalation. Net price 400-dose vial = £2.73.

Dose: by aerosol inhalation, 80–240 micrograms (1–3 puffs); do not repeat within 30 minutes and not more than 8 times in 24 hours

COUNSELLING. Advise patients as above

PoM **Medihaler-iso Forte**® (Riker)

Aerosol inhalation, isoprenaline sulphate 400 micrograms/metered inhalation. Net price 400-dose vial = £3.17.

Note. Not recommended therefore no dose stated

ORCIPRENALINE SULPHATE

Indications: reversible airways obstruction

Cautions; Side-effects: see under Salbutamol (section 3.1.1.1) and notes above

Dose: by mouth, 20 mg 4 times daily; CHILD up to 1 year 5–10 mg 3 times daily, 1–3 years 5–

10 mg 4 times daily, 3–12 years 40–60 mg daily in divided doses

By aerosol inhalation, 670–1340 micrograms (1–2 puffs) repeated if necessary after not less than 30 minutes to a max. of 8.04 mg (12 puffs) daily; CHILD up to 6 years 670 micrograms (1 puff) up to 4 times daily, 6–12 years 670–1340 micrograms (1–2 puffs) up to 4 times daily

PoM **Alupent**® (Boehringer Ingelheim)
Tablets, scored, orciprenaline sulphate 20 mg. Net price 20 = 67p
Syrup, sugar-free, orciprenaline sulphate 10 mg/5 ml. Diluents syrup or sorbitol solution, life of diluted syrup 14 days. Net price 100 ml = 69p
Aerosol inhalation, orciprenaline sulphate 670 micrograms/metered inhalation. Net price 300-dose vial with mouthpiece = £3.22; refill vial = £2.66.
COUNSELLING. Advise patients not to exceed prescribed dose and to follow manufacturer's directions

3.1.2   Anticholinergic bronchodilators

These drugs have traditionally been regarded as more effective in relieving bronchoconstriction associated with chronic bronchitis. Of this group, **ipratropium** (Atrovent®) may provide some bronchodilation in patients with chronic bronchitis who fail to respond to the selective beta$_2$-adrenoceptor stimulants (section 3.1.1.1). Unlike the other anticholinergic drugs, side-effects are rare and it does not increase sputum viscosity or affect mucociliary clearance of sputum. The aerosol inhalation has a slower onset of action than that of the beta$_2$-adrenoceptor stimulants, with a maximum effect 30–60 minutes after use; its duration of action is longer than that of beta$_2$-adrenoceptor stimulants following inhalation and bronchodilatation can usually be maintained with treatment three times a day.

The other atropine-like bronchodilators are now rarely used and often have unpleasant side-effects which limit their usefulness. They should be avoided, particularly in children, because although they reduce bronchial secretions, sputum viscosity may be increased and this can lead to blockage of the smaller airways.

IPRATROPIUM BROMIDE
Indications: reversible airways obstruction, particularly in chronic bronchitis
Cautions: glaucoma (standard doses unlikely to be harmful); prostatic hypertrophy
Side-effects: dry mouth occasionally reported; rarely urinary retention, constipation
Dose: see below

PoM **Atrovent**® (Boehringer Ingelheim)
Aerosol inhalation, ipratropium bromide 18 micrograms/metered inhalation. Net price 200-dose unit = £4.21
Dose: by aerosol inhalation, 18–36 micrograms (1–2 puffs), in early treatment up to 72 micrograms (4 puffs) at a time, 3–4 times daily; CHILD up to 6 years 18 micrograms (1 puff) 3 times daily, 6–12 years 18–36 micrograms (1–2 puffs) 3 times daily

COUNSELLING. Advise patient not to exceed prescribed dose and to follow manufacturer's directions

Nebuliser solution, isotonic, ipratropium bromide 250 micrograms/ml (0.025%); net price 10 × 2-ml unit-dose vials (preservative-free), = £3.76. If dilution is necessary use only sterile sodium chloride solution 0.9%
Dose: by inhalation of nebulised solution, 100–500 micrograms (0.4–2 ml of a 0.025% solution) up to 4 times daily; CHILD 3–14 years 100–500 micrograms up to 3 times daily. Dilution of solution is adjusted according to equipment and length of administration
Note. Because paradoxical bronchospasm may occur, treatment should always be initiated in hospital and be subject to close medical supervision during the first week. Bottles of nebuliser solution (which contained preservative) have been discontinued to reduce the risk; unit-dose vials are preservative-free.

PoM **Atrovent Forte**® (Boehringer Ingelheim)
Aerosol inhalation, ipratropium bromide 36 micrograms/metered inhalation. Net price 200-dose unit = £4.91
Dose: by aerosol inhalation 36–72 micrograms (1–2 puffs) 3–4 times daily; CHILD 6–12 years 36 micrograms (1 puff) 3 times daily
COUNSELLING. Advise patient not to exceed prescribed dose and to follow manufacturer's directions

3.1.3   Theophylline

With the introduction of the beta$_2$-adrenoceptor stimulants (section 3.1.1.1), the use of *rapid-release* oral aminophylline and theophylline preparations declined because of the high incidence of side-effects associated with rapid absorption. However, there has been a revival of interest in these drugs since the introduction of *sustained-release* preparations which are usually able to produce adequate plasma concentrations for up to 12 hours. These sustained-release preparations are all equally effective but due to different pharmacokinetic profiles are not interchangeable without retitration of dosage.

Theophylline is metabolised in the liver and there is considerable variation in its half-life in healthy non-smokers, which is even more marked in smokers, in patients with hepatic impairment or heart failure, or if other drugs are taken concurrently. The half-life is *increased* in heart failure, cirrhosis, viral infections, and by drugs such as cimetidine, ciprofloxacin, erythromycin, and oral contraceptives. The half-life is *decreased* in smokers and in heavy drinkers, and by drugs such as phenytoin, carbamazepine, rifampicin, and barbiturates.

These differences in half-life are important because theophylline has a narrow margin between the therapeutic and toxic dose. In most subjects plasma concentrations of between 10 and 20 mg/litre are required for satisfactory bronchodilatation. Side-effects can occur with concentrations below 20 mg/litre and are common at concentrations above 30–40 mg/litre.

Theophylline *sustained-release* preparations

when given as a single dose at night have a useful role in controlling nocturnal asthma and early morning wheezing. They have replaced aminophylline suppositories which cause proctitis and can show an unpredictable response. Recent studies suggest that theophylline has an additive effect when used in conjunction with beta$_2$-adrenoceptor stimulants, though combination may increase the risk of arrhythmias in certain situations.

Choline theophyllinate is a modification of theophylline. There is no evidence that it is better tolerated than the sustained-release preparations.

Aminophylline, a mixture of theophylline with ethylenediamine, is 20 times more soluble than theophylline alone, which is an advantage for the injection but not for the tablets.

The use of aminophylline *injection*, given intravenously, is of established value in the treatment of severe attacks of asthma and is still preferred by many prescribers to intravenous treatment with the selective beta$_2$-adrenoceptor stimulants (section 3.1.1.1). Plasma concentrations should be monitored, particularly if patients have previously been taking oral xanthine preparations, as serious side-effects such as convulsions and arrhythmias can occasionally occur before the appearance of other symptoms of toxicity.

Aminophylline injection was formerly used in the treatment of left ventricular failure but has been superseded by diuretics (see sections 2.2.1 and 2.2.2) and the opioid analgesics (see section 4.7.2) for this purpose. However, it may have a role in patients with heart failure who are also suffering from asthma and bronchitis, where opioids are contra-indicated, though care is needed in using aminophylline in patients with increased myocardial excitability.

AMINOPHYLLINE
Indications: reversible airways obstruction, status asthmaticus, left ventricular failure
Cautions: see notes above; also liver disease (reduce dose), epilepsy, breast-feeding, cardiac disease, elderly patients, fever
Side-effects: tachycardia, palpitations, nausea, gastro-intestinal disturbances, insomnia, arrhythmias, and convulsions especially if given rapidly by intravenous injection; use of suppositories for more than a few days may cause proctitis; intramuscular injection is painful (this route is therefore not used)
Dose: by mouth, 100–300 mg, 3–4 times daily, after food; for doses of sustained-release preparations, see under preparations (next page)
By slow intravenous injection (over 20 minutes), 250–500 mg (5 mg/kg) when necessary; maintenance, if required, in patients not previously treated with xanthines, 500 micrograms/kg/hour *by slow intravenous infusion*
CHILD, *by slow intravenous injection* (over 20 minutes), 5 mg/kg; maintenance, if required, in patients not previously treated with xanthines, 6 months–9 years 1 mg/kg/hour, 10–16 years 800 micrograms/kg/hour *by slow intravenous infusion*

By rectum in suppositories, 360 mg once or twice daily; CHILD, once or twice daily, up to 1 year 12.5–25 mg, 1–5 years 50–100 mg, 6–12 years 100–200 mg (now rarely used, see notes above)
Note. Plasma theophylline concentration for optimum response 10–20 mg/litre (55–110 micromol/litre)

Aminophylline (Non-proprietary)
Tablets, aminophylline 100 mg, net price 20 = 33p. Label: 21
PoM *Injection,* aminophylline 25 mg/ml, net price 10-ml amp = 44p; 250 mg/ml, 2-ml amp = 27p
Suppositories, aminophylline 50, 100, 150, 180, and 360 mg.
Available from Macarthys and Penn (special order)
Note. Aminophylline suppositories cause proctitis and show an unpredictable response; they are now rarely used

With antacid
Theodrox® (Riker)
Tablets, aminophylline 195 mg, dried aluminium hydroxide gel 260 mg. Net price 20 = 31p. Label: 21
Dose: 1 tablet 3 times daily, after food; max. 1–2 tablets 4 times daily.

Sustained-release preparations
Note. The Council of the Pharmaceutical Society of Great Britain advises pharmacists that if a general practitioner prescribes a sustained-release, oral theophylline preparation without specifying a brand name, the pharmacist should contact the prescriber and agree the brand to be dispensed. Additionally, it is essential that a patient discharged from hospital should be maintained on the brand on which that patient was stabilised as an in-patient.
Phyllocontin Continus® (Napp)
Tablets, s/r, yellow, f/c, aminophylline 225 mg. Net price 20 = £1.13. Label: 25
Dose: 1 tablet twice daily initially, increased after 1 week to 2 tablets twice daily
Forte tablets, s/r, yellow, f/c, aminophylline 350 mg. Net price 60 = £5.45. Label: 25
Note. Forte tablets are for smokers and other patients with decreased theophylline half-life (see notes above).
Tablets, paediatric, s/r, pale yellow, aminophylline 100 mg. Net price 20 = 68p. Label: 25
Dose: 6 mg/kg twice daily initially, increased after 1 week to 12 mg/kg twice daily

CHOLINE THEOPHYLLINATE
Indications: reversible airways obstruction
Cautions; Side-effects: see under Aminophylline
Dose: by mouth, 100–400 mg 2–4 times daily preferably after food; CHILD, 3 times daily, 3–5 years 62.5–125 mg, 6–12 years 100 mg
Note. Plasma theophylline concentration for optimum response 10–20 mg/litre (55–110 micromol/litre)

Choledyl® (P-D)
Tablets, pink, compression coated, choline theophyllinate 100 mg. Net price 20 = 39p
Tablets, yellow, compression coated, choline theophyllinate 200 mg. Net price 20 = 54p
Syrup, yellow, choline theophyllinate 62.5 mg/5 ml. Diluent syrup (without preservative), life

of diluted syrup 14 days. Net price 100 ml = £1.15

Sustained-release preparations
(see advice on p. 119)
Sabidal SR 270® (Zyma)
Tablets, s/r, light yellow, choline theophyllinate 424 mg. Net price 20 = £1.54. Label: 25
Dose: 1 tablet twice daily initially, increased after 3 days to 1 in the morning and 2 at night

THEOPHYLLINE
Indications: reversible airways obstruction
Cautions; Side-effects: see under Aminophylline. Drug interactions: see Appendix 1 (sections 3, 4.2)
Dose: see below
Note. Plasma theophylline concentration for optimum response 10–20 mg/litre (55–110 micromol/litre)

Biophylline® (Delandale)
Syrup, yellow, sugar-free, theophylline hydrate 125 mg (as sodium glycinate)/5 ml. Net price 250 ml = £3.77. Label: 21
Dose: 125–250 mg 3–4 times daily; CHILD 2–6 years 62.5 mg, 7–12 years 62.5–125 mg, 3–4 times daily

▼ PoM **Labophylline®** (LAB)
Injection, theophylline 20 mg/ml, lysine 12.2 mg/ml. Net price 10-ml amp = 23p
Dose: in patients not previously treated with xanthines, *by slow intravenous injection* (over 20 minutes) initially 200 mg, *or by intravenous infusion* 4 mg/kg; maintenance if required, 500 micrograms/kg/hour for 12 hours, then 400 micrograms/kg/hour; CHILD *by slow intravenous injection* (over 20 minutes) 4 mg/kg initially

Nuelin® (Riker)
Tablets, scored, theophylline 125 mg. Net price 20 = 75p. Label: 21
Dose: 125 mg 3–4 times daily after food, increased to 250 mg if required; CHILD 7–12 years 62.5–125 mg 3–4 times daily
Liquid, brown, theophylline 60 mg (as sodium glycinate)/5 ml. Diluent syrup, life of diluted liquid 14 days. Net price 100 ml = £1.01. Label: 21
Dose: 120–240 mg 3–4 times daily after food; CHILD 2–6 years 60–90 mg, 7–12 years 90–120 mg, 3–4 times daily

Sustained-release preparations
(see advice on p. 119)
Lasma® (Pharmax)
Tablets, s/r, scored, theophylline 300 mg. Net price 20 = £1.94. Label: 25
Dose: 300 mg every 12 hours *or* 600 mg every 24 hours (increased to 900 mg after 1 week in patients over 70 kg); adjust dose by 150-mg increments as required
Nuelin SA® (Riker)
Tablets, s/r, theophylline 175 mg. Net price 20 = £1.01. Label: 25
Dose: 175–350 mg every 12 hours; CHILD over 6 years 175 mg every 12 hours

Nuelin SA 250® (Riker)
Tablets, s/r, scored, theophylline 250 mg. Net price 20 = £1.42. Label: 25
Dose: 250–500 mg every 12 hours; CHILD over 6 years 125–250 mg every 12 hours
Pro-Vent® (Wellcome)
Capsules, s/r, white/clear, theophylline 300 mg. Net price 20 = £1.50. Label: 25
Dose: 300 mg every 12 hours, with a further 300 mg daily if required
Slo-Phyllin® (Lipha)
Capsules, s/r, white/clear, enclosing white pellets, theophylline 60 mg. Net price 20 = 72p. Label: 25 *or* counselling advised, see below
Capsules, s/r, brown/clear, enclosing white pellets, theophylline 125 mg. Net price 20 = 91p. Label: 25 *or* counselling advised, see below
Capsules, s/r, blue/clear, enclosing white pellets, theophylline 250 mg. Net price 20 = £1.13. Label: 25 *or* counselling advised, see below
Dose: 250–500 mg every 12 hours; CHILD, every 12 hours, 2–6 years 60–120 mg, 7–12 years 125–250 mg. Max. in adults and children over 9 years 13 mg/kg daily, children up to 9 years 24 mg/kg daily
COUNSELLING. Swallow whole with fluid *or* swallow enclosed granules with soft food (e.g. yoghurt)
Theo-Dur® (Astra)
Tablets, s/r, scored, theophylline 200 mg. Net price 20 = £1.24. Label: 25
Tablets, s/r, scored, theophylline 300 mg. Net price 20 = £1.80. Label: 25
Dose: 200–300 mg every 12 hours; CHILD up to 35 kg 100 mg, over 35 kg 200 mg, every 12 hours
Uniphyllin Continus® (Napp)
Tablets, s/r, scored, theophylline 400 mg. Net price 56-tab pack = £7.51. Label: 25
Dose: initially 400 mg daily, increased after 1 week to 600–800 mg daily
Paediatric tablets, s/r, scored, theophylline 200 mg. Net price 60 = £3.87. Label: 25
Dose: 9 mg/kg daily, increased after 1 week to 18 mg/kg daily

3.1.4 Compound bronchodilator preparations

Most compound bronchodilator preparations have no place in the management of patients with airways obstruction. Some include sedatives, intended to allay the anxiety associated with breathlessness, and should be avoided, particularly if they contain barbiturates, as they depress respiration. In general, patients are best treated with single-ingredient preparations, such as a selective beta$_2$-adrenoceptor stimulant (section 3.1.1.1) or ipratropium bromide (section 3.1.2), so that the dose of each drug can be adjusted. This flexibility is lost with combinations, although those in which both components are effective may occasionally have a role when compliance is a problem.

Solutions of adrenaline deteriorate rapidly on exposure to air; they are not recommended.

NHS PoM **Bricanyl Compound**® (Astra)
Tablets, guaiphenesin 100 mg, terbutaline sulphate
2.5 mg. Net price 20 = £1.05
Dose: 2 tablets 3 times daily

PoM **Bricanyl Expectorant**® (Astra)
Elixir, sugar-free, guaiphenesin 66.5 mg, terbutaline
sulphate 1.5 mg/5 ml. Diluent water for preparations,
life of diluted elixir 14 days. Net price 300 ml = £2·88
Dose: 10–15 ml 3 times daily

PoM **Bronchilator**® (Sterling Research)
Aerosol inhalation, isoetharine mesylate 350 micrograms,
phenylephrine hydrochloride 70 micrograms/metered
dose. Net price 250-dose unit = £10.18
Dose: 1–2 puffs repeated after 30 minutes if necessary;
max. 16 puffs daily

Brovon® (Torbet)
Inhalant spray, adrenaline 0.5%, atropine methonitrate
0.14%, papaverine hydrochloride 0.88%. Net price
20-ml bottle = £1.28; 50-ml bottle = £2.86; midget
inhaler = £4.62; reservoir and closure = £2.89; rubber
bulb = £1.46
Dose: 1–2 puffs twice daily and at night

CAM® (Rybar)
Mixture, green, butethamate citrate 4 mg, ephedrine
hydrochloride 4 mg/5 ml. Diluent syrup or water for
preparations, life of diluted mixture 14 days. Net price
100 ml = 70p
Dose: 20 ml 3–4 times daily; CHILD 1½–2 years 2.5 ml,
2–4 years 5 ml, over 4 years 10 ml, 3 times daily

PoM **Duo-Autohaler**® (Riker)
Aerosol inhalation, isoprenaline hydrochloride 160
micrograms, phenylephrine bitartrate 240 micrograms/
metered inhalation. Net price 400-dose breath-actuated
unit = £4.86; refill = £3.25
Note. Not recommended therefore no dose stated

PoM **Duovent**® (Boehringer Ingelheim)
Aerosol inhalation, fenoterol hydrobromide 90 micrograms, ipratropium bromide 36 micrograms/metered
inhalation. Net price 200-dose unit with mouthpiece =
£5.28 (extension tube also available)
Dose: 1–2 puffs 3–4 times daily; CHILD over 6 years
1 puff 3 times daily

PoM **Medihaler-duo**® (Riker)
Aerosol inhalation, isoprenaline hydrochloride 160
micrograms, phenylephrine bitartrate 240 micrograms/
metered inhalation. Net price 400-dose unit = £3.25
Note. Not recommended therefore no dose stated

Rybarvin Inhalant® (Rybar)
Spray solution, adrenaline 0.4%, atropine methonitrate
0.1%, benzocaine 0.08%, in saline vehicle. Net price
30 ml = £1.80. For use with Rybar no. 1 and no. 2
inhalers, net price (both) = £7.87

PoM **Tedral**® (P-D)
Tablets, ephedrine hydrochloride 24 mg, theophylline
120 mg. Net price 20 = 25p. Label: 21
Dose: 1 tablet every 4 hours after food
Elixir, yellow, sugar-free, ephedrine hydrochloride 6 mg,
theophylline 30 mg/5 ml. Diluent syrup, life of diluted
elixir 28 days. Net price 200 ml = 80p. Label: 21
Dose: 20 ml every 4 hours, after food; CHILD 2–5 years
5 ml, 6–10 years 10 ml

BRONCHODILATORS WITH SEDATIVES

CD **Franol**® (Winthrop)
Tablets, ephedrine hydrochloride 11 mg, phenobarbitone
8 mg, theophylline 120 mg. Net price 20 = 95p. Label:
21
Dose: 1 tablet 3–4 times daily after food

CD **Franol Plus**® (Winthrop)
Tablets, ephedrine sulphate 15 mg, phenobarbitone 8 mg,
theophylline 120 mg, thenyldiamine hydrochloride
10 mg. Net price 20 = £1.41. Label: 21
Dose: 1 tablet 3–4 times daily after food

3.2 Corticosteroids

Corticosteroids have been used in the treatment of asthma for many years. In recent years, with the introduction of corticosteroid inhalations, their use has increased and has been extended to the treatment of less severe and more chronic asthma, as the side-effects associated with systemic administration (see section 6.3.3) are much reduced. Corticosteroids are usually of no benefit in patients with chronic bronchitis and emphysema; some patients with asthma, however, may be clinically indistinguishable from those with chronic bronchitis except that they will respond to a trial course of corticosteroids.

The action of corticosteroids is not fully understood but it is probable that they provide relief by reducing bronchial mucosal inflammatory reactions such as oedema and hypersecretion of mucus.

INHALATION. Corticosteroid aerosol inhalations must be used regularly to obtain maximum benefit; alleviation of symptoms usually occurs 3 to 7 days after initiation. **Beclomethasone dipropionate** is most commonly used. A *high-dose inhaler* (Becloforte®) is available for patients who only have a partial response to the *standard inhaler* (Becotide®). The maximum recommended dose of 2 mg daily with the high-dose inhaler is associated with very slight adrenal suppression (see section 6.3.3), therefore patients on high doses should be given a steroid card and may need corticosteroid cover during an episode of infection or stress (e.g. an operation). Corticosteroids are better inhaled using spacing devices (e.g. Nebuhaler® or Volumatic®) which increase airway deposition and reduce oropharyngeal deposition, permitting a marked reduction in the incidence of candidiasis; these devices are bulky, but corticosteroids have a long half-life therefore most patients only need to use them morning and night. **Budesonide** (Pulmicort®) is very similar to beclomethasone dipropionate.

Dry powder inhalers (Becotide Rotacaps®) (see section 3.1.1 for description) may be tried in patients who are unable to use the aerosol inhalers.

Beclomethasone dipropionate *suspension for nebulisation* may be used for children who cannot manage either the aerosol inhalers or the dry powder inhalers. Because of its poor solubility it is relatively inefficient; a spacing device will allow a larger amount to be administered more effectively and can be used by some children as young as 2 years.

Maximum penetration of inhaled corticosteroid is facilitated if a beta$_2$-adrenoceptor stimulant drug such as salbutamol is inhaled beforehand; this is usual practice even in patients with only a mild degree of bronchospasm.

Patients who have been taking long-term oral corticosteroids can often be transferred to inhalation but the transfer must be done slowly, with gradual reduction in dose of oral corticosteroid, and at a time when the asthma is well controlled.

ORAL. *Acute attacks* of asthma should be treated with short courses of oral corticosteroids starting with a high dose, e.g. prednisolone 30 to 40 mg daily for a few days, gradually reduced once the attack has been controlled. Patients whose asthma has deteriorated rapidly usually respond quickly to corticosteroids, which can then be tailed down over a few days; more gradual reduction is necessary in those whose asthma has deteriorated gradually.

For use of corticosteroids in the emergency treatment of *severe acute asthma* see section 3.1.1.

In *chronic continuing asthma*, when all other anti-asthma drugs have failed, continued administration of oral corticosteroids may be necessary; in such cases high doses of inhaled corticosteroids should be continued so that oral requirements are reduced to a minimum. Oral corticosteroids should normally be taken as a single dose in the morning to reduce the disturbance to circadian cortisol secretion. Dosage should always be titrated to the lowest dose which controls symptoms. Regular monitored peak flow measurements often help both patient and doctor to adjust the dose optimally. Prednisolone is available as tablets of 1 mg as well as 5 mg, and the smaller tablets may conveniently be used to adjust the maintenance dosage to the minimum necessary.

Alternate-day administration has not been very successful in the management of asthma and patients tend to deteriorate during the second 24 hours. If an attempt is made to introduce this pulmonary function should be monitored carefully over the 48 hours.

Corticotrophin and **tetracosactrin** (see section 6.5.1) may occasionally be used instead of the corticosteroids. They may cause less growth inhibition in children but their value is limited by the variable and unpredictable therapeutic response and the waning of their effect with time.

BECLOMETHASONE DIPROPIONATE

Indications: chronic airways obstruction, especially in asthma not controlled by bronchodilators

Cautions: see notes above; also respiratory infection, active or quiescent tuberculosis

Side-effects: hoarseness; candidiasis of mouth or throat, usually only with large doses (reduced by using spacer, see notes above; responds to antifungal lozenges, see section 12.3.2, without discontinuation of therapy; rinsing the mouth with water after inhalation of a dose may also be helpful)

Dose: see below

Standard-dose inhalers

PoM **Becodisks®** (A&H)

Powder for inhalation, disks containing 8 blisters of beclomethasone dipropionate 100 micrograms/blister, net price pack of 14 × 8 = £10.99; 200 micrograms/blister, pack of 14 ×

8 = £20.90 (both with Diskhaler®). Label: 8, counselling advised, dose

Dose: by inhalation of powder, 400 micrograms twice daily *or* 200 micrograms 3–4 times daily; CHILD 100 micrograms 2–4 times daily

PoM **Becotide®** (A&H)

Rotacaps®, buff/clear, beclomethasone dipropionate 100 micrograms. Net price 20 = £1.51. Label: 8, counselling advised, dose

Rotacaps®, brown/clear, beclomethasone dipropionate 200 micrograms. Net price 20 = £2.87. Label: 8, counselling advised, dose

Dose: by inhalation of powder, 200 micrograms 3–4 times daily or 400 micrograms twice daily; max. 1 mg daily; CHILD 100 micrograms 2–4 times daily

Suspension for nebulisation, beclomethasone dipropionate 50 micrograms/ml. Net price 10 ml = £2.50. For use with respirator or nebuliser. May be diluted up to 50% with sterile physiological saline

Dose: by inhalation of nebulised suspension, CHILD up to 1 year 50 micrograms 2–4 times daily; 1–12 years 100 micrograms 2–4 times daily, adjusted according to response

Note. Unsuitable for adults because of large volumes required.

PoM **Becotide 50®** (A&H)

Aerosol inhalation, beclomethasone dipropionate 50 micrograms/metered inhalation. Net price 200-dose unit = £5.56. Label: 8, counselling advised, dose

Dose: by aerosol inhalation, 200 micrograms (4 puffs) twice daily *or* 100 micrograms (2 puffs) 3–4 times daily (in more severe cases initially 600–800 micrograms daily); CHILD 50–100 micrograms (1–2 puffs) 2–4 times daily

PoM **Becotide 100®** (A&H)

Aerosol inhalation, beclomethasone dipropionate 100 micrograms/metered inhalation. Net price 200-dose unit = £10.56. Label: 8, counselling advised, dose

Dose: by aerosol inhalation, 200 micrograms (2 puffs) twice daily *or* 100 micrograms (1 puff) 3–4 times daily (in more severe cases initially 600–800 micrograms daily)

High-dose inhalers

PoM **Becloforte®** (A&H)

Aerosol inhalation, beclomethasone dipropionate 250 micrograms/metered inhalation. Net price 200-dose unit = £23.10. Label: 8, counselling advised, dose, 10 steroid card

Dose: by aerosol inhalation, 500 micrograms (2 puffs) twice daily *or* 250 micrograms (1 puff) 4 times daily; if necessary may be increased to 500 micrograms 3–4 times daily

Compound preparations

▼ PoM **Ventide®** (A&H)

Aerosol inhalation, beclomethasone dipropionate 50 micrograms, salbutamol 100 micrograms/metered inhalation. Net price 200-dose unit = £8.02. Label: 8, counselling advised, dose

Dose: maintenance, 2 puffs 3–4 times daily; CHILD 1–2 puffs 2–4 times daily

---

Paediatric Rotacaps®, light grey/clear, beclomethasone dipropionate 100 micrograms, salbutamol (as sulphate) 200 micrograms. Net price 100 = £12.59. Label: 8, counselling advised, dose
Dose: by inhalation of powder, 1 Rotacap® 2–4 times daily
Rotacaps®, dark grey/clear, beclomethasone dipropionate 200 micrograms, salbutamol (as sulphate) 400 micrograms. Net price 100 = £22.83. Label: 8, counselling advised, dose
Dose: by inhalation of powder, 1 Rotacap® 2–4 times daily

Devices
Rotahaler® (A&H)
Breath actuated inhaler for use with Rotacaps. Net price = 78p
Volumatic® (A&H)
Inhaler, large-volume spacer device. For use with Ventolin, Becotide, Becloforte, and Ventide inhalers. Net price = £2.75

BETAMETHASONE VALERATE
Indications; Cautions; Side-effects: see under Beclomethasone Dipropionate
Dose: by aerosol inhalation, adults and children, initially 800 micrograms daily, usually as 200 micrograms (2 puffs) 4 times daily; reduced to the minimum effective dose

PoM **Bextasol**® (Glaxo)
Aerosol inhalation, betamethasone valerate 100 micrograms/metered inhalation. Net price 200-dose unit = £4.50. Label: 8, counselling advised, dose

---

BUDESONIDE
Indications; Cautions; Side-effects: see under Beclomethasone Dipropionate
Dose: by aerosol inhalation, initially 200 micrograms (1 puff Pulmicort) twice daily, adjusted according to response to minimum effective dose but not less than 200 micrograms daily; in severe asthma dose may be increased to 1.2 mg (6 puffs Pulmicort) daily; CHILD 50–200 micrograms (1–4 puffs Pulmicort LS) twice daily

Standard-dose inhalers
▼ PoM **Pulmicort LS**® (Astra)
Aerosol inhalation, budesonide 50 micrograms/metered inhalation. Net price 200-dose unit with standard or Spacer inhaler = £6.66; 200-dose refill for use with Nebuhaler or Spacer inhaler = £4.66. Label: 8, counselling advised, dose

High-dose inhalers
▼ PoM **Pulmicort**® (Astra)
Aerosol inhalation, budesonide 200 micrograms/metered inhalation. Net price 200-dose unit with standard or Spacer inhaler = £19.00; 200-dose refill for use with Nebuhaler or Spacer inhaler = £17.00; 100-dose unit with standard and Spacer inhaler = £10.16 (hosp. only); 100-

dose refill = £8.66 (hosp. only). Label: 8, counselling advised, dose, 10 steroid card

Devices
Nebuhaler® (Astra)
Inhaler, fitted with plastic cone and one-way valve. For use with Bricanyl and Pulmicort refill canisters. Net price = £4.75

3.3 Prophylaxis of asthma

Regular administration of prophylactic drugs can reduce the incidence of attacks and often allow dosage reduction of concurrent corticosteroids and bronchodilators. Prophylactic drugs are of no value in the treatment of acute attacks as their effects take some time to develop.

Sodium cromoglycate (Intal®) is the main drug of this group and is administered by inhalation. Its mode of action is not completely understood but it prevents release of pharmacological mediators of bronchospasm by stabilising mast-cell membranes and is of particular value in patients whose asthma has an allergic basis, although it may also be useful in some patients in whom an allergic basis has not been demonstrated. It may also be of value in the prevention of exercise-induced asthma. Children seem to respond better than adults to sodium cromoglycate but, as it is difficult to predict who will benefit, it is reasonable to try it in all patients whose asthma is poorly controlled with bronchodilators. Patients, and particularly children, should be given careful instruction on the use of sodium cromoglycate inhalations and it should be emphasised that regular administration is necessary, whether symptoms are present or not. Dose frequency is adjusted according to the patient's response but is usually 4 times daily. As improvement occurs this may be reduced if possible. When used to prevent attacks in exercise-induced asthma, sodium cromoglycate is administered half an hour before exercise as a single dose. Sodium cromoglycate should be discontinued after 4 weeks if there is no response but should be continued in patients who benefit.

Sodium cromoglycate has few side-effects. However, occasionally the dry powder inhalations may cause bronchospasm. In such patients, the best procedure is to use a selective beta$_2$-adrenoceptor stimulant inhalation such as salbutamol or terbutaline a few minutes before the sodium cromoglycate inhalation is given. There is **no** advantage in using the compound inhalation of sodium cromoglycate which contains isoprenaline (Intal Compound®) as isoprenaline has a less selective action; moreover, it may lead to the patient misusing the preparation for relieving bronchospasm rather than for its prophylactic effect. Sodium cromoglycate nebuliser solution is useful for those patients who cannot manage the dry powder inhaler and pressurised aerosols. It is conveniently used when individuals already possess and use a home nebuliser for bronchodilator therapy.

Nedocromil (Tilade®) is a recently introduced drug with a pharmacological action that is similar to that of sodium cromoglycate but wider ranging.

Ketotifen (Zaditen®) has an action said to resemble that of sodium cromoglycate. Although some studies have suggested that it has certain anti-asthma effects, in clinical practice it does not seem to have fulfilled its early promise in the majority of patients. It is given by mouth and, while this may be an advantage to patients who find inhalation difficult, ketotifen may have to be given for 4 weeks or more to achieve full prophylaxis. In addition, ketotifen is an antihistamine and as such may cause drowsiness. Doses for asthma prophylaxis and relief of allergy are similar.

There is some recent evidence that selective beta2-adrenoceptor stimulants may be used on a regular basis for prophylaxis (as opposed to bronchodilator effects). As a consequence a number of aerosols are being marketed which contain both a beta-adrenoceptor stimulant and a corticosteroid or an atropine derivative. While these are convenient and cheaper for the patient, they do not provide flexibility in dosage, and patient education is more difficult.

SODIUM CROMOGLYCATE

Indications: prophylaxis of asthma
Side-effects: coughing, transient bronchospasm, and throat irritation due to inhalation of powder (see also notes above)
Dose: see below

PoM **Intal**® (Fisons)
Aerosol inhalation, sodium cromoglycate 1 mg/ metered inhalation. Net price 200-dose unit = £12.13. Label: 8
　　Dose: by aerosol inhalation, adults and children, 2 mg (2 puffs) 4 times daily, increased in severe cases or during periods of risk to 6–8 times daily
Spincaps®, yellow/clear, sodium cromoglycate 20 mg. Net price 112-cap pack = £11.59. Label: 8
　　Dose: by inhalation of powder, adults and children, 20 mg 4 times daily, increased in severe cases to 8 times daily
Spinhaler insufflator® (for use with Intal and Intal Compound Spincaps). Net price £1.10
Nebuliser solution, sodium cromoglycate 10 mg/ ml. Net price 2-ml amp = 20p. For use with power-operated nebuliser
　　Dose: by inhalation of nebulised solution, adults and children, 20 mg 4 times daily, increased in severe cases to 6 times daily
▼ PoM **Intal 5**® (Fisons)
Aerosol inhalation, sodium cromoglycate 5 mg/metered inhalation. Net price 112-dose unit = £14.52. Label: 8
　　Dose: by aerosol inhalation, adults and children, 10 mg (2 puffs) 4 times daily initially; maintenance 5 mg (1 puff) 4 times daily
PoM **Intal Compound**® (Fisons)
Spincaps®, orange/clear, isoprenaline sulphate 100

micrograms, sodium cromoglycate 20 mg. Net price 112-cap pack = £9.17. Label: 8
Dose: see under Intal Spincaps

KETOTIFEN

Indications: see notes above
Cautions: may affect ability to drive or operate machinery and increase effects of alcohol; previous anti-asthmatic treatment should be continued for a minimum of 2 weeks after initiation of ketotifen treatment; avoid concomitant use with oral antidiabetic drugs (depressed thrombocyte count). Drug interactions: as for Antihistamines (section 3.4.1)
Side-effects: dry mouth, sedation
Dose: 1–2 mg twice daily with food; initial treatment in readily sedated patients 0.5–1 mg at night; CHILD over 2 years 1 mg twice daily

PoM **Zaditen**® (Sandoz)
Capsules, ketotifen 1 mg (as hydrogen fumarate). Net price 60 = £11.93. Label: 2, 8, 21
Tablets, off-white, scored, ketotifen 1 mg (as hydrogen fumarate). Net price 60 = £11.93. Label: 2, 8, 21
Elixir, ketotifen 1 mg (as hydrogen fumarate)/ 5 ml. Diluent syrup, life of diluted elixir 14 days. Net price 150 ml = £7.05. Label: 2, 8, 21

NEDOCROMIL SODIUM

Indications: prophylaxis of asthma
Side-effects: headache, nausea (both mild and transient); bitter taste
Dose: by aerosol inhalation, 4 mg (2 puffs) twice daily, increased to 4 times daily if necessary; CHILD under 12 years, not yet recommended

▼ PoM **Tilade**® (Fisons)
Aerosol inhalation, nedocromil sodium 2 mg/ metered inhalation. Net price 112-dose unit = £17.76. Label: 8

3.4　Allergic disorders

Drugs modifying allergic disorders are discussed under the following headings:
　3.4.1 Antihistamines
　3.4.2 Hyposensitisation
　3.4.3 Allergic emergencies

For the treatment of asthma see sections 3.1.1 and 3.2. For the treatment of hay fever by nasal application of corticosteroids and prophylaxis with sodium cromoglycate see section 12.2. For eye preparations see section 11.4. For the treatment of allergic skin conditions with topical corticosteroid preparations see section 13.4.

3.4.1　Antihistamines

All antihistamines are of potential value in the treatment of nasal allergies, particularly seasonal (hay fever) and may be of some value in vasomotor rhinitis. They reduce rhinorrhoea and sneezing but are usually less effective for nasal congestion.

Oral antihistamines are also of some value in preventing urticaria and are used to treat allergic rashes, pruritus, and insect bites and stings; they are also used in drug allergies. Injections of chlorpheniramine or promethazine are used as an adjunct to adrenaline in the emergency treatment of angioedema and anaphylaxis (section 3.4.3).

There is no evidence that any one of the older antihistamines is superior to any other and patients vary widely in their responses. Antihistamines differ somewhat in duration of action and incidence of side-effects (drowsiness and anticholinergic effects). Most are relatively short-acting but some, (e.g. promethazine) act for up to 12 hours. They all cause sedation but **promethazine**, **trimeprazine**, and **dimenhydrinate** may be more sedating whereas **chlorpheniramine**, **cyclizine**, and **mequitazine** may be less so.

Astemizole (Hismanal®), **oxatomide** (Tinset®), and **terfenadine** (Triludan®) are recently introduced antihistamines which appear to have some advantages over the older antihistamines. Astemizole and terfenadine cause less sedation and psychomotor impairment because they only penetrate the blood brain barrier to a slight extent (and for this reason do not alleviate pruritus of non-allergic origin). The drug interactions described in Appendix 1 apply to a lesser extent and they do not appear to potentiate the effects of alcohol.

Several antihistamines are described in other chapters (see Index).

DISADVANTAGES OF ANTIHISTAMINES. With most antihistamines drowsiness is a serious disadvantage; patients should be warned that their ability to drive or operate machinery may be impaired, and that the effects of alcohol may be increased. Other side-effects include headache, psychomotor impairment, anticholinergic effects such as urinary retention, dry mouth, blurred vision, and gastro-intestinal disturbances; occasional rashes and photosensitivity reactions have been reported; paradoxical stimulation may rarely occur, especially in high dosage or in children. Antihistamines should be used with caution in epilepsy, prostatic hypertrophy, glaucoma, and hepatic disease. Drug interactions: see Appendix 1 (sections *4.1, 4.6, 4.9*).

ASTEMIZOLE
Indications: symptomatic relief of allergy such as hay fever, urticaria
Cautions: see notes above; pregnancy (toxicity at high doses in *animal* studies)
Side-effects: see notes above; weight gain occurs infrequently; incidence of sedation is low; anticholinergic effects and psychomotor impairment have not been reported; ventricular arrhythmias have followed excessive dosage
Dose: 10 mg daily before food; initially up to 30 mg as a single daily dose can be given for a max. of 7 days, but thereafter the daily dose of

10 mg must **not** be exceeded; CHILD 6–12 years, half adult dose

▼ PoM **Hismanal**® (Janssen)
Tablets, scored, astemizole 10 mg. Net price 30 = £4.95. Label: 23
Suspension, sugar-free, astemizole 5 mg/5 ml. Net price 100 ml = £2.90. Label: 23

AZATADINE MALEATE
Indications: symptomatic relief of allergy such as hay fever, urticaria
Cautions; Side-effects: see notes above
Dose: 1 mg, increased if necessary to 2 mg, twice daily; CHILD 1–6 years 250 micrograms twice daily, 6–12 years 0.5–1 mg twice daily

Optimine® (Kirby-Warrick)
Tablets, scored, azatadine maleate 1 mg. Net price 56-tab pack = £4.48. Label: 2
Syrup, azatadine maleate 500 micrograms/5 ml. Diluent syrup, life of diluted syrup 28 days. Net price 120 ml = £1.43. Label: 2

BROMPHENIRAMINE MALEATE
Indications: symptomatic relief of allergy such as hay fever, urticaria
Cautions; Side-effects: see notes above
Dose: 4–8 mg 3–4 times daily; CHILD up to 3 years 0.4–1 mg/kg daily in 4 divided doses, 3–6 years 2 mg 3–4 times daily, 6–12 years 2–4 mg 3–4 times daily

Dimotane® (Robins)
Tablets, peach, scored, brompheniramine maleate 4 mg. Net price 20 = 70p. Label: 2
Elixir, yellow-green, brompheniramine maleate 2 mg/5 ml. Diluent syrup, life of diluted elixir 14 days. Net price 100 ml = 84p. Label: 2
Dimotane LA® (Robins)
Tablets, s/r, peach, s/c, brompheniramine maleate 12 mg. Net price 20 = £1.05. Label: 2, 25
Dose: 12–24 mg twice daily; CHILD 6–12 years 12 mg at bedtime, increased if necessary to 12 mg twice daily

CHLORPHENIRAMINE MALEATE
Indications: symptomatic relief of allergy such as hay fever, urticaria; emergency treatment of anaphylactic reactions (section 3.4.3)
Cautions; Side-effects: see notes above. Injections may be irritant and cause transitory hypotension or CNS stimulation
Dose: by mouth, 4 mg 3–4 times daily; CHILD up to 1 year 1 mg twice daily, 1–5 years 1–2 mg 3 times daily, 6–12 years 2–4 mg 3–4 times daily
By subcutaneous or intramuscular injection, 10–20 mg, repeated if required; max. 40 mg in 24 hours
By slow intravenous injection over 1 minute, 10–20 mg diluted in syringe with 5–10 ml blood

Chlorpheniramine Tablets, chlorpheniramine maleate 4 mg. Net price 20 = 18p. Label: 2

Alunex® (Steinhard)
Tablets, yellow, scored, chlorpheniramine maleate 4 mg. Net price 20 = 16p. Label: 2

Piriton® (A&H)
Tablets, ivory, chlorpheniramine maleate 4 mg. Net price 20 = 19p. Label: 2
Spandets® (= tablets s/r), ivory/white, chlorpheniramine maleate 12 mg. Net price 20 = 53p. Label: 2, 25
Dose: 12 mg every 8–12 hours; CHILD over 12 years 12 mg daily
Syrup, chlorpheniramine maleate 2 mg/5 ml. Diluent syrup (without preservative), life of diluted syrup 14 days. Net price 150 ml = 29p. Label: 2
PoM *Injection*, chlorpheniramine maleate 10 mg/ml. Net price 1-ml amp = 12p

CINNARIZINE
See section 4.6

CLEMASTINE
Indications: symptomatic relief of allergy such as hay fever, urticaria
Cautions; Side-effects: see notes above
Dose: 1 mg twice daily; CHILD up to 12 years 0.5–1 mg twice daily

Tavegil® (Sandoz)
Tablets, scored, clemastine 1 mg (as hydrogen fumarate). Net price 50 = £2.10. Label: 2
Elixir, sugar-free, clemastine 500 micrograms (as hydrogen fumarate)/5 ml. Diluent syrup or sorbitol solution, life of diluted elixir 14 days. Net price 150 ml = 98p. Label: 2
Note. A proprietary brand of clemastine hydrogen fumarate (Aller-eze®) is on sale to the public

CYCLIZINE
See section 4.6

CYPROHEPTADINE HYDROCHLORIDE
Indications: symptomatic relief of allergy such as hay fever, urticaria; stimulation of appetite
Cautions; Side-effects: see notes above
Dose: allergy, 4–20 mg daily in 3–4 divided doses, max. 32 mg daily; CHILD 2–6 years 2 mg 3 times daily, max. 12 mg daily; 7–14 years 4 mg 3 times daily, max. 16 mg daily
Migraine, 4 mg with a further 4 mg after 30 minutes if necessary; maintenance, 4 mg every 4–6 hours
Stimulation of appetite, 4 mg 3 times daily *or* 12 mg in the evening; CHILD not recommended

Periactin® (MSD)
Tablets, scored, cyproheptadine hydrochloride 4 mg. Net price 20 = 57p. Label: 2
Syrup, yellow, cyproheptadine hydrochloride 2 mg/5 ml. Diluent syrup, life of diluted syrup 14 days. Net price 200 ml = £1.27. Label: 2

DIMETHINDENE MALEATE
Indications: symptomatic relief of allergy such as hay fever, urticaria
Cautions; Side-effects: see notes above

Fenostil Retard® (Zyma)
Tablets, s/r, greyish-white, dimethindene maleate 2.5 mg. Net price 20 = 57p. Label: 2, 25
Dose: 2.5 mg twice daily

DIPHENYLPYRALINE HYDROCHLORIDE
Indications: symptomatic relief of allergy such as hay fever, urticaria
Cautions; Side-effects: see notes above

Histryl® (SK&F)
Spansule®(= capsules s/r), pink/clear, enclosing pink and white pellets, diphenylpyraline hydrochloride 5 mg. Net price 20 = 53p. Label: 2, 25
Dose: 5–10 mg twice daily
Paediatric Spansule® (= capsules s/r), pink/clear, enclosing pink and white pellets, diphenylpyraline 2.5 mg. Net price 20 = 41p. Label: 1, 25
Dose: CHILD over 7 years 2.5 mg twice daily

Lergoban® (Riker)
Tablets, s/r, diphenylpyraline hydrochloride 5 mg. Net price 20 = 60p. Label: 2, 25
Dose: 5–10 mg twice daily; CHILD over 10 years 5 mg twice daily

HYDROXYZINE HYDROCHLORIDE
See section 4.1.2

KETOTIFEN
See section 3.3

MEBHYDROLIN
Indications: symptomatic relief of allergy such as hay fever, urticaria
Cautions: see notes above
Side-effects: see notes above; also reversible granulocytopenia occurs rarely
Dose: 50–100 mg 3 times daily; CHILD, daily in divided doses, up to 2 years 50–100 mg, 2–5 years 50–150 mg, 6–12 years 100–200 mg

PoM **Fabahistin®** (Bayer)
Tablets, orange, s/c, mebhydrolin 50 mg. Net price 20 = 68p. Label: 2
Suspension, orange, mebhydrolin 50 mg (as napadisylate)/5 ml. Diluents tragacanth mucilage for 5 days storage, *or* carmellose sodium 0.5% and methyl hydroxybenzoate 0.07% in purified water, freshly boiled and cooled, for longer storage. Net price 100 ml = 89p. Label: 2

MEQUITAZINE
Indications: symptomatic relief of allergy such as hay fever, urticaria
Cautions; Side-effects: see notes above
Dose: 5 mg twice daily

PoM **Primalan**® (M&B)
Tablets, mequitazine 5 mg. Net price 50 = £4.80.
Label: 2

OXATOMIDE

Indications: symptomatic relief of allergy such as
hay fever, food allergy, urticaria
Cautions; Side-effects: see notes above. Drowsiness most common; increased appetite with
weight gain may occur above 120 mg daily
Dose: 30 mg twice daily after food, increased if
necessary to 60 mg twice daily; CHILD 5–14 years
15–30 mg twice daily

▼ PoM **Tinset**® (Janssen)
Tablets, scored, oxatomide 30 mg. Net price 25 =
£3.70. Label: 2, 21

PHENINDAMINE TARTRATE

Indications: symptomatic relief of allergy such as
hay fever, urticaria
Cautions; Side-effects: see notes above; may
cause mild CNS stimulation
Dose: 25–50 mg up to 4 times daily; CHILD over
10 years 25 mg 1–3 times daily

Thephorin® (Sinclair)
Tablets, s/c, phenindamine tartrate 25 mg. Net
price 20 = 73p. Label: 2

PHENIRAMINE MALEATE

Indications: symptomatic relief of allergy such as
hay fever, urticaria
Cautions; Side-effects: see notes above

Daneral SA® (Hoechst)
Tablets, s/r, pink, s/c, pheniramine maleate
75 mg. Net price 50 = £4.35. Label: 2, 25
Dose: 75–150 mg at night or 75 mg night and
morning

PROMETHAZINE HYDROCHLORIDE

Indications: symptomatic relief of allergy such as
hay fever, urticaria, emergency treatment of
anaphylactic reactions (section 3.4.3)
For use in premedication see section 15.1.4.2;
sedation see section 4.1.1
Cautions; Side-effects: see notes above; intramuscular injection may be painful
Dose: by mouth, 20–50 mg daily in divided doses
or as a single dose at night; max. 75 mg daily;
CHILD 1–5 years 5–15 mg, 6–10 years 10–25 mg
daily
By deep intramuscular injection, 25–50 mg; max.
100 mg; CHILD 5–10 years 6.25–12.5 mg
By slow intravenous injection in emergencies,
25–50 mg, max. 100 mg, as a solution containing
2.5 mg/ml in water for injections

Phenergan® (M&B)
Tablets, blue, f/c, promethazine hydrochloride
10 mg. Net price 20 = 28p. Label: 2
Tablets, blue, f/c, promethazine hydrochloride
25 mg. Net price 20 = 44p. Label: 2

Elixir, golden, promethazine hydrochloride
5 mg/5 ml. Diluent syrup, life of diluted elixir
14 days. Net price 100 ml = 50p. Label: 2
PoM *Injection*, promethazine hydrochloride
25 mg/ml. Net price 1-ml amp = 26p; 2-ml
amp = 32p
Note. A proprietary brand of promethazine hydrochloride tablets 20 mg (Sominex®) is on sale to the
public for the treatment of occasional insomnia in adults

TERFENADINE

Indications: symptomatic relief of allergy such as
hay fever, urticaria (see notes above)
Side-effects: see notes above; incidence of sedation is low; anticholinergic effects and psychomotor impairment have not been reported;
possibly associated with hair loss
Dose: 60 mg twice daily (for hay fever, 120 mg
may be taken in the morning); CHILD 6–12 years
30 mg

▼ **Triludan**® (Merrell)
Tablets, scored, terfenadine 60 mg. Net price
20 = £1.89
Suspension, terfenadine 30 mg/5 ml. Diluent
syrup, life of diluted suspension 14 days (in
refrigerator). Net price 120 ml = £2.40

TRIMEPRAZINE TARTRATE

Indications: symptomatic relief of allergy, particularly pruritus
For use in premedication, see section 15.1.4.2
Cautions; Side-effects: see notes above
Dose: 10 mg 2–3 times daily, increased if necessary to max. 100 mg daily; elderly 10 mg 1–2
times daily; CHILD 2.5–5 mg 3–4 times daily

PoM **Vallergan**® (M&B)
Tablets, blue, f/c, trimeprazine tartrate 10 mg.
Net price 20 = 65p. Label: 2
Syrup, straw coloured, trimeprazine tartrate
7.5 mg/5 ml. Diluent syrup, life of diluted syrup
14 days. Net price 100 ml = 78p. Label: 2
Syrup forte, pale yellow, trimeprazine tartrate
30 mg/5 ml. Diluent as above. Net price
100 ml = £1.68. Label: 2
Note. For use of Vallergan Forte Syrup see section
15.1.4.2

TRIPROLIDINE HYDROCHLORIDE

Indications: symptomatic relief of allergy such as
hay fever, urticaria
Cautions; Side-effects: see notes above
Dose: 2.5–5 mg 3 times daily (in severe allergy,
initial dose 5–7.5 mg, then 2.5–5 mg every 4
hours); CHILD, 3 times daily, up to 1 year 1 mg,
1–5 years 2 mg, 6–12 years 3 mg

Actidil® (Wellcome)
Tablets, scored, triprolidine hydrochloride
2.5 mg. Net price 20 = £1.19. Label: 2
Elixir, orange, triprolidine hydrochloride
2 mg/5 ml. Diluent syrup, life of diluted elixir
14 days. Net price 100 ml = 99p. Label: 2

Pro-Actidil® (Wellcome)
Tablets, s/r, white/pink/blue, triprolidine hydrochloride 10 mg. Net price 20 = £3.70. Label: 2, 25
Dose: 10 mg early evening increased to 20 mg daily when necessary; CHILD over 10 years 10 mg daily

3.4.2   Hyposensitisation

Except for wasp and bee sting allergy the value of specific hyposensitisation is uncertain. Most atopic (allergic) patients are sensitive to a wide range of allergens hence hyposensitisation with an extract of a single allergen is usually no more than partially successful. Furthermore, diagnostic skin tests are unreliable and can only be used in conjunction with a detailed history of allergen exposure.

Hyposensitisation with a mixture of several allergens combined in a single solution is **not** recommended because there is no evidence that such mixtures are effective.

Patients with seasonal or perennial rhinitis due to pollen or house dust mite seem to derive most benefit from hyposensitisation and nose and eye symptoms may be reduced by about half, though the duration of benefit is unknown. The value of hyposensitisation in patients with allergic asthma and eczema is uncertain but the majority do not benefit and there is a greater risk of anaphylaxis in patients with asthma (see below).

Where it is decided to undertake specific hyposensitisation, graded injections of increasing concentration are administered, usually every 1 to 2 weeks and usually over a period of about 10 weeks. Courses for pollen hyposensitisation (hay fever) are given preseasonally, usually beginning in January to ensure the course is completed before commencement of the grass pollen season. Courses are usually repeated for 2 to 3 consecutive years. *Maintenance courses* are also available and are usually recommended for house dust mite allergy. They consist of booster injections administered at gradually increasing time intervals (4–6 weeks) after the initial treatment course.

CSM Warning. The CSM has warned that since 1980, in the UK alone, 11 patients, most of whom were young, have died from anaphylaxis caused by allergen extract desensitising vaccines; patients with asthma appear to be particularly susceptible. The CSM is not aware of such problems when these allergens are used for diagnostic purposes (skin testing). Although some vaccines can prevent anaphylactic reactions (e.g. to bee stings) the effectiveness of the others is controversial. The CSM therefore recommends that it is important for doctors to balance carefully the known risks of desensitising vaccines against potential benefits before embarking on treatment. *Such treatment should only be carried out where facilities for full cardiorespiratory resuscitation are immediately available, and patients should be kept under medical observation for at least 2 hours after treatment.*

For details of the management of anaphylactic shock, see section 3.4.3.

ALLERGEN EXTRACT VACCINES

Each set usually contains vials for the administration of graded amounts to patients undergoing hyposensitisation. Maintenance sets containing vials at the highest strength are also available. Manufacturer's literature must be consulted for details of allergens, vial strengths, and administration

Indications: hypersensitivity to one or more common allergens (see notes above)
Cautions: see notes above including CSM warning; manufacturers recommend that patients should be warned not to eat a heavy meal before the injection
Contra-indications: pregnancy, febrile conditions, acute asthma
Side-effects: allergic reactions, especially in small children
Dose: by subcutaneous injection, see manufacturer's literature; very sensitive patients may be given an antihistamine tablet one hour before the injection

Pollen allergy (hay fever) preparations
PoM **Alavac-P®** (Bencard)
    Product discontinued
PoM **Allpyral-G®** (Dome/Hollister-Stier)
    Prepared from 5 varieties of common grass pollen. Net price treatment set = £23.73
▼ PoM **Conjuvac Two Grass®** (Dome/Hollister-Stier)
    Prepared from Timothy (*Phleum pratense*) and Cocksfoot (*Dactylis glomerata*). Net price treatment set = £29.30
PoM **Pollinex®** (Bencard)
    Product discontinued
▼ PoM **Spectralgen Single Species®**
(Pharmacia)
    Prepared from any one of 7 varieties common grasses or trees. Net price treatment set = £45.41–£61.20
▼ PoM **Spectralgen 4 Grass Mix®** (Pharmacia)
    Prepared from 4 varieties of common grasses. Net price treatment set = £64.99
▼ PoM **Spectralgen 3 Tree Mix®** (Pharmacia)
    Prepared from 3 varieties of common trees. Net price treatment set = £63.06

House dust mite allergy preparations
PoM **Allpyral D. pteronyssinus®** (Dome/Hollister-Stier)
    Prepared from *D. pteronyssinus*. Net price treatment set = £31.41
PoM **Allpyral-Mite   Fortified   House   Dust®**
(Dome/Hollister-Stier)
    Prepared from mite-fortified house dust (*Dermatophagoides* spp.). Net price treatment set = £31.41

▼ PoM **Conjuvac Mite**® (Dome/Hollister-Stier)
Prepared from the house dust mite (*D. pteronyssinus*). Net price treatment set = £42.00

PoM **Migen**® (Bencard)
Product discontinued

Specific allergy preparations

PoM **Alavac-S**® (Bencard)
Product discontinued

PoM **Allpyral-Specific**® (Dome/Hollister-Stier)
Prepared from specific allergens to which patient is sensitive. Net price treatment set = £26.47

PoM **SDV**® (Bencard)
Product discontinued

Wasp and bee venom allergy preparations

▼ PoM **Albay Pure Venom**® (Dome/Hollister-Stier)
Bee venom extract (*Apis mellifera*) or wasp venom extract (*Vespula* spp.). Net price treatment set = £29.30 (bee), £34.18 (wasp)

PoM **Pharmalgen**® (Pharmacia)
Bee venom extract (*Apis mellifera*) or wasp venom extract (*Vespula* spp.). Net price treatment set = £44.16 (bee), £56.76 (wasp)

3.4.3 Allergic emergencies

Anaphylactic shock requires prompt energetic treatment of laryngeal oedema, bronchospasm, and hypotension. It is relatively uncommon and is usually precipitated by blood products, vaccines, insect stings, and certain drugs such as antibiotics, iron injections, anti-inflammatory analgesics, heparin, hyposensitising (allergen) preparations, and neuromuscular blocking drugs. It is more likely to occur after parenteral administration and atopic individuals are particularly susceptible.

First-line treatment includes restoration of blood pressure, laying the patient flat, raising the feet, and administration of **adrenaline** injection. This is usually given intramuscularly in a dose of 0.5–1 mg (0.5–1 ml adrenaline injection 1 in 1000), repeated every 10 minutes until improvement occurs; several times the usual dose may be given if the patient is unconscious. Antihistamines, e.g. **chlorpheniramine**, given by slow intravenous injection (section 3.4.1), are a useful adjunctive treatment. This is given after adrenaline injection and continued for 24 to 48 hours to prevent relapse.

Continuing deterioration requires further treatment including intravenous fluids (see section 9.2.2), intravenous aminophylline (section 3.1.3) or a nebulised beta$_2$-adrenoceptor stimulant (such as salbutamol or terbutaline, section 3.1.1.1), oxygen, assisted respiration, and possibly emergency tracheostomy.

Intravenous **corticosteroids** are of secondary value in anaphylactic shock as their onset of action is delayed for several hours but they should be used to prevent further deterioration in severely affected patients (see section 6.3.4).

Some patients with severe allergy to insect stings are encouraged to carry adrenaline inhalations (Medihaler-epi®) or pre-filled adrenaline syringes for emergency administration during periods of risk.

Angioedema is dangerous when it affects respiration. If obstruction is present, adrenaline injection as well as intravenous corticosteroids should be given as described above; antihistamine injections are also helpful. Tracheal intubation as well as other measures may also be necessary.

ADRENALINE

Indications: reversible airways obstruction, emergency treatment of acute anaphylaxis

Cautions: hyperthyroidism, diabetes mellitus, ischaemic heart disease, hypertension, elderly patients; avoid intravenous use with tricyclic antidepressants, digoxin, or quinidine because of increased risk of arrhythmias. Drug interactions: see Appendix 1 (sections *2.4*, *2.7*, *15*)

Side-effects: anxiety, tremor, tachycardia, arrhythmias, dry mouth, cold extremities (seldom troublesome when given by aerosol inhalation, but tolerance and increased viscosity of bronchial secretions occur)

Dose: acute airways obstruction, as a single dose, *by subcutaneous or intramuscular injection*, 200–500 micrograms, repeated at intervals of 15–30 minutes; CHILD 10 micrograms/kg; max. 500 micrograms as a single dose

Acute anaphylaxis, *by intramuscular injection*, 0.5–1 mg (0.5–1 ml of 1 in 1000), repeated as necessary; CHILD, 10 micrograms/kg (0.01 ml/kg of 1 in 1000), max. 500 micrograms (0.5 ml of 1 in 1000), *or* 3–5 months 0.05 ml of 1 in 1000, 6–11 months 0.075 ml, 1 year 0.1 ml, 5 years 0.25 ml, 12 years 0.5 ml

PoM **Adrenaline Injection,** adrenaline 1 in 1000 (adrenaline 1 mg/ml as acid tartrate). Net price 0.5-ml amp = 27p; 1-ml amp = 28p

PoM **Medihaler-epi**® (Riker)
Aerosol inhalation, adrenaline acid tartrate 280 micrograms/metered inhalation. Net price 400-dose unit = £2.73
Dose: by aerosol inhalation, adjunct to anaphylaxis treatment only, min. of 20 puffs

PoM **Min-i-Jet Adrenaline**® (IMS)
Injection, adrenaline 1 in 1000 (1 mg/ml as hydrochloride). Net price 0.5-ml = £2.45; 1-ml = £2.32 (both disposable syringe)

3.5 Respiratory stimulants

Respiratory stimulants (analeptic drugs) have a limited place in the treatment of ventilatory failure in patients with chronic obstructive airways disease. They are effective only when given by intravenous injection or infusion and have a short duration of action. Their use has largely been replaced by ventilatory support. However, occasionally when the latter is contra-indicated and in patients with hypercapnic respiratory failure who are becoming drowsy or comatose, respiratory stimulants in the short term may arouse patients sufficiently to co-operate and clear their secretions.

Respiratory stimulants may be harmful in respiratory failure since they stimulate non-respiratory as well as respiratory muscles. They should only be given under **expert supervision** in hospital and must be combined with active physiotherapy. There is at present no oral respiratory stimulant available for long-term use in chronic respiratory failure.

Doxapram (Dopram®) is given by continuous intravenous infusion in a dosage of 2 mg per minute. Frequent arterial blood gas studies and pH measurements are necessary during treatment to ensure the correct dosage. Doxapram probably has a greater safety margin than nikethamide, which used to be the drug of choice. **Nikethamide** is given by regular bolus injection, in doses of 0.5 to 1 g (2 to 4 ml), into the drip tubing of an intravenous infusion. This may arouse patients with carbon dioxide narcosis sufficiently to co-operate with supervised coughing. However, the effective dose is close to that causing toxic effects, especially convulsions.

Ethamivan (Clairvan®) has properties similar to those of nikethamide.

Respiratory stimulants such as ethamivan and nikethamide have no place whatsoever in the management of asphyxia in the newborn.

DOXAPRAM HYDROCHLORIDE

Indications: see notes above; for postoperative use see section 15.1.7

Cautions: epilepsy, patients taking MAOIs; see also notes above

Contra-indications: severe hypertension, status asthmaticus, coronary artery disease, thyrotoxicosis

Side-effects: increase in blood pressure and heart rate, dizziness, perineal warmth

Dose: by intravenous infusion, 1.5–4 mg per minute according to patient's response

By intravenous injection—see section 15.1.7

PoM **Dopram®** (Robins)
   Intravenous infusion, doxapram hydrochloride 2 mg/ml in glucose 5%. Net price 500-ml bottle = £20.88

NIKETHAMIDE

Indications: see notes above

Cautions: see notes above, severe hypertension, ischaemic heart disease

Contra-indications: respiratory failure due to neurological disease or drug overdose; status asthmaticus, coronary artery disease, thyrotoxicosis

Side-effects: nausea, restlessness, convulsions, dizziness, tremor, vasoconstriction, arrhythmias

Dose: by slow intravenous injection, 0.5–1 g repeated at intervals of 15–30 minutes as necessary

PoM **Nikethamide Injection,** nikethamide 250 mg/ ml. Net price 2-ml amp = 57p

ETHAMIVAN

Indications; Cautions; Contra-indications; Side-effects: see under Nikethamide and notes above

Dose: by intravenous injection, 100 mg, repeated when necessary

PoM **Clairvan®** (Sinclair)
   Oral solution, ethamivan 50 mg/ml (5%) in ethyl alcohol 25%. Net price 5-ml dropper bottle = £5.25
   Note. Use of this paediatric preparation is not recommended (see notes above)
   Injection, ethamivan 50 mg/ml (5%). Net price 2-ml amp = £1.37

3.6   Oxygen

Oxygen should be regarded as a drug. It is prescribed for hypoxaemic patients to increase alveolar oxygen tension and decrease the work of breathing necessary to maintain a given arterial oxygen tension. The concentration depends on the condition being treated; an inappropriate concentration may have serious or even lethal effects.

High concentration oxygen therapy, with concentrations of up to 60% for short periods, is safe in conditions such as pneumonia, pulmonary thromboembolism, and fibrosing alveolitis. In such conditions a low arterial plasma P_aO_2 is usually associated with low or normal arterial plasma P_aCO_2 therefore there is little risk of hypoventilation and carbon dioxide retention.

In severe acute asthma, the arterial plasma P_aCO_2 is initially subnormal but as asthma deteriorates may rise steeply (particularly in children). These patients usually require high concentrations of oxygen and if the P_aCO_2 remains high despite other treatment intermittent positive pressure ventilation needs to be considered urgently. Where facilities for blood gas measurements are not immediately available, for example while transferring the patient to hospital, 35% to 50% oxygen delivered through a conventional mask is recommended. Exceptionally, asthma is diagnosed in patients with a long history of chronic bronchitis and probable respiratory failure; in these patients a lower concentration (24% to 28%) may be needed to limit oxygen-induced reduction of respiratory drive.

Low concentration oxygen therapy (controlled oxygen therapy) is reserved for patients with ventilatory failure due to chronic obstructive airways disease or other causes. The concentration should not exceed 28% and in some patients a concentration above 24% may be excessive. The aim is to provide the patient with just enough oxygen to correct hypoxaemia without worsening pre-existing carbon dioxide retention and respiratory acidosis. Treatment should be initiated in hospital as repeated blood gas measurements are required to estimate the correct concentration.

DOMICILIARY OXYGEN. Oxygen should only be prescribed for patients in the home after careful evaluation in hospital by respiratory experts; it should never be prescribed on a placebo basis.

Oxygen may be prescribed for *intermittent* use in a variety of respiratory conditions. It is used in patients with hypoxaemia of short duration, for example asthma, when the condition is likely to recur over months or years. Such patients are usually supplied with cylinders.

Alternatively, intermittent oxygen may be prescribed for patients with advanced irreversible respiratory disorders to increase mobility and capacity for exercise and to ease discomfort, for example in chronic obstructive bronchitis, emphysema, widespread fibrosis, and primary or thromboembolic pulmonary hypertension. These patients may be prescribed portable equipment through the hospital service, refillable from cylinders in the home.

Long-term administration of oxygen (at least 15 hours daily) may be prescribed on an elective basis in an attempt to prolong survival in patients with severe chronic obstructive airways disease with cor pulmonale.

DHSS guidelines suggest that this treatment should be reserved for patients who fulfil the following criteria:

$P_aO_2 < 7.3$ kPa; $P_aCO_2 > 6$ kPa;
$FEV_1 < 1.5$ litre and FVC < 2 litre

The measurements should be stable on two occasions at least three weeks apart after the patient has received appropriate bronchodilator therapy.

Less information is available on long-term oxygen in patients with a similar degree of hypoxaemia and airflow obstruction but no hypercapnia; the DHSS suggests that these patients should not be denied this form of treatment but the effects of long-term therapy have not yet been assessed completely.

Increased respiratory depression from low concentrations of oxygen is seldom a problem in patients with stable respiratory failure although it may occur during exacerbations; patients and relatives should be warned to call for medical help if drowsiness or confusion occur.

Patients should be advised of the fire risks when receiving therapy.

The DHSS recommends that patients prescribed long-term oxygen should be provided with a concentrator. Oxygen concentrators are more economical for patients requiring oxygen for long periods, and in England and Wales are now prescribable on the NHS on a regional tendering basis.

Long-term oxygen treatment is very demanding. Before a concentrator is installed patients must be prepared to take oxygen for 15 hours a day. To provide oxygen for 15 hours a day at a rate of 2 litres per minute requires ten 'F' size oxygen cylinders a week.

Under the NHS oxygen may be supplied by chemist contractors as cylinders. Oxygen flow can be adjusted as the cylinders are equipped with an oxygen flow meter with 'medium' (2 litres/minute) and 'high' (4 litres/minute) settings. Patients are supplied with either constant or variable performance masks. The Intersurgical 010 28% or Ventimask Mk III 28% are constant performance masks and provide a nearly constant supply of oxygen (28%) over a wide range irrespective of the patient's breathing pattern. The variable performance masks include the Intersurgical 005 Mask and the MC Mask; the concentration of oxygen supplied to the patient varies with the rate of flow of oxygen and also with the patient's breathing pattern; they are generally used in patients who require oxygen concentrations below 28%.

3.7 Mucolytics

Mucolytics are often prescribed to facilitate expectoration by reducing sputum viscosity in chronic asthma and bronchitis. Few patients, however, have been shown to derive much benefit from them although they do render sputum less viscid.

Tyloxapol is probably no more effective than water or steam inhalation, which in itself, with postural drainage, is good expectorant therapy in bronchiectasis and some chronic bronchitics.

Acetylcysteine (Fabrol®), **carbocisteine** (Mucodyne®), and **methylcysteine** (Visclair®) are given by mouth.

INHALATIONAL MUCOLYTICS

TYLOXAPOL
Indications: reduction of sputum viscosity
Side-effects: occasional febrile reactions
Dose: by inhalation of a nebulised solution, continuous treatment using an Oxygenaire atomiser 144–360 ml (180–450 mg) over 24 hours *or* intermittent treatment 6–20 ml of a 0.125% solution (7.5–25 mg) over a period of 24 hours divided into 3–4 doses inhaled over 20 minutes; concentration adjusted to equipment and oxygen flow rate

Alevaire® (Winthrop)
Solution, tyloxapol 0.125% (1.25 mg/ml). Net price 60 ml = £6.95; 200 ml = £14.52
Note. Brass or copper apparatus should not be used

ORAL MUCOLYTICS

ACETYLCYSTEINE
Indications: reduction of sputum viscosity
Side-effects: occasional gastro-intestinal irritation, headache, urticaria, tinnitus, and sensitivity

Dose: adults and children over 6 years, 200 mg in water 3 times daily, usually for 5–10 days but if necessary may be extended to 6 months or longer; CHILD up to 2 years 200 mg daily, 2–6 years 200 mg twice daily

NHS * ▼ PoM **Acetylcysteine Granules,** acetylcysteine 200 mg/sachet. Net price 30 sachets = £5.75. Label: 13
* except for abdominal complications associated with cystic fibrosis and endorsed 'S3B' ('S2B' in Scotland)
NHS ▼ PoM **Fabrol®** (Zyma)
Granules, yellow, acetylcysteine 200 mg/sachet. Net price 30 sachets = £5.75. Label: 13

CARBOCISTEINE

Indications: reduction of sputum viscosity
Side-effects: occasional gastro-intestinal irritation, rashes
Dose: 750 mg 3 times daily initially, then 1.5 g daily in divided doses; CHILD 2–5 years 62.5–125 mg 4 times daily, 6–12 years 250 mg 3 times daily

NHS * PoM **Carbocisteine Capsules,** carbocisteine 375 mg. Net price 20 = £2.13
NHS * PoM **Carbocisteine Tablets,** carbocisteine 375 mg. Net price 20 = £2.98
NHS * PoM **Carbocisteine Syrup,** carbocisteine 125 mg/5 ml. Diluent syrup, life of diluted syrup 14 days, net price 100 ml = £1.17; 250 mg/5 ml, 100 ml = £1.50
* except, for patients under the age of 18 years, any condition which, through damage or disease, affects the airways and has required a tracheostomy and endorsed 'S3B' ('S2B' in Scotland)

NHS PoM **Mucodyne®** (Rorer)
Capsules, yellow, carbocisteine 375 mg. Net price 30 = £3.20
Syrup, amber-coloured, carbocisteine 250 mg/5 ml. Diluent syrup (without preservative), life of diluted syrup 14 days. Net price 300 ml = £4.50
Paediatric syrup, red, carbocisteine 125 mg/5 ml. Diluent as above. Net price 300 ml = £3.50

METHYLCYSTEINE HYDROCHLORIDE

Indications: reduction of sputum viscosity
Dose: 100–200 mg 3–4 times daily before meals reduced to 200 mg twice daily after 6 weeks; CHILD over 5 years 100 mg 3 times daily
Prophylaxis, 100–200 mg 2–3 times every other day during winter months

NHS **Visclair®** (Sinclair)
Tablets, yellow, s/c, e/c, methylcysteine hydrochloride 100 mg. Net price 20 = £2.74. Label: 5, 22, 25

3.8   Aromatic inhalations

Inhalations containing volatile substances such as eucalyptus oil are traditionally used and although the vapour may contain little of the additive it encourages deliberate inspiration of warm moist air which is often comforting in bronchitis. Inhalations are also used for the relief of nasal obstruction in acute rhinitis or sinusitis.

CHILDREN. The use of strong aromatic decongestants (applied as rubs or to pillows) could be hazardous to infants less than one month of age, since in certain circumstances, apnoea could be induced. Mothers with young infants in whom nasal obstruction with mucus is a problem can readily be taught appropriate techniques of suction aspiration.

Benzoin Tincture, Compound, balsamic acids approx. 4.5%. Net price 50 ml = 26p. Label: 15
Directions for use: add one teaspoonful to a pint of hot, not boiling, water and inhale the vapour
NHS **Menthol and Benzoin Inhalation,** menthol 2%, in benzoin inhalation (see Formulary). Net price 50 ml = 31p. Label: 15
Directions for use: as above
Menthol and Eucalyptus Inhalation, (see Formulary). Net price 50 ml = 18p
Directions for use: as above
NHS **Karvol®** (Crookes Products)
Inhalation capsules, menthol 35.9 mg, with chlorbutol, cinnamon oil, pine oil, terpineol, and thymol. Net price 10 = 66p
Directions for use: inhale vapour from contents of 1 capsule expressed into handkerchief or a pint of hot, not boiling, water

3.9   Antitussives

3.9.1 Cough suppressants
3.9.2 Expectorant, demulcent, and compound cough preparations

3.9.1   Cough suppressants

The drawbacks of prescribing cough suppressants are rarely outweighed by the benefits of treatment and only occasionally are they useful, as, for example, if sleep is disturbed by a dry cough. Cough suppressants may cause sputum retention and this may be harmful in patients with chronic bronchitis and bronchiectasis. Though commonly used in acute bronchitis and pneumonia they can be harmful; such conditions are best treated by prompt administration of antibacterial drugs (see section 5.1, Table 1).

Cough suppressants such as codeine, dextromethorphan, and pholcodine are seldom sufficiently potent to be effective and all tend to cause constipation.

CHILDREN. The use of cough suppressants containing codeine or similar opioid analgesics is not generally recommended in children and should be avoided altogether in those under 1 year of age.

CODEINE PHOSPHATE

Indications: dry or painful cough
Cautions: asthma; hepatic and renal impairment; history of drug abuse; see also notes above and

section 4.7.2. Drug interactions: see Appendix 1 (sections *2.3*, *4.1*, *4.3*, *4.6*)
Contra-indications: liver disease, ventilatory failure
Side-effects: constipation, in large doses respiratory depression

Codeine Linctus, codeine phosphate 15 mg/5 ml. Net price 100 ml = 35p
Dose: 5–10 ml 3–4 times daily
Codeine Linctus, Diabetic, codeine phosphate 15 mg/5 ml. Net price 100 ml = 68p
Dose: 5–10 ml 3–4 times daily
Note. The title 'Diabetic Codeine Linctus' may be used for a preparation that complies with the requirements of the BP monograph for Codeine Linctus and that is formulated with a vehicle appropriate for administration to diabetics.
Codeine Linctus, Paediatric, codeine phosphate 3 mg/5 ml (see Formulary). Net price 100 ml = 18p
Dose: CHILD 1–5 years 5 ml 3–4 times daily
Note. Sugar-free versions are available; they conform to the BP 1988 description
Galcodine® (Galen)
Linctus, orange, sugar-free, codeine phosphate 15 mg/5 ml. Diluent water for preparations, life of diluted linctus 14 days. Net price 100 ml = 29p
Dose: see under Codeine Linctus
Paediatric linctus, orange-red, sugar-free, codeine phosphate 3 mg/5 ml. Diluent as above. Net price 100 ml = 17p
Dose: see under Codeine Linctus, Paediatric

ISOAMINILE CITRATE
Indications: dry or painful cough
Cautions: see notes above
Side-effects: occasionally constipation, dizziness, nausea
Dose: see below

PoM **Isoaminile Linctus,** isoaminile citrate 40 mg/5 ml. Diluent syrup, life of diluted linctus 14 days. Net price 150 ml = £1.88
Dose: 5 ml 3–5 times daily; CHILD, 2.5–5 ml
NHS PoM **Dimyril**® (Fisons)
Linctus, red, isoaminile citrate 40 mg/5 ml. Diluent syrup, life of diluted linctus 14 days. Net price 150 ml = £1.88

NOSCAPINE
Indications: dry or painful cough
Cautions; Contra-indications; Side-effects: see under Codeine Phosphate
Dose: 15–30 mg 3–4 times daily; CHILD, 2–5 years 2–5 mg, 6–12 years 6–12 mg

NHS **Noscapine Linctus,** noscapine 15 mg/5 ml. Net price 100 ml = 62p

PHOLCODINE
Indications: dry or painful cough
Cautions; Contra-indications; Side-effects: see under Codeine Phosphate

Pholcodine Linctus, pholcodine 5 mg/5 ml. Net price 100 ml = 29p
Dose: 5–10 ml 3–4 times daily
Pholcodine Linctus, Strong, pholcodine 10 mg/5 ml. Net price 100 ml = 46p
Dose: 5 ml 3–4 times daily
Galenphol® (Galen)
Linctus, red, sugar-free, pholcodine 5 mg/5 ml. Diluent water for preparations, life of diluted linctus 14 days. Net price 100 ml = 24p
Dose: see under Pholcodine Linctus
Linctus, strong, orange-red, sugar-free, pholcodine 10 mg/5 ml. Diluent as above. Net price 100 ml = 41p
Dose: see under Pholcodine Linctus, Strong
Paediatric linctus, orange, sugar-free, pholcodine 2 mg/5 ml. Diluent as above. Net price 100 ml = 17p
Dose: CHILD 1–5 years 5–10 ml 3 times daily; 6–12 years 10 ml
Pavacol-D® (Boehringer Ingelheim)
Mixture, brown, sugar-free, pholcodine 5 mg/5 ml. Diluent sorbitol solution, life of diluted mixture 14 days. Net price 100 ml = 48p
Dose: 5–10 ml when required; CHILD 1–2 years 2.5 ml 3–4 times daily, 3–5 years 5 ml 3 times daily, 6–12 years 5 ml 4–5 times daily

TERMINAL CARE

Diamorphine and methadone are effective cough suppressants; they are given in linctuses to control distressful cough in terminal lung cancer although morphine is now preferred (see Terminal Care, p. 13). In other circumstances they are contra-indicated because they induce sputum retention and ventilatory failure as well as causing opioid dependence.

DIAMORPHINE HYDROCHLORIDE
Indications: dry or painful cough in terminal disease
Cautions; Contra-indications; Side-effects: see notes in section 4.7.2; more potent than morphine
Dose: see below

CD **Diamorphine Linctus,** diamorphine hydrochloride 3 mg/5 ml (see Formulary). Net price 100 ml = 93p. Label: 2
Dose: 2.5–10 ml every 4 hours

METHADONE HYDROCHLORIDE
Indications: dry or painful cough in terminal disease
Cautions; Contra-indications; Side-effects: see notes in section 4.7.2; longer-acting than morphine therefore effects may be cumulative
Dose: see below

CD **Methadone Linctus,** methadone hydrochloride 2 mg/5 ml in a suitable vehicle with a tolu flavour. Net price 100 ml = 86p. Label: 2
Dose: 2.5–5 ml every 4–6 hours, reduced to twice daily on prolonged use

3.9.2   Expectorant, demulcent, and compound cough preparations

The prescriber is often called upon to prescribe such preparations for minor respiratory disorders. Although there is no scientific basis for prescribing any of the preparations listed in this section, it may be that a harmless expectorant such as ammonia and ipecacuanha mixture or a demulcent such as simple linctus has a useful placebo role. Certainly this is preferable to the indiscriminate prescribing of antibiotics.

Expectorants are claimed to promote expulsion of bronchial secretions but there is no evidence that any drug, whether given by mouth, injection, or inhalation can specifically facilitate expectoration by stimulation or augmentation of the cough reflex.

Sub-emetic doses of expectorants such as ammonium chloride, ipecacuanha, and squill are commonly used to treat cough on the basis that emetic doses of these substances can without doubt expel mucus at the same time as provoking retching and vomiting by gastric irritation, but the assumption that sub-emetic doses can also promote expectoration is a myth. However, a simple expectorant mixture may serve a useful placebo function and has the advantage of being inexpensive. Expectorants are included in many compound preparations but the use of such mixtures should be avoided. Mucolytics (section 3.7) and inhalations (section 3.8) are also claimed to facilitate expectoration.

Demulcent cough preparations contain soothing substances such as syrup or glycerol and certainly some patients believe that such preparations relieve a dry irritating cough. Preparations such as **simple linctus** have the advantage of being harmless and inexpensive and **paediatric simple linctus** is particularly useful in children.

Compound cough preparations have no place in the treatment of respiratory disorders. Many of them contain an unnecessarily large number of ingredients, often in subtherapeutic doses, and often with similar therapeutic properties. Other preparations contain ingredients which have opposing effects, in particular the inclusion of expectorants together with antihistamines, sedatives, cough suppressants, bronchodilators, and sympathomimetics. Such preparations are to be **deprecated** not only as irrational but also for administering a large number of drugs to patients in inappropriate dosage and in excess of their needs; for example, the sedative effect of antihistamines may lead to carbon dioxide retention in patients with chronic bronchitis or emphysema. It is therefore best to prescribe one of the simple cough mixtures recommended above and if any other component is needed it may then be prescribed separately, tailored to the needs of the patient, and dosage adjusted accordingly.

CHILDREN. The use of cough suppressants containing codeine or similar opioid analgesics is not generally recommended in children and should be avoided altogether in those under 1 year of age.

NHS **Ammonia and Ipecacuanha Mixture** (see Formulary). Net price 100 ml = 12p
Dose: 10–20 ml 3–4 times daily

NHS **Ammonium Chloride and Morphine Mixture** (see Formulary). Net price 100 ml = 14p
Dose: 10–20 ml 3–4 times daily

NHS **Ipecacuanha and Morphine Mixture** (see Formulary). Net price 100 ml = 12p
Dose: 10 ml 3–4 times daily

Simple Linctus (see Formulary). Net price 100 ml = 16p
Dose: 5 ml 3–4 times daily

Simple Linctus, Paediatric (see Formulary). Net price 100 ml = 16p
Dose: CHILD, 5–10 ml 3–4 times daily

NHS **Squill Linctus, Opiate**, Gee's Linctus (see Formulary). Net price 100 ml = 23p
Dose: 5 ml 3–4 times daily

NHS **Squill Linctus, Opiate, Paediatric** (see Formulary). Net price 100 ml = 26p
Dose: 5–10 ml 3–4 times daily

NHS **Tolu Linctus, Compound, Paediatric.** Net price 100 ml = 45p
Dose: CHILD, 5–10 ml 3–4 times daily

NHS **Actifed Compound Linctus**® (Wellcome)
Linctus, red, dextromethorphan hydrobromide 10 mg, pseudoephedrine hydrochloride 30 mg, triprolidine hydrochloride 1.25 mg/5 ml. Diluent syrup, life of diluted linctus 14 days. Net price 100 ml = 85p; 200 ml = £1.69. Label: 2
Dose: 10 ml 3 times daily; CHILD 2–5 years 2.5 ml, 6–12 years 5 ml

NHS **Actifed Expectorant**® (Wellcome)
Elixir, orange, guaiphenesin 100 mg, pseudoephedrine hydrochloride 30 mg, triprolidine hydrochloride 1.25 mg/5 ml. Diluent syrup, life of diluted elixir 14 days. Net price 100 ml = 85p; 200 ml = £1.69. Label: 2
Dose: 10 ml 3 times daily; CHILD 2–5 years 2.5 ml, 6–12 years 5 ml

NHS **Benylin Expectorant**® (W-L)
Syrup, red, ammonium chloride 135 mg, diphenhydramine hydrochloride 14 mg, menthol 1.1 mg, sodium citrate 57 mg/5 ml. Diluent syrup, life of diluted syrup 14 days. Net price 125 ml = 86p; 300 ml = £2.07. Label: 2
Dose: 5–10 ml every 2–3 hours; CHILD 1–5 years 2.5 ml, 6–12 years 5 ml every 3–4 hours

NHS **Benylin Paediatric**® (W-L)
Syrup, red, diphenhydramine hydrochloride 7 mg, menthol 550 micrograms, sodium citrate 28.5 mg/5 ml. Diluent syrup, life of diluted syrup 14 days. Net price 125 ml = 93p; 300 ml = £1.60. Label: 1
Dose: CHILD 1–5 years 5 ml, 6–12 years 10 ml every hours

NHS **Benylin with Codeine**® (W-L)
Syrup, red, codeine phosphate 5.7 mg, diphenhydramine hydrochloride 14 mg, menthol 1.1 mg, sodium citrate 57 mg/5 ml. Diluent syrup, life of diluted syrup 14 days. Net price 300 ml = £2.49. Label: 2
Dose: 10 ml every 3–4 hours; CHILD 1–5 years 2.5 ml, 6–12 years 5 ml

NHS **Copholco**® (Fisons)
Linctus, brown, pholcodine 5.63 mg, cineole 0.0026 ml, menthol 1.41 mg, terpin hydrate 2.82 mg/5 ml. Do not dilute. Net price 100 ml = 79p
Dose: 10 ml 4–5 times daily; CHILD over 5 years 2.5–5 ml

NHS **Davenol**® (Wyeth)
Linctus, orange, carbinoxamine maleate 2 mg, ephedrine hydrochloride 7 mg, pholcodine 4 mg/5 ml. Diluent syrup (without preservative), life of diluted linctus 15 days. Net price 100 ml = 43p. Label: 2
Dose: 5–10 ml 3–4 times daily; CHILD over 1 year up to 5 ml

NHS **Dimotane Expectorant**® (Robins)
Elixir, pink, brompheniramine maleate 2 mg, guai-phenesin 100 mg, phenylephrine hydrochloride 5 mg, phenylpropanolamine hydrochloride 5 mg/5 ml. Diluent syrup, life of diluted elixir 14 days. Net price 100 ml = £1.10. Label: 2
Dose: 5–10 ml 3–4 times daily; CHILD 2–3 years 1–2.5 ml, 3–5 years 2.5–5 ml, 6–12 years 5 ml

NHS **Dimotane Co**® (Robins)
Elixir, pink, sugar-free, brompheniramine maleate 2 mg, codeine phosphate 10 mg, pseudoephedrine hydro-chloride 30 mg/5 ml. Diluent 70% glycerol, life of diluted elixir 14 days. Net price 100 ml = £1.10. Label: 2
Dose: 10 ml 3 times daily; CHILD 6–12 years 7.5 ml

NHS **Dimotane Co Paediatric**® (Robins)
Elixir, pink, sugar-free, brompheniramine maleate 2 mg, codeine phosphate 3 mg, pseudoephedrine hydrochloride 15 mg/5 ml. Diluent as above. Net price 100 ml = £1·04. Label: 1
Dose: CHILD 2–3 years 5 ml, 4–6 years 10 ml, 7–12 years 15 ml, 3 times daily

NHS **Expulin**® (Galen)
Linctus, yellow, sugar-free, chlorpheniramine maleate 2 mg, pseudoephedrine hydrochloride 15 mg, phol-codine 5 mg, menthol 1.1 mg/5 ml. Net price 100 ml = 92p. Label: 2
Dose: 10 ml 4 times daily; CHILD 2–6 years 2.5–5 ml, 6–12 years 5–10 ml
Paediatric linctus, pink, sugar-free, chlorpheniramine maleate 1 mg, pholcodine 2 mg, menthol 1.1 mg/5 ml. Net price 100 ml = 86p. Label: 1
Dose: CHILD 1–3 years 5 ml, 3–10 years 10 ml, 2–3 times daily

NHS **Guanor Expectorant**® (RP Drugs)
Syrup, red, ammonium chloride 135 mg, diphen-hydramine hydrochloride 14 mg, menthol 1.1 mg, sodium citrate 57 mg/5 ml. Net price 100 ml = 26p. Label: 2
Dose: 5–10 ml every 2–3 hours; CHILD 1–5 years 2.5 ml, 6–12 years 5 ml, every 3–4 hours

NHS **Histalix**® (Wallace Mfg)
Syrup, ammonium chloride 135 mg, diphenhydramine hydrochloride 14 mg, menthol 1.1 mg, sodium citrate 57 mg/5 ml. Net price 100 ml = £1.06. Label: 2
Dose: 5–10 ml every 3 hours; CHILD 2.5–5 ml

NHS **Lotussin**® (Searle)
Linctus, amber, dextromethorphan hydrobromide 6.25 mg, diphenhydramine hydrochloride 5 mg, eph-edrine hydrochloride 7.5 mg, guaiphenesin 50 mg/5 ml. Diluent syrup, life of diluted linctus 14 days. Net price 100 ml = 92p. Label: 2
Dose: 10 ml 3 times daily; CHILD 1–5 years 2.5–5 ml, 6–12 years 5–10 ml

NHS **Noradran**® (Norma)
Syrup, diphenhydramine hydrochloride 5 mg, dipro-phylline 50 mg, ephedrine hydrochloride 7.5 mg, guai-phenesin 25 mg/5 ml. Net price 150 ml = 81p. Label: 2
Dose: 10 ml every 4 hours; CHILD over 5 years 5 ml

NHS **Phensedyl**® (M&B)
Linctus, orange-brown, codeine phosphate 9 mg, eph-edrine hydrochloride 7.2 mg, promethazine hydro-chloride 3.6 mg/5 ml. Diluent syrup, life of diluted linctus 14 days. Net price 100 ml = £1.19. Label: 2
Dose: 5–10 ml 2–3 times daily; CHILD 2–5 years 2.5 ml, 5–10 years 2.5–5 ml

Pholcomed® (Medo)
NHS *Linctus*, red, papaverine hydrochloride 1.25 mg, pholcodine 5 mg/5 ml. Diluent syrup, life of diluted linctus 14 days. Net price 100 ml = 37p
Dose: 10–15 ml 3–4 times daily after food; CHILD 1–2 years 2.5 ml, over 2 years 5 ml

Pholcomed D® (Medo)
Linctus, red, ingredients as for Pholcomed but without sugar. Diluent purified water, freshly boiled and cooled,

life of diluted linctus 14 days. Net price 125 ml = 79p; 300 ml = £1.90

NHS **Pholcomed Expectorant**® (Medo)
Syrup, red, guaiphenesin 62.5 mg, methylephedrine hydrochloride 625 micrograms/5 ml. Net price 100 ml = 48p
Dose: 10–20 ml 3 times daily; CHILD 2.5–5 ml

NHS **Pholcomed Forte**® (Medo)
Linctus, red, papaverine hydrochloride 5 mg, pholcodine 19 mg/5 ml. Diluent syrup, life of diluted linctus 14 days. Net price 100 ml = 87p
Dose: 5 ml 3 times daily

NHS **Pholcomed Forte Diabetic**® (Medo)
Linctus, red, ingredients as for Pholcomed Forte but without sugar. Diluent purified water, freshly boiled and cooled, life of diluted linctus 14 days. Net price 125 ml = £1.30

NHS **Pholtex**® (Riker)
Mixture, s/r, orange, sugar-free, phenyltoloxamine 10 mg, pholcodine 15 mg/5 ml, as resin complexes. Diluent syrup or tragacanth mucilage, life of diluted mixture 14 days. Net price 100 ml = 86p. Label: 2
Dose: 5 ml 2–3 times daily; CHILD 2.5–5 ml

NHS **Sudafed Expectorant**® (Calmic)
Syrup, red, guaiphenesin 100 mg, pseudoephedrine hydrochloride 30 mg/5 ml. Diluent syrup, life of diluted syrup 14 days. Net price 100 ml = 99p
Dose: 10 ml 3 times daily; CHILD 2–5 years 2.5 ml, 6–12 years 5 ml

NHS **Tancolin**® (Ashe)
Linctus (paediatric), orange, ascorbic acid 12.35 mg, cit-ric acid 45.85 mg, dextromethorphan hydrobromide 2.62 mg, glycerol 655 mg, sodium citrate 99.56 mg/5 ml. Net price 100 ml = 84p
Dose: CHILD 1–3 years 5 ml, 4–5 years 10 ml, 6–12 years 15 ml, 3 times daily

NHS **Tercoda**® (Sinclair)
Elixir, yellow, codeine phosphate 8 mg, terpin hydrate 8 mg/5 ml. Net price 100 ml = 96p
Dose: 5–10 ml 3 times daily

NHS **Terpoin**® (Hough)
Elixir, yellow, codeine phosphate 15 mg/5 ml with cine-ole and menthol. Net price 100 ml = £1.46
Dose: 5 ml every 3 hours

NHS **Tixylix**® (Intercare)
Linctus, blackcurrant, pholcodine 1.5 mg (as citrate), promethazine hydrochloride 1.5 mg/5 ml. Net price 100 ml = 93p. Label: 1 *or* 2
Dose: 10–20 ml 3 times daily; CHILD 3–5 years 5 ml, 6–10 years 5–10 ml, 2–3 times daily

3.10 Systemic nasal decongestants

These preparations are of doubtful value but unlike the preparations for local application (see section 12.2.2) they do not give rise to rebound nasal congestion. They contain sympatho-mimetics, and should therefore be **avoided** in patients with hypertension, hyperthyroidism, cor-onary heart disease, or diabetes, and in patients taking monoamine-oxidase inhibitors. Drug inter-actions: see Appendix 1 (sections *2.4*, *2.5*, *4.3*) Many of the preparations also contain anti-histamines which may cause drowsiness and affect ability to drive or operate machinery.

Ephedrine Preparations
Section 3.1.1.2

NHS **Actifed**® (Wellcome)
Tablets, scored, pseudoephedrine hydrochloride 60 mg,

triprolidine hydrochloride 2.5 mg. Net price 12 = 73p.
Label: 2
Dose: 1 tablet 3 times daily
Syrup, yellow, pseudoephedrine hydrochloride 30 mg,
triprolidine hydrochloride 1.25 mg/5 ml. Diluent syrup,
life of diluted syrup 14 days. Net price 100 ml = 87p.
Label: 2
Dose: 10 ml 3 times daily; CHILD 2–5 years 2.5 ml, 6–12
years 5 ml

NHS **Benylin Decongestant**® (W-L)
Syrup, yellow, diphenhydramine hydrochloride 14 mg,
menthol 1.1 mg, pseudoephedrine hydrochloride 10 mg,
sodium citrate 57 mg/5 ml. Diluent syrup, life of diluted
syrup 14 days. Net price 300 ml = £1.96. Label: 2
Dose: 10 ml 4 times daily; CHILD 1–5 years 2.5 ml, 6–12
years 5 ml

Dimotane Plus® (Robins)
Liquid, brown, sugar-free, brompheniramine maleate
4 mg, pseudoephedrine hydrochloride 30 mg/5 ml.
Diluent glycerol 70%, life of diluted liquid 14 days. Net
price 100 ml = 76p. Label: 2
Dose: 10 ml 3 times daily; CHILD 6–12 years 5 ml
Paediatric liquid, brown, sugar-free, brompheniramine
maleate 2 mg, pseudoephedrine hydrochloride 15 mg/
5 ml. Diluent as above. Net price 100 ml = 69p. Label:
1
Dose: CHILD 2–6 years 5 ml, 6–12 years 10 ml, 3 times
daily

NHS **Dimotapp**® (Robins)
Elixir, red-brown, sugar-free, brompheniramine maleate
4 mg, phenylephrine hydrochloride 5 mg, phenylpropanolamine hydrochloride 5 mg/5 ml. Diluent syrup,
life of diluted elixir 14 days. Net price 100 ml = 98p.
Label: 2
Dose: 5–10 ml 3–4 times daily; CHILD 6–12 years 5 ml
Paediatric elixir, red-brown, sugar-free, brompheniramine maleate 1 mg, phenylephrine hydrochloride
2.5 mg, phenylpropanolamine hydrochloride 2.5 mg/
5 ml. Diluent as above. Net price 100 ml = 92p. Label:
1
Dose: CHILD 2–5 years 2.5–10 ml, 6–12 years 10 ml, 3–
4 times daily

NHS **Dimotapp LA**® (Robins)
Tablets, s/r, brown, s/c, brompheniramine maleate
12 mg, phenylephrine hydrochloride 15 mg, phenylpropanolamine hydrochloride 15 mg. Net price 20 =
£1.30. Label: 2, 25, counselling advised, gluten
Dose: 1–2 tablets twice daily

NHS **Eskornade**® (SK&F)
Spansule® (= capsules s/r), grey/clear, enclosing red,
grey, and white pellets, diphenylpyraline hydrochloride
5 mg, phenylpropanolamine hydrochloride 50 mg. Net
price 30 = £2.32. Label: 2, 25
Dose: 1 capsule twice daily
Syrup, green, sugar-free, diphenylpyraline hydrochloride
1.5 mg, phenylpropanolamine hydrochloride 12.5 mg/
5 ml. Diluent syrup or sorbitol solution, life of diluted
syrup 14 days. Net price 150 ml = £2.08. Label: 2
Dose: 10 ml up to 4 times daily; CHILD 2–5 years 2.5 ml,
6–12 years 5 ml, up to 4 times daily

NHS **Expurhin**® (Galen)
Paediatric linctus, orange, sugar-free, chlorpheniramine
maleate 1 mg, ephedrine hydrochloride 4 mg, menthol
1.1 mg/5 ml. Net price 100 ml = 86p. Label: 1

Dose: CHILD 1–5 years 5–10 ml 3 times daily, 6–12 years
10–15 ml

Galpseud® (Galen)
Tablets, pseudoephedrine hydrochloride 60 mg. Net
price 20 = 53p
Dose: 1 tablet 3 times daily
Linctus, orange, sugar-free, pseudoephedrine hydrochloride 30 mg/5 ml. Diluent water for preparations, life
of diluted linctus 14 days. Net price 100 ml = 40p
Dose: 10 ml 3 times daily; CHILD 2–6 years 2.5 ml, 6–12
years 5 ml

Haymine® (Pharmax)
Tablets, s/r, yellow, chlorpheniramine maleate 10 mg
ephedrine hydrochloride 15 mg. Net price 30 = £2.23
Label: 2, 25
Dose: 1 tablet 1–2 times daily

Sudafed® (Calmic)
Tablets, s/c, pseudoephedrine hydrochloride 60 mg
Net price 20 = £1.07
Dose: 1 tablet 3 times daily
Elixir, pink, pseudoephedrine hydrochloride 30 mg/5 ml
Diluent syrup, life of diluted elixir 14 days. Net price
100 ml = 86p
Dose: 10 ml 3 times daily; CHILD 2–5 years 2.5 ml, 6–12
years 5 ml

PoM **Sudafed SA**® (Calmic)
Capsules, s/r, red/clear, pseudoephedrine hydrochloride
120 mg. Net price 20 = £1.32. Label: 25
Dose: 1 capsule every 12 hours

NHS **Sudafed-Co**® (Calmic)
Tablets, scored, paracetamol 500 mg, pseudoephedrine
hydrochloride 60 mg. Net price 12 = 76p
Dose: 1 tablet 3 times daily; CHILD 6–12 years, half
tablet

NHS **Triogesic**® (Beecham)
Tablets, pink, scored, paracetamol 500 mg, phenylpropanolamine hydrochloride 12.5 mg. Net price 30 =
£1.13
Dose: 1–2 tablets every 4 hours, max. 6 daily; CHILD
over 12 years 1 tablet every 4 hours, max. 4 daily
Elixir, red, sugar-free, paracetamol 125 mg, phenyl
propanolamine hydrochloride 3 mg/5 ml. Net price
100 ml = 96p
Dose: 20 ml every 4 hours, max. 120 ml daily; CHILD
over 12 years 15 ml every 4 hours, max. 75 ml

NHS **Triominic**® (Beecham)
Tablets, yellow, pheniramine maleate 25 mg, phenylpropanolamine hydrochloride 25 mg. Net price 30 =
£1.13. Label: 2
Dose: 1 tablet every 6–8 hours, max. 3 daily
Syrup, orange, pheniramine maleate 12.5 mg, phenylpropanolamine hydrochloride 12.5 mg/5 ml. Net price
100 ml = 96p. Label: 2
Dose: 10 ml up to 3 times daily; CHILD over 12 years
5 ml up to 4 times daily

NHS **Uniflu with Gregovite C**® (Unigreg)
Tablets, composite pack of pairs of tablets: Uniflu *tablets*
magenta, s/c, caffeine 30 mg, codeine phosphate 10 mg,
diphenhydramine hydrochloride 15 mg, paracetamol
500 mg, phenylephrine hydrochloride 10 mg; Gregovite
C *tablets*, yellow, chewable, ascorbic acid 300 mg. Net
price 6 of each tablet = 79p; or 12 of each tablet =
£1.30. Label: 2
Dose: 1 of each tablet every 6 hours

4: Drugs acting on the
CENTRAL NERVOUS SYSTEM

In this chapter, drug treatments are discussed under the following headings:

4.1 Hypnotics and anxiolytics
4.2 Drugs used in psychoses and related disorders
4.3 Antidepressant drugs
4.4 Central nervous stimulants
4.5 Appetite suppressants
4.6 Drugs used in nausea and vertigo
4.7 Analgesics
4.8 Antiepileptics
4.9 Drugs used in parkinsonism and related disorders
4.10 Drugs used in alcoholism and cigarette smoking

4.1 Hypnotics and anxiolytics

4.1.1 Hypnotics
4.1.2 Anxiolytics
4.1.3 Barbiturates and methyprylone

For peri-operative sedation see section 15.1.4.

Most anxiolytics ('sedatives') will induce sleep when given in large doses at night and most hypnotics will sedate when given in divided doses during the day. Prescribing of these drugs is widespread but dependence (either physical or psychological) and tolerance to their effects occurs. This may lead to difficulty in withdrawing the drug after the patient has been taking it regularly for more than a few weeks (see Dependence and Withdrawal, below). Hypnotics and anxiolytics should not therefore be prescribed indiscriminately and should, instead, be reserved for short courses to alleviate acute conditions after causal factors have been established.

Prescribing of more than one anxiolytic or hypnotic at the same time is **not** recommended. It may constitute a hazard and there is no evidence that side-effects are minimised.

Benzodiazepines are the most commonly used anxiolytics and hypnotics; barbiturates (section 4.1.3) are no longer recommended.

Benzodiazepines have fewer side-effects than barbiturates and are much less dangerous in

overdosage. They are also less likely to interact with other drugs because, unlike barbiturates, they do not induce liver microsomal enzymes.

Side-effects of benzodiazepines are generally mild and include drowsiness and ataxia (particularly in the elderly).

A paradoxical increase in hostility and aggression may be reported by patients taking benzodiazepines. The effects range from talkativeness and excitement, to aggressive and anti-social acts. Adjustment of the dose (up or down) usually attenuates the impulses. Increased anxiety and perceptual disorders are other paradoxical effects. Increased hostility and aggression after barbiturates and alcohol usually indicates intoxication.

DEPENDENCE AND WITHDRAWAL. Compared with other anxiolytics and hypnotics, especially the barbiturates, the benzodiazepine withdrawal syndrome may be delayed in onset (but less so with those that are short-acting); it may also last longer (8 to 10 days). It is characterised by insomnia, anxiety, loss of appetite and body weight, tremor, perspiration, and perceptual disturbances. These symptoms may be similar to the original complaint and encourage further prescribing; some symptoms may continue for weeks or months.

Withdrawal of a benzodiazepine following either high dosage or long-term administration should be gradual as abrupt withdrawal may produce confusion, toxic psychosis, convulsions, or a condition resembling delirium tremens. It is important to note however that withdrawal symptoms can also occur following administration of therapeutic doses for short periods of time.

DRIVING. Hypnotics and anxiolytics may impair judgement and increase reaction time, and so affect ability to drive or operate machinery; they increase the effects of alcohol. Moreover the hangover effects of a night dose may impair driving on the following day.

4.1.1 Hypnotics

Before a hypnotic is prescribed the cause of the insomnia should be established and, where possible, underlying factors should be treated. However, it should be noted that some patients have unrealistic sleep expectations, and others understate their alcohol consumption which is often the cause of the insomnia.

Transient insomnia may occur in those who normally sleep well and may be due to extraneous factors such as noise, shift work, and jet lag. If a hypnotic is indicated one that is rapidly eliminated should be chosen, and only one or two doses should be given.

Short-term insomnia is usually related to an emotional problem or serious medical illness. It

CSM advice.
1. Benzodiazepines are indicated for the short-term relief (two to four weeks only) of anxiety that is severe, disabling or subjecting the individual to unacceptable distress, occurring alone or in association with insomnia or short-term psychosomatic, organic or psychotic illness.
2. The use of benzodiazepines to treat short-term 'mild' anxiety is inappropriate and unsuitable.
3. Benzodiazepines should be used to treat insomnia only when it is severe, disabling, or subjecting the individual to extreme distress.

may last for a few weeks, and may recur; a hypnotic can be useful but should not be given for more than three weeks (preferably only one week). Intermittent use is desirable with omission of some doses. A rapidly eliminated drug is generally appropriate.

Chronic insomnia is rarely benefited by hypnotics and is more often due to mild dependence caused by injudicious prescribing. Psychiatric disorders such as anxiety, depression, and abuse of drugs and alcohol are common causes. Sleep disturbance is very common in depressive illness and early wakening is often a useful pointer. The underlying psychiatric complaint should be treated, adapting the drug regimen to alleviate insomnia. For example, amitriptyline, prescribed for depression, will also help to promote sleep if it is taken at night. Other causes of insomnia include daytime cat-napping and physical causes such as pain, pruritus, and dyspnoea.

Hypnotics should **not** be prescribed indiscriminately and routine prescribing, especially in hospitals, is undesirable though commonplace. Ideally, they should be reserved for short courses in the acutely distressed. Tolerance to their effects develops within 3 to 14 days of continuous use and long-term efficacy cannot be assured. A major drawback of long-term use is that withdrawal causes rebound insomnia and precipitates a withdrawal syndrome (section 4.1).

Where prolonged administration is unavoidable hypnotics should be discontinued as soon as feasible and the patient warned that sleep may be disturbed for a few days before normal rhythm is re-established; broken sleep with vivid dreams and increased REM (rapid eye movement) may persist for several weeks. This represents a mild form of dependence even if clinical doses are used.

For drug interactions of hypnotics, see Appendix 1 (sections *2.5*, 4.1).

CHILDREN. The prescribing of hypnotics to children, except for occasional use such as for night terrors and somnambulism, is not justified.

ELDERLY. Hypnotics should be avoided in the elderly, who are at risk of becoming ataxic and confused and so liable to fall and injure themselves.

BENZODIAZEPINES

Benzodiazepines used as hypnotics include **nitrazepam, flunitrazepam**, and **flurazepam** which have a prolonged action and may give rise to residual effects on the following day; repeated doses tend to be cumulative.

Loprazolam, lormetazepam, temazepam, and **triazolam** act for a shorter time and they have little or no hangover effect. Withdrawal phenomena however are more common with the short-acting benzodiazepines.

Benzodiazepine anxiolytics such as **diazepam** (section 4.1.2) given as a single dose at night may also be used as hypnotics.

NITRAZEPAM
Indications: insomnia (short-term use)
Cautions: respiratory disease, muscle weakness, history of drug abuse, marked personality disorder, pregnancy, breast-feeding; reduce dose in elderly and debilitated, and in hepatic and renal impairment; avoid prolonged use (and abrupt withdrawal thereafter). Drug interactions: see Appendix 1 (sections *2.5*, *4.1*, *4.8*, *4.9*)
DRIVING. Drowsiness may persist the next day and affect performance of skilled tasks (e.g. driving); effects of alcohol enhanced
Contra-indications: respiratory depression; acute pulmonary insufficiency
Side-effects: drowsiness and lightheadedness the next day; confusion and ataxia (especially in the elderly); dependence. See also under Diazepam (section 4.1.2)
Dose: 5–10 mg (elderly patients 2.5–5 mg), 30 minutes before bedtime

PoM **Nitrazepam** (Non-proprietary)
Tablets, nitrazepam 5 mg, net price 20 = 7p; 10 mg, 20 = 38p. Label: 19
Mixture, nitrazepam 2.5 mg/5 ml. Diluent syrup, life of diluted mixture 14 days. Net price 150 ml = £3.36. Label: 19
NHS PoM **Mogadon**® (Roche)
Capsules, purple/black, nitrazepam 5 mg. Net price 20 = 85p. Label: 19
Tablets, scored, nitrazepam 5 mg. Net price 20 = 85p. Label: 19
NHS PoM **Nitrados**® (Berk)
Tablets, scored, nitrazepam 5 mg. Net price 20 = 26p. Label: 19
NHS PoM **Noctesed**® (Unimed)
Tablets, scored, nitrazepam 5 mg. Net price 20 = 31p. Label: 19
NHS PoM **Somnite**® (Norgine)
Suspension, off-white, nitrazepam 2.5 mg/5 ml. Diluent syrup, life of diluted suspension 14 days. Net price 150 ml = £3.36. Label: 19
NHS PoM **Surem**® (Galen)
Capsules, mauve/grey, nitrazepam 5 mg. Net price 20 = 26p. Label: 19
NHS PoM **Unisomnia**® (Unigreg)
Tablets, scored, nitrazepam 5 mg. Net price 20 = 46p. Label: 19

FLUNITRAZEPAM
Indications: insomnia (short-term use)
Cautions; Contra-indications; Side-effects: see under Nitrazepam
Dose: 0.5–1 mg (elderly patients 500 micrograms) 30 minutes before bedtime; severe insomnia, 1–2 mg

NHS PoM **Rohypnol**® (Roche)
Tablets, purple, f/c, scored, flunitrazepam 1 mg. Net price 30 = £2.78. Label: 19

FLURAZEPAM

Indications: insomnia (short-term use)
Cautions; Contra-indications; Side-effects: see under Nitrazepam
Dose: 15–30 mg (elderly patients 15 mg) 30 minutes before bedtime

NHS PoM **Dalmane**® (Roche)
Capsules (as hydrochloride), 15 mg (grey/yellow), net price 20 = £1.31; 30 mg (black/grey), 20 = £1.70. Label: 19

NHS PoM **Paxane**® (Steinhard)
Capsules (as hydrochloride), 15 mg (green/grey), net price 20 = 82p; 30 mg (green/black), 20 = £1.10. Label: 19

LOPRAZOLAM

Indications: insomnia (short-term use)
Cautions; Contra-indications; Side-effects: see under Nitrazepam
Dose: 1 mg at bedtime, increased to 1.5 or 2 mg if required (max. 1 mg in elderly or debilitated patients)

▼ PoM **Loprazolam Tablets,** loprazolam 1 mg (as mesylate). Net price 20 = £1.20. Label: 19

NHS ▼ PoM **Dormonoct**® (Roussel)
Tablets, yellow, scored, loprazolam 1 mg (as mesylate). Net price 20 = £1.20. Label: 19

LORMETAZEPAM

Indications: insomnia (short-term use)
Cautions; Contra-indications; Side-effects: see under Nitrazepam; shorter acting, hence preferable in elderly and less drowsiness next day, but withdrawal phenomena more common with short-acting benzodiazepines
Dose: 1 mg (elderly patients 500 micrograms) at bedtime

▼ PoM **Lormetazepam Tablets,** lormetazepam 500 micrograms, net price 20 = 84p; 1 mg, 20 = £1.09. Label: 19

TEMAZEPAM

Indications: insomnia (short-term use); see also section 15.1.4 for peri-operative use
Cautions; Contra-indications; Side-effects: see under Nitrazepam; shorter acting, hence preferable in elderly and less drowsiness next day, but withdrawal phenomena more common with short-acting benzodiazepines
Dose: 10–30 mg (elderly patients 5–15 mg), increasing in severe insomnia to 60 mg, immediately before bedtime

Note. Absorption of temazepam from hard gelatin capsules and from tablets may be slower than from soft gelatin capsules.

PoM **Temazepam** (Non-proprietary)
Capsules (soft gelatin), temazepam 10 mg, net price 20 = 47p; 15 mg, 20 = £1.44; 20 mg, 20 = 82p; 30 mg, 20 = £2.28. Label: 19

Capsules (hard gelatin), temazepam 10 mg, net price 20 = 22p; 20 mg, 20 = 36p. Label: 19
Tablets, temazepam 10 mg, net price 20 = 39p; 20 mg, 20 = 69p. Label: 19
Elixir, temazepam 10 mg/5 ml; diluent glycerol, life of diluted elixir 14 days; net price 100 ml = £2.28. Label: 19

PoM **Temazepam Planpak** (Farmitalia Carlo Erba)
Capsules (soft gelatin), all green, 14 capsules each of temazepam 2 mg, 5 mg, and 10 mg. Net price per pack = £8.57. Label: 19
Dose: withdrawal, 1 capsule at bedtime, commencing with highest strength and finishing with lowest

NHS PoM **Normison**® (Wyeth)
Capsules (soft gelatin), both yellow, temazepam 10 mg, net price 20 = 83p; 20 mg, 20 = £1.35. Label: 19

TRIAZOLAM

Indications: insomnia (short-term use)
Cautions; Contra-indications; Side-effects: see under Nitrazepam; shorter acting, hence preferable in elderly and less drowsiness next day, but withdrawal phenomena more common with short-acting benzodiazepines
Dose: 250 micrograms (elderly patients 125 micrograms) 15–30 minutes before bedtime

PoM **Triazolam Tablets,** triazolam 125 micrograms, net price 20 = £1.15; 250 micrograms, 20 = £1.55. Label: 19

NHS PoM **Halcion**® (Upjohn)
Tablets, both scored, triazolam 125 micrograms (lavender), net price 20 = £1.15; 250 micrograms (blue), 20 = £1.55. Label: 19

CHLORAL AND DERIVATIVES

Chloral hydrate and chloral derivatives are useful hypnotics for children (but see notes above). There is no convincing evidence that they are particularly useful in the elderly. **Dichloralphenazone** and **triclofos sodium** cause fewer gastrointestinal upsets than chloral hydrate.

CHLORAL HYDRATE

Indications: insomnia (short-term use)
Cautions: respiratory disease, history of drug abuse, marked personality disorder, pregnancy, breast-feeding; reduce dose in elderly and debilitated; avoid prolonged use (and abrupt withdrawal thereafter); avoid contact with skin and mucous membranes. Drug interactions: see Appendix 1 (sections *2.5*, *2.8C*, *4.1*)
DRIVING. Drowsiness may persist the next day and affect performance of skilled tasks (e.g. driving); effects of alcohol enhanced
Contra-indications: severe cardiac disease, gastritis, marked hepatic or renal impairment
Side-effects: gastric irritation; *occasionally:* rashes, headache, ketonuria, excitement, delirium; dependence and renal damage on prolonged use

---

Cautionary label wordings, see inside back cover

Prices are **net**, see p. 1

Dose: insomnia, 0.5–1 g (max. 2 g), 15–30 minutes before bedtime; CHILD 30–50 mg/kg up to a max. single dose of 1 g
Sedation, 250 mg 3 times daily

PoM **Chloral Mixture,** chloral hydrate 500 mg/5 ml (see Formulary). Net price 100 ml = 14p. Label: 19, 27
Dose: insomnia, 5–20 ml; CHILD 1–5 years 2.5–5 ml, 6–12 years 5–10 ml, taken well diluted with water 15–30 minutes before bedtime

PoM **Chloral Elixir, Paediatric,** chloral hydrate 200 mg/5 ml (see Formulary). Net price 100 ml = 43p. Label: 1, 27
Dose: up to 1 year 5 ml, well diluted with water

PoM **Noctec**® (Squibb)
Capsules, red, chloral hydrate 500 mg. Net price 20 = 76p. Label: 19, 27

DICHLORALPHENAZONE

Indications: insomnia (short-term use)
Cautions; Contra-indications; Side-effects: see under Chloral Hydrate; less gastric irritation; contra-indicated in porphyria. Drug interactions: see Appendix 1 (sections *2.5, 2.8A,* 4.1, 7)
Dose: insomnia, 1.3–1.95 g (2–3 tablets) with water 20 minutes before bedtime; CHILD up to 1 year 112.5–225 mg (2.5–5 ml elixir) 1–5 years 225–450 mg (5–10 ml elixir), 6–12 years 450–900 mg (10–20 ml elixir) taken well diluted with water 20 minutes before bedtime

PoM **Welldorm**® (S&N Pharm.)
Tablets, purple, f/c, dichloralphenazone 650 mg. Net price 30 = £1.70. Label: 19, 27
Elixir, red, dichloralphenazone 225 mg/5 ml. Diluent syrup, life of diluted elixir 14 days. Net price 150 ml = £1.48. Label: 19, 27

TRICLOFOS SODIUM

Indications: insomnia (short-term use)
Cautions; Contra-indications; Side-effects: see under Chloral Hydrate; less gastric irritation
Dose: 1–2 g 30 minutes before bedtime; CHILD up to 1 year 100–250 mg, 1–5 years 250–500 mg, 6–12 years 0.5–1 g

PoM **Triclofos Elixir,** triclofos sodium 500 mg/5 ml. Net price 100 ml = £2.83. Label: 19

OTHER HYPNOTICS

Chlormethiazole may be a useful hypnotic for elderly patients because of its freedom from hangover but, as with all hypnotics, routine administration is undesirable and dependence occurs occasionally. It is used in the treatment of acute withdrawal symptoms in alcoholics but to minimise the risk of dependence administration should be limited to 9 days under inpatient supervision.

Promethazine is popular for use in children (but see notes above).

Alcohol is a poor hypnotic as its diuretic action interferes with sleep during the latter part of the night. With chronic use, alcohol disturbs sleep patterns and causes insomnia. For drug interactions, see Appendix 1 (sections *2.5, 2.8B, 4.1, 4.3, 5.1, 6.1, 8, 13*).

CHLORMETHIAZOLE EDISYLATE

Indications: see under Dose
Cautions: cardiac and respiratory disease, history of drug abuse, marked personality disorder, pregnancy, breast-feeding; reduce dose in elderly and debilitated, and in hepatic and renal impairment; avoid prolonged use (and abrupt withdrawal thereafter); during intravenous infusion the sleep induced may quickly lapse into deep unconsciousness and patients must be observed constantly; see also section 4.8.2. Drug interactions: see Appendix 1 (sections *2.5,* 4.1)
Contra-indications: acute pulmonary insufficiency; alcoholics who continue to drink
Side-effects: sneezing, conjunctival irritation, headache, gastro-intestinal disturbances; rarely, confusion. On intravenous infusion in high doses, cardiovascular and respiratory depression and localised thrombophlebitis
Dose: by mouth, severe insomnia in the elderly, 1–2 capsules at bedtime
Restlessness and agitation in the elderly, 1 capsule 3 times daily
Alcohol withdrawal, initially 2–4 capsules, repeated if necessary; day 1, 9–12 capsules; day 2, 6–8 capsules; day 3, 4–6 capsules, then gradually reduced over days 4–6; capsules given in 3–4 divided doses; treatment for not more than 9 days
Note. For an equivalent therapeutic effect 1 capsule = 5 ml elixir
By intravenous infusion, acute alcohol withdrawal, 40–100 ml (320–800 mg) initially as 0.8% solution over 5–10 minutes and the infusion rate then adjusted according to response *or* 30–50 ml (240–400 mg) initially as a 0.8% solution at a rate of about 60 drops (4 ml)/minute, until drowsy, reduced to 10–15 drops/minute, then adjusted according to response

PoM **Heminevrin**® (Astra)
Capsules, grey-brown, chlormethiazole base 192 mg in an oily basis. Net price 20 = £1.48. Label: 19
Syrup, sugar-free, chlormethiazole edisylate 250 mg/5 ml. Diluent water for preparations, life of diluted syrup 14 days. Net price 100 ml = £1.24. Label: 19
Intravenous infusion 0.8%, chlormethiazole edisylate 8 mg/ml. Net price 500-ml bottle = £5.25

PROMETHAZINE HYDROCHLORIDE

Indications: insomnia (short-term use)
Cautions; Side-effects: see section 3.4.1
Dose: by mouth, 25 mg at bedtime increased to 50 mg if necessary; CHILD 1–5 years 15–20 mg, 5–10 years 20–25 mg, at bedtime

---

Preparations
See section 3.4.1

4.1.2   Anxiolytics

Benzodiazepine anxiolytics can be effective in alleviating definite anxiety states and they are widely prescribed. Although there is a tendency to prescribe these drugs to almost anyone with stress-related symptoms, unhappiness, or minor physical disease, their use in many situations is unjustified. In particular, they should not be used to treat depression, phobic or obsessional states, or chronic psychosis. In bereavement, psychological adjustment may be inhibited by benzodiazepines. In children anxiolytic treatment should be used only to relieve acute anxiety (and related insomnia) caused by fear e.g. before surgery.

Anxiolytic treatment should be limited to the lowest possible dose for the shortest possible time (see CSM advice, section 4.1). Dependence is particularly likely in patients with a history of alcoholism or drug abuse and in patients with marked personality disorders.

Anxiolytics, particularly the benzodiazepines, have been termed 'minor tranquillisers'. This term is misleading because not only do they differ markedly from the antipsychotic drugs ('major tranquillisers') but their use is by no means minor. Antipsychotics, in low doses, are also sometimes used in severe anxiety for their sedative action but long-term use should be avoided in view of a possible risk of tardive dyskinesia (section 4.2.1).

BENZODIAZEPINES

Benzodiazepines are indicated for the short-term relief of severe anxiety but long-term use should be avoided (see notes above). Diazepam, alprazolam, bromazepam, chlordiazepoxide, clobazam, clorazepate, ketazolam and medazepam have a sustained action. Shorter-acting compounds such as **lorazepam** and **oxazepam** may be preferred in patients with hepatic impairment but they carry a greater risk of withdrawal symptoms; they may be appropriate for relieving persistent or severe phobic panic attacks but should only be used under specialist supervision.

Diazepam or lorazepam, are very occasionally administered intravenously for the control of severe panic. This route is the most rapid but the procedure is not without risk (section 4.8.2) and should be used only when alternative measures have failed. The intramuscular route has no advantage over the oral route.

Benzodiazepines are also used in the treatment of alcohol withdrawal (section 4.10).

DIAZEPAM

Indications: short-term use in anxiety or insomnia, adjunct in acute alcohol withdrawal; epilepsy (section 4.8); muscle spasm see section 10.2.2; peri-operative use see section 15.1.4.2
Cautions: respiratory disease, muscle weakness, history of drug abuse, marked personality disorder, pregnancy, breast-feeding; reduce dose in elderly and debilitated, and in hepatic and renal impairment; avoid prolonged use (and abrupt withdrawal thereafter); special precautions for intravenous injection (section 4.8.2). Drug interactions: see Appendix 1 (sections *2.5*, 4.1, *4.8, 4.9*)
DRIVING. Drowsiness may affect performance of skilled tasks (e.g. driving); effects of alcohol enhanced
Contra-indications: respiratory depression; acute pulmonary insufficiency
Side-effects: drowsiness and lightheadedness the next day; confusion and ataxia (especially in the elderly); dependence; *occasionally:* headache, hypotension, salivation changes, rashes, visual disturbances, changes in libido, urinary retention; on intravenous injection, pain, thrombophlebitis
Dose: by mouth, anxiety, 2 mg 3 times daily increased in severe anxiety to 15–30 mg daily in divided doses (elderly half adult dose)
Insomnia, 5–15 mg at bedtime
CHILD night terrors and somnambulism, 1–5 mg at bedtime
By intramuscular injection or slow intravenous injection (at a rate of not more than 5 mg/minute), for severe anxiety, control of acute panic attacks, and acute alcohol withdrawal, 10 mg, repeated if necessary after 4 hours
Note. Only use intramuscular route when oral and intravenous routes not possible
By intravenous infusion—section 4.8.2
By rectum as rectal solution, for acute anxiety and agitation, adults and children over 3 years 10 mg (elderly 5 mg), repeated after 5 minutes if necessary; CHILD 1–3 years, 5 mg

PoM **Diazepam** (Non-proprietary)
Capsules, diazepam 2 mg, net price 20 = 12p; 5 mg, 20 = 18p. Label: 2 *or* 19
Tablets, diazepam 2 and 5 mg, net price (both), 20 = 2p; 10 mg, 20 = 5p. Label: 2 *or* 19
Elixir, diazepam 2 mg/5 ml. Diluent syrup or sorbitol solution, life of diluted elixir 14 days. Net price 100 ml = £1.10. Label: 2 *or* 19
NHS PoM **Alupram**® (Steinhard)
Tablets, all scored, diazepam 2 mg, net price 20 = 16p; 5 mg (yellow), 20 = 24p; 10 mg (blue), 20 = 36p. Label: 2 *or* 19
NHS PoM **Atensine**® (Berk)
Tablets, all scored, diazepam 2 mg, net price 20 = 8p; 5 mg (yellow), 20 = 10p; 10 mg (blue), 20 = 22p. Label: 2 *or* 19
PoM **Diazemuls**® (KabiVitrum)
Injection (emulsion), diazepam 5 mg/ml. For intravenous injection or infusion. Net price 2-ml amp = 44p
NHS PoM **Evacalm**® (Unimed)
Tablets, both scored, diazepam 2 mg, net price 20 = 9p; 5 mg (yellow), 20 = 14p. Label: 2 *or* 19
NHS PoM **Solis**® (Galen)
Capsules, diazepam 2 mg (violet/turquoise), net price 20 = 12p; 5 mg (violet/mauve), 20 = 18p. Label: 2 *or* 19

PoM **Stesolid**® (CP)
Injection, diazepam 5 mg/ml. Do not dilute (except for intravenous infusion). Net price 2-ml amp = 25p
Rectal tubes (= rectal solution), diazepam 2 mg/ml. Net price 5 × 2.5-ml (5 mg) tubes = £4.50
Rectal tubes (= rectal solution), diazepam 4 mg/ml. Net price 5 × 2.5-ml (10 mg) tubes = £5.60
NHS PoM **Tensium**® (DDSA)
Tablets, all scored, diazepam 2 mg, net price 20 = 8p; 5 mg (yellow), 20 = 10p; 10 mg (blue), 20 = 21p. Label: 2 *or* 19
PoM **Valium**® (Roche)
NHS *Capsules*, diazepam 2 mg (blue/white), net price 20 = 28p; 5 mg (blue/yellow), 20 = 42p. Label: 2 *or* 19
NHS *Tablets*, all scored, diazepam 2 mg, net price 20 = 28p; 5 mg (yellow), 20 = 42p; 10 mg (blue), 20 = 85p. Label: 2 *or* 19
NHS *Syrup*, pink, sugar-free, diazepam 2 mg/5 ml. Diluent sorbitol solution, life of diluted syrup 14 days. Net price 100 ml = £1.27. Label: 2 *or* 19
Injection, diazepam 5 mg/ml. Do not dilute (except for intravenous infusion). Net price 2-ml amp = 26p
Suppositories, diazepam 10 mg, net price 5 = £1.00. Label: 2 *or* 19

ALPRAZOLAM

Indications: anxiety (short-term use)
Cautions; Contra-indications; Side-effects: see under Diazepam
Dose: 250–500 micrograms 3 times daily (elderly or debilitated patients 250 micrograms 2–3 times daily), increased if necessary to a total of 3 mg daily

NHS ▼ PoM **Xanax**® (Upjohn)
Tablets, both scored, alprazolam 250 micrograms, net price 20 = 72p; 500 micrograms (pink), 20 = £1.39. Label: 2

BROMAZEPAM

Indications: anxiety (short-term use)
Cautions; Contra-indications; Side-effects: see under Diazepam
Dose: 3–18 mg daily in divided doses; elderly patients half adult dose; max. (in hospitalised patients) 60 mg daily in divided doses

NHS ▼ PoM **Lexotan**® (Roche)
Tablets, both scored, bromazepam 1.5 mg (lilac), net price 60 = £4.04; 3 mg (pink), 60 = £4.73. Label: 2

CHLORDIAZEPOXIDE

Indications: anxiety (short-term use), adjunct in acute alcohol withdrawal
Cautions; Contra-indications; Side-effects: see under Diazepam
Dose: anxiety, 10 mg 3 times daily increased in severe anxiety to 100 mg daily in divided doses (elderly half adult dose)
Note. The doses stated above refer equally to chlordiazepoxide and to its hydrochloride

PoM **Chlordiazepoxide Capsules,** chlordiazepoxide hydrochloride 5 mg, net price 20 = 28p; 10 mg, 20 = 35p. Label: 2
PoM **Chlordiazepoxide Hydrochloride Tablets,** chlordiazepoxide hydrochloride 5 mg, net price 20 = 20p; 10 mg, 20 = 22p; 25 mg, 20 = 44p. Label: 2
PoM **Chlordiazepoxide Tablets,** chlordiazepoxide 5 mg, net price 20 = 28p; 10 mg, 20 = 35p; 25 mg, 20 = 71p. Label: 2
PoM **Librium**® (Roche)
NHS *Capsules*, chlordiazepoxide hydrochloride 5 mg (green/yellow), net price 20 = 28p; 10 mg (green/black), 20 = 35p. Label: 2
NHS *Tablets*, all green, f/c, chlordiazepoxide 5 mg, net price 20 = 28p; 10 mg, 20 = 35p; 25 mg, 20 = 75p. Label: 2

CLOBAZAM

Indications: anxiety (short-term use); adjunct in epilepsy
Cautions; Contra-indications; Side-effects: see under Diazepam
Dose: 20–30 mg daily in divided doses or as a single dose at bedtime, increased in severe anxiety (in hospitalised patients) to a max. of 60 mg daily in divided doses; elderly and debilitated patients 20 mg daily; CHILD over 3 years, up to half adult dose
Epilepsy, 20–30 mg daily; max. 60 mg daily

NHS * PoM **Clobazam Capsules,** clobazam 10 mg. Net price 20 caps = £1.29. Label: 2 *or* 19
NHS PoM **Frisium**® (Hoechst)
Capsules, blue, clobazam 10 mg. Net price 20 = £1.29. Label: 2 *or* 19
* except for epilepsy and endorsed 'S3B' ('S2B' in Scotland)

CLORAZEPATE DIPOTASSIUM

Indications: anxiety (short-term use)
Cautions; Contra-indications; Side-effects: see under Diazepam
Dose: 7.5–22.5 mg daily in 2–3 divided doses *or* a single dose of 15 mg at bedtime (elderly half adult dose)

NHS PoM **Tranxene**® (Boehringer Ingelheim)
Capsules, clorazepate dipotassium 7.5 mg (maroon/grey), net price 20 = £1.22; 15 mg (pink/grey), 20 = £1.39. Label: 2 *or* 19

KETAZOLAM

Indications: anxiety (short-term use)
Cautions; Contra-indications; Side-effects: see under Diazepam
Dose: initially 30 mg (elderly patients 15 mg) at bedtime, adjusted according to the response; usual range 15–60 mg daily as a single dose at bedtime *or* in divided doses

NHS PoM **Anxon**® (Beecham)
Capsules, both dark pink/light pink, ketazolam 15 mg, net price 20 = £1.77; 30 mg, 20 = £3.03. Label: 2 *or* 19

LORAZEPAM

Indications: short-term use in anxiety or insomnia; status epilepticus (section 4.8.2); peri-operative (section 15.1.4.2)

Cautions; Contra-indications; Side-effects: see under Diazepam; short acting hence preferable in elderly and less drowsiness next day, but withdrawal phenomena more common with short-acting benzodiazepines

Dose: by mouth, anxiety, 1–4 mg daily in divided doses (elderly half adult dose)

Insomnia, 1–4 mg at bedtime

By intramuscular or slow intravenous injection, for the control of acute panic attacks, 25–30 micrograms/kg every 6 hours if necessary

Note. Only use intramuscular route when oral and intravenous routes not possible

PoM **Lorazepam Tablets,** lorazepam 1 mg, net price 20 = 22p; 2.5 mg, 20 = 36p. Label: 2 *or* 19

NHS PoM **Almazine**® (Steinhard)
Tablets, both scored, lorazepam 1 mg (green), net price 20 = 34p; 2.5 mg (pink), 20 = 53p. Label: 2 *or* 19

PoM **Ativan**® (Wyeth)
NHS *Tablets,* both scored, lorazepam 1 mg (blue), net price 20 = 44p; 2.5 mg (yellow), 20 = 70p. Label: 2 *or* 19

▼ *Injection,* lorazepam 4 mg/ml. Net price 1-ml amp = 36p. For intramuscular injection it should be diluted with an equal volume of water for injections or sodium chloride intravenous infusion 0.9%

MEDAZEPAM

Indications: anxiety (short-term use)

Cautions; Contra-indications; Side-effects: see under Diazepam

Dose: anxiety, 15–30 mg daily in divided doses, increased in severe anxiety to max. 40 mg daily in divided doses (elderly half adult dose)

NHS PoM **Nobrium**® (Roche)
Capsules, medazepam 5 mg (orange/yellow), net price 20 = 51p; 10 mg (orange/black), 20 = 76p. Label: 2

OXAZEPAM

Indications: anxiety (short-term use)

Cautions; Contra-indications; Side-effects: see under Diazepam; short acting hence preferable in elderly and less drowsiness next day, but withdrawal phenomena more common with short-acting benzodiazepines

Dose: anxiety, 15–30 mg (elderly patients 10–20 mg) 3–4 times daily

PoM **Oxazepam** (Non-proprietary)
Capsules, oxazepam 30 mg, net price 20 = 33p. Label: 2
Tablets, oxazepam 10 mg, net price 20 = 24p; 15 mg, 20 = 27p; 30 mg, 20 = 33p. Label: 2

NHS PoM **Oxanid**® (Steinhard)
Tablets, oxazepam 10 mg, net price 20 = 29p; 15 mg, 20 = 32p; 30 mg, 20 = 33p. Label: 2

OTHER DRUGS FOR ANXIETY

Buspirone is a new drug for the treatment of anxiety; its mode of action is not fully understood and response to treatment may take up to 2 weeks. It does not alleviate the symptoms of benzodiazepine withdrawal. Therefore a patient taking a benzodiazepine should not be transferred directly to buspirone but must first have the benzodiazepine withdrawn gradually. The dependence and abuse liability of buspirone has not yet been established.

Meprobamate is **less effective** than the benzodiazepines, more hazardous in overdosage, and can also induce dependence.

Beta-blockers (e.g. propranolol, oxprenolol) (see section 2.4) do not affect psychological symptoms, such as worry, tension, and fear, but they do reduce autonomic symptoms, such as palpitations, sweating, and tremor; they do not reduce non-autonomic symptoms, such as muscle tension. Beta-blockers are therefore indicated for patients with predominantly somatic symptoms; this, in turn, may prevent the onset of worry and fear. Patients with predominantly psychological symptoms may obtain no benefit.

BUSPIRONE HYDROCHLORIDE

Indications: anxiety (short-term use)

Cautions: does not alleviate benzodiazepine withdrawal, see notes above; history of hepatic or renal impairment. Drug interactions: see Appendix 1 (section *4.3*)

Contra-indications: epilepsy, severe hepatic or renal impairment, pregnancy, MAOIs

Side-effects: nausea, dizziness, headache, nervousness, lightheadedness, excitement; rarely tachycardia, palpitations, chest pain, drowsiness, confusion, dry mouth, fatigue, and sweating

Dose: initially 5 mg 2–3 times daily, increased as necessary every 2–3 days; usual range 15–30 mg daily in divided doses; max. 45 mg daily (30 mg in elderly)

COUNSELLING. May affect reactions and during initial stages patients should exercise caution while driving; effects of alcohol during early stages may be unpredictable

▼ PoM **Buspar**® (Bristol-Myers)
Tablets, buspirone hydrochloride 5 mg. Net price 100 = £32.00. Counselling advised, see above

CHLORMEZANONE

Indications: short-term use in anxiety or insomnia; muscle spasm (but see section 10.2.2)

Cautions: respiratory disease, muscle weakness, history of drug abuse, marked personality disorder, pregnancy, breast-feeding; reduce dose in elderly and debilitated, and in hepatic and renal impairment; avoid prolonged use (and

abrupt withdrawal thereafter). Drug interactions: see Appendix 1 (sections *2.5*, 4.1)
DRIVING. Drowsiness may persist the next day and
affect performance of skilled tasks (e.g. driving); effects
of alcohol enhanced
Contra-indications: acute pulmonary insufficiency; respiratory depression
Side-effects: drowsiness and lethargy, dizziness,
nausea, headache, dry mouth, rashes;
cholestatic jaundice reported
Dose: 200 mg 3–4 times daily *or* 400 mg at
bedtime; elderly patients half adult dose

PoM **Trancopal**® (Winthrop)
Tablets, yellow, chlormezanone 200 mg. Net
price 20 = £1.66. Label: 2 *or* 19

HYDROXYZINE HYDROCHLORIDE
Indications: anxiety (short-term use)
Cautions; Side-effects: see under Antihistamines
(section 3.4.1)
Dose: 50–100 mg 4 times daily

PoM **Atarax**® (Pfizer)
Tablets, both s/c, hydroxyzine hydrochloride
10 mg (orange), net price 20 = 36p; 25 mg
(green), 20 = 73p. Label: 2
Syrup, hydroxyzine hydrochloride 10 mg/5 ml.
Diluent syrup, life of diluted syrup 14 days. Net
price 150 ml = 85p. Label: 2

MEPROBAMATE
Indications: short-term use in anxiety, but see
notes above
Cautions: respiratory disease, muscle weakness,
epilepsy (may induce seizures), history of drug
abuse, marked personality disorder, pregnancy; reduce dose in elderly and debilitated, and in hepatic and renal impairment;
avoid prolonged use, abrupt withdrawal may
precipitate convulsions. Drug interactions: see
Appendix 1 (sections *2.5*, 4.1)
Contra-indications: acute pulmonary insufficiency; respiratory depression; porphyria;
breast-feeding
Side-effects: see under Diazepam, but the incidence is greater and drowsiness is the most
common side-effect. Also gastro-intestinal disturbances, hypotension, paraesthesia, weakness, CNS effects which include headache,
paradoxical excitement, disturbances of vision;
rarely agranulocytosis and rashes
Dose: 400 mg 3–4 times daily; elderly patients
half adult dose or less

CD **Equanil**® (Wyeth)
Tablets, meprobamate 200 mg, net price 20 = 15p;
400 mg (scored), 20 = 22p. Label: 2
CD **Meprate**® (DDSA)
Tablets, meprobamate 400 mg. Net price 20 = 13p.
Label: 2
CD **Tenavoid**® (Leo)
Tablets, orange, f/c, meprobamate 200 mg, bendro-
fluazide 3 mg. Net price 24 = £1.84. Label: 2
Dose: premenstrual syndrome, combination not rec-
ommended therefore dose not stated

4.1.3   Barbiturates and methyprylone
The intermediate-acting **barbiturates** and **methyprylone** (Noludar®) only have a place in the treatment of severe intractable insomnia in patients
already taking barbiturates; they should be
avoided in the elderly. The long-acting barbiturates phenobarbitone and methylphenobarbitone are of value in epilepsy (section 4.8.1) but
their use as sedatives is unjustified. The short-
acting barbiturates, methohexitone and thiopentone, are used in anaesthesia (section 15.1.1).

BARBITURATES
Indications: severe intractable insomnia in patients
already taking barbiturates
Cautions: avoid use where possible; dependence and
tolerance readily occur; abrupt withdrawal may precipitate a serious withdrawal syndrome (rebound insomnia, anxiety, tremor, dizziness, nausea, fits, and
delirium); repeated doses are cumulative and may lead
to excessive sedation; may affect ability to drive or
operate machinery and increase the effects of alcohol;
caution in respiratory disease, renal disease, hepatic
impairment. Drug interactions: see Appendix 1 (sections *2.8A*, *3*, *4.3*, *5.1*, *6.3*, *7*)
Contra-indications: insomnia caused by pain; porphyria;
pregnancy; breast-feeding; avoid in children, elderly
and debilitated patients, also patients with a history of
drug or alcohol abuse
Side-effects: hangover with drowsiness, dizziness, ataxia,
respiratory depression, hypersensitivity reactions,
headache, particularly in elderly; paradoxical excitement and confusion occasionally precedes sleep

CD **Amytal**® (Lilly)
Tablets, amylobarbitone 15 mg, net price 20 = 14p;
30 mg, 20 = 18p; 50 mg, 20 = 23p; 100 mg, 20 = 41p;
200 mg (scored), 20 = 84p. Label: 19
Dose: 100–200 mg 30 minutes before bedtime
CD **Phanodorm**® (Winthrop)
Tablets, cyclobarbitone calcium 200 mg. Net price 20 =
£1.72. Label: 19
Dose: 100–400 mg 30 minutes before bedtime
CD **Sodium Amytal**® (Lilly)
Capsules, both blue, amylobarbitone sodium 60 mg, net
price 20 = 36p; 200 mg, 20 = 75p. Label: 19
Tablets, amylobarbitone sodium 60 mg, net price 20 =
33p; 200 mg, 20 = 61p. Label: 19
Dose: 60–200 mg 15–30 minutes before bedtime
Injection, powder for reconstitution, amylobarbitone
sodium. Net price 250-mg vial = £2.83; 500-mg vial =
£3.18
Dose: by intramuscular or slow intravenous injection,
sedation in severely agitated patients, 0.25–1 g daily;
max. single dose, intramuscular 500 mg, intravenous 1 g
CD **Soneryl**® (M&B)
Tablets, pink, scored, butobarbitone 100 mg. Net price
20 = 18p. Label: 19
Dose: 100–200 mg 30 minutes before bedtime
Quinalbarbitone
Note. Quinalbarbitone has been transferred from sched-
ule 3 to schedule 2 of the Misuse of Drugs Regulations
1985; receipt and supply must therefore be recorded in
the CD register.
CD **Seconal Sodium**® (Lilly)
Capsules, both orange, quinalbarbitone sodium 50 mg,
net price 20 = 71p; 100 mg, 20 = £1.02. Label: 19
Dose: 50–100 mg 30 minutes before bedtime
CD **Tuinal**® (Lilly)
Capsules, orange/blue, amylobarbitone sodium 50 mg,
quinalbarbitone sodium 50 mg. Net price 20 = 52p.
Label: 19
Dose: 1–2 capsules 15–30 minutes before bedtime

METHYPRYLONE

Indications; Cautions; Contra-indications; Side-effects: see under Barbiturates

Dose: 200–400 mg 15 minutes before bedtime

CD Noludar ® (Roche)

Tablets, scored, methyprylone 200 mg. Net price 20 = 68p. Label: 19

4.2   Drugs used in psychoses and related disorders

4.2.1   Antipsychotic drugs
4.2.2   Antipsychotic depot injections
4.2.3   Lithium salts

4.2.1   Antipsychotic drugs

Antipsychotic drugs are also known as 'neuro-leptics' and (misleadingly) as 'major tranquill-isers'. Antipsychotic drugs generally tranquillise without impairing consciousness and without causing paradoxical excitement but they should not be regarded merely as tranquillisers. For con-ditions such as schizophrenia the tranquillising effect is of secondary importance.

In the short term they are used to quieten disturbed patients whatever the underlying psy-chopathology, which may be brain damage, mania, toxic delirium, agitated depression, or acute behavioural disturbance.

They are used to alleviate severe anxiety but this too should be a short-term measure. Some antipsychotic drugs (e.g. chlorpromazine, thior-idazine, flupenthixol) also have an antidepressant effect while others may exacerbate depression (e.g. fluphenazine, pimozide, pipothiazine).

SCHIZOPHRENIA. Antipsychotic drugs relieve florid psychotic symptoms such as thought disorder, hal-lucinations, and delusions, and prevent relapse. They are usually less effective in apathetic with-drawn patients.

Sometimes they appear to have an activating influence. For example, large doses of chlor-promazine may restore an acutely ill schizo-phrenic to normal activity and social behaviour who was previously withdrawn or even mute and akinetic. Patients with acute schizophrenia gen-erally respond better than those with chronic symptoms.

Long-term treatment of a patient with a definite diagnosis of schizophrenia may be necessary even after the first episode of illness in order to prevent the manifest illness from becoming chronic. With-drawal of drug treatment requires careful sur-veillance because the patient who appears well on medication may suffer a disastrous relapse if treatment is withdrawn inappropriately. In addition the need for continuation of treatment may not become immediately evident because

relapse is often delayed for several weeks after cessation of treatment.

Antipsychotic drugs are considered to act by interfering with dopaminergic transmission in the brain by blocking dopamine receptors and may give rise to the extrapyramidal effects described below, and also to hyperprolactinaemia. Anti-psychotic drugs also affect cholinergic, alpha-adrenergic, histaminergic, and tryptaminergic (serotonergic) receptors.

SIDE-EFFECTS. Extrapyramidal symptoms are the most troublesome. They are caused most fre-quently by the piperazine phenothiazines (flu-phenazine, perphenazine, prochlorperazine, and trifluoperazine), the butyrophenones (ben-peridol, droperidol, haloperidol, and trifluperi-dol), and the depot preparations. They are easy to recognise but cannot be accurately predicted because they depend partly on the dose and partly on the type of drug, and on patient susceptibility. They consist of parkinsonian symptoms (including tremor) which may occur gradually, dystonia (abnormal face and body movements) which may appear after only a few doses, akathisia (rest-lessness) which may resemble an exacerbation of the condition being treated, and tardive dyski-nesia (which usually takes longer to develop).

Parkinsonian symptoms remit if the drug is withdrawn and may be suppressed by the adminis-tration of **anticholinergic** drugs (section 4.9.2). Routine administration of such drugs is **not** jus-tified as not all patients are affected and because tardive dyskinesia may be unmasked or worsened by them. Furthermore, these drugs are sometimes abused for their mood-altering effects. Tardive dyskinesia is of particular concern because it may be irreversible on withdrawing therapy and treat-ment may be ineffective. It occurs fairly fre-quently in patients (especially the elderly) on long-term therapy and with high dosage, and the treatment of such patients must be carefully and regularly reviewed. Tardive dyskinesia may also occur occasionally after short-term treatment with low dosage. 'Drug holidays' (temporary dis-continuation of drugs for perhaps 1 month in every 6) have been advocated. Theoretically this is an attractive approach to preventing tardive dyskinesia, but may jeopardise the patient's clini-cal condition.

Hypotension and interference with temperature regulation are dose-related side-effects and are liable to cause dangerous falls and hypothermia in the elderly; very serious consideration should be given before prescribing these drugs for patients over 70 years of age.

Neuroleptic malignant syndrome (hyperther-mia, fluctuating level of consciousness, muscular rigidity and autonomic dysfunction with pallor, tachycardia, labile blood pressure, sweating, and urinary incontinence) is a rare but potentially fatal side-effect of some drugs. Drugs for which it has been reported in the UK include haloperidol, chlorpromazine, and flupenthixol decanoate. Discontinuation of drug therapy is essential as there is no proven effective treatment and the syndrome, which usually lasts for 5–10 days after drug discontinuation, may be unduly prolonged if depot preparations have been used.

CLASSIFICATION OF ANTIPSYCHOTICS. The **phenothiazine** derivatives can be divided into 3 main groups.

Group 1: chlorpromazine, methotrimeprazine, and promazine, generally characterised by pronounced sedative effects and moderate anticholinergic and extrapyramidal side-effects.

Group 2: pericyazine, pipothiazine, and thioridazine, generally characterised by moderate sedative effects, marked anticholinergic effects, but fewer extrapyramidal side-effects than groups 1 or 3.

Group 3: fluphenazine, perphenazine, prochlorperazine, and trifluoperazine, generally characterised by fewer sedative effects, fewer anticholinergic effects, but more pronounced extrapyramidal side-effects than groups 1 and 2.

Drugs of other chemical groups tend to resemble the phenothiazines of *group 3.* They include the **butyrophenones** (benperidol, droperidol, haloperidol, and trifluperidol); **diphenylbutylpiperidines** (fluspirilene and pimozide); **thioxanthenes** (flupenthixol and zuclopenthixol); and **oxypertine**.

CHOICE. As indicated above, the various drugs differ somewhat in predominant actions and side-effects. Selection is influenced by the degree of sedation required and the patient's susceptibility to extrapyramidal side-effects. However, the differences between antipsychotic drugs are less important than the great variability in patient response; moreover, tolerance to these secondary effects usually develops.

Prescribing of more than one antipsychotic for the same indication is **not** recommended; it may constitute a hazard and there is no significant evidence that side-effects are minimised.

Chlorpromazine is widely used. It has a marked sedating effect and is particularly useful for treating violent patients without causing stupor. Agitated states in the elderly can be controlled without confusion, a dose of 25 mg usually being adequate.

Flupenthixol and **pimozide** are less sedating than chlorpromazine.

Sulpiride is structurally distinct from other antipsychotic drugs. In high doses it controls florid positive symptoms, but in lower doses it has an alerting effect on apathetic withdrawn schizophrenics; further reductions in dosage increase this alerting effect.

Fluphenazine, haloperidol, and **trifluoperazine** are also of value but their use is limited by the high incidence of extrapyramidal symptoms. Haloperidol may be preferred for the rapid control of hyperactive psychotic states.

Thioridazine is popular for treating the elderly as there is a reduced incidence of extrapyramidal symptoms.

Promazine is not sufficiently active to be used as an antipsychotic drug but may be of value in elderly patients with minor psychiatric problems.

OTHER USES. **Chlorpromazine** and **prochlorperazine** are effective drugs for the relief of nausea and vomiting (section 4.6), and hiccups. **Haloperidol** is used as adjunctive treatment in choreas and stuttering (section 4.9.3). **Benperidol** is used in deviant and antisocial sexual behaviour but its value is not established.

> DOSAGE. In some patients it is necessary to raise the dose of an antipsychotic drug above that which is normally recommended. This should be done with caution and under specialist supervision.
> *Once-daily dose.* After an initial period of stabilisation, in most patients, the long half-life of antipsychotic drugs allows the total daily dose to be given as a single dose.

CHLORPROMAZINE HYDROCHLORIDE

WARNING. Owing to the risk of contact sensitisation, pharmacists, nurses, and other health workers should avoid direct contact with chlorpromazine; tablets should not be crushed and solutions should be handled with care

Indications: schizophrenia and related psychoses, tranquillisation and emergency control in behavioural disturbances; short-term adjunctive treatment of severe anxiety, terminal disease, intractable hiccup

Cautions: cardiovascular disease, respiratory disease, phaeochromocytoma, parkinsonism, epilepsy, acute infections, pregnancy, breast-feeding, renal and hepatic impairment, history of jaundice, leucopenia; hypothyroidism, myasthenia gravis, prostatic hypertrophy; caution in elderly particularly in very hot or very cold weather. Avoid drugs which depress leucopoiesis. Initially, sedation may affect the ability to drive or operate machinery and increase the effects of alcohol. On prolonged use examinations for eye defects and abnormal skin pigmentation are required. Avoid abrupt withdrawal. Patients should remain supine for 30 minutes after intramuscular injection. Drug interactions of phenothiazine derivatives: see Appendix 1 (sections *2.5, 4.1, 4.2, 4.2, 4.3, 4.8, 4.9, 6.7, 15*)

Contra-indications: coma caused by CNS depressants; bone-marrow depression; closed-angle glaucoma

Side-effects: extrapyramidal symptoms (reversed by dose reduction or anticholinergic drugs) and, on prolonged administration, occasionally tardive dyskinesia; hypothermia (occasionally pyrexia), drowsiness, apathy, pallor, nightmares, insomnia, depression, and, more rarely, agitation. Anticholinergic symptoms such as dry mouth, nasal congestion, constipation, difficulty with micturition, and blurred vision; cardiovascular symptoms such as hypotension and arrhythmias; endocrine effects such as menstrual disturbances, galactorrhoea, gynaecomastia, impotence, and weight gain; sensitivity reactions such as agranulocytosis, leucopenia, leucocytosis, and haemolytic anaemia, photosensitisation, contact sensitisation, rashes, and jaundice; lupus erythematosus-like syndrome reported. With prolonged high dosage, corneal and lens opacities and purplish pigmentation of the skin, cornea, conjunctiva, and retina. Intramuscular injection may be painful, cause hypotension and tachycardia (see Cautions), and give rise to nodule formation

Dose: by mouth, psychoses and severe anxiety, initially 25 mg 3 times daily (*or* 75 mg at night), adjusted according to response, to usual maintenance dose of 75–300 mg daily (but up to 1 g daily may be required in psychoses); CHILD 1–5 years 500 micrograms/kg every 4–6 hours (max. 40 mg daily); 6–12 years ⅓–½ adult dose (max. 75 mg daily)

Elderly and debilitated patients, ⅓–½ adult dose Intractable hiccup, 25–50 mg 3–4 times daily

By deep intramuscular injection, (for relief of acute symptoms), 25–50 mg every 6–8 hours; CHILD, as dose by mouth

By rectum in suppositories, chlorpromazine 100 mg every 6–8 hours

Note. For equivalent therapeutic effect 100 mg chlorpromazine base given *rectally* as a suppository ≡ 20–25 mg chlorpromazine hydrochloride *by intramuscular injection* ≡ 40–50 mg of chlorpromazine base or hydrochloride *by mouth*

PoM Chlorpromazine (Non-proprietary)
Tablets, chlorpromazine hydrochloride 10 mg, net price 20 = 11p; 25 mg, 20 = 14p; 50 mg, 20 = 33p; 100 mg, 20 = 62p. Label: 2
Elixir, chlorpromazine hydrochloride 25 mg/ 5 ml. Net price 100 ml = 26p. Label: 2

PoM Chloractil® (DDSA)
Tablets, s/c, chlorpromazine hydrochloride 25 mg, net price 20 = 14p; 50 mg, 20 = 27p; 100 mg, 20 = 50p. Label: 2

PoM Largactil® (M&B)
Tablets, all off-white, f/c, chlorpromazine hydrochloride 10 mg. Net price 20 = 11p; 25 mg, 20 = 17p; 50 mg, 20 = 33p; 100 mg, 20 = 61p. Label: 2
Syrup, brown, chlorpromazine hydrochloride 25 mg/5 ml. Diluent syrup (without preservative), life of diluted syrup 14 days. Net price 100 ml = 26p. Label: 2
Suspension forte, orange, sugar-free, chlorpromazine hydrochloride 100 mg (as embonate)/5 ml. Diluent syrup (without preservative), life of diluted suspension 7 days. Net price 100 ml = £1.14. Label: 2
Injection, chlorpromazine hydrochloride 25 mg/ml. Net price 2-ml amp = 27p
Suppositories, chlorpromazine 100 mg. Net price 10 = £1.84. Label: 2

BENPERIDOL
Indications: control of deviant and antisocial sexual behaviour (but see notes above)

Cautions; Contra-indications; Side-effects: see under Haloperidol; avoid in children
Dose: 0.25–1.5 mg daily in divided doses, adjusted according to the response; elderly, initially half adult dose

PoM Anquil® (Janssen)
Tablets, benperidol 250 micrograms. Net price 20 = £2.44. Label: 2

DROPERIDOL
Indications: tranquillisation and emergency control in psychoses, particularly mania, and in behavioural disturbances; chemotherapy-induced nausea and vomiting. Peri-operative use see section 15.1.4.2
Cautions; Contra-indications; Side-effects: see under Haloperidol
Dose: by mouth, 5–20 mg repeated every 4–8 hours if necessary (elderly, initially half adult dose); CHILD, 0.5–1 mg daily
By intramuscular injection, up to 10 mg repeated every 4–6 hours if necessary (elderly, initially half adult dose); CHILD, 0.5–1 mg daily
By intravenous injection, 5–15 mg repeated every 4–6 hours if necessary (elderly, initially half adult dose)
Cancer chemotherapy, *by intramuscular or intravenous injection*, 1–10 mg 30 minutes before starting therapy, followed by *continuous intravenous infusion* of 1–3 mg/hour *or* 1–5 mg by *intramuscular or intravenous injection* every 1–6 hours as necessary; CHILD *by intramuscular or intravenous injection*, 20–75 micrograms/kg

PoM Droleptan® (Janssen)
Tablets, yellow, scored, droperidol 10 mg. Net price 20 = £3.30. Label: 2
Oral liquid, sugar-free, droperidol 1 mg/ml. Diluent purified water, freshly boiled and cooled, life of diluted liquid 14 days. Net price 100 ml (with graduated cap) = £3.00; 500 ml = £14.25. Label: 2
Injection, droperidol 5 mg/ml. Net price 2-ml amp = 70p

FLUPENTHIXOL
Indications: schizophrenia and related psychoses, particularly with apathy and withdrawal but not mania or psychomotor hyperactivity; short-term adjunctive treatment of severe anxiety. For use in depression see section 4.3.4
Cautions; Contra-indications; Side-effects: see under Chlorpromazine Hydrochloride but less sedating; extrapyramidal symptoms are more frequent (25% of patients) and tardive dyskinesia also occurs. Oral administration may cause restlessness and insomnia. Avoid in children, senile confusional states, excitable and overactive patients
Dose: initially 3–9 mg twice daily adjusted according to the response; max. 18 mg daily

PoM **Depixol**® (Lundbeck)

Tablets, yellow, s/c, flupenthixol 3 mg (as dihydrochloride). Net price 20 = £2.59. Label: 2

Depot injection (flupenthixol decanoate): section 4.2.2

Fluanxol (depression), see section 4.3.4

FLUPHENAZINE HYDROCHLORIDE

Indications: schizophrenia and related psychoses, tranquillisation in behavioural disturbances, short-term adjunctive treatment of severe anxiety

Cautions; Contra-indications; Side-effects: see under Chlorpromazine Hydrochloride, but less sedating and fewer anticholinergic or hypotensive symptoms. Extrapyramidal symptoms, particularly dystonic reactions and akathisia, are more frequent. Avoid in depression; avoid in children

Dose: psychoses initially 2.5–10 mg daily in 2–3 divided doses, adjusted according to the response to a max. of 20 mg daily

Severe anxiety, initially 1 mg twice daily, increased as necessary to 4 mg daily

PoM **Moditen**® (Squibb)

Tablets, all s/c, fluphenazine hydrochloride 1 mg (pink), net price 20 = £1.09; 2.5 mg (yellow), 20 = £1.36; 5 mg, 20 = £1.82. Label: 2

Depot injections (fluphenazine decanoate): section 4.2.2

HALOPERIDOL

Indications: schizophrenia and related psychoses, particularly mania; tranquillisation and emergency control in behavioural disturbances; short-term adjunctive treatment of severe anxiety; motor tics, hiccups (section 4.9.3)

Cautions; Contra-indications; Side-effects: see under Chlorpromazine Hydrochloride but less sedating, and fewer anticholinergic or hypotensive symptoms. Extrapyramidal symptoms, particularly dystonic reactions and akathisia are more frequent especially in thyrotoxic patients. Rarely, alterations in liver function, gastrointestinal disturbances, and weight loss. Caution in depression. Avoid in basal ganglia disease. Drug interactions: see Appendix 1 (sections 2.5, 4.2, 4.2, 4.9, 6.7)

Dose: by mouth, psychoses, initially 1.5–20 mg daily in divided doses, gradually increased to 100 mg (and occasionally 200 mg) daily in severely disturbed patients; CHILD initially 25–50 micrograms/kg daily to a max. of 10 mg; adolescents up to 30 mg daily (exceptionally 60 mg)

Severe anxiety, adults 500 micrograms twice daily

By intramuscular injection, 2–10 mg (increasing to 30 mg for emergency control) then 5 mg up to every hour if necessary (intervals of 4–6 hours may be satisfactory)

PoM **Haloperidol** (Non-proprietary)

Tablets, haloperidol 1.5 mg, net price 20 = 22p; 5 mg, 20 = 45p; 10 mg, 20 = £1.58; 20 mg, 20 = £2.30. Label: 2

PoM **Dozic**® (RP Drugs)

Oral liquid, sugar-free, haloperidol 1 mg/ml. Net price 100 ml (with pipette) = £5.00. Label: 2

Oral liquid, sugar-free, haloperidol 2 mg/ml. Net price 100 ml (with pipette) = £5.50. Label: 2

PoM **Fortunan**® (Steinhard)

Tablets, haloperidol 500 micrograms, net price 20 = 44p; 1.5 mg (scored), 20 = 83p; 5 mg (green, scored), 20 = £2.25; 10 mg (pink, scored), 20 = £3.80; 20 mg (scored), 20 = £7.47. Label: 2

PoM **Haldol**® (Janssen)

Tablets, both scored, haloperidol 5 mg (blue), net price 20 = £1.69; 10 mg (yellow), 20 = £3.30. Label: 2

Oral liquid, sugar-free, haloperidol 2 mg/ml. Diluent purified water, freshly boiled and cooled, life of diluted liquid 14 days. Net price 100 ml (with pipette) = £5.21. Label: 2

Oral liquid concentrate, sugar-free, haloperidol 10 mg/ml. Diluent purified water, freshly boiled and cooled, life of diluted concentrate 14 days. Alternatively, purified water, freshly boiled and cooled, containing 0.05% of methyl hydroxybenzoate and 0.005% of propyl hydroxybenzoate, life of diluted concentrate 2 months. Net price 100 ml = £22.84. Label: 2

Injection, haloperidol 5 mg/ml. Net price 1-ml amp = 33p; 2-ml amp = 63p

Depot injection (haloperidol decanoate): section 4.2.2

PoM **Serenace**® (Searle)

Capsules, green, haloperidol 500 micrograms. Net price 20 = 67p. Label: 2

Tablets, all scored, haloperidol 1.5 mg, net price 20 = £1.19; 5 mg (pink), 20 = £3.36; 10 mg (pale pink), 20 = £6.02; 20 mg (dark pink), 20 = £10.85. Label: 2

Oral liquid, sugar-free, haloperidol 2 mg/ml. Diluent syrup or purified water, freshly boiled and cooled, or syrup for dilutions containing 1% or less of the elixir, life of diluted elixir 2 months. Net price 100 ml = £8.99. Label: 2

Injection, haloperidol 5 mg/ml, net price 1-ml amp = 59p; 10 mg/ml, 2-ml amp = £2.03

METHOTRIMEPRAZINE

Indications: schizophrenia and related psychoses, adjunctive treatment in terminal care (including management of pain and associated restlessness, distress or vomiting)

Cautions; Contra-indications; Side-effects: see under Chlorpromazine Hydrochloride but more sedating. Postural hypotension may occur; caution in patients over 50 years

Dose: by mouth, initially 25–50 mg daily in divided doses increased as necessary; bedpatients initially 100–200 mg daily in 3 divided doses, increased if necessary to 1 g daily

By intramuscular or intravenous injection, adjunct in terminal care, 12.5–25 mg (severe agitation up to 50 mg) every 6–8 hours if necessary

By continuous subcutaneous infusion, adjunct in terminal care (via syringe driver), 25–200 mg daily (over 24-hour period), diluted in a suitable volume of sodium chloride 0.9% injection

PoM **Nozinan**® (M&B)
Injection, methotrimeprazine hydrochloride 25 mg/ml. Net price 1-ml amp = £1.00

PoM **Veractil**® (M&B)
Tablets, varnished, scored, methotrimeprazine maleate 25 mg. Net price 20 = £1.72. Label: 2

OXYPERTINE

Indications: schizophrenia and related psychoses, particularly with apathy and withdrawal, also suitable in mania and psychomotor hyperactivity; tranquillisation in behavioural disturbances; short-term adjunctive treatment of severe anxiety

Cautions; Side-effects: see under Chlorpromazine Hydrochloride, but extrapyramidal symptoms may occur less frequently. With low doses agitation and hyperactivity occur and with high doses sedation. Occasionally gastro-intestinal disturbances, photophobia, and rashes may occur. Drug interactions: see Appendix 1 (section *4.3*)

Dose: psychoses, initially 80–120 mg daily in divided doses adjusted according to the response; max. 300 mg daily

Severe anxiety, initially 10 mg 3–4 times daily preferably after food

PoM **Integrin**® (Sterling Research)
Capsules, oxypertine 10 mg. Net price 20 = £1.68. Label: 2
Tablets, scored, oxypertine 40 mg. Net price 20 = £5.25. Label: 2

PERICYAZINE

Indications: tranquillisation in behavioural disturbances, schizophrenia and related psychoses, short-term adjunctive treatment of severe anxiety

Cautions; Contra-indications; Side-effects: see under Chlorpromazine Hydrochloride, but more sedating; hypotension commonly occurs when treatment is initiated

Dose: psychoses, initially 15–30 mg (elderly patients 5–10 mg) daily divided into 2 doses, taking the larger dose at bedtime, adjusted according to the response; severely disturbed hospital patients, initially 75 mg daily; CHILD (severe mental or behavioural disorders only), initially, 500 micrograms daily for 10-kg child, increased by 1 mg for each additional 5 kg to max. total daily dose of 10 mg; max. maintenance should not exceed twice initial dose

PoM **Neulactil**® (M&B)
Tablets, all yellow, scored, pericyazine 2.5 mg, net price 20 = 43p; 10 mg, 20 = £1.15; 25 mg, 20 = £3.19. Label: 2

Syrup forte, brown, pericyazine 10 mg/5 ml. Diluent syrup, life of diluted syrup 14 days. Net price 100 ml = £2.35. Label: 2

PERPHENAZINE

Indications: schizophrenia and related psychoses, tranquillisation and emergency control in behavioural disturbances, short-term adjunctive treatment of severe anxiety, terminal disease, intractable hiccup

Cautions; Contra-indications; Side-effects: see under Chlorpromazine Hydrochloride, but it is less sedating; extrapyramidal symptoms, especially dystonia, are more frequent, particularly at high dosage. Avoid in children

Dose: by mouth, initially 4 mg 3 times daily adjusted according to the response; max. 24 mg daily; elderly patients quarter to half adult dose

By intramuscular injection (for relief of acute symptoms), 5–10 mg, followed if necessary by 5 mg every 6 hours; elderly patients quarter to half adult dose

PoM **Fentazin**® (A&H)
Tablets, both s/c, perphenazine 2 mg, net price 20 = 52p; 4 mg, 20 = 62p. Label: 2
Injection, perphenazine 5 mg/ml. Net price 1-ml amp = 15p

PIMOZIDE

Indications: see under Dose
Cautions; Side-effects: see under Chlorpromazine Hydrochloride, but less sedating
Dose: schizophrenia, paranoid psychoses, initially 20 mg daily, adjusted according to response; max. 60 mg daily; prevention of relapse, initially 8 mg daily (usual range 2–20 mg daily)

Monosymptomatic hypochondriacal psychosis, initially 4 mg daily, adjusted according to response; max. 16 mg daily

Mania, hypomania, and psychomotor agitation, initially 20 mg daily adjusted according to response; max. 60 mg daily
ELDERLY ½ usual starting dose

PoM **Orap**® (Janssen)
Tablets, all scored, pimozide 2 mg, net price 20 = £2.27; 4 mg (green), 20 = £4.40; 10 mg, 20 = £10.16. Label: 2

PROCHLORPERAZINE

Indications: schizophrenia and related psychoses, short-term adjunctive treatment of severe anxiety; see also section 4.6

Cautions; Contra-indications; Side-effects: see under Chlorpromazine Hydrochloride, but it is less sedating although extrapyramidal symptoms, particularly dystonic reactions, are more frequent especially with doses above 40 mg daily; tardive dyskinesia also occurs. Avoid in children (but see section 4.6 for use as anti-emetic)

Dose: by mouth, prochlorperazine maleate or mesylate, psychoses, 12.5 mg twice daily for 7 days adjusted to 75–100 mg daily according to response
Severe anxiety, 15–20 mg daily in divided doses; max. 40 mg daily
By deep intramuscular injection, psychoses, prochlorperazine mesylate 12.5–25 mg 2–3 times daily
By rectum in suppositories, psychoses, the equivalent of prochlorperazine maleate 25 mg 2–3 times daily

Preparations
Section 4.6

PROMAZINE HYDROCHLORIDE
Indications: agitation, particularly in the elderly, short-term adjunctive treatment of severe anxiety; terminal disease
Cautions; Contra-indications; Side-effects: see under Chlorpromazine Hydrochloride
Dose: by mouth, 25–200 mg 4 times daily, adjusted according to response
By intramuscular injection, 50 mg (25 mg in elderly or debilitated patients), repeated if necessary after 6–8 hours

PoM **Sparine**® (Wyeth)
Suspension, yellow, promazine hydrochloride 50 mg (as embonate)/5 ml. Diluent syrup, life of diluted suspension 14 days. Net price 150 ml = £1.44. Label: 2. Unsuitable for children
Injection, promazine hydrochloride 50 mg/ml. Net price 1-ml amp = 26p; 2-ml amp = 37p

SULPIRIDE
Indications: schizophrenia
Cautions; Contra-indications; Side-effects: see under Chlorpromazine Hydrochloride; also contra-indicated in phaeochromocytoma; reduce dose in renal impairment
Dose: 200–400 mg twice daily; max. 800 mg daily in patients with predominantly negative symptoms, and 2.4 g daily in patients with mainly positive symptoms; elderly, initially 50–100 mg

▼ PoM **Dolmatil**® (Squibb)
Tablets, scored, sulpiride 200 mg. Net price 20 = £4.20. Label: 2
▼ PoM **Sulpitil**® (Tillotts)
Tablets, scored, sulpiride 200 mg. Net price 20 = £4.11; 28 = £5.75. Label: 2

THIORIDAZINE
Indications: schizophrenia and related psychoses, tranquillisation and emergency control in behavioural disturbances, agitation in elderly patients, short-term adjunctive treatment of severe anxiety
Cautions; Contra-indications; Side-effects: see under Chlorpromazine Hydrochloride, but less

sedating and extrapyramidal symptoms and hypothermia rarely occur; more likely to induce hypotension. Caution in depression. Pigmentary retinopathy (with reduced visual acuity, brownish colouring of vision, and impaired night vision) occurs rarely with high doses. Sexual dysfunction, particularly retrograde ejaculation, may occur
Dose: psychoses, 150–600 mg daily (initially in divided doses); max. 800 mg daily for up to 4 weeks
Moderate to severe non-psychotic emotional disturbances, 75–200 mg daily
Anxiety, agitation, and restlessness in the elderly, 30–100 mg daily
CHILD (severe mental or behavioural problems only) under 5 years 1 mg/kg daily, 5–12 years 75–150 mg daily (in severe cases, up to 300 mg daily)

PoM **Thioridazine** (Non-proprietary)
Tablets, thioridazine hydrochloride 25 mg, net price 20 = 31p; 50 mg, 20 = 58p; 100 mg, 20 = £1.10. Label: 2
PoM **Melleril**® (Sandoz)
Tablets, all f/c, thioridazine hydrochloride 10 mg, net price 20 = 23p; 25 mg, 20 = 32p; 50 mg, 20 = 61p; 100 mg, 20 = £1.16. Label: 2
Suspension 25 mg/5 ml, thioridazine 25 mg/5 ml. Net price 100 ml = 58p. Label: 2
Suspension 100 mg/5 ml, thioridazine 100 mg/5 ml. Net price 100 ml = £2.13. Label: 2
These suspensions should not be diluted but the two preparations may be mixed with each other to provide intermediate doses
Syrup, orange, thioridazine 25 mg (as hydrochloride)/5 ml. Diluent syrup or sorbitol solution 70%, life of diluted syrup 14 days. Net price 100 ml = 59p. Label: 2

TRIFLUOPERAZINE
Indications: schizophrenia and related psychoses, tranquillisation in behavioural disturbances, short-term adjunctive treatment of severe anxiety
Cautions; Contra-indications; Side-effects: see under Chlorpromazine Hydrochloride but less sedating, and hypotension, hypothermia, and anticholinergic side-effects occur less frequently. Extrapyramidal symptoms, particularly dystonic reactions and akathisia, are more frequent (particularly when the daily dose exceeds 6 mg). Caution in children
Dose: by mouth, psychoses, initially 5 mg twice daily, *or* 10 mg daily in slow-release form, increased by 5 mg after 1 week, then at intervals of 3 days, according to the response; CHILD up to 12 years, initially up to 5 mg daily in divided doses, adjusted according to response, age, and body-weight
Severe anxiety, 2–4 mg daily in divided doses *or* 2–4 mg daily in slow-release form, increased if necessary to 6 mg daily; CHILD 3–5 years up to 1 mg, 6–12 years up to 4 mg daily in divided doses

By deep intramuscular injection (for acute symptoms), 1–3 mg daily in divided doses to a max. of 6 mg daily; CHILD 50 micrograms/kg daily in divided doses

PoM **Stelazine®** (SK&F)
Tablets, both blue, s/c, trifluoperazine (as hydrochloride) 1 mg, net price 20 = 34p; 5 mg, 20 = 48p. Label: 2
Spansule® (=capsules s/r), all clear/yellow, enclosing dark blue, light blue, and white pellets, trifluoperazine (as hydrochloride) 2 mg, net price 20 = 78p; 10 mg, 20 = £1.08; 15 mg, 20 = £1.61. Label: 2, 25
Syrup, yellow, sugar-free, trifluoperazine 1 mg (as hydrochloride)/5 ml. Diluent syrup, life of diluted syrup 14 days. Net price 100 ml = 60p. Label: 2
Liquid concentrate, yellow, trifluoperazine 10 mg (as hydrochloride)/ml for dilution before use. Diluent syrup or water for preparations, life of diluted liquid 12 weeks or 1 week respectively (hosp. only)
Injection, trifluoperazine 1 mg (as hydrochloride)/ml. Net price 1-ml amp = 42p

TRIFLUPERIDOL
Indications: schizophrenia and related psychoses, particularly mania
Cautions; Contra-indications; Side-effects: see under Haloperidol
Dose: initially 500 micrograms daily, adjusted by 500 micrograms every 3–4 days according to the response; max. 6–8 mg daily; CHILD 6–12 years initially 250 micrograms, adjusted according to the response; max. 2 mg daily

PoM **Triperidol®** (Lagap)
Tablets, both scored, trifluperidol 500 micrograms, net price 20 = £1.12; 1 mg, 20 = £1.57. Label: 2

ZUCLOPENTHIXOL DIHYDROCHLORIDE
Indications: schizophrenia and related psychoses, particularly when associated with agitated, aggressive, or hostile behaviour
Cautions; Contra-indications; Side-effects: see under Chlorpromazine Hydrochloride; should not be used in apathetic or withdrawn states; avoid in children
Dose: initially 20–30 mg daily in divided doses, increasing to a max. of 150 mg daily if necessary; usual maintenance dose 20–50 mg daily

▼ PoM **Clopixol®** (Lundbeck)
Tablets, all f/c, zuclopenthixol (as dihydrochloride) 2 mg (pink), net price 20 = 61p; 10 mg (light brown), 20 = £1.50; 25 mg (brown), 20 = £3.00. Label: 2
Depot injection (zuclopenthixol decanoate): section 4.2.2

4.2.2 Antipsychotic depot injections

For maintenance therapy, long-acting depot injections of antipsychotic drugs are used because they are more convenient than oral preparations and ensure better patient compliance. However, they may give rise to a higher incidence of extrapyramidal reactions than oral preparations.

ADMINISTRATION. Depot antipsychotics are administered by deep intramuscular injection at intervals of 1 to 4 weeks. Patients should first be given a small test-dose as undesirable side-effects are prolonged. In general not more than 2–3 ml of oily injection should be administered at any one site.

Individual responses to neuroleptic drugs are very variable and to achieve optimum effect, dosage and dosage interval must be titrated according to the patient's response.

CHOICE. There is no clear-cut division in the usage of these drugs, but **zuclopenthixol** may be suitable for the treatment of agitated or aggressive patients whereas **flupenthixol** can cause over-excitement in such patients. **Fluspirilene** (Redeptin®) has a shorter duration of action than the other depot injections. The incidence of extra-pyramidal reactions is similar for all these drugs.

CAUTIONS. Treatment requires careful monitoring for optimum effect; extrapyramidal symptoms occur frequently. When transferring from oral to depot therapy, dosage by mouth should be gradually phased out. Caution in arteriosclerosis.

CONTRA-INDICATIONS. Do not use in children, confusional states, coma caused by CNS depressants, parkinsonism, intolerance to antipsychotics.

SIDE-EFFECTS. Pain may occur at injection site and occasionally erythema, swelling, and nodules. For side-effects of specific antipsychotics see under the relevant monograph.

FLUPENTHIXOL DECANOATE
Indications: maintenance in schizophrenia and related psychoses
Cautions; Contra-indications; Side-effects: see under Chlorpromazine Hydrochloride (section 4.2.1) and notes above, but it may have a mood elevating effect. Extrapyramidal symptoms usually appear 1–3 days after administration and continue for about 5 days but may be delayed. With high doses, periodic blood counts are advisable. An alternative antipsychotic drug may be necessary if symptoms such as aggression or agitation appear
Dose: by deep intramuscular injection into the gluteal muscle, test dose 20 mg, then after 5–10 days 20–40 mg repeated at intervals of 2–4 weeks, adjusted according to the response; max. 400 mg weekly

PoM **Depixol®** (Lundbeck)
Injection (oily), flupenthixol decanoate 20 mg/ml. Net price 1-ml amp = £1.55; 1-ml

syringe = £1.70;   2-ml   amp = £2.60;   2-ml
syringe = £2.75; 10-ml vial = £14.74
PoM **Depixol Conc.**® (Lundbeck)
Injection (oily), flupenthixol decanoate
100 mg/ml. Net price 0.5-ml amp = £3.25; 1-ml
amp = £5.95; 5-ml vial = £28.27

FLUPHENAZINE DECANOATE

Indications: maintenance in schizophrenia and
related psychoses
Cautions; Contra-indications; Side-effects: see
under Chlorpromazine Hydrochloride (section
4.2.1) and notes above. Extrapyramidal symptoms usually appear a few hours after the dose
has been administered and continue for about
2 days but may be delayed. Contra-indicated in
severely depressed states
Dose: by deep intramuscular injection into the
gluteal muscle, test dose 12.5 mg (6.25 mg in
elderly patients), then after 4–7 days 12.5–
100 mg repeated at intervals of 14–40 days,
adjusted according to the response

PoM **Modecate**® (Squibb)
Injection (oily), fluphenazine decanoate
25 mg/ml. Net price 0.5-ml amp = £1.45; 1-ml
amp = £2.52; 1-ml syringe = £2.79; 2-ml amp =
£4.97; 2-ml syringe = £5.05; 10-ml vial = £24.05
PoM **Modecate Concentrate**® (Squibb)
Injection (oily), fluphenazine decanoate 100 mg/
ml. Net price 0.5-ml amp = £5.00; 1-ml amp =
£9.77

FLUPHENAZINE ENANTHATE

*Indications; Cautions; Contra-indications; Side-
effects:* see under Fluphenazine Decanoate but
it has less prolonged effect and higher incidence
of extrapyramidal symptoms
Dose: by deep intramuscular injection into the
gluteal muscle, test dose 12.5 mg (6.25 mg in
elderly patients), then after 4–7 days 12.5–
100 mg repeated at intervals of 10–21 days,
adjusted according to the response

PoM **Moditen Enanthate**® (Squibb)
Injection (oily), fluphenazine enanthate
25 mg/ml. Net price 1-ml amp = £3.00

FLUSPIRILENE

Indications: maintenance in schizophrenia and
related psychoses
Cautions; Contra-indications; Side-effects: see
under Chlorpromazine Hydrochloride (section
4.2.1) and notes above, but less sedating. Extrapyramidal symptoms usually appear 6–12 hours
after the dose and continue for about 48 hours
but may be delayed. Common side-effects are
restlessness and sweating. With prolonged use,
tissue damage (subcutaneous nodules) may
occur at injection site
Dose: by deep intramuscular injection, 2 mg,
increased by 2 mg at weekly intervals, according
to the response; usual maintenance dose 2–8 mg
weekly; max. 20 mg weekly

PoM **Redeptin**® (SK&F)
Injection (aqueous suspension), fluspirilene
2 mg/ml. Net price 1-ml amp = 90p; 3-ml
amp = £1.59; 6-ml vial = £2.76

HALOPERIDOL DECANOATE

Indications: maintenance in schizophrenia and
related psychoses
Cautions; Contra-indications; Side-effects: see
under Haloperidol (section 4.2.1) and notes
above
Dose: by deep intramuscular injection into the
gluteal muscle, initially 50 mg every 4 weeks, if
necessary increasing after 2 weeks by 50-mg
increments to 300 mg every 4 weeks; higher
doses may be needed in some patients; elderly,
initially 12.5–25 mg every 4 weeks

▼ PoM **Haldol Decanoate**® (Janssen)
Injection (oily), haloperidol 50 mg (as
decanoate)/ml. Net price 1-ml amp = £3.12
Injection (oily), haloperidol 100 mg (as
decanoate)/ml. Net price 1-ml amp = £4.80

PIPOTHIAZINE PALMITATE

Indications: maintenance in schizophrenia and
related psychoses
Cautions; Contra-indications; Side-effects: see
under Chlorpromazine Hydrochloride (section
4.2.1) and notes above
Dose: by deep intramuscular injection into the
gluteal muscle, test dose 25 mg, then a further
25–50 mg after 4–7 days, then adjusted according to the response at intervals of 4 weeks; usual
maintenance range 50–100 mg (max. 200 mg)
every 4 weeks

▼ PoM **Piportil Depot**® (M&B)
Injection (oily), pipothiazine palmitate 50 mg/
ml. Net price 1-ml amp = £5.98; 2-ml amp =
£9.78

ZUCLOPENTHIXOL DECANOATE

Indications: maintenance in schizophrenia and
related psychoses, particularly with aggression
and agitation
Cautions; Contra-indications; Side-effects: see
under Chlorpromazine Hydrochloride (section
4.2.1) and notes above, but it is less sedating
Dose: by deep intramuscular injection into the
gluteal muscle, test dose 100 mg, then after 7–
28 days 100–200 mg or more, followed by 200–
400 mg repeated at intervals of 2–4 weeks,
adjusted according to the response; max.
600 mg weekly

PoM **Clopixol**® (Lundbeck)
Injection (oily), zuclopenthixol decanoate
200 mg/ml. Net price 1-ml amp = £3.01; 10-ml
vial = £28.63
▼ PoM **Clopixol Conc.**® (Lundbeck)
Injection (oily), zuclopenthixol decanoate
500 mg/ml. Net price 1-ml amp with needle =
£7.25

4.2.3 Lithium salts

Lithium salts are used for their mood-regulating action in the treatment of manic illness and in the prevention of manic and depressive illnesses. Lithium treatment quietens the overactive euphoric patient. The decision to give prophylactic treatment usually requires specialist advice, and must be based on careful consideration of the likelihood of recurrence in the individual patient, and the benefit weighed against the risks. Lithium treatment is unsuitable for children.

Treatment should be discontinued only if relief from affective illness is absent or insignificant.

In the initial stages supplementary treatment with **antipsychotic drugs** (section 4.2.1) is usually required because it may take a few days for lithium to exert its effect. High doses of haloperidol, fluphenazine, or flupenthixol may be hazardous when used with lithium; irreversible toxic encephalopathy has been reported.

Lithium salts have a narrow therapeutic/toxic ratio and should therefore not be prescribed unless facilities for monitoring plasma concentrations are available. Patients should be carefully selected. Doses are adjusted to achieve plasma concentrations of 0.6 to 1.2 mmol Li^+/litre (lower end of the range for maintenance therapy and elderly patients) on samples taken 12 hours after the preceding dose. Overdosage, usually with plasma concentrations over 1.5 mmol Li^+/litre, may be fatal and toxic effects include tremor, ataxia, dysarthria, nystagmus, renal impairment, and convulsions. If these potentially hazardous signs occur, treatment should be stopped, plasma-lithium concentrations redetermined, and steps taken to reverse lithium toxicity.

Lithium toxicity is made worse by sodium depletion. In particular concurrent use of diuretics that inhibit the uptake of sodium by the distal tubule, with compensatory increase in reabsorption by the proximal tubule (e.g. thiazides), is hazardous and should be avoided. In mild cases withdrawal of lithium and administration of generous amounts of sodium and fluid will reverse the toxicity. Plasma concentrations in excess of 2.0 mmol Li^+/litre require emergency treatment as indicated under Emergency Treatment of Poisoning. When toxic concentrations are reached there may be a delay of 1 or 2 days before maximum toxicity occurs.

In long-term use, therapeutic concentrations of lithium have been thought to cause histological and functional changes in the kidney. The significance of such changes is not clear but is of sufficient concern to discourage long-term use of lithium unless it is definitely indicated. Patients should therefore be maintained on lithium treatment after 3–5 years only if, on assessment, benefit persists. Conventional and sustained-release tablets are available but it should be noted that **different preparations vary widely in bioavailability** and a change in the formulation used requires the same precautions as initiation of treatment. There seem few if any reasons for preferring one or other of the simple salts of lithium; the carbonate has been the more widely used but the citrate is also available.

LITHIUM CARBONATE

Indications: treatment and prophylaxis of mania, manic-depressive illness, and recurrent depression (see also notes above); aggressive or self-mutilating behaviour

Cautions: plasma concentrations must be measured regularly (every month on stabilised regimens), and thyroid function monitored; maintain adequate sodium and fluid intake. Avoid in renal impairment, cardiac disease, and conditions with sodium imbalance such as Addison's disease (dose adjustment may be necessary in diarrhoea, vomiting, and heavy sweating). Caution in pregnancy, breast-feeding, elderly patients (reduce dose), diuretic treatment, myasthenia gravis. Drug interactions: see Appendix 1 (sections 4.2, *6.1*, *10*, *15*)

Side-effects: gastro-intestinal disturbances, fine tremor, polyuria and polydipsia (may disappear with continued treatment); also weight gain and oedema (may respond to dose reduction). Signs of lithium intoxication are blurred vision, increasing gastro-intestinal disturbances (anorexia, vomiting, diarrhoea), increasing CNS disturbances (mild drowsiness and sluggishness increasing to giddiness with ataxia, coarse tremor, lack of co-ordination, dysarthria) require withdrawal of treatment. With severe overdosage (plasma concentrations above 2 mmol/litre) hyperreflexia and hyperextension of limbs, convulsions, toxic psychoses, syncope, oliguria, circulatory failure, coma, and occasionally, death. Goitre, raised antidiuretic hormone concentration, hypothyroidism, hypokalaemia, ECG changes, exacerbation of psoriasis, and kidney changes may also occur

Dose: initially 0.25–2 g daily, adjusted to achieve a plasma concentration of 0.6–1.2 mmol Li^+/litre by tests on samples taken 12 hours after the preceding dose on the fourth or seventh day of treatment, then weekly until dosage has remained constant for 4 weeks and monthly thereafter; daily doses are usually divided (sustained-release preparations normally given twice daily)

COUNSELLING. Patients should maintain an adequate fluid intake and should avoid dietary changes which might reduce or increase sodium intake

PoM **Camcolit 250**® (Norgine)
Tablets, f/c, scored, lithium carbonate 250 mg (6.8 mmol Li^+). Net price 20 = 48p. Counselling advised, see above

PoM **Camcolit 400**® (Norgine)
Tablets, s/r, f/c, scored, lithium carbonate 400 mg (10.8 mmol Li^+). Net price 20 = 61p. Label: 25, counselling advised, see above

PoM **Liskonum**® (SK&F)
Tablets, s/r, f/c, scored, lithium carbonate 450 mg (12.2 mmol Li^+). Net price 20 = 78p. Label: 25, counselling advised, see above

PoM **Phasal**® (Lagap)

Tablets, s/r, lithium carbonate 300 mg (8.1 mmol Li⁺). Net price 20 = 80p. Label: 25, counselling advised, see above

PoM **Priadel**® (Delandale)

Tablets, both s/r, scored, lithium carbonate 200 mg (5.4 mmol Li⁺), net price 20 = 51p; 400 mg (10.8 mmol Li⁺), 20 = 62p. Label: 25, counselling advised, not to be swallowed with hot drinks, see also above

LITHIUM CITRATE

Indications; Cautions; Side-effects: see under Lithium Carbonate and notes above

Dose: 564 mg twice daily adjusting dose to achieve plasma concentrations of 0.6–1.2 mmol Li⁺/litre as described under Lithium Carbonate

▼ PoM **Litarex**® (CP)

Tablets, s/r, lithium citrate 564 mg (6 mmol Li⁺). Net price 20 = 72p. Label: 25, counselling advised, see under Lithium Carbonate

4.3   Antidepressant drugs

4.3.1 Tricyclic and related antidepressant drugs

4.3.2 Monoamine-oxidase inhibitors (MAOIs)

4.3.3 Combined antidepressant preparations

4.3.4 Other antidepressant drugs

Tricyclic and related antidepressants (antidepressives) are the drugs of choice in the treatment of depressive illness, unless it is so severe that electroconvulsive therapy is immediately indicated. They are preferred to MAOIs because they are more effective antidepressants and do not show the dangerous interactions with some foods and drugs that are characteristic of the MAOIs. **Lithium** (section 4.2.3) has a mood-regulating action and is used specifically in the treatment of manic depressive illnesses.

Prescribing more than one antidepressant of the tricyclic type is **not** recommended. It may constitute a hazard and there is no evidence that side-effects are minimised.

Mixtures of antidepressants with tranquillisers are in section 4.3.3; they are **not** recommended.

Other drugs used to treat depression (flupenthixol and tryptophan) are in section 4.3.4.

It should be noted that although anxiety is often present in depressive illness and may be the presenting symptom, the use of antipsychotics or anxiolytics may mask the true diagnosis. They should therefore be used with caution though they are useful adjuncts in agitated depression.

DRUG INTERACTIONS. See Appendix 1 (sections *2.5*, *4.1*, *4.8*, *4.9*) and under individual entries.

4.3.1   Tricyclic and related antidepressant drugs

The term 'tricyclic' is misleading as there are now 1-, 2-, and 4-ring structured drugs with broadly similar properties.

These drugs are most effective for treating moderate to severe endogenous depression associated with psychomotor and physiological changes such as loss of appetite and sleep disturbances; improvement in sleep is usually the first benefit of therapy. Since there may be an interval of 2 to 4 weeks before the antidepressant action takes place electroconvulsive treatment may be required in severe depression when delay is hazardous or intolerable.

DOSAGE. About 10 to 20% of patients fail to respond to tricyclic and related antidepressant drugs and inadequate plasma concentrations may account for some of these failures. It is important to achieve plasma concentrations which are sufficiently high for effective treatment but not high enough to cause toxic effects. Low doses should be used for initial treatment in the elderly (see under Side-effects, below).

MANAGEMENT. The patient's condition must be checked frequently, especially in the early weeks of treatment, to detect any suicidal tendencies. Limited quantities of antidepressant drugs should be prescribed at any one time as they are dangerous in overdosage. Some of the newer drugs, for example mianserin and trazodone seem less dangerous in overdose than the older tricyclics.

Treatment should be continued for 2 to 4 weeks before suppression of symptoms can be expected and thereafter should be maintained at the optimum level for at least another month before any attempt is made at dose reduction. Treatment should not be withdrawn prematurely, otherwise symptoms are likely to recur. The natural history of depressive illness suggests that remission usually occurs after 3 months to a year or more and some patients appear to benefit from maintenance therapy with about half the therapeutic dosage for several months to prevent relapse. It may be appropriate during the early stages of treatment to add a hypnotic (section 4.1.1) to correct the sleeping pattern or an anxiolytic (section 4.1.2) to allay anxiety or agitation.

CHOICE. Antidepressant drugs can be roughly divided into those with additional sedative properties, for example **amitriptyline**, and those with less, for example **imipramine**. Agitated and anxious patients tend to respond best to the sedative compounds whereas withdrawn and apathetic patients will often obtain most benefit from less sedating compounds.

Amitriptyline may be given in divided doses or the entire daily dose may be given at night to promote sleep and avoid daytime drowsiness. **Imipramine** can also be given once daily but as it has a much less sedative action there is less need.

Imipramine and amitriptyline are well established and relatively safe and effective, but nevertheless have more marked anticholinergic or cardiac side-effects than some of the newer compounds (**doxepin**, **lofepramine**, **mianserin**, **trazodone**, and **viloxazine**); this may be important in individual patients.

Antidepressants with **sedative** properties include amitriptyline (Tryptizol®, Lentizol® etc.), dothiepin (Prothiaden®), doxepin (Sinequan®), maprotiline (Ludiomil®), mianserin (Bolvidon®, Norval®), trazodone (Molipaxin®), and trimipramine (Surmontil®).

Less sedative antidepressants include butriptyline (Evadyne®), clomipramine (Anafranil®), desipramine (Pertofran®), imipramine (Tofranil® etc.), iprindole (Prondol®), lofepramine (Gamanil®), nortriptyline (Allegron®, Aventyl®), and viloxazine (Vivalan®). Protriptyline has a **stimulant** action.

NOCTURNAL ENURESIS IN CHILDREN. Certain tricyclic antidepressants (**amitriptyline**, **imipramine** and less often **nortriptyline**) are used for the treatment of *nocturnal enuresis* in children (see section 7.4.2). Drug treatment should be reserved for children over 7 years of age and used only after other simple measures have failed.

SIDE-EFFECTS. Arrhythmias and heart block occasionally follow the use of tricyclic antidepressants, particularly amitriptyline, and may be a factor in the sudden death of patients with cardiac disease. Although the use of the older tricyclic antidepressants has been associated with reports of convulsions and of hepatic and haematological reactions, the frequency of these side-effects appears to be much higher, and deaths have been reported, with the newer non-tricyclic antidepressants. In particular, mianserin has been associated with haematological and hepatic reactions and maprotiline has been associated with convulsions. Patients being treated with these drugs therefore require careful supervision. In the case of **mianserin** a full **blood count** is recommended every 4 weeks during the first 3 months of treatment; subsequent clinical monitoring should continue and treatment should be stopped and a full blood count obtained if fever, sore throat, stomatitis, or other signs of infection develop. Nomifensine (Merital®) has now been withdrawn.

Other side-effects of tricyclic and related antidepressants include drowsiness, dry mouth, blurred vision, constipation, urinary retention, and sweating, attributed to anticholinergic activity. The patient should be encouraged to persist with treatment as some tolerance to these side-effects seems to develop. They are further reduced if low doses are given initially and then gradually increased.

This gradual introduction of treatment is particularly important in the elderly, who, because of the hypotensive effects of these drugs, are prone to attacks of dizziness or even syncope. The tricyclic and related antidepressants should be prescribed with caution in epilepsy as they lower the convulsive threshold.

Neuroleptic malignant syndrome (section 4.2.1) may, very rarely, arise in the course of antidepressant treatment.

HYPERTENSIVE PATIENTS. Antidepressants may interfere with antihypertensive therapy. They diminish the action of bethanidine, clonidine, debrisoquine, and guanethidine. Beta-adrenoceptor blocking drugs may be used in conjunction with antidepressants as this combination does not interact.

LACK OF RESPONSE. In patients who do not respond to antidepressants, the diagnosis, dosage, compliance, and possible continuation of psychosocial or physical aggravating causes should all be carefully reviewed; other drug treatment may be successful. The patient may respond to low-dose **flupenthixol** (Fluanxol®, section 4.3.4) or MAOIs (section 4.3.2). **Tryptophan** (section 4.3.4) appears to benefit some patients when given alone or as adjunctive therapy.

ONCE-DAILY DOSE. In most patients the long half-life of tricyclic antidepressant drugs allows once-daily administration, usually at night.

TRICYCLIC ANTIDEPRESSANTS

AMITRIPTYLINE HYDROCHLORIDE

Indications: depressive illness, particularly where sedation is required; nocturnal enuresis in children (see section 7.4.2)

Cautions: initially, sedation may affect the ability to drive or operate machinery; effects of alcohol may be increased; diabetes, cardiac disease (particularly with arrhythmias, see contra-indications below), epilepsy, pregnancy, hepatic impairment, thyroid disease, psychoses (may aggravate mania), glaucoma, urinary retention. Avoid abrupt cessation of therapy. Also caution in anaesthesia (increased risk of arrhythmias). See notes above for nocturnal enuresis. Drug interactions: see Appendix 1 (sections 2.5, 2.6, 2.7, 4.3, 4.3)

Contra-indications: recent myocardial infarction, heart block, mania

Side-effects: dry mouth, sedation, blurred vision, constipation, nausea, difficulty with micturition (due to anticholinergic action). Other common side-effects are cardiovascular (arrhythmias, postural hypotension, tachycardia, syncope, particularly with high doses), sweating, tremor, rashes, behavioural disturbances (particularly children), hypomania, confusion (particularly elderly), interference with sexual function, blood sugar and weight changes. Less common, black tongue, paralytic ileus, convulsions, agranulocytosis, leucopenia, eosinophilia, purpura, thrombocytopenia, and jaundice

Dose: by mouth, initially 50–75 mg (elderly and adolescents 25–50 mg) daily in divided doses *or* as a single dose at bedtime increased gradually as necessary to a max. of 150–200 mg; usual maintenance 50–100 mg daily

Nocturnal enuresis, CHILD 7–10 years 10–20 mg, 11–16 years 25–50 mg at night; max. period of treatment (including gradual withdrawal) should not exceed 3 months

By intramuscular or intravenous injection, 10–20 mg 4 times daily

PoM **Amitriptyline Tablets,** f/c or s/c, amitriptyline hydrochloride 10 mg, net price 20 = 22p; 25 mg, 20 = 8p; 50 mg, 20 = 56p. Label: 2

PoM **Domical**® (Berk)
Tablets, all f/c, amitriptyline hydrochloride 10 mg (blue), net price 20 = 22p; 25 mg (orange), 20 = 19p; 50 mg (red-brown), 20 = 59p. Label: 2

PoM **Elavil**® (DDSA)
Tablets, both f/c, amitriptyline hydrochloride 10 mg (blue), net price 20 = 13p; 25 mg (yellow), 20 = 17p. Label: 2

PoM **Lentizol**® (P-D)
Capsules, s/r, both enclosing white pellets, amitriptyline hydrochloride 25 mg (pink), net price 20 = 81p; 50 mg (pink/red), 20 = £1.52. Label: 2, 25

PoM **Tryptizol**® (Morson)
Capsules, s/r, orange, amitriptyline hydrochloride 75 mg. Net price 20 = £1.78. Label: 2, 25

Tablets, all f/c, amitriptyline hydrochloride 10 mg (blue), net price 20 = 22p; 25 mg (yellow), 20 = 46p; 50 mg (brown), 20 = 95p. Label: 2

Mixture, pink, sugar-free, amitriptyline 10 mg (as embonate)/5 ml. Diluent syrup, life of diluted mixture 14 days. Net price 100 ml = 91p. Label: 2

Injection, amitriptyline hydrochloride 10 mg/ml. Net price 10-ml vial = 47p

BUTRIPTYLINE
Indications: depressive illness
Cautions; Contra-indications; Side-effects: see under Amitriptyline Hydrochloride, but less sedating.
Dose: 25 mg 3 times daily, increased gradually as necessary to a max. of 150 mg; usual maintenance dose 25 mg 3 times daily

PoM **Evadyne**® (Wyeth)
Tablets, both f/c, butriptyline (as hydrochloride) 25 mg (orange), net price 20 = 77p; 50 mg (pink), 20 = £1.35. Label: 2

CLOMIPRAMINE HYDROCHLORIDE
Indications: depressive illness, adjunctive treatment of phobic and obsessional states; cataplexy associated with narcolepsy
Cautions; Contra-indications; Side-effects: see under Amitriptyline Hydrochloride. Postural hypotension may occur on intravenous infusion
Dose: by mouth, initially 10 mg daily, increased gradually as necessary to 30–150 mg or more in severe depression and phobic and obsessional states, in divided doses or as a single dose at bedtime; elderly patients 10 mg daily, up to 30–75 mg
By intramuscular injection, up to 150 mg daily

By intravenous infusion, initially to assess tolerance, 25–50 mg, then usually about 100 mg daily for 7–10 days

PoM **Anafranil**® (Geigy)
Capsules, clomipramine hydrochloride 10 mg (yellow/caramel), net price 20 = 69p; 25 mg (orange/caramel), 20 = £1.36; 50 mg (blue/caramel), 20 = £2.59. Label: 2
Syrup, orange, clomipramine hydrochloride 25 mg/5 ml. Diluent purified water, freshly boiled and cooled; for dilutions below 15 mg/5 ml equal parts of syrup and tragacanth mucilage (freshly prepared), life of diluted syrup 7 days. Net price 150 ml = £6.18. Label: 2
Injection, clomipramine hydrochloride 12.5 mg/ml. Net price 2-ml amp = 40p

PoM **Anafranil SR**® (Geigy)
Tablets, s/r, pink, f/c, clomipramine hydrochloride 75 mg. Net price 20 = £4.90. Label: 2, 25

DESIPRAMINE HYDROCHLORIDE
Indications: depressive illness
Cautions; Contra-indications; Side-effects: see under Amitriptyline Hydrochloride, but less sedating. Drug interactions: see Appendix 1 (section 4.3)
Dose: 75 mg (elderly patients 25 mg) daily in divided doses or as a single dose at bedtime, increased as necessary to a max. of 200 mg

PoM **Pertofran**® (Geigy)
Tablets, pink, s/c, desipramine hydrochloride 25 mg. Net price 20 = 71p. Label: 2

DOTHIEPIN HYDROCHLORIDE
Indications: depressive illness, particularly where sedation is required
Cautions; Contra-indications; Side-effects: see under Amitriptyline Hydrochloride
Dose: initially 75 mg (elderly patients 50–75 mg) daily in divided doses *or* as a single dose at bedtime, increased gradually as necessary to 150 mg daily; up to 225 mg daily in hospital patients

PoM **Prothiaden**® (Boots)
Capsules, red/brown, dothiepin hydrochloride 25 mg. Net price 20 = 96p. Label: 2
Tablets, red, s/c, dothiepin hydrochloride 75 mg. Net price 14 = £2.00. Label: 2

DOXEPIN
Indications: depressive illness, particularly where sedation is required
Cautions; Contra-indications; Side-effects: see under Amitriptyline Hydrochloride
Dose: initially 75 mg (elderly patients 10– 50 mg) daily in 3 divided doses, increased gradually to a max. of 300 mg daily in divided doses; range 30–300 mg daily; up to 100 mg may be given as a single dose at bedtime

PoM **Sinequan**® (Pfizer)
Capsules, doxepin (as hydrochloride) 10 mg
(orange), net price 20 = 37p; 25 mg (orange/
blue), 20 = 53p; 50 mg (blue), 20 = 93p; 75 mg
(yellow/blue), 20 = £1.47. Label: 2

IMIPRAMINE HYDROCHLORIDE
Indications: depressive illness; nocturnal
enuresis in children (see section 7.4.2)
Cautions; Contra-indications; Side-effects: see
under Amitriptyline Hydrochloride, but less
sedating. Drug interactions: see Appendix 1
(section 4.3)
Dose: initially 75 mg daily in divided doses
increased gradually to 200 mg (up to 225 mg or
more in hospital patients); up to 150 mg may
be given as a single dose at bedtime; elderly
patients 10–25 mg 1–3 times daily
Nocturnal enuresis, CHILD 7 years 25 mg, 8–
11 years 25–50 mg, over 11 years 50–75 mg at
bedtime; max. period of treatment (including
gradual withdrawal) not to exceed 3 months

PoM **Imipramine Tablets**, s/c, imipramine hydrochloride 10 mg, net price 20 = 14p; 25 mg, 20 =
13p. Label: 2
PoM **Praminil**® (DDSA)
Tablets, both s/c, imipramine hydrochloride
10 mg (brownish-pink), net price 20 = 28p;
25 mg (brown), 20 = 55p. Label: 2
PoM **Tofranil**® (Geigy)
Tablets, both red-brown, s/c, imipramine hydrochloride 10 mg, net price 20 = 33p; 25 mg, 20 =
63p. Label: 2
Syrup, imipramine hydrochloride 25 mg/5 ml.
Diluent purified water, freshly boiled and
cooled; for dilutions below 15 mg/5 ml equal
parts of syrup and tragacanth mucilage (freshly
prepared), life of diluted syrup 14 days. Net
price 150 ml = £2.70. Label: 2

LOFEPRAMINE
Indications: depressive illness
Cautions; Contra-indications; Side-effects: see
under Amitriptyline Hydrochloride, but less
sedating
Dose: 140–210 mg daily in divided doses

▼ PoM **Gamanil**® (Merck)
Tablets, lacquer-coated, brown-violet, lofepramine 70 mg (as hydrochloride). Net price 14-
tab pack = £2.49. Label: 2

NORTRIPTYLINE
Indications: depressive illness; nocturnal
enuresis in children (see section 7.4.2)
Cautions; Contra-indications; Side-effects: see
under Amitriptyline Hydrochloride but less
sedating. Drug interactions: see Appendix 1
(section 4.3)
Dose: initially 20–40 mg daily in divided doses,
increased gradually as necessary to a max. of
100 mg daily; usual maintenance dose 30–75 mg
daily

Nocturnal enuresis, CHILD 7 years 10 mg, 8–
11 years 10–20 mg, over 11 years 25–35 mg,
at night; max period of treatment (including
gradual withdrawal) should not exceed 3
months

PoM **Allegron**® (Dista)
Tablets, nortriptyline (as hydrochloride) 10 mg,
net price 20 = 55p; 25 mg (orange, scored),
20 = £1.10. Label: 2
PoM **Aventyl**® (Lilly)
Capsules, both yellow/white, nortriptyline (as
hydrochloride) 10 mg, net price 20 = 55p;
25 mg, 20 = £1.10. Label: 2
Liquid, sugar-free, nortriptyline 10 mg (as
hydrochloride)/5 ml. Diluent syrup, life of
diluted liquid 14 days. Net price 120 ml = £1.03.
Label: 2

PROTRIPTYLINE HYDROCHLORIDE
Indications: depressive illness, particularly with
apathy and withdrawal
Cautions; Contra-indications; Side-effects: see
under Amitriptyline Hydrochloride but less
sedating; anxiety, agitation, tachycardia, and
hypotension more common; rashes associated
with photosensitisation (avoid direct sunlight);
caution in elderly, particularly when daily dose
exceeds 20 mg
Dose: initially 10 mg 3–4 times daily (elderly 5 mg
3 times daily initially) if insomnia not after
4 p.m.; usual range 15–60 mg daily

PoM **Concordin**® (MSD)
Tablets, both f/c, protriptyline hydrochloride
5 mg (pink), net price 20 = 37p; 10 mg, 20 =
54p. Label: 2, 11

TRIMIPRAMINE
Indications: depressive illness, particularly where
sedation is required
Cautions; Contra-indications; Side-effects: see
under Amitriptyline Hydrochloride
Dose: 50–75 mg daily as a single dose 2 hours
before bedtime *or* as 25 mg midday and 50 mg
evening, increased as necessary to max. of
300 mg daily; usual maintenance dose 75–
150 mg daily
ELDERLY 10–25 mg 3 times daily initially, half
adult maintenance dose may be sufficient

PoM **Surmontil**® (M&B)
Capsules, green/white, trimipramine 50 mg (as
maleate). Net price 20 = £2.69. Label: 2
Tablets, both compression coated, trimipramine
(as maleate) 10 mg, net price 20 = 81p; 25 mg,
20 = £1.34. Label: 2

RELATED ANTIDEPRESSANTS

IPRINDOLE
Indications: depressive illness
Cautions; Contra-indications; Side-effects: see
under Amitriptyline Hydrochloride, but less
sedating. Caution in liver disease; jaundice,

---

although rare, may develop, usually in the first 14 days

Dose: initially 15–30 mg 3 times daily, increased gradually to max. of 60 mg 3 times daily; usual maintenance 30 mg 3 times daily

PoM **Prondol**® (Wyeth)
Tablets, both yellow, iprindole (as hydrochloride), 15 mg, net price 20 = 42p; 30 mg, 20 = 82p. Label: 2

MAPROTILINE HYDROCHLORIDE
Indications: depressive illness, particularly where sedation is required
Cautions; Contra-indications; Side-effects: see under Amitriptyline Hydrochloride, but anticholinergic effects occur less frequently. Rashes commonly occur and there is an increased risk of convulsions at higher dosage
Dose: initially 25–75 mg (elderly patients 30 mg) daily in 3 divided doses *or* as a single dose at bedtime, increased gradually as necessary to a max. of 150 mg daily

PoM **Ludiomil**® (Ciba)
Tablets, all f/c, maprotiline hydrochloride 10 mg (pale orange), net price 20 = 60p; 25 mg (greyish-red), 20 = £1.10; 50 mg (light orange), 20 = £2.15; 75 mg (brownish-orange), 28-tab pack = £4.40. Label: 2

MIANSERIN HYDROCHLORIDE
Indications: depressive illness, particularly where sedation is required
Cautions; Contra-indications; Side-effects: see under Amitriptyline; leucopenia, agranulocytosis and aplastic anaemia (particularly in the elderly); jaundice; arthritis, arthralgia; influenza-like syndrome may occur; **blood counts needed, p. 155**
Fewer and milder anticholinergic and cardiovascular effects; many interactions of tricyclic antidepressants absent
Dose: initially 30–40 mg (elderly patients 30 mg) daily in divided doses *or* as a single dose at bedtime, increased gradually as necessary; usual dose range 30–90 mg, max. 200 mg daily in divided doses

PoM **Bolvidon**® (Organon)
Tablets, all f/c, mianserin hydrochloride 10 mg, net price 30-tab pack = £1.94; 20 mg, 14-tab pack = £1.83; 30 mg, 14-tab pack = £2.75. Label: 2, 25
PoM **Norval**® (Bencard)
Tablets, all orange, f/c, mianserin hydrochloride 10 mg, net price 20 = £1.29; 20 mg, 20 = £2.59; 30 mg, 20 = £3.88. Label: 2, 25

TRAZODONE HYDROCHLORIDE
Indications: depressive illness, particularly where sedation is required
Cautions; Contra-indications; Side-effects: see under Amitriptyline Hydrochloride but fewer anticholinergic and cardiovascular effects; rarely priapism
Dose: initially 150 mg (elderly 100 mg) daily in divided doses after food *or* as a single dose at bedtime; may be increased to 200–300 mg daily; hospital patients up to max. 600 mg daily in divided doses

PoM **Molipaxin**® (Roussel)
Capsules, trazodone hydrochloride 50 mg (violet/green), net price 20 = £3.41; 100 mg (violet/fawn), 20 = £5.88. Label: 2, 21
Tablets, pink, f/c, trazodone hydrochloride 150 mg. Net price 30 = £10.30. Label: 2, 21
Liquid, sugar-free, trazodone hydrochloride 50 mg/5 ml. Net price 150 ml = £6.41. Label: 2, 21

VILOXAZINE HYDROCHLORIDE
Indications: depressive illness
Cautions; Contra-indications; Side-effects: see under Amitriptyline Hydrochloride, but less sedating and anticholinergic and cardiovascular side-effects are fewer and milder; nausea and headache may occur. Drug interactions: see Appendix 1 (sections *3, 4.8*)
Dose: 300 mg daily (preferably as 200 mg in the morning and 100 mg at midday), increased gradually as necessary; max. 400 mg daily; last dose not later than 6 p.m.
ELDERLY 100 mg daily initially, half adult maintenance dose may be sufficient

PoM **Vivalan**® (ICI)
Tablets, yellow, f/c, viloxazine 50 mg (as hydrochloride). Net price 20 = £1.27. Label: 2

4.3.2   Monoamine-oxidase inhibitors (MAOIs)
Monoamine-oxidase inhibitors are used much less frequently than tricyclic and related antidepressants because of the dangers of dietary and drug interactions and the fact that it is easier to prescribe MAOIs when tricyclic antidepressants have been unsuccessful than vice versa. **Tranylcypromine** (Parnate®) is the most **hazardous** of the MAOIs because of its stimulant action. The drugs of choice are **phenelzine** or **isocarboxazid** which are less stimulant and therefore safer.

Phobic patients and depressed patients with atypical, hypochondriacal, or hysterical features are said to respond best to MAOIs. However, MAOIs should be tried in any patients who are refractory to treatment with other antidepressants as there is occasionally a dramatic response. Response to treatment may be delayed for 3 weeks or more and may take an additional 1 or 2 weeks to become maximal.

MAOIs inhibit monoamine oxidase, thereby causing an accumulation of amine neurotransmitters. The metabolism of some amine drugs such as sympathomimetics is also inhibited and their pressor action may therefore be potentiated. The pressor effect of the tyramine present in some foods may also be dangerously potentiated.

Sympathomimetics are present in many proprietary cough mixtures and decongestant nasal drops. See Appendix 1 (section 4.3) and Treatment Card. These interactions may cause a dangerous rise in blood pressure. An early warning symptom may be a throbbing headache. The danger of interaction persists for up to 14 days after treatment with MAOIs is discontinued. Treatment cards which list the necessary precautions are distributed by the Pharmaceutical Society and given to patients at pharmacies etc.

Tricyclic and related antidepressants should **not** be given to patients for 14 days after treatment with MAOIs has been discontinued. Some psychiatrists use selected tricyclics in conjunction with MAOIs but this is hazardous, indeed potentially lethal, except in experienced hands and there is no evidence that the combination is more effective than when either constituent is used alone. The combination of tranylcypromine with clomipramine is particularly **dangerous**.

Note. For other interactions with monoamine-oxidase inhibitors including those with opioid analgesics, see Appendix 1 (section 4.3).

PHENELZINE

Indications: depressive illness
Cautions: may affect mental concentration and ability to drive or operate machinery. Avoid abrupt discontinuation of treatment, certain

---

TREATMENT CARD

Carry this card with you at all times. Show it to any doctor who may treat you other than the doctor who prescribed this medicine, and to your dentist if you require dental treatment.

INSTRUCTIONS TO PATIENTS

Please read carefully
While taking this medicine and for 14 days after your treatment finishes you must observe the following simple instructions:-

1 Do not eat CHEESE, PICKLED HERRING OR BROAD BEAN PODS.
2 Do not eat or drink BOVRIL, OXO, MARMITE or ANY SIMILAR MEAT OR YEAST EXTRACT.
3 Eat only FRESH foods and avoid food that you suspect could be stale or 'going off'. This is especially important with meat, fish, poultry or offal. Avoid game.
4 Do not take any other MEDICINES (including tablets, capsules, nose drops, inhalations or suppositories) whether purchased by you or previously prescribed by your doctor, without first consulting your doctor or your pharmacist.
   NB *Treatment for coughs and colds, pain relievers, tonics and laxatives are medicines.*
5 Avoid alcoholic drinks.

Keep a careful note of any food or drink that disagrees with you, avoid it and tell your doctor.
Report any unusual or severe symptoms to your doctor and follow any other advice given by him.

| M.A.O.I. | Prepared by The Pharmaceutical Society and the British Medical Association on behalf of the Health Departments of the United Kingdom. |

Printed in UK for HMSO D8919816 5/85 12773   33383

---

drugs and foods (see Treatment Card above). Avoid in elderly and debilitated patients. Drug interactions: see Appendix 1 (sections 4.3, *6.1*)
Contra-indications: hepatic, cardiovascular, or cerebrovascular disease, phaeochromocytoma, epilepsy, children
Side-effects: dizziness, postural hypotension, less commonly agitation, headache, tremor, constipation, dry mouth, blurred vision, difficulty in micturition, liver damage, rashes, psychotic episodes in susceptible patients; severe hypertensive reactions to certain drugs and foods
Dose: 15 mg 3 times daily, increased if necessary to 4 times daily after 2 weeks, then reduced gradually to lowest possible maintenance dose

PoM **Nardil**® (P-D)
Tablets, orange, f/c, phenelzine 15 mg (as sulphate). Net price 20 = £1.18. Label: 3, 10 MAOI card
Note. Nardil tablets are now gluten-free

ISOCARBOXAZID

Indications: depressive illness
Cautions;   Contra-indications: see under Phenelzine
Side-effects: see under Phenelzine; rarely anaemia, hepatitis, peripheral oedema, and rashes
Dose: initially up to 30 mg daily in single or divided doses; usual maintenance dose 10–20 mg daily

PoM **Marplan**® (Roche)
Tablets, pink, scored, isocarboxazid 10 mg. Net price 20 = 39p. Label: 3, 10 MAOI card

TRANYLCYPROMINE

Indications: depressive illness
Cautions;   Contra-indications: see under Phenelzine;   also   contra-indicated   in hyperthyroidism
Side-effects: insomnia, dizziness, muscular weakness, dry mouth, hypotension; hypertensive crises with throbbing headache requiring discontinuation of treatment occur more frequently than with other MAOIs; liver damage occurs less frequently than with phenelzine
Dose: initially 10 mg twice daily not later than 3 p.m., increasing the second daily dose to 20 mg after 1 week if necessary; usual maintenance dose 10 mg daily

PoM **Parnate**® (SK&F)
Tablets, red, s/c, tranylcypromine 10 mg (as sulphate). Net price 20 = 91p. Label: 3, 10 MAOI card

4.3.3 Compound antidepressant preparations

Antipsychotic drugs such as the phenothiazine derivatives or anxiolytics such as the benzodiazepines can be usefully given with antidepressants but the use of preparations listed below is **not** recommended because the dosage of the individual components should be adjusted separately to be appropriate for the individual patient. Whereas antidepressants are given continuously over several months, the phenothiazines and benzodiazepines are usually prescribed intermittently in the lowest effective dosage.

NHS PoM **Limbitrol 5**® (Roche)
Capsules, pink/green, amitriptyline 12.5 mg (as hydrochloride), chlordiazepoxide 5 mg. Net price 20 = 95p. Label: 2

NHS PoM **Limbitrol 10**® (Roche)
Capsules, pink/dark green, amitriptyline 25 mg (as hydrochloride), chlordiazepoxide 10 mg. Net price 20 = £1.38. Label: 2

PoM **Motipress**® (Squibb)
Tablets, yellow, s/c, fluphenazine hydrochloride 1.5 mg, nortriptyline 30 mg (as hydrochloride). Net price 28-tab pack = £2.90. Label: 2

PoM **Motival**® (Squibb)
Tablets, pink, s/c, fluphenazine hydrochloride 500 micrograms, nortriptyline 10 mg (as hydrochloride). Net price 20 = 70p. Label: 2

PoM **Parstelin**® (SK&F)
Tablets, green, s/c, tranylcypromine 10 mg (as sulphate), trifluoperazine 1 mg (as hydrochloride). Net price 20 = 93p. Label: 3, 10 MAOI card
Caution: contains MAOI

PoM **Triptafen**® (A&H)
Tablets, pink, s/c, amitriptyline hydrochloride 25 mg, perphenazine 2 mg. Net price 20 = 54p. Label: 2

PoM **Triptafen-M**® (A&H)
Tablets, pink, s/c, amitriptyline hydrochloride 10 mg, perphenazine 2 mg. Net price 20 = 48p. Label: 2

4.3.4   Other antidepressant drugs

Flupenthixol (Fluanxol®) has antidepressant properties, and low doses (1.5 to 3 mg daily) are given by mouth for this purpose. Its advantage over the tricyclic and related antidepressants is that, with the low doses employed, side-effects are fewer and overdosage less toxic. It should be withdrawn if there has been no response after 1 week at maximum dosage.

Tryptophan appears to benefit some patients when given alone or as adjunctive therapy. Its antidepressant effect may take up to 4 weeks to develop. Preparations containing pyridoxine are unsuitable for patients taking levodopa.

Fluvoxamine is a non-sedative antidepressant with few anticholinergic effects and low cardiotoxicity. However, it has a high incidence of gastro-intestinal side-effects (nausea and vomiting) and may exacerbate agitation and insomnia.

FLUPENTHIXOL

Indications: depressive illness. For use in psychoses, see section 4.2.1
Cautions: cardiovascular disease (including cardiac disorders and cerebral arteriosclerosis), senile confusional states, parkinsonism, renal and hepatic disease; avoid in excitable and overactive patients
Side-effects: restlessness, insomnia, rarely extrapyramidal symptoms

Dose: initially 1 mg (elderly patients 500 micrograms) in the morning, increased after 1 week to 2 mg (elderly patients 1 mg) if necessary. Max. 3 mg (elderly patients 2 mg) daily, doses above 2 mg (elderly patients 1 mg) being divided in 2 portions, the second given before 4 p.m.

Depixol (psychoses), see section 4.2.1
PoM **Fluanxol**® (Lundbeck)
Tablets, red, s/c, flupenthixol 500 micrograms (as dihydrochloride). Net price 20 = £1.18. Label: 2
Tablets, red, s/c, flupenthixol 1 mg (as dihydrochloride). Net price 20 = £2.39. Label: 2

FLUVOXAMINE MALEATE

Indications: depressive illness
Cautions: renal and hepatic impairment; effects of alcohol may be increased. Drug interactions: see Appendix 1 (sections *2.8C*, *4.3*)
Contra-indications: history of epilepsy
Side-effects: nausea and vomiting, drowsiness, agitation, headache, anorexia, tremor; constipation; bradycardia; convulsions
Dose: 100–200 mg daily (up to 100 mg as single dose in evening); max. 300 mg daily

▼ PoM **Faverin**® (Duphar)
Tablets, e/c, yellow, fluvoxamine maleate 50 mg. Net price 60 = £25.00. Label: 2, 5, 25

TRYPTOPHAN

Indications: mild to moderate depressive illness, (alone); more severe depressive illness (in conjunction with other antidepressants)
Cautions: active bladder disease, disorders of tryptophan metabolism. May initially affect ability to drive or operate machinery. Reduce dose when used in conjunction with MAOIs and discontinue if blurred vision or headache occur during tryptophan/MAOI therapy. Drug interactions: see Appendix 1 (section *4.3*)
Side-effects: nausea, drowsiness, headache
Dose: 1–2 g 3 times daily, preferably after meals. In conjunction with a monoamine-oxidase inhibitor, 500 mg daily for 1 week, gradually increased

PoM **Optimax**® (Merck)
Tablets, yellow, f/c, scored, L-tryptophan 500 mg, pyridoxine hydrochloride 5 mg, ascorbic acid 10 mg. Net price 20 = £1.82. Label: 2
Powder, L-tryptophan 1 g, pyridoxine hydrochloride 10 mg, ascorbic acid 20 mg/6 g. Net price 20 × 6-g sachets = £5.11. Label: 2, 13
PoM **Optimax WV**® (Merck)
Tablets, yellow, f/c, scored, L-tryptophan 500 mg. Net price 20 = £1.94. Label: 2
PoM **Pacitron**® (Rorer)
Tablets, orange, f/c, L-tryptophan 500 mg. Net price 20 = £1.87. Label: 2

4.4 Central nervous stimulants

4.4.1 Weak central nervous stimulants
4.4.2 Amphetamines and cocaine

Central nervous system stimulants have very few indications and in particular, should **not** be used to treat depression, obesity, senility, debility, or for relief of fatigue.

4.4.1 Weak central nervous stimulants

Caffeine is a weak stimulant present in tea and coffee. It is included in many analgesic preparations (section 4.7.1.1) but does not contribute to their analgesic or anti-inflammatory effect. Over-indulgence may lead to a state of anxiety.

Pemoline is a weak central nervous system stimulant that has been advocated for the management of hyperactive children. The same general reservations apply as for amphetamines (section 4.4.2) and treatment should be carried out only under specialist supervision.

PEMOLINE

Indications: hyperkinesia in children (under specialist supervision)
Cautions: cardiovascular disease, insomnia. Drug interactions: see Appendix 1 (section *4.3*)
Contra-indications: glaucoma, extrapyramidal disorders, hyperexcitable states (thyrotoxicosis)
Side-effects: insomnia, tachycardia, agitation
Dose: CHILD over 6 years, 10–20 mg in the morning and afternoon

PoM **Volital**® (LAB)
Tablets, scored, pemoline 20 mg. Net price 20 = 56p

STIMULANT WITH VITAMINS

Prolintane is contained in a preparation with vitamins; it is **not** recommended.
NHS PoM **Villescon**® (Boehringer Ingelheim)
Tablets, orange, s/c, prolintane hydrochloride 10 mg with vitamins B group and C. Net price 20 = 75p
  Dose: 1 tablet twice daily before 4 p.m. for 1–2 weeks but see notes above
Liquid, red, prolintane hydrochloride 2.5 mg/5 ml with vitamins B group and C. Diluent water for preparations, life of diluted liquid 14 days. Net price 100 ml = 45p
  Dose: 10 ml twice daily before 4 p.m. for 1–2 weeks but see notes above

4.4.2 Amphetamines and cocaine

The amphetamines have a limited field of usefulness and their use should be **discouraged** as they may cause dependence and psychotic states.

Patients with narcolepsy may derive benefit from treatment with amphetamines.

Amphetamines have been advocated for the management of hyperactive children; beneficial effects have been described. However, they must be used very selectively as they retard growth

and the effect of long-term therapy has not been evaluated.

Amphetamines have **no place** in the management of **depression** or **obesity**.

DEXAMPHETAMINE SULPHATE

Indications: narcolepsy, hyperkinesia in children (under specialist supervision)
Cautions: anorexia, insomnia, impaired renal function, unstable personality. Drug interactions: see Appendix 1 (sections *2.4*, *4.3*)
Contra-indications: cardiovascular disease, hyperexcitable states (thyrotoxicosis), glaucoma, extrapyramidal disorders
Side-effects: dependence and tolerance occur readily, also agitation, restlessness, insomnia, headache, dizziness, tremor, personality change, anorexia, arrhythmias, dry mouth, diarrhoea, or constipation. In children, anorexia, weight loss, growth inhibition, and tearfulness. Large doses cause disorientation and aggression, leading to paranoid psychosis, convulsions, and coma
Dose: narcolepsy, 10 mg daily in divided doses gradually increased to a max. of 60 mg daily
  Hyperkinesia, CHILD 3–5 years 2.5 mg in the morning gradually increased to a max. of 20 mg daily; 6–12 years 5–10 mg in the morning, gradually increased to a max. of 40 mg daily in 2 divided doses

CD **Dexedrine**® (SK&F)
Tablets, yellow, scored, dexamphetamine sulphate 5 mg. Net price 20 = 15p

COCAINE

Cocaine is a drug of addiction which causes central nervous stimulation. Its clinical use is mainly as a topical local anaesthetic (see sections 11.7 and 15.2). It has been included in analgesic elixirs for the relief of pain in terminal care (section 4.7.2) but this use is obsolescent.

4.5 Appetite suppressants

4.5.1 Bulk-forming drugs
4.5.2 Centrally acting appetite suppressants

The development of obesity appears to be multi-factorial. Aggravating factors may be depression or other psychosocial problems or drug treatment.

The main treatment of the obese patient is an appropriate diet, carefully explained to the patient, with support and encouragement from the doctor. Attendance at groups (for example 'weight-watchers') helps some individuals. Drugs can play only a limited role and should never be used as the sole element of treatment; their effects tend to be disappointing.

4.5.1 Bulk-forming drugs

The most commonly used bulk-forming drug is **methylcellulose**. It is claimed to reduce intake by producing feelings of satiety but there is little evidence to support this claim.

Prices are **net**, see p. 1

METHYLCELLULOSE
Indications: obesity
Cautions: maintain adequate fluid intake
Contra-indications: gastro-intestinal obstruction
Side-effects: flatulence, abdominal distension, intestinal obstruction

Celevac® (Boehringer Ingelheim)
Tablets, pink, methylcellulose '450' 500 mg. Net price 20 = 16p. Label: 22, 24, 27, counselling advised, administration
Dose: 3 tablets, chewed or crushed, with a tumblerful of liquid half an hour before food or when hungry

Cellucon® (Medo)
Tablets, buff, methylcellulose '2500' 500 mg. Net price 20 = 16p. Label: 22, 24, 27, counselling advised, administration
Dose: 1–4 tablets, chewed or crushed, with a tumblerful of liquid half an hour before food or when hungry

Nilstim® (De Witt)
Tablets, green, cellulose (microcrystalline) 220 mg, methylcellulose '2500' 400 mg. Net price 20 = 21p. Label: 22, 24, 27, counselling advised, administration
Dose: 2 tablets, chewed or crushed, with a tumblerful of liquid 15 minutes before the 2 main meals or when hungry

STERCULIA
Indications; Cautions; Side-effects: see under Methylcellulose

Prefil® (Norgine)
Granules, brown, coated, sterculia 55%. Net price 200 g = £1.92. Label: 22, 27, counselling advised, administration
Dose: two 5-ml spoonfuls followed by a tumblerful of liquid ½–1 hour before food, reduced in patients accustomed to a low-residue diet

4.5.2   Centrally acting appetite suppressants

Centrally acting appetite suppressants are of no real value in the treatment of obesity since they do not improve the long-term outlook. They are sympathomimetics and most have a pronounced stimulant effect on the central nervous system.

Use of the amphetamine-like drugs **diethylpropion, mazindol,** and **phentermine** is **not** justified as any possible benefits are outweighed by the risks involved; abuse, particularly of diethylpropion, is an increasing problem.

Although **fenfluramine** is also related to amphetamine, in standard doses it has a sedative rather than a stimulant effect. Nevertheless, abuse has occurred and abrupt withdrawal may induce depression. It should preferably be avoided but may be considered for short-term adjunctive

treatment in selected patients with severe obesity, given close support and supervision. It should **not** be given to patients with a past history of drug abuse or psychiatric illness and is **not recommended** for periods of treatment beyond 3 to 6 months. It should **not** be used for cosmetic reasons in mild to moderate obesity.

Thyroid hormones have no place in the treatment of obesity except in hypothyroid patients.

CHILDREN. These drugs should be avoided in children because of the possibility of growth suppression.

DIETHYLPROPION HYDROCHLORIDE
Indications: see notes above
Cautions: cardiovascular disease, peptic ulceration, epilepsy, depression, diabetes. Drug interactions: see Appendix 1 (sections *2.5, 4.3*)
Contra-indications: glaucoma, hyperthyroidism, unstable personality
Side-effects: headache, rashes, dependence; less common, insomnia, increased nervousness, psychosis, hallucinations, tachycardia, constipation; rarely, gynaecomastia

CD Apisate® (Wyeth)
Tablets, s/r, yellow, diethylpropion hydrochloride 75 mg, thiamine hydrochloride 5 mg, pyridoxine hydrochloride 2 mg, riboflavine 4 mg, nicotinamide 30 mg. Net price 20 = 52p. Label: 25, counselling, impaired reactions
Dose: 1 tablet mid-morning; max. period of treatment should not exceed 8 weeks

CD Tenuate Dospan® (Merrell)
Tablets, s/r, scored, diethylpropion hydrochloride 75 mg. Net price 20 = 63p. Label: 25, counselling, impaired reactions
Dose: 1 tablet mid-morning; max period of treatment should not exceed 8 weeks
Note. Must be prescribed as 'Tenuate Dospan Tablets'.

FENFLURAMINE HYDROCHLORIDE
Indications: see notes above
Cautions: dependence reported, depression on sudden withdrawal. Drug interactions: see Appendix 1 (sections *2.5, 4.3*)
COUNSELLING. Drowsiness may affect performance of skilled tasks (e.g. driving); effects of alcohol enhanced
Contra-indications: history of depressive illness, drug or alcohol abuse; personality disorders; epilepsy
Side-effects: diarrhoea and other gastro-intestinal disturbances; drowsiness, dizziness, and lethargy; also dry mouth, headache, sleep disturbances, depression, visual disorders, hypotension, urinary frequency, impotence and loss of libido; rarely rashes, blood disorders, reversible pulmonary hypertension
Dose: see below

PoM **Ponderax®** (Servier)
Pacaps® (= capsules s/r), clear/blue, enclosing white pellets, fenfluramine hydrochloride 60 mg. Net price 20 = £2.42. Label: 2, 25
Dose: 1–2 capsules daily, preferably before breakfast; max. period of treatment should not exceed 6 months

MAZINDOL

Indications: see notes above

Cautions; Contra-indications; Side-effects: see under Diethylpropion Hydrochloride. Avoid in peptic ulceration. Drug interactions: see Appendix 1 (section 2.5)

Dose: 2 mg after breakfast for up to 12 weeks

CD Teronac® (Sandoz)
Tablets, scored, mazindol 2 mg. Net price 20 = £2.01. Counselling advised, impaired reactions

PHENTERMINE

Indications: see notes above

Cautions; Contra-indications; Side-effects: see under Diethylpropion Hydrochloride

Dose: 15–30 mg before breakfast; max. period of treatment should not exceed 8 weeks

CD Duromine® (Riker)
Capsules, both s/r, phentermine (as resin complex) 15 mg (green/grey), net price 30 = £1.30; 30 mg (maroon/grey), 30 = £1.72. Label: 25
CD Ionamin® (Lipha)
Capsules, both s/r, phentermine (as resin complex) 15 mg (grey/yellow), net price 20 = 99p; 30 mg (yellow), 20 = £1.26. Label: 25

4.6   Drugs used in nausea and vertigo

Drug treatment of nausea and vertigo is discussed under the following headings:
    Vestibular disorders
    Vomiting of pregnancy
    Symptomatic relief of nausea from underlying disease

Anti-emetics should be prescribed only when the cause of vomiting is known, particularly in children, otherwise the symptomatic relief that they produce may delay diagnosis. Anti-emetics are unnecessary and sometimes harmful when the cause can be treated, e.g. as in diabetic keto-acidosis, or in excessive digoxin or antiepileptic dosage.

If antinauseant drug treatment is indicated the choice of drug depends on the aetiology of vomiting.

VESTIBULAR DISORDERS

Anti-emetics may be required in motion sickness, Ménière's disease, positional vertigo, labyrinthitis, and operative manipulation of the otovestibular apparatus. **Hyoscine** and the **antihistamines**, which act on the vomiting centre, are the drugs of choice. If possible they should be administered prophylactically at least 30 minutes before the emetic stimulus. Patients should be **warned** that these compounds may cause drowsiness, impair driving performance, and enhance the effects of alcohol and central nervous depressants.

MOTION SICKNESS. The most effective drug for the prevention of motion sickness is **hyoscine**. Adverse effects (drowsiness, blurred vision, dry mouth, urinary retention) are more frequent than with the **antihistamines** but are not generally prominent at the doses employed.

Antihistamines such as **cinnarizine, cyclizine, dimenhydrinate,** and **promethazine** are slightly less effective but generally better tolerated. There is no evidence that one antihistamine is superior to another but their duration of action and incidence of adverse effects (drowsiness and anticholinergic effects) differ. If a sedative effect is desired promethazine and dimenhydrinate are useful, but generally a less sedating antihistamine like cyclizine or cinnarizine is preferred. To prevent motion sickness the first dose is usually taken half an hour (2 hours for cinnarizine) before the start of the journey. Metoclopramide and the phenothiazine derivatives (except promethazine), which act selectively on the chemoreceptor trigger zone, are ineffective in motion sickness.

OTHER LABYRINTHINE DISORDERS. Vertigo and nausea associated with Ménière's disease and middle-ear surgery disorders may be difficult to treat. **Hyoscine, antihistamines,** and **phenothiazine derivatives** (such as prochlorperazine and thiethylperazine) are effective in the prophylaxis and treatment of such conditions. **Betahistine** and **cinnarizine** have been promoted as specific treatment for Ménière's disease. In the acute attack **cyclizine, prochlorperazine,** or **thiethylperazine** may be given rectally or by intramuscular injection.

Treatment of vertigo in its chronic forms is seldom fully effective but antihistamines (such as dimenhydrinate) or phenothiazine derivatives (such as prochlorperazine) may help.

For advice to avoid the inappropriate prescribing of drugs (notably phenothiazines) for dizziness in the elderly, see Prescribing for the Elderly, p. 12.

VOMITING OF PREGNANCY

Nausea in the first trimester of pregnancy does **not** require drug therapy. On rare occasions if vomiting is severe, an antihistamine or a phenothiazine derivative (promethazine or thiethylperazine) may be required. If symptoms have not settled in 24 to 48 hours then a specialist opinion should be sought.

SYMPTOMATIC RELIEF OF NAUSEA FROM UNDERLYING DISEASE

The **phenothiazine derivatives** are dopamine antagonists and act centrally by blocking the chemoreceptor trigger zone. In low doses they are the drugs of choice for the prophylaxis and treatment of nausea and vomiting associated with uraemia, diffuse neoplastic disease, radiation sickness, and the emesis caused by drugs such as opioid analgesics, general anaesthetics, and cytotoxic drugs. Rectal or parenteral administration is required if the vomiting has already started. **Prochlorperazine, perphenazine, trifluoperazine**, and **thiethylperazine** are less sedating than chlorpromazine but severe dystonic reactions sometimes occur, especially in children.

Metoclopramide is an effective anti-emetic with a spectrum of activity closely resembling that of the phenothiazine derivatives but it has a peripheral action on the gut in addition to its central effect and therefore may be superior to the phenothiazine derivatives in the emesis associated with gastroduodenal, hepatic, and biliary disease. The high-dose preparation is of value in the prevention of nausea and vomiting associated with cytotoxic drug therapy. Acute dystonic reactions may occur, particularly with children and young women, but they are less frequent than with phenothiazine derivatives.

Domperidone (Motilium®) is used for the relief of nausea and vomiting, especially when associated with cytotoxic drug therapy. It has the advantage over metoclopramide and the phenothiazine derivatives of being less likely to cause central effects such as sedation and dystonic reactions because it does not readily cross the blood-brain barrier. It may be given for the treatment of levodopa- and bromocriptine-induced vomiting in parkinsonism (section 4.9.1). Domperidone acts at the chemoreceptor trigger zone and so is unlikely to be effective in motion sickness and other vestibular disorders.

Antihistamines are active in most of these conditions, but are not usually drugs of choice.

Nabilone (Cesamet®) is a synthetic cannabinoid with anti-emetic properties, reported to be superior to prochlorperazine. It is beneficial in the relief of nausea and vomiting associated with cytotoxic drug therapy. Side-effects (more frequent than with prochlorperazine) occur in about half of patients given standard doses. Repeated use should be avoided because of possible neurotoxic effects.

BETAHISTINE HYDROCHLORIDE
Indications: vertigo and hearing disturbances in Ménière's disease
Cautions: asthma, peptic ulcer. Drug interactions: see Appendix 1 (section 4.6)
Contra-indications: phaeochromocytoma
Side-effects: nausea; rarely headache, rashes
Dose: 8–16 mg 3 times daily, after food, increased as necessary to a max. of 48 mg daily

PoM **Serc®** (Duphar)
Tablets, scored, betahistine hydrochloride 8 mg. Net price 20 = £2.15. Label: 21

CHLORPROMAZINE HYDROCHLORIDE
Indications: nausea and vomiting of terminal illness (where other drugs have failed or are not available)

Cautions; Contra-indications; Side-effects: see section 4.2.1
Dose: by mouth, 10–25 mg every 4–6 hours
By deep intramuscular injection 25 mg initially then 25–50 mg every 3–4 hours until vomiting stops
By rectum in suppositories, chlorpromazine 100 mg every 6–8 hours

Preparations
Section 4.2.1

CINNARIZINE
Indications: vestibular disorders, such as vertigo, tinnitus, nausea, and vomiting in Ménière's disease; motion sickness
Cautions; Side-effects: see under Cyclizine
Dose: vestibular disorders, 30 mg 3 times daily; CHILD 5–12 years ½ adult dose
Motion sickness, 30 mg 2 hours before travel then 15 mg every 8 hours during journey if necessary; CHILD 5–12 years ½ adult dose

Stugeron® (Janssen)
Tablets, scored, cinnarizine 15 mg. Net price 20 = 80p. Label: 2
Note. A proprietary brand of cinnarizine 15 mg tablets (Marzine RF®) is on sale to the public for travel sickness
Stugeron Forte: see section 2.6.3

CYCLIZINE
Indications: nausea, vomiting, vertigo, motion sickness, labyrinthine disorders
Cautions; Side-effects: drowsiness, occasional dry mouth and blurred vision; see also section 3.4.1 (Disadvantages of Antihistamines). Drug interactions: see Appendix 1 (sections *4.1, 4.6, 4.9*)
DRIVING. Drowsiness may affect performance of skilled tasks (e.g. driving); effects of alcohol enhanced
Dose: by mouth, cyclizine hydrochloride 50 mg 3 times daily; CHILD 1–10 years 25 mg 3 times daily
By intramuscular or intravenous injection, adults and children over 10 years, cyclizine lactate 50 mg 3 times daily

Valoid® (Calmic)
Tablets, scored, cyclizine hydrochloride 50 mg. Net price 20 = 69p. Label: 2
PoM *Injection*, cyclizine lactate 50 mg/ml. Net price 1-ml amp = 39p

DIMENHYDRINATE
Indications: nausea, vomiting, vertigo, motion sickness, labyrinthine disorders
Cautions; Side-effects: see under Cyclizine
Dose: 50–100 mg 2–3 times daily; CHILD 1–6 years 12.5–25 mg, 7–12 years 25–50 mg 2–3 times daily

Dramamine® (Searle)
Tablets, scored, dimenhydrinate 50 mg. Net price 20 = 93p. Label: 2

DOMPERIDONE
Indications: nausea and vomiting, particularly in

gastro-intestinal disorders or during treatment with cytotoxic drugs

Cautions: reduce dose in renal impairment. Drug interactions: see Appendix 1 (sections *4.6, 6.7*)

Contra-indications: chronic administration; routine postoperative administration

Side-effects: raised prolactin concentrations (possible galactorrhoea)

Dose: by mouth, 10–20 mg every 4–8 hours; CHILD, nausea and vomiting following cytotoxic therapy or radiotherapy, 200–400 micrograms/kg

By rectum, 60 mg every 4–8 hours; CHILD, 30–120 mg daily

▼ PoM **Evoxin**® (Sterling Research)
Tablets, f/c, domperidone 10 mg (as maleate). Net price 30 = £3.26
Suppositories, domperidone 30 mg. Net price 10 = £2.64

PoM **Motilium**® (Janssen)
Tablets, f/c, domperidone 10 mg (as maleate). Net price 20 = £2.17
Suspension, sugar-free, domperidone 5 mg/5 ml. Net price 200 ml = £1.80
Suppositories, domperidone 30 mg. Net price 10 = £2.64

DROPERIDOL
Section 4.2.1

HYOSCINE HYDROBROMIDE
(Scopolamine)

Indications: nausea, vomiting, vertigo, labyrinthine disorders, motion sickness

Cautions: elderly, urinary retention, cardiovascular disease, paralytic ileus, pyloric stenosis

Contra-indications: glaucoma

Side-effects: drowsiness, dry mouth, dizziness, blurred vision, difficulty with micturition

Dose: motion sickness, *by mouth,* 300 micrograms 30 minutes before start of journey followed by 300 micrograms every 6 hours if required; max. 3 doses in 24 hours; CHILD 4–10 years 75–150 micrograms, over 10 years 150–300 micrograms

By subcutaneous or intramuscular injection, 200 micrograms

PoM **Hyoscine** (Non-proprietary)
Tablets, hyoscine hydrobromide 300 micrograms, net price 20 = 23p; 600 micrograms, 20 = 41p. Label: 2
Injection, hyoscine hydrobromide 400 micrograms/ml, net price 1-ml amp = 74p; 600 micrograms/ml, 1-ml amp = 74p

METOCLOPRAMIDE HYDROCHLORIDE

Indications: adults, nausea and vomiting, particularly in gastro-intestinal disorders and treatment with cytotoxics or radiotherapy; gastro-intestinal—section 1.2; migraine—section 4.7.4.1

PATIENTS UNDER 20 YEARS. Use restricted to severe intractable vomiting of known cause, vomiting of radiotherapy and cytotoxics, aid to gastro-intestinal intubation, pre-medication

Cautions: renal impairment; caution in elderly, in young adults, and in children (measure dose accurately, preferably with a pipette); may mask underlying disorders such as cerebral irritation; avoid for 3–4 days following gastrointestinal surgery. Drug interactions: see Appendix 1 (sections *2.5, 4.2,* 4.6, *4.7, 4.9, 6.7*)

Side-effects: extrapyramidal (especially in children/young adults), hyperprolactinaemia, occasionally tardive dyskinesia on prolonged administration, may cause acute hypertensive response in phaeochromocytoma

Dose: by mouth, or by intramuscular or intravenous injection, 10 mg (5 mg in young adults 15–19 years under 60 kg) 3 times daily; CHILD up to 1 year 1 mg twice daily, 1–3 years 1 mg 2–3 times daily, 3–5 years 2 mg 2–3 times daily, 5–9 years 2.5 mg 3 times daily, 9–14 years 5 mg 3 times daily

Note. Daily dose of metoclopramide should not normally exceed 500 micrograms/kg, particularly for children and young adults (restricted use, see above)

For radiological examinations, as a single dose *by intramuscular or intravenous injection* 5–10 minutes before examination, 10–20 mg (10 mg in young adults 15–19 years); CHILD under 3 years 1 mg, 3–5 years 2 mg, 5–9 years 2.5 mg, 9–14 years 5 mg

By continuous intravenous infusion (preferred method), initially (before starting chemotherapy), 2–4 mg/kg over 15–30 minutes, then 3–5 mg/kg over 8–12 hours; max. in 24 hours, 10 mg/kg

By intermittent intravenous infusion, initially (before starting chemotherapy), up to 2 mg/kg over at least 15 minutes then up to 2 mg/kg over at least 15 minutes every 2 hours; max. in 24 hours, 10 mg/kg

PoM **Metoclopramide** (Non-proprietary)
Tablets, metoclopramide 10 mg, net price 20 = 43p
PoM **Maxolon**® (Beecham)
Tablets, scored, metoclopramide hydrochloride 10 mg. Net price 20 tabs = £1.77
Syrup, yellow, sugar-free, metoclopramide hydrochloride 5 mg/5 ml. Diluent purified water, freshly boiled and cooled, life of diluted syrup 14 days. Net price 100 ml = £1.52
Paediatric liquid, yellow, sugar-free, metoclopramide hydrochloride 1 mg/ml. Diluent as above. Net price 15 ml with pipette = £1.37. Counselling advised, use of pipette
Injection, metoclopramide hydrochloride 5 mg/ml. Net price 2-ml amp = 24p
▼ PoM **Maxolon High Dose**® (Beecham)
Injection, metoclopramide hydrochloride 5 mg/ml. Net price 20-ml amp = £2.43. For dilution and use as an intravenous infusion in nausea and vomiting associated with cytotoxic chemotherapy only
PoM **Metox**® (Steinhard)
Tablets, scored, metoclopramide hydrochloride 10 mg. Net price 20 = £1.71

PoM **Metramid**® (Nicholas)
Tablets, scored, metoclopramide hydrochloride 10 mg. Net price 20 = £1.03

PoM **Mygdalon**® (DDSA)
Tablets, scored, metoclopramide hydrochloride 10 mg. Net price 20 = 88p

PoM **Parmid**® (Lagap)
Tablets, scored, metoclopramide hydrochloride 10 mg. Net price 20 = 39p
Syrup, metoclopramide hydrochloride 5 mg/5 ml. Net price 100 ml = £1.05
Injection, metoclopramide hydrochloride 5 mg/ml. Net price 2-ml amp = 17p

PoM **Primperan**® (Berk)
Tablets, scored, metoclopramide hydrochloride 10 mg. Net price 20 = 97p
Syrup, lime, sugar-free, metoclopramide hydrochloride 5 mg/5 ml. Diluent syrup, life of diluted syrup 14 days. Net price 100 ml = £1.05
Injection, metoclopramide hydrochloride 5 mg/ml. Net price 2-ml amp = 17p

Sustained-release preparations
▼ PoM **Gastrobid Continus**® (Napp)
Tablets, s/r, metoclopramide hydrochloride 15 mg. Net price 28 = £4.03. Label: 25
Dose: patients over 20 years, 1 tablet twice daily
Caution: unsuitable for patients under 20 years
▼ PoM **Gastromax**® (Farmitalia Carlo Erba)
Capsules, s/r, orange/yellow, enclosing white to light beige pellets, metoclopramide hydrochloride 30 mg. Net price 28 = £11.20. Label: 22, 25
Dose: patients over 20 years, 1 capsule daily
Caution: unsuitable for patients under 20 years

NABILONE

Indications: nausea and vomiting caused by cytotoxic drugs
Cautions: may affect ability to drive or operate machinery and increase effects of alcohol; severe hepatic impairment; history of psychosis
Side-effects: drowsiness, postural hypotension, tachycardia, dry mouth, decreased appetite, abdominal cramps; also confusion, disorientation, euphoria, hallucinations, psychosis, depression, headache, blurred vision, tremors, decreased concentration and co-ordination
Dose: 1–2 mg twice daily throughout each cycle of cytotoxic therapy and, if necessary, for 24 hours after the last dose of each cycle; max. 6 mg daily. The first dose should be taken the night before initiation of cytotoxic treatment, and the second dose 1–3 hours before the first dose of cytotoxic drug

▼ PoM **Cesamet**® (Lilly)
Capsules, blue/white, nabilone 1 mg. Net price 20 = £35.29 (Hosp. only). Label: 2

PERPHENAZINE

Indications: severe nausea, vomiting (see notes above)
Cautions; Contra-indications; Side-effects: see section 4.2.1
Dose: by mouth, 2–4 mg 3 times daily, according to response; max. 24 mg daily (chemotherapy-induced)

By intramuscular injection, 5–10 mg initially, then 5 mg every 6 hours, max. 15 mg in 24 hours

Preparations
Section 4.2.1

PROCHLORPERAZINE

Indications: severe nausea, vomiting, vertigo, labyrinthine disorders, cytotoxic therapy (see notes above)
Cautions; Contra-indications: see under Chlorpromazine Hydrochloride (section 4.2.1). Avoid in children weighing less than 10 kg
Side-effects: dry mouth, drowsiness, which may affect the ability to drive or operate machinery or increase the CNS depressant effect of alcohol. Side-effects are rare with anti-emetic doses, but with high doses extrapyramidal symptoms may occur, particularly in children, elderly, and debilitated patients
Dose: by mouth, nausea and vomiting, prochlorperazine maleate or mesylate, acute attack, 20 mg initially then 10 mg after 2 hours; prevention 5–10 mg 2–3 times daily; CHILD (over 10 kg only) 250 micrograms/kg 2–3 times daily Labyrinthine disorders, 5 mg 3 times daily, gradually increased if necessary to 30 mg daily in divided doses, then reduced after several weeks to 5–10 mg daily
By deep intramuscular injection, 12.5 mg when required followed if necessary after 6 hours by an oral dose, as above
By rectum in suppositories, 25 mg followed if necessary after 6 hours by oral dose, as above

PoM **Stemetil**® (M&B)
Tablets, prochlorperazine maleate 5 mg (off-white), net price 20 = 62p; 25 mg (scored), 20 = £1.78. Label: 2
Syrup, straw-coloured, prochlorperazine mesylate 5 mg/5 ml. Diluent syrup, life of diluted syrup 14 days. Net price 100 ml = £1.46. Label: 2
Eff sachets, granules, effervescent, sugar-free, prochlorperazine mesylate 5 mg/sachet. Net price 21 sachets = £2.97. Label: 2, 13
Injection, prochlorperazine mesylate 12.5 mg/ml. Net price 1-ml amp = 31p; 2-ml amp = 39p
Suppositories, prochlorperazine maleate (as prochlorperazine), 5 mg, net price 10 = £4.00; 25 mg, 10 = £5.26; Label: 2

PoM **Vertigon**® (SK&F)
Spansule® (= capsules s/r), both clear/purple, enclosing yellowish-green and white pellets, prochlorperazine (as maleate), 10 mg, net price 20 = 75p; 15 mg, 20 = 91p. Label: 2, 25
Dose: initially 10–15 mg once or twice daily. Maintenance 10–15 mg daily

Buccal preparation
PoM **Buccastem**® (R&C)
Tablets (buccal), pale yellow, prochlorperazine maleate 3 mg. Net price 4 × 15-tab pack = £6.90. Label: 2, counselling advised, administration, see under Dose below

Dose: 1–2 tablets twice daily; tablets are placed high between upper lip and gum and left to dissolve

PROMETHAZINE HYDROCHLORIDE
Indications: nausea, vomiting, vertigo, labyrinthine disorders, motion sickness
Cautions; Side-effects: see under Cyclizine but more sedating; intramuscular injection may be painful
Dose: by mouth, 25–50 mg daily in single or divided doses; max. 75 mg
CHILD, motion sickness prevention, 1–5 years, 5 mg at night and following morning; 5–10 years, 10 mg at night and following morning
By deep intramuscular injection, 25–50 mg when necessary; CHILD 6–12 years 6.25–12.5 mg
By slow intravenous injection, section 3.4.1

Preparations
See section 3.4.1

PROMETHAZINE THEOCLATE
Indications: nausea, vertigo, labyrinthine disorders, motion sickness (acts longer than the hydrochloride)
Cautions; Side-effects: see under Cyclizine but more sedating
Dose: 25–75 mg, max. 100 mg, daily; CHILD 5–10 years 12.5–37.5 mg daily
Motion sickness prevention, 25 mg at bedtime on night before travelling *or* 25 mg 1–2 hours before travelling; CHILD 5–10 years half adult dose
For severe vomiting in pregnancy, 25 mg at bedtime, increased if necessary to a max. of 100 mg daily (but see also Vomiting of Pregnancy in notes above)

Avomine® (M&B)
Tablets, scored, promethazine theoclate 25 mg. Net price 10-tab pack = 30p. Label: 2

THIETHYLPERAZINE
Indications: severe nausea, vomiting, vertigo, labyrinthine disorders, cytotoxic therapy (see notes above)
Cautions; Contra-indications; Side-effects: see under Chlorpromazine Hydrochloride (section 4.2.1); young adults particularly susceptible to extrapyramidal effects; avoid in children under 15 years
Dose: by mouth, thiethylperazine maleate 10 mg 2–3 times daily
By intramuscular injection, thiethylperazine [base] 6.5 mg
By rectum in suppositories, thiethylperazine 6.5 mg night and morning
Note: Thiethylperazine 6.5 mg ≡ thiethylperazine maleate 10.86 mg ≡ thiethylperazine maleate 10.28 mg

PoM Torecan® (Sandoz)
Tablets, s/c, thiethylperazine *maleate* 10 mg. Net price 20 = 57p. Label: 2
Injection, thiethylperazine 6.5 mg (as *malate*)/ml. Net price 1-ml amp = 18p

Suppositories, thiethylperazine 6.5 mg (as *maleate*). Net price 6 = £1.09. Label: 2

TRIFLUOPERAZINE
Indications: severe nausea and vomiting (see notes above)
Cautions; Contra-indications; Side-effects: see section 4.2.1. Side-effects occur infrequently with anti-emetic doses
Dose: by mouth, 2–4 mg daily in divided doses *or* as a single dose of a sustained-release preparation; max. 6 mg daily; CHILD 3–5 years up to 1 mg daily, 6–12 years up to 4 mg daily
By deep intramuscular injection, 1–3 mg daily in divided doses

Preparations
Section 4.2.1

4.7 Analgesics
4.7.1 Non-opioid analgesics
4.7.1.1 Compound analgesic preparations
4.7.2 Opioid analgesics
4.7.3 Trigeminal neuralgia
4.7.4 Antimigraine drugs
4.7.4.1 Treatment of the acute migraine attack
4.7.4.2 Prophylaxis of migraine

Analgesic requirements may be profoundly affected by the attitude of both the patient and the prescriber to the pain; in many cases where analgesics might normally have been given, a placebo has provided substantial relief. For advice on pain relief in terminal care see Prescribing in Terminal Care, p. 13.

4.7.1 Non-opioid analgesics
The non-opioid drugs, aspirin and paracetamol, are particularly suited to the relief of pain in musculoskeletal conditions, whereas the opioid analgesics are more suited for the relief of severe pain of visceral origin.

Aspirin is the analgesic of choice for headache, transient musculoskeletal pain, and dysmenorrhoea. It also has anti-inflammatory properties which may be useful, and is an antipyretic. Aspirin tablets or dispersible aspirin tablets are adequate for most purposes as they act rapidly and are inexpensive.

Gastric irritation may be a problem; it is minimised by taking the dose after food. Numerous formulations are available which improve gastric tolerance, such as aloxiprin and enteric-coated aspirin (Nu-Seals®). Some of these preparations have a slow onset of action and are therefore unsuitable for single-dose analgesic use though their prolonged action may be useful for the relief of night pain.

Paracetamol is similar in efficacy to aspirin, but has no demonstrable anti-inflammatory activity; it is less irritant to the stomach. Overdosage with paracetamol is particularly dangerous as it may cause hepatic damage which is sometimes not apparent for 4 to 6 days. **Benorylate** is an aspirin–paracetamol ester which releases paracetamol slowly and so hepatotoxicity in overdosage may be reduced.

Nefopam (Acupan®) may have a place in the relief of persistent pain unresponsive to other non-opioid analgesics. It causes little or no respiratory depression, but sympathomimetic side-effects may be troublesome.

Anti-inflammatory analgesics (see section 10.1.1) are particularly useful for the treatment of patients with chronic disease accompanied by pain and inflammation. Some of them are also used in the short-term treatment of mild to moderate pain including transient musculoskeletal pain. They are also suitable for the relief of pain in *dysmenorrhoea* and to treat pain caused by *secondary bone tumours*, many of which produce lysis of bone and release prostaglandins (see Prescribing in Terminal Care, p. 13).

> **CSM advice.**
> The CSM has considered available evidence on possible links between Reye's syndrome and aspirin use by feverish children, and recommends that aspirin should no longer be given to children aged under 12 years, unless specifically indicated, e.g. for juvenile rheumatoid arthritis. It is therefore important to advise families that aspirin is not, on the evidence now available, a suitable medicine for children with minor illnesses. Paracetamol (see below) is an effective alternative treatment for fever in children.

ASPIRIN

Indications: mild to moderate pain, pyrexia (see notes above); see also section 10.1.1
Cautions: asthma, impaired renal or hepatic function, dehydration, pregnancy. Drug interactions: see Appendix 1 (sections *2.2, 2.8, 2.8E, 4.7, 4.8, 8, 10, 11*)
Contra-indications: children under 12 years and in breast-feeding (Reye's syndrome, see notes above); gastro-intestinal ulceration, haemophilia, concurrent anticoagulant therapy
Side-effects: generally mild and infrequent but high incidence of gastro-intestinal irritation with slight asymptomatic blood loss, increased bleeding time, bronchospasm and skin reactions in hypersensitive patients. Prolonged administration, see section 10.1.1
Dose: 300–900 mg every 4–6 hours when necessary; max. 4 g daily

Aspirin Tablets, aspirin 300 mg. Net price 20 = 8p. Label: 21
Aspirin Tablets, Dispersible, aspirin 300 mg. Net price 20 = 9p. Label: 13, 21
Note. From 1st December 1988 Soluble Aspirin Tablets BP will be the title of dispersible aspirin tablets which effervesce on addition of water
Aspirin Tablets, Dispersible, Low Dose, aspirin 75 mg. Net price 20 = 10p. Label: 13, 21
Note. For use as an antiplatelet drug (see section 2.9)
NHS Aspergum® (Plough)
Tablets, chewing gum, s/c, aspirin 227 mg. Net price 20 = 77p. Label: 21

Dose: 1–2 tablets chewed every 4–6 hours when necessary; max. 8 daily; CHILD 12–14 years up to 5 tablets daily
NHS Claradin® (Nicholas)
Tablets, effervescent, scored, aspirin 300 mg. Net price 20 = 27p. Label: 13, 21
NHS Laboprin® (LAB)
Tablets, mottled white/brown, aspirin 300 mg with lysine 245 mg. Net price 24 = £1.30. Label: 21
Palaprin Forte® (Nicholas)
Tablets, orange, scored, aloxiprin[1] 600 mg = aspirin 500 mg. To be taken dispersed in water, chewed, sucked, or swallowed whole. Net price 20 = 50p. Label: 12, 21
Dose: ½–2 tablets up to 4 times daily; max. 8 daily
[1] Aloxiprin is a polymeric condensation product of aluminium oxide and aspirin
NHS Paynocil® (Beecham)
Tablets, scored, aspirin 600 mg, glycine 300 mg. To be dissolved on the tongue. Net price 30 = 90p. Label: 21, 24
NHS Solprin® (R&C)
Tablets, dispersible, aspirin 300 mg. Net price 20 = 8p. Label: 13, 21

Preparations for intestinal release
Caprin® (Sinclair)
Tablets, s/r, pink, aspirin 324 mg (for intestinal release). Net price 20 = 42p. Label: 25
Dose: 1–4 tablets 3–4 times daily
Nu-Seals Aspirin® (Lilly)
Tablets, both red, e/c, aspirin 300 mg, net price 20 = 59p; 600 mg, 20 = £1.00. Label: 5, 25

Compound preparations, section 4.7.1.1

PARACETAMOL

Indications: mild to moderate pain, pyrexia
Cautions: hepatic impairment, alcoholism. Drug interactions: see Appendix 1 (section 4.7)
Side-effects: liver damage on prolonged use or overdosage
Dose: 0.5–1 g every 4–6 hours to a max. of 4 g daily; CHILD up to 1 year 60–120 mg, 1–5 years 120–250 mg, 6–12 years 250–500 mg; these doses may be repeated every 4–6 hours when necessary (max. of 4 doses in 24 hours)

Paracetamol (Non-proprietary)
Tablets, paracetamol 500 mg. Net price 20 = 9p. Label: 29
Soluble tablets (= Dispersible tablets), paracetamol 500 mg. Net price 12 = 24p. Label: 13, 29
Paediatric Elixir, paracetamol 120 mg/5 ml. Net price 100 ml = 47p
Note. Sugar-free versions are available and can be ordered by specifying 'sugar-free' on the prescription.
Oral Suspension 120 mg/5 ml (= Paediatric Mixture), paracetamol 120 mg/5 ml. Net price 100 ml = 43p
Note. BP 1988 (official from 1st December 1988) directs that when Paracetamol Paediatric Mixture is prescribed and no strength is stated Paracetamol Oral Suspension 120 mg/5 ml should be dispensed.

Oral Suspension 250 mg/5 ml (= Mixture), paracetamol 250 mg/5 ml. Net price 100 ml = 99p
Calpol® (Calmic)
Infant suspension, pink, paracetamol 120 mg/5 ml. Net price 100 ml = 80p
NHS *Six plus suspension*, orange, paracetamol 250 mg/5 ml. Net price 100 ml = 99p
Disprol® (R&C)
Paediatric suspension, yellow, sugar-free, paracetamol 120 mg/5 ml. Net price 100 ml = 43p
Paldesic® (RP Drugs)
Syrup, paracetamol 120 mg/5 ml. Net price 60 ml = 17p
Panadol® (Winthrop)
NHS *Caplets®* (= tablets), paracetamol 500 mg. Net price 20 = 44p. Label: 29
NHS *Tablets*, paracetamol 500 mg. Net price 20 = 18p. Label: 29
Elixir, red, sugar-free, paracetamol 120 mg/5 ml. Net price 60 ml = 43p
NHS **Panadol Soluble®** (Winthrop)
Tablets, effervescent, scored, paracetamol 500 mg. Net price 12 = 24p. Label: 13, 29
Panaleve® (Leo)
Elixir, yellow, sugar-free, paracetamol 120 mg/5 ml. Net price 100 ml = 70p
Salzone® (Wallace Mfg)
Syrup, paracetamol 120 mg/5 ml. Diluent syrup, life of diluted syrup 14 days. Net price 75 ml = 82p

With methionine
NHS ▼ **Pameton®** (Winthrop)
Tablets, paracetamol 500 mg, DL-methionine 250 mg. Net price 60-tab pack = £2.76. Label: 29
Dose: 2 tablets when required up to 4 times daily; CHILD 6–12 years ½–1 tablet when required; not more often than every 4 hours and max. of 4 doses in 24 hours

Compound preparations, section 4.7.1.1

BENORYLATE

(Aspirin-paracetamol ester)
Indications: mild to moderate pain; pyrexia; see also section 10.1.1
Cautions; Contra-indications; Side-effects: see under Aspirin and under Paracetamol. Side-effects resemble aspirin rather than paracetamol but tolerance is better and hepatotoxicity may be less than with paracetamol. Patients should be advised against taking analgesics containing aspirin or paracetamol
Note. Preparations containing aspirin are now contra-indicated in children under 12 years of age owing to an association with Reye's syndrome, see notes above
Dose: 1.5–2 g every 8 hours, preferably after food

Preparations
See section 10.1.1

DIFLUNISAL

Indications: mild to moderate pain; see also section 10.1.1

Cautions; Contra-indications; Side-effects: see section 10.1.1. Tablets should be swallowed whole
Dose: 250–500 mg twice daily preferably after food

Preparations
See section 10.1.1

FENOPROFEN

Indications: mild to moderate pain, pyrexia; see also section 10.1.1
Cautions; Contra-indications; Side-effects: See section 10.1.1
Dose: 200–400 mg 3–4 times daily, after food; max. 3 g daily

PoM **Progesic®** (Lilly)
Tablets, yellow, fenoprofen 200 mg (as calcium salt). Net price 20 = £1.84. Label: 21
Fenopron: see section 10.1.1

IBUPROFEN

Indications: mild to moderate pain; see also section 10.1.1
Cautions; Side-effects: see section 10.1.1
Dose: 1.2–1.8 g daily in divided doses, preferably after food, increased if necessary to a max. of 2.4 g daily; CHILD, see section 10.1.1

Preparations
See section 10.1.1

MEFENAMIC ACID

Indications: mild to moderate pain, pyrexia in children; menorrhagia; see also section 10.1.1
Cautions; Contra-indications; Side-effects: see section 10.1.1; exclude pathological conditions before treating menorrhagia
Dose: 500 mg 3 times daily after food; CHILD over 6 months 25 mg/kg daily in divided doses for not longer than 7 days, except in juvenile chronic arthritis (Still's disease)

Preparations
See section 10.1.1

NAPROXEN SODIUM

Indications: mild to moderate pain; see also Naproxen, section 10.1.1
Cautions; Side-effects: see section 10.1.1
Dose: 550 mg initially, then 275 mg 6–8 hourly when necessary, preferably after food
Note. 275 mg naproxen sodium ≡ 250 mg naproxen but the sodium salt has a more rapid action

Naprosyn: see section 10.1.1
PoM **Synflex®** (Syntex)
Tablets, orange, naproxen sodium 275 mg. Net price 20 = £2.22. Label: 21

NEFOPAM HYDROCHLORIDE

Indications: moderate pain
Cautions: hepatic disease, glaucoma, urinary retention

Contra-indications: convulsive disorders, myocardial infarction

Side-effects: nausea, nervousness, insomnia, dry mouth; less frequently blurred vision, drowsiness, sweating, tachycardia, headache, may colour urine

Dose: by mouth, initially 60 mg 3 times daily, adjusted according to response; usual range 30–90 mg 3 times daily

By intramuscular injection, 20 mg every 6 hours

Note. Nefopam hydrochloride 20 mg by injection ≡ 60 mg by mouth

▼ PoM **Acupan®** (Riker)

Tablets, f/c, nefopam hydrochloride 30 mg. Net price 20 = £2.97. Label: 14

Injection, nefopam hydrochloride 20 mg/ml. Net price 1-ml amp = 85p

4.7.1.1 COMPOUND ANALGESIC PREPARATIONS

Compound analgesic preparations of, for example, aspirin, paracetamol, and codeine are **not** recommended. Single-ingredient preparations should be prescribed in preference because compound preparations rarely have any advantage; they may increase the cost of treatment unnecessarily and complicate the treatment of overdosage. The dangers of co-proxamol (dextropropoxyphene-paracetamol) overdosage are described in section 4.7.2.

It is even more desirable to **avoid** mixtures of analgesics with laxatives, antihistamines, or hypnotics; the individual components should be prescribed separately so that the dose of each can be adjusted as appropriate.

Analgesic preparations containing muscle relaxants are discussed in section 10.2.2.

Caffeine is a weak stimulant that is often included, in small doses, in analgesic preparations. It does not contribute to the analgesic or anti-inflammatory effect of the preparation and may possibly aggravate the gastric irritation caused by aspirin. Moreover, in excessive dosage or on withdrawal caffeine may itself induce headache.

NEW NAMES FOR COMPOUND ANALGESICS. Following the exclusion of certain proprietary analgesics from NHS prescribing the following approved names have been adopted:

Co-codamol Compounded preparations of codeine phosphate and paracetamol in the proportions 2 parts to 125 parts

Co-codaprin Compounded preparations of codeine phosphate and aspirin in the proportions 1 part to 50 parts

Co-dydramol Compounded preparations of dihydrocodeine tartrate and paracetamol in the proportions 1 part to 50 parts

Co-proxamol Compounded preparations of dextropropoxyphene hydrochloride and paracetamol in the proportions 1 part to 10 parts

Aspirin, Paracetamol, and Codeine Tablets, aspirin 250 mg, paracetamol 250 mg, codeine phosphate 6.8 mg. Net price 20 = 60p. Label: 21, 29

Dose: 1–2 tablets every 4–6 hours when necessary

Co-codamol Tablets and **Dispersible Tablets.** When co-codamol tablets or dispersible tablets are prescribed and no strength is stated tablets, or dispersible tablets, respectively, containing codeine phosphate 8 mg and paracetamol 500 mg should be dispensed. Net price, co-codamol tablets, 20 = 28p; dispersible tablets, 20 = 45p. Label: co-codamol tablets, 29; dispersible tablets, 13, 29

Dose: 1–2 tablets every 4–6 hours when necessary; max. 8 tablets daily

Co-codaprin Tablets and **Dispersible Tablets.** When co-codaprin tablets or dispersible tablets are prescribed and no strength is stated tablets, or dispersible tablets, respectively, containing aspirin 400 mg and codeine phosphate 8 mg should be dispensed. Net price co-codaprin tablets, 20 = 24p; dispersible tablets, 20 = 31p. Label: co-codaprin tablets, 21; dispersible tablets, 13, 21

Dose: 1–2 tablets every 4–6 hours when necessary; max. 8 tablets daily

PoM **Co-dydramol Tablets.** When co-dydramol tablets are prescribed and no strength is stated tablets containing dihydrocodeine tartrate 10 mg and paracetamol 500 mg should be dispensed. Net price 20 = 33p. Label: 21, 29

Dose: 1–2 tablets every 4–6 hours when necessary; max. 8 tablets daily

PoM **Co-proxamol Tablets.** When co-proxamol tablets are prescribed and no strength is stated tablets containing dextropropoxyphene hydrochloride 32.5 mg and paracetamol 325 mg should be dispensed. Net price 20 = 28p. Label: 2, 10 patient information leaflet, 29

Dose: 2 tablets 3–4 times daily; max. 8 tablets daily

NHS **Antoin®** (Cox Pharmaceuticals)

Dispersible tablets, scored, aspirin 400 mg, codeine phosphate 5 mg, caffeine citrate 15 mg. Net price 20 = 44p. Label: 13, 21

Dose: 1–2 tablets in water 3–4 times daily; max. 10 tablets daily

PoM **Aspav®** (Cox Pharmaceuticals)

Dispersible tablets, aspirin 500 mg, papaveretum 10 mg. Net price 20 = £1.15. Label: 13, 21

Dose: 1–2 tablets in water every 4–6 hours if necessary; max. 8 tablets daily

NHS **Cafadol®** (Typharm)

Tablets, yellow, scored, paracetamol 500 mg, caffeine 30 mg. Net price 20 = 38p. Label: 29

Dose: 2 tablets every 3–4 hours, max. 8 tablets daily; CHILD 5–12 years 1 tablet

NHS **Codis®** (R&C)

Dispersible tablets, co-codaprin 408 mg (codeine phosphate 8 mg, aspirin 400 mg). Net price 20 = 28p. Label: 13, 21

Dose: 1–2 tablets in water every 4 hours, max. 8 tablets daily

NHS PoM **Distalgesic®** (Dista)

Tablets, f/c, co-proxamol 357.5 mg (dextropropoxyphene hydrochloride 32.5 mg, paracetamol 325 mg). Net price 20 = 28p. Label: 2, 10 patient information leaflet, 29

Dose: 2 tablets 3–4 times daily; max. 8 tablets daily

NHS CD **Equagesic®** (Wyeth)

Tablets, pink/white/yellow, ethoheptazine citrate 75 mg, meprobamate 150 mg, aspirin 250 mg. Net price 20 = 46p. Label: 2, 21

Dose: muscle pain, 1–2 tablets 3–4 times daily

NHS **Femerital®** (MCP)

Tablets, scored, ambucetamide 100 mg, paracetamol 250 mg. Net price 20 = 46p. Label: 29

Dose: dysmenorrhoea, 1–2 tablets 3 times daily starting 2 days before menstruation

NHS **Hypon®** (Calmic)
Tablets, yellow, aspirin 325 mg, caffeine 10 mg, codeine phosphate 5 mg. Net price 20 = 39p. Label: 21
Dose: 2 tablets every 4 hours, max. 12 tablets daily

NHS PoM **Lobak®** (Sterling Research)
Tablets, scored, chlormezanone 100 mg, paracetamol 450 mg. Net price 20 = £2.79. Label: 2, 29
Dose: muscle pain, 1–2 tablets 3 times daily, max. 8 tablets daily

NHS **Medised®** (Martindale, tabs; Panpharma, susp)
Tablets, scored, paracetamol 500 mg, promethazine hydrochloride 10 mg. Net price 12 = 60p. Label: 2, 29
Dose: 2 tablets (usually at night), repeated if necessary every 4 hours; max. 8 tablets daily
Suspension (= mixture), paracetamol 120 mg, promethazine hydrochloride 2.5 mg/5 ml. Net price 140 ml = £1.04. Label: 1
Note. The doses recommended by the manufacturer have been excluded because the combination is not recommended

NHS **Medocodene®** (Medo)
Tablets, yellow, scored, co-codamol 508 mg (paracetamol 500 mg, codeine phosphate 8 mg). Net price 20 = 46p. Label: 29
Dose: 1–2 tablets every 4 hours, max. 8 tablets daily; CHILD 6–12 years ½–1 tablet

NHS **Neurodyne®** (Fisons)
Capsules, co-codamol 508 mg (paracetamol 500 mg, codeine phosphate 8 mg). Net price 20 = 70p. Label: 29
Dose: 1–2 capsules every 4 hours, max. 8 capsules daily

NHS PoM **Norgesic®** (Riker)
Tablets, scored, orphenadrine citrate 35 mg, paracetamol 450 mg. Net price 20 = 72p. Label: 29
Dose: muscle pain, 2 tablets 3 times daily

NHS **Panadeine®** (Winthrop)
Tablets, scored, co-codamol 508 mg (codeine phosphate 8 mg, paracetamol 500 mg). Net price 20 = 43p. Label: 29
Dose: 2 tablets up to 4 times daily; CHILD 7–12 years ½–1 tablet

NHS **Panadeine Soluble®** (Winthrop)
Effervescent tablets, co-codamol 508 mg (codeine phosphate 8 mg, paracetamol 500 mg). Net price 20 = 42p. Label: 13, 29
Dose: 2 tablets in water up to 4 times daily; CHILD 7–12 years ½–1 tablet

NHS **Paracodol®** (Fisons)
Effervescent tablets, co-codamol 508 mg (paracetamol 500 mg, codeine phosphate 8 mg). Net price 20 = 51p. Label: 13, 29
Dose: 1–2 tablets in water every 4–6 hours, max. 8 tablets daily; CHILD 6–12 years ½–1 tablet, max. 4 tablets daily

NHS **Parahypon®** (Calmic)
Tablets, pink, scored, paracetamol 500 mg, codeine phosphate 5 mg, caffeine 10 mg. Net price 20 = 68p. Label: 29
Dose: 2 tablets up to 4 times daily; CHILD 6–12 years 1 tablet up to 4 times daily

NHS **Parake®** (Galen)
Tablets, co-codamol 508 mg (paracetamol 500 mg, codeine phosphate 8 mg). Net price 20 = 28p. Label: 29
Dose: 2 tablets every 4 hours, max. 8 tablets daily

NHS PoM **Paramol®** (DF)
Tablets, scored, co-dydramol 510 mg (paracetamol 500 mg, dihydrocodeine tartrate 10 mg). Net price 20 = 33p. Label: 21, 29
Dose: 1 tablet every 4 hours, max. 8 tablets daily

NHS **Pardale®** (Martindale)
Tablets, scored, paracetamol 400 mg, codeine phosphate 9 mg, caffeine hydrate 10 mg. Net price 20 = 73p. Label: 29
Dose: 1–2 tablets 3–4 times daily, max. 8 tablets daily

NHS **Pharmidone®** (Farmitalia Carlo Erba)
Tablets, yellow, scored, codeine phosphate 10 mg,

diphenhydramine hydrochloride 5 mg, paracetamol 400 mg, caffeine 50 mg. Net price 12 = 48p. Label: 2, 29
Dose: 1–2 tablets every 4 hours, max. 8 tablets daily

NHS **Propain®** (Panpharma)
Tablets, yellow, scored, codeine phosphate 10 mg, diphenhydramine hydrochloride 5 mg, paracetamol 400 mg, caffeine 50 mg. Net price 20 = 96p. Label: 2, 29
Dose: 1–2 tablets every 4 hours, max. 8 tablets daily

NHS PoM **Robaxisal Forte®** (Robins)
Tablets, pink/white, scored, methocarbamol 400 mg, aspirin 325 mg. Net price 20 = £1.15. Label: 2, 21
Dose: muscle pain, 2 tablets 4 times daily

NHS **Solpadeine®** (Sterling Research)
Effervescent tablets, paracetamol 500 mg, codeine phosphate 8 mg, caffeine 30 mg. Contains 18.5 mmol Na$^+$/tablet; avoid in renal impairment. Net price 20 = 73p. Label: 13, 29
Dose: 2 tablets in water 3–4 times daily; CHILD 7–12 years ½–1 tablet

NHS **Syndol®** (Merrell)
Tablets, yellow, scored, paracetamol 450 mg, codeine phosphate 10 mg, doxylamine succinate 5 mg, caffeine 30 mg. Net price 20 = £1.15. Label: 2, 29
Dose: 1–2 tablets every 4–6 hours, max. 8 tablets daily

NHS **Unigesic®** (Unimed)
Capsules, grey/yellow, paracetamol 500 mg, caffeine 30 mg. Net price 20 = £2.00. Label: 29
Dose: 1–2 capsules every 4 hours, max. 8 capsules daily

NHS **Veganin®** (W-L)
Tablets, scored, aspirin 250 mg, paracetamol 250 mg, codeine phosphate 6.8 mg. Net price 20 = 60p. Label: 21, 29
Dose: 1–2 tablets every 3–4 hours, max. 8 tablets daily

HIGHER OPIOID CONTENT

The following preparations have a higher opioid analgesic content than most compound analgesic preparations. For cautions and side-effects, see section 4.7.2.

NHS PoM **Doloxene Compound®** (Lilly)
Capsules, grey/red, dextropropoxyphene napsylate 100 mg, aspirin 375 mg, caffeine 30 mg. Net price 20 = £1.12. Label: 2, 21
Dose: 1 capsule 3–4 times daily; max. 4 capsules daily

NHS CD **Fortagesic®** (Sterling Research)
Tablets, pentazocine 15 mg (as hydrochloride), paracetamol 500 mg. Net price 20 = £1.40. Label: 2, 21, 29
Dose: 2 tablets up to 4 times daily; CHILD 7–12 years 1 tablet every 4 hours, max. 4 tablets daily

NHS PoM **Panadeine Forte®** (Winthrop)
Tablets, red, f/c, codeine phosphate 15 mg, paracetamol 500 mg. Net price 20 = 87p. Label: 2, 29
Dose: 2 tablets up to 4 times daily

PoM **Tylex®** (Ortho-Cilag)
Capsules, paracetamol 500 mg, codeine phosphate 30 mg. Net price 100 = £7.95. Label: 2
Dose: 1–2 capsules every 4 hours; max. 6 daily

4.7.2 Opioid analgesics

Opioid analgesics (narcotic analgesics) are used to relieve moderate to severe pain particularly of visceral origin. When used for acute pain repeated administration may cause dependence and tolerance. However, this is no deterrent in the control of pain in terminal illness, for guidelines see Prescribing in Terminal Care, p. 13.

CAUTIONS. In general all opioid analgesics should be used with caution, if at all, in patients taking monoamine-oxidase inhibitors and those with hypotension, hypothyroidism, asthma, decreased respiratory reserve, hepatic and renal impairment, and during pregnancy and breast-feeding. They should be prescribed with caution in patients with a history of drug abuse; there is an increasing problem of drug abuse with dextropropoxyphene compound preparations (co-proxamol). They should also be avoided in patients with raised intracranial pressure or head injury since, in addition to interfering with respiration, they affect pupillary responses, vital for neurological assessment. Dosage should be reduced in elderly and debilitated patients. In the control of pain in terminal illness, these cautions should not necessarily be a deterrent to the use of opioid analgesics.

SIDE-EFFECTS. Opioid analgesics share many side-effects though qualitative and quantitative differences exist. They all cause constipation (by reduction of intestinal motility), respiratory depression, cough suppression, urinary retention, nausea, and tolerance, and are all liable to cause dependence. They may also cause drowsiness. Injections may cause local pain and tissue damage.

CHOICE. **Morphine** remains the most valuable opioid analgesic for severe pain although it frequently causes nausea and vomiting. It may also confer a state of euphoria and mental detachment. Morphine is the standard against which other opioid analgesics are compared.

The initial dose depends largely on the patient's previous treatment. To replace a weak opioid analgesic, 5–10 mg of morphine should be prescribed, for an intermediate one, 10 mg, and for a strong one, 20 mg or more. If the first dose of morphine is no more effective than the previous medicine it should be increased by 50%. MST Continus® is a slow-release preparation which can be given twice daily. The starting dose is usually 10 to 20 mg twice daily, but the dose can be increased (maintaining the twice daily administration) until pain control is achieved.

Concurrent administration of small doses of phenothiazine derivatives (section 4.6) reduces the tendency to nausea and vomiting. Preparations containing morphine with an anti-emetic such as cyclizine (Cyclimorph®) are available but are not recommended as overdosage of the anti-emetic may result when they are used in regular regimens in terminal care.

Morphine is often formulated as an elixir for oral use (see below).

Mixed opium alkaloids such as **papaveretum** (see section 15.1.4.1) do not appear to have any advantage over morphine.

Buprenorphine (Temgesic®) is suitable for sublingual or parenteral use but like pentazocine has both opioid agonist and antagonist properties and may precipitate withdrawal symptoms, including pain, in patients dependent on other opioids. It has a much longer duration of action than morphine and sublingually is an effective analgesic for 8 to 12 hours. Vomiting may be a problem but it is thought to have a low dependence potential. Unlike most opioid analgesics its

effects are only partially reversed by naloxone but doxapram (Dopram®) may be used to reverse profound respiratory depression.

Codeine is used for the relief of mild to moderate pain but is too constipating for long-term use.

Dextromoramide (Palfium®) and **dipipanone** are less sedating than morphine and have a short duration of action. Diconal® is the only preparation of dipipanone available; like Cyclimorph® (above) it contains an anti-emetic and is therefore not suitable for regular regimens in terminal care.

Dextropropoxyphene given alone is a very mild analgesic and is somewhat less potent than codeine. Combinations of dextropropoxyphene and paracetamol (co-proxamol) or aspirin have a more powerful effect. However the chief disadvantage of combinations with paracetamol is that overdosage, which may be deliberate and combined with alcohol, is complicated by respiratory depression and acute heart failure due to dextropropoxyphene and hepatotoxicity due to paracetamol. Rapid treatment, as described under Emergency Treatment of Poisoning, is essential.

Diamorphine (heroin) is a powerful opioid analgesic. It is more likely to produce euphoria and addiction than morphine but causes relatively less nausea, constipation, and hypotension. The greater solubility of diamorphine hydrochloride allows effective doses to be injected in smaller volumes and this is important in the emaciated patient. In the case of mixtures for oral use those containing morphine are now preferred (see below).

Dihydrocodeine (DF 118®) is similar in potency to codeine. It is suitable for use in ambulant patients with moderate pain but may cause dizziness and constipation. It may be given by mouth or by injection. A slow-release preparation of dihydrocodeine (DHC Continus®) which can be given twice daily is now available.

Meptazinol (Meptid®) is claimed to have a low incidence of respiratory depression. It has a reported length of action of 2 to 7 hours with onset within 15 minutes, but there is an incidence of nausea and vomiting.

Methadone (Physeptone®) and **levorphanol** (Dromoran®) are less sedating than morphine and act for longer periods. In prolonged use, methadone should not be administered more often than twice daily to avoid the risk of accumulation and narcotic overdosage.

Nalbuphine (Nubain®) is a new analgesic equipotent with morphine for pain relief, but which may have fewer side-effects and less abuse potential. Nausea and vomiting occur less than with other narcotics but respiratory depression is similar to that with morphine.

Oxycodone is used as the pectinate in suppositories (special order, Boots) for the control of moderate to severe pain in terminal care.

Pentazocine (Fortral®) has both agonist and antagonist properties and should be avoided in patients dependent on other opioid analgesics as withdrawal symptoms including pain may be precipitated. By injection it is more potent than di-hydrocodeine or codeine, but hallucinations and thought disturbances may occur. It should be avoided after myocardial infarction as it may increase pulmonary and aortic blood pressure as well as cardiac work.

Pethidine produces a prompt but short-lasting analgesia and even in high doses it is a less potent analgesic than morphine. It is unsuitable for the relief of pain in terminal disease. It is used for analgesia in labour; in the neonate it is associated with less respiratory depression than other opioid analgesics probably because its pharmacological actions are, in general, weaker. See also section 15.1.4.1 (peri-operative use).

Phenazocine (Narphen®) is also effective in severe pain. It is particularly useful in biliary colic as it has less tendency to increase biliary pressure than other opioid analgesics. It may be administered sublingually if nausea and vomiting are a problem.

Diphenoxylate (with atropine as Lomotil®) is discussed in section 1.4.2. **Fentanyl** (Sublimaze®) and **phenoperidine** (Operidine®) are discussed in section 15.1.4.

ADDICTS. Although caution is necessary addicts (and ex-addicts) may be treated with analgesics in the same way as other people when there is a real clinical need. Doctors are reminded that they do not require a special licence to prescribe opioid analgesics for addicts for relief of pain due to organic disease or injury. For details, see p. 7.

MORPHINE SALTS

Indications: see notes above; acute pulmonary oedema; see also section 15.1.4 for peri-operative use

Cautions; Contra-indications; Side-effects: see notes above. Drug interactions: see Appendix 1 (sections *2.3, 4.1, 4.3, 4.6*)

Dose: acute pain, *by subcutaneous or intramuscular injection,* 10 mg every 4 hours if necessary (15 mg for heavier well-muscled patients); CHILD up to 1 month 150 micrograms/kg, 1–12 months 200 micrograms/kg, 1–5 years 2.5–5 mg, 6–12 years 5–10 mg

By slow intravenous injection, ¼–½ corresponding intramuscular dose

Myocardial infarction, *by slow intravenous injection* (2 mg/minute), 10 mg followed by a further 5–10 mg if necessary; elderly or frail patients, reduce dose by half

Acute pulmonary oedema, *by slow intravenous injection* (2 mg/minute) 5–10 mg

Chronic pain, *by mouth or by subcutaneous or intramuscular injection,* 5–20 mg regularly every 4 hours; dose may be increased according to needs; oral dose should be approximately double corresponding intramuscular dose and triple to quadruple corresponding intramuscular *diamorphine* dose (see also Prescribing in Terminal Care, p. 13); *by rectum,* as suppositories, 15–30 mg equally every 4 hours
Note. The doses stated above refer equally to morphine hydrochloride, sulphate, and tartrate

CD **Morphine Sulphate Injection,** morphine sulphate 10, 15, and 30 mg/ml, net price 1- and 2-ml amp (all) = 35–62p

CD **Morphine Suppositories,** morphine hydrochloride or sulphate 15 mg, net price 12 suppos = £3.52; 30 mg, 12 = £5.51. Label: 2.
Note. Both the strength of the suppositories and the morphine salt contained in them must be specified by the prescriber

CD **Opium Tincture,** morphine 1% (10 mg/ml). Net price 10 ml = 27p. Label: 2
Dose: 1–2 ml; CHILD 1–5 years 0.25–0.5 ml, 6–12 years 0.5–1 ml

CD **Cyclimorph-10®** (Calmic)
Injection, morphine tartrate 10 mg, cyclizine tartrate 50 mg/ml. Net price 1-ml amp = 78p
Dose: by subcutaneous, intramuscular, or intravenous injection, 1 ml, repeated not more often than 4-hourly, with not more than 3 doses in any 24-hour period; CHILD 1–5 years 0.25–0.5 ml as a single dose, 6–12 years 0.5–1 ml as a single dose

CD **Cyclimorph-15®** (Calmic)
Injection, morphine tartrate 15 mg, cyclizine tartrate 50 mg/ml. Net price 1-ml amp = 81p
Dose: by subcutaneous, intramuscular, or intravenous injection, 1 ml, repeated not more often than 4-hourly, with not more than 3 doses in any 24-hour period

CD **Duromorph®** (LAB)
Injection, s/r, morphine 64 mg/ml (aqueous suspension). Net price 1-ml amp = £1.25
Dose: by subcutaneous or intramuscular injection, in terminal pain, 1–1.5 ml every 9 hours

CD **MST Continus®** (Napp)
Tablets, s/r, brown, f/c, morphine sulphate 10 mg. Net price 20 = £2.57. Label: 2, 25
Tablets, s/r, purple, f/c, morphine sulphate 30 mg. Net price 20 = £6.16. Label: 2, 25
Tablets, s/r, orange, f/c, morphine sulphate 60 mg. Net price 20 = £12.02. Label: 2, 25
Tablets, s/r, grey, f/c, morphine sulphate 100 mg. Net price 20 = £19.03. Label: 2, 25
Dose: initially 10–20 mg twice daily, adjusted according to response
Note. Must be prescribed as 'MST Continus Tablets'.

CD **Nepenthe** (Evans)
Oral solution (= elixir), brown, anhydrous morphine 8.4 mg/ml (500 micrograms from opium tincture, 7.9 mg from morphine). Diluent syrup, life of diluted elixir 4 weeks. Net price 100 ml = £9.11. Label: 2
Dose: 1–2 ml, repeated not more often than every 4 hours when necessary; CHILD 6–12 years 0.5–1 ml, as a single dose
Note. This product must always be diluted when being dispensed.
CAUTION. *Nepenthe Oral Solution may become concentrated through evaporation of the solvent. It should be stored in a cool place in the original airtight container. If evaporation occurs during storage the solution should not be used because of risk of overdosage.*
Injection, anhydrous morphine 8.4 mg/ml (500 micrograms from papaveretum, 7.9 mg from morphine hydrochloride). Net price 0.5-ml amp = 99p
Dose: by subcutaneous or intramuscular injection, 1–2 ml, repeated not more often than every 4 hours when necessary; CHILD 6–12 years 0.5–1 ml as a single dose

PoM **Oramorph®** (Boehringer Ingelheim)
Oral solution, morphine sulphate 10 mg/5 ml.

Diluent freshly boiled and cooled purified water, life of diluted solution 14 days. Net price 100 ml = £2.31; 500 ml = £9.24. Label: 2

CD *Concentrated oral solution*, sugar-free, morphine sulphate 100 mg/5 ml. Net price 30 ml = £6.16; 120 ml = £23.00 (both with calibrated dropper). Label: 2

MORPHINE ANALGESIC ELIXIRS

Those containing diamorphine are also included here.

Both **morphine** and **diamorphine** are suitable for oral use in the relief of pain in terminal care; morphine is now preferred (see Prescribing in Terminal Care, p. 13).

Simple Elixirs

Simple elixirs of **morphine** or **diamorphine** should be prescribed by writing the formula in full, for example:

Morphine hydrochloride 5 mg
Chloroform water to 5 ml

Note. The total quantity of preparation to be supplied should be added in both words and figures, together with the other details required for controlled drug prescriptions (see Controlled Drugs and Drug Dependence, p. 7). It is usual to adjust the strength so that the dose volume is 5 or 10 ml. These simple elixirs are now generally preferred to the traditional compound elixirs given below.

Compound Elixirs

These are the traditional 'Brompton Cocktail' elixirs and are no longer recommended.

CD Diamorphine and Cocaine Elixir (see Formulary). Net price 100 ml = £1.66. Label: 2
CD Diamorphine, Cocaine, and Chlorpromazine Elixir (see Formulary). Net price 100 ml = £1.69. Label: 2
* **Morphine and Cocaine Elixir** (see Formulary). Net price 100 ml = £1.61. Label: 2
* **Morphine, Cocaine, and Chlorpromazine Elixir** (see Formulary). Net price 100 ml = £1.64. Label: 2
*PoM or CD according to cocaine and morphine content.

BUPRENORPHINE

Indications: moderate to severe pain
Cautions; Contra-indications; Side-effects: see notes above, but side-effects are less marked than for morphine, the risk of dependence is lower, and it may give rise to mild withdrawal symptoms in cases of opioid dependence. Commonest side-effects are drowsiness, nausea, vomiting, dizziness, and sweating; rarely respiratory depression. Effects only partially reversed by naloxone. Drug interactions: see Appendix 1 (sections *2.3, 4.1, 4.3, 4.6*)
Dose: by sublingual administration, initially 200 micrograms every 8 hours, increasing if necessary to 200–400 micrograms every 6–8 hours
By intramuscular or slow intravenous injection, 300–600 micrograms every 6–8 hours

PoM **Temgesic**® (R&C)
Tablets (sublingual), buprenorphine 200 micrograms (as hydrochloride). Net price 20 = £2.40. Label: 2, 26

Injection, buprenorphine 300 micrograms (as hydrochloride)/ml. Net price 1-ml amp = 55p; 2-ml amp = 99p

CODEINE PHOSPHATE

Indications: mild to moderate pain
Cautions: see notes above; avoid in children under 1 year. In therapeutic doses codeine is less liable than morphine to produce adverse effects. Drug interactions: see Appendix 1 (sections *2.3, 4.1, 4.3, 4.6*)
Contra-indications: respiratory depression
Side-effects: tolerance and dependence, particularly on injection, sedation, dizziness, nausea, constipation; may enhance the effects of alcohol
Dose: by mouth, 30–60 mg every 4 hours when necessary, to a max. of 200 mg daily; CHILD 1–12 years, 3 mg/kg daily in divided doses
By intramuscular injection, up to 30 mg when necessary

PoM **Codeine Phosphate Tablets**, codeine phosphate 15 mg, net price 20 = 38p; 30 mg, 20 = 39p; 60 mg, 20 = £1.22. Label: 2
Note. As for schedule 2 controlled drugs, travellers needing to take codeine phosphate preparations abroad may require a doctor's letter explaining why they are necessary.

Codeine Phosphate Syrup, codeine phosphate 25 mg/5 ml. Net price 100 ml = 76p. Label: 2
CD Codeine Phosphate Injection, codeine phosphate 60 mg/ml. Net price 1-ml amp = 84p
Compound preparations, section 4.7.1.1

DEXTROMORAMIDE

Indications: severe pain, particularly exacerbations in terminal disease
Cautions; Contra-indications; Side-effects: see notes above; less sedating than morphine and development of tolerance and dependence slower; only short duration of action (2–3 hours); avoid in obstetric analgesia (increased risk of neonatal depression). Drug interactions: see Appendix 1 (sections *2.3, 4.1, 4.3, 4.6*)
Dose: by mouth, 5 mg increasing to 20 mg, when required
By subcutaneous or intramuscular injection, 5 mg increasing to 15 mg, when required
By rectum in suppositories, 10 mg when required

CD Palfium® (MCP)
Tablets, both scored, dextromoramide (as tartrate) 5 mg, net price 20 = £1.59; 10 mg (peach), 20 = £3.15. Label: 2
Injection, dextromoramide 5 mg (as tartrate)/ml. Net price 1-ml amp = 20p
Injection, dextromoramide 10 mg (as tartrate)/ml. Net price 1-ml amp = 24p
Suppositories, dextromoramide 10 mg (as tartrate). Net price 10 = £2.35. Label: 2

DEXTROPROPOXYPHENE HYDROCHLORIDE

Indications: mild to moderate pain

Cautions: see notes above and under Codeine Phosphate. Drug interactions: see Appendix 1 (sections *2.8C*, *4.8*); see also under Codeine Phosphate

Side-effects: see under Codeine Phosphate; with daily doses above 720 mg toxic psychoses and convulsions may occur; CSM reports occasional hepatotoxicity

Dose: 65 mg every 6–8 hours when necessary
Note. 65 mg dextropropoxyphene hydrochloride = 100 mg dextropropoxyphene napsylate

PoM **Dextropropoxyphene Capsules,** the equivalent of dextropropoxyphene hydrochloride 65 mg (as napsylate). Net price 20 = 99p. Label: 2

NHS PoM **Doloxene**® (Lilly)
Capsules, orange, the equivalent of dextropropoxyphene hydrochloride 65 mg (as napsylate). Net price 20 = 99p. Label: 2

DIAMORPHINE HYDROCHLORIDE

Indications: see notes above; acute pulmonary oedema

Cautions; Contra-indications; Side-effects: see notes above but more potent than morphine. Drug interactions: see Appendix 1 (sections *2.3, 4.1, 4.3, 4.6*)

Dose: acute pain, *by subcutaneous or intramuscular injection*, 5 mg repeated every 4 hours if necessary (up to 10 mg for heavier well-muscled patients)

By slow intravenous injection, $\frac{1}{4}$–$\frac{1}{2}$ corresponding intramuscular dose

Myocardial infarction, *by slow intravenous injection* (1 mg/minute), 5 mg followed by a further 2.5–5 mg if necessary; elderly or frail patients, reduce dose by half

Acute pulmonary oedema, *by slow intravenous injection* (1 mg/minute) 2.5–5 mg

Chronic pain, *by mouth or by subcutaneous or intramuscular injection*, 5–10 mg regularly every 4 hours; dose may be increased according to needs; intramuscular dose should be approximately $\frac{1}{2}$ corresponding oral dose, and $\frac{1}{4}$–$\frac{1}{3}$ corresponding oral *morphine* dose; see also Prescribing in Terminal Care, p. 13

CD **Diamorphine Tablets,** diamorphine hydrochloride 10 mg (for oral administration). Net price 20 = 91p. Label: 2

CD **Diamorphine Injection,** powder for reconstitution, diamorphine hydrochloride. Net price 5-mg amp = 85p, 10-mg amp = 98p, 30-mg amp = £1.12, 100-mg amp = £3.49, 500-mg amp = £16.60

Diamorphine Analgesic Elixirs
See under Morphine Salts

DIHYDROCODEINE TARTRATE

Indications: moderate to severe pain
Cautions; Side-effects: see notes above and under Codeine Phosphate

Dose: by mouth, 30 mg every 4–6 hours when necessary, after food; CHILD over 4 years 0.5–1 mg/kg

By deep subcutaneous or intramuscular injection, up to 50 mg every 4–6 hours

PoM **Dihydrocodeine** (Non-proprietary)
Tablets, dihydrocodeine tartrate 30 mg. Net price 20 = 62p. Label: 2, 21
Elixir, dihydrocodeine tartrate 10 mg/5 ml. Net price 150 ml = £1.28. Label: 2, 21
CD Injection, dihydrocodeine tartrate 50 mg/ml. Net price 1-ml amp = 30p

NHS **DF 118**® (DF)
PoM Tablets, dihydrocodeine tartrate 30 mg. Net price 20 = 62p. Label: 2, 21
PoM Elixir, brown, dihydrocodeine tartrate 10 mg/5 ml. Diluent syrup (without preservative or preserved with *p*-hydroxybenzoic acid), life of diluted elixir 14 days. Net price 150 ml = £1.28. Label: 2, 21
CD Injection, dihydrocodeine tartrate 50 mg/ml. Net price 1-ml amp = 30p

PoM **DHC Continus** (Napp)
Tablets, s/r, scored, dihydrocodeine tartrate 60 mg. Net price 56 = £6.74. Label: 2, 25
Dose: for relief of moderately severe pain in cancer, 1 tablet twice daily
Compound preparations, section 4.7.1.1

DIPIPANONE HYDROCHLORIDE

Indications: moderate to severe pain
Cautions; Contra-indications; Side-effects: see notes above but less sedating than morphine. Drug interactions: see Appendix 1 (sections *2.3, 4.1, 4.3, 4.6*)

CD **Diconal**® (Calmic)
Tablets, pink, scored, dipipanone hydrochloride 10 mg, cyclizine hydrochloride 30 mg. Net price 20 = £1.86. Label: 2
Dose: 1 tablet gradually increased to 3 tablets every 6 hours

LEVORPHANOL TARTRATE

Indications: severe pain, see notes above
Cautions; Contra-indications; Side-effects: see notes above. Drug interactions: see Appendix 1 (sections *2.3, 4.1, 4.3, 4.6*)
Dose: by mouth, 1.5–4.5 mg 1–2 times daily
By subcutaneous or intramuscular injection, 2–4 mg, repeated when necessary
By slow intravenous injection, 1–2 mg, repeated when necessary

CD **Dromoran**® (Roche)
Tablets, levorphanol tartrate 1.5 mg. Net price 20 = 97p. Label: 2
Injection, levorphanol tartrate 2 mg/ml. Net price 1-ml amp = 25p

MEPTAZINOL

Indications: moderate to severe pain, including postoperative and obstetric pain and renal colic

---

Cautions; Contra-indications; Side-effects: see
under Buprenorphine. Drug interactions: see
Appendix 1 (sections *2.3, 4.1, 4.3, 4.6*)
Dose: by mouth, 200 mg every 3–6 hours as
required
By intramuscular injection, 75–100 mg every 2–
4 hours if necessary; obstetric analgesia, 100–
150 mg according to patient's weight (2 mg/kg)
By slow intravenous injection, 50–100 mg every
2–4 hours if necessary

▼ PoM **Meptid**® (Wyeth)
Tablets, orange, f/c, meptazinol 200 mg. Net
price 20 = £2.85. Label: 2
Injection, meptazinol 100 mg (as hydrochloride)/ml. Net price 1-ml amp = 79p

METHADONE HYDROCHLORIDE
Indications: severe pain, see notes above
Cautions; Contra-indications; Side-effects: see
notes above, but less sedating than morphine.
Drug interactions: see Appendix 1 (sections
2.3, 4.1, 4.3, 4.6, 4.7)
*Dose: by mouth or by subcutaneous or intra-
muscular injection,* 5–10 mg every 6–8 hours,
adjusted according to response

Methadone Linctus, see section 3.9.1
Methadone Mixture 1 mg/1 ml, see Preparations for Drug Dependence, p. 9

CD **Physeptone**® (Calmic)
Tablets, scored, methadone hydrochloride 5 mg.
Net price 20 = 76p. Label: 2
Injection, methadone hydrochloride 10 mg/ml.
Net price 1-ml amp = 53p

NALBUPHINE HYDROCHLORIDE
Indications: moderate to severe pain; peri-operative analgesia
Cautions; Contra-indications; Side-effects: see
notes above. Drug interactions: see Appendix
1 (sections *2.3, 4.1, 4.3, 4.6*)
*Dose: by subcutaneous, intramuscular, or intra-
venous injection,* 10–20 mg every 3–6 hours,
adjusted as required
Myocardial infarction, *by slow intravenous
injection,* 10–20 mg repeated after 30 minutes if
necessary

▼ PoM **Nubain**® (Du Pont)
Injection, nalbuphine hydrochloride 10 mg/ml.
Net price 1-ml amp = 75p; 2-ml amp = £1.16

PAPAVERETUM
See section 15.1.4.1

PENTAZOCINE
Indications: moderate to severe pain
Cautions; Side-effects: see notes above and under
Codeine Phosphate. Occasionally hallucinations occur. Avoid in patients dependent on
opioid analgesics and in arterial or pulmonary
hypertension and heart failure

Dose: by mouth, pentazocine hydrochloride
50 mg every 3–4 hours after food (range 25–
100 mg); CHILD 6–12 years 25 mg
*By subcutaneous, intramuscular, or intravenous
injection,* moderate pain, pentazocine 30 mg,
severe pain 45–60 mg every 3–4 hours when
necessary; CHILD over 1 year, by subcutaneous
or intramuscular injection, up to 1 mg/kg, by
intravenous injection up to 500 micrograms/kg
By rectum in suppositories, pentazocine 50 mg
up to 4 times daily

CD **Pentazocine** (Non-proprietary)
Capsules, pentazocine hydrochloride 50 mg. Net
price 20 = £3.40. Label: 2, 21
Tablets, pentazocine hydrochloride 25 mg. Net
price 20 = £1.65. Label: 2, 21
Injection, pentazocine 30 mg (as lactate)/ml. Net
price 1-ml amp = 61p; 2-ml amp = £1.17
Suppositories, pentazocine 50 mg (as lactate).
Net price 20 = £7.20. Label: 2
NHS CD **Fortral**® (Sterling Research)
Capsules, grey/yellow, pentazocine hydro-
chloride 50 mg. Net price 20 = £3.40. Label: 2,
21
Tablets, f/c, pentazocine hydrochloride 25 mg.
Net price 20 = £1.60. Label: 2, 21
Injection, pentazocine 30 mg (as lactate)/ml. Net
price 1-ml amp = 61p; 2-ml amp = £1.17
Suppositories, pentazocine 50 mg (as lactate).
Net price 20 = £7.22. Label: 2

PETHIDINE HYDROCHLORIDE
Indications: moderate to severe pain, obstetric
analgesia
Cautions; Contra-indications; Side-effects: see
notes above, but less constipating than
morphine. Avoid in severe renal impairment
Drug interactions: see Appendix 1 (sections
2.3, 4.1, 4.3, 4.6, 4.7)
Dose: by mouth, 50–150 mg every 4 hours; CHILD
0.5–2 mg/kg
By subcutaneous or intramuscular injection, 25–
100 mg, repeated after 4 hours; CHILD, *by intramuscular injection,* 0.5–2 mg/kg
By slow intravenous injection, 25–50 mg
repeated after 4 hours
Obstetric analgesia, *by subcutaneous or intramuscular injection,* 50–100 mg, repeated 1–3
hours later if necessary; max. 400 mg in 24 hours

CD **Pethidine** (Non-proprietary)
Tablets, pethidine hydrochloride 25 mg, net price
20 = 35p; 50 mg, 20 = 39p. Label: 2
Injection, pethidine hydrochloride 50 mg/ml.
Net price 1-ml amp = 11p; 2-ml amp = 14p
10 mg/ml see section 15.1.4.1
CD **Pamergan P100**® (Martindale)
Injection, pethidine hydrochloride 50 mg, promethazine hydrochloride 25 mg/ml. Net price
2-ml amp = 35p
Dose: by intramuscular injection, for obstetric
analgesia, 1–2 ml every 4 hours if necessary;
severe pain, 1–2 ml every 4–6 hours if necessary

PHENAZOCINE HYDROBROMIDE

Indications: severe pain, biliary or pancreatic pain

Cautions; Contra-indications; Side-effects: see notes above, but less sedating than morphine. Drug interactions: see Appendix 1 (sections *2.3, 4.1, 4.3, 4.6*)

Dose: by mouth or sublingually, 5 mg every 4–6 hours when necessary; single doses may be increased to 20 mg

CD **Narphen**® (S&N Pharm.)
Tablets, scored, phenazocine hydrobromide 5 mg. Net price 20 = £2.28. Label: 2

4.7.3   Trigeminal neuralgia

Carbamazepine (section 4.8.1), taken during the acute stages of trigeminal neuralgia, reduces the frequency and severity of attacks if given continuously. It has no effect on other forms of headache. A dose of 100 mg once or twice a day should be given initially and the dose slowly increased until the best response is obtained; most patients require 200 mg 3–4 times daily but a few may require an increased total daily dosage of up to 1.6 g. Plasma concentrations should be monitored when high doses are given. Occasionally extreme dizziness is encountered which is a further reason for starting treatment with a small dose and increasing it slowly.

Some cases of trigeminal neuralgia respond to **phenytoin** (section 4.8.1) given alone or in conjunction with carbamazepine. A combination of phenytoin and carbamazepine is only required in very refractory cases or in those unable to tolerate high doses of carbamazepine.

4.7.4   Antimigraine drugs

These drugs are discussed under treatment of the acute migraine attack (section 4.7.4.1) and prophylaxis of migraine (section 4.7.4.2).

4.7.4.1   TREATMENT OF THE ACUTE MIGRAINE ATTACK

Most migraine headaches respond to analgesics such as **aspirin** or **paracetamol** (section 4.7.1) but as peristalsis is often reduced during migraine attacks the medication may not be sufficiently well absorbed to be effective; dispersible or effervescent preparations should therefore preferably be used.

Ergotamine is used in patients who do not respond to analgesics. It relieves migraine headache by constricting cranial arteries but visual and other prodromal symptoms are not affected and vomiting may be made worse. This can be relieved by the addition of an **anti-emetic** (see below).

The value of ergotamine is limited by difficulties in absorption and by its side-effects, particularly nausea, vomiting, abdominal pain, and muscular cramps. In some patients repeated administration may cause habituation. Rarely headache may be provoked, either by chronic overdosage or by rapid withdrawal of the drug. Doses of 6 to 8 mg per attack and 10 to 12 mg per week should be **not** be exceeded. Ergotamine treatment should be **not** repeated at intervals of less than 4 days and it should **never** be prescribed prophylactically; it should not be given to patients with hemiplegic migraine.

There are various ergotamine preparations designed to improve absorption and best results are obtained when the dose is given early in an attack. An aerosol form (Medihaler-Ergotamine®) is acceptable to some patients. Sublingual ergotamine (Lingraine®) probably has no advantage over oral treatment.

Dihydroergotamine (Dihydergot®) is less effective than ergotamine and is of doubtful value.

Anti-emetics (section 4.6), such as **metoclopramide** by mouth or, if vomiting is likely, by intramuscular injection, or the phenothiazine and antihistamine anti-emetics, relieve the nausea associated with migraine attacks. Prochlorperazine may be given rectally if vomiting is a problem. Metoclopramide has the added advantage of promoting gastric emptying and normal peristalsis. A single dose should be given at the onset of symptoms. Oral analgesic preparations containing metoclopramide are available.

Diazepam and similar anxiolytics (section 4.1.2) may be useful adjuvant medication to counteract muscle spasm and anxiety often present in a migraine attack.

ANALGESICS—see section 4.7.1

ANALGESICS WITH ANTI-EMETICS

Migraleve® (International Labs)
Tablets, all f/c, *pink tablets*, buclizine hydrochloride 6.25 mg, paracetamol 500 mg, codeine phosphate 8 mg; *yellow tablets*, paracetamol 500 mg, codeine phosphate 8 mg. Net price 16 tabs (pink) + 8 tabs (yellow) = £2.14; 24 pink = £2.33; 24 yellow = £1.98. Label: 17
Dose: 2 pink tablets at onset of attack, or if it is imminent then 2 yellow tablets every 4 hours if necessary; max. in 24 hours 2 pink and 6 yellow; CHILD 10–14 years, half adult dose

PoM **Migravess**® (Bayer)
Tablets, effervescent, scored, metoclopramide hydrochloride 5 mg, aspirin 325 mg. Net price 20 = £2.40. Label: 13, 17
Forte tablets, effervescent, scored, metoclopramide hydrochloride 5 mg, aspirin 450 mg. Net price 20 = £3.29. Label: 13, 17
Dose: tablets or forte tablets, 2 dissolved in water at onset of attack then every 4 hours when necessary; max. 6 tablets in 24 hours; CHILD 12–15 years, half adult dose

PoM **Paramax**® (Beecham)
Tablets, scored, paracetamol 500 mg, metoclopramide hydrochloride 5 mg. Net price 20 = £1.68. Label: 17
Sachets, effervescent powder, sugar-free, the contents of 1 sachet = 1 tablet; to be dissolved in ¼ tumblerful of liquid before administration. Net price 30 sachets = £3.42. Label: 13, 17

Dose: 1–2 tablets or sachets at onset of attack then every 4 hours when necessary to a max. of 6 in 24 hours; CHILD max. in 24 hours 12–14 years 3 tablets or sachets, 15–20 years 5 tablets or sachets

ERGOTAMINE TARTRATE

Indications: acute attacks of migraine and migraine variants unresponsive to analgesics
Cautions: withdraw treatment immediately if numbness or tingling of extremities develops; should not be used for migraine prophylaxis. Drug interactions: see Appendix 1 (sections 2.4, 4.7)
Contra-indications: peripheral vascular disease, coronary heart disease, obliterative vascular disease and Raynaud's syndrome, hepatic or renal impairment, sepsis, severe or inadequately controlled hypertension, pregnancy, breast-feeding
Side-effects: headache, nausea, vomiting, and abdominal pain; repeated high dosage may cause ergotism with gangrene and confusion

PoM **Cafergot**® (Sandoz)
Tablets, ergotamine tartrate 1 mg, caffeine 100 mg. Net price 20 = 91p. Label: 18, counselling advised, dosage
Dose: 1–2 tablets at onset; max. 4 tablets in 24 hours; not to be repeated at intervals of less than 4 days; max. 10 tablets weekly
Suppositories, ergotamine tartrate 2 mg, caffeine 100 mg. Net price 6 = £1.00. Label: 18, counselling advised, dosage
Dose: 1 suppository at onset; max. 2 in 24 hours and 5 weekly
PoM **Lingraine**® (Winthrop)
Tablets (for sublingual use), green, ergotamine tartrate 2 mg. Net price 12 = £6.03. Label: 18, 26, counselling advised, dosage
Dose: 1 tablet at onset repeated after 30 minutes if necessary; max. 3 daily and 6 weekly
PoM **Medihaler-Ergotamine**® (Riker)
Aerosol inhalation (oral), ergotamine tartrate 360 micrograms/metered inhalation. Net price 75-dose unit = £3.44. Label: 18, counselling advised, dosage
Dose: 360 micrograms repeated every 5 minutes if necessary; max. 6 inhalations daily and 15 inhalations weekly
PoM **Migril**® (Wellcome)
Tablets, scored, ergotamine tartrate 2 mg, cyclizine hydrochloride 50 mg, caffeine hydrate 100 mg. Net price 20 = £7.16. Label: 2, 18, counselling advised, dosage
Dose: 1–2 tablets at onset, followed after 30 minutes by ½–1 tablet, repeated every 30 minutes if necessary; max. 4 tablets per attack and 6 tablets weekly

DIHYDROERGOTAMINE MESYLATE

Indications: migraine attack unresponsive to analgesics

Cautions; Contra-indications; Side-effects: see under Ergotamine Tartrate, as well as numbness and tingling of extremities, precordial pain reported; also contra-indicated in shock; avoid intra-arterial injection
Dose: by subcutaneous or intramuscular injection, 1 mg repeated once after 30–60 minutes if necessary; max. 3 mg daily and 6 mg weekly

PoM **Dihydergot**® (Sandoz)
Injection, dihydroergotamine mesylate 1 mg/ml. Net price 1-ml amp = 21p

ISOMETHEPTENE MUCATE

Indications: migraine attack
Cautions: cardiovascular disease. Drug interactions: see Appendix 1 (section 4.3)
Contra-indications: glaucoma; patients on monoamine-oxidase inhibitors or within 2 weeks of MAOI therapy
Side-effects: dizziness, circulatory disturbances

PoM **Midrid**® (Carnrick)
Capsules, red, isometheptene mucate 65 mg, dichloralphenazone 100 mg, paracetamol 325 mg. Net price 20 = £2.72. Label: 2, 17
Dose: migraine, 2 capsules at onset of attack, followed by 1 capsule every hour if necessary; max. 5 capsules in 12 hours
Note. With effect from 1st August 1988 Midrid® has been reformulated omitting the dichloralphenazone; the new formulation will not be PoM.

4.7.4.2 PROPHYLAXIS OF MIGRAINE

Where attacks are frequent, search should be made for provocative factors such as stress or diet (chocolate, cheese, alcohol, etc.). Benzodiazepines should be avoided because of the risk of dependence. In patients with more than one attack a month, one of three prophylactic agents may be tried: pizotifen, beta-blockers, or tricyclic antidepressants (even when the patient is not obviously depressed). Oral contraceptives may precipitate or worsen migraine; patients reporting a sharp increase in frequency of migraine or focal features should be recommended alternative contraceptive measures.

Pizotifen (Sanomigran®) is an antihistamine and antiserotonergic drug structurally related to the tricyclic antidepressants. It affords good prophylaxis but may cause weight gain. To avoid undue drowsiness treatment may be started at 500 micrograms at night and gradually increased to 3 mg; it is rarely necessary to exceed this dose.

Beta-blockers. Propranolol, metoprolol, nadolol, and timolol (see section 2.4) are all effective. Propranolol is the most commonly used in an initial dose of 40 mg 2 to 3 times daily by mouth. Beta-blockers may also be given as a single dose of a long-acting preparation. The value of beta-blockers is limited by their contra-indications (see section 2.4) and by interaction with ergotamine (see Appendix 1, section 2.4).

Tricyclic antidepressants may usefully be prescribed in a dose, for example, of amitriptyline 10 mg at night, increasing to a maintenance dose of 50 to 75 mg at night.

There is recent evidence that the calcium-channel blockers (see section 2.6.2), e.g. verapamil (Cordilox® etc.) and nifedipine (Adalat®) may be useful in migraine prophylaxis.

Cyproheptadine, an antihistamine with serotonin-antagonist and calcium channel-blocking properties, may also be tried in refractory cases. **Clonidine** (Dixarit®) is probably little better than placebo and may aggravate depression or produce insomnia. **Methysergide** (Deseril®) has dangerous side-effects (retroperitoneal fibrosis and fibrosis of the heart valves and pleura); it should only be administered under hospital supervision.

CLONIDINE HYDROCHLORIDE

Indications: prevention of recurrent migraine, vascular headache, menopausal flushing
Cautions: depressive illness, concurrent antihypertensive therapy. Drug interactions: see Appendix 1 (section 2.5)
Side-effects: dry mouth, sedation, dizziness, nausea, nocturnal restlessness; occasionally rashes
Dose: 50 micrograms twice daily, increased after 2 weeks to 75 micrograms twice daily if necessary

PoM **Dixarit**® (Boehringer Ingelheim)
Tablets, blue, s/c, clonidine hydrochloride 25 micrograms. Net price 20 = £1.09
Catapres (hypertension), see section 2.5.2

METHYSERGIDE

Indications: prevention of severe recurrent migraine and cluster headache in patients who are refractory to other treatment and whose lives are seriously disrupted (hospital supervision only, see notes above)
Cautions: history of peptic ulceration; avoid abrupt withdrawal of treatment; withdraw for reassessment after 6 months (see also notes above)
Contra-indications: renal, hepatic, pulmonary, and cardiovascular disease, collagen disease, cellulitis, urinary tract disorders, cachectic or septic conditions, pregnancy, breast-feeding
Side-effects: nausea, heartburn, abdominal discomfort, drowsiness, and dizziness occur frequently in initial treatment; psychic reactions, insomnia, oedema, cramps, arterial spasm, paraesthesias of extremities, postural hypotension, and tachycardia also occur. Retroperitoneal and other abnormal fibrotic reactions may occur on prolonged administration, requiring immediate withdrawal of treatment
Dose: 1 mg at bedtime, gradually increased to 1–2 mg 2–3 times daily with food (see notes above)
Carcinoid syndrome, usual range, 12–20 mg daily (hospital supervision)

PoM **Deseril**® (Sandoz)
Tablets, s/c, methysergide 1 mg (as maleate). Net price 20 = £1.83. Label: 2, 21

PIZOTIFEN

Indications: prevention of vascular headache including classical migraine, common migraine, and cluster headache
Cautions: may affect the ability to drive or operate machinery and increase effects of alcohol. Drug interactions: see Appendix 1 (section 2.5)
Contra-indications: urinary retention; closed-angle glaucoma
Side-effects: anticholinergic effects, drowsiness, weight gain; occasionally nausea, dizziness, muscle pain
Dose: 1.5 mg at night *or* 500 micrograms 3 times daily but see also notes above, adjusted according to response within the usual range 0.5–3 mg daily; max. single dose 3 mg, max. daily dose 6 mg; CHILD up to 1.5 mg daily; max. single dose at night 1 mg

PoM **Sanomigran**® (Sandoz)
Tablets, both ivory-yellow, s/c, pizotifen (as hydrogen malate), 500 micrograms, net price 20 = £1.60; 1.5 mg, 28 = £7.98. Label: 2
Elixir, pizotifen 250 micrograms (as hydrogen malate)/5 ml. Net price 100 ml = £1.41. Label: 2

4.8 Antiepileptics

In this section drugs are discussed under the following subsections:
4.8.1 Control of epilepsy
4.8.2 Drugs used in status epilepticus
4.8.3 Febrile convulsions

4.8.1 Control of epilepsy

The object of treatment is to prevent the occurrence of seizures by maintaining an effective plasma concentration of the drug. Careful adjustment of doses is necessary, starting with low doses and increasing gradually until fits are controlled or there are overdose effects.

The frequency of administration is determined by the plasma half-life, and should be kept as low as possible to encourage better patient compliance. Most antiepileptics, when used in average dosage, may be given twice daily. Phenobarbitone and sometimes phenytoin, which have long half-lives, may often be given as a daily dose at bedtime. However, with large doses, some antiepileptics may need to be administered 3 times daily to avoid adverse effects associated with high peak plasma concentrations. Young children metabolise antiepileptics more rapidly than adults and therefore require more frequent dose and a higher dose per kilogram body-weight.

Therapy with several drugs concurrently should be avoided. Patients are best controlled with one antiepileptic. Combinations of drugs have been used on the grounds that their therapeutic effects were additive while their individual toxicity was reduced but there is no evidence for this. In fact, toxicity may be enhanced with combination therapy. A second drug should only be added to the regimen if seizures continue despite high plasma concentrations or toxic effects. The use of more than two antiepileptics is rarely justified.

Another disadvantage of multiple therapy is that drug interactions occur between the various antiepileptics (see Appendix 1, section 4.8) and other drugs. Because of liver enzyme induction, phenobarbitone, phenytoin, primidone, and carbamazepine may increase each other's metabolism and reduce plasma concentrations. The reduction of carbamazepine concentration by concurrent phenytoin administration is a most important example. Moreover, it is illogical to combine primidone and phenobarbitone as the former is largely metabolised to phenobarbitone in the liver, which is responsible for most, if not all, of its antiepileptic action.

Compound preparations of antiepileptics in fixed proportions are particularly undesirable because the dose of each antiepileptic should be adjusted separately; there are no longer any on the UK market.

Abrupt withdrawal of antiepileptics, particularly the barbiturates and benzodiazepines, should be avoided, as this may precipitate severe rebound seizures. Reduction in dosage should be carried out in stages and, in the case of the barbiturates, the withdrawal process may take months. The changeover from one antiepileptic drug regimen to another should be made cautiously.

The decision to withdraw all antiepileptics from a seizure-free patient, and its timing, is often difficult and may depend on individual patient factors.

DRIVING. Patients suffering from epilepsy may drive a motor vehicle (but not a heavy goods or public service vehicle) provided that they have had a fit-free period of two years or, if subject to attacks only while asleep, have established a three-year period of asleep attacks without awake attacks. Patients affected by drowsiness should not drive or operate machinery.

PREGNANCY AND BREAST-FEEDING. During pregnancy, plasma concentrations of antiepileptics should be frequently monitored as they may fall, particularly in the later stages. There is an increased risk of teratogenicity associated with the use of anticonvulsant drugs but, generally, prescribing in pregnancy should follow the same principles as that in non-pregnant patients. Breast-feeding is acceptable with all antiepileptic drugs, taken in normal doses, with the possible exception of the barbiturates. See under Prescribing in Pregnancy (p. 27) and Prescribing during Breast-feeding (p. 32).

Drug treatment is usually independent of the aetiology but does vary according to the type of seizure. It is discussed under the headings tonic-clonic (grand mal) seizures; partial (focal) seiz-

ures; absence seizures (petit mal); myoclonic seizures (myoclonic jerks), atypical absence, atonic and tonic seizures (all in section 4.8.1); status epilepticus (section 4.8.2); and febrile convulsions (section 4.8.3).

TONIC-CLONIC (GRAND MAL) AND PARTIAL (FOCAL) SEIZURES

The drugs of choice for tonic-clonic seizures occurring as part of a syndrome of primary generalised epilepsy are carbamazepine, phenytoin, and sodium valproate. Phenobarbitone and primidone are also effective but may be more sedating.

Partial epilepsy is more difficult to control. Carbamazepine and phenytoin are the drugs of choice for secondary generalised tonic-clonic seizures and for partial seizures themselves, but sodium valproate may be less effective. Phenobarbitone and primidone are also effective but, once again, are likely to be more sedating. Second-line drugs for both tonic-clonic and partial seizures include clonazepam, clobazam, and acetazolamide.

Phenytoin (Epanutin®) is effective in tonic-clonic and partial seizures. It has a narrow therapeutic index and the relationship between dose and plasma concentration is non-linear; small dosage increases in some patients may produce large rises in plasma concentrations with acute toxic side-effects. Monitoring of plasma concentration greatly assists dosage adjustment. A few missed doses or a small change in drug absorption may result in a marked change in plasma concentration.

Phenytoin may cause coarse facies, acne, hirsutism, and gingival hyperplasia and for these reasons may be particularly undesirable in adolescent patients.

Carbamazepine (Tegretol®) is a drug of choice for simple and complex partial seizures and for tonic-clonic seizures regardless of whether they are primary or secondary to a focal discharge. It has a wider therapeutic index than phenytoin and the relationship between dose and plasma concentration is linear, but monitoring of plasma concentrations may be helpful in determining optimum dosage. It has generally fewer side-effects than phenytoin or the barbiturates, but reversible blurring of vision, dizziness, and unsteadiness are dose-related, and may be dose-limiting. These side-effects may be reduced by altering the timing of medication. It is essential to initiate carbamazepine therapy at a low dose and build this up over one or two weeks.

Phenobarbitone is an effective drug but may be sedative in adults and cause behavioural disturbances and hyperkinesia in children. Rebound seizures may be a problem on withdrawal. Monitoring plasma concentrations is less useful than with other drugs because tolerance occurs. **Methylphenobarbitone** is largely converted to phenobarbitone in the liver and has no advantages. **Primidone** (Mysoline®) is largely converted to phenobarbitone in the body and this is probably responsible for its antiepileptic action. A small starting dose (125 mg) is essential, and the drug should be introduced over several weeks.

Sodium valproate (Epilim®) is effective in controlling tonic-clonic seizures, particularly in primary generalised epilepsy. Plasma concentrations are not a useful index of efficacy, therefore routine monitoring is unhelpful. The drug has widespread metabolic effects, and may have dose-related side-effects. There has been recent concern over severe hepatic or pancreatic toxicity, although these effects are rare.

Clonazepam (Rivotril®) is occasionally used in tonic-clonic or partial seizures, but its sedative side-effects may be prominent. **Clobazam** (Frisium®) may be used as adjunctive therapy in the treatment of epilepsy (section 4.1.2), but the effectiveness of these and other **benzodiazepines** may wane considerably after weeks or months of continuous therapy.

ABSENCE SEIZURES (PETIT MAL)

Ethosuximide (Emeside®, Zarontin®) and **sodium valproate** (Epilim®) are the drugs of choice in simple absence seizures. Sodium valproate is also highly effective in treating the tonic-clonic seizures which may co-exist with absence seizures in primary generalised epilepsy. Monitoring plasma-ethosuximide concentrations is helpful in determining optimum dosage.

MYOCLONIC SEIZURES (MYOCLONIC JERKS)

Myoclonic seizures occur in a variety of syndromes, and response to treatment varies considerably. **Sodium valproate** (Epilim®) is the drug of choice and **clonazepam** (Rivotril®), **ethosuximide** (Emeside®, Zarontin®), and other antiepileptic drugs may be used.

ATYPICAL ABSENCE, ATONIC, AND TONIC SEIZURES

These seizure types are usually seen in childhood, in specific epileptic syndromes, or associated with cerebral damage or mental retardation. They may respond poorly to the traditional drugs. **Phenytoin** (Epanutin®), **sodium valproate** (Epilim®), **clonazepam** (Rivotril®), and **ethosuximide** (Emeside®, Zarontin®), and **phenobarbitone** may be tried. Other second-line antiepileptic drugs are occasionally helpful, including acetazolamide (Diamox®) and corticosteroids.

ACETAZOLAMIDE

Indications: see notes above
Cautions; Side-effects: see section 11.6
Dose: 0.25–1 g daily in divided doses; CHILD 125–750 mg daily

Preparations
Section 11.6

CARBAMAZEPINE

Indications: all forms of epilepsy except absence seizures; trigeminal neuralgia (section 4.7.3)

Cautions: see notes above; hepatic impairment; pregnancy and breast-feeding (see notes above). Drug interactions: see Appendix 1 (sections *2.8A*, *3*, *4.2*, *4.8*, *4.8*, *5.1*, *6.2*, *6.3*, *7*)
Contra-indications: previous sensitivity to carbamazepine, atrioventricular conduction abnormalities; porphyrias; patients on monamine-oxidase inhibitors or within 2 weeks of MAOI therapy (theoretical grounds only)
Side-effects: gastro-intestinal disturbances, dizziness, drowsiness, visual disturbances (especially double vision and often associated with peak plasma concentrations); a generalised erythematous rash may occur in about 3% of patients; leucopenia and other blood disorders have occurred rarely
Dose: initially, 100–200 mg 1–2 times daily, increased slowly to a usual dose of 0.8–1.2 g daily according to the patient's needs; in some cases 1.6 g (or even 1.8 g) daily may be needed; CHILD daily in divided doses, up to one year 100–200 mg, 1–5 years 200–400 mg, 5–10 years 400–600 mg, 10–15 years 0.6–1 g
Prophylaxis of manic depressive psychosis unresponsive to lithium, initially, 400 mg daily in divided doses increased until symptoms controlled; usual range 400–600 mg daily; max. 1.6 g daily
Note. Plasma concentration for optimum response 4–12 mg/litre (20–50 micromol/litre)

PoM **Carbamazepine Tablets,** carbamazepine 100 mg, net price 20 = 53p; 200 mg, 20 = 99p; 400 mg, 20 = £2.01
PoM **Tegretol®** (Geigy)
Tablets, all scored, carbamazepine 100 mg, net price 20 = 60p; 200 mg, 20 = £1.11; 400 mg, 20 = £2.26
Liquid, sugar-free, carbamazepine 100 mg/5 ml. Diluent tragacanth mucilage for 1 + 1 dilution, life of diluted liquid 14 days. Net price 100 ml = £1.84

CLONAZEPAM

Indications: all forms of epilepsy. For status epilepticus see section 4.8.2
Cautions: may affect the ability to drive or operate machinery and increase the effects of alcohol; breast-feeding; see notes above. Drug interactions: see Appendix 1 (section 4.8)
Side-effects: drowsiness, fatigue, dizziness, muscle hypotonia, hypersalivation in infants, paradoxical aggression, irritability and mental changes
Dose: 1 mg, initially at night for 4 nights, increased over 2–4 weeks to a usual daily maintenance dose of 4–8 mg; CHILD up to 1 year 250 micrograms increased as above to 0.5–1 mg, 1–5 years 250 micrograms increased to 1–3 mg, 6–12 years 500 micrograms increased to 3–6 mg

PoM **Rivotril®** (Roche)
Tablets, both scored, clonazepam 500 micrograms (beige), net price 20 = 77p; 2 mg, 20 = £1.60. Label: 2

ETHOSUXIMIDE

Indications: absence seizures
Cautions: see notes above. Drug interactions: see Appendix 1 (section 4.8)
Contra-indications: porphyrias
Side-effects: gastro-intestinal disturbances, drowsiness, dizziness, ataxia, headache, depression, and mild euphoria. Psychotic states, rashes, liver changes, and haematological disorders such as leucopenia and agranulocytosis occur rarely
Dose: initially, 500 mg daily, increased according to patient's needs by 250 mg at intervals of 4–7 days to a max. of 2 g daily; CHILD up to 6 years 250 mg daily, over 6 years 500 mg, increased gradually to a max. of 1 g daily
Note. Plasma concentration for optimum response 40–100 mg/litre (300–700 micromol/litre)

PoM **Emeside**® (LAB)
Capsules, orange, ethosuximide 250 mg. Net price 20 = £1.25. Label: 2
Syrup, black currant or orange, ethosuximide 250 mg/5 ml. Diluent syrup, life of diluted syrup 14 days. Net price 100 ml = £1.60. Label: 2
PoM **Zarontin**® (P-D)
Capsules, orange, ethosuximide 250 mg. Net price 20 = £1.46. Label: 2
Syrup, red, ethosuximide 250 mg/5 ml. Diluent syrup, life of diluted syrup 14 days. Net price 100 ml = £1.78. Label: 2

METHYLPHENOBARBITONE

Indications: tonic-clonic and partial seizures
Cautions; Contra-indications; Side-effects: see under Phenobarbitone
Dose: 100–600 mg daily, according to the patient's needs

CD **Prominal**® (Winthrop)
Tablets, methylphenobarbitone 30 mg, net price 20 = 63p; 60 mg, 20 = 83p; 200 mg, 20 = £1.78. Label: 2

PHENOBARBITONE

Indications: all forms of epilepsy except absence seizures. For status epilepticus see section 4.8.2
Cautions: elderly, children, impaired renal or hepatic function, severe respiratory depression, pregnancy and breast-feeding (see notes above); avoid sudden withdrawal; see also notes above and Barbiturates (section 4.1.3). Drug interactions: see Appendix 1 (sections 2.1, 2.8A, 4.3, 4.8, 4.8, 5.1, 5.2, 6.3, 7, 8)
Contra-indications: porphyrias
Side-effects: drowsiness, lethargy, mental depression, ataxia and allergic skin reactions; paradoxical excitement, restlessness and confusion in the elderly and hyperkinesia in children; megaloblastic anaemia (may be treated with folic acid)
Dose: by mouth, 60–180 mg at night; CHILD 5–8 mg/kg daily (febrile convulsions, see 4.8.3)
By intramuscular or intravenous injection, 50–200 mg, repeated after 6 hours if necessary; max. 600 mg daily

Note. For therapeutic purposes phenobarbitone and phenobarbitone sodium may be considered equivalent in effect. Plasma concentration for optimum response 15–40 mg/litre (60–180 micromol/litre)

CD **Phenobarbitone Tablets,** phenobarbitone 15 mg, net price 20 = 6p; 30 mg, 20 = 7p; 60 mg, 20 = 10p; 100 mg, 20 = 18p. Label: 2
CD **Phenobarbitone Sodium Tablets,** phenobarbitone sodium 30 mg, net price 20 = 13p; 60 mg, 20 = 29p. Label: 2
CD **Phenobarbitone Elixir,** phenobarbitone 15 mg/5 ml. Net price 100 ml = 52p. Label: 2
CD **Phenobarbitone Injection,** phenobarbitone sodium 200 mg/ml in propylene glycol 90% and water for injections 10%. Net price 1-ml amp = 40p
CD **Gardenal Sodium**® (M&B)
Injection, phenobarbitone sodium 200 mg/ml. Net price 1-ml amp = 28p
CD **Luminal**® (Winthrop)
Tablets, phenobarbitone 15 mg, net price 20 = 26p; 30 mg, 20 = 22p; 60 mg, 20 = 45p. Label: 2

PHENYTOIN

Indications: all forms of epilepsy except absence seizures
Cautions: hepatic impairment (reduce dose), change-over from other drugs should be made cautiously; avoid sudden withdrawal; see also notes above. Drug interactions: see Appendix 1 (sections 2.1, 2.3, 2.8D, 3, 4.2, 4.3, 4.8, 4.8, 5.1, 5.2, 6.2, 6.3, 7, 8)
Contra-indications: porphyrias
Side-effects: nausea, vomiting, mental confusion, dizziness, headache, tremor, insomnia occur commonly. Ataxia, slurred speech, nystagmus and blurred vision are signs of overdosage. Skin eruptions (sometimes severe), coarse facies, acne and hirsutism, fever and hepatitis; lupus erythematosus, erythema multiforme; lymphadenopathy; gingival hypertrophy and tenderness; rarely haematological effects, including megaloblastic anaemia (folate deficiency), leucopenia, thrombocytopenia, agranulocytosis, and aplastic anaemia. Plasma calcium may be lowered (rickets and osteomalacia)
Dose: by mouth, daily as a single dose or 2 divided doses, with water, 150–300 mg increased gradually to 600 mg according to the patient's needs; CHILD 5–8 mg/kg daily in 1 or 2 doses
By intravenous injection—section 4.8.2
Note. Plasma concentration for optimum response 10–20 mg/litre (40–80 micromol/litre)

Phenytoin and phenytoin sodium
Note. Phenytoin 100 mg = phenytoin sodium 108 mg
PoM **Phenytoin Tablets,** s/c, phenytoin sodium 50 mg, net price 20 = 14p; 100 mg, 20 = 14p
Note. Owing to variation in bioavailability different brands of phenytoin tablets may not be interchangeable with one another.
PoM **Epanutin**® (P-D)
Capsules, phenytoin sodium 25 mg (white/

---

purple), net price 20 = 39p; 50 mg (white/pink), 20 = 40p; 100 mg (white/orange), 20 = 43p
Infatabs® (= tablets, chewable), yellow, scored, phenytoin 50 mg. Net price 20 = £1.10. Label: 24
Suspension, red, phenytoin 30 mg/5 ml. Diluent syrup, life of diluted suspension 14 days. Net price 100 ml = 64p
Injection, section 4.8.2

PRIMIDONE

Indications: all forms of epilepsy except absence seizures
Cautions; Contra-indications; Side-effects: see under Phenobarbitone. Drowsiness, ataxia, nausea, visual disturbances, and rashes, particularly at first, usually reversible on continued administration. Drug interactions: see Appendix 1 (sections *2.3, 2.8A, 4.3*, 4.8, *4.8, 6.3*, 7)
Dose: initially, 125 mg daily at bedtime, increased by 125 mg every 3 days to 500 mg daily in 2 divided doses then increased by 250 mg every 3 days to a max. of 1.5 g daily in divided doses; CHILD 20–30 mg/kg daily in 2 divided doses
Note. Monitor plasma concentrations of derived phenobarbitone. Optimum range as for phenobarbitone.

PoM **Mysoline**® (ICI)
Tablets, scored, primidone 250 mg. Net price 20 = 26p. Label: 2
Oral suspension, primidone 250 mg/5 ml. Diluent propyl hydroxybenzoate 0.015%, methyl hydroxybenzoate 0.15%, carmellose sodium '50' 1%, sucrose 20%, in freshly boiled and cooled purified water. Net price 250 ml = 75p. Label: 2

SODIUM VALPROATE

Indications: all forms of epilepsy
Cautions: in patients most at risk (e.g. children and those with history of liver disease) monitor liver function in first 6 months; pregnancy and breast-feeding (see notes above); monitor platelet function before major surgery; may give false-positive urine tests for ketones in diabetes mellitus; see also notes above. Drug interactions: see Appendix 1 (sections 4.8, *4.8*)
Contra-indications: active liver disease
Side-effects: gastric irritation, nausea; hyperammonaemia, increased appetite and weight gain; transient hair loss (regrowth may be curly), oedema, thrombocytopenia, and inhibition of platelet aggregation; impaired hepatic function leading rarely to fatal hepatic failure (see Cautions—withdraw treatment immediately if vomiting, anorexia, jaundice, drowsiness, or loss of seizure control occurs); rarely pancreatitis (estimate plasma amylase in acute abdominal pain)
Dose: initially, 600 mg daily in divided doses, preferably after food, increasing by 200 mg/day at 3-day intervals to a max. of 2.5 g daily in divided doses, according to the patient's needs; CHILD up to 20 kg (about 4 years), initially 20 mg/kg daily in divided doses increased

gradually to a max. of 40 mg/kg daily; over 20 kg, initially 400 mg daily in divided doses increased gradually to 30 mg/kg daily, according to the patient's needs

PoM **Epilim**® (Labaz)
Tablets (crushable), scored, sodium valproate 100 mg. Net price 20 = 80p
Tablets, both e/c, lilac, sodium valproate 200 mg, net price 20 = £1.32; 500 mg, 20 = £3.29. Label: 5, 25
Liquid, red, sugar-free, sodium valproate 200 mg/5 ml. Net price 100 ml = £2.02
Syrup, red, sodium valproate 200 mg/5 ml. Diluent syrup (without preservative), life of diluted syrup 14 days. Net price 100 ml = £2.02

4.8.2 Drugs used in status epilepticus

Major status epilepticus should be treated first with intravenous **diazepam** or **clonazepam** (Rivotril®) but they should be used with caution because of the risk of respiratory depression; there may be a high incidence of venous thrombophlebitis. Intramuscular injection is unsatisfactory as the drugs are too slowly absorbed. When diazepam is given intravenously the risk of thrombophlebitis is minimised by using an emulsion (Diazemuls®). If intravenous administration is not possible, diazepam may be given as a rectal solution (Stesolid®). Absorption from suppositories is too slow for treatment of status epilepticus.

If status epilepticus continues or returns, **chlormethiazole** (Heminevrin®) may be given by intravenous infusion. Chlormethiazole has a short half-life, and the rate of infusion can be titrated against the patient's clinical condition. It does, however, cause respiratory depression. Alternatively **phenytoin sodium** may be given by slow intravenous injection, with ECG monitoring at a rate of not more than 50 mg/minute (in adults) to a maximum of 1 g followed by the maintenance dosage. Intramuscular use of phenytoin is not recommended (absorption is slow and erratic) and intravenous infusion is not recommended (precipitates).

Paraldehyde also remains a valuable drug. It is usually given by deep intramuscular injection but may be given rectally. In some specialist centres, with intensive care facilities, it is also given, with caution, by intravenous injection diluted with sodium chloride intravenous infusion. When given by intramuscular injection, paraldehyde causes little respiratory depression and is therefore useful where facilities for resuscitation are poor.

Phenobarbitone sodium (section 4.8.1) is occasionally used but it is less satisfactory for urgent treatment because of its slow metabolism.

Lorazepam is rarely used for status epilepticus.

DIAZEPAM

Indications: status epilepticus; convulsions due to poisoning (see Emergency Treatment of Poisoning)

Cautions; Side-effects: see section 4.1.2. When given intravenously facilities for reversing respiratory depression with mechanical ventilation should be at hand

Dose: by slow intravenous injection, as a 0.5% solution or emulsion, 10–20 mg at a rate of 0.5 ml (2.5 mg) per 30 seconds, repeated if necessary after 30–60 minutes; may be followed by *slow intravenous infusion* to a max. of 3 mg/kg over 24 hours; CHILD 200–300 micrograms/kg

By rectum in solution, adults and children over 3 years 10 mg; CHILD 1–3 years and elderly patients 5 mg; repeat after 5 minutes if necessary

PoM **Diazemuls**® (KabiVitrum)
Injection (emulsion), diazepam 5 mg/ml (0.5%). See Appendix 2. Net price 2-ml amp = 44p

PoM **Stesolid**® (CP)
Injection, diazepam 5 mg/ml (0.5%). See Appendix 2. Net price 2-ml amp = 25p
Rectal tubes (= rectal solution), diazepam 2 mg/ml. Net price 5 × 2.5-ml (5 mg) tubes = £4.50
Rectal tubes (= rectal solution), diazepam 4 mg/ml. Net price 5 × 2.5-ml (10 mg) tubes = £5.60

PoM **Valium**® (Roche)
Injection, diazepam 5 mg/ml (0.5%) in solvent. See Appendix 2. Net price 2-ml amp = 26p
Oral preparations, section 4.1.2

CLONAZEPAM

Indications: status epilepticus
Cautions; Side-effects: see section 4.8.1. Hypotension and apnoea may occur and resuscitation facilities must be available
Dose: by slow intravenous injection or infusion, 1 mg over 30 seconds; CHILD all ages, 500 micrograms

PoM **Rivotril**® (Roche)
Injection, clonazepam 1 mg/ml in solvent, for dilution with 1 ml water for injections immediately before injection or as described in Appendix 2. Net price 1-ml amp (with 1 ml water for injections) = 62p
Oral preparations, section 4.8.1

CHLORMETHIAZOLE EDISYLATE

Indications: status epilepticus
Cautions: obstructive pulmonary disease; during continuous infusion the sleep induced may quickly lapse into deep unconsciousness and patients must be observed constantly; see also section 4.1.1
Side-effects: tingling in the nose, sneezing, conjunctival irritation, headache, slight hypotension, respiratory depression, local thrombophlebitis at site of continuous infusion; see also section 4.1.1
Dose: by intravenous infusion, as a 0.8% solution, initially, 40–100 ml (320–800 mg) at a rate of 60–150 drops per minute then continued if necessary at a reduced rate adjusted according to the patient's condition (see notes above)

Note. Special care on prolonged administration since accumulation may occur

PoM **Heminevrin**® (Astra)
Intravenous infusion 0.8%, chlormethiazole edisylate 8 mg/ml. Net price 500-ml bottle = £5.25
Oral preparations, section 4.1.1

LORAZEPAM

Indications: status epilepticus
Cautions; Side-effects: see section 4.1.2
Dose: by intravenous injection, 4 mg; CHILD 2 mg

Preparations
    Section 4.1.2

PARALDEHYDE

Indications: status epilepticus
Cautions: bronchopulmonary disease, hepatic impairment
Side-effects: rashes; injections are painful
Dose: by deep intramuscular injection, as a single dose, 5–10 ml; not more than 5 ml at any one site; CHILD up to 3 months 0.5 ml, 3–6 months 1 ml, 6–12 months 1.5 ml, 1–2 years 2 ml, 3–5 years 3–4 ml, 6–12 years 5–6 ml
By slow intravenous injection, diluted with several times its volume of sodium chloride intravenous infusion 0.9%, up to 4–5 ml (specialist centres only, see notes above)
By rectum, 5–10 ml, administered as a 10% enema in physiological saline; CHILD as for intramuscular dose
Note. Do not use paraldehyde if it has a brownish colour or an odour of acetic acid. Avoid contact with rubber and plastics.

PoM **Paraldehyde Injection,** sterile paraldehyde. Net price 5-ml amp = £1.95; 10-ml amp = £2.52

PHENYTOIN SODIUM

Indications: status epilepticus; prophylaxis of seizures in neurosurgery
Cautions; Side-effects: see under Phenytoin Sodium, section 4.8.1. Do not give with lignocaine hydrochloride. Injection solutions are alkaline and may be irritant. May cause hypotension, asystole, bradycardia, and confusion. Resuscitation facilities must be available
Contra-indications: should not be given intravenously in patients with bradycardia, supraventricular tachycardias, or heart block
Dose: by slow intravenous injection, status epilepticus, 13–15 mg/kg at a rate not exceeding 50 mg per minute, as a loading dose (see also notes above). Maintenance doses of about 100 mg should be given thereafter at intervals of every 6 hours, monitored by measurement of plasma concentrations; rate and dose reduced according to weight
By intramuscular injection, not recommended (see notes above)

PoM **Epanutin Ready Mixed Parenteral**® (P-D)
Injection, phenytoin sodium 50 mg/ml with pro-

pylene glycol 40% and alcohol 10% in water for injections. Net price 5-ml amp = £3.65

Oral preparations, section 4.8.1

4.8.3 Febrile convulsions

Brief febrile convulsions need only simple treatment such as tepid sponging or bathing, or antipyretic medication, e.g. **paracetamol** (section 4.7.1.1). *Prolonged febrile convulsions* (those lasting 15 minutes or longer), *recurrent convulsions*, or those occurring in a child at known risk must be treated more actively, as there is the possibility of resulting brain damage. **Diazepam** is the drug of choice given either by slow intravenous injection in a dose of 250 micrograms/kg (as Diazemuls®, section 4.8.2) or preferably rectally in solution (Stesolid®, section 4.8.2) in a dose of 500 micrograms/kg, repeated if necessary. The rectal route is preferred as satisfactory absorption is achieved within minutes and administration is much easier. Suppositories are not suitable because absorption is too slow.

Intermittent prophylaxis (i.e. the anticonvulsant administered at the onset of fever) is possible in only a small proportion of children. Again **diazepam** is the treatment of choice, orally or rectally.

The exact role of continuous prophylaxis in children at risk from prolonged or complex febrile convulsions is controversial. It is probably indicated in only a small proportion of children, including those whose first seizure occurred at under 14 months or who have pre-existing neurological abnormalities or who have had previous prolonged or focal convulsions. Either **phenobarbitone** (3 to 4 mg/kg daily) or **sodium valproate** (20 mg/kg daily) (section 4.8.1) may be given.

4.9 Drugs used in parkinsonism and related disorders

4.9.1 Dopaminergic drugs used in parkinsonism

4.9.2 Anticholinergic drugs used in parkinsonism

4.9.3 Drugs used in essential tremor, chorea, tics, and related disorders

In idiopathic Parkinson's disease, progressive degeneration of pigment-containing cells of the substantia nigra leads to deficiency of the inhibitory neurotransmitter dopamine. This, in turn, results in a neurohumoral imbalance in the basal ganglia, causing the characteristic signs and symptoms of the illness to appear. The pathogenesis of this process is still obscure and current therapy aims simply to correct the imbalance. Although this approach fails to prevent the progression of the disease, it greatly improves the quality and expectancy of life of most patients.

Levodopa, used in conjunction with **dopa-decarboxylase inhibitors** (section 4.9.1), is the treatment of choice for patients disabled by idiopathic Parkinson's disease. It is less effective in patients

with post-encephalitic parkinsonism and should be avoided in neuroleptic-induced parkinsonism.

Parkinsonism caused by generalised degenerative brain disease does not normally respond to levodopa.

Anticholinergic drugs (section 4.9.2) are the other main class of drugs used in Parkinson's disease. They are less effective than levodopa in idiopathic Parkinson's disease although they often usefully supplement its action. Patients with mild symptoms may be treated with anticholinergic drugs before they are eventually transferred to levodopa therapy as symptoms progress. Anticholinergic drugs have value in treating drug-induced parkinsonism or in patients with post-encephalitic parkinsonism.

Other antiparkinsonian drugs include amantadine and bromocriptine (section 4.9.1).

The patient should be advised at the outset of the limitations of treatment and possible side-effects. About 10 to 20% of patients are unresponsive to treatment.

For drug interactions of antiparkinsonian drugs, see Appendix 1 (section 4.9).

THE ELDERLY. Antiparkinsonian drugs carry a special risk of inducing confusion in the elderly. It is therefore particularly important to initiate treatment with low doses and to use small increments.

4.9.1 Dopaminergic drugs used in parkinsonism

Levodopa is the treatment of choice for disabled patients. It is least valuable in elderly patients and in those with long-standing disease who may not tolerate a dose large enough to overcome their deficit. It is also less valuable in patients with post-encephalitic disease who are particularly susceptible to the side-effects.

Levodopa, the amino-acid precursor of dopamine, acts mainly by replenishing depleted striatal dopamine. It improves bradykinesia and rigidity more than tremor. It is generally administered in conjunction with an extra-cerebral dopa-decarboxylase inhibitor (**carbidopa**, as in Sinemet® or **benserazide**, as in Madopar®) which prevents the peripheral degradation of levodopa to dopamine.

The presence of the inhibitor enables the effective dose of levodopa to be greatly reduced, while peripheral side-effects such as nausea and vomiting and cardiovascular effects are minimised. There is less delay in onset of therapeutic effect and a smoother clinical response is obtained. A disadvantage is that there is an increased incidence of abnormal involuntary movements. When Sinemet® is used in low dosage the dose of carbidopa may be insufficient to achieve full inhibition of extracerebral dopa-decarboxylase; Sinemet-Plus® (containing 25 mg of carbidopa for each 100 mg of levodopa) should then be used so that the daily dose of carbidopa is at least 75 mg. This will ensure maximum effectiveness of the levodopa with a minimum of adverse peripheral effects.

Treatment with levodopa should be initiated with low doses and gradually increased, by small increments, at intervals of 2 to 3 days. (It is rarely necessary to exceed a daily dose of 1 gram when levodopa is used in conjunction with a dopa-decarboxylase inhibitor.) When titrated in this way the final dose is usually a compromise between increased mobility and dose-limiting side-effects. Intervals between doses may be critical and should be chosen to suit the needs of the individual patient. Nausea and vomiting are rarely dose-limiting if levodopa is given in this way but doses should be taken after meals. Domperidone may be useful in controlling vomiting (section 4.6). The most frequent dose-limiting side-effects of levodopa are involuntary movements and psychiatric complications.

Treatment with levodopa should not be discontinued abruptly. As the patient ages, the maintenance dose may need to be reduced. When substituting the combined levodopa-decarboxylase inhibitor preparations for levodopa alone, treatment should be discontinued for 12 hours before starting therapy with the combined preparation.

During the first 6 to 18 months of levodopa therapy there may be a slow improvement in the response of the patient which is maintained for $1\frac{1}{2}$ to 2 years; thereafter a slow decline may occur. Particularly troublesome is the 'on-off' effect the incidence of which increases as the treatment progresses. This is characterised by fluctuations in performance with normal performance during the 'on' period and weakness and akinesia lasting for 2 to 4 hours during the 'off' period.

Monoamine-oxidase inhibitors must be withdrawn at least 14 days before treatment. Close observation is especially necessary in patients with dementia or with a past history of psychiatric illness, open-angle glaucoma, or skin melanoma. Antipsychotic drugs should not be administered concurrently.

Selegiline (Eldepryl®) is a recently-introduced monoamine-oxidase-B inhibitor used in severe parkinsonism in conjunction with levodopa to reduce 'end-of-dose' akinesia. Unlike other monoamine-oxidase inhibitors, it does not cause episodes of hypertension.

Bromocriptine (Parlodel®) acts by direct stimulation of surviving dopamine receptors. Although effective, it has no advantages over levodopa. Its use should be restricted to the treatment of previously untreated disabled patients and those who despite careful titration cannot tolerate levodopa. Its use is often restricted by its side-effects and when used with levodopa, abnormal involuntary movements and confusional states are common. The doses of the two drugs should be balanced for optimum effect.

Amantadine (Symmetrel®) has modest anti-parkinsonian effects. It improves mild bradykinetic disabilities as well as tremor and rigidity. Unfortunately only a small proportion of patients derive much benefit from this drug and tolerance to its effects occurs. However it has the advantage of being relatively free from side-effects.

LEVODOPA

Indications: parkinsonism (but not drug-induced extrapyramidal symptoms), see notes above

Cautions: pulmonary disease, peptic ulceration, cardiovascular disease, diabetes, open-angle glaucoma, skin melanoma, psychiatric illness. In prolonged therapy, psychiatric, hepatic, haematological, renal, and cardiovascular surveillance is advisable. Discontinue treatment 8 hours before surgery (increased risk of arrhythmias). Warn patients who benefit from therapy to resume normal activities gradually. Drug interactions: see Appendix 1 (sections 2.5, 4.3, 4.9, 15)

Contra-indications: closed-angle glaucoma

Side-effects: anorexia, nausea, insomnia, agitation, postural hypotension, dizziness, tachycardia, arrhythmias, discoloration of urine and other body fluids, rarely hypersensitivity; abnormal involuntary movements and psychiatric symptoms which include hypomania and psychosis may be dose-limiting, occasionally depression reported

Dose: initially 125–500 mg daily in divided doses after meals, increased according to response (see notes above)

PoM **Levodopa Capsules,** levodopa 125 mg, net price 20 = 24p; 250 mg, 20 = 47p; 500 mg, 20 = 92p. Label: 14, 21

PoM **Levodopa Tablets,** levodopa 500 mg. Net price 20 = £1.34. Label: 14, 21

PoM **Brocadopa®** (Brocades)
Capsules, levodopa 125 mg, net price 20 = 24p; 250 mg, 20 = 47p; 500 mg, 20 = 92p. Label: 14, 21

PoM **Larodopa®** (Roche)
Tablets, scored, levodopa 500 mg. Net price 20 = £1.34. Label: 14, 21

LEVODOPA WITH BENSERAZIDE

Indications; Cautions; Contra-indications; Side-effects: see under Levodopa and notes above

Dose: expressed as levodopa, initially 50–100 mg twice daily, adjusted according to response; usual maintenance dose 400–800 mg daily in divided doses after meals

Note. When transferring patients from levodopa 3 capsules Madopar 125® should be substituted for 2 g levodopa

PoM **Madopar®** (Roche)
Capsules 62.5, blue/grey, levodopa 50 mg, benserazide 12.5 mg (as hydrochloride). Net price 20 = £1.41. Label: 14, 21, 25

Capsules 125, blue/pink, levodopa 100 mg, benserazide 25 mg (as hydrochloride). Net price 20 = £2.50. Label: 14, 21, 25

Capsules 250, blue/caramel, levodopa 200 mg, benserazide 50 mg (as hydrochloride). Net price 20 = £4.16. Label: 14, 21, 25

Dispersible tablets 62.5, scored, levodopa 50 mg, benserazide 12.5 mg (as hydrochloride). Net price 20 = £1.51. Label: 14, 21, counselling advised, administration, see below

---

Dispersible tablets 125, scored, levodopa 100 mg, benserazide 25 mg (as hydrochloride). Net price 20 = £2.72. Label: 14, 21, counselling advised, administration, see below
Note. The tablets may be dispersed in water or orange squash or swallowed whole

LEVODOPA WITH CARBIDOPA

Indications; Cautions; Contra-indications; Side-effects: see under Levodopa and notes above
Dose: expressed as levodopa, initially 100–125 mg 3–4 times daily adjusted according to response; usual maintenance dose 0.75–1.5 g daily in divided doses after food. See also under Sinemet-Plus®
Note. When transferring patients from levodopa, 3 tablets Sinemet-275 should be substituted for 4 g levodopa

PoM **Sinemet**® (MSD)
Tablets (Sinemet-110), blue, scored, levodopa 100 mg, carbidopa 10 mg (as monohydrate). Net price 20 = £1.71. Label: 14, 21
Tablets (Sinemet-275), blue, scored, levodopa 250 mg, carbidopa 25 mg (as monohydrate). Net price 20 = £3.57. Label: 14, 21
PoM **Sinemet LS**® (MSD)
Tablets, yellow, scored, levodopa 50 mg, carbidopa 12.5 mg (as monohydrate). Net price 84 = £6.87. Label: 14, 21
Dose: initially 1 tablet 3 times daily, adjusted according to response; see also Sinemet Plus®, 2 tablets Sinemet LS® ≡ 1 tablet Sinemet Plus®
PoM **Sinemet-Plus**® (MSD)
Tablets, yellow, scored, levodopa 100 mg, carbidopa 25 mg (as monohydrate). Net price 20 = £2.52. Label: 14, 21
Dose: initially 1 tablet 3 times daily, adjusted according to response to 8 daily in divided doses; larger doses by gradual substitution of Sinemet for Sinemet-Plus

AMANTADINE HYDROCHLORIDE

Indications: parkinsonism (but not drug-induced extrapyramidal symptoms)
Cautions: cardiovascular, hepatic, or renal disease, recurrent eczema, psychosis, elderly patients, breast-feeding. Avoid abrupt discontinuation of treatment. Drug interactions: see Appendix 1 (section *4.9*)
Contra-indications: epilepsy, gastric ulceration
Side-effects: nervousness, inability to concentrate, insomnia, dizziness, gastro-intestinal disturbances, skin discoloration, dry mouth, peripheral oedema; rarely leucopenia
Dose: 100 mg daily increased if necessary to 100 mg twice daily (not later than 4 p.m.), usually in conjunction with other treatment
COUNSELLING. Second dose not later than 4 p.m.

PoM **Symmetrel**® (Geigy)
Capsules, brownish-red, amantadine hydrochloride 100 mg. Net price 20 = £3.22
Syrup, amantadine hydrochloride 50 mg/5 ml. Diluent syrup, life of diluted syrup 4 weeks. Net price 150 ml = £3.02

BROMOCRIPTINE

Indications: parkinsonism (but not drug-induced extrapyramidal symptoms)
Cautions; Side-effects: see section 6.7.1
Dose: first week 1–1.25 mg at night, second week 2–2.5 mg at night, third week 2.5 mg twice daily, then 3 times daily increasing by 2.5 mg every 3–14 days according to response to a usual range of 10–40 mg daily; taken with food
COUNSELLING. Hypotensive reactions may be disturbing in some patients during the first few days of treatment and particular care should be exercised when driving vehicles or operating machinery; tolerance to bromocriptine reduced by alcohol

PoM **Parlodel**® (Sandoz)
Tablets, both scored, bromocriptine (as mesylate), 1 mg, net price 20 = £2.65; 2.5 mg, 20 = £5.13. Label: 21, counselling advised, see above
Capsules, bromocriptine (as mesylate), 5 mg (blue/white), net price 20 = £10.06; 10 mg, 20 = £18.62. Label: 21, counselling advised, see above
Parkinson's disease starter pack, in 4 separate containers, 7 tablets, scored, bromocriptine 1 mg (as mesylate); 7, 14 and 21 tablets, scored, bromocriptine 2.5 mg (as mesylate). Net price per pack = £13.00. Label: 10, 21, counselling advised, dosage schedule

SELEGILINE

Indications: adjunct in Parkinson's disease treated with levodopa, particularly in patients who have developed 'end-of-dose' akinesia
Cautions: side-effects of levodopa may be increased, concurrent levodopa dosage may need to be reduced by 20–50%
Side-effects: hypotension, nausea and vomiting, confusion, agitation
Dose: initially 5 mg in the morning, increasing to 10 mg if necessary

▼ PoM **Eldepryl**® (Britannia)
Tablets, scored, selegiline hydrochloride 5 mg. Net price 20 = £9.30

4.9.2 Anticholinergic drugs used in parkinsonism

These drugs exert their antiparkinsonian effect by correcting the relative cholinergic excess which is thought to occur in parkinsonism as a result of dopamine deficiency. In most patients their effects are only moderate, reducing tremor and rigidity to some effect but without significant action on bradykinesia. Anticholinergics (more correctly termed 'antimuscarinics') exert a synergistic effect when used with levodopa and are also useful in reducing sialorrhoea.

They may be used as first-line drugs in mild cases, particularly with tremor or rigidity, or as adjunctive therapy with levodopa. The anticholinergic drugs also reduce the symptoms of drug-induced parkinsonism as seen, for example, with antipsychotic drugs (section 4.2.1) but there is no justification for giving them simultaneously with antipsychotics unless parkinsonian side-effects occur. Tardive dyskinesia is not improved by the anticholinergic drugs and may be made worse.

No important differences exist between the many synthetic drugs available but certain patients appear to tolerate one preparation better than another. Doses may be taken before food if dry mouth is troublesome, or after food if gastro-intestinal symptoms predominate.

The most commonly used drugs are **orphenadrine hydrochloride** (Disipal®) and **benzhexol** (Artane®). **Benztropine** (Cogentin®) and **procyclidine** (Kemadrin®) are also used. Benztropine is similar to benzhexol but is excreted more slowly; changes in dose therefore need to be carried out very gradually. Both procyclidine and benztropine may be given parenterally and are effective emergency treatment for acute drug-induced dystonic reactions which may be severe.

BENZHEXOL HYDROCHLORIDE

Indications: parkinsonism; drug-induced extra-pyramidal symptoms
Cautions: urinary retention, glaucoma, cardiovascular disease, hepatic or renal impairment; avoid abrupt discontinuation of treatment; drugs of this type liable to abuse (section 4.2.1). Drug interactions of anticholinergic drugs: see Appendix 1 (sections *2.3, 4.2, 4.6, 4.9, 5.2*)
Side-effects: dry mouth, gastro-intestinal disturbances, dizziness, blurred vision; less commonly tachycardia, hypersensitivity, nervousness, and with high doses in susceptible patients, mental confusion, excitement, and psychiatric disturbances which may necessitate discontinuation of treatment
Dose: 1 mg daily, gradually increased; usual maintenance dose 5–15 mg daily in 3–4 divided doses

PoM **Benzhexol** (Non-proprietary)
Tablets, benzhexol hydrochloride 2 mg, net price 20 = 31p; 5 mg, 20 = 63p. Counselling advised, before or after food (see notes above)
PoM **Artane**® (Lederle)
Tablets, both scored, benzhexol hydrochloride 2 mg, net price 20 = 32p; 5 mg, 20 = 65p. Counselling advised, before or after food (see notes above)
Sustets® (= capsules s/r), blue-green, benzhexol hydrochloride 5 mg. Net price 20 = £1.09. Label: 25, counselling advised, before or after food (see notes above)
Dose: 1–3 capsules daily in divided doses or as a single dose in the morning
PoM **Bentex**® (Steinhard)
Tablets, both scored, benzhexol hydrochloride 2 mg, net price 20 = 31p; 5 mg, 20 = 63p. Counselling advised, before or after food (see notes above)
PoM **Broflex**® (Bio-Medical)
Syrup, pink, benzhexol hydrochloride 5 mg/5 ml. Diluent syrup, life of diluted syrup

14 days. Net price 100 ml = 79p. Counselling advised, before or after food (see notes above)

ORPHENADRINE HYDROCHLORIDE

Indications: parkinsonism; drug-induced extra-pyramidal symptoms
Cautions; Contra-indications; Side-effects: see under Benzhexol Hydrochloride, but more euphoric; may cause insomnia; less effective in controlling tremor
Dose: by mouth, adults and children, daily in divided doses, 150 mg gradually increased; max. 400 mg daily
By intramuscular injection, adults and children, 20–40 mg when necessary

PoM **Biorphen**® (Bio-Medical)
Elixir, sugar-free, orphenadrine hydrochloride 25 mg/5 ml. Net price 100 ml = 84p
PoM **Disipal**® (Brocades)
Tablets, yellow, s/c, orphenadrine hydrochloride 50 mg. Net price 20 = 30p
Injection, orphenadrine hydrochloride 20 mg/ml. Net price 2-ml amp = 31p

BENZTROPINE MESYLATE

Indications: parkinsonism, drug-induced extra-pyramidal symptoms
Cautions; Contra-indications; Side-effects: see under Benzhexol Hydrochloride, but causes sedation rather than stimulation; persons affected should not drive or operate machinery; avoid alcohol (CNS depression); avoid in children under 3 years
Dose: by mouth, 0.5–1 mg daily usually at bedtime, gradually increased; max. 6 mg daily; usual maintenance dose 1–4 mg daily in single or divided doses
By intramuscular or intravenous injection, 1–2 mg, repeated if symptoms reappear

PoM **Cogentin**® (MSD)
Tablets, scored, benztropine mesylate 2 mg. Net price 20 = 29p. Label: 2
Injection, benztropine mesylate 1 mg/ml. Net price 2-ml amp = 77p

BIPERIDEN

Indications: parkinsonism, drug-induced extra-pyramidal symptoms
Cautions; Contra-indications; Side-effects: see under Benzhexol Hydrochloride, but may cause drowsiness; persons affected should not drive or operate machinery; injection may cause hypotension
Dose: by mouth, biperiden hydrochloride 1 mg twice daily, gradually increased if necessary; usual maintenance dose 2–6 mg daily in divided doses
By intramuscular or slow intravenous injection, biperiden lactate 5–20 mg daily in divided doses

PoM **Akineton**® (Abbott)
Tablets, scored, biperiden hydrochloride 2 mg. Net price 20 = 47p. Label: 2

Injection, biperiden lactate 5 mg/ml. Net price
1-ml amp = 35p

METHIXENE HYDROCHLORIDE

Indications: parkinsonism, drug-induced extrapyramidal symptoms, senile tremor, more
effective in controlling tremor than rigidity
Cautions; Contra-indications; Side-effects: see
under Benzhexol Hydrochloride
Dose: 2.5 mg 3 times daily gradually increased;
usual maintenance dose 15–60 mg (elderly
patients 15–30 mg) daily in divided doses

PoM **Tremonil**® (Sandoz)
Tablets, scored, methixene hydrochloride 5 mg.
Net price 20 = 68p. Label: 2

PROCYCLIDINE HYDROCHLORIDE

Indications: parkinsonism, drug-induced extrapyramidal symptoms
Cautions; Contra-indications; Side-effects: see
under Benzhexol Hydrochloride
Dose: by mouth, 2.5 mg 3 times daily, gradually
increased if necessary; usual max. 30 mg daily
Acute dystonia, *by intravenous injection*, 5 mg
(usually effective within 5 minutes); an
occasional patient may need 10 mg or more and
may require up to half an hour to obtain relief
Note. The intramuscular route can also be used
although not currently on the manufacturer's data sheet

PoM **Procyclidine** (Non-proprietary)
Tablets, procyclidine hydrochloride 5 mg. Net
price 20 = 85p
PoM **Arpicolin**® (RP Drugs)
Syrup procyclidine hydrochloride 2.5 mg/5 ml,
net price 100 ml = 96p; 5 mg/5 ml, 100 ml =
£1.74
PoM **Kemadrin**® (Wellcome)
Tablets, scored, procyclidine hydrochloride
5 mg. Net price 20 = £1.10
Injection, procyclidine hydrochloride 5 mg/ml.
Net price 2-ml amp = £1.18

4.9.3   Drugs used in essential tremor, chorea, tics, and related disorders

Tetrabenazine (Nitoman®) is mainly used to control movement disorders in Huntington's chorea
and related disorders. It may act by depleting
nerve endings of dopamine. It has useful action
in only a proportion of patients and its use may
be limited by the development of depression.

Haloperidol may be useful in improving motor
tics, stuttering, hiccup, and symptoms of Gilles
de la Tourette syndrome and related choreas.
Pimozide (section 4.2.1) and more recently clonidine (section 4.7.4.2) and sulpiride (section
4.2.1), are also used in Gilles de la Tourette
syndrome. **Benzhexol** (section 4.9.2) at high
dosage may also improve some movement
disorders. It is sometimes necessary to build the
dose up over many weeks, to a maximum of 20 to
30 mg daily. Other antipsychotic drugs such as
chlorpromazine and **perphenazine** are used to
relieve intractable hiccup (section 4.2.1).

Propranolol or another beta-adrenoceptor
blocking drug (see section 2.4) may be useful in
treating essential tremor or tremors associated
with anxiety or thyrotoxicosis. Propranolol is
given in a dosage of 40 mg 2 or 3 times daily,
increased if necessary; 80 to 160 mg daily is usually
required for maintenance.

HALOPERIDOL

Indications: motor tics, stuttering, adjunctive
treatment in choreas and Gilles de la Tourette
syndrome
Cautions; Contra-indications; Side-effects: see
section 4.2.1
Dose: by mouth, 0.5–1.5 mg 3 times daily
adjusted according to the response; 10 mg daily
or more may occasionally be necessary in Gilles
de la Tourette syndrome; CHILD, stuttering 50
micrograms/kg daily, Gilles de la Tourette syndrome up to 10 mg daily

Preparations
Section 4.2.1

TETRABENAZINE

Indications: movement disorders due to Huntington's chorea, senile chorea, and related
neurological conditions
Cautions: drug interactions: see Appendix 1
(sections *4.2, 4.3, 4.9*)
Side-effects: drowsiness, gastro-intestinal disturbances, depression, extrapyramidal
dysfunction
Dose: initially 25 mg 3 times daily, gradually
increased (elderly patients 12.5 mg daily,
increasing to 3 times daily if necessary); max.
200 mg daily

PoM **Nitoman**® (Roche)
Tablets, pale yellow-buff, scored, tetrabenazine
25 mg. Net price 20 = 93p. Label: 2

4.10   Drugs used in alcoholism and cigarette smoking

Disulfiram (Antabuse®) is used as an adjunct
to the treatment of alcoholism. It gives rise to
extremely unpleasant systemic reactions after the
ingestion of even small amounts of alcohol
because it leads to accumulation of acetaldehyde
in the body. Reactions include flushing of the face,
throbbing headache, palpitations, tachycardia,
nausea, vomiting, and, with large doses of alcohol,
arrhythmias, hypotension, and collapse. Even the
small amounts of alcohol included in many oral
medicines may be sufficient to precipitate a
reaction. It may be advisable for patients to carry
a card warning of the danger of administration of
alcohol. For drug interactions of disulfiram see
Appendix 1 (sections *2.8B, 4.1, 4.3, 4.8, 5.1*).

For use of chlormethiazole in withdrawal treatment see section 4.1.1 and for use of benzodiazepines see section 4.1.2.

ALCOHOLISM

DISULFIRAM

Indications: adjunct in the treatment of chronic alcoholism (under specialist supervision)

Cautions: ensure that alcohol not consumed for at least 12 hours before initiating treatment; see also notes above; variable and occasionally severe reactions on alcohol challenge; hepatic or renal impairment, respiratory disease, diabetes mellitus, epilepsy. Drug interactions: see Appendix 1 (sections *2.8B, 4.1, 4.3, 4.8, 5.1*)

ALCOHOL REACTION. Patients should be warned of unpredictable and occasionally severe nature of disulfiram-alcohol interactions. Reactions can occur in 10 minutes and last several hours (may require intensive supportive therapy). Patients should not ingest alcohol at all and should be warned of possible presence of alcohol in liquid medicines

Contra-indications: cardiac failure, coronary artery disease, psychosis and drug addiction, pregnancy

Side-effects: initially drowsiness and fatigue; nausea, vomiting, halitosis, reduced libido; rarely psychotic reactions (depression, paranoia, schizophrenia, mania), allergic dermatitis, peripheral neuritis, hepatic cell damage

Dose: 800 mg as a single dose on first day, reducing over 5 days to 100–200 mg daily; may be continued for up to 1 year

PoM **Antabuse 200**® (CP)
Tablets, scored, disulfiram 200 mg. Net price 20 = £4.60. Label: 2

SMOKING

NHS ▼ PoM **Nicorette**® (Lundbeck)
Chewing gum, sugar-free, nicotine (as resin) 2 mg, net price, pack of 105 = £5.56; 4 mg, 105 = £8.54.

Dose: nicotine replacement, initially one 2-mg piece to be chewed slowly for approx. 30 minutes, when urge to smoke occurs; patients needing more than 15 pieces daily may need the 4-mg strength.

5: Drugs used in the treatment of
INFECTIONS

In this chapter, drug treatment is discussed under the following headings:

5.1   Antibacterial drugs

CHOICE OF A SUITABLE DRUG. Before selecting an antibiotic the clinician must first consider two factors—the patient and the known or likely causative organism. Factors related to the patient which must be considered include history of allergy, renal and hepatic function, resistance to infection (i.e. whether immunocompromised), ability to tolerate drugs by mouth, severity of illness, ethnic origin, age and, if female, whether pregnant, breast-feeding or taking an oral contraceptive.

The known or likely organism and its antibiotic sensitivity, in association with the above factors, will suggest one or more antibiotics, the final choice depending on the microbiological, pharmacological, and toxicological properties.

An example of a rational approach to the selection of an antibiotic is treatment of a urinary-tract infection in a patient complaining of nausea in early pregnancy. The organism is reported as being resistant to ampicillin but sensitive to nitrofurantoin (can cause nausea), gentamicin (can only be given by injection and best avoided in pregnancy), tetracycline and co-trimoxazole (both contra-indicated in pregnancy), and cephalexin. The safest antibiotics in pregnancy are the penicillins and cephalosporins; therefore, cephalexin would be indicated for this patient.

The principles involved in selection of an antibiotic must allow for a number of variables including changing renal and hepatic function, increasing bacterial resistance, and new information on side-effects. Duration of therapy, dosage, and route of administration depend on site, type and severity of infection.

ANTIBIOTIC POLICIES. Many health authorities now place limits on the antibiotics that may be used in their hospitals, to achieve reasonable economy consistent with adequate cover, and to reduce the development of resistant organisms. An authority may indicate a range of drugs for general use, and permit treatment with other drugs only on the advice of the microbiologist or physician responsible for the control of infectious diseases.

BEFORE STARTING THERAPY. The following precepts should be considered before starting:

Viral infections should not be treated with antibiotics.

Samples should be taken for culture and sensitivity testing; **'blind'** prescribing of an antibiotic for a patient ill with unexplained pyrexia usually leads to further difficulty in establishing the diagnosis.

An up-to-date knowledge of **prevalent organisms** and their current sensitivity is of great help in choosing an antibiotic before bacteriological confirmation is available.

The **dose** of an antibiotic will vary according to a number of factors including age, weight, renal function, and severity of infection. The prescribing of the so-called 'standard' dose in serious infections may result in failure of treatment or even death of the patient. Most antibiotics are rapidly excreted from the body and should be administered every 6 hours for the treatment of serious infections. Less severe infections as seen in general practice usually respond to administration every 8 hours. Agents with prolonged plasma half-lives such as trimethoprim need only be given every 12 hours. The aminoglycoside antibiotics should not be given more frequently than every 8 hours and the interval between doses must be increased in patients with renal failure.

The **route** of administration of an antibiotic will often depend on the severity of the infection. Life-threatening infections require intravenous therapy. Whenever possible painful intramuscular injections should be avoided in children.

Duration of therapy depends on the nature of the infection and the response to treatment. Courses should not be unduly prolonged as they are wasteful and may lead to side-effects. However, in certain infections such as endocarditis or tuberculosis it is necessary to continue treatment for relatively long periods. Conversely a single dose of an antibiotic may cure uncomplicated urinary-tract infections.

Suggested treatment is shown in Table 1. When the pathogen has been isolated treatment may be changed to a more appropriate antibiotic if necessary. If no bacterium is cultured the antibiotic can be continued or stopped on clinical grounds. Infections for which prophylaxis is useful are listed in Table 2.

Table 1. Summary of antibacterial therapy

Infection	Suggested antibacterial	Comment
1: Gastro-intestinal system		
Gastro-enteritis	Antibiotic not usually indicated	Frequently nonbacterial aetiology
Bacillary dysentery	Antibiotic usually not indicated	Co-trimoxazole (or trimethoprim) in severe illness
Campylobacter enteritis	Erythromycin	
Invasive salmonellosis	Co-trimoxazole *or* ampicillin[1]	
Typhoid fever	Chloramphenicol *or* co-trimoxazole *or* amoxycillin	
Biliary-tract infection	Gentamicin *or* a cephalosporin	
Peritonitis	Gentamicin + metronidazole (*or* clindamycin)	
Peritoneal dialysis-associated peritonitis	Vancomycin + gentamicin added to dialysis fluid	Discontinue either gentamicin or vancomycin when sensitivity known; treat for 5–10 days
2: Cardiovascular system		
Endocarditis caused by:		
Staphylococcus aureus	Flucloxacillin[1] + fusidic acid (*or* gentamicin)	Treat for at least 4 weeks
Streptococci with reduced sensitivity to penicillin e.g. *Streptococcus faecalis*	Benzylpenicillin + low-dose gentamicin (i.e. 60–80 mg twice daily)	Treat for at least 4 weeks
Penicillin-sensitive streptococci (e.g. viridans streptococci)	Benzylpenicillin + low-dose gentamicin (i.e. 60–80 mg twice daily)	Treat for 4 weeks; stop gentamicin after 2 weeks if organism fully sensitive to penicillin. Oral amoxycillin may be substituted for benzylpenicillin after 2 weeks
3: Respiratory system		
Haemophilus epiglottitis	Chloramphenicol	Give intravenously
Exacerbations of chronic bronchitis	Ampicillin[1] *or* co-trimoxazole (*or* trimethoprim) *or* erythromycin *or* tetracycline	Note that 20% of pneumococci and some *Haemophilus influenzae* strains are tetracycline-resistant
Pneumonia:		
Previously healthy chest	Benzylpenicillin *or* ampicillin[1]	Add flucloxacillin[1] if *Staphylococcus* suspected e.g. in influenza or measles; use erythromycin if *Legionella* infection is suspected
Previously unhealthy chest	Flucloxacillin[1] + ampicillin[1] (*or* co-trimoxazole *or* erythromycin)	Substitute erythromycin for flucloxacillin if *Legionella* infection is suspected
4: Central nervous system		
Meningitis caused by:		
Meningococcus	Benzylpenicillin	Intrathecal therapy not necessary
Pneumococcus	Benzylpenicillin	
Haemophilus influenzae	Chloramphenicol	
7: Genital system		
Syphilis	Procaine penicillin (*or* tetracycline *or* erythromycin if penicillin-allergic)	Treat for 10–21 days
Gonorrhoea	Procaine penicillin with probenecid *or* ampicillin[1] with probenecid (*or* co-trimoxazole, spectinomycin, *or* cefuroxime if penicillin-allergic)	Single-dose treatment
Non-gonococcal urethritis	Tetracycline	Treat for 10–21 days
Pelvic inflammatory disease	Metronidazole + doxycycline	Not active against all causative organisms; remember gonorrhoea
Urinary tract		
Acute pyelonephritis or prostatitis	Co-trimoxazole (*or* trimethoprim) *or* gentamicin *or* cephalosporin	Do not give co-trimoxazole (*or* trimethoprim) in pregnancy. Treat prostatitis with co-trimoxazole (*or* trimethoprim) for 4 weeks

Table 1. Summary of antibacterial therapy (*continued*)

Infection	Suggested antibacterial	Comment
'Lower' UTI	Trimethoprim *or* ampicillin[1] *or* nitrofurantoin *or* oral cephalosporin	
9: Blood Septicaemia Initial 'blind' therapy	Aminoglycoside + a penicillin *or* a cephalosporin alone *In immunocompromised,* aminoglycoside + a broad-spectrum penicillin *or* a 'third generation' cephalosporin alone	Choice of agents depends on local bacterial resistance patterns and clinical presentation; add metronidazole if anaerobic infection suspected
10: Musculoskeletal system Osteomyelitis and septic arthritis	Clindamycin *or* flucloxacillin[1] + fusidic acid. If *Haemophilus influenzae* give ampicillin[1] *or* co-trimoxazole	Under 5 years of age may be *H. influenzae* Treat acute disease for at least 6 weeks and chronic infection for at least 12 weeks
11: Eye Purulent conjunctivitis	Chloramphenicol *or* gentamicin eye-drops	
12: Ear, nose, and oropharynx Dental infections	Amoxycillin (*or* ampicillin ester)	Metronidazole for anaerobic infections *or* those not responding to amoxycillin
Sinusitis	Erythromycin *or* co-trimoxazole	
Otitis media	Benzylpenicillin Phenoxymethylpenicillin Amoxycillin (*or* ampicillin ester) if under 5 years (*or* erythromycin if penicillin-allergic)	Initial i/m therapy (if possible) with benzylpenicillin, then oral therapy with phenoxymethylpenicillin Under 5 years of age may be *Haemophilus influenzae*
Tonsillitis	Benzylpenicillin Phenoxymethylpenicillin (*or* erythromycin if penicillin-allergic)	Initial i/m therapy (in severe infection) with benzylpenicillin, then oral therapy with phenoxymethylpenicillin. Most infections are caused by viruses
13: Skin Impetigo	Topical chlortetracycline *or* oral flucloxacillin[1] if systemic toxicity	
Erysipelas	Benzylpenicillin Phenoxymethylpenicillin	Initial i/m therapy (if possible) with benzylpenicillin, then oral therapy with phenoxymethylpenicillin
Cellulitis	Flucloxacillin[1] (*or* erythromycin if penicillin-allergic)	
Acne	Tetracycline	Treat for at least 3–4 months

[1]Where ampicillin is suggested in the table amoxycillin or an ester of ampicillin may be used, and where flucloxacillin is suggested cloxacillin may be used.

Table 2. Summary of antibacterial prophylaxis

Infection	Antibacterial and adult dose
Prevention of recurrence of rheumatic fever	Phenoxymethylpenicillin 500 mg daily *or* sulphadimidine 500 mg daily (250 mg for children)
Prevention of secondary case of meningococcal meningitis	Rifampicin 600 mg every 12 hours for 2 days; CHILD 10 mg/kg (3 months–1 year, 5 mg/kg) every 12 hours for 2 days; *or* sulphadimidine (if strain known to be sensitive) 1 g every 12 hours for 2 days; CHILD 500 mg (3 months–1 year, 250 mg) every 12 hours for 2 days
Prevention of secondary case of diphtheria in non-immune patient	Erythromycin 500 mg every 6 hours for 5 days

Cautionary label wordings, see inside back cover

Prices are **net**, see p. 1

Table 2. Summary of antibacterial prophylaxis (*continued*)

Infection	Antibacterial and adult dose
Prevention of endocarditis in patients with heart-valve lesion, septal defect, patent ductus, or prosthetic valve	*Dental procedures under local anaesthesia*, including patients with a prosthetic heart valve but not those who have had endocarditis, oral amoxycillin 3 g 1 hour before procedure *or* if penicillin-allergic, oral erythromycin 1.5 g (as stearate) 1 hour before procedure, then 500 mg 6 hours later; patients who have had endocarditis, amoxycillin + gentamicin, as under general anaesthesia
Note. High-dose 3-g amoxycillin regimens are now considered suitable for patients who have received penicillins in the preceding month	*Dental procedures under general anaesthesia*, no special risk, *either* i/m amoxycillin 1 g before induction, then oral amoxycillin 500 mg 6 hours later *or* oral amoxycillin 3 g 4 hours before induction then oral amoxycillin 3 g as soon as possible after procedure *or* oral amoxycillin 3 g + oral probenecid 1 g 4 hours before procedure; special risk (patients with a prosthetic heart valve or who have had endocarditis), i/m amoxycillin 1 g + i/m gentamicin 1.5 mg/kg immediately before induction, then oral amoxycillin 500 mg 6 hours later; patients who are penicillin-allergic, i/v vancomycin 1 g over 60 minutes then i/v gentamicin 1.5 mg/kg before induction
	Genito-urinary and colonic procedures, i/m amoxycillin 1 g + i/m gentamicin 1.5 mg/kg immediately before induction, then oral or i/m amoxycillin 500 mg 6 hours later *or* if penicillin-allergic, i/v vancomycin 1 g over 60 minutes then i/v gentamicin 1.5 mg/kg immediately before induction; metronidazole may also be added
Prevention of gas-gangrene in high lower-limb amputations or following major trauma	Benzylpenicillin 300–600 mg every 6 hours for 5 days; *or* procaine penicillin 2.4 g every 12 hours for 5 days; *or* if penicillin-allergic give metronidazole 500 mg every 6 hours
Prevention of tuberculosis in susceptible close contacts	Isoniazid 300 mg daily for 6–12 months; CHILD, isoniazid 5–10 mg/kg daily
Prevention of infection in abdominal surgery	
Operations on stomach or oesophagus for carcinoma, or cholecystectomy in patients with possibly infected bile	Single immediate pre-operative dose of gentamicin *or* a cephalosporin
Resections of colon and rectum for carcinoma, and resections in inflammatory bowel disease	Single immediate pre-operative dose of gentamicin + metronidazole
Hysterectomy	Metronidazole as suppository *or* single i/v dose

5.1.1 Penicillins

5.1.1.1 Benzylpenicillin and phenoxymethyl-penicillin
5.1.1.2 Penicillinase-resistant penicillins
5.1.1.3 Broad-spectrum penicillins
5.1.1.4 Antipseudomonal penicillins
5.1.1.5 Mecillinams

The penicillins are bactericidal and act by interfering with bacterial cell wall synthesis. They diffuse well into body tissues and fluids, but penetration into the cerebrospinal fluid is poor except when the meninges are inflamed. They are excreted in the urine in therapeutic concentrations. Probenecid blocks the renal tubular excretion of the penicillins, producing higher and more prolonged plasma concentrations. (For suggested doses see section 10.1.4)

The most important side-effect of the penicillins is hypersensitivity, which causes rashes and, occasionally, anaphylaxis, which can be fatal. Patients who are allergic to one penicillin will be allergic to all as the hypersensitivity is related to the basic penicillin structure. A rare but serious toxic effect of the penicillins is encephalopathy

due to cerebral irritation. This may result from excessively high doses but can also develop with normal doses given to patients with renal failure. Encephalopathy may follow intrathecal injection of the penicillins and this route of administration is best **avoided**, unless absolutely necessary, as chemical irritation of the brain can produce convulsions and sometimes death.

A second problem relating to high doses of penicillin, or normal doses given to patients with renal failure, is the accumulation of electrolyte since most injectable penicillins contain either sodium or potassium.

Diarrhoea frequently occurs during oral penicillin therapy. It is commonest with ampicillin and its derivatives, which can also cause pseudomembranous colitis.

UNITS. International units are no longer used for penicillins and all doses are stated in milligrams.

5.1.1.1 BENZYLPENICILLIN AND PHENOXYMETHYLPENICILLIN

Benzylpenicillin (Penicillin G, Crystapen®), the first of the penicillins, remains an important and

---

useful antibiotic; it is inactivated by bacterial penicillinases (beta-lactamases). It is the drug of choice for streptococcal, pneumococcal, gonococcal, and meningococcal infections and also for actinomycosis, anthrax, diphtheria, gas-gangrene, syphilis, tetanus, yaws, and treatment of Lyme disease in children. Pneumococci and gonococci have recently been isolated which have decreased sensitivity to penicillin. Benzylpenicillin is inactivated by gastric acid and absorption from the gut is low; therefore it is best given by injection. Benzylpenicillin may cause convulsions after high doses by intravenous injection or in renal failure.

Procaine penicillin (Depocillin®) is a sparingly soluble salt of benzylpenicillin. It is used in intramuscular depot preparations which provide therapeutic tissue concentrations for up to 24 hours. It is commonly used for the treatment of syphilis and gonorrhoea.

Benethamine penicillin is a benzylpenicillin salt with very low solubility giving a prolonged action after intramuscular injection, though producing low plasma concentrations; it is used, with soluble and procaine penicillin, in Triplopen®.

Phenoxymethylpenicillin (Penicillin V) has a similar antibacterial spectrum to benzylpenicillin, but is less active. It is gastric acid-stable, so is suitable for oral administration. It should not be used for serious infections because absorption can be unpredictable and plasma concentrations variable. It is indicated principally for respiratory-tract infections in children, for streptococcal tonsillitis, and for continuing treatment after one or more injections of benzylpenicillin when clinical response has begun. It should not be used for meningococcal or gonococcal infections. Phenoxymethylpenicillin is used for prophylaxis against streptococcal infections following rheumatic fever.

Phenethicillin has similar antibacterial activity, but is no more effective than phenoxymethylpenicillin.

BENZYLPENICILLIN
(Penicillin G)

Indications: tonsillitis, otitis media, erysipelas, streptococcal endocarditis, meningococcal and pneumococcal meningitis, prophylaxis in limb amputation
Cautions: history of allergy; renal impairment
Contra-indications: penicillin hypersensitivity
Side-effects: sensitivity reactions including urticaria, fever, joint pains; angioedema; anaphylactic shock in hypersensitive patients; diarrhoea after administration by mouth
Dose: by intramuscular injection or slow intravenous injection or infusion, 0.6–1.2 g daily in 2–4 divided doses, increased if necessary to 2.4 g daily; NEONATE, 30 mg/kg daily (in 2 divided doses in the first few days of life then in 3–4 divided doses); CHILD 1 month–12 years, 10–20 mg/kg daily in 4 divided doses
Bacterial endocarditis, *by slow intravenous injection or infusion,* up to 7.2 g daily in divided doses

Meningitis, *by slow intravenous injection or infusion,* NEONATE, 60–90 mg/kg daily in 3–4 divided doses; CHILD 1 month–12 years, 20–40 mg/kg daily in 4 divided doses
Prophylaxis in limb amputation, section 5.1, Table 2

PoM **Crystapen**® (Glaxo)
Injection, powder for reconstitution, benzyl-penicillin sodium (unbuffered). Net price 300-mg vial = 8p; 600-mg vial = 12p
Injection, powder for reconstitution, benzyl-penicillin sodium (buffered). Net price 3-g vial = 39p; 6-g vial = 64p

BENETHAMINE PENICILLIN
Indications: penicillin-sensitive infections; prophylaxis
Cautions; Contra-indications; Side-effects: see under Benzylpenicillin

PoM **Triplopen**® (Glaxo)
Injection, powder for reconstitution, benethamine penicillin 475 mg, procaine penicillin 250 mg, benzylpenicillin sodium 300 mg. Net price per vial = 40p
Dose: by deep intramuscular injection, 1 vial every 2–3 days

BENZATHINE PENICILLIN
Indications: penicillin-sensitive infections
Cautions; Contra-indications; Side-effects: see under Benzylpenicillin
Dose: see below

PoM **Penidural**® (Wyeth)
Suspension (= mixture), pink, benzathine penicillin 229 mg/5 ml. Diluent syrup, life of diluted mixture 14 days. Net price 100 ml = £1.86. Label: 9
Dose: 10 ml 3–4 times daily; CHILD 5 ml 3–4 times daily
Paediatric drops, pink, benzathine penicillin 115 mg/ml. Net price 10 ml = £2.04. Label: 9, counselling advised, use of pipette
Dose: CHILD up to 5 years, 1–2 dropperfuls (approx. 77–154 mg) 3–4 times daily

PHENETHICILLIN
Indications: penicillin-sensitive infections
Cautions; Contra-indications; Side-effects: see under Benzylpenicillin
Dose: 250 mg every 6 hours, at least 30 minutes before food; CHILD, under 2 years ¼ adult dose, 2–10 years ½ adult dose

PoM **Broxil**® (Beecham)
Capsules, black/ivory, phenethicillin 250 mg (as potassium salt). Net price 20 = £1.86. Label: 9, 23
Syrup, phenethicillin 125 mg (as potassium salt)/5 ml when reconstituted with water for preparations. Diluent syrup, life of diluted syrup 7 days. Net price 100 ml = £1.74. Label: 9, 23

PHENOXYMETHYLPENICILLIN
(Penicillin V)

Indications: tonsillitis, otitis media, erysipelas, rheumatic fever prophylaxis

Cautions; Contra-indications; Side-effects: see under Benzylpenicillin. Drug interactions: see Appendix 1 (section 5.1)

Dose: 250–500 mg every 6 hours, at least 30 minutes before food; CHILD, every 6 hours, up to 1 year 62.5 mg, 1–5 years 125 mg, 6–12 years 250 mg

PoM **Phenoxymethylpenicillin** (Non-proprietary)
Capsules, phenoxymethylpenicillin (as potassium salt) 250 mg. Label: 9, 23
Tablets, phenoxymethylpenicillin (as potassium salt) 125 mg and 250 mg. Label: 9, 23
Elixir, phenoxymethylpenicillin 62.5 mg (as potassium salt)/5 ml when reconstituted with water for preparations. Diluent syrup, life of diluted elixir 7 days. Label: 9, 23
Elixir, phenoxymethylpenicillin 125 mg (as potassium salt)/5 ml when reconstituted with water for preparations. Diluent as above. Label: 9, 23
Elixir, phenoxymethylpenicillin 250 mg (as potassium salt)/5 ml when reconstituted with water for preparations. Diluent as above. Label: 9, 23

PoM **Apsin VK**® (APS)
Tablets, f/c, scored, phenoxymethylpenicillin 250 mg (as potassium salt). Net price 20 = 41p. Label: 9, 23
Syrup, orange, phenoxymethylpenicillin 125 mg (as potassium salt)/5 ml when reconstituted with water for preparations. Diluent syrup, life of diluted syrup 7 days. Net price 100 ml = 66p. Label: 9, 23
Syrup, orange, phenoxymethylpenicillin 250 mg (as potassium salt)/5 ml when reconstituted with water for preparations. Diluent as above. Net price 100 ml = £1.01. Label: 9, 23

PoM **Distaquaine V-K**® (Dista)
Tablets, both scored, phenoxymethylpenicillin (as potassium salt) 125 mg, net price 20 = 21p; 250 mg, 20 = 36p. Label: 9, 23
Elixir, orange, phenoxymethylpenicillin 62.5 mg (as potassium salt)/5 ml when reconstituted with water for preparations. Diluent syrup, life of diluted elixir 7 days. Net price 100 ml = 44p. Label: 9, 23
Syrup, orange, phenoxymethylpenicillin 125 mg (as potassium salt)/5 ml when reconstituted with water for preparations. Diluent as above. Net price 100 ml = 58p. Label: 9, 23
Syrup, orange, phenoxymethylpenicillin 250 mg (as potassium salt)/5 ml when reconstituted with water for preparations. Diluent as above. Net price 100 ml = £1.06. Label: 9, 23

PoM **Econocil VK**® (DDSA)
Capsules, pink, phenoxymethylpenicillin 250 mg (as potassium salt). Net price 20 = 37p. Label: 9, 23
Tablets, phenoxymethylpenicillin (as potassium salt) 125 mg, net price 20 = 14p; 250 mg, 20 = 26p. Label: 9, 23

PoM **Stabillin V-K**® (Boots)
Tablets, phenoxymethylpenicillin 250 mg (as potassium salt). Net price 20 = 22p. Label: 9, 23
Elixir, phenoxymethylpenicillin 62.5 mg (as potassium salt)/5 ml when reconstituted with water for preparations. Diluent syrup, life of diluted elixir 7 days. Net price 100 ml = 40p. Label: 9, 23
Elixir, phenoxymethylpenicillin 125 mg (as potassium salt)/5 ml when reconstituted with water for preparations. Diluent as above. Net price 100 ml = 50p. Label: 9, 23
Elixir, phenoxymethylpenicillin 250 mg (as potassium salt)/5 ml when reconstituted with water for preparations. Diluent as above. Net price 100 ml = 80p. Label: 9, 23

PoM **V-Cil-K**® (Lilly)
Capsules, pink, phenoxymethylpenicillin 250 mg (as potassium salt). Net price 20 = 47p. Label: 9, 23
Tablets, phenoxymethylpenicillin (as potassium salt) 125 mg, net price 20 = 21p; 250 mg, 20 = 36p. Label: 9, 23
Paediatric syrup, phenoxymethylpenicillin 62.5 mg (as potassium salt)/5 ml when reconstituted with water for preparations. Diluent syrup, life of diluted syrup 7 days. Net price 100 ml = 44p. Label: 9, 23
Paediatric syrup, phenoxymethylpenicillin 125 mg (as potassium salt)/5 ml when reconstituted with water for preparations. Diluent as above. Net price 100 ml = 58p. Label: 9, 23
Syrup, phenoxymethylpenicillin 250 mg (as potassium salt)/5 ml when reconstituted with water for preparations. Diluent as above. Net price 100 ml = £1.06. Label: 9, 23

PROCAINE PENICILLIN

Indications: gas-gangrene following amputation; syphilis, gonorrhoea

Cautions; Contra-indications; Side-effects: see under Benzylpenicillin; **not** for intravenous administration

Dose: by intramuscular injection, 300 mg 1–2 times daily
Gonorrhoea, men, 2.4 g; women, 4.8 g as a single dose
Syphilis, 600 mg daily for at least 10 days; up to 1.2 g daily for heavier patients
See also section 5.1, Table 1

PoM **Bicillin**® (Brocades)
Injection, powder for reconstitution, procaine penicillin 3 g, benzylpenicillin sodium 600 mg. Net price per multidose vial = 33p
Dose: when reconstituted with 7.5 ml water for injections, 1 ml 1–2 times daily by intramuscular injection

PoM **Depocillin**® (Brocades)
Injection, powder for reconstitution, procaine penicillin. Net price 3-g multidose vial = 28p

---

5.1.1.2 PENICILLINASE-RESISTANT PENICILLINS

Most staphylococci are now resistant to benzylpenicillin because they produce penicillinases. **Cloxacillin** and **flucloxacillin**, however, are not inactivated by these enzymes and are thus effective in infections caused by penicillin-resistant *Staphylococci*, which is the sole indication for their use. They are acid-stable and can, therefore, be given by mouth as well as by injection.

Flucloxacillin is better absorbed from the gut than cloxacillin and is, therefore, to be preferred for oral therapy.

Methicillin (Celbenin®) is also effective against penicillin-resistant *Staph. aureus*, but can only be given by injection because it is not acid-stable and is now seldom used.

Staph. aureus strains resistant to methicillin and cloxacillin have emerged in some hospitals; some of these organisms are only sensitive to vancomycin (section 5.1.7).

CLOXACILLIN

Indications: infections due to penicillinase-producing staphylococci

Cautions; Contra-indications; Side-effects: see under Benzylpenicillin (section 5.1.1.1)

Dose: by mouth, 500 mg every 6 hours, at least 30 minutes before food

By intramuscular injection, 250 mg every 4–6 hours

By intravenous injection or infusion, 500 mg every 4–6 hours

Doses may be doubled in severe infections

CHILD, any route, under 2 years ¼ adult dose; 2–10 years ½ adult dose

PoM **Orbenin**® (Beecham)
Capsules, orange/black, cloxacillin 250 mg (as sodium salt). Net price 20 = £3.64. Label: 9, 23
Capsules, orange/black, cloxacillin 500 mg (as sodium salt). Net price 20 = £7.29. Label: 9, 23
Syrup, cloxacillin 125 mg (as sodium salt)/5 ml when reconstituted with water for preparations. Diluent syrup, life of diluted syrup 7 days. Net price 100 ml = £3.16. Label: 9, 23
Injection, powder for reconstitution, cloxacillin (as sodium salt). Net price 250-mg vial = 93p; 500-mg vial = £1.86; also available as 1-g vial

FLUCLOXACILLIN

Indications: infections due to penicillinase-producing staphylococci

Cautions; Contra-indications; Side-effects: see under Benzylpenicillin (section 5.1.1.1)

Dose: by mouth, 250 mg every 6 hours, at least 30 minutes before food

By intramuscular injection, 250 mg every 6 hours

By slow intravenous injection or infusion, 0.25–1 g every 6 hours

Doses may be doubled in severe infections

CHILD, any route, under 2 years ¼ adult dose; 2–10 years ½ adult dose

PoM **Flucloxacillin** (Non-proprietary)
Capsules, flucloxacillin (as sodium salt) 250 mg, net price 20 = £2.70; 500 mg, 20 = £5.60. Label: 9, 23
Elixir, flucloxacillin (as sodium salt) 125 mg/5 ml. Net price 100 ml = £3.32. Label: 9, 23
PoM **Floxapen**® (Beecham)
Capsules, both black/caramel, flucloxacillin (as sodium salt) 250 mg, net price 20 = £4.02; 500 mg, 20 = £8.04. Label: 9, 23
Syrup, flucloxacillin 125 mg (as magnesium salt)/5 ml when reconstituted with water for preparations. Diluent syrup, life of diluted syrup 14 days. Net price 100 ml = £3.32. Label: 9, 23
Syrup forte, flucloxacillin 250 mg (as magnesium salt)/5 ml when reconstituted with water for preparations. Diluent as above. Net price 100 ml = £6.64. Label: 9, 23
Injection, powder for reconstitution, flucloxacillin (as sodium salt). Net price 250-mg vial = 93p; 500-mg vial = £1.86; 1-g vial = £3.71
PoM **Ladropen**® (Berk)
Capsules, both brown/orange, flucloxacillin (as sodium salt) 250 mg, net price 20 = £3.45; 500 mg, 20 = £6.91. Label: 9, 23
PoM **Stafoxil**® (Brocades)
Capsules, both cream/brown, flucloxacillin (as sodium salt) 250 mg, net price 28 = £3.78; 500 mg, 28 = £7.84. Label: 9, 23
PoM **Staphlipen**® (Lederle)
Capsules, both brown/grey, flucloxacillin (as sodium salt) 250 mg, net price 20 = £2.70; 500 mg, 20 = £5.60. Label: 9, 23
Injection, powder for reconstitution, flucloxacillin (as sodium salt). Net price 250-mg vial = 93p; 500-mg vial = £1.86; 1-g vial = £3.71

METHICILLIN SODIUM

Indications: infections due to penicillinase-producing staphylococci

Cautions; Contra-indications; Side-effects: see under Benzylpenicillin (section 5.1.1.1)

Dose: by intramuscular injection or slow intravenous injection or infusion, 1 g every 4–6 hours

PoM **Celbenin**® (Beecham)
Injection, powder for reconstitution, methicillin sodium. Net price 1-g vial = £1.88

5.1.1.3 BROAD-SPECTRUM PENICILLINS

Ampicillin (Penbritin®) is active against certain Gram-positive and Gram-negative organisms but is inactivated by penicillinases including those produced by *Staphylococcus aureus* and by common Gram-negative bacilli such as *Escherichia coli*. Almost all staphylococci, one-third of *E. coli* strains and up to one-tenth of *Haemophilus influenzae* strains are now resistant. Ampicillin should therefore not be used for the 'blind' treatment of infections, especially in hospital patients.

Ampicillin is well excreted in the bile and urine. It is principally indicated for the treatment of exacerbations of chronic bronchitis and middle ear infections, both of which are usually due to *Streptococcus pneumoniae* and *H. influenzae*, and for urinary-tract infections and gonorrhoea.

Ampicillin can be given by mouth but less than half the dose is absorbed, and absorption is further decreased by the presence of food in the gut. Higher plasma concentrations are obtained with the ampicillin esters **bacampicillin** (Ambaxin®), **pivampicillin** (Pondocillin®), and **talampicillin** (Talpen®); their absorption is little affected by the presence of food, and the incidence of diarrhoea is less than with ampicillin. These antibiotics should be given every 8 hours for moderate or severe infections, especially outside the renal tract.

Maculopapular rashes commonly occur with ampicillin (and amoxycillin) but are not usually related to true penicillin allergy. They almost always occur in patients with glandular fever or chronic lymphatic leukaemia who are given these antibiotics.

Amoxycillin (Amoxil®) is a derivative of ampicillin which differs by only one hydroxyl group and has a similar antibacterial spectrum. It is, however, better absorbed when given by mouth, producing higher plasma and tissue concentrations; unlike ampicillin, absorption is not affected by the presence of food in the stomach.

Augmentin® consists of amoxycillin with the beta-lactamase inhibitor **clavulanic acid**. Clavulanic acid itself has no significant antibacterial activity but, by inactivating penicillinases, it makes the product active against penicillinase-producing bacteria that are resistant to amoxycillin. These include most *Staph. aureus*, one-third of *E. coli* strains, and up to 10% of *H. influenzae* strains, as well as many *Bacteroides* and *Klebsiella* spp.

Ciclacillin (Calthor®) is another derivative of ampicillin. It is less active than ampicillin but, like amoxycillin, is better absorbed from the gastrointestinal tract.

Mezlocillin (Baypen®) is a ureidopenicillin which is active against certain ampicillin-resistant bacteria. However, like ampicillin, it is inactivated by beta-lactamases. It possesses anti-pseudomonal activity.

AMOXYCILLIN

Indications: see under Ampicillin; also typhoid fever and dental prophylaxis

Cautions; Contra-indications; Side-effects: see under Benzylpenicillin (section 5.1.1.1); also erythematous rashes in glandular fever and chronic lymphatic leukaemia; reduce dose in renal impairment

Dose: by mouth, 250 mg every 8 hours, doubled in severe infections; CHILD up to 10 years, 125 mg every 8 hours, doubled in severe infections

Severe or recurrent purulent respiratory infection, 3 g every 12 hours

Dental prophylaxis, section 5.1, Table 2

Short-course oral therapy

Dental abscess, 3 g repeated after 8 hours

Urinary-tract infections, 3 g repeated after 10–12 hours

Gonorrhoea, single dose of 3 g

Otitis media, CHILD 3–10 years, 750 mg twice daily for 2 days

By intramuscular injection, 500 mg every 8 hours; CHILD, 50–100 mg/kg daily in divided doses

By intravenous injection or infusion. 500 mg every 8 hours increased to 1 g every 6 hours; CHILD, 50–100 mg/kg daily in divided doses

PoM **Amoxycillin** (Non-proprietary)

Capsules, amoxycillin (as trihydrate) 250 mg, net price 20 = £2.74; 500 mg, 20 = £5.40. Label: 9

Mixture, amoxycillin (as trihydrate) for reconstitution with water for preparations, 125 mg/5 ml, net price 100 ml = £1.74; 250 mg/5 ml, 100 ml = £3.23. Label: 9.

PoM **Almodan**® (Berk)

Capsules, both yellow/brown, amoxycillin (as sodium salt) 250 mg, net price 20 = £3.31; 500 mg, 20 = £6.62. Label: 9

Syrup, amoxycillin (as trihydrate) for reconstitution with water for preparations, 125 mg/5 ml, net price 100 ml = £1.88; 250 mg/5 ml, 100 ml = £3.76. Label: 9

Injection, powder for reconstitution, amoxycillin (as sodium salt), 250-mg vial, net price = 39p; 500-mg vial = 71p

PoM **Amoxil**® (Bencard)

Capsules, both maroon/gold, amoxycillin (as trihydrate), 250 mg, net price 20 = £3.39; 500 mg, 20 = £6.78. Label: 9

Dispersible tablets, sugar-free, amoxycillin 500 mg (as trihydrate). Net price 20 = £7.27. Label: 9, 13

Syrup SF, both sugar-free, amoxycillin (as trihydrate) for reconstitution with water for preparations, 125 mg/5 ml, net price 100 ml = £2.00; 250 mg/5 ml, 100 ml = £4.00. Diluent water for preparations, life of diluted preparation 14 days. Label: 9

Paediatric suspension, amoxycillin 125 mg (as trihydrate)/1.25 ml when reconstituted with water for preparations. Net price 20 ml = £3.00. Label: 9, counselling advised, use of pipette

Sachets SF, powder, sugar-free, amoxycillin 750 mg (as trihydrate)/sachet, net price 4 sachets = £2.60. 3 g/sachet, 2 sachets = £4.30. Label: 9, 13

Injection, powder for reconstitution, amoxycillin (as sodium salt). Net price 250-mg vial = 40p; 500-mg vial = 73p; 1-g vial = £1.46

With clavulanic acid

▼ PoM **Augmentin**® (Beecham)

Tablets, f/c, amoxycillin 250 mg (as trihydrate), clavulanic acid 125 mg (as potassium salt). Net price 20 = £5.80. Label: 9

Dose: 1 tablet every 8 hours, increased to 2 tablets in severe infections

Dispersible tablets, sugar-free, amoxycillin 250 mg (as trihydrate), clavulanic acid 125 mg (as potassium salt). Net price 20 = £6.51. Label: 9, 13

Dose: see under tablets above

Junior suspension, sugar-free, amoxycillin 125 mg (as trihydrate), clavulanic acid 62 mg (as potassium salt)/5 ml when reconstituted with water for preparations. Net price 100 ml = £3.55. Label: 9

Dose: CHILD 6–12 years, 5 ml every 8 hours, increased to 10 ml in severe infections

Paediatric suspension, sugar-free, amoxycillin 125 mg (as trihydrate), clavulanic acid 31 mg (as potassium salt)/5 ml when reconstituted with water for preparations. Diluent not more than an equal volume of water for preparations, life of diluted suspension 7 days. Net price 100 ml = £2.80. Label: 9

Dose: CHILD 3–8 months, 1.25 ml every 8 hours; 9 months–2 years, 2.5 ml every 8 hours; 3–6 years, 5 ml every 8 hours, increased to 10 ml in severe infections

Injection 600 mg, powder for preparing intravenous injections, amoxycillin 500 mg (as sodium salt), clavulanic acid 100 mg (as potassium salt). Net price per vial = £1.35

Injection 1.2 g, powder for preparing intravenous injections, amoxycillin 1 g (as sodium salt), clavulanic acid 200 mg (as potassium salt). Net price per vial = £2.70

Dose: by slow intravenous injection or infusion, 1.2 g vial every 8 hours, increased to every 6 hours in more serious infections; CHILD 30 mg/kg every 8 hours (every 12 hours in neonates)

AMPICILLIN

Indications: urinary-tract infections, otitis media, chronic bronchitis, invasive salmonellosis, gonorrhoea

Cautions; Contra-indications; Side-effects: see under Benzylpenicillin (section 5.1.1.1); also erythematous rashes in glandular fever and chronic lymphatic leukaemia; reduce dose in renal impairment. Drug interactions: see Appendix 1 (section 7)

Dose: by mouth, 0.25–1 g every 6 hours, at least 30 minutes before food

Gonorrhoea, 2 g as a single dose with probenecid 1 g; repeated for women

Urinary-tract infections, 500 mg every 8 hours

By intramuscular injection or intravenous injection or infusion, 500 mg every 4–6 hours; higher doses in meningitis

CHILD under 10 years, any route, ½ adult dose

PoM **Ampicillin** (Non-proprietary)

Capsules, ampicillin 250 mg, net price 20 = 67p; 500 mg, 20 = £1.45. Label: 9, 23

Mixture, ampicillin 125 mg/5 ml when reconstituted with water for preparations. Diluent syrup, life of diluted mixture 7 days, net price 100 ml = 76p; 250 mg/5 ml, 100 ml = £1.23. Label: 9, 23

PoM **Amfipen**® (Brocades)

Capsules, both red/grey, ampicillin 250 mg, net price 20 = 84p; 500 mg, 20 = £1.76. Label: 9, 23

Syrup, pink, ampicillin 125 mg/5 ml when reconstituted with water for preparations. Net price 100 ml = 76p. Label: 9, 23

Syrup forte (= strong mixture), pink, ampicillin 250 mg/5 ml when reconstituted with water for preparations. Net price 100 ml = £1.23. Label: 9, 23

Injection, powder for reconstitution, ampicillin (as sodium salt). Net price 250-mg vial = 31p; 500-mg vial = 62p

PoM **Penbritin**® (Beecham)

Capsules, both black/red, ampicillin (as trihydrate) 250 mg, net price 20 = £1.42; 500 mg, 20 = £2.85. Label: 9, 23

Syrup, ampicillin 125 mg (as trihydrate)/5 ml when reconstituted with water for preparations. Diluent syrup, life of diluted mixture 7 days. Net price 100 ml = £1.09. Label: 9, 23

Syrup forte, ampicillin 250 mg (as trihydrate)/5 ml when reconstituted with water for preparations. Diluent as above. Net price 100 ml = £2.17. Label: 9, 23

Paediatric suspension, pink, ampicillin 125 mg (as trihydrate)/1.25 ml. Net price 25 ml = £2.03. Label: 9, 23, counselling advised, use of pipette

Injection, powder for reconstitution, ampicillin (as sodium salt). Net price 250-mg vial = 33p; 500-mg vial = 67p

PoM **Vidopen**® (Berk)

Capsules, both pink/red, ampicillin (as trihydrate) 250 mg, net price 20 = 84p; 500 mg, 20 = £1.72. Label: 9, 23

Syrup, pink, ampicillin 125 mg (as trihydrate)/5 ml when reconstituted with water for preparations. Diluent syrup, life of diluted mixture 7 days. Net price 100 ml = 76p. Label: 9, 23

Syrup forte, pink, ampicillin 250 mg (as trihydrate)/5 ml when reconstituted with water for preparations. Diluent as above. Net price 100 ml = £1.23. Label: 9, 23

With penicillinase-resistant penicillins

PoM **Ampiclox**® (Beecham)

Injection, ampicillin 250 mg (as sodium salt), cloxacillin 250 mg (as sodium salt). Net price per vial = £1.36

Dose: by intramuscular injection or intravenous injection or infusion, 1–2 vials every 4–6 hours; CHILD up to 2 years ¼ adult dose, 2–10 years ½ adult dose

PoM **Ampiclox Neonatal**® (Beecham)

Suspension, sugar-free, ampicillin 60 mg (as trihydrate), cloxacillin 30 mg (as sodium salt)/0.6 ml when reconstituted with water for preparations. Net price 10 ml = £2.06. Label: 9, counselling advised, use of pipette

Dose: 0.6 ml every 4 hours

Injection, powder for reconstitution, ampicillin 50 mg (as sodium salt), cloxacillin 25 mg (as sodium salt). Net price per vial = 43p

Dose: by intramuscular injection or intravenous injection or infusion, 1 vial every 8 hours

PoM **Flu-Amp**® (Generics)

Capsules, grey/blue, ampicillin 250 mg (as trihydrate), flucloxacillin 250 mg (as sodium salt). Net price 20 = £4.00. Label: 9, 23

Dose: 1 capsule every 6 hours

PoM **Magnapen**® (Beecham)

Capsules, black/turquoise, ampicillin 250 mg (as trihydrate), flucloxacillin 250 mg (as sodium salt). Net price 20 = £4.23. Label: 9, 23

Dose: 1 capsule every 6 hours

Syrup, ampicillin 125 mg (as trihydrate), flucloxacillin 125 mg (as magnesium salt)/5 ml when reconstituted with water for preparations. Diluent syrup, life of diluted syrup 14 days. Net price 100 ml = £3.44. Label: 9, 23

Dose: 10 ml every 6 hours; CHILD up to 2 years ¼ adult dose, 2–10 years ½ adult dose

Injection 500 mg, powder for reconstitution, ampicillin 250 mg (as sodium salt), flucloxacillin 250 mg (as sodium salt). Net price per vial = £1.10

Dose: by intramuscular injection or intravenous injection or infusion, 1 vial every 6 hours; CHILD up to 2 years ¼ adult dose, 2–10 years ½ adult dose; doses may be doubled in severe infections

Injection 1 g, powder for reconstitution, ampicillin 500 mg (as sodium salt), flucloxacillin 500 mg (as sodium salt). Net price per vial = £2.20

BACAMPICILLIN HYDROCHLORIDE

Indications: see under Ampicillin

Cautions; Contra-indications; Side-effects: see under Benzylpenicillin (section 5.1.1.1); also erythematous rashes in glandular fever and chronic lymphatic leukaemia; avoid in severe liver disease and renal impairment

Dose: 400 mg 2–3 times daily, doubled in severe infections

▼ PoM **Ambaxin**® (Upjohn)

Tablets, scored, bacampicillin hydrochloride 400 mg. Net price 20 = £5.77. Label: 9

CICLACILLIN

Indications: bronchitis, urinary-tract infections, soft-tissue infections

Cautions; Contra-indications; Side-effects: see under Benzylpenicillin (section 5.1.1.1); also erythematous rashes in glandular fever and chronic lymphatic leukaemia

Dose: 250–500 mg every 6 hours; longer interval between doses in renal impairment

PoM **Calthor** (Wyeth)

Tablets, both scored, ciclacillin 250 mg, net price 20 = £2.32; 500 mg, 20 = £4.64. Label: 9

Suspension, pink, ciclacillin 125 mg/5 ml when reconstituted with water for preparations. Diluent syrup, life of diluted suspension 7 days. Net price 120 ml = £2.01. Label: 9

Suspension, ciclacillin 250 mg/5 ml when reconstituted with water for preparations. Diluent as above. Net price 120 ml = £3.40. Label: 9

MEZLOCILLIN

Indications: Gram-positive and Gram-negative infections (including enteric bacilli); see also notes above.

Cautions; Contra-indications; Side-effects: see under Benzylpenicillin (section 5.1.1.1); increase interval between doses in renal impairment

Dose: by intravenous injection, 2 g every 6–8 hours

By intravenous infusion, in serious infections, 5 g every 6–8 hours

By intramuscular injection, 0.5–2 g

PoM **Baypen**® (Bayer)

Injection, powder for reconstitution, mezlocillin (as sodium salt). Net price 500-mg vial = £1.20; 1-g vial = £1.85; 2-g vial = £3.36

Infusion, powder for reconstitution, mezlocillin (as sodium salt). Net price 5-g vial = £7.64 (also available with 50 ml water for injections and transfer needle)

PIVAMPICILLIN

Indications: see under Ampicillin

Cautions; Contra-indications; Side-effects: see under Benzylpenicillin (section 5.1.1.1); also erythematous rashes in chronic lymphatic leukaemia; liver- and kidney-function tests required in long-term use; avoid in severe liver disease and renal impairment. Drug interactions: see Appendix 1 (section 5.1)

Dose: 500 mg every 12 hours, doubled in severe infections; CHILD up to 1 year 40–60 mg/kg daily in 2–3 divided doses; 1–5 years 350–525 mg daily; 6–10 years 525–700 mg daily

▼ PoM **Pondocillin**® (Leo)

Tablets, f/c, pivampicillin 500 mg. Net price 20 = £4.22. Label: 5, 9

Suspension, sugar-free, pivampicillin 175 mg/5 ml when reconstituted with water for preparations. Net price 50 ml = £1.76; 100 ml = £2.84. Label: 5, 9

Sachets, granules, off-white, pivampicillin 175 mg/sachet. Net price 20 sachets = £3.96. Label: 5, 9, 13

With pivmecillinam

▼ PoM **Miraxid**® (Fisons)

Tablets, f/c, pivampicillin 125 mg, pivmecillinam hydrochloride 100 mg. Net price 20 = £2.59. Label: 9, 21, 27, counselling advised, posture (see below)

Dose: 2 tablets twice daily, increased to 3 tablets twice daily for severe infections; CHILD 6–10 years 1 tablet twice daily

450 Tablets, f/c, pivampicillin 250 mg, pivmecillinam hydrochloride 200 mg. Net price 20 = £5.06. Label: 9, 21, 27, counselling advised, posture (see below)

Dose: 1 tablet twice daily, increased to 2 tablets twice daily for severe infections

COUNSELLING. Tablets should be swallowed whole with plenty of fluid during meals while sitting or standing

Paediatric suspension, pivampicillin 62.5 mg, pivmecillinam 46.2 mg/unit-dose sachet. Net price 10 sachets = £2.70. Label: 9, 13, 21
Dose: under 6 years 1 sachet twice daily increased to 2 sachets twice daily for severe infections, 6–10 years 2 sachets twice daily increased to 3 sachets twice daily for severe infections

▼ PoM **Pondocillin Plus®** (Leo)
Tablets, f/c, pivampicillin 250 mg, pivmecillinam hydrochloride 200 mg. Net price 20 = £5.98. Label: 9, 21, 27, counselling advised, posture (see below)
Dose: 1 tablet twice daily, increased to 2 tablets twice daily for severe infections
COUNSELLING. Tablets should be swallowed whole with plenty of fluid during meals while sitting or standing

TALAMPICILLIN HYDROCHLORIDE
Indications: see under Ampicillin
Cautions; Contra-indications; Side-effects: see under Benzylpenicillin (section 5.1.1.1); avoid in severe hepatic or renal impairment; also erythematous rashes in glandular fever and chronic lymphatic leukaemia
Dose: 250–500 mg every 8 hours

PoM **Talpen®** (Beecham)
Tablets, red, f/c, talampicillin hydrochloride 250 mg. Net price 20 = £2.99. Label: 9
Syrup (= mixture), talampicillin hydrochloride 125 mg (as napsylate)/5 ml when reconstituted with water for preparations. Diluent syrup, life of diluted mixture 7 days. Net price 100 ml = £2.13. Label: 9

5.1.1.4 ANTIPSEUDOMONAL PENICILLINS

The carboxypenicillins, **carbenicillin** (Pyopen®) and **ticarcillin** (Ticar®), are principally indicated for the treatment of serious infections caused by *Pseudomonas aeruginosa* although they also have activity against certain other Gram-negative bacilli including *Proteus* spp. and *Bacteroides fragilis*. Carbenicillin has been replaced by ticarcillin which is more active against these organisms.
Timentin®, which consists of ticarcillin and clavulanic acid (section 5.1.1.3), is active against penicillinase-producing bacteria that are resistant to ticarcillin.
The ureidopenicillins, **azlocillin** (Securopen®) and **piperacillin** (Pipril®), have a broad spectrum of activity and are both more active than ticarcillin against *Ps. aeruginosa*.
For *Pseudomonas* septicaemias (especially in neutropenic patients or those with endocarditis) these antipseudomonal penicillins should be given with an aminoglycoside (e.g. gentamicin or tobramycin, section 5.1.4) as there is a synergistic effect. Penicillins and aminoglycosides must not, however, be mixed in the same syringe or infusion.

Carfecillin (Uticillin®), an ester of carbenicillin, unlike the parent drug, is not inactivated when given by mouth. Concentrations of carbenicillin released into the blood are low but concentrations in the urine may be sufficient to treat *Pseudomonas* and *Proteus* infections of the lower urinary tract.

AZLOCILLIN
Indications: infections due to *Pseudomonas aeruginosa*, see notes above
Cautions; Contra-indications; Side-effects: see under Benzylpenicillin (section 5.1.1.1); also longer dose interval in renal impairment
Dose: by intravenous injection, 2 g every 8 hours
By intravenous infusion, in serious infections, 5 g every 8 hours

PoM **Securopen®** (Bayer)
Injection, powder for reconstitution, azlocillin (as sodium salt). Net price 500-mg vial = £1.62; 1-g vial = £3.21; 2-g vial = £5.02
Infusion, powder for reconstitution, azlocillin (as sodium salt). Net price 5-g vial = £11·80 (also available with 50 ml water for injections and transfer needle)

CARBENICILLIN
Indications: infections due to *Pseudomonas aeruginosa* and *Proteus* spp., see notes above
Cautions; Contra-indications: see under Benzylpenicillin (section 5.1.1.1); reduce dose in renal impairment
Side-effects: see under Benzylpenicillin (section 5.1.1.1); also hypokalaemia, alteration in platelet function
Dose: by slow intravenous injection or rapid infusion, severe systemic infections, 5 g every 4–6 hours; CHILD 250–400 mg/kg daily in divided doses
By intramuscular injection, urinary-tract infections, 2 g every 6 hours; CHILD 50–100 mg/kg daily in divided doses

PoM **Pyopen®** (Beecham)
Injection, powder for reconstitution, carbenicillin (as sodium salt). Net price 1-g vial = £1.54; 5-g vial = £7.50

CARFECILLIN SODIUM
Indications: urinary-tract infections due to *Pseudomonas* and *Proteus* spp.
Cautions; Contra-indications; Side-effects: see under Benzylpenicillin (section 5.1.1.1)
Dose: 0.5–1 g 3 times daily

PoM **Uticillin®** (Beecham)
Tablets, carfecillin sodium 500 mg. Net price 20 = £7.08. Label: 9

PIPERACILLIN
Indications: infections due to *Pseudomonas aeruginosa*, see notes above
Cautions; Contra-indications; Side-effects: see under Benzylpenicillin (section 5.1.1.1);

increase interval between doses in moderate or severe renal impairment

Dose: by intramuscular injection or slow intravenous injection or infusion, 100–150 mg/kg daily (in divided doses), increased to 200–300 mg/kg daily in severe infections, and to at least 16 g/day in life-threatening infections; single doses over 2 g intravenous route only

▼ PoM **Pipril**® (Lederle)
Injection, powder for reconstitution, piperacillin (as sodium salt). Net price 1-g vial = £3.07; 2-g vial = £6.08; 4-g vial = £12.01
Infusion, powder for reconstitution, piperacillin 4 g (as sodium salt), with 50-ml bottle water for injections and transfer needle. Net price complete unit = £12.80

TICARCILLIN

Indications: infections due to *Pseudomonas* and *Proteus* spp, see notes above.
Cautions; Contra-indications; Side-effects: see under Benzylpenicillin (section 5.1.1.1)
Dose: by slow intravenous injection over 3–4 minutes *or by intravenous infusion* over 30–40 minutes, 15–20 g daily in divided doses; CHILD 200–300 mg/kg daily in divided doses
Urinary-tract infections, *by intramuscular or slow intravenous injection*, 3–4 g daily in divided doses; CHILD 50–100 mg/kg daily in divided doses

PoM **Ticar**® (Beecham)
Injection, powder for reconstitution, ticarcillin (as sodium salt). Net price 1-g vial = £1.68; 3-g vial = £4.10; 5-g vial = £6.84
Infusion, powder for reconstitution, ticarcillin 5 g (as sodium salt) in infusion bottle, with transfer needle and diluent. Net price complete unit = £8.03

With clavulanic acid
▼ PoM **Timentin**® (Beecham)
Injection 800 mg, powder for reconstitution, ticarcillin 750 mg (as sodium salt), clavulanic acid 50 mg (as potassium salt). Net price per vial = £1.81
Injection 1.6 g, powder for reconstitution, ticarcillin 1.5 g (as sodium salt), clavulanic acid 100 mg (as potassium salt). Net price per vial = £2.65
Injection 3.2 g, powder for reconstitution, ticarcillin 3 g (as sodium salt), clavulanic acid 200 mg (as potassium salt). Net price per vial = £5.29
Dose: by intravenous infusion, 3.2 g every 6–8 hours increased to every 4 hours in more severe infections; CHILD 80 mg/kg every 6–8 hours (every 12 hours in neonates)

5.1.1.5   MECILLINAMS

Mecillinam (Selexidin®) and **pivmecillinam** (Selexid®) have significant activity against many Gram-negative bacteria including salmonellae, but excluding *Ps. aeruginosa*. Pivmecillinam is

given by mouth and subsequently hydrolysed to mecillinam, which is the active agent and must itself be given by injection.

MECILLINAM

Indications: severe infections due to Gram-negative enteric bacteria
Cautions; Contra-indications; Side-effects: see under Benzylpenicillin (section 5.1.1.1); liver- and kidney-function tests on long-term use
Dose: by intramuscular injection or slow intravenous injection or infusion, 5–15 mg/kg every 6–8 hours

PoM **Selexidin**® (Leo)
Injection, powder for reconstitution, mecillinam. Net price 200-mg vial = 61p; 400-mg vial = £1.22

PIVMECILLINAM

Indications: see under Dose below
Cautions; Contra-indications; Side-effects: see under Benzylpenicillin (section 5.1.1.1); also liver- and kidney-function tests required in long-term use
Dose: acute uncomplicated cystitis, 400 mg initially, then 200 mg every 8 hours for 3 days (10-tab pack)
Chronic or recurrent bacteriuria, 400 mg every 6–8 hours
Salmonellosis, 1.2–2.4 g daily for 14 days (14–28 days for carriers)
COUNSELLING. Tablets should be swallowed whole with plenty of fluid during meals while sitting or standing

PoM **Selexid**® (Leo)
Tablets, f/c, pivmecillinam hydrochloride 200 mg. Net price 10-tab pack = £2.32, 20 = £4.48. Label: 9, 21, 27, counselling advised, posture (see Dose above)
Suspension, granules, pivmecillinam 100 mg/single-dose sachet. Net price 20 sachets = £4.03. Label: 9, 13, 21

With pivampicillin
see under Pivampicillin (section 5.1.1.3)

5.1.2   Cephalosporins, cephamycins and other beta-lactam antibiotics

Antibiotics discussed in this section include the cephalosporins such as cefotaxime, ceftazidime, cefuroxime, cephalexin, and cephradine, and latamoxef disodium, the cephamycin cefoxitin, and the monobactam, aztreonam.

CEPHALOSPORINS AND CEPHAMYCINS

The cephalosporins are broad-spectrum antibiotics but in spite of the number of cephalosporins currently available there are few absolute indications for their use. All have a similar antibacterial spectrum although individual agents have differing activity against certain organisms. The pharmacology of the cephalosporins is similar to that of the penicillins, excretion being principally renal and blocked by probenecid.

The principal side-effect of the cephalosporins is hypersensitivity and about 10% of penicillin-sensitive patients will also be allergic to the cephalosporins. Haemorrhage due to interference with blood clotting factors has been associated with several cephalosporins and there have been recent reports of severe bleeding in patients receiving latamoxef, particularly in elderly or debilitated patients. For drug interactions of the cephalosporins see Appendix 1 (section 5.1).

One of the first cephalosporins was **cephalothin** which is less active and less stable than the newer cephalosporins. It has been replaced by the newer cephalosporins, **cephradine** (Velosef®), **cephazolin** (Kefzol®).

The oral cephalosporins, **cephalexin** (Ceporex®, Keflex®), **cephradine** (Velosef®), **cefaclor** (Distaclor®), and **cefadroxil** (Baxan®) have a similar antimicrobial spectrum. They are useful for urinary-tract infections which do not respond to other drugs or which occur in pregnancy. Cefaclor has good activity against *Haemophilus influenzae*, but is associated with protracted skin reactions especially in children. Although cefadroxil has a longer half-life than the other cephalosporins it should still be given at intervals of 8 hours if the infection is of moderate severity; it has poor activity against *H. infuenzae*.

Cefuroxime (Zinacef®) and **cephamandole** (Kefadol®) are 'second generation' cephalosporins and are less susceptible than the other cephalosporins to inactivation by penicillinases. They are, therefore, active against certain bacteria which are resistant to the other drugs and have greater activity against *H. influenzae* and *Neisseria gonorrhoeae*.

Cefotaxime (Claforan®), **ceftazidime** (Fortum®), **ceftizoxime** (Cefizox®) and **latamoxef** (Moxalactam®) are 'third generation' cephalosporins with greater activity than the 'second generation' cephalosporins against certain Gram-negative bacteria. However, they are less active than cefuroxime and cephamandole against Gram-positive bacteria, most notably *Staphylococcus aureus*. Their broad antibacterial spectrum may encourage superinfection with resistant bacteria or fungi.

Cefsulodin (Monaspor®) and **ceftazidime** (Fortum®) have good activity against *Pseudomonas*. Ceftazidime is also active against other Gram-negative bacteria. Cefsulodin has a very much narrower spectrum and should be used only for pseudomonal infections.

Cefoxitin (Mefoxin®), a cephamycin antibiotic, is active against bowel flora including *Bacteroides fragilis* and because of this it has been recommended for the treatment of abdominal sepsis such as peritonitis.

CEFACLOR

Indications: infections due to sensitive Gram-positive and Gram-negative bacteria, but see notes above

Cautions: penicillin sensitivity; renal impairment; false positive urinary glucose (if tested for reducing substances) and false positive Coombs' test. Drug interactions: see Appendix 1 (section 5.1)

Contra-indications: cephalosporin hypersensitivity

Side-effects: allergic reactions including urticaria and rashes; hypersensitivity reactions including anaphylaxis; nausea, vomiting, diarrhoea

Dose: 250 mg every 8 hours, doubled for severe infections; max. 4 g daily; CHILD, 20 mg/kg daily in divided doses, doubled for severe infections, max. 1 g daily; *or* under 1 year, 62.5 mg three times daily; 1–5 years, 125 mg; over 5 years, 250 mg

PoM **Distaclor**® (Dista)

Capsules, violet/white, cefaclor 250 mg. Net price 20 = £7.41. Label: 9

Suspension, pink, cefaclor 125 mg/5 ml when reconstituted with water for preparations. Diluent water for preparations or syrup, life of diluted suspension 14 days. Net price 100 ml = £3.60. Label: 9

Suspension, pink, cefaclor 250 mg/5 ml when reconstituted with water for preparations. Diluent as above. Net price 100 ml = £6.72. Label: 9

CEFADROXIL

Indications: see under Cefaclor; see also notes above

Cautions; Contra-indications; Side-effects: see under Cefaclor

Dose: patients over 40 kg, 0.5–1 g twice daily (but see also notes above); skin, soft tissue, and simple urinary-tract infections, 1 g daily; CHILD under 1 year, 25 mg/kg daily in divided doses; 1–6 years, 250 mg twice daily; over 6 years, 500 mg twice daily

PoM **Baxan**® (Bristol-Myers)

Capsules, cefadroxil 500 mg (as monohydrate). Net price 20 = £6.50. Label: 9

Suspension (= mixture), cefadroxil 125 mg (as monohydrate)/5 ml when reconstituted with water for preparations. Net price 60 ml = £1.75. Label: 9

Suspension (= mixture), cefadroxil 250 mg (as monohydrate)/5 ml when reconstituted with water for preparations. Net price 60 ml = £3.48. Label: 9

Suspension (= mixture), cefadroxil 500 mg (as monohydrate)/5 ml when reconstituted with water for preparations. Net price 60 ml = £5.21. Label: 9

CEFOTAXIME

Indications: see under Cefaclor; surgical prophylaxis; see also notes above

Cautions; Contra-indications; Side-effects: see under Cefaclor

Dose: by intramuscular or intravenous injection, 1 g every 12 hours; in moderate to serious infection 1 g every 8 hours; life-threatening infection 2 g every 8 hours; exceptionally, for life-threatening infections due to organisms less sensitive to cefotaxime, up to 12 g daily

Gonorrhoea 1 g as a single dose

In severe renal impairment, doses to be halved after initial dose of 1 g. NEONATE, 50 mg/kg daily in 2–4 divided doses; in severe infections 150–200 mg/kg daily. CHILD, 100–150 mg/kg daily in 2–4 divided doses; in severe infections, up to 200 mg/kg daily

By intravenous infusion, 1–2 g over 20–60 minutes

PoM **Claforan**® (Roussel)

Injection, powder for reconstitution, cefotaxime (as sodium salt). Net price 500-mg vial = £2.48; 1-g vial = £4.95; 2-g vial = £9.90

CEFOXITIN

Indications: see under Cefaclor; surgical prophylaxis; more active against Gram-negative bacteria

Cautions; Contra-indications; Side-effects: see under Cefaclor

Dose: by intramuscular injection or slow intravenous injection or infusion, 1–2 g every 6–8 hours, increased in severe infections; max. 12 g daily; CHILD up to 1 week 20–40 mg/kg every 12 hours; 1–4 weeks 20–40 mg/kg every 8 hours; over 1 month 20–40 mg/kg every 6–8 hours

PoM **Mefoxin**® (MSD)

Injection, powder for reconstitution, cefoxitin (as sodium salt). Net price 1-g vial = £4.92; 2-g vial = £9.84

CEFSULODIN SODIUM

Indications: infections due to sensitive strains of *Ps. aeruginosa;* surgical prophylaxis

Cautions; Contra-indications; Side-effects: see under Cefaclor

Dose: by intramuscular or intravenous injection, 1–4 g daily in 2–4 divided doses; CHILD 20–50 mg/kg daily

▼ PoM **Monaspor**® (Ciba)

Injection, powder for reconstitution, cefsulodin sodium. Net price 500-mg vial = £5.65; 1-g vial = £11.30

CEFTAZIDIME

Indications: see under Cefaclor; see also notes above

Cautions; Contra-indications; Side-effects: see under Cefaclor

Dose: by intramuscular injection or intravenous injection or infusion, 1 g every 8 hours *or* 2 g every 12 hours; 2 g every 8–12 hours in severe infections; single doses over 1 g intravenous route only; CHILD, up to 2 months 25–60 mg/kg

daily in 2 divided doses, over 2 months 30–100 mg/kg daily in 2–3 divided doses; up to 150 mg/kg daily if immunocompromised or meningitis; intravenous route recommended for children

Urinary-tract and less serious infections, 0.5–1 g every 12 hours

Pseudomonal lung infection in cystic fibrosis, ADULT with normal renal function 100–150 mg/kg daily in 3 divided doses; CHILD up to 150 mg/kg daily; intravenous route recommended for children

PoM **Fortum**® (Glaxo)

Injection, powder for reconstitution, ceftazidime (as pentahydrate), with sodium carbonate. Net price 250-mg vial = £2.48; 500-mg vial = £4.95; 1-g vial = £9.90; 2-g vial (for injection and for infusion) = £19.80

CEFTIZOXIME

Indications: see Cefaclor; also notes above

Cautions; Contra-indications; Side-effects: see under Cefaclor

Dose: by intramuscular injection or slow intravenous injection or infusion, up to 8 g daily, in divided doses; CHILD over 3 months 30–60 mg/kg daily in divided doses, increased to 100–150 mg/kg daily for severe infections

Gonorrhoea, *by intramuscular injection,* 1 g as a single dose

Urinary-tract infections, *by intramuscular or slow intravenous injection or infusion,* 0.5–1 g every 12 hours

PoM **Cefizox**® (Wellcome)

Injection, powder for reconstitution, ceftizoxime (as sodium salt). Net price 500-mg vial = £2.76; 1-g vial = £5.50; 2-g vial = £11.00

CEFUROXIME

Indications: see under Cefaclor; surgical prophylaxis; more active against *H. influenzae* and *N. gonorrhoeae*

Cautions; Contra-indications; Side-effects: see under Cefaclor

Dose: by mouth (as cefuroxime axetil), 250 mg twice daily, doubled in bronchitis and pneumonia

Urinary-tract infection, 125 mg twice daily, doubled in pyelonephritis

Gonorrhoea, 1 g as a single dose

CHILD over 5 years, 125 mg twice daily, if necessary doubled in otitis media

By intramuscular injection or intravenous injection or infusion, 750 mg every 6–8 hours; 1.5 g every 6–8 hours in severe infections; single doses over 750 mg intravenous route only

CHILD, 30–100 mg/kg daily in 3–4 divided doses (2–3 divided doses in neonates)

Gonorrhoea, 1.5 g as a single dose by intramuscular injection (divided between 2 sites)

Surgical prophylaxis, 1.5 g by intravenous injection at induction; may be supplemented with 750 mg intramuscularly 8 and 16 hours later

---

(abdominal, pelvic, and orthopaedic operations) *or* followed by 750 mg intramuscularly every 8 hours for further 24–48 hours (cardiac, pulmonary, oesophageal, and vascular operations)
Meningitis, 3 g intravenously every 8 hours; CHILD, 200–240 mg/kg daily (in 3–4 divided doses) reduced to 100 mg/kg daily after 3 days or on clinical improvement; NEONATE, 100 mg/ kg daily reduced to 50 mg/kg daily

PoM **Zinacef**® (Glaxo)
Injection, powder for reconstitution, cefuroxime (as sodium salt). Net price 250-mg vial = 88p; 750-mg vial = £2.64; 1.5-g vial = £5.29

▼ PoM **Zinnat**® (Glaxo)
Tablets, both f/c, cefuroxime 125 mg (as cefuroxime axetil), net price 14-tab pack = £6.30; 250 mg, 14-tab pack = £12.60. Label: 9, 21, 25

CEPHALEXIN

Indications: see under Cefaclor
Cautions; Contra-indications; Side-effects: see under Cefaclor
Dose: 250 mg every 6 hours *or* 500 mg every 8–12 hours; CHILD, 25 mg/kg daily in divided doses, doubled for severe infections, max. 100 mg/kg daily; *or* under 1 year, 125 mg every 12 hours; 1–5 years, 125 mg every 8 hours; 6–12 years, 250 mg every 8 hours

PoM **Ceporex**® (Glaxo)
Capsules, both caramel/grey, cephalexin 250 mg, net price 20 = £3.00; 500 mg, 20 = £6.23. Label: 9
Tablets, both pink, f/c, cephalexin 250 mg, net price 20 = £3.00; 500 mg, 20 = £6.23. Label: 9
Paediatric drops, orange, cephalexin 125 mg/ 1.25 ml when reconstituted with water for preparations. Net price 10 ml = £1.38. Label: 9, counselling advised, use of pipette
Suspension, both yellow, cephalexin 125 mg/ 5 ml, net price 100 ml = £1.59; 250 mg/5 ml, 100 ml = £3.19. Do not dilute. Label: 9
Syrup, orange, cephalexin for reconstitution with water for preparations, 125 mg/5 ml, net price 100 ml = £1.59; 250 mg/5 ml, 100 ml = £3.19; 500 mg/5 ml, 100 ml = £6.19. Diluent water for preparations, life of diluted syrup 7 days. Label: 9

PoM **Keflex**® (Lilly)
Capsules, cephalexin 250 mg (green/white), net price 20 = £3.00; 500 mg (green), 20 = £6.23. Label: 9
Tablets, both peach, cephalexin 250 mg, net price 20 = £3.00; 500 mg, 20 = £6.23. Label: 9
Suspension, cephalexin for reconstitution with water for preparations, 125 mg/5 ml (pink), net price 100 ml = £1.59; 250 mg/5 ml (orange), 100 ml = £3.19. Diluent syrup, life of diluted suspension 10 days. Label: 9

PoM **Keflex-C**® (Lilly)
Chewable tablets, pale yellow, cephalexin 250 mg. Net price 15 = £3.64. Label: 9, 24

CEPHALOTHIN

Indications: see under Cefaclor; surgical prophylaxis
Cautions; Contra-indications; Side-effects: see under Cefaclor. Drug interactions: see Appendix 1 (section 5.1)
Dose: by intravenous injection or infusion, 1 g every 4–6 hours; max. 12 g daily; CHILD, 80–160 mg/kg daily in divided doses

PoM **Keflin**® (Lilly)
Injection, powder for reconstitution, cephalothin (as sodium salt). Net price 1-g vial = £2.28

CEPHAMANDOLE

Indications: see under Cefaclor; surgical prophylaxis
Cautions; Contra-indications; Side-effects: see under Cefaclor. Drug interactions: see Appendix 1 (section 5.1)
Dose: by deep intramuscular injection or intravenous injection or infusion, 0.5–2 g every 4–8 hours; CHILD, 50–100 mg/kg daily in divided doses

PoM **Kefadol**® (Dista)
Injection, powder for reconstitution, cephamandole (as nafate) with sodium carbonate. Net price 500-mg vial = £2.04; 1-g vial = £3.90; 2-g vial = £7.51 (hosp. only)

CEPHAZOLIN

Indications: see under Cefaclor; surgical prophylaxis
Cautions; Contra-indications; Side-effects: see under Cefaclor
Dose: by intramuscular injection or intravenous injection or infusion, 0.5–1 g every 6–12 hours; CHILD, 25–50 mg/kg daily (in divided doses), increased to 100 mg/kg daily in severe infections

PoM **Kefzol**® (Lilly)
Injection, powder for reconstitution, cephazolin (as sodium salt). Net price 500-mg vial = £2.45; 1-g vial = £4.63

CEPHRADINE

Indications: see under Cefaclor; surgical prophylaxis
Cautions; Contra-indications; Side-effects: see under Cefaclor
Dose: by mouth, 250–500 mg every 6 hours *or* 0.5–1 g every 12 hours; CHILD, 25–50 mg/kg daily in divided doses
By intramuscular injection or intravenous injection or infusion, 0.5–1 g every 6 hours, increased to 8 g daily in severe infections; CHILD, 50–100 mg/kg daily in 4 divided doses

PoM **Velosef**® (Squibb)
Capsules, cephradine 250 mg (orange/blue), net price 20 = £3.42; 500 mg, 20 = £7.00. Label: 9
Syrup, cephradine 250 mg/5 ml when reconstituted with water for preparations. Diluent

syrup, life of diluted syrup 7 days. Net price 100 ml = £4.22. Label: 9

Injection, powder for reconstitution, cephradine. Net price 500-mg vial = 99p; 1-g vial = £1.95

LATAMOXEF DISODIUM

Indications: see notes above

Cautions: see under Cefaclor; also hypoprothrombinaemia (administer prophylactic vitamin K 10 mg per week, avoid high-dose heparin and oral anticoagulants) and thrombocytopenia (monitor bleeding time in patients receiving more than 4 g daily for longer than 3 days); hepatic impairment; poor nutritional status; disulfiram-like reaction with alcohol. Drug interactions: see Appendix 1 (sections *2.8B*, 5.1)

Side-effects: hypersensitivity reactions; haematological effects including eosinophilia, reversible leucopenia, thrombocytopenia, and decreased prothrombin; rarely diarrhoea

Dose: by deep intramuscular injection or intravenous injection or infusion, 0.25–2 g every 12 hours, increased to max. of 4 g every 8 hours in severe infections but see Cautions; INFANT up to 1 week, 25 mg/kg every 12 hours; 1–4 weeks, 25 mg/kg every 8 hours; CHILD, 50 mg/kg every 12 hours. Doses may be doubled in severe infections

▼ PoM **Moxalactam**® (Lilly)

Injection, powder for reconstitution, latamoxef disodium. Net price 500-mg vial = £3.96; 1-g vial = £7.91; 2-g vial = £15.82

OTHER BETA-LACTAM ANTIBIOTICS

Aztreonam (Azactam®) is a monocyclic beta-lactam ('monobactam') antibiotic with an antibacterial spectrum limited to Gram-negative aerobic bacteria including *Pseudomonas aeruginosa*, *Neisseria gonorrhoeae*, and *Haemophilus influenzae*. Side-effects are similar to those of the other beta-lactams although aztreonam may be less likely to cause hypersensitivity in penicillin-sensitive patients.

AZTREONAM

Indications: Gram-negative infections including *Pseudomonas aeruginosa* and *Haemophilus influenzae*

Cautions: hypersensitivity to beta-lactam antibiotics; hepatic impairment; reduce dose in renal impairment. Drug interactions: see Appendix 1 (section *2.8B*)

Contra-indications: aztreonam hypersensitivity; pregnancy and breast-feeding

Side-effects: nausea, vomiting, diarrhoea, abdominal cramps; mouth ulcers, altered taste; jaundice and hepatitis; blood disorders (including thrombocytopenia and neutropenia); urticaria and rashes

Dose: by intramuscular injection or intravenous injection or infusion: 1 g every 8 hours *or* 2 g every 12 hours; 2 g every 6–8 hours for severe

infections; single doses over 1 g intravenous route only

Urinary-tract infections, 0.5–1 g every 8–12 hours

Gonorrhoea/cystitis,   *by   intramuscular injection*, 1 g as a single dose

▼ PoM **Azactam**® (Squibb)

Injection, powder for reconstitution, aztreonam. Net price 500-mg vial = £4.48; 1-g vial = £8.95; 2-g vial and 2-g bottle (for preparing infusion) (both) = £17.90

5.1.3   Tetracyclines

The tetracyclines are broad-spectrum antibiotics whose usefulness has decreased as a result of increasing bacterial resistance. They remain, however, the treatment of choice for infections caused by chlamydia (causing trachoma, psittacosis, salpingitis, urethritis, and lymphogranuloma venereum), rickettsia (including Q-fever), mycoplasma (respiratory and genital tract infections), brucella, and the spirochaete, *Borrelia burgdorferi* (Lyme disease). They are also used for the treatment of exacerbations of chronic bronchitis because of their activity against *Haemophilus influenzae*. They are also used in acne and in destructive (refractory) periodontal disease.

Microbiologically, there is little to choose between the various tetracyclines, the only exception being **minocycline** (Minocin®) which has a broader spectrum, is active against *Neisseria meningitidis* and has been used for meningococcal prophylaxis; however it may cause dizziness and vertigo.

The tetracyclines are deposited in growing bone and teeth (being bound to calcium) causing staining and occasionally dental hypoplasia, and should **not** be given to children under 12 years or to pregnant women. With the exception of **doxycycline** (Vibramycin®) and **minocycline** the tetracyclines may exacerbate renal failure and should **not** be given to patients with kidney disease. Absorption of tetracyclines is decreased by milk (except doxycycline and minocycline), antacids, and calcium, iron, and magnesium salts.

TETRACYCLINE

Indications: exacerbations of chronic bronchitis; infections due to brucella, chlamydia, mycoplasma, and rickettsia; acne vulgaris

Cautions: breast-feeding; rarely causes photosensitivity. Avoid intravenous administration in hepatic impairment. Drug interactions: see Appendix 1 (sections *2.8C*, 5.1, 7, 9)

Contra-indications: renal failure, pregnancy, children under 12 years of age

Side-effects: nausea, vomiting, diarrhoea; superinfection with resistant organisms; rarely allergic reactions

Dose: by mouth, 250–500 mg every 6 hours Acne, see section 13.6

Early syphilis, 500 mg 4 times daily for 14 days Non-gonococcal urethritis, 500 mg 4 times daily for 10–21 days

---

By intramuscular injection, 100 mg every 8–12 hours, or every 4–6 hours in severe infections
By intravenous infusion, 500 mg every 12 hours; max. 2 g daily

PoM **Tetracycline Tablets,** f/c or s/c, tetracycline hydrochloride 250 mg. Net price 20 = 29p. Label: 7, 9, 23

PoM **Achromycin**® (Lederle)
Capsules, orange, tetracycline hydrochloride 250 mg. Net price 20 = 95p. Label: 7, 9, 23
Tablets, orange, f/c, tetracycline hydrochloride 250 mg. Net price 20 = 67p. Label: 7, 9, 23
Syrup, red, tetracycline hydrochloride 125 mg (as tetracycline)/5 ml. Net price 100 ml = £1.66. Label: 7, 9, 23. Diluent syrup, life of diluted syrup 14 days
Note. Stains teeth; avoid in children under 12 years of age
Intramuscular injection, powder for reconstitution, tetracycline hydrochloride 100 mg, procaine hydrochloride 40 mg. Net price per vial = £1.09
Intravenous injection, powder for reconstitution, tetracycline hydrochloride. Net price 250-mg vial = £1.27; 500-mg vial = £2.03

PoM **Achromycin V**® (Lederle)
Capsules, pink, tetracycline hydrochloride 250 mg (as tetracycline) with buffer. Net price 20 = £2.27. Label: 7, 9, 23

PoM **Sustamycin**® (MCP)
Capsules, s/r, blue, tetracycline hydrochloride 250 mg. Net price 20 = £2.08. Label: 7, 9, 23, 25
Dose: 2 capsules initially, then 1 every 12 hours

PoM **Tetrabid-Organon**® (Organon)
Capsules, s/r, purple/yellow, tetracycline hydrochloride 250 mg. Net price 20 = £2.42. Label: 7, 9, 23, 25
Dose: 2 capsules initially, then 1 every 12 hours; acne, 1 daily

PoM **Tetrachel**® (Berk)
Capsules, orange, tetracycline hydrochloride 250 mg. Net price 20 = 29p. Label: 7, 9, 23
Tablets, orange, f/c, tetracycline hydrochloride 250 mg. Net price 20 = 27p. Label: 7, 9, 23

PoM **Tetrex**® (Bristol-Myers)
Capsules, yellow/orange, tetracycline 250 mg (as phosphate complex). Net price 20 = £1.82. Label: 7, 9, 23

Compound preparations

PoM **Chymocyclar**® (Rorer)
Capsules, pink, tetracycline hydrochloride 250 mg, pancreatic enzymes (trypsin and chymotrypsin) 50 000 Armour units. Net price 20 = £2.77. Label: 7, 9, 23, 25

PoM **Deteclo**® (Lederle)
Tablets, blue, f/c, tetracycline hydrochloride 115.4 mg, chlortetracycline hydrochloride 115.4 mg, demeclocycline hydrochloride 69.2 mg. Net price 20 = £2.54. Label: 7, 9, 11, 23
Dose: 1 tablet every 12 hours; 3–4 tablets daily in more severe infections

PoM **Mysteclin**® (Squibb)
Tablets, orange, s/c, tetracycline hydrochloride 250 mg, nystatin 250 000 units. Net price 20 = £1.29. Label: 7, 9, 23

Syrup, yellow, tetracycline 125 mg (as hydrochloride), amphotericin 25 mg/5 ml. Net price 100 ml = £1.22. Label: 7, 9, 23
Note. Tetracycline stains teeth; avoid in children under 12 years of age

CHLORTETRACYCLINE HYDROCHLORIDE
Indications: see under Tetracycline
Cautions; Contra-indications; Side-effects: see under Tetracycline
Dose: 250–500 mg every 6 hours

PoM **Aureomycin**® (Lederle)
Capsules, yellow, chlortetracycline hydrochloride 250 mg. Net price 20 = £2.36. Label: 7, 9, 23

CLOMOCYCLINE SODIUM
Indications: see under Tetracycline
Cautions; Contra-indications; Side-effects: see under Tetracycline
Dose: 170–340 mg every 6–8 hours

PoM **Megaclor**® (Pharmax)
Capsules, red, clomocycline sodium 170 mg. Net price 20 = £1.96. Label: 7, 9, 23

DEMECLOCYCLINE HYDROCHLORIDE
Indications: see under Tetracycline; also inappropriate secretion of antidiuretic hormone, section 6.5.2
Cautions; Contra-indications; Side-effects: see under Tetracycline, but photosensitivity is more common
Dose: 150 mg every 6 hours *or* 300 mg every 12 hours

PoM **Ledermycin**® (Lederle)
Capsules, red, demeclocycline hydrochloride 150 mg. Net price 20 = £4.24. Label: 7, 9, 11, 23
Tablets, red, f/c, demeclocycline hydrochloride 300 mg. Net price 20 = £8.43. Label: 7, 9, 11, 23

DOXYCYCLINE
Indications: see under Tetracycline; also chronic prostatitis
Cautions; Contra-indications; Side-effects: see under Tetracycline, but may be used in renal impairment
Dose: 200 mg on first day, then 100 mg daily
Acne, 50 mg daily for 6–12 weeks or longer

PoM **Nordox**® (Panpharma)
Capsules, green, doxycycline 100 mg (as hydrochloride). Net price 10-tab pack = £4.66. Label: 6, 9, 27

PoM **Vibramycin**® (Pfizer)
Capsules, green/ivory, doxycycline 50 mg (as hydrochloride). Net price 28-tab pack = £7.74. Label: 6, 9, 27
Capsules, green, doxycycline 100 mg (as hydrochloride). Net price 20 = £10.00. Label: 6, 9, 27

Syrup, sugar-free, red, doxycycline 50 mg (as calcium chelate)/5 ml. Diluent syrup, life of diluted preparation 14 days. Net price 30 ml = £1.55. Label: 6, 9

Note. Stains teeth; avoid in children under 12 years of age

PoM **Vibramycin-D**® (Pfizer)

Dispersible tablets, off-white, doxycycline 100 mg. Net price 10 = £6.15. Label: 6, 9, 13

LYMECYCLINE

Indications: see under Tetracycline
Cautions; Contra-indications; Side-effects: see under Tetracycline
Dose: 408 mg every 12 hours

PoM **Tetralysal 300**® (Farmitalia Carlo Erba)

Capsules, lymecycline 408 mg (= tetracycline 300 mg). Net price 20 = £2.76. Label: 7, 9, 23

MINOCYCLINE

Indications: see under Tetracycline; also meningococcal carrier state
Cautions; Contra-indications: see under Tetracycline, but may be used in renal impairment
Side-effects: see under Tetracycline; also dizziness and vertigo (more common in women)
Dose: 100 mg twice daily
Acne, 50 mg twice daily (minimum course of 6 weeks)

PoM **Minocin**® (Lederle)

Tablets, beige, f/c, minocycline 50 mg (as hydrochloride). Net price 28-tab calendar pack = £7.84. Label: 6, 9
Tablets, orange, f/c, minocycline 100 mg (as hydrochloride). Net price 20 = £11.19. Label: 6, 9

OXYTETRACYCLINE

Indications: see under Tetracycline
Cautions; Contra-indications; Side-effects: see under Tetracycline
Dose: 250–500 mg every 6 hours

PoM **Oxytetracycline** (Non-proprietary)

Capsules, oxytetracycline hydrochloride 250 mg, net price 20 = 44p; oxytetracycline 250 mg (as hydrochloride), net price 20 = 69p. Label: 7, 9, 23
Tablets, f/c or s/c, oxytetracycline dihydrate 250 mg, net price 20 = 24p; oxytetracycline 250 mg (as dihydrate), net price 20 = 66p. Label: 7, 9, 23
Mixture, oxytetracycline (as calcium salt) 125 mg/5 ml. Net price 100 ml = £1.32. Label: 7, 9, 23

Note. Stains teeth; avoid in children under 12 years of age

PoM **Berkmycen**® (Berk)

Tablets, yellow, f/c, oxytetracycline dihydrate 250 mg. Net price 20 = 24p. Label: 7, 9, 23

PoM **Imperacin**® (ICI)

Tablets, yellow, f/c, oxytetracycline dihydrate 250 mg. Net price 20 = 36p. Label: 7, 9, 23

PoM **Terramycin**® (Pfizer)

Capsules, yellow, oxytetracycline 250 mg (as hydrochloride). Net price 20 = 69p. Label: 7, 9, 23
Tablets, yellow, s/c, oxytetracycline 250 mg (as dihydrate). Net price 20 = 66p. Label: 7, 9, 23

PoM **Unimycin**® (Unigreg)

Capsules, yellow/red, oxytetracycline hydrochloride 250 mg. Net price 20 = 44p. Label: 7, 9, 23

5.1.4   Aminoglycosides

This group includes amikacin, gentamicin, kanamycin, neomycin, netilmicin, streptomycin, and tobramycin. All are bactericidal and active against some Gram-positive and many Gram-negative organisms. Amikacin, gentamicin, and tobramycin are also active against *Pseudomonas aeruginosa*; streptomycin is active against *Mycobacterium tuberculosis* and is now almost entirely reserved for tuberculosis (section 5.1.9).

The aminoglycosides are not absorbed from the gut (although there is a risk of absorption in inflammatory bowel disease and liver failure) and must, therefore, be given by injection to treat systemic infections.

Excretion is principally via the kidney and accumulation occurs in renal impairment.

Most side-effects of this group of antibiotics are dose-related therefore care must be taken with dosage and whenever possible treatment should not exceed 7 days. The important side-effects are ototoxicity, and to a lesser degree nephrotoxicity; they occur most commonly in the elderly and in patients with renal failure.

If there is impairment of renal function (or high pre-dose plasma concentrations) the interval between doses must be increased; if the renal impairment is severe the dose itself should be reduced as well.

Aminoglycosides may impair neuromuscular transmission and should not be given to patients with myasthenia gravis; large doses given during surgery have been responsible for a transient myasthenic syndrome in patients with normal neuromuscular function.

Aminoglycosides should not be given with potentially ototoxic diuretics (e.g. frusemide and ethacrynic acid); if concurrent use is unavoidable

---

PLASMA CONCENTRATIONS. Plasma concentration monitoring avoids both excessive and sub-therapeutic concentrations, thus preventing toxicity and, at the same time, ensuring efficacy.

If possible plasma concentrations of aminoglycosides should be measured in all patients and **must** be determined if high doses are being given, if there is renal impairment, or if treatment lasts longer than 7 days.

Note. Plasma concentrations should be measured approximately one hour after intravenous or intramuscular injection, and also just before the next dose. One-hour concentrations of **gentamicin** should not exceed 10 mg/litre while the pre-dose (trough) concentrations should be less than 2 mg/litre.

---

administration of the aminoglycoside and of the diuretic should be separated by as long a period as practicable.

Gentamicin is the most important of the aminoglycosides and is widely used for the treatment of serious infections. It is the aminoglycoside of choice in the UK. It has a broad spectrum but is inactive against anaerobes and has poor activity against haemolytic streptococci and pneumococci. When used for the 'blind' therapy of undiagnosed serious infections it is usually given in conjunction with a penicillin and/or metronidazole.

The daily dose is up to 5 mg/kg given in divided doses every 8 hours (if renal function is normal); whenever possible treatment should not exceed 7 days. Higher doses are occasionally indicated for serious infections, especially in the neonate or the compromised host. A lower dose of 80 mg twice daily (60 mg for lighter or elderly patients) in association with benzylpenicillin is sufficient for endocarditis due to oral streptococci (often termed *Streptococcus viridans*) and gut streptococci.

Amikacin (Amikin®) is a derivative of kanamycin and has one important advantage over gentamicin in that it is stable to 8 of the 9 classified aminoglycoside-inactivating enzymes whereas gentamicin is inactivated by 5. It is principally indicated for the treatment of serious infections caused by Gram-negative bacilli which are resistant to gentamicin, and is given by intramuscular or intravenous injection.

Kanamycin (Kannasyn®) has been replaced by gentamicin as the drug of first choice for serious infections caused by Gram-negative bacilli.

Netilmicin (Netillin®) has similar activity to gentamicin, but is claimed to cause less ototoxicity and nephrotoxicity. It is active against a number of gentamicin-resistant Gram-negative bacilli but is less active against *Ps. aeruginosa* than gentamicin or tobramycin.

Tobramycin (Nebcin®) is similar to gentamicin. It is slightly more active against *Ps. aeruginosa* but shows less activity against certain other Gram-negative bacteria. Tobramycin is claimed to be less toxic than gentamicin.

Neomycin is too toxic for parenteral administration and can only be used for infections of the skin or mucous membranes or to reduce the bacterial population of the colon prior to bowel surgery or in hepatic failure. Oral administration may lead to malabsorption. Small amounts of neomycin may be absorbed from the gut in patients with hepatic failure and, as these patients may also be uraemic, cumulation may occur with resultant ototoxicity. **Framycetin** is almost identical with neomycin in its actions and uses.

PREGNANCY. Where possible, the aminoglycosides should be avoided in pregnancy as they cross the placenta and can cause fetal eighth nerve damage.

GENTAMICIN

Indications: septicaemia and neonatal sepsis; meningitis and other CNS infections; biliary tract infection, acute pyelonephritis or prostatitis, endocarditis caused by *Strep. viridans* or *faecalis* (with a penicillin)

Cautions: increase dose interval in renal impairment (see below). Drug interactions: see Appendix 1 (sections 5.1, *5.1*, *8*, *10*, *15*)

Contra-indications: pregnancy, myasthenia gravis

Side-effects: vestibular damage, reversible nephrotoxicity; rarely, hypomagnesaemia on prolonged therapy, pseudomembraneous colitis; see also notes above

Dose: by intramuscular injection or slow intravenous injection or infusion, 2–5 mg/kg daily, in divided doses every 8 hours. In renal impairment the interval between successive doses should be increased to 12 hours when the creatinine clearance is 30–70 ml/minute, 24 hours for 10–30 ml/minute, 48 hours for 5–10 ml/minute, and 3–4 days after dialysis for less than 5 ml/minute

CHILD, up to 2 weeks, 3 mg/kg every 12 hours; 2 weeks–12 years, 2 mg/kg every 8 hours

By intrathecal injection, 1 mg daily, with 2–4 mg/kg daily *by intramuscular injection* in divided doses every 8 hours

Endocarditis prophylaxis in dentistry, see section 5.1, table 2

PoM **Cidomycin®** (Roussel)
Injection, gentamicin 40 mg (as sulphate)/ml. Net price 2-ml amp or vial = £1.59
Injection, gentamicin 80 mg (as sulphate)/ml. Net price 2-ml amp = £3.18
Paediatric injection, gentamicin 10 mg (as sulphate)/ml. Net price 2-ml vial = 67p
Intrathecal injection, gentamicin 5 mg (as sulphate)/ml. Net price 1-ml amp = 79p

PoM **Genticin®** (Nicholas)
Injection, gentamicin 40 mg (as sulphate)/ml. Net price 2-ml amp or vial = £1.58
Paediatric injection, gentamicin 10 mg (as sulphate)/ml. Net price 2-ml vial = 66p

PoM **Lugacin®** (Lagap)
Injection, gentamicin 40 mg (as sulphate)/ml. Net price 2-ml amp = £1.27

AMIKACIN

Indications: serious Gram-negative infections resistant to gentamicin

Cautions; Contra-indications; Side-effects: see under Gentamicin

Dose: by intramuscular injection or slow intravenous injection or infusion, 15 mg/kg daily in 2 divided doses

PoM **Amikin®** (Bristol-Myers)
Injection, amikacin 250 mg (as sulphate)/ml. Net price 2-ml vial = £10.14
Paediatric injection, amikacin 50 mg (as sulphate)/ml. Net price 2-ml vial = £2.36

FRAMYCETIN SULPHATE

Indications: see under Neomycin Sulphate

Cautions; Contra-indications; Side-effects: see under Gentamicin
Dose: by mouth, 2–4 g daily

PoM **Soframycin**® (Roussel)
Tablets, scored, framycetin sulphate 250 mg. Net price 20 = £6.01

KANAMYCIN

Indications: serious Gram-negative infections resistant to gentamicin
Cautions; Contra-indications; Side-effects: see under Gentamicin
Dose: by intramuscular injection, 250 mg every 6 hours *or* 500 mg every 12 hours
By slow intravenous infusion, 15–30 mg/kg daily in divided doses every 8–12 hours

PoM **Kannasyn**® (Winthrop)
Solution (for injection), kanamycin 250 mg (as sulphate)/ml. Net price 4-ml vial = £19.27
Powder (for preparing injections), kanamycin (as acid sulphate). Net price 1-g vial = £19.27

NEOMYCIN SULPHATE

Indications: bowel sterilisation prior to surgery
Cautions; Contra-indications; Side-effects: see under Gentamicin; avoid in renal impairment. Drug interactions: see Appendix 1 (sections 2.8, 2.8C, 5.1, 15)
Dose: by mouth, 1 g every 4 hours

PoM **Neomycin Elixir,** neomycin sulphate 100 mg/5 ml. Net price 100 ml = 60p
PoM **Nivemycin**® (Boots)
Tablets, neomycin sulphate 500 mg. Net price 20 = £1.88
Elixir, neomycin sulphate 100 mg/5 ml. Net price 100 ml = 60p

NETILMICIN

Indications: serious Gram-negative infections resistant to gentamicin
Cautions; Contra-indications; Side-effects: see under Gentamicin
Dose: by intramuscular injection or intravenous injection or infusion, 4–6 mg/kg daily, in divided doses every 8 or 12 hours; in severe infections, up to 7.5 mg/kg daily in divided doses every 8 hours (usually for 48 hours)
INFANT age up to 1 week, 3 mg/kg every 12 hours; age over 1 week, 2.5–3 mg/kg every 8 hours; CHILD 2–2.5 mg/kg every 8 hours

▼ PoM **Netillin**® (Kirby-Warrick)
Injection, netilmicin 10 mg (as sulphate)/ml. Net price 1.5-ml amp = £1.49
Injection, netilmicin 50 mg (as sulphate)/ml. Net price 1-ml amp = £2.21
Injection, netilmicin 100 mg (as sulphate)/ml. Net price 1-ml amp = £2.88; 1.5-ml amp or vial = £4.11

TOBRAMYCIN

Indications: see under Gentamicin and notes above
Cautions; Contra-indications; Side-effects: see under Gentamicin
Dose: by intramuscular injection or intravenous injection or infusion, 3–5 mg/kg daily in divided doses every 8 hours; INFANT age up to 1 week 2 mg/kg twice daily; age over 1 week 2–2.5 mg/kg every 8 hours

PoM **Nebcin**® (Lilly)
Injection, tobramycin 10 mg (as sulphate)/ml. Net price 2-ml vial = £1.08
Injection, tobramycin 40 mg (as sulphate)/ml. Net price 1-ml vial = £1.46; 2-ml vial = £2.63

5.1.5   Erythromycin

Erythromycin has a similar, although not identical, antibacterial spectrum to that of penicillin and is thus an alternative in penicillin-allergic patients. Indications include respiratory infections in children, whooping-cough, legionnaires' disease, and campylobacter enteritis. It has activity against gut anaerobes and has been used with neomycin for prophylaxis prior to bowel surgery. It is active against many penicillin-resistant staphylococci, and also chlamydia and mycoplasmas.

Erythromycin, if given for more than 14 days, may occasionally cause cholestatic jaundice.

ERYTHROMYCIN

Indications: alternative to penicillin in hypersensitive patients; sinusitis, diphtheria and whooping cough prophylaxis; legionnaires' disease; chronic prostatitis; acne vulgaris (see section 13.6)
Cautions: hepatic impairment. Drug interactions: see Appendix 1 (sections 2.1, 2.8B, 3, 4.7, 4.8, 8)
Contra-indications: estolate contra-indicated in liver disease
Side-effects: nausea, vomiting, diarrhoea after large doses
Dose: by mouth, 250–500 mg every 6 hours *or* 0.5–1 g every 12 hours; up to 4 g daily in severe infections; CHILD up to 2 years 125 mg every 6 hours, 2–8 years 250 mg every 6 hours, doses doubled for severe infections
Acne, see section 13.6
Early syphilis, 500 mg 4 times daily for 14 days
By intravenous infusion, 2 g daily in divided doses, increased to 4 g in severe infections; CHILD, 25–50 mg/kg daily in divided doses
Bolus injection not recommended

PoM **Erythromycin Tablets,** e/c, erythromycin 250 mg, net price 20 = 86p; 500 mg, 20 = £1.97. Label: 5, 9, 25
Note. Erythromycin Tablets are not recommended for the dental prophylaxis of bacterial endocarditis; Erythromycin Stearate Tablets should be specified

---

PoM **Erythromycin Stearate Tablets**, erythromycin 250 and 500 mg (both as stearate). Label: 9

PoM **Arpimycin**® (RP Drugs)
Mixture, pink, erythromycin 125 mg (as ethyl succinate)/5 ml when reconstituted with water for preparations. Diluent syrup, life of diluted mixture 7 days. Net price 100 ml = £1.36. Label: 9
Mixture, pink, erythromycin 250 mg (as ethyl succinate)/5 ml when reconstituted with water for preparations. Diluent as above. Net price 100 ml = £2.03. Label: 9
Mixture, pink, erythromycin 500 mg (as ethyl succinate)/5 ml when reconstituted with water for preparations. Diluent as above. Net price 100 ml = £3.85. Label: 9

PoM **Erycen**® (Berk)
Tablets, both orange, e/c, f/c, erythromycin 250 mg, net price 20 = 97p; 500 mg, 20 = £2.41. Label: 5, 9, 25

▼ PoM **Erymax**® (P-D)
Capsules, opaque orange/clear orange, enclosing orange and white e/c pellets, erythromycin 250 mg. Net price 20 = £3.67. Label: 5, 9, 25
Dose: 1 every 6 hours *or* 2 every 12 hours; acne, 1 twice daily then 1 daily after 1 month

PoM **Erythrocin**® (Abbott)
Tablets, both f/c, erythromycin (as stearate), 250 mg, net price 20 = £2.13; 500 mg, 20 = £4.48, 56-tab 'acne pack' = £12.54. Label: 9
Intravenous injection, powder for reconstitution, erythromycin (as lactobionate). Net price 1-g vial = £6.85

PoM **Erythrolar**® (Lagap)
Tablets, both pink, f/c, erythromycin (as stearate), 250 mg, net price 20 = £1.70; 500 mg, 20 = £3.51. Label: 9
Suspension (= mixture), erythromycin 250 mg (as ethyl succinate)/5 ml when reconstituted with water for preparations. Diluent syrup, life of diluted mixture 5 days. Net price 100 ml = £2.13. Label: 9

PoM **Erythromid**® (Abbott)
Tablets, orange, e/c, f/c, erythromycin 250 mg. Net price 20 = 86p. Label: 5, 9, 25

PoM **Erythromid DS**® (Abbott)
Tablets, e/c, f/c, erythromycin 500 mg. Net price 20 = £1.94. Label: 5, 9, 25

PoM **Erythroped**® (Abbott)
Suspension PI (= paediatric mixture), erythromycin 125 mg (as ethyl succinate)/5 ml when reconstituted with water for preparations. Diluent syrup, life of diluted mixture 5 days. Net price 100 ml = £1.48. Label: 9
Suspension (= mixture), erythromycin 250 mg (as ethyl succinate)/5 ml when reconstituted with water for preparations. Diluent as above. Net price 100 ml = £2.23. Label: 9
Sugar-free granules, erythromycin 250 mg (as ethyl succinate)/sachet. Net price 20 sachets = £5.60. Label: 9, 13
Suspension forte (= strong mixture), erythromycin 500 mg (as ethyl succinate)/5 ml when reconstituted with water for preparations.

Diluent as above. Net price 100 ml = £4.26. Label: 9

PoM **Erythroped A**® (Abbott)
Tablets, yellow, f/c, erythromycin 500 mg (as ethyl succinate). Net price 20 = £3.91. Label: 9
Granules, erythromycin 1 g (as ethyl succinate)/sachet. Net price 14 sachets = £6.82. Label: 9, 13

PoM **Ilosone**® (Dista)
Capsules, ivory/red, erythromycin 250 mg (as estolate). Net price 20 = £3.52. Label: 9
Tablets, pink, erythromycin 500 mg (as estolate). Net price 20 = £7.18. Label: 9
Suspension (= mixture), orange, erythromycin 125 mg (as estolate)/5 ml. Diluent syrup, life of diluted mixture 14 days. Net price 100 ml = £2.51. Label: 9
Suspension forte (= strong mixture), orange, erythromycin 250 mg (as estolate)/5 ml. Diluent as above. Net price 100 ml = £4.89. Label: 9

5.1.6 Clindamycin and lincomycin

These antibiotics have only a limited use because of their serious side-effects.

Clindamycin (Dalacin C®), which is more active and better absorbed from the gut, has generally replaced **lincomycin** (Lincocin®).

They are active against Gram-positive cocci, including penicillin-resistant staphylococci and also against many anaerobes, especially *Bacteroides fragilis*. They are well concentrated in bone and excreted in bile and urine.

Clindamycin is recommended for staphylococcal bone and joint infections, and intra-abdominal sepsis.

The most serious toxic effect of clindamycin and lincomycin is pseudomembranous colitis which may be fatal and is commonest in middle-aged and elderly females, especially following operation. This complication may occur with most antibiotics but is more frequently seen with clindamycin and is due to a toxin produced by *Clostridium difficile*, an anaerobic organism resistant to many antibiotics including clindamycin. It is sensitive to vancomycin (section 5.1.7) and metronidazole (section 5.1.11) administered by mouth.

CLINDAMYCIN

Indications: staphylococcal bone and joint infections, peritonitis
Cautions: discontinue immediately if diarrhoea or colitis develops; impaired hepatic or renal function. Drug interactions: see Appendix 1 (sections *10*, *15*)
Contra-indications: diarrhoeal states
Side-effects: diarrhoea (discontinue treatment), nausea, vomiting, pseudomembranous colitis
Dose: by mouth, 150–300 mg every 6 hours; up to 450 mg every 6 hours in severe infections; CHILD, 3–6 mg/kg every 6 hours
COUNSELLING. Patients should discontinue immediately and contact doctor if diarrhoea develops; capsules should be swallowed with a glass of water.

By intramuscular injection or slow intravenous infusion, 0.6–2.7 g daily in 2–4 divided doses; CHILD, 15–40 mg/kg daily in 3–4 divided doses

PoM **Dalacin C®** (Upjohn)
Capsules, clindamycin (as hydrochloride) 75 mg (lavender), net price 20 = £4.92; 150 mg, (lavender/maroon), 20 = £9.07. Label: 9, 27, counselling advised, see above (diarrhoea)
Paediatric suspension, pink, clindamycin 75 mg (as palmitate hydrochloride)/5 ml when reconstituted with water for preparations. Diluent water for preparations, life of diluted suspension 14 days. Net price 100 ml = £6.62. Label: 9, 27, counselling advised, see above (diarrhoea)
Injection, clindamycin 150 mg (as phosphate)/ml. Net price 2-ml amp = £5.17; 4-ml amp = £10.29

LINCOMYCIN

Indications: see under Clindamycin, also notes above
Cautions; Contra-indications; Side-effects: see under Clindamycin. Drug interactions: see Appendix 1 (sections 5.1, *10*, *15*)
Dose: by mouth, 500 mg every 6–8 hours
By intramuscular injection, 600 mg every 12–24 hours
By slow intravenous infusion, 600 mg every 8–12 hours

PoM **Lincocin®** (Upjohn)
Capsules, blue, lincomycin 500 mg (as hydrochloride). Net price 20 = £11.55. Label: 9, 23, counselling advised, see above (diarrhoea)
Syrup, red, lincomycin 250 mg (as hydrochloride)/5 ml. Diluent syrup, life of diluted syrup 14 days. Net price 100 ml = £7.55. Label: 9, 23, counselling advised, see above (diarrhoea)
Injection, lincomycin 300 mg (as hydrochloride)/ml. Net price 2-ml amp = £2.64

5.1.7   Some other antibiotics

Antibacterials discussed in this section include chloramphenicol, colistin, fusidic acid, polymyxin B, spectinomycin, and vancomycin.

Chloramphenicol is a potent, potentially toxic, broad-spectrum antibiotic which should be reserved for the treatment of life-threatening infections, particularly those caused by *Haemophilus influenzae*, and also for typhoid fever.

Its toxicity renders it unsuitable for systemic use except in the circumstances indicated above.

Eye-drops of chloramphenicol (see section 11.3.1) are useful for the treatment of bacterial conjunctivitis.

CHLORAMPHENICOL

Indications: see notes above
Cautions: avoid repeated courses and prolonged treatment; reduce doses in hepatic or renal impairment; periodic blood counts required; interferes with development of immunity; may cause 'grey syndrome' in neonates (monitor plasma concentrations). Drug interactions: see Appendix 1 (sections *2.8B*, *4.8*, 5.1, *6.1*)
Contra-indications: pregnancy, breast-feeding
Side-effects: leucopenia, thrombocytopenia, irreversible aplastic anaemia, peripheral neuritis, optic neuritis, erythema multiforme, nausea, vomiting, diarrhoea
Dose: by mouth, 500 mg every 6 hours
By intravenous injection or infusion, 50 mg/kg daily in divided doses; CHILD, haemophilus epiglottitis and pyogenic meningitis, 50–100 mg/kg daily in divided doses (high dosages decreased as soon as clinically indicated); INFANTS under 2 weeks 25 mg/kg daily in divided doses, under 1 year 50 mg/kg daily in divided doses
Note. Plasma concentration monitoring required in neonates and preferred also in those under 4 years of age; recommended plasma concentration 15–25 mg/litre

PoM **Chloromycetin®** (P-D)
Capsules, white/grey, chloramphenicol 250 mg. Net price 20 = £1.55
Suspension, chloramphenicol 125 mg (as palmitate)/5 ml. Diluent syrup, life of diluted suspension 14 days. Net price 100 ml = £3.63
Injection, powder for reconstitution, chloramphenicol (as sodium succinate). Net price 300 mg vial = £5.16; 1.2-g vial = £4.42

PoM **Kemicetine®** (Farmitalia Carlo Erba)
Injection, powder for reconstitution, chloramphenicol (as sodium succinate). Net price 1-g vial = 66p

Colistin is a polymyxin active against Gram-negative organisms including *Ps. aeruginosa*.

It is **not** absorbed when given by mouth but is sometimes prescribed in infantile gastro-enteritis (but see section 1.4) and used topically for skin infection and as ear drops. It is also used in bowel sterilisation regimens in neutropenic patients. For use in bladder irrigation see section 7.4.4.

COLISTIN

Indications: see notes above
Cautions: reduce dose in renal impairment. Drug interactions: see Appendix 1 (section *15*)
Contra-indications: myasthenia gravis
Side-effects: perioral paraesthesia, vertigo, muscle weakness, apnoea
Dose: by mouth, 1.5–3 million units every 8 hours
By intramuscular injection or intravenous injection or infusion, 2 million units every 8 hours

PoM **Colomycin®** (Pharmax)
Tablets, scored, colistin sulphate 1.5 million units. Net price 20 = £25.19
Syrup, pink, colistin sulphate 250 000 units/5 ml when reconstituted with water for preparations. Diluent syrup, life of diluted syrup 14 days. Net price 80 ml = £3.75

Injection, powder for reconstitution, colistin sulphomethate sodium. Net price 500 000-unit vial = £1.23; 1 million-unit vial = £1.81

Fusidic acid and its salts are narrow-spectrum antibiotics. The only indication for their use is in infections caused by penicillin-resistant staphylococci, especially osteomyelitis, as they are well concentrated in bone; a second antistaphylococcal antibiotic is usually required.

SODIUM FUSIDATE

Indications: see notes above
Cautions: liver-function tests required
Side-effects: nausea, vomiting, rashes, reversible jaundice, especially after high dosage or rapid infusion (withdraw therapy if persistent)
Dose: by mouth, 500 mg every 8 hours
By slow intravenous infusion, 500 mg over 6 hours, 3 times daily

PoM **Fucidin**® (Leo)
Tablets, e/c, sodium fusidate 250 mg. Net price 20 = £13.48. Label: 5, 9, 25
Suspension, orange, fusidic acid 250 mg (≡ sodium fusidate 175 mg)/5 ml. Do not dilute. Net price 25 ml = £7.54. Label: 9, 21
Intravenous infusion, powder for reconstitution, diethanolamine fusidate 580 mg (≡ sodium fusidate 500 mg), with buffer. Net price per vial (with diluent) = £4.51

Polymyxin B sulphate is effective against Gram-negative organisms, particularly *Ps. aeruginosa*. It is a toxic antibiotic and there are very few indications for its use. For use in bladder irrigation see section 7.4.4.

POLYMYXIN B SULPHATE

Indications: see notes above
Cautions: impaired renal function. Drug interactions: see Appendix 1 (section *15*)
Contra-indications: myasthenia gravis
Side-effects: circumoral and peripheral paraesthesia; haematuria, proteinuria, tubular necrosis; vertigo, muscle weakness, apnoea
Dose: by slow intravenous infusion, 15 000–25 000 units/kg daily in divided doses

PoM **Aerosporin**® (Calmic)
Injection, powder for reconstitution, polymyxin B sulphate. Net price 500 000-unit vial = £9.32
PoM **Polybactrin**® (Calmic)
Soluble GU, powder for reconstitution, polymyxin B sulphate 75 000 units, neomycin sulphate 20 000 units, bacitracin 1000 units. For bladder irrigation. Net price per vial = £4.47

Spectinomycin is active against Gram-negative organisms, including *N. gonorrhoeae*. Its only indication is the treatment of gonorrhoea caused by penicillin-resistant organisms or in a penicillin-allergic patient.

SPECTINOMYCIN

Indications: see notes above
Side-effects: nausea, vomiting, dizziness, urticaria, fever
Dose: by deep intramuscular injection, 2 g; up to 4 g in difficult-to-treat cases and areas of resistance

PoM **Trobicin**® (Upjohn)
Injection, powder for reconstitution, spectinomycin (as hydrochloride). Net price 2-g vial (with diluent) = £8.16

Vancomycin is a bactericidal antibiotic. It is the drug of choice for antibiotic-associated pseudomembranous colitis, for which it is given by mouth; a dose of 125 mg every 6 hours for 7 to 10 days is considered to be adequate. It also has a limited use by the intravenous route in the prophylaxis and treatment of endocarditis and other serious infections caused by Gram-positive cocci including multi-resistant staphylococci. It has a relatively long plasma half-life of approximately 6 hours therefore administration every 12 hours is usually adequate; plasma concentrations should be monitored (especially in patients with renal impairment). It is ototoxic and nephrotoxic.

VANCOMYCIN

Indications: see notes above
Cautions: extravasation at injection site may cause necrosis and thrombophlebitis, blood counts and liver- and kidney-function tests required. Drug interactions: see Appendix 1 (sections 5.1, *5.1*)
Contra-indications: if possible avoid parenteral administration in patients with renal impairment or a history of deafness
Side-effects: after parenteral administration nausea, chills, fever, urticaria, rashes, 'red man' syndrome (on rapid intravenous injection), eosinophilia, tinnitus (discontinue use), renal impairment
Dose: by mouth, 125 mg every 6 hours for 7–10 days, see notes above
By intravenous infusion, 500 mg over 60 minutes every 6 hours *or* 1 g every 12 hours
Endocarditis prophylaxis in dentistry, see section 5.1, table 2

PoM **Vancocin**® (Lilly)
Matrigel capsules, vancomycin hydrochloride 125 mg (blue/peach), net price 20 = £63.08; 250 mg (blue/grey), 20 = £126.16
Powder (for oral use), vancomycin hydrochloride. Net price 10-g bottle = £261.23
Injection, powder for reconstitution, vancomycin (as hydrochloride). Net price 500-mg vial = £13.36

5.1.8 Sulphonamides and trimethoprim

The importance of the sulphonamides as chemotherapeutic agents has decreased as a result of

---

increasing bacterial resistance and their replacement by antibiotics which are generally more active and less toxic.

The principal indication for sulphonamides used alone is urinary-tract infections caused by sensitive organisms.

The addition of the folic acid antagonist trimethoprim to sulphamethoxazole (co-trimoxazole) increases the activity of the sulphonamide against certain bacteria.

Indications for **co-trimoxazole** (Bactrim®, Septrin® etc.) include urinary-tract infections, prostatitis, exacerbations of chronic bronchitis, invasive salmonella infections, brucellosis, and *Pneumocystis carinii* infections. Pentamidine is also effective for *Pneumocystis* pneumonia (section 5.4.8).

Trimethoprim is increasingly being used alone for the treatment of urinary- and respiratory-tract infections. Side-effects are less than with co-trimoxazole especially in older patients.

Side-effects of the sulphonamides include rashes, which are common, the Stevens-Johnson syndrome (erythema multiforme), renal failure (especially with the less soluble preparations), and blood dyscrasias, notably marrow depression and agranulocytosis.

Side-effects of co-trimoxazole are similar to those of the sulphonamides but a particular watch should be kept for haematological effects and special care should be taken in patients who may be folate deficient such as the elderly and chronic sick. There have been recent reports of deaths in patients over the age of 65 years being treated with co-trimoxazole and almost certainly associated with the sulphonamide component. For this reason co-trimoxazole should not be prescribed in the elderly unless there is no acceptable alternative. The effect on the fetus is unknown and the drugs should not be used in pregnancy.

The **longer-acting sulphonamide**, sulfametopyrazine which is usually highly bound to plasma proteins, has the advantage of requiring less frequent administration, but toxic effects due to accumulation are more likely to occur.

The **poorly-absorbed sulphonamides** (calcium sulphaloxate and sulphaguanidine) have been widely used for the treatment of intestinal infections and pre-operative bowel preparation but can no longer be recommended for these indications (for use in acute and chronic diarrhoeas see sections 1.4.3 and 1.5).

For *topical preparations* of sulphonamides used in the treatment of burns see section 13.10.1.1.

CO-TRIMOXAZOLE

A mixture of sulphamethoxazole 5 parts, trimethoprim 1 part

Indications: invasive salmonellosis, typhoid fever, bone and joint infections due to *H. influenzae*, urinary-tract infections, sinusitis, exacerbations of chronic bronchitis, gonorrhoea in penicillin-allergic patients

Cautions: blood counts in prolonged treatment, maintain adequate fluid intake, renal impairment, breast-feeding; photosensitivity; elderly patients (see notes above). Drug interactions: see Appendix 1 (sections *2.8B, 4.8, 6.1, 8, 15*)

Contra-indications: pregnancy, infants under 6 weeks (risk of kernicterus), renal or hepatic failure, jaundice, blood disorders

Side-effects: nausea, vomiting, rashes, erythema multiforme, epidermal necrolysis, eosinophilia, agranulocytosis, granulocytopenia, purpura, leucopenia; megaloblastic anaemia due to trimethoprim

Dose: by mouth, 960 mg every 12 hours, increased to 1.44 g in severe infections; 480 mg every 12 hours if treated for more than 14 days; CHILD, every 12 hours, 6 weeks to 5 months, 120 mg; 6 months to 5 years, 240 mg; 6–12 years, 480 mg

Gonorrhoea, 1.92 g every 12 hours for 2 days, or 2.4 g followed by a further dose of 2.4 g after 8 hours

High-dose therapy for *Pneumocystis carinii* infections, 120 mg/kg daily in divided doses

By intramuscular injection or intravenous infusion, 960 mg every 12 hours

Note: 480 mg of co-trimoxazole consists of sulphamethoxazole 400 mg and trimethoprim 80 mg

PoM **Co-trimoxazole Tablets,** co-trimoxazole 480 mg. Net price 20 = 88p. Label: 9

PoM **Co-trimoxazole Tablets, Dispersible,** co-trimoxazole 480 mg. Net price 20 = £1.30. Label: 9, 13

PoM **Co-trimoxazole Tablets, Double-strength,** co-trimoxazole 960 mg. Net price 20 = £2.62. Label: 9

PoM **Co-trimoxazole Tablets, Double-strength, Dispersible,** co-trimoxazole 960 mg. Label: 9, 13

PoM **Co-trimoxazole Tablets, Paediatric,** co-trimoxazole 120 mg. Net price 20 = 56p. Label: 9

PoM **Co-trimoxazole Mixture,** co-trimoxazole 480 mg/5 ml. Diluent syrup, life of diluted mixture 14 days. Net price 100 ml = £3·14. Label: 9

PoM **Co-trimoxazole Mixture, Paediatric,** co-trimoxazole 240 mg/5 ml. Diluent as above. Net price 100 ml = £1·96. Label: 9

PoM **Co-trimoxazole Intramuscular Injection,** co-trimoxazole 320 mg/ml in solvent. 3-ml amp

PoM **Co-trimoxazole Solution, Strong Sterile,** co-trimoxazole 96 mg/ml. **Co-trimoxazole Intravenous Infusion** is prepared by diluting this solution with 25 to 35 times its volume of glucose intravenous infusion 5% or sodium chloride intravenous infusion 0.9% before use. Net price 5-ml amp = £1.08; 10-ml amp = £2.02

PoM **Bactrim®** (Roche)

Drapsules® (= tablets), orange, f/c, co-trimoxazole 480 mg. Net price 20 = £2.15. Label: 9

Tablets (dispersible), yellow, scored, co-trimoxazole 480 mg. Net price 20 = £2.15. Label: 9, 13

Double-strength tablets, scored, co-trimoxazole 960 mg. Net price 20 = £3.38. Label: 9

Paediatric tablets, co-trimoxazole 120 mg. Net price 20 = 61p. Label: 9

Adult suspension (= mixture), yellow, co-trimoxazole 480 mg/5 ml. Diluent syrup, life of diluted mixture 14 days. Net price 100 ml = £2.86. Label: 9

Paediatric syrup, sugar-free, yellow, co-trimoxazole 240 mg/5 ml. Diluent as above. Net price 100 ml = £1.99. Label: 9

Intramuscular injection, co-trimoxazole 320 mg/ml. Net price 3-ml amp = £1.64

Intravenous infusion, co-trimoxazole 96 mg/ml. To be diluted before use. Net price 5-ml amp = £1.07 (Hosp. only)

PoM **Chemotrim**® (RP Drugs)

Paediatric suspension (= paediatric mixture), pale pink, co-trimoxazole 240 mg/5 ml. Diluent syrup, life of diluted mixture 14 days. Net price 125 ml = £1.90. Label: 9

PoM **Comox**® (Norton)

Tablets, scored, co-trimoxazole 480 mg. Net price 20 = £2.13. Label: 9

Dispersible tablets, orange, co-trimoxazole 480 mg. Net price 20 = £2.08. Label: 9, 13

Forte tablets, scored, co-trimoxazole 960 mg. Net price 20 = £3.15. Label: 9

Paediatric suspension (= paediatric mixture), pink, co-trimoxazole 240 mg/5 ml. Net price 100 ml = £1.60. Label: 9

PoM **Fectrim**® (DDSA)

Tablets (dispersible), co-trimoxazole 480 mg. Net price 20 = £1.60. Label: 9, 13

Forte tablets (dispersible), co-trimoxazole 960 mg. Net price 20 = £2.50. Label: 9, 13

Paediatric tablets, co-trimoxazole 120 mg. Net price 20 = 46p. Label: 9

PoM **Laratrim**® (Lagap)

Tablets, co-trimoxazole 480 mg. Net price 20 = 84p. Label: 9

Forte tablets, co-trimoxazole 960 mg. Net price 20 = £2.34. Label: 9

Adult suspension, co-trimoxazole 480 mg/5 ml. Diluent syrup, life of diluted suspension 14 days. Net price 100 ml = £2.27. Label: 9

Paediatric suspension, co-trimoxazole 240 mg/5 ml. Net price 100 ml = £1.40. Label: 9

PoM **Septrin**® (Wellcome)

Tablets, co-trimoxazole 480 mg. Net price 20 = £2.51. Label: 9

Dispersible tablets, orange, sugar-free, co-trimoxazole 480 mg. Net price 20 = £2.67. Label: 9, 13

Forte tablets, scored, co-trimoxazole 960 mg. Net price 20 = £4.19. Label: 9

Paediatric dispersible tablets, orange, co-trimoxazole 120 mg. Net price 20 = 84p. Label: 9, 13

Adult suspension (= mixture), co-trimoxazole 480 mg/5 ml. Diluent syrup, life of diluted mixture 14 days. Net price 100 ml = £3.94. Label: 9

Paediatric suspension (= paediatric mixture), sugar-free, co-trimoxazole 240 mg/5 ml. Diluent syrup or sorbitol solution 70%, life of diluted suspension 14 days. Net price 100 ml = £2.18. Label: 9

Intramuscular injection, co-trimoxazole 320 mg/ml. Net price 3-ml amp = £2.25

Intravenous infusion, co-trimoxazole 96 mg/ml. To be diluted before use. Net price 5-ml amp = £1.32

CALCIUM SULPHALOXATE

Indications: see notes on poorly-absorbed sulphonamides

Cautions; Contra-indications; Side-effects: see under Co-trimoxazole; side-effects less common because of limited absorption

Dose: 1 g every 8 hours

PoM **Enteromide**® (Consolidated)

Tablets, calcium sulphaloxate 500 mg. Net price 20 = £1.06

SULFAMETOPYRAZINE

Indications: urinary-tract infections, chronic bronchitis

Cautions; Contra-indications; Side-effects: see under Co-trimoxazole

Dose: 2 g once weekly

PoM **Kelfizine W**® (Farmitalia Carlo Erba)

Tablets, sulfametopyrazine 2 g. Tablets to be taken in water. Net price 1 = £1.13. Label: 9, 13

SULPHADIAZINE

Indications: meningococcal meningitis

Cautions; Contra-indications; Side-effects: see under Co-trimoxazole; avoid in severe renal impairment

Dose: by intramuscular injection or intravenous infusion, 1–1.5 g every 4 hours for 2 days, followed by oral treatment

PoM **Sulphadiazine Tablets**, sulphadiazine 500 mg. Net price 20 = £1.17. Label: 9, 27

PoM **Sulphadiazine Injection**, sulphadiazine 250 mg (as sodium salt)/ml. Net price 4-ml amp = 67p

SULPHADIMIDINE

Indications: urinary-tract infections; meningococcal meningitis prophylaxis (see Table 2)

Cautions; Contra-indications; Side-effects: see under Co-trimoxazole

Dose: by mouth or by intravenous or intramuscular injection, 2 g initially, then 0.5–1 g every 6–8 hours

PoM **Sulphadimidine Tablets**, sulphadimidine 500 mg. Net price 20 = £1.10. Label: 9, 27

PoM **Sulphamezathine**® (ICI)

Injection, sulphadimidine sodium 333 mg/ml. Net price 3-ml (1-g) amp = 23p

SULPHAGUANIDINE

Indications: see notes on poorly-absorbed sulphonamides

Cautions; Contra-indications; Side-effects: see
under Co-trimoxazole; rashes frequent
Dose: 3 g every 6–8 hours for 3 days

PoM **Sulphaguanidine Tablets,** sulphaguanidine 500 mg.
Net price 20 = 77p. Label: 9

SULPHAUREA
Indications: urinary-tract infections
Cautions; Contra-indications; Side-effects: see
under Co-trimoxazole

PoM **Uromide**® (Consolidated)
Tablets, yellow, sulphaurea 500 mg, phenazopyridine
hydrochloride 50 mg. Net price 20 = 71p. Label: 9, 14,
22

TRIMETHOPRIM
Indications: urinary-tract infections, acute and
chronic bronchitis
Cautions: reduce dose in moderate renal impairment, predisposition to folate deficiency, blood
counts required on long-term therapy. Drug
interactions: see Appendix 1 (section *8*)
Contra-indications: severe renal impairment,
pregnancy, neonates
Side-effects: gastro-intestinal disturbances
including nausea and vomiting, pruritus,
rashes, depression of haemopoiesis
Dose: by mouth, acute infections, 200 mg every
12 hours; urinary-tract infections, 300 mg daily
or 200 mg twice daily; chronic infections and
prophylaxis, 100 mg at night; CHILD, twice daily,
2–5 months 25 mg, 6 months–5 years 50 mg, 6–
12 years 100 mg
By slow intravenous injection or infusion, 150–
250 mg every 12 hours; CHILD under 12 years,
6–9 mg/kg daily in 2–3 divided doses

PoM **Trimethoprim** (Non-proprietary)
Tablets, trimethoprim 100 mg, net price 20 =
60p; 200 mg, 20 tabs = 89p; 300 mg, 20 =
£8.81. Label: 9
Mixture, trimethoprim 50 mg/5 ml. Diluents, see
below. Label: 9
Injection, trimethoprim 20 mg (as lactate)/ml. 5-
ml amp
PoM **Ipral**® (Squibb)
Tablets, trimethoprim 100 mg, net price 20 =
80p; 200 mg, 20 = £1.71. Label: 9
Paediatric suspension, sugar-free, trimethoprim
50 mg/5 ml. Diluents sorbitol solution, syrup,
or water for preparations, life of diluted sus-
pension 14 days. Net price 100 ml = £1.38.
Label: 9
PoM **Monotrim**® (Duphar)
Tablets, both scored, trimethoprim 100 mg, net
price 20 = 82p; 200 mg, 20 = £1.44. Label: 9
Suspension, sugar-free, trimethoprim 50 mg/
5 ml. Diluents sorbitol solution or water for
preparations, life of diluted suspension 14 days.
Net price 100 ml = £1.36. Label: 9
Injection, trimethoprim 20 mg (as lactate)/ml.
Net price 5-ml amp = 68p

PoM **Syraprim**® (Wellcome)
Tablets, both scored, trimethoprim 100 mg, net
price 20 = £2.98; 300 mg, 20 = £8.81. Label: 9
Injection, trimethoprim 20 mg (as lactate)/ml.
Net price 5-ml amp = £1.25
PoM **Tiempe**® (DDSA)
Tablets, trimethoprim 100 mg, net price 20 =
78p; 200 mg, 20 = £1.40. Label: 9
PoM **Trimogal**® (Lagap)
Tablets, trimethoprim 100 mg, net price 20 =
59p; 200 mg, 20 = 86p. Label: 9
PoM **Trimopan**® (Berk)
Tablets, both scored, trimethoprim 100 mg, net
price 20 = 97p; 200 mg, 14-tab pack = £1.34.
Label: 9
Suspension, sugar-free, trimethoprim 50 mg/
5 ml. Diluent syrup, life of diluted suspension
14 days. Net price 100 ml = £1.37. Label: 9

5.1.9   Antituberculous drugs
The treatment of tuberculosis has two phases—
an *initial phase* using at least three drugs and a
continuation phase with two drugs.

Treatment requires specialised knowledge,
particularly where the organisms are resistant to
the first-line drugs isoniazid, rifampicin, streptomycin, and ethambutol, or where the disease
involves non-respiratory organs.

The treatment outlined below reflects current
practice in the UK; variations occur in other
countries

INITIAL PHASE. The concurrent use of at least three
drugs during the initial phase is designed to reduce
the population of viable bacteria as rapidly as
possible and to minimise the risk of ineffective
treatment in those patients infected by drug-resist-
ant bacteria. Treatment of choice for the initial
phase is the daily use of isoniazid, rifampicin, and
pyrazinamide possibly supplemented by either
ethambutol or streptomycin. These drugs should
be continued for 8 weeks.

CONTINUATION PHASE. After the initial phase,
treatment is continued with isoniazid and rifampicin (in the absence of contra-indications).
Pyrazinamide is ineffective after the first two or
three months and should be stopped after that
time. Ethambutol and streptomycin should only
be given under special circumstances; they are
less effective than isoniazid and rifampicin, and
need to be given for longer and are significantly
more toxic. Treatment under full supervision with
high-dose isoniazid (15 mg/kg) and rifampicin
(600–900 mg) twice weekly is as effective as
unsupervised therapy.

DURATION OF TREATMENT. The duration of treatment depends on the combination of drugs used.
Where isoniazid and rifampicin are given daily
throughout treatment a *9-month course* is sufficient for patients with respiratory disease regardless of its extent. If in the initial phase

pyrazinamide is included with isoniazid and rifampicin, which are then used in the continuation phase, a total of *6 months treatment* gives equally good results.

> Major causes of treatment failure are incorrect prescribing by the physician and inadequate compliance by the patient. It is important to avoid both excessive and inadequate dosage.

Isoniazid (Rimifon®) is cheap and highly effective. Its only common side-effect is peripheral neuropathy which is more likely to occur when high dosage is used (as in meningitis) or where there are pre-existing risk factors. In these circumstances pyridoxine 10 mg daily should be given prophylactically from the start of treatment. Other side-effects such as hepatitis and psychosis are rare.

Streptomycin is given intramuscularly in a standard dose of 1 g daily, reduced to 500 to 750 mg in small patients or those over the age of 40 years. Measurement of plasma drug concentrations should be performed, particularly in patients with impaired renal function in whom streptomycin must be used with great care. Side-effects increase after a cumulative dose of 100 g, which should only be exceeded in exceptional circumstances.

Rifampicin (Rifadin®, Rimactane®) is an essential component of any short-course regimen. It should be given in a single daily dose of 450 mg in adults of less than 50 kg and 600 mg in those above that weight.

During the first two months of rifampicin administration transient disturbance of liver function with elevated serum transaminases is common but generally does not require interruption of treatment. Occasionally more serious liver toxicity requires a change of treatment particularly in those with pre-existing liver disease.

On intermittent treatment six toxicity syndromes have been recognised—influenzal, abdominal, and respiratory symptoms, shock, renal failure, and thrombocytopenic purpura—and can occur in 20 to 30% of patients.

Rifampicin induces hepatic enzymes which accelerate the metabolism of several drugs including oestrogens, corticosteroids, sulphonylureas, and anticoagulants. The effectiveness of oral contraceptives is reduced and, where appropriate, alternative family planning advice should be offered.

Ethambutol (Myambutol®) is used in conjunction with isoniazid or rifampicin. Side-effects are largely confined to visual disturbances in the form of loss of acuity, colour blindness, and restriction of visual fields. These toxic effects are more common where excessive dosage is used or the patient's renal function is impaired, in which case the drug should be **avoided**. The earliest features of ocular toxicity are subjective and patients should be advised to report any visual disturbance immediately. Early discontinuation of the drug is almost always followed by recovery of eyesight. Patients who cannot understand warnings about visual side-effects should, if possible, be given an alternative drug. In particular, ethambutol should be **avoided** in children until they are at least 6 years old and capable of reporting symptomatic visual changes accurately.

Ophthalmic examination should be performed prior to treatment and at intervals during treatment.

Pyrazinamide (Zinamide®) is a bactericidal drug active against *Mycobacterium tuberculosis* but not *M. bovis*; it exerts its main effect only in the first two months. It is particularly useful in tuberculous meningitis because of good meningeal penetration.

Second-line drugs available for infections caused by resistant organisms, or when first-line drugs cause unacceptable side-effects, include capreomycin (Capastat®), cycloserine, and prothionamide (no longer on UK market).

CAPREOMYCIN

Indications: tuberculosis resistant to first-line drugs

Cautions: renal, hepatic, or auditory impairment; breast-feeding; do not give with streptomycin or other ototoxic drugs

Contra-indications: pregnancy

Side-effects: hypersensitivity reactions including urticaria and rashes, changes in liver function, renal damage, hearing loss with tinnitus and vertigo, pain and induration at injection site

Dose: by intramuscular injection, 1 g daily (not more than 20 mg/kg)

PoM **Capastat®** (Dista)
Injection, powder for reconstitution, capreomycin sulphate 1 million units (capreomycin approx. 1 g). Net price per vial = £1.52

CYCLOSERINE

Indications: tuberculosis resistant to first-line drugs

Cautions: reduce dose in renal impairment

Contra-indications: epilepsy, depression, severe anxiety, psychotic states, alcoholism

Side-effects: mainly neurological, including headache, dizziness, vertigo, drowsiness, convulsions; allergic rashes

Dose: usually 250 mg every 12 hours; max. 1 g daily

PoM **Cycloserine** (Lilly)
Capsules, cycloserine 125 mg, net price 20 = £5.13; 250 mg, 20 = £9.46. Label: 2, 8

ETHAMBUTOL HYDROCHLORIDE

Indications: tuberculosis, in combination with other drugs

Cautions: warn patients to report visual changes—see notes above

Contra-indications: renal impairment; young children (see notes), elderly patients, optic neuritis, poor vision

Side-effects: optic neuritis, red/green colour blindness, peripheral neuritis

Dose: 15 mg/kg daily; CHILD over 6 years, 25 mg/kg daily for 60 days, followed by 15 mg/kg daily

PoM **Myambutol**® (Lederle)
Tablets, ethambutol hydrochloride 100 mg (yellow), net price 20 = £1.45; 400 mg (grey), 20 = £5.23. Label: 8

PoM **Mynah 200**® (Lederle)
Tablets, ethambutol hydrochloride 200 mg, isoniazid 100 mg. Net price 20 = £3.16. Label: 8, 23

PoM **Mynah 250**® (Lederle)
Tablets, yellow, ethambutol hydrochloride 250 mg, isoniazid 100 mg. Net price 20 = £3.92. Label: 8, 23

PoM **Mynah 300**® (Lederle)
Tablets, orange, ethambutol hydrochloride 300 mg, isoniazid 100 mg. Net price 20 = £4.68. Label: 8, 23

PoM **Mynah 365**® (Lederle)
Tablets, pink, ethambutol hydrochloride 365 mg, isoniazid 100 mg. Net price 20 = £5.67. Label: 8, 23

ISONIAZID

Indications: tuberculosis, in combination with other drugs; prophylaxis—section 5.1, Table 2

Cautions: impaired liver and kidney function, epilepsy, alcoholism, breast-feeding. Drug interactions: see Appendix 1 (section *4.8*)

Contra-indications: drug-induced liver disease

Side-effects: nausea, vomiting, hypersensitivity reactions including rashes, peripheral neuritis with high doses (pyridoxine prophylaxis, see notes above), convulsions, psychotic episodes, agranulocytosis; hepatitis (especially over age of 35)

Dose: by mouth or intramuscular injection, pulmonary tuberculosis, 300 mg daily *or* up to 1 g (14 mg/kg) twice weekly; CHILD 6 mg/kg daily
Tuberculous meningitis, 10 mg/kg daily

PoM **Isoniazid Tablets,** isoniazid 50 mg, net price 20 = 26p; 100 mg, 20 = 26p. Label: 8, 22

PoM **Isoniazid Elixir,** isoniazid 50 mg/5 ml (see Formulary). Net price 100 ml = 30p. Label: 8, 22

PoM **Rimifon**® (Roche)
Injection, isoniazid 25 mg/ml. Net price 2-ml amp = 9p

PYRAZINAMIDE

Indications: tuberculosis in combination with other drugs

Cautions: impaired renal function, diabetes, gout. Drug interactions: see Appendix 1 (section *10*)

Contra-indications: liver damage

Side-effects: hepatotoxicity including fever, anorexia, hepatomegaly, jaundice, liver failure;

nausea, vomiting, arthralgia, sideroblastic anaemia, urticaria

Dose: 20–35 mg/kg daily in 3–4 divided doses; max. 3 g daily

PoM **Zinamide**® (MSD)
Tablets, scored, pyrazinamide 500 mg. Net price 20 = £1.44. Label: 8

RIFAMPICIN

Indications: tuberculosis, in combination with other drugs; leprosy (section 5.1.10)

Cautions: reduce dose in hepatic impairment; alcoholism, pregnancy; advise patients on oral contraceptives to use additional means; discolours soft contact lenses. See also notes above. Drug interactions: see Appendix 1 (sections *1*, *2.1*, *2.3*, *2.4*, *2.8A*, *3*, *4.2*, *4.7*, *4.8*, *5.1*, *5.1*, *5.2*, *6.1*, *6.3*, *7*, *8*)

Contra-indications: jaundice

Side-effects: gastro-intestinal symptoms including anorexia, nausea, vomiting, diarrhoea; influenzal syndrome (mainly on intermittent therapy) with chills, fever, dizziness, bone pain; respiratory symptoms including shortness of breath; collapse and shock; acute renal failure; thrombocytopenic purpura; hepatic reactions with alterations of liver function, jaundice; urticaria and rashes; urine, saliva, and other body secretions coloured orange-red

Dose: 450–600 mg (about 10 mg/kg) daily preferably before breakfast; CHILD up to 20 mg/kg daily to a max. of 600 mg
Dose in hepatic impairment should not exceed 8 mg/kg daily

PoM **Rifadin**® (Merrell)
Capsules, rifampicin 150 mg (blue/red), net price 20 = £3.82; 300 mg (red), 20 = £7.64. Label: 8, 14, 22, counselling advised, see lenses above
Syrup, red, rifampicin 100 mg/5 ml. Do not dilute. Net price 120 ml = £3.71. Label: 8, 14, 22, counselling advised, see lenses above
Intravenous infusion, powder for reconstitution, rifampicin. Net price 600-mg vial (with solvent) = £8.00

PoM **Rimactane**® (Ciba)
Capsules, rifampicin 150 mg (red), net price 20 = £3.82; 300 mg (red/brown), 20 = £7.64. Label: 8, 14, 22, counselling advised, see lenses above
Syrup, red, rifampicin 100 mg/5 ml. Do not dilute. Net price 100 ml = £3.09. Label: 8, 14, 22, counselling advised, see lenses above
Intravenous infusion, powder for reconstitution, rifampicin. Net price 300-mg vial (with diluent) = £8.09

Combined preparations
PoM **Rifater**® (Merrell)
Tablets, pink-beige, s/c, rifampicin 120 mg, isoniazid 50 mg, pyrazinamide 300 mg. Net price 20 = £4.40. Label: 8, 14, 22, counselling advised, see lenses above
Dose: initial treatment of pulmonary tuberculosis, patients up to 40 kg 3 tablets daily, 40–49 kg 4 tablets daily, 50–64 kg 5 tablets daily,

---

65 kg or more, 6 tablets daily; not suitable for use in children

PoM **Rifinah 150**® (Merrell)
Tablets, pink, rifampicin 150 mg, isoniazid 100 mg. Net price 21-tab pack = £4.15. Label: 8, 14, 22, counselling advised, see lenses above
Dose: patients under 50 kg, 3 tablets daily, preferably before breakfast

PoM **Rifinah 300**® (Merrell)
Tablets, orange, rifampicin 300 mg, isoniazid 150 mg. Net price 14-tab pack = £5.48. Label: 8, 14, 22, counselling advised, see lenses above
Dose: patients over 50 kg, 2 tablets daily, preferably before breakfast

PoM **Rimactazid 150**® (Ciba)
Tablets, pink, s/c, rifampicin 150 mg, isoniazid 100 mg. Net price 21-tab pack = £4.15. Label: 8, 14, 22, counselling advised, see lenses above
Dose: patients under 50 kg, 3 tablets daily, preferably before breakfast

PoM **Rimactazid 300**® (Ciba)
Tablets, orange, s/c, rifampicin 300 mg, isoniazid 150 mg. Net price 14-tab pack = £5.48. Label: 8, 14, 22, counselling advised, see lenses above
Dose: patients over 50 kg, 2 tablets daily, preferably before breakfast

STREPTOMYCIN

Indications: tuberculosis, in combination with other drugs
Cautions; Contra-indications; Side-effects: see under Aminoglycosides, section 5.1.4; also hypersensitivity reactions, paraesthesia of mouth
Dose: by intramuscular injection, 1 g daily; in patients over 40 years, 750 mg; in small patients, 500 mg; cumulative dose should not normally exceed 100 g, see notes above

PoM **Streptomycin Sulphate** (Evans)
Injection, powder for reconstitution, streptomycin (as sulphate). Net price 1-g vial = £1.02

5.1.10 Antileprotic drugs

Advice from a member of the Panel of Leprosy Opinion is essential for the treatment of leprosy (Hansen's disease). Details of the Panel can be found in *Memorandum on Leprosy*, DHSS, London, H. M. Stationery Office, 1977 [in Scotland, NHS Circular 1978(GEN)44].

For over twenty years the mainstay of leprosy treatment was dapsone monotherapy but resistance to dapsone became an increasing concern. A World Health Organization Study Group has made recommendations to overcome this problem of dapsone resistance and to prevent the emergence of resistance to other antileprotic drugs. These recommendations are based on the same principles as those determining the chemotherapy of tuberculosis. Drugs advocated are **dapsone**, **rifampicin**, and **clofazimine** and, secondarily ethionamide or prothionamide (which are not marketed in the UK).

For treatment purposes leprosy patients are divided into those suffering from multibacillary leprosy (lepromatous, borderline-lepromatous, and borderline leprosy) and those suffering from paucibacillary leprosy (borderline-tuberculoid, tuberculoid, and indeterminate). A three-drug regimen is recommended for the former group and a two-drug regimen for the latter. These regimens are as follows:

Multibacillary leprosy (3-drug regimen)

Rifampicin	600 mg once-monthly, supervised (450 mg for those weighing less than 35 kg)
Dapsone	100 mg daily, self-administered
Clofazimine	300 mg once-monthly, supervised, *and* 50 mg daily, self-administered

(*or*, if clofazimine unacceptable, ethionamide or prothionamide 250–375 mg daily, self-administered).

Treatment should be given for at least 2 years and be continued, wherever possible, up to smear negativity. It should be continued unchanged during lepromatous lepra reactions which, if severe, should receive their own specific treatment (e.g. prednisolone or increased clofazimine dosage).

Paucibacillary leprosy (2-drug regimen)

Rifampicin	600 mg once-monthly, supervised (450 mg for those weighing less than 35 kg)
Dapsone	100 mg daily, self-administered

Treatment should be given for 6 months. If treatment is interrupted the regimen should be recommenced where it was left off to complete the full course.

Neither the multibacillary nor the paucibacillary antileprosy regimen is sufficient to treat active pulmonary tuberculosis, therefore patients who also have active pulmonary tuberculosis should be given an appropriate course of antitubercular chemotherapy in addition to the antileprosy regimen.

These WHO regimens are widely applicable throughout the world, with minor variations in different areas.

DAPSONE

Indications: leprosy, dermatitis herpetiformis
Cautions: cardiac or pulmonary disease; pregnancy; breast-feeding. Drug interactions: see Appendix 1 (section 5.1)
Side-effects: (dose-related and uncommon at doses used for leprosy), neuropathy, allergic dermatitis, anorexia, nausea, vomiting, headache, insomnia, tachycardia, anaemia, hepatitis, agranulocytosis
Dose: leprosy, 1–2 mg/kg daily, see notes above
Dermatitis herpetiformis, see specialist literature

PoM **Dapsone Tablets,** dapsone 50 mg, net price 20 = 37p; 100 mg, 20 = 69p. Label: 8

CLOFAZIMINE

Indications: leprosy

Cautions: hepatic and renal impairment—function tests required

Side-effects: nausea, giddiness, headache, and diarrhoea with high doses, red coloration of skin and urine, blue-black discoloration of lesions

Dose: leprosy, see notes above

Lepromatous lepra reactions, dosage increased to 300 mg daily for 3 months

PoM **Lamprene**® (Geigy)

Capsules, brown, clofazimine 100 mg. Net price 20 = £1.65. Label: 8, 14, 21

5.1.11 Metronidazole and tinidazole

Metronidazole (Flagyl® etc.) is an antimicrobial drug with high activity against anaerobic bacteria and protozoa. Indications include surgical and gynaecological sepsis in which its activity against colonic anaerobes, especially *Bacteroides fragilis*, is important, trichomonal vaginitis (section 5.4.3), non-specific vaginitis (*Gardnerella vaginalis* infections), and *Entamoeba histolytica* and *Giardia lamblia* infections (section 5.4.2). Metronidazole is effective in the treatment of pseudomembranous colitis in a dose of 400 mg by mouth three times daily. Side-effects are uncommon but neuropathy can occur during prolonged therapy. Gastro-intestinal disturbances may be minimised by taking tablets with or after food, but the mixture (which contains metronidazole benzoate) should be taken at least 1 hour before food.

Tinidazole (Fasigyn®) is similar to metronidazole but has a longer plasma half-life, thus allowing less frequent administration.

METRONIDAZOLE

Indications: see notes above

Cautions: disulfiram-like reaction with alcohol, hepatic impairment; pregnancy and breast-feeding (manufacturer advises avoidance of high-dose regimens). Drug interactions: see Appendix 1 (section *2.8B, 4.8*, 5.1)

Side-effects: nausea, vomiting and gastro-intestinal disturbances, drowsiness, headache, rashes, leucopenia, darkening of urine, peripheral neuropathy in prolonged treatment, dizziness, ataxia, transient epileptiform seizures with high doses

Dose: anaerobic infections, *by mouth*, 400 mg every 8 hours; *by rectum*, 1 g every 8 hours for 3 days, then 1 g every 12 hours; *by intravenous infusion*, 500 mg every 8 hours for up to 7 days; CHILD, any route, 7.5 mg/kg every 8 hours

Non-specific vaginitis, *by mouth*, 400 mg twice daily for 7 days *or* 2 g as a single dose

Trichomoniasis, *by mouth*, 200 mg every 8 hours for 7 days, *or* 800 mg in the morning and 1.2 g at night for 2 days, *or* 2 g as a single dose

Amoebiasis, *by mouth*, 800 mg every 8 hours for 5 days

Giardiasis, *by mouth*, 2 g daily for 3 days

Acute ulcerative gingivitis, see section 12.3.2

PoM **Metronidazole** (Non-proprietary)

Tablets, metronidazole 200 mg, net price 20 = 58p; 400 mg, 20 = £1.39. Label: 4, 9, 21, 25

Intravenous infusion, metronidazole 5 mg/ml. Net price 100-ml vial = £3.65

Suppositories, metronidazole 500 mg, net price 10 = £4.50; 1 g, 10 = £7.00. Label: 4, 9

PoM **Elyzol**® (CP)

Suppositories, metronidazole 500 mg, net price 10 = £4.50; 1 g, 10 = £7.00. Label: 4

PoM **Flagyl**® (M&B)

Tablets, both f/c, ivory, metronidazole 200 mg, net price 20 = £1.34; 400 mg, 20 = £3.61. Label: 4, 9, 21, 25

Intravenous infusion, metronidazole 5 mg/ml. Net price 20-ml amp = £1.87; 100-ml bottle = £4.34; 100-ml Viaflex® bag = £4.78

Suppositories, metronidazole 500 mg, net price 10 = £6.33; 1 g, 10 = £9.61. Label: 4, 9

PoM **Flagyl S**® (M&B)

Suspension, metronidazole 200 mg (as benzoate)/5 ml. Diluent syrup, life of diluted suspension 14 days. Net price 100 ml = £4.13. Label: 4, 9, 23

PoM **Flagyl Compak**® (M&B)

Treatment pack, tablets, off-white, f/c, metronidazole 200 mg, with pessaries, yellow, nystatin 100000 units. Net price 21 tablets and 14 pessaries (with applicator) = £3.10

Dose: for mixed trichomonal and candidal infections, 1 tablet 3 times daily for 7 days and 1 pessary inserted twice daily for 7 days *or* 1 at night for 14 nights

PoM **Metrolyl**® (Lagap)

Tablets, both scored, metronidazole 200 mg, net price 20 = 56p; 400 mg, 20 = £1.25. Label: 4, 9, 21, 25

Intravenous infusion, metronidazole 5 mg/ml. Net price 100-ml vial = £3.65; 100-ml Steriflex® bag = £4.05

Suppositories, metronidazole 500 mg, net price 10 = £4.25; 1 g, 10 = £6.80. Label: 4, 9

PoM **Nidazol**® (Steinhard)

Tablets, scored, metronidazole 200 mg. Net price 20 = £1.73. Label: 4, 9, 21, 25

PoM **Zadstat**® (Lederle)

Tablets, scored, metronidazole 200 mg. Net price 20 = 56p. Label: 4, 9, 21, 25

Intravenous infusion, metronidazole 5 mg/ml. Net price 100-ml Steriflex Minipack® = £4.62

Suppositories, metronidazole 500 mg, net price 10 = £4.25; 1 g, 10 = £6.80. Label: 4, 9

TINIDAZOLE

Indications: anaerobic bacterial and protozoal infections

Cautions; Side-effects: see under Metronidazole

Dose: by mouth, 2 g initially, followed by 1 g daily *or* 500 mg twice daily, usually for 5–6 days

Non-specific vaginitis, trichomoniasis, giardiasis and ulcerative gingivitis, a single 2-g dose; CHILD single dose of 50–75 mg/kg

---

Intestinal amoebiasis, 2 g daily for 2–3 days; CHILD 50–60 mg/kg daily for 3 days.

Amoebic involvement of liver, 1.5–2 g daily for 3–5 days; CHILD 50–60 mg/kg daily for 5 days

Abdominal surgery prophylaxis, a single 2-g dose approximately 12 hours before surgery

By intravenous infusion, 800 mg daily until treatment by mouth can be given

Abdominal surgery prophylaxis, 1.6 g as a single pre-operative dose *or* in 2 divided doses (just before surgery and no later than 12 hours after)

PoM **Fasigyn**® (Pfizer)
Tablets, f/c, tinidazole 500 mg. Net price 20 = £11.50. Label: 4, 9, 21, 25
Intravenous infusion, tinidazole 2 mg/ml. Net price 400-ml bottle = £19.20; 800-ml bottle = £38.40

5.1.12 4-Quinolones

Antibacterials discussed in this section include ciprofloxacin, acrosoxacin, and the urinary antiseptics cinoxicin and nalidixic acid.

Acrosoxacin is used only in the treatment of gonorrhoea in patients allergic to penicillins or who have strains resistant to penicillins and other antibiotics.

Nalidixic acid and **cinoxacin** are effective in uncomplicated urinary-tract infections.

Ciprofloxacin is a recently introduced 4-quinolone derivative which is active against both Gram-positive and Gram-negative bacteria. It is particularly active against Gram-negative bacteria, including salmonella, shigellae, campylobacter, neisseria, and pseudomonas. It only has moderate activity against Gram-positive bacteria such as *Streptococcus pneumoniae* and *Streptococcus faecalis*. It is active against chlamydia and some mycobacteria. Most anaerobic organisms are not susceptible. Indications for ciprofloxacin include infections of the respiratory and urinary tracts, and of the gastro-intestinal system, and gonorrhoea and septicaemia caused by sensitive organisms. Whenever possible, ciprofloxacin should be reserved for the treatment of infections caused by organisms resistant to standard drugs.

CSM warning. Ciprofloxacin increases plasma theophylline concentrations. If concomitant use is essential, the dose of theophylline should be reduced and plasma concentrations should be closely monitored to avoid toxicity.

ACROSOXACIN

(Rosoxacin)
Indications: gonorrhoea
Cautions: impaired renal or hepatic function; patient's ability to drive or operate machinery may be impaired; avoid frequent repeat doses in patients under 18 years (lesions in weight-bearing joints of young *animals*)
Side-effects: dizziness, drowsiness, headache, gastro-intestinal disturbances

Dose: 300 mg as a single dose on an empty stomach

PoM **Eradacin**® (Sterling Research)
Capsules, red/yellow, acrosoxacin 150 mg. Net price 2 caps = £2.90. Label: 2, 23

CINOXACIN

Indications: urinary-tract infections
Cautions: moderately impaired renal function
Contra-indications: severe renal impairment
Side-effects: gastro-intestinal symptoms including anorexia, nausea, vomiting, cramps, diarrhoea; hypersensitivity reactions including urticaria, rashes, peripheral and oral oedema; dizziness, headache, photophobia, tinnitus, perineal burning, changes in liver-function tests
Dose: 500 mg every 12 hours; prophylaxis, 500 mg at night

PoM **Cinobac**® (Lilly)
Capsules, green/orange, cinoxacin 500 mg. Net price 14 = £9.17. Label: 9

CIPROFLOXACIN

Indications: Gram-negative and Gram-positive infections, see notes above
Cautions: epilepsy; excessive alkalinity of urine, inadequate fluid intake (risk of crystalluria); renal impairment; pregnancy and breast-feeding (arthropathy in *animal* studies); not recommended in children or growing adolescents. Drug interactions: see Appendix 1 (sections *3*, 5.1)
Side-effects: nausea, vomiting, diarrhoea, dyspepsia, abdominal pain; dizziness, headache, fatigue, confusion, convulsions; rashes, pruritus, joint pain, photosensitivity; increases in liver enzymes (particularly in those with previous liver damage) and in serum bilirubin, urea, or creatinine
Dose: by mouth, 250–750 mg twice daily
Urinary-tract infections, 250–500 mg twice daily
Gonorrhoea, 250 mg as a single dose
By intravenous infusion (over 30–60 minutes), 200 mg twice daily
Urinary-tract infections, 100 mg twice daily
Gonorrhoea, 100 mg as a single dose

▼ PoM **Ciproxin**® (Baypharm)
Tablets, f/c, ciprofloxacin (as hydrochloride) 250 mg. Net price 20 = £15.00. Label: 5, 9, 25
Intravenous infusion, ciprofloxacin 2 mg (as lactate)/ml. Net price 50-ml bottle = £12.00; 100-ml bottle = £24.00

NALIDIXIC ACID

Indications: urinary-tract infections
Cautions: impaired renal or hepatic function, pregnancy (arthropathy in *animal* studies), breast-feeding, avoid strong sunlight, interference with tests using copper salts (e.g. Benedict's test). Drug interactions: see Appendix 1 (sections *2.8C*, 5.1)

Contra-indications: infants under 3 months, epilepsy, CNS lesions

Side-effects: gastro-intestinal disturbances including nausea, vomiting, diarrhoea; hae-molysis in G6PD deficiency; allergic reactions including urticaria, rashes, fever, arthralgia, eosinophilia; also myalgia, muscle weakness, phototoxicity, jaundice, visual disturbances, convulsions

Dose: 1 g every 6 hours for 7 days, reducing to 500 mg every 6 hours

PoM **Mictral**® (Winthrop)

Granules, effervescent, nalidixic acid 660 mg, sodium citrate 3.75 g/sachet (Na$^+$ 41 mmol/sachet). Net price 9 sachets = £4.65. Label: 9, 11, 13

Dose: 1 sachet in water 3 times daily for 3 days

PoM **Negram**® (Sterling Research)

Tablets, beige, nalidixic acid 500 mg. Net price 20 = £4.07. Label: 9, 11

Suspension, pink, sugar-free, nalidixic acid 300 mg/5 ml. Diluent syrup, life of diluted mixture 14 days. Net price 100 ml = £7.30. Label: 9, 11

PoM **Uriben**® (RP Drugs)

Suspension, pink, nalidixic acid 300 mg/5 ml. Diluent syrup, life of diluted suspension 14 days. Net price 100 ml = £4.50. Label: 9, 11

5.1.13   Urinary-tract infections

Urinary-tract infection commonly implies a functional or anatomical disorder of the urinary tract. Most of the organisms involved are bowel commensals, the commonest being *Escherichia coli*. *Proteus*, micrococci, coliforms, and faecal streptococci are also prevalent. *Pseudomonas* and *Klebsiella* spp. may be derived from hospital bacterial flora and *Staphylococcus epidermidis* may occur following catheterisation or instrumentation. Chlamydia are intracellular bacteria which may cause urethritis in males or cervicitis in females.

Urinary infection in pregnancy is often asymptomatic but requires prompt treatment to prevent progression to pyelonephritis. Penicillins, cephalosporins, and nitrofurantoin are safe in pregnancy but co-trimoxazole and sulphonamides, and tetracyclines should be avoided.

In uncomplicated infections ampicillin (section 5.1.1.3), co-trimoxazole and trimethoprim (section 5.1.8), nitrofurantoin, and nalidixic acid (section 5.1.12) are all effective. Hexamine should **not** be used as it is only bacteriostatic, requires acidification of the urine, and frequently causes side-effects. Chronic prostatitis is very difficult to eradicate and requires a lipid-soluble antibiotic to penetrate prostatic tissue. Long-term treatment may be needed using various antibiotics in rotation; these include co-trimoxazole, erythromycin (section 5.1.5), and doxycycline (section 5.1.3).

Where infection is localised and associated with the presence of a urinary catheter, the use of a simple bladder instillation is often effective (see section 7.4.4).

Although aseptic instrumentation of the urinary tract does not require antibiotic cover (except in patients with heart-valve lesions) a parenteral bactericidal agent such as gentamicin (section 5.1.4) or a cephalosporin (section 5.1.2) is necessary should bacteraemia or septicaemia occur.

Noxythiolin (see section 7.4.4) is a topical antimicrobial agent with antibacterial and antifungal properties.

In renal failure, impaired renal function will cause accumulation of many antibiotics or their metabolites with resultant toxicity. Drugs to be avoided include tetracyclines, hexamine, and nitrofurantoin. Peritoneal dialysis or haemodialysis is often able to remove the drug and supplementary doses can be given later. Aminoglycosides are more successfully cleared by haemodialysis; they should be used with great caution in renal failure. Adequacy of dosage of any drug should be accurately checked by plasma concentrations.

NITROFURANTOIN

Indications: urinary-tract infections

Cautions: ineffective in alkaline urine. Drug interactions: see Appendix 1 (section 5.1)

Contra-indications: impaired renal function, infants less than 1 month old, G6PD deficiency

Side-effects: nausea, vomiting, rashes, peripheral neuropathy, pulmonary infiltration, allergic liver damage

Dose: 100 mg every 6 hours with food

PoM **Furadantin**® (Norwich Eaton)

Tablets, all yellow, scored, nitrofurantoin 50 mg, net price 20 = £1.47; 100 mg, 20 = £2.77. Label: 9, 14, 21

Suspension, yellow, sugar-free, nitrofurantoin 25 mg/5 ml. Do not dilute. Net price 300 ml = £4.50. Label: 9, 14, 21

PoM **Macrodantin**® (Norwich Eaton)

Capsules, nitrofurantoin 50 mg (yellow/white), net price 20 = £1.98; 100 mg (yellow), 20 = £3.59. Label: 9, 14, 21

PoM **Urantoin**® (DDSA)

Tablets, all yellow, scored, nitrofurantoin 50 mg, net price 20 = 75p; 100 mg, 20 = £1.34. Label: 9, 14, 21

HEXAMINE

(Methenamine)

Indications: see notes above

Cautions: urine must be acidic

Contra-indications: impaired renal and hepatic function, dehydration, metabolic acidosis

Side-effects: gastro-intestinal disturbances, frequent and painful micturition, bladder irritation, haematuria, proteinuria, rashes

Dose: hexamine hippurate, 1 g every 12 hours

Hiprex® (Riker)

Tablets, scored, hexamine hippurate 1 g. Net price 20 = £1.41. Label: 9

5.2 Antifungal drugs

It is important to remember that fungal infections are frequently associated with a defect in host resistance which should, if possible, be corrected otherwise drug therapy may fail. Similarly, treatment of dermatophyte infection may be unsuccessful until the animal source has been removed or controlled.

Amphotericin (Fungilin®) is not absorbed from the gut and is the only polyene antibiotic which can be given parenterally. It is the most important drug for the treatment of systemic fungal infections and is active against most fungi and yeasts. It is highly protein bound and penetrates poorly into body fluids and tissues. Amphotericin is a toxic drug and side-effects are common.

Flucytosine (Alcobon®) is a synthetic antifungal drug which is only active against yeasts and has been used for the treatment of systemic candidiasis, cryptococcosis, and torulopsosis. It is well absorbed from the gut and distributed widely in the body. Side-effects are uncommon but bone-marrow depression can occur and weekly blood counts are necessary during prolonged therapy. It can be given with amphotericin and synergy has been demonstrated. Resistance to flucytosine is not uncommon and can develop during therapy; sensitivity testing is, therefore, essential before treatment.

Griseofulvin is selectively concentrated in keratin and is the drug of choice for widespread or intractable dermatophyte infections. It is well absorbed from the gut but is inactive when applied topically. It is more effective in skin than in nail infections and treatment must be continued for several weeks or even months. Side-effects are uncommon. For topical applications for localised infections see section 13.10.2.

The imidazole group of antifungal drugs includes clotrimazole, econazole, ketoconazole, and miconazole. The imidazoles are active against a wide range of fungi and yeasts (excluding aspergillosis). The main indications for their use at present are vaginal candidiasis and dermatophyte infections. **Miconazole** is also available for oral and parenteral administration, but the injection contains polyethoxylated castor oil, which may give rise to hypersensitivity reactions. **Ketoconazole** (Nizoral®) is significantly better absorbed after oral administration than the other imidazoles, but has been associated with fatal hepatotoxicity. The CSM has advised that prescribers should weigh the potential benefits of ketoconazole treatment against the liver damage risk and should carefully monitor patients both clinically and biochemically. It should not be given for superficial fungal infections unless topically applied antifungal agents (or griseofulvin) have failed or are contra-indicated because of local hypersensitivity reactions. The imidazoles are not effective in aspergillosis infections.

Nystatin (Nystan®) is a polyene antibiotic which is not absorbed when given by mouth and is too toxic for parenteral use. It is active against a number of yeasts and fungi but is principally used for *Candida albicans* infections of skin and mucous membranes. It is also used in the treatment of intestinal candidiasis.

For antifungal preparations used in genital infections see section 7.2.2 and in skin infections, see section 13.10.2. For use in bladder irrigation see section 7.4.4.

AMPHOTERICIN

Indications: See under Dose
Cautions: when given parenterally, renal-function tests required, frequent change of injection site, avoid use with other nephrotoxic drugs. Drug interactions: see Appendix 1 (section 8)
Side-effects: when given parenterally, fever, anorexia, nausea, vomiting, hypokalaemia, nephrotoxicity, tinnitus
Dose: by mouth, intestinal candidiasis, 100–200 mg every 6 hours
By intravenous infusion, systemic fungal infections, 250 micrograms/kg daily, gradually increased if tolerated to 1 mg/kg daily; max. in severely ill patients 1.5 mg/kg daily or on alternate days

PoM **Fungilin**® (Squibb)
Tablets, yellow, scored, amphotericin 100 mg. Net price 20 = £2.70. Label: 9
Lozenges—see section 12.3.2
Suspension, yellow, sugar-free, amphotericin 100 mg/ml. Do not dilute. Net price 12 ml = £2.10. Label: 9, counselling advised, use of pipette
PoM **Fungizone**® (Squibb)
Intravenous infusion, powder for reconstitution, amphotericin (as sodium deoxycholate complex). Net price 50-mg vial = £2.90

FLUCYTOSINE

Indications: systemic yeast infections
Cautions: renal and hepatic impairment, blood disorders, liver-function tests and blood counts required, plasma concentrations monitored in renal impairment; pregnancy, breast-feeding
Side-effects: nausea, vomiting, diarrhoea, rashes, thrombocytopenia, leucopenia
Dose: by mouth or intravenous infusion, 100–200 mg/kg daily in 4 divided doses; reduce dose in renal impairment

PoM **Alcobon**® (Roche)
Tablets, scored, flucytosine 500 mg. Net price 20 = £8.72 (Hosp. only)
Intravenous infusion, flucytosine 10 mg/ml. Net price 250-ml infusion bottle and giving set = £15.33 (Hosp. only)

GRISEOFULVIN

Indications: dermatophyte infections of the skin, scalp, hair and nails, where topical therapy has failed or is inappropriate

Cautions: rarely aggravation or precipitation of systemic lupus erythematosus. Drug interactions: see Appendix 1 (sections *2.8A*, 5.2, 7)

Contra-indications: liver failure, porphyria; pregnancy

Side-effects: headache, nausea, vomiting, rashes, photosensitivity

Dose: 0.5–1 g daily, in divided doses or as a single dose; CHILD, 10 mg/kg daily in divided doses or as a single dose

PoM **Fulcin®** (ICI)
Tablets, scored, griseofulvin 125 mg. Net price 20 = 49p. Label: 9, 21
Tablets, f/c, griseofulvin 500 mg. Net price 20 = £1.91. Label: 9, 21
Suspension (= mixture), brown, griseofulvin 125 mg/5 ml. Diluent syrup, life of diluted mixture 14 days. Net price 100 ml = 94p. Label: 9, 21

PoM **Grisovin®** (Glaxo)
Tablets, f/c, griseofulvin 125 mg. Net price 20 = 47p. Label: 9, 21
Tablets, f/c, griseofulvin 500 mg. Net price 20 = £1.75. Label: 9, 21

KETOCONAZOLE

Indications: systemic mycoses, serious chronic resistant mucocutaneous candidiasis, serious resistant gastro-intestinal mycoses, chronic resistant vaginal candidiasis, resistant dermatophyte infections of skin or finger nails (not toe nails); prophylaxis of mycoses in immunosuppressed patients

Contra-indications: hepatic impairment

Cautions: pregnancy (teratogenicity in *animal* studies). Drug interactions: see Appendix 1 (sections *2.8B*, *4.8*, 5.2, 8)

Side-effects: rarely nausea, rashes, pruritus; fatal liver damage—for CSM advice see notes above

Dose: 200 mg once daily with food, usually for 14 days; if response inadequate continue until at least 1 week after symptoms have cleared and cultures become negative; max. 400 mg daily. CHILD, 3 mg/kg daily
Chronic resistant vaginal candidiasis, 400 mg daily with food for 5 days

PoM **Nizoral®** (Janssen)
Tablets, scored, ketoconazole 200 mg. Net price 20 = £9.51. Label: 5, 9, 21
Suspension (= mixture), pink, ketoconazole 100 mg/5 ml. Net price 100 ml = £6.51. Label: 5, 9, 21

MICONAZOLE

Indications: see under Dose

Cautions: change infusion site to avoid phlebitis; pregnancy. Drug interactions: see Appendix 1 (sections *2.8B*, *4.8*, *6.1*)

Side-effects: nausea and vomiting, pruritus, rashes

Dose: by mouth, oral and intestinal fungal infections, 250 mg every 6 hours for 10 days or up to 2 days after symptoms clear

By intravenous infusion, systemic fungal infections, initially, 600 mg every 8 hours; CHILD max. 15 mg/kg every 8 hours up to 40 mg/kg day

Daktarin® (Janssen)
PoM *Tablets*, scored, miconazole 250 mg. Net price 20 = £14.89. Label: 9, 21
Note. Can be sucked for oral treatment
Oral gel, sugar-free, miconazole 25 mg/ml. Net price 40 g = £2.50. Label: 9, counselling advised, hold in mouth, after food
Dose: oral and intestinal fungal infections, 5 10 ml 4 times daily; CHILD under 2 years, 2.5 m twice daily, 2–6 years, 5 ml twice daily, over years, 5 ml 4 times daily
PoM *Intravenous solution*, miconazole 10 mg/ml
For dilution and use as an infusion. Net price 20-ml amp = £1.47 (Hosp. only)
Note. Contains polyethoxylated castor oil which ha been associated with anaphylaxis

NATAMYCIN

Indications: fungal infections of lungs and respiratory tract
Dose: by inhalation, 2.5 mg every 8 hours

PoM **Pimafucin®** (Brocades)
Oral suspension—see section 12.3.2
Suspension for inhalation, natamycin 25 mg/ml
Net price 20 ml = £3.70

NYSTATIN

Indications: candidiasis

Side-effects: nausea, vomiting, diarrhoea at hig doses

Dose: by mouth, intestinal candidiasis 500 00 units every 6 hours, doubled in severe infec tions; CHILD 100 000 units 4 times daily
For use as a mouth-wash in oral candidiasis, se section 12.3.2

PoM **Nystan®** (Squibb)
Tablets, brown, s/c, nystatin 500 000 units. Ne price 20 = £1.60. Label: 9
Pastilles—see section 12.3.2
Suspension, yellow, nystatin 100 000 units/m Do not dilute. Measure with pipette. Net pric 30 ml with pipette = £2.27. Label: 9, coun selling advised, use of pipette
Suspension, gluten-, lactose-, and sugar-free nystatin 100 000 units/ml when reconstitute with water for preparations. Measure wi pipette. Net price 24 ml with pipette = £1.6 Label: 9, counselling advised, use of pipette

PoM **Nystatin-Dome®** (Lagap)
Suspension, yellow, nystatin 100 000 units/m Net price 30 ml with 1-ml spoon = £2.36 Label: 9, counselling advised, use of 1-ml spoo

5.3 Antiviral drugs

The specific therapy of virus infections is generall unsatisfactory and treatment is, therefore, pr

---

marily symptomatic. Fortunately, the majority of infections resolve spontaneously.

Acyclovir is active against herpes viruses but does not eradicate them. Uses include the treatment of varicella/zoster and herpes simplex infections of the skin and mucous membranes, including initial and recurrent genital herpes. It is only active if started at the onset of infection. It can be life-saving in herpes simplex and varicella/zoster infections in the immunocompromised; it is also used in the immunocompromised for prevention of recurrence and prophylaxis. See also 11.3.1 (eye) and 13.10.3 (skin, including herpes labialis).

Idoxuridine is active against herpes viruses; it is too toxic for systemic administration, a problem with many antiviral drugs, but has been used in the treatment of herpes simplex lesions of the skin, eye, and external genitalia with variable results. Idoxuridine is also used for the topical treatment of shingles, in which it is claimed to reduce the duration of pain and lessen the incidence of post-herpetic neuralgia. However, to be effective, it must be applied early in the illness as soon as the first skin lesions appear. See also 11.3.1 (eye) and 13.10.3 (skin).

Amantadine (Symmetrel®), given by mouth, has been used for the prophylaxis of influenza A infections and for the treatment of shingles.

Vidarabine (Vira-A®) is used in immunosuppressed patients for the treatment of serious infections caused by herpes viruses; these include varicella (chickenpox), zoster (shingles), and herpes simplex infections. See also 11.3.1 (eye).

Inosine pranobex (Imunovir®) is also used for herpes simplex infections; its effectiveness has not been established.

Tribavirin (Virazid®) inhibits a wide range of DNA and RNA viruses. It is given by inhalation for the treatment of severe bronchiolitis caused by the respiratory syncytial virus in infants, especially when they have other serious diseases.

ACYCLOVIR

Indications: herpes simplex and varicella/zoster
Cautions: maintain adequate hydration; reduce dose in renal impairment; pregnancy. Drug interactions: see Appendix 1 (section 5.3)
Side-effects: rashes; gastro-intestinal disturbances; rises in bilirubin and liver-related enzymes, increases in blood urea and creatinine, decreases in haematological indices, headache, neurological reactions, fatigue
Dose: *by mouth*,
Herpes simplex, treatment, 200 mg (400 mg in the immunocompromised) 5 times daily, usually for 5 days; CHILD under 2 years, ½ adult dose, over 2 years, adult dose
Prevention of recurrence, 200 mg 4 times daily *or* 400 mg twice daily possibly reduced to 200 mg 2 or 3 times daily and interrupted every 6–12 months
Prophylaxis in the immunocompromised, 200–400 mg 4 times daily; CHILD under 2 years, ½ adult dose, over 2 years, adult dose

Herpes zoster, 800 mg 5 times daily for 7 days
By slow intravenous infusion, 5 mg/kg over 1 hour, repeated every 8 hours; doubled in zoster in the immunocompromised, and in simplex encephalitis; CHILD 3 months–12 years, 250 mg/m² doubled in the immunocompromised and in simplex encephalitis

▼ PoM **Zovirax**® (Wellcome)
Tablets, blue, acyclovir 200 mg. Net price 25 = £25.00. Label: 9
Tablets, pink, acyclovir 400 mg. Net price 70-tab pack = £119.00. Label: 9
Suspension, off-white, sugar-free, acyclovir 200 mg/5 ml. Diluent syrup or sorbitol solution for 1 + 1 dilution, life of diluted mixture 28 days. Net price 125 ml = £25.00. Label: 9
Intravenous infusion, powder for reconstitution, acyclovir (as sodium salt). Net price 250-mg vial = £9.75

AMANTADINE HYDROCHLORIDE

Indications: see under Dose
Cautions; Contra-indications; Side-effects: see section 4.9.1
Dose: herpes zoster, 100 mg twice daily for 14 days, if necessary extended for a further 14 days for post-herpetic neuralgia
Influenza A₂, treatment, 100 mg twice daily for 5–7 days; prophylaxis 100 mg twice daily for as long as required (usually 7–10 days); CHILD 10–15 years, 100 mg daily
COUNSELLING. Second dose not later than 4 p.m.

PoM **Symmetrel**® (Geigy)
Capsules, brown, amantadine hydrochloride 100 mg. Net price 20 = £3.22
Syrup (= elixir), amantadine hydrochloride 50 mg/5 ml. Diluent syrup, life of diluted elixir 28 days. Net price 150 ml = £3.02

INOSINE PRANOBEX

Indications: see under Dose
Cautions: avoid in renal impairment; history of gout or hyperuricaemia
Side-effects: reversible increases in serum and urinary uric acid
Dose: mucocutaneous herpes simplex, 1 g 4 times daily for 7–14 days
Adjunctive treatment of genital warts, 1 g 3 times daily for 14–28 days

▼ PoM **Imunovir**® (Leo)
Tablets, inosine pranobex 500 mg. Net price 20 = £7.45. Label: 9

TRIBAVIRIN
(Ribavirin)

Indications: severe respiratory syncytial virus bronchiolitis in infants and children
Cautions: maintain standard supportive respiratory and fluid management therapy; monitor equipment for precipitation
Contra-indications: pregnancy

Side-effects: reticulocytosis; also worsening respiration, bacterial pneumonia, and pneumothorax reported
Dose: by aerosol inhalation or nebulisation (via small particle aerosol generator) of solution containing 20 mg/ml for 12–18 hours for at least 3 days; max. 7 days

▼ PoM **Virazid®** (Britannia)
Inhalation, tribavirin 6 g for reconstitution with 300 ml water for injections. Net price 3 × 6 g vials = £585.00

VIDARABINE

Indications: chickenpox and herpes zoster infections in immunosuppressed patients
Cautions: reduce dose in renal impairment; blood counts required; pregnancy (toxicity in *animal* studies)
Side-effects: anorexia, nausea, vomiting, diarrhoea; tremor, ataxia, dizziness, confusion; decreased haematocrit, white cell count, and platelet count
Dose: by slow intravenous infusion, 10 mg/kg daily for at least 5 days

PoM **Vira-A®** (P-D)
Injection, vidarabine 200 mg/ml. For dilution and use as an infusion. Net price 5-ml vial = £37.38

AIDS

ZIDOVUDINE
(Azidothymidine, AZT)
Indications: serious manifestations of human immunodeficiency virus (HIV) infections in patients with acquired immunodeficiency syndrome (AIDS) or AIDS-related complex
Cautions: haematological toxicity (blood tests required at least every 2 weeks for first 3 months then at least once a month thereafter)—dose to be adjusted according to manufacturer's literature if anaemia or myelosuppression; renal and hepatic impairment; elderly
Contra-indications: abnormally low neutrophil counts or haemoglobin values (see literature)
Side-effects: most frequent and serious, anaemia (often requiring transfusion), neutropenia, and leucopenia; also include, nausea and vomiting, anorexia, abdominal pain, headache, rashes, fever, myalgia, paraesthesia, and insomnia
Dose: 200–300 mg every 4 hours (i.e. 6 times daily, including night dose); dosage more accurately calculated as 3.5 mg/kg every 4 hours

▼ PoM **Retrovir®** (Wellcome)
Capsules, white/blue band, zidovudine 100 mg, net price 100 = £114.60; 250 mg (blue/white), 40-cap pack = £114·60

5.4   Antiprotozoal drugs
5.4.1   Antimalarials
5.4.2   Amoebicides

5.4.3   Trichomonacides
5.4.4   Antigiardial drugs
5.4.5   Leishmaniacides
5.4.6   Trypanocides
5.4.7   Drugs for toxoplasmosis
5.4.8   Drugs for pneumocystis pneumonia

Advice on specific problems available from:

Birmingham	021-772 4311
Glasgow	041-946 7120 Extn 247
Liverpool	051-708 9393
London	01-387 4411 (treatment)
	01-636 8636 Extn 212 (prophylaxis)
	01-636 7921 (recorded advice)

5.4.1   Antimalarials

TREATMENT

BENIGN MALARIAS
Benign malaria is usually caused by *Plasmodium vivax* and less commonly by *P. ovale* and *P. malariae.*

Chloroquine is the drug of choice for the treatment of benign malarias.

The adult dosage regimen for chloroquine is an initial dose of 600 mg (of base) followed by a single dose of 300 mg after 6 to 8 hours, followed by a single dose of 300 mg on each of the next 2 days (approximate total cumulative dose of 25 mg/kg of base).

Chloroquine alone is adequate for *P. malariae* infections but in the case of *P. vivax* and *P. ovale,* a *radical cure* (to destroy parasites in the liver and thus prevent relapses) is required. This is achieved with **primaquine**[1] in an adult dosage of 15 mg (of base) daily for 14 to 21 days given after the chloroquine.

CHILDREN. Children are given an initial dose of chloroquine 10 mg/kg (of base) followed by a single dose of 5 mg/kg after 6–8 hours, then a single dose of 5 mg/kg on each of the following 2 days.

For a *radical cure* children are then given primaquine[1] in a dose of 250 micrograms/kg (of base) daily.

FALCIPARUM MALARIA
Falciparum malaria (malignant malaria) is caused by *Plasmodium falciparum.*

Many strains of *P. falciparum* are now resistant to chloroquine. Where the sensitivity is uncertain treatment should be given as for chloroquine-resistant strains.

---

1. Before starting primaquine the blood should be tested for glucose-6-phosphate dehydrogenase (G6PD) activity as the drug can cause haemolysis in patients who are deficient in the enzyme. If the patient is G6PD deficient primaquine, in a dose for adults of 30 mg once a week for 8 weeks, has been found useful and without undue harmful effects.

CHLOROQUINE-SENSITIVE STRAINS. Chloroquine is effective by mouth in the dosage schedule outlined under benign malarias (above).

If the patient with a chloroquine-sensitive infection is seriously ill, chloroquine is given by intravenous infusion[1]. The adult dosage is chloroquine 5 mg/kg (of base) infused over 4 hours and repeated at intervals of 12 hours. Oral therapy is instituted as soon as possible to complete the course; the total cumulative dose for the course should be 25 mg/kg of base.

Intravenous infusion of quinine (see below) is also suitable for chloroquine-sensitive infections and should be used in preference to chloroquine if the sensitivity of the infective strain is uncertain or if the infection 'breaks through' chloroquine prophylaxis.

CHILDREN. *Oral.* The dose of chloroquine by mouth is as the children's doses for benign malarias (above).
Parenteral. The dose of chloroquine by intravenous infusion is 5 mg/kg (of base) given at intervals of 12 hours, as for adults.

CHLOROQUINE-RESISTANT STRAINS. These strains are becoming increasingly common particularly in South-east Asia including the Indian subcontinent, Central and South America, and Central, East, and West Africa.

Quinine is effective by mouth in an adult dosage of 600 mg (of salt[2]) every 8 hours for 7 days.

Following (or together with) the course of quinine adults should be given a single dose of 3 tablets of **Fansidar**®. Some chloroquine-resistant strains are now also resistant to Fansidar®; in these cases **tetracycline** seems to be effective but expert advice should be sought since other drugs, such as mefloquine, may be available. Tetracycline is given in a dose of 250 mg every 6 hours for 7 days.

If the patient with chloroquine-resistant infection is seriously ill, **quinine**[3] should be given by intravenous infusion over 4 hours in a loading dose of 20 mg/kg of salt[2] followed by a maintenance dose of 10 mg/kg of salt[2] over 4 hours every 8 hours until the patient can swallow tablets to complete the 7-day course. (**Important: the loading dose should not be used if the patient has received quinine or mefloquine during the previous 12 hours; if parenteral treatment is required for more than 72 hours the maintenance dose should be reduced by a third, i.e. to 6.7 mg/kg of salt[2]).

Following (or together with) the course of quinine the patient should be given Fansidar® or tetracycline as above.

CHILDREN. *Oral.* Quinine is well tolerated by children although the salts are bitter; the dose is 10 mg/kg of salt[2] every 8 hours for 7 days, as for adults. Doses of Fansidar® (given after quinine) are reduced as follows for children: up to 4 years ½ tablet, 5 to 6 years 1 tablet, 7 to 9 years 1½ tablets, 10 to 14 years 2 tablets.
Parenteral. The dose of quinine by intravenous infusion is calculated on a mg/kg basis as for adults (see above).

CHEMOPROPHYLAXIS

The chemoprophylaxis of malaria is becoming more complex as a result of drug resistance, and varies for different areas of the world. The choice of drug must take into consideration the following 5 criteria:

(i) the level of malaria transmission,
(ii) the risk of exposure,
(iii) the efficacy of the recommended drugs,
(iv) the side-effects of the drugs,
(v) the age of the patient.

The most important point to remember is that **prophylaxis is relative and not absolute**, and that breakthrough can occur with any of the drugs recommended anywhere in the world. The importance of personal protection, e.g. use of mosquito nets, repellants etc. is emphasised.

Prophylaxis should be started one week before travel into an endemic area (or if not possible at earliest opportunity up to 1 or 2 days before travel); it should be continued for at least 4 weeks after leaving.

For **North Africa** and the **Middle East**, give chloroquine 300 mg (as the base) once weekly or proguanil 200 mg daily.

For the **Indian subcontinent**, **China**, **East**, **Central**, and **West Africa**, **Central** and **South America**, give proguanil 200 mg daily together with chloroquine 300 mg (as the base) once weekly.

For malarious areas of **South-east Asia**, **Western Pacific**, and **Oceania** the use of Maloprim® 1 tablet once weekly together with chloroquine 300 mg (as the base) once weekly seems justified in the light of present evidence.

CHEMOPROPHYLAXIS IN CHILDREN. Doses for chloroquine and proguanil are reduced as follows:

Age of child	Fraction of adult dose
Under 6 weeks	one-eighth
6 weeks–1 year	one-quarter
1–5 years	one-half
6–12 years	three-quarters
over 12 years	adult dose

Note. These doses reflect the current views of UK experts in malaria.

Specialist advice should be obtained for use of Maloprim® in children.

Prophylaxis is required in breast-fed infants; although antimalarials are excreted in milk, the amounts are too variable to give reliable protection.

1. If intravenous infusion is not feasible, chloroquine may be given by intramuscular injection in a dosage of 3.5 mg/kg (of base) repeated at intervals of 8 hours until oral therapy is possible.
2. Valid for quinine hydrochloride, dihydrochloride, and sulphate; not valid for quinine bisulphate which contains a correspondingly smaller amount of quinine.
3. If quinine is not available quinidine may be given by intravenous infusion in a dose of 7.5 mg/kg (of base) but cardiotoxicity is more likely.

PoM[1] *Syrup* (= elixir), red, chloroquine sulphate 68 mg/5 ml. Diluent syrup, life of diluted elixir 14 days. Net price 60 ml = £1.25. Label: 5

PoM *Injection*, chloroquine 40 mg (as sulphate)/ ml. Net price 5-ml amp = 45p

[1]*Note.* Can be sold to the public provided it is licensed and labelled for the prophylaxis of malaria

CHEMOPROPHYLAXIS IN PREGNANCY. Chloroquine and proguanil may be given in usual doses in areas where *P. falciparum* strains are sensitive. The centres listed in section 5.4 should be consulted for advice on prophylaxis in resistant areas.

TREATMENT COURSES. Travellers to areas of chloroquine-resistance who are unlikely to have easy access to medical care should carry a treatment course of 3 tablets of Fansidar® which should be taken (in a single dose) at the first sign of fever. Travellers to chloroquine-resistant areas such as East Africa, South-east Asia, Western Pacific, and Oceania should preferably carry a treatment course of quinine tablets, 600 mg (of salt[2]) every 8 hours for 5 days. Self-medication should be **avoided** if medical help is accessible; prophylaxis should be continued during and after the attack.

AMODIAQUINE

Indications: not recommended in the UK, see Cautions
Cautions: see under Chloroquine; **not** recommended for chemoprophylaxis owing to high incidence of agranulocytosis
Side-effects: nausea, vomiting, diarrhoea, lethargy; agranulocytosis and other blood disorders, hepatitis, peripheral neuropathy; on prolonged treatment corneal deposits, blue-grey pigmentation of skin, finger nails, hard palate

PoM **Camoquin®** (P-D)
Tablets, yellow, f/c, scored, amodiaquine 200 mg (as hydrochloride). Net price 20 = £1.08

CHLOROQUINE

Indications: chemoprophylaxis and treatment of malaria; amoebiasis
Cautions: impaired renal or hepatic function, psoriasis, porphyria, ocular examinations in long-term treatment. Drug interactions: see Appendix 1 (sections 5.4, *10*)
Side-effects: headache, nausea, vomiting, diarrhoea, rashes; pruritus; rarely psychotic episodes, convulsions; corneal and retinal changes with prolonged high dosage (may be irreversible)
Dose: see notes above
Note. Chloroquine base 150 mg ≡ chloroquine sulphate 200 mg ≡ chloroquine phosphate 250 mg (approx.)

PoM[1] **Avloclor®** (ICI)
Tablets, scored, chloroquine phosphate 250 mg. Net price 20-tab pack = 62p. Label: 5
PoM[1] **Malarivon®** (Wallace Mfg)
Syrup (= elixir), chloroquine phosphate 80 mg/ 5 ml. Net price 75 ml = 98p. Label: 5
Nivaquine® (M&B)
PoM[1] *Tablets*, f/c, yellow, scored, chloroquine sulphate 200 mg. Net price 20 = 74p. Label: 5

2. Valid for quinine hydrochloride, dihydrochloride, and sulphate; not valid for quinine bisulphate which contains a correspondingly smaller amount of quinine.

PRIMAQUINE

Indications: eradication of benign malaria
Cautions: see notes above; pregnancy
Side-effects: anorexia, nausea, vomiting, jaundice; less commonly bone-marrow depression, methaemoglobinaemia, haemolytic anaemia
Dose: see notes above

Primaquine Tablets, s/c, primaquine 7.5 mg (as phosphate). Net price 20 = 12p

PROGUANIL HYDROCHLORIDE

Indications: chemoprophylaxis of malaria
Cautions: renal impairment
Side-effects: mild gastric intolerance
Dose: see notes above

Paludrine® (ICI)
Tablets, scored, proguanil hydrochloride 100 mg. Net price 20 = 23p. Label: 21

PYRIMETHAMINE

Indications: see notes above
Cautions: hepatic or renal impairment, folate supplements in pregnancy, blood counts required with high doses. Drug interactions: see Appendix 1 (section *8*)
Side-effects: depression of haemopoiesis with prolonged treatment, rashes

Daraprim® (Wellcome)
Tablets, scored, pyrimethamine 25 mg. Net price 20 = £1.00
Dose: not recommended alone
▼ PoM **Fansidar®** (Roche)
Tablets, scored, pyrimethamine 25 mg, sulfadoxine 500 mg. Net price 20 = £3.89
Dose: treatment, see notes above
Chemoprophylaxis, not recommended by UK experts.
PoM **Maloprim®** (Wellcome)
Tablets, scored, pyrimethamine 12.5 mg, dapsone 100 mg. Net price 20 = £1.25
Dose: limited use, see Chemoprophylaxis (above).

QUININE

Indications: falciparum malaria
Cautions: atrial fibrillation, conduction defects, heart block, pregnancy. Drug interactions: see Appendix 1 (sections *2.1*, *5.4*)
Contra-indications: haemoglobinuria, optic neuritis
Side-effects: cinchonism, including tinnitus, headache, nausea, abdominal pain, rashes, visual disturbances (including temporary blindness), confusion; hypersensitivity reactions including angioedema
Dose: see notes above

Note. Quinine (anhydrous base) 100 mg

= quinine bisulphate 169 mg
= quinine dihydrochloride 122 mg
= quinine hydrochloride 122 mg
= quinine sulphate 121 mg

Tablets containing quinine bisulphate 300 mg are available but provide correspondingly smaller amounts of quinine than the dihydrochloride, hydrochloride, or sulphate

PoM **Quinine Dihydrochloride Tablets,** quinine dihydrochloride 300 mg. Net price 20 = £2.01
PoM **Quinine Hydrochloride Tablets,** quinine hydrochloride 300 mg. Net price 20 = £1.84
PoM **Quinine Sulphate Tablets,** s/c or f/c, quinine sulphate 125 mg. Net price 20 = 50p
PoM **Quinine Sulphate Tablets,** s/c or f/c, quinine sulphate 200 mg, net price 20 = 70p; 300 mg, 20 = 72p
PoM **Quinine Dihydrochloride Injection,** quinine dihydrochloride 300 mg/ml. For dilution with physiological saline and use as an infusion. 1- and 2-ml amps

Available from Macarthys and Penn (both special order) or from specialist centres (see p. 226)
Note. Intravenous injection of quinine is so hazardous that it has been superseded by infusion

5.4.2 Amoebicides

Metronidazole (section 5.1.11) is the drug of choice for acute invasive *amoebic dysentery* for it is very effective against vegetative amoebae in ulcers at a dosage of 800 mg three times daily for 5 days. It is also effective against amoebae which may have migrated to the liver. It is given either for 10 days, or for 5 days followed by a 10-day course of diloxanide furoate. It is relatively ineffective in chronic intestinal amoebiasis in which only cysts are present in the stool.

Diloxanide furoate (Furamide®) is the drug of choice in chronic infections in which only cysts and not vegetative forms of *Entamoeba histolytica* are present in the faeces. It is relatively free from toxic effects in therapeutic doses and the usual course is of 10 days, given alone for chronic infections or following 5 days of metronidazole in acute dysenteric infections.

For the treatment of *amoebic abscesses* of the liver **metronidazole** is effective in doses of 400 mg 3 times daily for 5–10 days and the course may be repeated after 2 weeks if necessary.

Tinidazole is also an effective amoebicide, for doses in intestinal amoebiasis and amoebic involvement in the liver, see section 5.1.11.

If metronidazole or tinidazole are not available emetine may be used but its side-effects are more marked. Diloxanide is not effective against hepatic amoebiasis, but a 10-day course should be given at the completion of metronidazole, tinidazole, or emetine treatment to destroy any amoeba in the gut.

Chloroquine (section 5.4.1) is also used for hepatic amoebiasis and for adults a dosage of 600 mg (base) daily for 5 days followed by 300 mg (base)

daily for 14 to 21 days is effective but is slower and less certain in its action than metronidazole. A 10-day course of diloxanide should be given at the completion of chloroquine treatment. For abscesses containing more than 100 ml of pus (i.e. approximately 6 to 10 cm in diameter) aspiration carried out in conjunction with drug therapy will greatly reduce the period of disability.

Emetine hydrochloride and **emetine and bismuth iodide** have now been largely replaced by metronidazole (or tinidazole) and are rarely used for they cause more nausea and have a smaller margin of safety between the therapeutic and the cardiotoxic dose.

DILOXANIDE FUROATE

Indications: chronic amoebiasis—see notes above
Side-effects: flatulence, vomiting, urticaria, pruritus
Dose: 500 mg every 8 hours for 10 days—see notes above

PoM **Furamide®** (Boots)
Tablets, scored, diloxanide furoate 500 mg. Net price 30 = £2.12. Label: 9
PoM **Entamizole®** (Boots)
Tablets, off-white, diloxanide furoate 250 mg, metronidazole 200 mg. Net price 30 = £5.69. Label: 4, 9, 21, 25
Dose: amoebiasis, 2 tablets 3 times daily for 5 days; CHILD 5–12 years ½–1 tablet, according to age, for 5 days
Treatment may be extended to 10 days in refractory cases; not suitable for prophylactic use

5.4.3 Trichomonacides

Metronidazole (section 5.1.11) is the treatment of choice for *Trichomonas vaginalis* infection.

If metronidazole is ineffective, **nimorazole** (Naxogin®) may be tried; it is usually given as a single 2-g dose, with food. A further 2-g dose may be given if there is no clinical improvement.

Alcohol should be avoided during treatment with both metronidazole and nimorazole.

NIMORAZOLE

Indications: trichomoniasis (acute ulcerative gingivitis, see section 12.3.2)
Contra-indications: active CNS disease, severe renal failure
Side-effects: nausea, vomiting, rashes, vertigo, drowsiness, ataxia (discontinue treatment), intolerance to alcohol
Dose: see notes above

Naxogin 500® (Farmitalia Carlo Erba)
Tablets, scored, nimorazole 500 mg. Net price 4 = 49p. Label: 4, 21

5.4.4 Antigiardial drugs

Metronidazole (section 5.1.11) is the treatment of choice for *Giardia lamblia* infections, given by mouth in a dosage of 2 g daily for 3 days, 200 mg every 8 hours for 14 days or 400 mg every 8 hours for 7 days.

Alternative treatments are **tinidazole** (section 5.1.11) 2 g as a single dose or **mepacrine hydrochloride** 100 mg every 8 hours for 5–8 days.

5.4.5 Leishmaniacides

Cutaneous leishmaniasis frequently heals spontaneously without specific treatment. If the skin lesions are extensive or unsightly, treatment is indicated, as it is in visceral leishmaniasis (kala-azar).

Sodium stibogluconate (Pentostam®), an organic pentavalent antimony compound, is the treatment of choice. The dose is 10 mg/kg daily for 30 days by intramuscular or intravenous injection. Skin lesions are treated for 10 days.

Pentamidine isethionate (section 5.4.8) has been used in antimony-resistant visceral leishmaniasis, but although the initial response is often good, the relapse rate is high; it is associated with serious side-effects.

SODIUM STIBOGLUCONATE

Indications: leishmaniasis

Cautions: intravenous injections must be given slowly and stopped if coughing or substernal pain develops

Contra-indications: pneumonia, myocarditis, nephritis, hepatitis

Side-effects: anorexia, vomiting, coughing, substernal pain

Dose: see notes above

PoM **Pentostam**® (Wellcome)
Injection, sodium stibogluconate equivalent to pentavalent antimony 100 mg/ml. Net price 100-ml bottle = £45.92

5.4.6 Trypanocides

The prophylaxis and treatment of trypanosomiasis is difficult and differs according to the strain of organism. Expert advice should therefore be obtained.

5.4.7 Drugs for toxoplasmosis

Most infections caused by *Toxoplasma gondii* are self-limiting, and treatment is not necessary. Exceptions are patients with eye involvement, and those who are immunosuppressed. The treatment of choice is a combination of pyrimethamine and a sulphonamide, given for several weeks. Pyrimethamine is a folate antagonist, and adverse reactions to this combination are relatively common.

5.4.8 Drugs for Pneumocystis pneumonia

Pneumonia caused by *Pneumocystis carinii* occurs in immunosuppressed or severely debilitated patients. It is the commonest cause of pneumonia in AIDS. **Co-trimoxazole** (section 5.1.8) is the drug of choice for the treatment of pneumocystis pneumonia. **Pentamidine isethionate** is an alternative to co-trimoxazole and is particularly indicated for patients with a history of adverse reactions to, or who have not responded to, co-trimoxazole. It is a potentially toxic drug that can cause severe hypotension during or immediately after administration; it should only be administered by those experienced in its use.

PENTAMIDINE ISETHIONATE

Indications: See under Dose (should only be given by experienced personnel and manufacturer's literature should be studied with care)

Cautions: risk of severe hypotension following administration (establish baseline blood pressure and administer with patient lying down; monitor blood pressure closely during administration, and at regular intervals, until treatment concluded); hepatic and renal impairment; hypertension or hypotension; hyperglycaemia or hypoglycaemia; leucopenia, thrombocytopenia, or anaemia; carry out laboratory monitoring for all functions according to manufacturer's literature

Side-effects: severe reactions, sometimes fatal, due to hypotension, hypoglycaemia, pancreatitis, and cardiac arrhythmias, leucopenia, thrombocytopenia, acute renal failure, hypocalcaemia; also reported: azotaemia, abnormal liver-function tests, leucopenia, anaemia, thrombocytopenia, hyperkalaemia, nausea and vomiting, hypotension, dizziness, syncope, flushing, hypoglycaemia, hyperglycaemia, rash, and taste disturbances

Local reactions range from discomfort and pain to induration, abscess formation, and muscle necrosis

Dose: Pneumocystis carinii pneumonia, preferably *by intravenous infusion*, 4 mg/kg daily for at least 14 days (reduced according to manufacturer's literature in renal impairment)

Visceral leishmaniasis (Kala-azar), preferably by *intramuscular injection*, 3–4 mg/kg on alternate days to max. total of 10 injections; course may be repeated if necessary

Cutaneous leishmaniasis, *by deep intramuscular injection*, 3–4 mg/kg once or twice weekly until condition resolves

Trypanosomiasis, *by deep intramuscular injection or intravenous infusion*, 4 mg/kg daily or on alternate days to total of 7–10 injections
Note. Direct bolus intravenous injection should be avoided whenever possible and **never** given rapidly; intramuscular injections should be deep and preferably given into the buttock

PoM **Pentamidine isethionate** (M&B)
Injection, powder for reconstitution, pentamidine isethionate. Net price 300-mg vial = £12·00

5.5 Anthelmintics

5.5.1 Drugs for threadworms
5.5.2 Ascaricides
5.5.3 Taenicides
5.5.4 Drugs for hookworms
5.5.5 Schistosomicides
5.5.6 Filaricides
5.5.7 Drugs for guinea worms
5.5.8 Drugs for strongyloidiasis

Advice on prophylaxis and treatment of helminth infections is available from:

Birmingham	021-772 4311
Glasgow	041-946 7120 Extn 247
Liverpool	051-708 9393
London	01-387 4411 (treatment)
	01-636 8636 Extn 212 (prophylaxis)

5.5.1 Drugs for threadworms
(pinworms, *Enterobius vermicularis*)

Anthelmintics are relatively ineffective in thread-worm infections, and their use should be combined with hygienic measures to break the cycle of auto-infection. All members of the family require treatment.

Adult threadworms do not live for longer than 6 weeks and for development of fresh worms, ova must be swallowed and exposed to the action of digestive juices in the upper intestinal tract. Direct multiplication of worms does not take place in the large bowel. Adult female worms lay ova on the peri-anal skin and cause pruritus by so doing; scratching the area then leads to ova being transmitted on fingers to the mouth, often via food eaten with unwashed hands. Washing the hands and fingers with the aid of a nail brush before each meal and after each visit to the toilet is essential. A bath taken immediately after rising will remove ova laid during the night and limit their dissemination.

Mebendazole (Vermox®) in a single dose of 100 mg is the drug of choice for patients of all ages over 2 years.

Piperazine salts including the citrate and phosphate are used. Piperazine may be given in doses equivalent to the following quantities of piperazine hydrate: up to 2 years 50–75 mg/kg, 2–4 years 750 mg, 5–12 years 1.5 g, adults and children over 12 years 2 g. These doses are given daily for 7 days. A further 7-day course may be given if necessary after an interval of 1 week.

Pyrantel (Combantrin®) given as a single dose of 10 mg/kg (max. 1 g) is equally effective.

MEBENDAZOLE
Indications: threadworm, roundworm, whipworm, and hookworm infections
Cautions: pregnancy (toxicity in *rats*)
Contra-indications: children under 2 years
Side-effects: rarely abdominal pain, diarrhoea
Dose: see notes above and sections 5.5.2, 5.5.4, and 5.5.8.

PoM **Vermox®** (Janssen)
Tablets, pink, scored, chewable, mebendazole 100 mg. Net price 6-tab pack = £1.57
Suspension (= mixture), mebendazole 100 mg/ 5 ml. Net price 30 ml = £1.82

PIPERAZINE
Indications: threadworm and roundworm infections
Cautions: impaired renal function, psychiatric states, neurological disease
Contra-indications: epilepsy, renal failure, liver disease
Side-effects: nausea, vomiting, diarrhoea, urticaria; rarely dizziness, paraesthesia, muscular incoordination
Dose: see notes above
Note. 100 mg piperazine hydrate ≡ 125 mg piperazine citrate ≡ 104 mg piperazine phosphate

Antepar® (Wellcome)
Tablets, yellow, scored, piperazine hydrate 500 mg (as phosphate). Net price 28 = £2.86. Label: 24
Elixir, orange, piperazine hydrate 750 mg/5 ml (as hydrate and citrate). Diluent syrup, life of diluted elixir 14 days. Net price 100 ml = £1.95
Pripsen® (R&C)
Oral powder, cream, piperazine phosphate 4 g and sennosides 15.3 mg/sachet. Net price 2 sachets = £1.66. Label: 13
Dose: stirred into a small glass of milk or water, adults and children over 6 years, 1 sachet; INFANTS 3 months–1 year, 5 ml powder; CHILD 1–6 years, 10 ml powder. Repeat after 14 days

5.5.2 Ascaricides
(common roundworm infections)

***Levamisole** is very effective against ascaris and is generally considered to be the drug of choice. It is very well tolerated; mild nausea or vomiting has been reported in about 1% of treated patients; it is given as a single dose of 120–150 mg in adults.

Mebendazole (section 5.5.1) is also active against *Ascaris lumbricoides*; the usual dose is 100 mg twice daily for 3 days. **Pyrantel** (Combantrin®) is also an effective broad-spectrum anthelmintic and a single dose of 10 mg/kg (max. 1 g) is usually sufficient to eradicate ascaris; it may occasionally produce mild nausea but experience shows it to be a very safe drug. **Piperazine** may also be given in a single dose equivalent to 4 g of piperazine hydrate.

PYRANTEL
Indications: roundworm, threadworm, and hookworm infections
Cautions: liver disease
Side-effects: see notes above

Dose: ADULT and CHILD over 6 months, *Ascaris lumbricoides* alone, a single dose of 5 mg/kg; mixed infections involving *Ascaris lumbricoides*, single dose of 10 mg/kg
Hookworm—section 5.5.4
Threadworms—section 5.5.1

PoM **Combantrin**® (Pfizer)
Tablets, orange, pyrantel 125 mg (as embonate). Net price 6 = 64p

5.5.3   Taenicides
(tapeworms)

Niclosamide (Yomesan®) is the most widely used drug for tapeworm infections and side-effects are limited to occasional gastro-intestinal upset, light-headedness, and pruritus. Fears of developing cysticercosis in *Taenia solium* infections have proved unfounded. All the same, it is wise to anticipate this possibility by using an anti-emetic on wakening.

*Praziquantel is as effective as niclosamide and is given as a single dose of 10–20 mg/kg after a light breakfast.

NICLOSAMIDE

Indications: tapeworm infections—see notes above and under Dose
Side-effects: gastro-intestinal discomfort
Dose: 2 g after a light breakfast, followed by a purgative after 2 hours; CHILD up to 2 years, 500 mg, 2–6 years, 1 g
T. saginata and *Diphyllobothrium latum*, as for *T. solium* but half the dose may be taken after breakfast and the remainder one hour later
Hymenolepsis nana, 2 g on first day, then 1 g daily for next 6 days; CHILD up to 2 years, quarter adult dose; 2–6 years, half adult dose
COUNSELLING. To be chewed thoroughly and washed down with water or taken crushed in water

Yomesan® (Bayer)
Tablets, yellow, chewable, niclosamide 500 mg. Net price 4 = £1.41. Label: 4, 24, 27, counselling advised, administration

5.5.4   Drugs for hookworms
(ancylostomiasis, necatoriasis)

Hookworms live in the upper small intestine and draw blood from the point of their attachment to their host. An iron-deficiency anaemia may thereby be produced and, if present, effective treatment of the infection requires not only expulsion of the worms but treatment of the anaemia.
Bephenium is widely used and its side-effects are limited to occasional nausea and vomiting. A single dose of 2.5 g is given and repeated after 1–2 days. It is thought to be more effective against *Ancylostoma duodenale* than against *Necator americanus*. **Pyrantel** (section 5.5.2) is very effective against hookworms and, like bephenium, has side-effects limited to occasional nausea and

vomiting. The usual dose is 10 mg/kg (max. 1 g) given as a single dose.
Mebendazole (section 5.5.1) has a useful broad-spectrum activity, and is effective against hookworms; the usual dose is 100 mg twice daily for 3 days.
Tetrachloroethylene is still widely used in the tropics for hookworm infection. It is best administered in a suspension rather than in capsules so that effective action of the drug on the worms in the upper intestine can be assured; the usual dose is 2.5 to 5 ml. Alcohol and fatty foods should be avoided following treatment with tetrachloroethylene as they increase its absorption and therefore hepatotoxicity. Toxic effects are rare but occasionally nausea and headache or drowsiness may be experienced. It should be avoided in debilitated patients or young children.
Thiabendazole (section 5.5.8) and *levamisole are also used.

BEPHENIUM

Indications: roundworm   and   hookworm infections
Side-effects: nausea, vomiting, diarrhoea, headache, vertigo
Dose: see notes above

Alcopar® (Wellcome)
Granules, yellow/green, bephenium 2.5 g (as hydroxynaphthoate)/sachet. Net price per sachet = 57p. Label: 13

5.5.5   Schistosomicides
(bilharziasis)

Adult *Schistosoma haematobium* worms live in the genito-urinary veins and adult *S. mansoni* in those of the colon and mesentery. *S. japonicum* is more widely distributed in veins of the alimentary tract and portal system.
*Praziquantel (Biltricide®) is effective against all human schistosomes. The dose is 40 mg/kg as a single oral dose (60 mg/kg in 3 divided doses on one day for *S. japonicum* infections). No serious toxic effects have been reported. Of all the available schistosomicides, it has the most attractive combination of effectiveness, broad-spectrum activity, and low toxicity.
Oxamniquine (Vansil® *Pfizer*) is effective against *S. mansoni* infections only. It is a quinoline compound given by mouth in doses of 15–30 mg/kg daily for 1 to 3 days. It can occasionally cause epileptic fits.
*Metriphonate (Bilarcil®) is an organophosphorus compound which is only effective against *S. haematobium* infections. It is given by mouth in 3 doses of 7.5 mg/kg at intervals of 2 weeks. As it reduces plasma-cholinesterase concentrations it should be used with caution in patients likely to be frequently exposed to organophosphorus insecticides.
Hycanthone, lucanthone, niridazole, and stibocaptate have now been superseded.

5.5.6 Filaricides

Diethylcarbamazine (Banocide®) is highly effective against microfilariae and adults of *Loa loa* and of *Wuchereria bancrofti* and against the microfilariae of *Onchocerca volvulus*. It has no effect against adult *O. volvulus*. The destruction of the microfilariae is associated with release of antigens and a resulting allergic response. Headache, nausea, and sometimes vomiting are complained of and in onchocerciasis the filarial dermatitis is temporarily aggravated and conjunctivitis and punctate keratitis temporarily increased; the main danger is that acute iritis may develop. Antihistamines may be helpful in controlling these reactions but topical or systemic corticosteroids may be required for the skin irritation and ocular reactions in severely affected patients.

With the object of limiting allergic responses in onchocerciasis, diethylcarbamazine treatment is commenced with a dose of 1 mg/kg bodyweight, gradually increased over 3 days to 6 mg/kg daily in divided doses; this dosage is maintained for 21 days. Close medical supervision is necessary particularly in the early phase of treatment. Diethylcarbamazine has never been a satisfactory treatment for onchocerciasis since symptoms recur when treatment is stopped.

In very persistent cases **suramin** may be used for it is active against adult worms although it has little action on microfilariae. It is nephrotoxic and it is for this reason that its use is usually withheld except in chronically relapsing cases. When used, a preliminary test dose of 200 mg is administered intravenously and if well tolerated is followed by an increasing weekly dose of 0.4, 0.6, 0.8, and 1 g dissolved in 10 ml of water for injections given intravenously. The whole course of treatment lasts 5 weeks. It is important to ensure that the urine is free from albumin and casts which if present contra-indicate further suramin treatment.

***Ivermectin** is very effective in onchocerciasis and it is now the drug of choice. A single dose of 150 micrograms/kg by mouth produces a prolonged reduction in microfilarial levels with fewer reactions than diethylcarbamazine; annual retreatment must be given until the adult worms die out.

DIETHYLCARBAMAZINE CITRATE
Indications: filariasis
Cautions; Side-effects: see notes above
Dose: see notes above

Banocide® (Wellcome)
Tablets, scored, diethylcarbamazine citrate 50 mg. Net price 20 = 71p. Label: 9

5.5.7 Drugs for guinea worms
(dracontiasis)

Guinea worms, *Dracunculus medinensis*, may be killed and their removal from the tissues facilitated by a course of *niridazole (formerly marketed as Ambilhar®). Use of niridazole does not obviate the concomitant need for sterile dressing of the ulcer caused by a guinea worm and for its extraction, wherever possible, under sterile conditions. In India, niridazole has been reported as effective at a dosage of 200 mg twice daily for 7 days. **Metronidazole** has also been reported to be effective in a dose of 400 mg three times daily for 5 days.

5.5.8 Drugs for strongyloidiasis

Adult *Strongyloides stercoralis* live in the gut and produce larvae which penetrate the gut wall and invade the tissues, setting up a cycle of auto-infection. **Thiabendazole** is the drug of choice, at a dosage of 25 mg/kg every 12 hours for 3 days. **Mebendazole** is also effective, given in 3 courses of 100 mg twice daily for 3 days at intervals of 2 weeks.

THIABENDAZOLE
Indications: strongyloidiasis, cutaneous and visceral larva migrans, dracontiasis, symptoms of trichinosis; threadworm when mixed with any of the above infestations; refractory hookworm, whipworm, or roundworm
Cautions: hepatic or renal impairment, if drowsiness occurs warn patients not to drive, discontinue if hypersensitivity reactions occur
Side-effects: anorexia, nausea, vomiting, dizziness, diarrhoea, headache, pruritus, drowsiness; hypersensitivity reactions including fever, chills, angioedema, rashes, erythema multiforme; rarely tinnitus, collapse, parenchymal liver damage
Dose: see notes above

Mintezol® (MSD)
Tablets, orange, chewable, thiabendazole 500 mg. Net price 6 = 52p. Label: 3, 21, 24

---

*Not on UK market

6: Drugs used in the treatment of disorders of the
ENDOCRINE SYSTEM

In this chapter, drug treatment is discussed under the following headings:

6.1 Drugs used in diabetes
6.2 Thyroid and antithyroid drugs
6.3 Corticosteroids
6.4 Sex hormones
6.5 Hypothalamic and pituitary hormones
6.6 Drugs affecting bone metabolism
6.7 Other endocrine drugs

6.1 Drugs used in diabetes

Two groups of drugs are used in the treatment of diabetes, insulin preparations (section 6.1.1) and oral antidiabetic drugs (section 6.1.2).

The treatment of diabetic ketoacidosis or hyperosmolar non-ketotic 'coma' (section 6.1.3), hypoglycaemia (section 6.1.4), and diabetic neuropathy (section 6.1.5) are also discussed.

6.1.1 Insulin

6.1.1.1 Short-acting insulin preparations
6.1.1.2 Intermediate- and long-acting insulin preparations

Insulin plays a key role in the body's regulation of carbohydrate, fat, and protein metabolism. Diabetes mellitus is due to a deficiency in insulin synthesis and secretion. Patients are generally described as insulin-dependent diabetics (Type 1) or non-insulin-dependent diabetics (Type 2), although many of the latter need insulin to maintain satisfactory control.

Insulin is a polypeptide hormone of complex structure. It is extracted from beef or pork pancreas and purified by crystallisation; it can also be made biosynthetically by recombinant DNA technology using *Escherichia coli* or semisynthetically by enzymatic modification of porcine material (see under Human Insulins, below). All insulin preparations are to a greater or lesser extent immunogenic in man but immunological resistance to insulin action is uncommon.

Insulin is inactivated by gastro-intestinal enzymes, and must therefore be given by injection; the subcutaneous route is ideal for most circumstances. It is usually injected into the upper arms, thighs, buttocks, or abdomen; there may be increased absorption from a limb site if the limb is used in strenuous exercise. Insulin is usually administered using a syringe and needle but portable injection devices (e.g. NovoPen®, Penject®) which hold one of the soluble insulins in cartridge form and meter the required dose are rapidly growing in popularity; they permit greater freedom even though injections may be needed 3 or 4 times daily.

Insulin can also be given by continuous subcutaneous infusion using soluble forms of insulin in an infusion pump. This technique now has an established place in the treatment of diabetes, and provides continuous basal insulin infusion with preprandial boosts. Its chief benefit is the considerable improvement in quality of life enjoyed by some patients, and, at times, the elimination of troublesome hypoglycaemia. There is, at present, only slender evidence of a beneficial effect on diabetic complications, and no proof of harmful effects. It is unsuitable for emotionally or psychiatrically disturbed patients, and thus does not provide a general solution for 'brittle' diabetics. There are many disadvantages to this technique, especially the tendency to rapid development of ketoacidosis, together with the bulkiness of the apparatus, risk of mechanical failure, difficulties with vigorous physical activities, some tendency to gain weight, and sometimes problems from skin sepsis. Patients using it must be well-motivated, reliable, and able to monitor their own blood glucose, and must have access to expert advice both day and night.

When treating diabetic ketoacidosis (section 6.1.3), insulin should be given by intravenous or intramuscular injection, since absorption from subcutaneous depots may be slow and erratic.

Minor allergic reactions at the sites of injections during the first few weeks of treatment are uncommon, usually transient and require no treatment.

CHOICE OF TREATMENT. About 25% of diabetics require insulin treatment; apart from those presenting in ketoacidosis, insulin is needed by most of those with a rapid onset of symptoms, weight loss, weakness, and sometimes vomiting, often associated with ketonuria. The majority of those who are obese can be managed by restriction of carbohydrate or energy intake alone or with the subsequent administration of oral hypoglycaemic drugs. Most children require insulin from the outset.

MANAGEMENT OF DIABETIC PATIENTS. The aim of treatment is to achieve the best possible control of plasma glucose without disabling hypoglycaemia, and close co-operation is needed between the patient and the medical team. Mixtures of available insulin preparations may be required and these combinations have to be worked out for the individual patient. Insulin requirements may be affected by variations in lifestyle, infection, and steroids, and sometimes by a very small amount when the oral contraceptive pill is taken. In pregnancy insulin requirements should be assessed frequently by an experienced diabetic physician.

The energy and carbohydrate intake must be adequate to allow normal growth and development but obesity must be avoided. The carbohydrate intake must be regulated in those patients on insulin and should be distributed throughout the day. Fine control of plasma glucose can be achieved by moving portions of carbohydrate from one meal to another without altering the total intake.

Insulin doses are determined on an individual basis, by gradually increasing the dose but avoiding troublesome hypoglycaemic reactions.

There are 3 main types of insulin preparations:
1. those of **short** duration which have a relatively rapid onset of action, namely soluble forms of insulin;
2. those with an **intermediate** action, e.g. Isophane Insulin Injection and Insulin Zinc Suspension; and
3. those whose action is slower in onset and lasts for **long** periods, e.g. Ultratard insulin.

The duration of action of different insulin preparations varies considerably from one patient to another, and needs to be assessed for every individual. The durations of action indicated below are only approximations. The type of insulin used and its dose and frequency of administration depend on the particular needs of the patient. Most patients are best started on insulins of intermediate action twice daily and a short-acting insulin can later be added to cover any hyperglycaemia which may follow breakfast or evening meal.

Table 1: Some recommended insulin regimens

Insulin	Regimen
1. Short-acting insulin mixed with Intermediate-acting insulin	twice daily (before meals)
2. Short-acting insulin mixed with Intermediate-acting insulin	before breakfast
Short-acting insulin	before evening meal
Intermediate-acting insulin	bedtime
3. Short-acting insulin	three times daily (before breakfast, mid-day and evening meal)
Intermediate-acting insulin	bedtime
4. Short-acting insulin mixed with Intermediate-acting insulin	before breakfast (sufficient in some cases)

HUMAN INSULINS. There are differences in the amino-acid sequence in animal and human insulins, and until recently all available insulins reflected the sequence in the animal (ox or pig) from which they had been prepared. Recently insulin of human sequence prepared by modification of porcine material (emp) or biosynthetically (crb or prb) has become available. Preparations of human sequence insulin should theoretically be less immunogenic, but in trials no real advantage has been shown.

Hypoglycaemia is a potential hazard when the type of insulin is changed, expecially when converting from beef to human insulin. The conversion from beef to human sequence insulin should always be undertaken with specialist advice; it is usual to reduce the total dose by about 10%, with careful monitoring for the first few days. When changing from porcine to human sequence insulin, a dose change is not usually needed, but careful monitoring is advised.

UNITS. The word 'unit' should **not** be abbreviated.

6.1.1.1 SHORT-ACTING INSULIN PREPARATIONS

Neutral Insulin Injection is the form of short-acting insulin now used by most patients. For maintenance regimens it is usual to inject it 15 to 30 minutes before meals.

Acid Insulin Injection has now been discontinued.

Short-acting insulins are the only appropriate forms of insulin for use in diabetic emergencies and at the time of surgical operations. They have the great advantage that they can be given intravenously and intramuscularly, as well as subcutaneously. When injected subcutaneously, they have a rapid onset of action after 30 to 60 minutes, a peak action between 2 and 4 hours, and a duration of action of up to 8 hours. Human sequence preparations tend to have a more rapid onset and a shorter overall duration.

ACID INSULIN INJECTION
(Acid Insulin)
Note. This title and sub-title became official from 1 July 1987. When Insulin Injection or Soluble Insulin is prescribed or demanded, Neutral Insulin Injection should now be dispensed or supplied
  Indications: diabetes mellitus; diabetic ketoacidosis (section 6.1.3)
  Cautions: see notes above; reduce dose in renal impairment. Drug interactions: see Appendix 1 (section 6.1)
  Side-effects: see notes above; local reactions and lipo-atrophy at injection site; overdose causes hypoglycaemia
  Dose: by subcutaneous, intramuscular, or intravenous injection or intravenous infusion, according to patient's requirements

Hypurin Soluble® (CP)
Product discontinued

NEUTRAL INSULIN INJECTION
(Insulin, Injection; Soluble Insulin)
Note. Neutral Insulin Injection should be dispensed or supplied when Insulin Injection or Soluble Insulin is prescribed or demanded; title of Neutral Insulin Injection becomes Insulin Injection in BP 1988 (official from 1st December 1988)
  Indications: diabetes mellitus; diabetic ketoacidosis (section 6.1.3)
  Cautions; Side-effects; Dose: see under Acid Insulin Injection

Highly purified animal insulins
Neutral Insulin Injection (Evans)
Injection, neutral insulin (bovine, highly purified), 100 units/ml. Net price 10-ml vial = £5.35

Hypurin Neutral® (CP)
Injection, neutral insulin (bovine, highly purified) 100 units/ml. Net price 10-ml vial = £6.80

Velosulin® (Nordisk Wellcome)
Injection, neutral insulin (porcine, highly purified) 100 units/ml. Net price 10-ml vial = £7.13

▼ **Velosulin Cartridge**® (Nordisk Wellcome)
Injection (subcutaneous infusion only), neutral insulin (porcine, highly purified) 100 units/ml. Net price 5.7-ml cartridge vial (for use only in Nordisk Wellcome Infuser®) = £4.67

Human sequence insulins
▼ **Human Actrapid**® (Novo)
Injection, neutral insulin (human, emp) 100 units/ml. Net price 10-ml vial = £7.15
▼ **Human Actrapid Penfill**® (Novo)
Injection, neutral insulin (human, emp) 100 units/ml. Net price 5 × 1.5-ml cartridge for use only in NovoPen® device = £6.05
▼ **Human Velosulin**® (Nordisk Wellcome)
Injection, neutral insulin (human, emp) 100 units/ml. Net price 10-ml vial = £7.13
▼ **Humulin S**® (Lilly)
Injection, neutral insulin (human, prb) 100 units/ml. Net price 10-ml vial = £6.95

Injection devices
NHS **Nordisk Wellcome Infuser**® (Nordisk Wellcome)
Injection device, for use with Velosulin Cartridge®. Net price = £630.00
NHS **NovoPen**® (Novo)
Injection device, for use with Human Actrapid Penfill®. Price = £33.00
NHS **Penject**® (Hypoguard)
Injection device, for use with a Becton Dickinson U100 1-ml syringe. Price = £20.00

6.1.1.2 INTERMEDIATE- AND LONG-ACTING INSULIN PREPARATIONS

When given by subcutaneous injection these preparations have an onset of action in approximately 1–2 hours, a maximal effect at 4–12 hours, and a duration of 16–35 hours. They are used to provide background levels in insulin regimens. Some are given twice daily in conjunction with the short-acting insulins, and others are given once daily, particularly in elderly patients. They can be mixed with neutral insulin in the syringe, essentially retaining the properties of the two components, although there may be some blunting of the initial effect of the soluble insulin component (especially on mixing with protamine zinc insulin, see below).

Isophane Insulin Injection is a suspension of insulin with protamine which is of particular value for initiation of twice-daily insulin regimens. Patients usually mix isophane with neutral insulin but ready-mixed preparations may be appropriate.

Biphasic Insulin Injection (Rapitard MC®) is a ready-mixed insulin suitable for twice-daily injection.

Insulin Zinc Suspension (Amorphous) has an intermediate duration of action and **Insulin Zinc Suspension (Crystalline)** a more prolonged duration of action. These preparations may be used independently or in **Insulin Zinc Suspension** (30% amorphous, 70% crystalline). The duration of action of these insulins may be modified for use in once-daily regimens, although insulin zinc suspension and insulin zinc suspension (amorphous) are usually given twice daily. Porcine and human insulin zinc suspensions have a shorter duration of action than bovine insulins of similar formulation.

Protamine Zinc Insulin is usually given once-daily in conjunction with a short-acting insulin. It has the drawback of binding with the short-acting insulins when mixed in the same syringe, and is now rarely used.

For some recommended insulin regimens see section 6.1.1, table 1.

BIPHASIC INSULIN INJECTION

A sterile suspension of crystals containing bovine insulin in a solution of porcine insulin
Indications: diabetes mellitus (intermediate acting)
Cautions; Side-effects: see under Acid Insulin Injection (section 6.1.1.1)
Dose: by subcutaneous injection, according to patient's requirements

Rapitard MC® (Novo)
Injection, biphasic insulin injection (highly purified) 100 units/ml. Net price 10-ml vial = £6.15

INSULIN ZINC SUSPENSION

(Insulin Zinc Suspension, Mixed; I.Z.S.)
Indications: diabetes mellitus (long acting)
Cautions; Side-effects: see under Acid Insulin Injection (section 6.1.1.1)
Dose: by subcutaneous injection, according to patient's requirements

Highly purified animal insulins
Insulin Zinc Suspension Lente (Evans)
Injection, insulin zinc suspension (bovine, highly purified) 100 units/ml. Net price 10-ml vial = £5.35

Hypurin Lente® (CP)
Injection, insulin zinc suspension (bovine, highly purified) 100 units/ml. Net price 10-ml vial = £6.90

Lentard MC® (Novo)
Injection, insulin zinc suspension (bovine and porcine, highly purified) 100 units/ml. Net price 10-ml vial = £6.15

Human sequence insulins
▼ **Human Monotard®** (Novo)
Injection, insulin zinc suspension (human, emp) 100 units/ml. Net price 10-ml vial = £7.15
▼ **Humulin Lente®** (Lilly)
Injection, insulin zinc suspension (human, prb) 100 units/ml. Net price 10-ml vial = £6.95

INSULIN ZINC SUSPENSION (AMORPHOUS)
(Amorph. I.Z.S.)
Indications: diabetes mellitus (intermediate acting)
Cautions; Side-effects: see under Acid Insulin Injection (section 6.1.1.1)
Dose: by subcutaneous injection, according to patient's requirements

Semitard MC® (Novo)
Injection, insulin zinc suspension (amorphous) (porcine, highly purified) 100 units/ml. Net price 10-ml vial = £6.68

INSULIN ZINC SUSPENSION (CRYSTALLINE)
(Cryst. I.Z.S.)
Indications: diabetes mellitus (duration of action, see below)
Cautions; Side-effects: see under Acid Insulin Injection (section 6.1.1.1)
Dose: by subcutaneous injection, according to patient's requirements

Human sequence insulins
Human Ultratard® (Novo) (long acting)
Injection, insulin zinc suspension, crystalline (human, emp) 100 units/ml. Net price 10-ml vial = £7.15
▼ **Humulin Zn®** (Lilly) (intermediate acting)
Injection, insulin zinc suspension, crystalline (human, prb) 100 units/ml. Net price 10-ml vial = £6.95

ISOPHANE INSULIN INJECTION
(Isophane Insulin (NPH); Isophane Protamine Insulin Injection)
Indications: diabetes mellitus (intermediate acting)
Cautions; Side-effects: see under Acid Insulin Injection (section 6.1.1.1); protamine may cause allergic reactions
Dose: by subcutaneous injection, according to patient's requirements

Highly purified animal insulins
Isophane Insulin Injection (Evans)
Injection, isophane insulin (bovine, highly purified) 100 units/ml. Net price 10-ml vial = £5.35
Hypurin Isophane® (CP)
Injection, isophane insulin (bovine, highly purified) 100 units/ml. Net price 10-ml vial = £6.90

Insulatard® (Nordisk Wellcome)
Injection, isophane insulin (porcine, highly purified) 100 units/ml. Net price 10-ml vial = £7.13

Mixed highly purified animal insulins
Initard 50/50® (Nordisk Wellcome)
Injection, isophane insulin (porcine, highly purified) 50%, neutral insulin (porcine, highly purified) 50%. 100 units/ml. Net price 10-ml vial = £7.13
Mixtard 30/70® (Nordisk Wellcome)
Injection, isophane insulin (porcine, highly purified) 70%, neutral insulin (porcine, highly purified) 30%. 100 units/ml. Net price 10-ml vial = £7.13

Human sequence insulins
▼ **Human Insulatard®** (Nordisk Wellcome)
Injection, isophane insulin (human, emp) 100 units/ml. Net price 10-ml vial = £6.95
▼ **Human Protaphane®** (Novo)
Injection, isophane insulin (human, emp) 100 units/ml. Net price 10-ml vial = £7.15
▼ **Humulin I®** (Lilly)
Injection, isophane insulin (human, prb) 100 units/ml. Net price 10-ml vial = £6.95

Mixed human sequence insulins
▼ **Human Actraphane®** (Novo)
Injection, isophane insulin (human, emp) 70%, neutral insulin (human, emp) 30%. 100 units/ml. Net price 10-ml vial = £7.15
▼ **Human Initard 50/50®** (Nordisk Wellcome)
Injection, isophane insulin (human, emp) 50%, neutral insulin (human, emp) 50%. 100 units/ml. Net price 10-ml vial = £6.95
▼ **Human Mixtard 30/70®** (Nordisk Wellcome)
Injection, isophane insulin (human, emp) 70%, neutral insulin (human, emp) 30%. 100 units/ml. Net price 10-ml vial = £6.95
▼ **Humulin M1®** (Lilly)
Injection, isophane insulin (human, prb) 90%, neutral insulin (human, prb) 10%. 100 units/ml. Net price 10-ml vial = £6.95
▼ **Humulin M2®** (Lilly)
Injection, isophane insulin (human, prb) 80%, neutral insulin (human, prb) 20%. 100 units/ml. Net price 10-ml vial = £6.95
▼ **Humulin M3®** (Lilly)
Injection, isophane insulin (human, prb) 70%, neutral insulin (human, prb) 30%. 100 units/ml. Net price 10-ml vial = £6.95
▼ **Humulin M4®** (Lilly)
Injection, isophane insulin (human, prb) 60%, neutral insulin (human, prb) 40%. 100 units/ml. Net price 10-ml vial = £6.95

PROTAMINE ZINC INSULIN INJECTION
Indications: diabetes mellitus (long acting)
Cautions; Side-effects: see under Acid Insulin Injection (section 6.1.1.1); protamine may cause allergic reactions; see also notes above
Dose: by subcutaneous injection, according to patient's requirements

---

Hypurin Protamine Zinc® (CP)
Injection, protamine zinc insulin (bovine, highly
purified) 100 units/ml. Net price 10-ml vial =
£7.40

6.1.2   Oral antidiabetic drugs

6.1.2.1 Sulphonylureas
6.1.2.2 Biguanides
6.1.2.3 Guar gum

Oral antidiabetic drugs should not be used until
patients have been shown not to respond
adequately to at least one month's restriction of
energy and carbohydrate intake. They should be
used to augment the effect of diet, and not to
replace it.

6.1.2.1   SULPHONYLUREAS AND RELATED DRUGS

The sulphonylureas act mainly by augmenting
insulin secretion and consequently are effective
only when some residual pancreatic beta-cell
activity is present. All may lead to hypoglycaemia
4 hours or more after food but this is usually an
indication of overdose. Hypoglycaemia is relatively uncommon and those most vulnerable are
elderly patients (in whom chlorpropamide should
not be used).

Tolbutamide (Rastinon®, etc.) has a short
duration of action and is usually given twice daily.
Chlorpropamide (Diabinese®, etc.) has a more
prolonged action, and need only be given once
daily. It may cause prolonged hypoglycaemia,
particularly in the elderly and in those with renal
disease, in whom it should not be used. A short-
acting drug such as tolbutamide is preferable in
the elderly.

Glibenclamide (Daonil®, Euglucon®, etc.) has
a duration between tolbutamide and chlorpropamide, but is usually given once daily. Other
sulphonylureas are acetohexamide (Dimelor®),
gliclazide (Diamicron®), glipizide (Glibenese®,
Minodiab®), gliquidone (Glurenorm®), and tolazamide (Tolanase®).

Glymidine (Gondafon®) is a related compound
which shows most of the properties of the
sulphonylureas. It may be tried cautiously in sulphonylurea hypersensitivity.

CAUTIONS AND CONTRA-INDICATIONS. These drugs
tend to encourage weight gain and should only be
prescribed if poor control and symptoms persist
despite adequate attempts at dieting. They should
not be used during breast-feeding, and caution is
needed in the elderly and those with renal failure
because of the hazard of hypoglycaemia. The
short-acting tolbutamide may be used in renal
impairment, as may gliquidone and gliclazide as
the latter are principally metabolised and inactivated in the liver.

Insulin therapy should be instituted temporarily
during intercurrent illness (such as myocardial
infarction, coma, infection, and trauma) and during surgery since control of diabetes with the
sulphonylureas is often inadequate in such
circumstances. Insulin therapy is also usually substituted during pregnancy. Sulphonylureas are
contra-indicated in the presence of ketoacidosis.
Drug interactions: see Appendix 1 (section 6.1).

SIDE-EFFECTS. These are generally mild and
infrequent and include gastro-intestinal disturbances and headache.

Chlorpropamide may cause facial flushing after
drinking alcohol; this effect is not normally wit-
nessed with other sulphonylureas.

Sensitivity reactions (usually in first 6–8 weeks
of therapy) include transient rashes which rarely
progress to erythema multiforme and exfoliative
dermatitis, fever, and jaundice; photosensitivity
has also rarely been reported with chlorpropamide. Blood disorders are rare but include
thrombocytopenia, agranulocytosis, and aplastic
anaemia.

ACETOHEXAMIDE
Indications: diabetes mellitus
Cautions; Contra-indications; Side-effects: see
  notes above. Drug interactions: see Appendix
  1 (section 6.1)
Dose: initially 0.25–1.5 g daily, adjusted according to response; up to 500 mg given as a single
  daily dose, higher doses divided

PoM **Dimelor®** (Lilly)
Tablets, yellow, scored, acetohexamide 500 mg.
Net price 20 = £1.08

CHLORPROPAMIDE
Indications: diabetes mellitus (for use in diabetes
  insipidus, see section 6.5.2)
Cautions; Contra-indications; Side-effects: see
  notes above. Drug interactions: see Appendix
  1 (sections 2.2, 6.1)
Dose: initially 250 mg daily (elderly patients 100–
  125 mg but avoid—see notes above), adjusted
  according to response; max. 500 mg daily; taken
  with breakfast

PoM **Chlorpropamide** (Non-proprietary)
Tablets, chlorpropamide 100 mg, net price 20 =
18p; 250 mg, 20 = 27p. Label: 4
PoM **Diabinese®** (Pfizer)
Tablets, scored, chlorpropamide 100 mg, net
price 20 = 40p; 250 mg, 20 = 88p. Label: 4
PoM **Glymese®** (DDSA)
Tablets, scored, chlorpropamide 250 mg. Net
price 20 = 56p. Label: 4

GLIBENCLAMIDE
Indications: diabetes mellitus
Cautions; Contra-indications; Side-effects: see
  notes above. Drug interactions: see Appendix
  1 (section 6.1).
Dose: initially 5 mg daily (elderly patients
  2.5 mg), adjusted according to response; max.
  15 mg daily; taken with breakfast

ᴾoM **Glibenclamide** (Non-proprietary)
Tablets, glibenclamide 2.5 mg, net price 20 =
62p; 5 mg, 20 = 68p

ᴾoM **Calabren**® (Berk)
Tablets, scored, glibenclamide 5 mg. Net price
20 = £1.02

ᴾoM **Daonil**® (Hoechst)
Tablets, scored, glibenclamide 5 mg. Net price
20 = £1.93

ᴼM **Semi-Daonil**® (Hoechst)
Tablets, scored, glibenclamide 2.5 mg. Net price
20 = £1.16

ᴼM **Euglucon**® (Roussel)
Tablets, glibenclamide 2.5 mg, net price 20 =
£1.16; 5 mg (scored), 20 = £1.93

ᴼM **Libanil**® (APS)
Tablets, glibenclamide 2.5 mg, net price 20 =
86p; 5 mg (scored), 20 = £1·01

ᴼM **Malix**® (Lagap)
Tablets, glibenclamide 2.5 mg, net price 20 =
58p; 5 mg, 20 = 60p

GLICLAZIDE
Indications: diabetes mellitus
Cautions; Contra-indications; Side-effects: see
notes above. Drug interactions: see Appendix
1 (section 6.1)
Dose: initially, 40–80 mg daily, adjusted according to response; up to 160 mg as a single dose,
with breakfast; higher doses divided; max.
320 mg daily

ᴼM **Diamicron**® (Servier)
Tablets, scored, gliclazide 80 mg. Net price 20 =
£2.16

GLIPIZIDE
Indications: diabetes mellitus
Cautions; Contra-indications; Side-effects: see
notes above. Drug interactions: see Appendix
1 (section 6.1)
Dose: initially 2.5–5 mg daily, adjusted according
to response; max. 40 mg daily; up to 15 mg
may be given as a single dose before breakfast;
higher doses divided

ᴼM **Glibenese**® (Pfizer)
Tablets, scored, glipizide 5 mg. Net price 20 =
£1.18

ᴼM **Minodiab**® (Farmitalia Carlo Erba)
Tablets, glipizide 2.5 mg, net price 20 = 93p;
5 mg (scored), 20 = £1.31

GLIQUIDONE
Indications: diabetes mellitus
Cautions; Contra-indications; Side-effects: see
notes above. Drug interactions: see Appendix
1 (section 6.1)
Dose: initially 15 mg daily before breakfast,
adjusted to 45–60 mg daily in 2 or 3 divided
doses; max. single dose 60 mg, max. daily dose
180 mg

ᴾoM **Glurenorm**® (Winthrop)
Tablets, scored, gliquidone 30 mg. Net price 20 =
£2.65

GLYMIDINE
Indications: diabetes mellitus
Cautions; Contra-indications; Side-effects: see
notes above. Drug interactions: see Appendix
1 (section 6.1)
Dose: initially 1–1.5 g daily, with breakfast,
adjusted according to response; max. 2 g daily
(1.5 g at breakfast and 500 mg in late afternoon)

ᴾoM **Gondafon**® (Schering)
Product discontinued

TOLAZAMIDE
Indications: diabetes mellitus
Cautions; Contra-indications; Side-effects: see
notes above. Drug interactions: see Appendix
1 (section 6.1)
Dose: initially 100–250 mg daily with breakfast
adjusted according to response; max. 1 g daily;
higher doses divided

ᴾoM **Tolanase**® (Upjohn)
Tablets, scored, tolazamide 100 mg. Net price
20 = £1.00
Tablets, scored, tolazamide 250 mg. Net price
20 = £2.18

TOLBUTAMIDE
Indications: diabetes mellitus
Cautions; Contra-indications; Side-effects: see
notes above. Drug interactions: see Appendix
1 (section 6.1)
Dose: 0.5–1.5 g (max. 2 g) daily in divided doses
(see notes above)

ᴾoM **Tolbutamide** (Non-proprietary)
Tablets, tolbutamide 500 mg. Net price 20 = 29p
ᴾoM **Glyconon**® (DDSA)
Tablets, scored, tolbutamide 500 mg. Net price
20 = 24p
ᴾoM **Rastinon**® (Hoechst)
Tablets, scored, tolbutamide 500 mg. Net price
20 = 65p

6.1.2.2 BIGUANIDES

Metformin (Glucophage®), the only available
biguanide, acts in a different way from the sulphonylureas, and is not interchangeable with
them. It exerts its effect mainly by decreasing
gluconeogenesis and by increasing peripheral utilisation of glucose, and is only effective in diabetics
with functioning pancreatic islet cells. Metformin
is used in the treatment of non-insulin-dependent
diabetics when strict dieting and sulphonylurea
treatment have failed to control diabetes,
especially in overweight patients, in whom it may,
if necessary, be used first. It does not exert a
hypoglycaemic action in non-diabetic subjects
unless given in overdose.

Metformin is not free from the hazard of lactic acidosis which, however, occurs almost exclusively in renal failure patients, in whom it should not be used.

METFORMIN HYDROCHLORIDE

Indications: diabetes mellitus (see notes above)
Cautions: see notes above. Drug interactions: see Appendix 1 (section 6.1)
Contra-indications: renal or hepatic failure, predisposition to lactic acidosis, heart failure, severe infection or trauma, dehydration, alcoholism; pregnancy, breast-feeding
Side-effects: anorexia, nausea, vomiting, diarrhoea (usually transient), lactic acidosis (withdraw treatment), decreased vitamin-B$_{12}$ absorption
Dose: 500 mg every 8 hours *or* 850 mg every 12 hours with or after food; max. 3 g daily in divided doses

PoM **Metformin** (Non-proprietary)
Tablets, metformin hydrochloride 500 mg, net price 20 = 48p; 850 mg, 20 = 80p. Label: 21
PoM **Glucophage**® (Lipha)
Tablets, f/c, metformin hydrochloride 500 mg, net price 20 = 48p; 850 mg, 20 = 80p. Label: 21
PoM **Orabet**® (Lagap)
Tablets, f/c, metformin hydrochloride 500 mg, net price 20 = 48p; 850 mg, 20 = 80p. Label: 21

6.1.2.3 GUAR GUM

Guar gum, if taken in adequate quantities, results in some reduction of postprandial plasma-glucose concentrations in diabetes mellitus, probably by retarding carbohydrate absorption. It is also used to relieve symptoms of the dumping syndrome.

Severe flatulence limits its use.

GUAR GUM

Indications: see notes above
Cautions: maintain adequate fluid intake. Drug interactions: see Appendix 1 (section *5.1*)
Contra-indications: gastro-intestinal obstruction
Side-effects: flatulence, abdominal distension, intestinal obstruction

Glucotard® (MCP)
Mini-tablets, guar gum 5 g/sachet. Net price 20 sachets = £2.15. Label: 27, counselling advised, food
Dose: 5 g up to 3 times daily immediately before main meals washed down in portions with 250 ml of fluid
Guarem® (Rybar)
Granules, ivory, sugar-free, guar gum 5 g/sachet. Net price 20 sachets = £2.50. Label: 13, counselling advised, food
Dose: 5 g stirred into 200 ml fluid 3 times daily immediately before main meals (or sprinkled on food and eaten accompanied by 200 ml fluid)

Guarina® (Norgine)
Granules, dispersible, guar gum 5 g/sachet. Net price 20 sachets = £2.98. Label: 13, counselling advised, food
Dose: 5 g stirred into 150 ml fluid immediately before main meals up to 3 times daily (or sprinkled on food and eaten accompanied by 150 ml of fluid)

6.1.3 Treatment of diabetic ketoacidosis

A clear solution (**acid insulin injection** or **neutral insulin injection**) is the only form of insulin that may be given intravenously and it should be used in the management of diabetic ketoacidotic and hyperosmolar nonketotic coma. It is preferable to use the type of insulin (highly purified or human sequence) that the patient has been using previously. It is necessary to achieve and to maintain an adequate plasma-insulin concentration until the metabolic disturbance is brought under control.

If a slow infusion pump is available, insulin is best given by the intravenous route; a single bolus (however large) will only achieve an adequate concentration for a short period of time. Adequate plasma concentrations are usually maintained with infusion rates of 6 units/hour for adults and 0.1 units/kg/hour for children. Insulin is diluted to 1 unit/ml (care in mixing: see Appendix 2).

If the response is judged inadequate the infusion rate may be doubled or quadrupled. When plasma glucose has fallen to 10 mmol/litre the rate of infusion can be dropped to about 0.02 units/kg/hour (1 to 2 units/hour for adults) and continued until the patient is ready to take food by mouth. The insulin infusion should not be stopped before subcutaneous insulin is started.

If facilities for administering insulin by continuous infusion are inadequate it may be given by intramuscular injection. Absorption of insulin after intramuscular administration is usually rapid but may be impaired in patients who are hypotensive or who have poor peripheral circulation. An initial loading dose of 20 units is followed by 6 units given every hour until the plasma glucose concentration is less than 10 mmol/litre. Doses are then given by intramuscular injection every 2 hours.

In the presence of hypotension and poor tissue perfusion the intravenous route of insulin administration is preferable. Depots of insulin may build up during treatment and late hypoglycaemia should be watched for and treated appropriately.

6.1.4 Treatment of hypoglycaemia

Initially, glucose or 3 or 4 lumps of sugar should be taken with a little water. If necessary, this may be repeated in 10 to 15 minutes.

If hypoglycaemia causes unconsciousness, up to 50 ml of **50% glucose intravenous infusion** should be given intravenously (see section 9.2.2).

Glucagon can be given as an alternative to parenteral glucose in hypoglycaemia. It is a polypeptide hormone produced by the alpha cells of the islets of Langerhans. Its action is to increase plasma glucose concentration by mobilising glycogen stored in the liver.

Glucagon is used to treat acute hypoglycaemic reactions and it has the advantage that it can be injected by any route (intramuscular, subcutaneous, or intravenous) in a dose of 1 mg (1 unit) in circumstances when an intravenous injection of glucose would be difficult or impossible to administer.

It may be issued to close relatives of insulin-treated patients for emergency use in hypoglycaemic attacks. It is often advisable to prescribe on an 'if necessary' basis to all hospitalised insulin-treated patients, so that it may be given rapidly by the nurses during an hypoglycaemic emergency. If not effective in 20 minutes intravenous glucose should be given.

GLUCAGON

Indications: acute hypoglycaemia
Cautions: see notes above. Ineffective in chronic hypoglycaemia, starvation, and adrenal insufficiency
Contra-indications: insulinoma, phaeochromocytoma, glucagonoma
Side-effects: nausea, vomiting, rarely hypersensitivity reactions
Dose: by subcutaneous, intramuscular, or intravenous injection, adults and children 0.5–1 unit repeated after 20 minutes if necessary
Note. 1 unit of glucagon = 1 mg of glucagon or glucagon hydrochloride

PoM **Glucagon Injection,** powder for reconstitution, glucagon (as hydrochloride, with lactose). Net price 1-unit vial (Lilly) = £4.30; (Novo) = £4.19; 10-unit vial (Novo) = £24.57 (all with diluent)

CHRONIC HYPOGLYCAEMIA

Diazoxide (Eudemine®), administered by mouth, is useful in the management of patients with chronic hypoglycaemia from excess endogenous insulin secretion, either from an islet cell tumour or islet cell hyperplasia. It has no place in the management of acute hypoglycaemia.

DIAZOXIDE

Indications: chronic intractable hypoglycaemia (for use in hypertensive crisis see section 2.5.1)
Cautions: ischaemic heart disease, pregnancy, labour, impaired renal function; haematological examinations and blood pressure monitoring required during prolonged treatment. Drug interactions: see Appendix 1 (section 6.1)
Side-effects: anorexia, nausea, vomiting, hyperuricaemia, hypotension, oedema, tachycardia, arrhythmias, extrapyramidal effects; hypertrichosis on prolonged treatment
Dose: by mouth, adults and children, initially 5 mg/kg daily in 2–3 divided doses

PoM **Eudemine®** (A&H)
Tablets, s/c, diazoxide 50 mg. Net price 20 = £1.62

6.1.5 Treatment of diabetic neuropathy

Optimal diabetic control is beneficial for the management of *painful neuropathy.* Most patients should be treated with insulin, and relief can probably be accelerated by continuous insulin infusion. **Non-opioid analgesics** such as aspirin and paracetamol (see section 4.7.1) are indicated. Relief may also be obtained with the **tricyclic antidepressants,** amitriptyline, imipramine, and nortriptyline (see section 4.3.1) with or without a low dose of **phenothiazine** (see section 4.2). **Carbamazepine** (see section 4.8.1) may be useful; phenytoin, mexiletine, and lignocaine have also been used but need further evaluation. In *autonomic neuropathy* diabetic diarrhoea can often be aborted by two or three doses of **tetracycline** 250 mg (see section 5.1.3). Otherwise **codeine phosphate** (see section 1.4.2) is the best agent, but all other antidiarrhoeal preparations can be tried.

In *postural hypotension* an increased salt intake and the use of the **mineralocorticoid** fludrocortisone 100 to 400 micrograms daily (see section 6.3.1) help by increasing plasma volume but uncomfortable oedema is a common side-effect. Fludrocortisone can also be combined with **flurbiprofen** (see section 10.1.1) and **ephedrine hydrochloride** (see section 3.1.1.2), and the intrinsic alpha-stimulant activity of the **beta-blocker** pindolol (see section 2.4) may help.

Gustatory sweating can be treated with **anticholinergics** (see section 1.2), poldine methylsulphate is the best but propantheline bromide may also be used; side-effects are common. **Ephedrine hydrochloride** 30 to 60 mg three times daily offers impressive relief in some patients with *neuropathic oedema.*

6.2 Thyroid and antithyroid drugs

6.2.1 Thyroid hormones
6.2.2 Antithyroid drugs

6.2.1 Thyroid hormones

Thyroid hormones are used in hypothyroidism (myxoedema), and also in diffuse non-toxic goitre, lymphadenoid goitre, and thyroid carcinoma. Neonatal hypothyroidism requires prompt treatment for normal development.

Thyroxine sodium (Eltroxin®) is the treatment of choice for maintenance therapy. The initial dose should not exceed 100 micrograms daily, preferably before breakfast, or 25 to 50 micrograms in elderly patients or those with cardiac disease, increased by 25 to 50 micrograms at intervals of 2 to 4 weeks. The usual maintenance dose to relieve hypothyroidism is 100 to 200 micrograms daily which can be administered as a single dose.

In infants a daily dose of 10 micrograms/kg up to a maximum of 50 micrograms daily should be given; subsequent therapy should reach 100 micrograms daily by 5 years and adult doses by 12 years, guided by clinical response, growth assessment, and measurements of plasma thyroxine and thyroid-stimulating hormone.

Liothyronine sodium (Tertroxin®) has a similar action to thyroxine but is more rapidly metabolised; 20 micrograms is equivalent to 100 micrograms of thyroxine. Its effects develop after a few hours and disappear within 24 to 48 hours of discontinuing treatment. It may be used in severe hypothyroid states when a rapid response is desired.

Liothyronine by intravenous injection is the treatment of choice in hypothyroid coma. Adjunctive therapy includes intravenous fluids, hydrocortisone, and antibiotics; assisted ventilation is often required.

Dried **thyroid** should **not** be used as its effects are unpredictable.

LIOTHYRONINE SODIUM
(L-Tri-iodothyronine sodium)
Indications: see notes above
Cautions: adrenal insufficiency. Drug interactions: see Appendix 1 (sections *2.8*, *2.8B*, *6.2*)
Contra-indications: angina, cardiovascular disorders
Side-effects: arrhythmias, anginal pain, tachycardia, cramps in skeletal muscles, headache, restlessness, excitability, flushing, sweating, diarrhoea, excessive weight loss
Dose: by mouth, initially 10–20 micrograms daily in 2–3 divided doses gradually increased to 20 micrograms 3 times daily; elderly patients should receive smaller initial doses, gradually increased; CHILD, adult dose reduced in proportion to body-weight
By slow intravenous injection, hypothyroid coma, 5-20 micrograms repeated 12-hourly or more frequently (4-hourly if necessary); alternatively 50 micrograms initially then 25 micrograms 8-hourly, reducing to 25 micrograms twice daily

PoM **Tertroxin**® (Glaxo)
Tablets, scored, liothyronine sodium 20 micrograms. Net price 20 = 18p
PoM **Triiodothyronine** (Glaxo)
Injection, powder for reconstitution, liothyronine sodium (with dextran). Net price 20-microgram amp = £3.60

THYROXINE SODIUM
Indications: hypothyroidism
Cautions; Contra-indications; Side-effects: see under Liothyronine Sodium; has a delayed effect and cumulative action
Dose: see notes above

PoM **Thyroxine** (Non-proprietary)
Tablets, thyroxine sodium 25 micrograms, net price 20 = 7p; 50 micrograms, 20 = 4p; 100 micrograms, 20 = 5p
PoM **Eltroxin**® (Glaxo)
Tablets, scored, thyroxine sodium 50 micrograms, net price 20 = 5p; 100 micrograms, 20 = 6p

6.2.2   Antithyroid drugs

Antithyroid drugs are used to prepare patients for thyroidectomy. They are also used for prolonged periods in the hope of inducing life-long remission. In the United Kingdom carbimazole is the most commonly used drug. Propylthiouracil may be used in patients who suffer sensitivity reactions to carbimazole as sensitivity is rarely displayed to both drugs. Both drugs act primarily by interfering with the synthesis of thyroid hormones.

Carbimazole (Neo-Mercazole®) should be given in a daily dose of 30 to 60 mg and maintained at this dose until the patient becomes euthyroid, usually 4 to 8 weeks; the dose may then be progressively reduced to a maintenance dose of between 5 and 15 mg daily; therapy is usually given for 18 months. Children may be given 15 mg daily, adjusted according to response. Rashes are common, and **propylthiouracil** may then be substituted. Pruritus and rashes can be treated with antihistamines without discontinuing therapy, whereas patients should be advised to report any sore throat immediately because of the rare complication of agranulocytosis.

Antithyroid drugs may be given once daily although divided doses are still commonly used. Over-treatment with the rapid development of hypothyroidism is not uncommon and should be avoided particularly during pregnancy since it can cause fetal goitre.

A combination of carbimazole, 20 to 60 mg daily with thyroxine, 50 to 150 micrograms daily, may be used in a *blocking-replacement regimen*; therapy is again usually given for 18 months. The blocking-replacement regimen is not suitable during pregnancy.

Unless operation or use of radioactive iodine is planned, treatment should be for at least a year.

Before partial thyroidectomy **iodine** may be given for 10 to 14 days in addition to carbimazole or propylthiouracil to assist control and reduce vascularity of the thyroid. Iodine should not be used for long-term treatment since its antithyroid action tends to diminish.

Radioactive sodium iodide (^{131}I) solution is used increasingly for the treatment of thyrotoxicosis at all ages, particularly where medical therapy or compliance is a problem, in patients with cardiac disease, and in patients who relapse after thyroidectomy.

Propranolol is useful for rapid relief of symptoms and may be used in conjunction with antithyroid drugs or as an adjunct to radioactive iodine treatment. In addition beta-blockers are useful in neonatal thyrotoxicosis and in supraventricular arrhythmias due to hyperthyroidism. Propranolol may be used in conjuction with iodine to prepare mildly thyrotoxic patients for operation but it is still preferable to render the patient euthyroid with carbimazole before surgery. Laboratory tests of thyroid function are not altered by beta-blockers. Most experience in treating thyrotoxicosis has been gained with propranolol but **nadolol** and **sotalol** are also of use. For doses and preparations see section 2.4.

Thyrotoxic crisis ('thyroid storm') requires emergency treatment with intravenous administration of fluids, propranolol (5 mg) and hydrocortisone (100 mg every 6 hours, as sodium phosphate or succinate), as well as oral iodine solution and carbimazole or propylthiouracil which may need to be administered by nasogastric tube.

For the use of **protirelin** in the diagnosis of hyperthyroidism see section 6.7.2.

PREGNANCY AND BREAST-FEEDING. Radioactive iodine therapy is contra-indicated during pregnancy. Propylthiouracil and carbimazole can be given. Both drugs cross the placenta and in high doses may cause fetal goitre and hypothyroidism. Rarely, carbimazole has been associated with aplasia cutis of the neonate.

Carbimazole and propylthiouracil transfer to breast milk but this does not preclude breast-feeding as long as neonatal development is closely monitored.

CARBIMAZOLE

Indications: hyperthyroidism
Cautions: large goitre; pregnancy, breast-feeding (see notes)
Side-effects: nausea, headache, rashes and pruritus, arthralgia; rarely alopecia, agranulocytosis, jaundice
Dose: see notes above

PoM **Neo-Mercazole 5**® (Nicholas)
Tablets, pink, scored, carbimazole 5 mg. Net price 20 = 42p
PoM **Neo-Mercazole 20**® (Nicholas)
Tablets, pink, carbimazole 20 mg. Net price 20 = £1.71

IODINE AND IODIDE

Indications: thyrotoxicosis (pre-operative)
Cautions: pregnancy, children; not for long-term treatment
Contra-indications: breast-feeding
Side-effects: hypersensitivity reactions including coryza-like symptoms, headache, lachrymation, conjunctivitis, pain in salivary glands, laryngitis, bronchitis, rashes; on prolonged treatment depression, insomnia, impotence; goitre in infants of mothers taking iodides

Aqueous Iodine Oral Solution (Lugol's Solution), iodine 5%, potassium iodide 10% in purified water, freshly boiled and cooled, total iodine 130 mg/ml. Net price 100 ml = £1.32. Label: 27
Dose: 0.1–0.3 ml 3 times daily well diluted with milk or water
Potassium Iodide Tablets (CP)
Tablets, potassium iodide 60 mg. Net price 20 = £1.12. Label: 27

PROPYLTHIOURACIL

Indications: hyperthyroidism
Cautions; Side-effects: see under Carbimazole; also rarely tendency to haemorrhage; reduce dose in renal impairment
Dose: 300–450 mg daily in divided doses

PoM **Propylthiouracil Tablets,** propylthiouracil 50 mg. Net price 20 = £1.20

6.3 Corticosteroids

6.3.1 Replacement therapy
6.3.2 Suppression of disease processes
6.3.3 Disadvantages of corticosteroids
6.3.4 Clinical management

6.3.1 Replacement therapy

The adrenal cortex normally secretes hydrocortisone (cortisol) which has predominantly glucocorticoid activity as well as weak mineralocorticoid actions. It also secretes the mineralocorticoid aldosterone.

In deficiency states, physiological replacement is best achieved with a combination of oral **hydrocortisone** (section 6.3.4) and the mineralocorticoid **fludrocortisone** (Florinef®); hydrocortisone alone does not usually provide sufficient mineralocorticoid activity for complete replacement. Cortisone is no longer used in replacement therapy.

Management with the more potent synthetic glucocorticoids such as prednisolone (with fludrocortisone) though practicable, offers no advantage. They tend to have less mineralocorticoid activity than hydrocortisone and their greater potency is only of advantage in the treatment of inflammatory and neoplastic disease.

In *Addison's disease* or following adrenalectomy, **hydrocortisone** 20 to 30 mg daily by mouth is usually required. This should be given in 2 doses, the larger in the morning and the smaller in the evening, mimicking the normal diurnal rhythm of cortisol secretion. The optimum daily dose should be determined for each individual on the basis of clinical response and also, if possible, by monitoring the plasma-cortisol concentration. Glucocorticoid therapy should be supplemented by fludrocortisone 50 to 300 micrograms daily.

In *acute adrenocortical insufficiency*, **hydrocortisone** is given intravenously (as sodium phosphate or succinate) in doses of 100 mg every 6 to 8 hours in sodium chloride intravenous infusion 0.9%.

In *hypopituitarism* glucocorticoids should be given as in adrenocortical insufficiency, but since the production of aldosterone is also regulated by the renin-angiotensin system a mineralocorticoid is not usually required. Additional replacement therapy with thyroxine (section 6.2.1) and sex hormones (section 6.4) should be given as indicated by the pattern of hormone deficiency that is present.

Corticosteroid cover for *adrenalectomy*, *hypophysectomy* or operations on patients on long-term treatment with corticosteroids is determined logically from the knowledge that in a normal person major stress will not lead to the secretion of more than 300 mg of cortisol in 24 hours. Once the stress is over, cortisol production rapidly returns to the usual level of approximately 20 mg per 24 hours. A simple way of mimicking this is to administer hydrocortisone, initially parenterally but changing to oral therapy once this is possible.

On the day of operation hydrocortisone 100 mg is given intramuscularly (as sodium phosphate or succinate) with the premedication, and repeated every 8 hours. In the absence of any complications, the dose can be halved every 24 hours until a normal maintenance dose of 25 mg per 24 hours is reached on the 5th postoperative day. In the case of adrenalectomy it is not necessary to start mineralocorticoid therapy immediately and this can be withheld until the patient can take tablets.

Dexamethasone and **betamethasone** have little if any mineralocorticoid action and their long duration of action makes them particularly suitable for suppressing corticotrophin secretion in *congenital adrenal hyperplasia* where the dose should be tailored to the individual by measurement of adrenal androgens and 17-hydroxyprogesterone. In common with all glucocorticoids their suppressive action on the hypothalamic-pituitary-adrenal axis is greatest and most prolonged when they are given at night. In normal subjects a single dose of 1 to 2 mg of dexamethasone at night, depending on weight, is sufficient to inhibit corticotrophin secretion for 24 hours. This is the basis of the 'overnight dexamethasone suppression test' for diagnosing Cushing's syndrome.

Although most types of *Cushing's syndrome* are treated surgically, that which occasionally accompanies carcinoma of the bronchus is not usually amenable to surgery. **Metyrapone** (section 6.7.2), which interferes directly with steroid synthesis in the adrenal glands, has been found helpful in controlling the symptoms of the disease; it is also used in other forms of Cushing's syndrome to prepare the patient for surgery. The dosages used are either low, and tailored to cortisol production, or high, in which case corticosteroid replacement therapy is also needed. Metyrapone should only be used under specialist advice.

See also trilostane (section 6.7.4) and aminoglutethimide (see section 8.3.4).

FLUDROCORTISONE ACETATE

Indications: mineralocorticoid replacement in adrenocortical insufficiency

Cautions; Contra-indications; Side-effects: section 6.3.3

Dose: adrenocortical insufficiency, 50–300 micrograms daily; CHILD 5 micrograms/kg daily

PoM **Florinef**® (Squibb)
Tablets, pink, scored, fludrocortisone acetate 100 micrograms. Net price 20 = 96p. Label: 10 steroid card

6.3.2 Suppression of disease processes

Betamethasone, dexamethasone, hydrocortisone, prednisolone, and prednisone are used for their anti-inflammatory effect; Table 2 shows equivalent anti-inflammatory doses.

Table 2: Equivalent Doses of Glucocorticoids

Drug	Equivalent anti-inflammatory dose (mg)
Betamethasone	0.75
Cortisone acetate	25
Dexamethasone	0.75
Hydrocortisone	20
Methylprednisolone	4
Prednisolone	5
Prednisone	5
Triamcinolone	4

High potency is of no advantage, though the effect on water and electrolyte retention is important. **Prednisolone** is the glucocorticoid most commonly used by mouth for continued treatment. **Prednisone** is only active after conversion in the body to prednisolone. **Betamethasone** and **dexamethasone** are as satisfactory. All must be given in divided doses for a continuous effect. Cortisone acetate and hydrocortisone are not used for inflammatory disease suppression, as they cause fluid retention owing to their higher mineralocorticoid content (section 6.3.1). Use can be made of the mineralocorticoid activity of fludrocortisone to treat postural hypotension in autonomic neuropathy (see section 6.1.5).

Very high doses of corticosteroids have been given by intravenous injection in *septic shock*. However a recent study (using methylprednisolone sodium succinate) did not demonstrate efficacy and, moreover, suggested a higher mortality in some subsets of patients given the high-dose corticosteroid therapy.

Betamethasone and dexamethasone are used in conditions when water retention would be a disadvantage, as for example in treating traumatic *cerebral oedema* with doses of 12 to 20 mg daily.

In acute hypersensitivity reactions such as *angioedema* of the upper respiratory tract and *anaphylactic shock*, corticosteroids are indicated as an adjunct to emergency treatment with adrenaline (see section 3.4.3). In such cases **hydrocortisone** (as sodium succinate or sodium phosphate) by intravenous injection in a dose of 100 to 300 mg may be required.

Corticosteroids are also indicated with broncho-dilator therapy in the emergency treatment of severe acute asthma (see section 3.1.1).

The action of corticosteroids in suppressing inflammatory reactions may be useful in conditions such as *rheumatoid arthritis*, *rheumatic fever*, *chronic active hepatitis*, *sarcoidosis*, *ulcerative colitis*, and *Crohn's disease*. The prognosis of serious conditions such as *systemic lupus erythematosus* and *polyarteritis nodosa* can be improved. The effects of the disease process may be suppressed and symptoms relieved, but the underlying condition is not cured, although it may ultimately burn itself out. It is usual to commence therapy in these conditions at fairly high dose, such as 40 to 60 mg prednisolone daily, and then to reduce the dose to the lowest commensurate with disease control. If serious side-effects occur in response to the large doses of corticosteroids required to suppress the disease process, it is sometimes possible to reduce the dose of corticosteroid by giving a small dose of an immunosuppressive drug (see section 8.2.1).

Because corticosteroids reduce antibody formation, they may be used to suppress or modify *allergic reactions*. This may benefit some types of *asthma* and *skin diseases*. It may also lead to remissions of acquired *haemolytic anaemia*, and some cases of the *nephrotic syndrome* and *thrombocytopenic purpura*.

For the use of the corticosteroids in the treatment of *reticuloses* and some types of *leukaemia*, see section 8.2.2.

Corticosteroids are extensively used on the skin, and also as aerosols, eye-drops, enemas, and intra-articular injections. The formulation here is of the greatest importance and partly determines the choice of drug. A potent drug such as betamethasone valerate may be more effective than a weaker one such as hydrocortisone, regardless of strength.

The use of corticosteroids in the treatment of many other disease processes is described elsewhere in the following sections:

colon and rectum, sections 1.5 and 1.7.2
asthma, section 3.2
rheumatic diseases, section 10.1.2
eye, section 11.4
otitis externa, section 12.1.1
allergic rhinitis, section 12.2.1
aphthous ulcers, section 12.3.1
skin, section 13.4

6.3.3 Disadvantages of corticosteroids

Overdosage or prolonged use may exaggerate some of the normal physiological actions of corticosteroids. Mineralocorticoid effects include hypertension, sodium and water retention, potassium loss, and muscle weakness. Glucocorticoid effects include diabetes and osteoporosis which is a danger, particularly in the elderly, as it may result in vertebral collapse. Mental disturbances may occur; a serious paranoid state or depression with risk of suicide may be induced, particularly in patients with a history of mental disorder.

Euphoria is frequently observed. Corticosteroid therapy is weakly linked with peptic ulceration; the use of soluble or enteric-coated preparations to reduce the risk is speculative only. Mineralocorticoid effects are most marked with fludrocortisone, but are significant with cortisone, hydrocortisone, corticotrophin, and tetracosactrin. Mineralocorticoid effects are negligible with the high potency glucocorticoids betamethasone, dexamethasone, methylprednisolone, and triamcinolone and occur only slightly with prednisolone and prednisone.

In children, administration of corticosteroids may result in suppression of growth. Corticosteroids given in high dosage during pregnancy may affect adrenal development in the child.

Modification of tissue reactions may result in spread of infection. Suppression of clinical signs may allow septicaemia or tuberculosis to reach an advanced stage before being recognised. Systemic corticosteroid therapy should be avoided in patients with psoriasis, as subsequent reduction in dose is commonly followed by a severe and persistent exacerbation.

ADRENAL SUPPRESSION. The administration of exogenous corticosteroids suppresses the secretion of corticotrophin and may lead to adrenal atrophy which can persist for years after stopping prolonged corticosteroid therapy; any illness or surgical emergency may then require further corticosteroid therapy to compensate for lack of sufficient adrenocortical response.

High doses of corticosteroids may cause Cushing's syndrome, with moon face, striae, and acne; it is usually reversible on withdrawal of treatment, but this must always be gradually tapered to avoid symptoms of acute adrenal insufficiency (see 'steroid card', section 6.3.4).

Drug interactions: see Appendix 1 (sections *2.2*, *2.5*, *4.7*, *6.1*, 6.3).

6.3.4 Clinical management

Corticosteroids should not be used unless the benefits justify the hazards and the lowest dose that will produce an acceptable response should be used. Dosage varies widely in different diseases and in different patients. Whenever possible local treatment with intra-articular injections, inhalations, eye-drops, or enemas should be used in preference to systemic treatment.

If the use of corticosteroids can save or prolong life, as in exfoliative dermatitis, pemphigus, or acute leukaemia, high doses must be given, as the complications of therapy are likely to be less serious than the effects of the disease itself.

When long-term corticosteroid therapy is used to relieve discomfort and disability in relatively benign chronic diseases such as rheumatoid arthritis the danger of treatment may become greater than the disabilities produced by the disease. To minimise side-effects the maintenance dose should be kept as low as possible, seldom exceeding the equivalent of 10 mg of prednisolone daily or ideally 5–6 mg daily (see also section 10.1.2.1).

When long-term treatment is to be discontinued, the dose should be reduced gradually over a period of several weeks or months depending on the dosage and duration of the therapy. Too rapid a reduction of corticosteroid dosage can lead to acute adrenal insufficiency, hypotension, and death. A number of minor withdrawal symptoms may also result such as rhinitis, conjunctivitis, loss of weight, and painful itchy nodules.

In an attempt to reduce pituitary-adrenal suppression in patients requiring long-term corticosteroid therapy, intermittent treatment has been used, either in short courses, or by giving the corticosteroid as a single (higher) dose on alternate days instead of daily. Alternate-day administration has not been very successful in the management of asthma (see section 3.2).

STEROID CARDS. Patients should carry cards giving details of their dosage and possible complications. These 'steroid cards' can be obtained from local Family Practitioner Committees or

> DHSS Printing and Stationery Unit
> Room 110
> North Fylde Central Office
> Norcross
> Blackpool FY5 3TA

In Scotland 'steroid cards' are available from Health Boards.

Pharmacists may obtain these cards from the Royal Pharmaceutical Society of Great Britain.

ANAESTHESIA. Anaesthetists must know whether a patient is taking or has been taking corticosteroids as adrenal suppression may cause a precipitous fall in blood pressure during anaesthesia or in the immediate postoperative period.

CHILDREN. In children the indications for corticosteroids are the same as for adults but risks are greater. The implications of starting these drugs are serious, and they should be used only when specifically indicated, in a minimal dosage, and for the shortest possible time. Prolonged or continuous treatment is rarely justified. Stunting of growth may be mitigated by giving corticotrophin, or by giving prednisolone as single doses on alternate days.

Stimulation of the adrenal cortex by **corticotrophin** or **tetracosactrin** has been used as an alternative to corticosteroids to control certain diseases but there is no close relationship between the dose producing satisfactory clinical improvement and the equivalent dose of oral corticosteroid producing the same degree of improvement.

BETAMETHASONE

Indications: suppression of inflammatory and allergic disorders; congenital adrenal hyperplasia (section 6.3.1); cerebral oedema (section 6.3.2)

I am a patient on—

STEROID
TREATMENT

which must not be stopped abruptly

and in the case of intercurrent illness may have to be increased

full details are available from the hospital or general → practitioners shown overleaf

STC1

INSTRUCTIONS

1 *DO NOT STOP taking the steroid drug except on medical advice. Always have a supply in reserve.*

2 *In case of feverish illness, accident, operation (emergency or otherwise), diarrhoea or vomiting the steroid treatment MUST be continued. Your doctor may wish you to have a LARGER DOSE or an INJECTION at such times.*

3 *If the tablets cause indigestion consult your doctor AT ONCE.*

4 *Always carry this card while receiving steroid treatment and show it to any doctor, dentist, nurse or midwife or anyone else who is giving you treatment.*

5 *After your treatment has finished you must still tell any doctor, dentist, nurse or midwife or anyone else who is giving you treatment that you have had steroid treatment.*

Cautions; Contra-indications; Side-effects: section 6.3.3

Dose: by mouth, 0.5–5 mg daily in divided doses
By intramuscular injection or slow intravenous injection or infusion, 4–20 mg, repeated up to 4 times in 24 hours; CHILD, *by slow intravenous injection*, up to 1 year 1 mg, 1–5 years 2 mg, 6–12 years 4 mg

PoM **Betnelan**® (Glaxo)
Tablets, scored, betamethasone 500 micrograms. Net price 20 = 69p. Label: 10 steroid card

PoM **Betnesol**® (Glaxo)
Tablets, pink, scored, soluble, betamethasone 500 micrograms (as sodium phosphate). Net price 20 = 64p. Label: 10 steroid card, 13
Injection, betamethasone 4 mg (as sodium phosphate)/ml. Net price 1-ml amp = 57p. Label: 10 steroid card

CORTISONE ACETATE
Indications: section 6.3.1
Cautions; Contra-indications; Side-effects: section 6.3.3
Dose: by mouth, replacement therapy, 25–37.5 mg daily in divided doses but see also section 6.3.1

PoM **Cortisone Acetate** (Non-proprietary)
Tablets, cortisone acetate 5 mg, net price 20 = 24p; 25 mg, 20 = 63p. Label: 10 steroid card

PoM **Cortelan**® (Glaxo)
Tablets, scored, cortisone acetate 25 mg. Net price 20 = 79p. Label: 10 steroid card

PoM **Cortistab**® (Boots)
Tablets, both scored, cortisone acetate 5 mg, net price 20 = 13p; 25 mg, 20 = 52p. Label: 10 steroid card

PoM **Cortisyl**® (Roussel)
Tablets, scored, cortisone acetate 25 mg. Net price 20 = £1.19. Label: 10 steroid card

DEXAMETHASONE
Indications: suppression of inflammatory and allergic disorders; shock; diagnosis of Cushing's disease, congenital adrenal hyperplasia (both section 6.3.1); cerebral oedema (section 6.3.2)
Cautions; Contra-indications; Side-effects: section 6.3.3; perineal irritation may follow intravenous administration of the phosphate ester
Dose: by mouth, 0.5–2 mg daily in divided doses; up to 15 mg daily in severe disease
Adrenal hyperplasia, 0.5–1.5 mg daily in divided doses
By intramuscular injection or slow intravenous injection or infusion, initially 0.5–20 mg; CHILD 200–500 micrograms/kg daily
Shock, *by intravenous injection or infusion*, 2–6 mg/kg, repeated if necessary after 2–6 hours (but see section 6.3.2)
Cerebral oedema, *by intravenous injection*, 10 mg initially, then 4 mg *by intramuscular injection* every 6 hours as required for 2–10 days
Note. 1.3 mg dexamethasone sodium phosphate ≡ 1.2 mg dexamethasone phosphate ≡ 1 mg dexamethasone

PoM **Decadron**® (MSD)
Tablets, scored, dexamethasone 500 micrograms. Net price 20 = 91p. Label: 10 steroid card
Injection, dexamethasone phosphate 4 mg/ml (as sodium salt) (= 3.33 mg dexamethasone/ml). Net price 2-ml vial = £1.76. Label: 10 steroid card

PoM **Decadron Shock-Pak**® (MSD)
Injection, dexamethasone 20 mg (as sodium phosphate)/ml. Net price 5-ml vial = £15.13. Label: 10 steroid card

PoM **Oradexon**® (Organon)
Tablets, dexamethasone 500 micrograms, net price 20 = 64p; 2 mg, 20 = £1.73. Label: 10 steroid card
Injection, dexamethasone 4 mg (as sodium phosphate)/ml. Net price 1-ml amp = 83p; 2-ml vial = £1.27. Label: 10 steroid card

HYDROCORTISONE
Indications: adrenocortical insufficiency (section 6.3.1); suppression of inflammatory and allergic disorders; shock (section 6.3.2)
Cautions; Contra-indications; Side-effects: section 6.3.3; perineal irritation may follow intravenous administration of the phosphate ester
Dose: by mouth, replacement therapy, 20–30 mg daily in divided doses—see section 6.3.1
By intramuscular injection or slow intravenous injection or infusion, 100–500 mg, 3–4 times in 24 hours or as required; CHILD *by slow intravenous injection* up to 1 year 25 mg, 1–5 years 50 mg, 6–12 years 100 mg
Shock—see section 6.3.2

Oral preparations

PoM **Hydrocortistab**® (Boots)
Tablets, scored, hydrocortisone 20 mg. Net price 20 = 56p. Label: 10 steroid card

PoM **Hydrocortone**® (MSD)
Tablets, scored, hydrocortisone 10 mg, net price 20 = 46p; 20 mg, 20 = 71p. Label: 10 steroid card

Parenteral preparations

PoM **Hydrocortisone Sodium Succinate** (Non-proprietary)
Injection, powder for reconstitution, hydrocortisone (as sodium succinate). Net price 100-mg vial (with 2-ml amp water for injections) = 60p; 500-mg vial = £1.92. Label: 10 steroid card

PoM **Efcortelan Soluble**® (Glaxo)
Injection, powder for reconstitution, hydrocortisone (as sodium succinate). Net price 100-mg vial (with 2-ml amp water for injections) = 67p. Label: 10 steroid card

PoM **Efcortesol**® (Glaxo)
Injection, hydrocortisone 100 mg (as sodium phosphate)/ml. Net price 1-ml amp = 75p; 5-ml amp = £3.40. Label: 10 steroid card

PoM **Solu-Cortef**® (Upjohn)
Injection, powder for reconstitution, hydrocortisone (as sodium succinate). Net price 100-mg vial (with 2-ml amp water for injec-

tions) = £1.02; without water for injections = 96p. Label: 10 steroid card

METHYLPREDNISOLONE

Indications: suppression of inflammatory and allergic disorders; shock; cerebral oedema
Cautions; Contra-indications; Side-effects: section 6.3.3
Dose: by mouth, in inflammatory disorders up to 16 mg daily in 4 divided doses preferably with food; in allergic disorders initially, up to 40 mg daily, in divided doses
By intramuscular injection or slow intravenous injection or infusion, up to 120 mg daily for up to 3 days
Shock, *by intravenous infusion,* up to 30 mg/kg (not septic shock, see section 6.3.2)

Oral preparations
PoM **Medrone**® (Upjohn)
Tablets, pink, scored, methylprednisolone 2 mg, net price 20 = £1.79; 4 mg, 20 = £3.44; 16 mg, 20 = £9.54. Label: 10 steroid card

Parenteral preparations
PoM **Min-I-Mix Methylprednisolone**® (IMS)
Injection, powder for reconstitution, methylprednisolone sodium succinate. Net price 0.5-g vial = £10.97; 1-g vial = £18.06. Label: 10 steroid card
PoM **Solu-Medrone**® (Upjohn)
Injection, powder for reconstitution, methylprednisolone (as sodium succinate). Net price 40-mg mix-o-vial = £1.32; 125-mg mix-o-vial = £3.96; 500-mg vial (with solvent) = £11.77; 1-g vial (with solvent) = £21.21; 2-g vial (with solvent) = £40.27. Label: 10 steroid card

Intramuscular depot
PoM **Depo-Medrone**® (Upjohn)
Injection (aqueous suspension), methylprednisolone acetate 40 mg/ml. Net price 1-ml vial = £2.59; 2-ml vial or syringe = £4.65; 5-ml vial = £10.40. Label: 10 steroid card
Dose: by deep intramuscular injection, 40–120 mg, repeated every 2–3 weeks if required

PREDNISOLONE

Indications: suppression of inflammatory and allergic disorders
Cautions; Contra-indications; Side-effects: section 6.3.3; perineal irritation may follow intravenous administration of the phosphate ester
Dose: by mouth, initially up to 30 mg daily in divided doses
By intravenous injection or infusion or intramuscular injection, prednisolone sodium phosphate, initially 4–60 mg daily in divided doses
By intramuscular injection, prednisolone acetate, 25–100 mg once or twice weekly

PoM **Prednisolone** (Non-proprietary)
Tablets, prednisolone 1 mg, net price 20 = 9p; 5 mg, 20 = 15p. Label: 10 steroid card

PoM **Codelsol**® (MSD)
Injection, prednisolone 16 mg (as sodium phosphate)/ml. Net price 2-ml vial = £1.39. Label: 10 steroid card
PoM **Deltacortril Enteric**® (Pfizer)
Tablets, both e/c, prednisolone 2.5 mg (brown), net price 20 = 19p; 5 mg (red), 20 = 36p. Label: 5, 10 steroid card, 25
PoM **Deltastab**® (Boots)
Tablets, scored, prednisolone 1 mg, net price 20 = 5p; 5 mg, 20 = 12p. Label: 10 steroid card
Injection (aqueous suspension), prednisolone acetate 25 mg/ml. Net price 5-ml vial = 90p. Label: 10 steroid card
PoM **Precortisyl**® (Roussel)
Tablets, prednisolone 1 mg, net price 20 = 7p; 5 mg (scored), 20 = 15p. Label: 10 steroid card
PoM **Precortisyl Forte**® (Roussel)
Tablets, scored, prednisolone 25 mg. Net price 20 = £1.56. Label: 10 steroid card
PoM **Prednesol**® (Glaxo)
Tablets, pink, scored, soluble, prednisolone 5 mg (as sodium phosphate). Net price 20 = £1.15. Label: 10 steroid card, 13
PoM **Sintisone**® (Farmitalia Carlo Erba)
Tablets, scored, prednisolone steaglate 6.65 mg (= prednisolone 5 mg). Net price 20 = £1.29. Label: 10 steroid card

PREDNISONE

Indications: suppression of inflammatory and allergic disorders
Cautions; Contra-indications; Side-effects: section 6.3.3. Avoid in liver disease
Dose: initially up to 30 mg daily

PoM **Prednisone** (Non-proprietary)
Tablets, prednisone 1 mg, net price 20 = 9p; 5 mg, 20 = 15p. Label: 10 steroid card
PoM **Decortisyl**® (Roussel)
Tablets, scored, prednisone 5 mg. Net price 20 = 15p. Label: 10 steroid card

TRIAMCINOLONE

Indications: suppression of inflammatory and allergic disorders
Cautions; Contra-indications; Side-effects: section 6.3.3. Triamcinolone in high dosage has a tendency to cause proximal myopathy and should be avoided in chronic therapy
Dose: by mouth, up to 24 mg daily in divided doses
By deep intramuscular injection, 40 mg of acetonide for depot effect, repeated at intervals according to the patient's response; max. single dose 100 mg

PoM **Kenalog**® (Squibb)
Injection (aqueous suspension), triamcinolone acetonide 40 mg/ml. Net price 1-ml vial = £1.70; 1-ml syringe = £2.11; 2-ml syringe = £3.66. Label: 10 steroid card
PoM **Ledercort**® (Lederle)
Tablets, blue, triamcinolone 2 mg. Net price 20 = £1.94. Label: 10 steroid card

Tablets, triamcinolone 4 mg. Net price 20 = £3.54. Label: 10 steroid card

6.4 Sex hormones

Sex hormones are described under the following section headings:
  6.4.1 Female sex hormones
  6.4.2 Male sex hormones and antagonists
  6.4.3 Anabolic steroids

6.4.1 Female sex hormones

There are two groups of female sex hormones, the oestrogens (section 6.4.1.1) and progestogens (section 6.4.1.2). Combined hormone preparations for menopausal symptoms are listed in section 6.4.1.3 and for menstrual disorders in section 6.4.1.4. Combined and other preparations for use as contraceptives are in sections 7.3.1 and 7.3.2.

6.4.1.1 OESTROGENS

Oestrogens are necessary for the development of female secondary sexual characteristics; they stimulate myometrial hypertrophy, with endometrial hyperplasia which may lead to withdrawal bleeding when treatment is stopped, and they promote cornification of the vagina. They are used as oral contraceptives (see section 7.3.1) with **progestogens** since oestrogens suppress ovulation and inhibit production of follicle-stimulating hormone (FSH) from the anterior pituitary gland. They may also be used with benefit in some neoplastic conditions (see section 8.3.1), particularly cancer of the prostate and some cases of breast cancer. Several gynaecological conditions also benefit from treatment with oestrogens but systemic administration is associated with an increased risk of thrombo-embolism and this should be borne in mind when they are prescribed. For a warning on oestrogens and elective surgery see Combined Oral Contraceptives, section 7.3.1.

Ethinyloestradiol is the oestrogen of choice for most conditions. The natural (as opposed to synthetic) oestrogens have not been shown to have any advantages. Since all oral preparations are subject to first-pass metabolism in the liver and intestine, subcutaneous or transdermal administration mimics more closely endogenous hormonal activity. Stilboestrol is used mainly in neoplastic conditions (see section 8.3.1).

MENOPAUSAL SYMPTOMS. Hormone replacement therapy is **not** routinely recommended in post-menopausal women but small doses of oestrogen given for long periods will diminish postmenopausal osteoporosis. Menopausal vasomotor symptoms and menopausal vaginitis and vulvitis can, if severe, justify treatment for a few months. Topical preparations (see section 7.2.1) are used to treat menopausal vaginitis and vulvitis; patients who do not respond require systemic treatment. The oestrogen can be given cyclically or continuously but in either case a progestogen should be added cyclically to prevent cystic hyperplasia of the endometrium and possible transformation to atypical aplasia and carcinoma. Quite low doses of progestogens have been shown to be effective (see section 6.4.1.3 for suitable combined preparations). The use of oestrogens alone is no longer recommended, except for short periods.

If the patient has had a hysterectomy the oestrogen is given continuously and cyclical addition of a progestogen is not necessary.

For long-term administration implants or dermal patches may be preferable (see above).

MENSTRUAL DISORDERS. Oestrogens are used in *hypogonadism* or *premature ovarian failure* to induce secondary sexual characteristics and to avoid the complications of oestrogen deficiency. Where long-term therapy is necessary they must be given in combination with cyclical progestogen therapy if the uterus is present (as indicated above).

Combined cyclical therapy is also useful in regulating *dysfunctional uterine bleeding* and relieving *spasmodic dysmenorrhoea*. For a suitable combined preparation see section 6.4.1.4; this may suppress ovulation, but where contraception is required a combined oral contraceptive (see section 7.3.1) should be used.

SUPPRESSION OF LACTATION. Oestrogens are no longer used to suppress lactation because of their association with thrombo-embolism, and **bromocriptine** (section 6.7.1) is used where necessary.

ETHINYLOESTRADIOL
Indications: see notes above
Cautions: prolonged exposure to unopposed oestrogens may increase risk of development of endometrial carcinoma (see notes above); pregnancy, breast-feeding, diabetes, epilepsy, hypertension, migraine, cardiac or renal disease, history of jaundice, wearing of contact lenses (may irritate); may interfere with results of thyroid-function tests and cortisol estimations by increasing concentrations of hormone-binding protein. Drug interactions: see Appendix 1 (sections *2.2*, *2.5*)
Contra-indications: oestrogen-dependent carcinoma, history of thrombo-embolism, hepatic impairment, endometriosis, porphyria, sickle-cell anaemia (but see also Oral Contraceptives), undiagnosed vaginal bleeding, history of herpes gestationis
Side-effects: nausea and vomiting, weight gain, breast enlargement and tenderness, withdrawal bleeding, sodium retention with oedema, changes in liver function, jaundice, rashes and chloasma, depression, headache, endometrial carcinoma in postmenopausal women
Dose: menopausal symptoms 10–20 micrograms daily continuously *or* for 21 days, repeated after 7 days, with progestogen from day 17 to day 26 of cycle (see notes above)

 Prices are **net**, see p. 1

Primary amenorrhoea, 10 micrograms on alternate days increasing to a max. of 50 micrograms daily continuously with a progestogen for the last 5 days of month
Hereditary haemorrhagic telangiectasia, 0.5–1 mg daily

Oestrogen-only preparations
PoM **Ethinyloestradiol Tablets,** ethinyloestradiol 10 micrograms, net price 20 = 44p; 50 micrograms, 20 = 60p; 1 mg, 20 = £1.71

Combined preparations, see section 6.4.1.3

OESTRADIOL

Indications: see notes above and under preparations
Cautions; Contra-indications; Side-effects: see under Ethinyloestradiol
Dose: see below

Oestrogen-only preparations
PoM **Oestradiol Implants** (Organon)
Implant, oestradiol 25 mg (duration 36 weeks), net price each = £4.67; 50 mg (duration 44 weeks), each = £9.34; 100 mg (duration 57 weeks), each = £19.66
Dose: by implantation, oestrogen replacement (with cyclical progestogen if uterus intact, see notes above), 25–100 mg as required (usually every 4–8 months)
PoM **Benztrone®** (Paines & Byrne)
Injection (oily), oestradiol benzoate 1 mg/ml, net price 1-ml amp = 31p; 5 mg/ml, 1-ml amp = 44p
Dose: by intramuscular injection, oestrogen replacement (with cyclical progestogen if uterus intact, see notes above), 1–5 mg every 14 days
▼ PoM **Estraderm TTS®** (Ciba)
25 Dressing (TTS 25), self-adhesive, releasing oestradiol approx. 25 micrograms/24 hours when in contact with skin. Net price 8 dressings = £6.30. Counselling advised, see below
50 Dressing (TTS 50), self-adhesive, releasing oestradiol approx. 50 micrograms/24 hours when in contact with skin. Net price 8 dressings = £6.95. Counselling advised, see below
100 Dressing (TTS 100), self-adhesive, releasing oestradiol approx. 100 micrograms/24 hours when in contact with skin. Net price 8 dressings = £7.65. Counselling advised, see below
Dose: for menopausal symptoms, 1 patch to be applied twice weekly on continuous basis together with a progestogen on 12 days a month (unless patient has had hysterectomy); therapy should be initiated with TTS 50 for first month, subsequently adjusted to lowest effective dose; max. one TTS 100 daily
COUNSELLING. Patch should be removed after 3–4 days and replaced with fresh patch on slightly different site; recommended sites: clean, dry, unbroken areas of skin on trunk below waistline; not to be applied on or near breasts

PoM **Hormonin®** (Carnrick)
Tablets, pink, scored, oestradiol 600 micrograms, oestriol 270 micrograms, oestrone 1.4 mg. Net price 20 = £1.10
Dose: menopausal symptoms (short-term), ½–1 tablet daily or 1 tablet on alternate days; can be given cyclically
PoM **Progynova®** (Schering)
Tablets, both s/c, oestradiol valerate 1 mg (beige), net price 21-tab pack = £1.98; 2 mg (blue), 21-tab pack = £1.98
Dose: menopausal symptoms (short-term), 1 mg daily for 21 days, with 7-day interval before next course; increased to 2 mg daily if required

Combined preparations, see section 6.4.1.3

OESTRIOL

Indications: see notes above and under preparations
Cautions; Contra-indications; Side-effects: see under Ethinyloestradiol
Dose: see below

Oestrogen-only preparations
PoM **Ovestin®** (Organon)
Tablets, oestriol 250 micrograms. Net price 20 = 48p. Label: 25
Dose: menopausal symptoms (short-term), 250–500 micrograms daily

Combined preparations, see section 6.4.1.3

OESTROGENS, CONJUGATED

Indications: see notes above and under preparations
Cautions; Contra-indications; Side-effects: see under Ethinyloestradiol
Dose: see below

Oestrogen-only preparations
PoM **Premarin®** (Wyeth)
Tablets, all s/c, conjugated oestrogens 625 micrograms (maroon), net price 20 = 90p; 21-tab pack = 94p; 1.25 mg (yellow), 20 = £1.46; 21-tab pack = £1.54; 2.5 mg (purple), 20 = £1.90
Dose: menopausal symptoms (with progestogen for 10–12 days per cycle if uterus intact), 0.625–1.25 mg daily for 21 days from 5th day of cycle, repeated after 7 days if necessary
Combined preparations, see section 6.4.1.3

PIPERAZINE OESTRONE SULPHATE

(Estropipate)
Indications: see notes above and under preparations
Cautions; Contra-indications; Side-effects: see under Ethinyloestradiol
Dose: see below

Oestrogen-only preparations
PoM **Harmogen®** (Abbott)
Tablets, peach, scored, piperazine oestrone sulphate 1.5 mg. Net price 20 = £1.58

Dose: menopausal symptoms (short-term), 1.5–4.5 mg daily in single or divided doses for 21–28 days, repeated after 5–7 days if necessary

6.4.1.2 PROGESTOGENS

Progestogens modify some of the effects of, and act mainly on tissues sensitised by, oestrogens; their effects are inhibited by oestrogen excess. There are two main groups of progestogen, the naturally occurring hormone *progesterone* and its analogues (allyloestrenol, dydrogesterone, hydroxyprogesterone, and medroxyprogesterone) and the *testosterone* analogues e.g. norethisterone. Progesterone and its analogues are less androgenic than the testosterone derivatives and neither progesterone nor dydrogesterone causes virilisation. Other synthetic derivatives are variably metabolised into testosterone and oestrogen; thus side-effects vary with the preparation and the dose.

Progestogens are useful in many menstrual disorders, including *severe dysmenorrhoea*, and *dysfunctional uterine bleeding*. **Norethisterone** and **dydrogesterone** are suitable and may be given alone on a cyclical basis during part of the menstrual cycle or in conjunction with oestrogens (section 6.4.1.1). Suitable preparations are listed in section 6.4.1.4. Alternatively the combined oral contraceptives (see section 7.3.1) may be used. See also bromocriptine (section 6.7.1).

Where *endometriosis* requires drug treatment, it usually responds to a progestogen, e.g. norethisterone, administered on a continuous basis. Alternatively, cyclical or continuous treatment with the oral contraceptives (see section 7.3.1) or danazol (section 6.7.3) may be given.

Progestogens have been widely advocated for the alleviation of *premenstrual symptoms* but the evidence is conflicting and no convincing physiological basis for such treatment has been shown. Progesterone (given as suppositories) and dydrogesterone are possibly more effective than norethisterone.

The progestogens desogestrel, ethynodiol, levonorgestrel[1], lynoestrenol, and norethisterone are used in combined oral and in progestogen-only *contraceptives* (see sections 7.3.1 and 7.3.2).

Progestogens are also used in conjunction with oestrogens in *hormone replacement therapy* in menopausal women (see section 6.4.1.3). See section 8.3.2 for use in *neoplastic disease*.

Progestogens have been used in *habitual abortion* but there is no evidence of benefit. If they are used for this purpose they should be of the true progesterone-derivative type, e.g. **hydroxyprogesterone hexanoate** to avoid any masculinisation of a female fetus.

ALLYLOESTRENOL

Indications: habitual abortion, but see notes above
Cautions; Contra-indications; Side-effects: see under Progesterone and notes above

Dose: habitual abortion, 5–10 mg daily for at least 16 weeks (but see notes above)

PoM **Gestanin**® (Organon)
Tablets, allyloestrenol 5 mg. Net price 20 = £1.99

DYDROGESTERONE

Indications: see under Dose and notes above
Cautions; Contra-indications; Side-effects: see under Progesterone and notes above; breakthrough bleeding may occur (increase dose)
Dose: endometriosis, 10 mg 2–3 times daily from 5th to 25th day of cycle or continuously
Infertility, irregular cycles, 10 mg twice daily from 11th to 25th day for at least 6 cycles
Habitual abortion, 10 mg twice daily from day 11 to day 25 of cycle until conception, then continuously until 20th week of pregnancy and gradually reduced (but see notes above)
Dysfunctional uterine bleeding, 10 mg twice daily (together with an oestrogen) for 5–7 days to arrest bleeding; 10 mg twice daily (together with an oestrogen) from 11th to 25th day of cycle to prevent bleeding
Dysmenorrhoea, 10 mg twice daily from 5th to 25th day of cycle
Amenorrhoea, 10 mg twice daily from 11th to 25th day of cycle with oestrogen therapy from 1st to 25th day of cycle
Premenstrual syndrome, 10 mg twice daily from 12th to 26th day of cycle increased if necessary (but see notes above)
Hormone replacement therapy, with continuous oestrogen therapy, 10 mg twice daily, for the first 12–14 days of each calendar month; with cyclical oestrogen, 10 mg twice daily for the last 12–14 days of each treatment cycle

PoM **Duphaston**® (Duphar)
Tablets, scored, dydrogesterone 10 mg. Net price 20 = £3.35

HYDROXYPROGESTERONE HEXANOATE

Indications: habitual abortion but see notes above
Cautions; Contra-indications; Side-effects: see under Progesterone and notes above
Dose: by intramuscular injection, 250–500 mg weekly during first half of pregnancy

PoM **Proluton* Depot**® (Schering)
Injection (oily), hydroxyprogesterone hexanoate 250 mg/ml. Net price 1-ml amp = £2.35; 2-ml amp = £3.69
*formerly Primolut Depot®

MEDROXYPROGESTERONE ACETATE

Indications: see under Dose; for use as a contraceptive, see section 7.3.2; for use in malignant disease, see section 8.3.2
Cautions; Contra-indications; Side-effects: see under Progesterone and notes above; disturbances of normal menstrual cycle and irregular bleeding may occur

---

[1]Levonorgestrel is the active isomer and has twice the potency of racemic norgestrel.   Prices are **net**, see p. 1

Dose: by mouth, 2.5–10 mg daily for 5–10 days beginning on 16th–21st day of cycle, repeated for 2 cycles in dysfunctional uterine bleeding and 3 cycles in secondary amenorrhoea

By deep intramuscular injection, endometriosis, 50 mg weekly or 100 mg every 2 weeks

▼ PoM **Depo-Provera**® (Upjohn)
Injection (aqueous suspension), medroxyprogesterone acetate 50 mg/ml. Net price 1-ml vial = £1.41; 3-ml vial = £3.79; 5-ml vial = £6.23

PoM **Provera**® (Upjohn)
Tablets, scored, medroxyprogesterone acetate 5 mg. Net price 20-tab pack = £2.58

NORETHISTERONE

Indications: see under Dose; for use as a contraceptive see sections 7.3.1 and 7.3.2

Cautions; Contra-indications; Side-effects: see under Progesterone but more virilising and greater incidence of liver disturbances and jaundice; avoid in pregnancy; exacerbation of epilepsy and migraine

Dose: endometriosis 10 mg daily starting on 5th day of cycle (increased if spotting occurs to 25 mg daily in divided doses to prevent breakthrough bleeding)

Dysfunctional uterine bleeding, menorrhagia, 5 mg 3 times daily for 10 days to arrest bleeding; to prevent bleeding 5 mg twice daily from 19th to 26th day

Dysmenorrhoea, 5 mg 3 times daily from 5th to 25th day for 3–4 cycles

Premenstrual syndrome, 10–15 mg daily from 19th to 26th day for several cycles (but see notes above)

Postponement of menstruation, 5 mg 3 times daily starting 3 days before anticipated onset

PoM **Primolut N**® (Schering)
Tablets, norethisterone 5 mg. Net price 20 = £1.92

PoM **Utovlan**® (Syntex)
Tablets, scored, norethisterone 5 mg. Net price 20 = £1.64

PROGESTERONE

Indications: see under Dose and notes above

Cautions: diabetes, breast-feeding, hypertension; liver, cardiac, or renal disease. Drug interactions: see Appendix 1 (section 8)

Contra-indications: undiagnosed vaginal bleeding, missed or incomplete abortion, history of thrombo-embolism, mammary carcinoma

Side-effects: acne, urticaria, oedema, weight gain, gastro-intestinal disturbances, changes in libido, breast discomfort, irregular menstrual cycles; rarely jaundice. Injection may be painful

Dose: by vagina or rectum, premenstrual syndrome, 200 mg daily to 400 mg twice daily starting at day 12–14 and continued until onset of menstruation (but see notes above); rectally if barrier methods of contraception are used, or if vaginal infection

By deep intramuscular injection, into buttock dysfunctional uterine bleeding, 5–10 mg daily for 5–10 days until 2 days before anticipated onset of menstruation

Embryo transfer, consult manufacturer's literature

PoM **Progesterone Implants** (Organon)
Implant, progesterone 100 mg. Net price each = £9.72

PoM **Cyclogest**® (Hoechst)
Suppositories, progesterone 200 mg, net price 20 = £7.20; 400 mg, 20 = £10.43

PoM **Gestone**® (Paines & Byrne)
Injection, progesterone 10 mg/ml, net price 1-ml amp = 28p; 25 mg/ml, 1-ml amp = 29p; 50 mg/ml, 1-ml amp = 38p, 2-ml amp = 50p

6.4.1.3 COMBINED PREPARATIONS FOR MENOPAUSAL SYMPTOMS

Note. The preparations in this section are unsuitable for use as oral contraceptives. Combined preparations are not necessary for women who have had a hysterectomy, who may receive oestrogen alone (section 6.4.1.1)

For *Cautions; Contra-indications; Side-effects:* see under Combined Oral Contraceptives, section 7.3.1

PoM **Cyclo-Progynova 1 mg**® (Schering)
Calendar pack, all s/c, 11 beige tablets, oestradiol valerate 1 mg; 10 brown tablets, oestradiol valerate 1 mg and norgestrel 500 micrograms (≡ levonorgestrel 250 micrograms). Net price per pack = £3.13
Dose: 1 beige tablet daily for 11 days, starting on 5th day of menstrual cycle or at any time if cycles have ceased or are infrequent, then 1 brown tablet daily for 10 days, followed by a 7-day interval

PoM **Cyclo-Progynova 2 mg**® (Schering)
Calendar pack, all s/c, 11 white tablets, oestradiol valerate 2 mg; 10 brown tablets, oestradiol valerate 2 mg and norgestrel 500 micrograms (≡ levonorgestrel 250 micrograms). Net price per pack = £3.11
Dose: see above, but starting with 1 white tablet daily

PoM **Menophase**® (Syntex)
Calendar pack, 5 pink tablets, mestranol 12.5 micrograms; 8 orange tablets, mestranol 25 micrograms; 2 yellow tablets, mestranol 50 micrograms; 3 green tablets, mestranol 25 micrograms and norethisterone 1 mg; 6 blue tablets, mestranol 30 micrograms and norethisterone 1.5 mg; 4 lavender tablets, mestranol 20 micrograms and norethisterone 750 micrograms. Net price per pack = £2.63
Dose: 1 tablet daily, starting with a pink tablet on Sunday, then in sequence (without interruption)

PoM Prempak-C 0.625® (Wyeth)
Calendar pack, all s/c, 28 maroon tablets, conjugated oestrogens 625 micrograms; 12 light brown tablets, norgestrel 150 micrograms (≡levonorgestrel 75 micrograms). Net price per pack = £3.77
Dose: 1 maroon tablet daily for 16 days, starting on 1st day of cycle or at any time if cycles have ceased or are infrequent, then 1 maroon and 1 brown tablet daily for 12 days. Subsequent courses should be repeated without interval

PoM Prempak-C 1.25® (Wyeth)
Calendar pack, all s/c, 28 yellow tablets, conjugated oestrogens 1.25 mg; 12 light brown tablets, norgestrel 150 micrograms (≡levonorgestrel 75 micrograms). Net price per pack = £3.77
Dose: see above, but starting with 1 yellow tablet daily

PoM Trisequens® (Novo)
Calendar pack, 12 blue tablets, oestradiol 2 mg, oestriol 1 mg; 10 white tablets, oestradiol 2 mg, oestriol 1 mg, norethisterone acetate 1 mg; 6 red tablets, oestradiol 1 mg, oestriol 500 micrograms. Net price per pack = £3.40
Dose: 1 blue tablet daily, starting on 5th day of menstrual cycle or at any time if cycles have ceased or are infrequent, then 1 tablet daily in sequence (without interruption)

6.4.1.4 COMBINED PREPARATIONS FOR MENSTRUAL DISORDERS

Cautions; Contra-indications; Side-effects: see under Combined Oral Contraceptives, section 7.3.1

PoM Controvlar® (Schering)
Tablets, pink, s/c, norethisterone acetate 3 mg, ethinyloestradiol 50 micrograms. Net price 21 = 90p
Dose: dysmenorrhoea, menstrual irregularities, menorrhagia, endometriosis, 1 tablet daily for 21 days, starting on 5th day of menstrual cycle, followed by a 7-day interval
Ovran and **Ovranette:** see section 7.3.1

6.4.2 Male sex hormones and antagonists

Androgens cause masculinisation; they may be used as replacement therapy in castrated adults and in those who are hypogonadal due to either pituitary or testicular disease. In the normal male they depress spermatogenesis and inhibit pituitary gonadotrophin secretion. Androgens also have an anabolic action which has led to the development of anabolic steroids (section 6.4.3).

Androgens are useless as a treatment of impotence and impaired spermatogenesis unless there is associated hypogonadism; they should not be given until the hypogonadism has been properly investigated. Treatment should be under expert supervision.

When given to patients with hypopituitarism they can lead to normal sexual development and potency but not fertility. If fertility is desired, the correct treatment is with chorionic gonadotrophin injection (HCG) and with menotrophin (FSH) (section 6.5.1) which will stimulate spermatogenesis as well as androgen production.

Caution should be used when androgens or chorionic gonadotrophin are used in treating boys with delayed puberty since the fusion of epiphyses is hastened and may result in short stature.

Androgens are still quite useful in occasional patients with disseminated carcinoma of the breast despite their masculinising effects. The synthetic anabolic steroids (such as nandrolone) which cause less masculinisation are usually preferred (see section 8.3.3).

Intramuscular depot preparations of **testosterone** are preferred for replacement therapy. Testosterone propionate (Virormone®) or alternatively Sustanon®, which consists of a mixture of testosterone esters and has a longer duration of action, may be used. Satisfactory replacement therapy can sometimes be obtained with 1 ml of Sustanon 250®, given by intramuscular injection once a month, although more frequent dose intervals are often necessary. Implants of testosterone have been superseded.

Of the orally active preparations, methyltestosterone is not generally used and other preparations are preferred because like the other 17α-alkyl derivatives of testosterone it can sometimes cause dose-related but reversible cholestatic jaundice. **Mesterolone** (Pro-Viron®) is not a 17α-alkyl derivative and is less toxic to the liver.

MESTEROLONE

Indications: hypogonadism
Cautions; Contra-indications; Side-effects: see under Testosterone
Dose: 25 mg 3–4 times daily for several months, reduced to 50–75 mg daily in divided doses for maintenance

PoM Pro-Viron® (Schering)
Tablets, scored, mesterolone 25 mg. Net price 20 = £3.16

METHYLTESTOSTERONE

Indications: hypogonadism
Cautions; Contra-indications; Side-effects: see under Testosterone; also dose-related cholestatic jaundice
Dose: initially 30–50 mg daily, in divided doses

PoM Methyltestosterone Tablets, methyltestosterone 5 mg, net price 20 = 65p; 10 mg, 20 = 99p; 25 mg, 20 = £1.90; 50 mg, 20 = £3.40

TESTOSTERONE

Indications: hypogonadism
Cautions: cardiac, renal, or hepatic impairment, circulatory failure, hypertension, epilepsy, migraine, thyroid disease, diabetes mellitus

---

Contra-indications: breast cancer in men, prostatic carcinoma, pregnancy, breast-feeding, nephrosis

Side-effects: oedema, increase in weight, hypercalcaemia, increased bone growth, priapism, premature closure of epiphyses in early puberty, prostatism in elderly patients, high doses cause virilism in women, and suppress spermatogenesis in men

Dose: by implantation, 200–600 mg; duration of effect 7–8 months

PoM **Testosterone Implants** (Organon)
Implant, testosterone 100 mg (duration 30 weeks), net price each = £4.44; 200 mg (duration 34 weeks), each = £8.24

TESTOSTERONE ESTERS

Indications; Cautions; Contra-indications; Side-effects: see under Testosterone

PoM **Primoteston Depot®** (Schering)
Injection (oily), testosterone enanthate 250 mg/ml. Net price 1-ml amp = £4.13
Dose: by intramuscular injection, initially 250 mg every 2–3 weeks; maintenance 250 mg every 3–6 weeks

PoM **Restandol®** (Organon)
Capsules, red-brown, testosterone undecanoate 40 mg in oily solution. Net price 20 = £5.26. Label: 21, 25
Dose: 120–160 mg daily for 2–3 weeks; maintenance 40–120 mg daily

PoM **Sustanon 100®** (Organon)
Injection (oily), testosterone propionate 20 mg, testosterone phenylpropionate 40 mg, and testosterone isocaproate 40 mg/ml. Net price 1-ml amp = £1.11
Dose: by deep intramuscular injection, 1 ml every 2 weeks

PoM **Sustanon 250®** (Organon)
Injection (oily), testosterone propionate 30 mg, testosterone phenylpropionate 60 mg, testosterone isocaproate 60 mg, and testosterone decanoate 100 mg/ml. Net price 1-ml amp = £2.61
Dose: by deep intramuscular injection, 1 ml every 2–4 weeks

PoM **Virormone®** (Paines & Byrne)
Injection, testosterone propionate 25 mg/ml, net price 1-ml amp = 32p; 50 mg/ml, 1-ml amp = 34p, 2-ml amp = 40p
Dose: by intramuscular injection, 10–50 mg 2–3 times weekly

ANTI-ANDROGENS

Cyproterone acetate (Androcur®) is an anti-androgen used in the treatment of severe hypersexuality and sexual deviation in the male; it inhibits spermatogenesis and produces reversible infertility. Abnormal sperm forms are produced. Cyproterone acetate is also used in the treatment of acne and hirsutism in women (see section 13.6) and in prostatic cancer (see section 8.3.4). As hepatic tumours have been produced in *animal*

studies, careful consideration should be given to the risk/benefit ratio before treatment.

CYPROTERONE ACETATE

Indications: see notes above

Cautions: impaired ability to drive and operate machinery; ineffective in chronic alcoholism; blood counts and monitor hepatic function, adrenocortical function and blood glucose regularly; diabetes mellitus, adrenocortical insufficiency, breast-feeding

Contra-indications: hepatic disease, malignant or wasting disease, severe depression, history of thrombo-embolic disorders; youths under 18 years (may arrest bone maturation and testicular development); these contra-indications do not apply in prostate cancer

Side-effects: fatigue and lassitude, weight gain, changes in hair pattern, gynaecomastia (rarely leading to galactorrhoea and benign breast nodules); rarely osteoporosis; inhibition of spermatogenesis (see notes above); liver abnormalities reported

Dose: male hypersexuality, 50 mg twice daily after food

PoM **Androcur®** (Schering)
Tablets, scored, cyproterone acetate 50 mg. Net price 20 = £12.64. Label: 2, 21

6.4.3   Anabolic steroids

All the anabolic steroids have some androgenic activity but they cause less virilisation than androgens in women. Their protein-building property led to the hope that they might be widely useful in medicine but this hope has not been realised. They have, for example, been given for osteoporosis in women and in cases of wasting. Their use as body builders or tonics is quite unjustified; they are abused by some athletes although no beneficial effect has been produced.

It is doubtful whether anabolic steroids should be used to increase height in children; apart from virilising properties, they may lead to premature closing of the epiphyses so that the eventual height is the same as or less than without treatment. Side-effects such as cholestatic jaundice may occur, particularly with the 17-α alkyl derivatives of testosterone (e.g. stanozolol) which should be **avoided** in hepatic impairment. Some anabolic steroids produce hepatic tumours in long-term use.

Anabolic steroids are also used in the treatment of some aplastic anaemias (see section 9.1.3), in the palliative treatment of breast cancer (see section 8.3.3), to reduce the itching of chronic biliary obstruction (see Prescribing in Terminal Care), and to stimulate fibrinolysis (see section 2.10).

NANDROLONE

Indications: protein synthesis after major surgery or chronic debilitating disease

Cautions: cardiac and renal impairment, circulatory failure, hypertension, diabetes mellitus, epilepsy, migraine; monitor skeletal maturation in young patients. Drug interactions: see Appendix 1 (sections *2.8*, *2.8B*)

Contra-indications: hepatic impairment, prostatic carcinoma, male breast carcinoma, pregnancy, porphyria

Side-effects: acne, oedema, virilism with high doses, hypercalcaemia, menstrual irregularities

Dose: see below

PoM **Deca-Durabolin**® (Organon)
Injection (oily), nandrolone decanoate 25 mg/ml, net price 1-ml amp = £1.75, 1-ml syringe = £1.88; 50 mg/ml, 1-ml amp = £3.37, 1-ml syringe = £3.57
 Dose: by deep intramuscular injection, 25–50 mg every 3 weeks
Deca-Durabolin 100®, see section 9.1.3

PoM **Durabolin**® (Organon)
Injection (oily), nandrolone phenylpropionate 25 mg/ml, net price = 86p, 1-ml syringe = 91p; 50 mg/ml, 1-ml syringe = £1.70
 Dose: by deep intramuscular injection, 25–50 mg weekly

STANOZOLOL

Indications: protein synthesis after major surgery or chronic debilitating disease; hereditary angio-oedema (for use in aplastic anaemia, see section 9.1.3; for use as a fibrinolytic, see section 2.10)

Cautions; Contra-indications; Side-effects: see under Nandrolone. Headache, euphoria, depression, cramp, and cholestatic jaundice occur occasionally

Dose: by mouth, anabolic effect, 5 mg daily
Hereditary angioedema, 2.5–10 mg to control attacks, reduced for maintenance
By deep intramuscular injection, 50 mg every 2–3 weeks

PoM **Stromba**® (Sterling Research)
Tablets, scored, stanozolol 5 mg. Net price 56-tab pack = £21.19
Injection (aqueous suspension), stanozolol 50 mg/ml. Net price 1-ml amp = £5.93

6.5 Hypothalamic and pituitary hormones and anti-oestrogens

Hypothalamic and pituitary hormones are described under the following section headings:
6.5.1 Hypothalamic and anterior pituitary hormones and anti-oestrogens
6.5.2 Posterior pituitary hormones and antagonists

Use of preparations in these sections requires detailed prior investigation of the patient and *should be reserved for specialist centres.*

6.5.1 Hypothalamic and anterior pituitary hormones and anti-oestrogens

ANTI-OESTROGENS

The anti-oestrogens **clomiphene**, **cyclofenil**, and **tamoxifen** are used in the treatment of female infertility due to secondary amenorrhoea (e.g. polycystic ovarian disease). They induce gonadotrophin release by occupying oestrogen receptors in the hypothalamus, thereby interfering with feedback mechanisms; chorionic gonadotrophin is sometimes used as an adjunct. Care is taken to avoid hyperstimulation and multiple pregnancies.

CLOMIPHENE CITRATE

Indications: anovulatory infertility—see notes above

Cautions: see notes above; polycystic ovary syndrome (cysts may enlarge during treatment), incidence of multiple births increased

Contra-indications: hepatic disease, ovarian cysts, endometrial carcinoma, pregnancy, abnormal uterine bleeding

Side-effects: visual disturbances (withdraw), ovarian hyperstimulation (withdraw), hot flushes, abdominal discomfort, occasionally nausea, vomiting, depression, insomnia, breast tenderness, weight gain, rashes, dizziness, hair loss

Dose: 50 mg daily for 5 days starting on 5th day of menstrual cycle or at any time if cycles have ceased
In absence of ovulation second course of 100 mg daily for 5 days may be given; most patients who are going to respond will do so to first course; 3 courses should constitute adequate therapeutic trial; long-term cyclical therapy not recommended

PoM **Clomid**® (Merrell)
Tablets, yellow, scored, clomiphene citrate 50 mg. Net price 20 = £6.73
PoM **Serophene**® (Serono)
Tablets, scored, clomiphene citrate 50 mg. Net price 20 tabs = £6.73

CYCLOFENIL

Indications: anovulatory infertility—see notes above

Contra-indications: see under Clomiphene Citrate

Side-effects: hot flushes, abdominal discomfort, nausea; rarely cholestatic jaundice

Dose: 200 mg twice daily for 10 days starting on 3rd day of natural or progesterone-induced bleeding, followed by 20 treatment-free days, repeated for at least 3 months

▼ PoM **Rehibin**® (Serono)
Tablets, scored, cyclofenil 100 mg. Net price 20 = £3.70

TAMOXIFEN
See section 8.3.4

ANTERIOR PITUITARY HORMONES

CORTICOTROPHINS
Corticotrophin and tetracosactrin are used mainly as diagnostic agents (see section 6.7.2). The long-acting depot forms (Synacthen Depot® etc.) have been used as alternatives to corticosteroids in conditions such as Crohn's disease or rheumatoid arthritis; the purported advantages being less adrenocortical suppression and less growth retardation (see section 6.3.4). Dosage may be adjusted on the basis of urinary free cortisol estimations.

CORTICOTROPHIN
(ACTH)
Indications: see notes above
Cautions; Contra-indications; Side-effects: see section 6.3.3; also caution in hypertension. Drug interactions: see Appendix 1 (sections *2.2, 2.5, 6.1,* 6.3)
Dose: by subcutaneous or intramuscular injection, depot preparations, initially 40–80 units daily, reduced according to response

PoM **Acthar Gel®** (Rorer)
Injection, corticotrophin (with gelatin) 20 units/ ml, net price 5-ml vial = £4.73; 40 units/ml, 2-ml vial = £3.39, 5-ml vial = £8.57; 80 units/ml, 5-ml vial = £16.68

TETRACOSACTRIN
Indications: see notes above
Cautions; Contra-indications; Side-effects: see section 6.3.3; hypersensitivity reactions may occur less frequently than with corticotrophin

PoM **Synacthen®** (Ciba)
Injection, tetracosactrin 250 micrograms (as acetate)/ml. Net price 1-ml amp = 93p
Dose: diagnostic, *by intramuscular injection,* 250 micrograms as a single dose
PoM **Synacthen Depot®** (Ciba)
Injection (aqueous suspension), tetracosactrin 1 mg (as acetate)/ml, with zinc phosphate complex. Net price 1-ml amp = £1.05; 2-ml vial = £1.92
Dose: by intramuscular injection, initially 1 mg daily (or every 12 hours in acute cases); subsequently reduced to 1 mg every 2–3 days, then 1 mg weekly (or 500 micrograms every 2–3 days); CHILD 1 month–2 years initially 250 micrograms daily, 2–5 years 250–500 micrograms, 5–12 years 0.25–1 mg, subsequently reduced to every 2–8 days

GONADOTROPHINS
Human **follicle-stimulating hormone** (FSH) (Pergonal®, etc.) is used in the treatment of infertile women with proven hypopituitarism or who have not responded to clomiphene; it is used in conjunction with **chorionic gonadotrophin** (HCG) (Gonadotraphon LH®, Profasi®). Treatment requires careful monitoring to avoid the ovarian

hyperstimulation syndrome and multiple pregnancy. The two gonadotrophins are also occasionally used in the treatment of oligospermia associated with hypopituitarism. There is no justification for their use in primary gonadal failure. Chorionic gonadotrophin has also been used in delayed puberty in the male to stimulate endogenous testosterone production, but has little advantage over testosterone (section 6.4.2).

CHORIONIC GONADOTROPHIN
(Human Chorionic Gonadotrophin; HCG)
Indications: see notes above
Cautions: see notes above; cardiac or renal impairment, asthma, epilepsy, migraine
Side-effects: oedema (particularly in males—reduce dose), headache, tiredness, mood changes, local reactions; sexual precocity with high doses; may aggravate ovarian hyperstimulation after menotrophin
Dose: by intramuscular injection, according to patient's requirements

PoM **Gonadotraphon LH®** (Paines & Byrne)
Injection, powder for reconstitution, human chorionic gonadotrophin. Net price 500-unit amp = 79p; 1000-unit amp = £1.00; 5000-unit amp = £2.97 (all with solvent)
PoM **Profasi®** (Serono)
Injection, powder for reconstitution, human chorionic gonadotrophin. Net price 500-unit amp = 69p; 1000-unit amp = 93p; 2000-unit amp = £1.75; 5000-unit amp = £3.08 (all with solvent)

FOLLICLE-STIMULATING   HORMONE (FSH)
Indications: see notes above
Cautions: ovarian cysts, adrenal or thyroid disorders, intracranial lesions
Side-effects: ovarian hyperstimulation, multiple pregnancy; local reactions (general sensitivity reactions with serum gonadotrophin)
Dose: by deep intramuscular injection, according to patient's response

PoM **Metrodin®** (Serono)
Injection, powder for reconstitution, urofollitrophin (from human menopausal urine) as human follicle-stimulating hormone 75 units, lactose 10 mg. Net price per amp (with solvent) = £14.70
PoM **Pergonal®** (Serono)
Injection, powder for reconstitution, menotrophin (from postmenopausal urine) as human follicle-stimulating hormone 75 units, human luteinising hormone 75 units, lactose 10 mg. Net price per amp (with solvent) = £8.90

GROWTH HORMONE
Growth hormone is used in the treatment of short stature due to growth hormone deficiency; only the human type is effective as growth hormone is species specific. Growth hormone of human origin (HGH; somatotrophin) has been replaced by a

growth hormone of human sequence, **somatrem** (Somatonorm®), produced using recombinant DNA technology.

SOMATREM
(Methionyl Human Growth Hormone)
Indications: see notes above
Cautions: only patients with open epiphyses should be treated; diabetes mellitus (adjustment of antidiabetic therapy may be necessary)
Side-effects: antibody formation; lipo-atrophy with subcutaneous injection (rotate sites)
Dose: 0.5 unit/kg weekly divided into 2 or 3 doses for *intramuscular injection* or divided into 6 or 7 doses for *subcutaneous injection*

▼ PoM **Somatonorm 4IU®** (KabiVitrum)
Injection, powder for preparing intramuscular injections, somatrem, with glycine and sodium phosphate. Net price 4-unit vial (with diluent) = £30.50

HYPOTHALAMIC HORMONES

Gonadorelin (gonadotrophin-releasing hormone, LH-RH) and **protirelin** (thyrotrophin-releasing hormone, TRH) are used mainly as diagnostic agents (section 6.7.2). Gonadorelin is also used for treatment of infertility, particularly in the female. Buserelin and goserelin, gonadotrophin-releasing hormone analogues, are indicated in metastatic prostate cancer (see section 8.3.4).

6.5.2 Posterior pituitary hormones and antagonists

POSTERIOR PITUITARY HORMONES

DIABETES INSIPIDUS. Vasopressin (antidiuretic hormone, ADH) is used in the treatment of *pituitary* ('cranial') *diabetes insipidus* as its analogues **lypressin** (Syntopressin®) or **desmopressin** (DDAVP). Dosage is tailored to produce a slight diuresis every 24 hours to avoid water intoxication. Treatment may be required for a limited period only in diabetes insipidus following trauma or pituitary surgery.

Desmopressin has a longer duration of action than vasopressin or lypressin; unlike vasopressin and lypressin it has no vasoconstrictor effect. It is given intranasally for maintenance therapy, and by injection in the postoperative period or in unconscious patients; the injection is also used for the diagnosis of diabetes insipidus (section 6.7.2).

In *nephrogenic* and *partial pituitary diabetes insipidus* benefit may be gained from the paradoxical antidiuretic effect of thiazides (see section 2.2.1) e.g. chlorthalidone 100 mg twice daily reduced to maintenance dose of 50 mg daily.

Chlorpropamide (section 6.1.2.1) is also useful in partial pituitary diabetes insipidus, and probably acts by sensitising the renal tubules to the action of remaining endogenous vasopressin; it is given in doses of up to 350 mg daily in adults and 200 mg daily in children, care being taken to avoid hypoglycaemia. Carbamazepine (see section 4.8.1) is also sometimes useful (in a dose of 200 mg once or twice daily); its mode of action may be similar to that of chlorpropamide.

OTHER USES. Desmopressin injection is also used to boost factor VIII concentrations on mild to moderate haemophilia.

Vasopressin infusion is used to control variceal bleeding in portal hypertension, prior to more definitive treatment and with variable results. Terlipressin (Glypressin®), a new derivative of vasopressin, is used similarly.

Oxytocin, another posterior pituitary hormone, is indicated in obstetrics (see section 7.1.1).

VASOPRESSIN
Indications: pituitary diabetes insipidus; bleeding from oesophageal varices
Cautions: heart failure, asthma, epilepsy, migraine; adjust fluid intake to avoid hyponatraemia and water intoxication
Contra-indications: vascular disease, chronic nephritis (until reasonable blood nitrogen concentrations attained)
Side-effects: pallor, nausea, belching, cramp, desire to defaecate, uterine cramps, hypersensitivity reactions, constriction of coronary arteries (may cause anginal attacks and myocardial ischaemia)
Dose: by subcutaneous or intramuscular injection, diabetes insipidus, 5–20 units every four hours
By intravenous infusion, variceal bleeding, 20 units over 15 minutes

Synthetic vasopressin
PoM **Pitressin®** (P-D)
Injection, argipressin (synthetic vasopressin) 20 units/ml. Net price 1-ml amp = 62p (Hosp. only)

DESMOPRESSIN
Indications: see under Dose; diagnostic procedures (section 6.7.2)
Cautions: see under Vasopressin; almost devoid of pressor activity and well tolerated
Dose: intranasally, pituitary diabetes insipidus (diagnosis), adults and children, 20 micrograms
Pituitary diabetes insipidus (treatment), adults and children, 10–20 micrograms once or twice daily
Primary nocturnal enuresis, adults and children over 7 years, 20 micrograms at bedtime, increased to 40 micrograms if necessary, for 28 days (long-term use not recommended)
By intramuscular or intravenous injection, pituitary diabetes insipidus, 1–4 micrograms daily; CHILD 400 nanograms

PoM **DDAVP®** (Ferring)
Intranasal solution, desmopressin 100 micrograms/ml. Net price 2.5-ml dropper bottle and catheter = £9.50
Injection, desmopressin 4 micrograms/ml. Net price 1-ml amp = £1.07

PoM **Desmospray**® (Ferring)
Nasal spray, desmopressin 10 micrograms/
metered spray. Net price 5-ml metered unit =
£19.92

LYPRESSIN

Indications: pituitary diabetes insipidus
Cautions; Contra-indications; Side-effects: see
under Vasopressin; less hypersensitivity; also
nasal congestion with ulceration of mucosa
Dose: intranasally, 2.5–10 units 3–7 times daily

PoM **Syntopressin**® (Sandoz)
Nasal spray, lypressin 50 units/ml, providing 2.5
units/squeeze. Net price 5-ml spray bottle =
£3.49

TERLIPRESSIN

Indications: bleeding from oesophageal varices
Cautions; Contra-indications; Side-effects: see
under Vasopressin, but effects are milder
Dose: by intravenous injection, 2 mg followed by
1 or 2 mg every 4 to 6 hours until bleeding is
controlled, for up to 72 hours

▼ PoM **Glypressin**® (Ferring)
Injection, terlipressin, powder for reconstitution.
Net price 1-mg vial with 5 ml diluent = £19.00
(Hosp. only)

ANTIDIURETIC HORMONE
ANTAGONISTS

Demeclocycline (see section 5.1.3) may be used in
the treatment of hyponatraemia resulting from
inappropriate secretion of antidiuretic hormone.
It is thought to act by directly blocking the renal
tubular effect of antidiuretic hormone. Initially
0.9 to 1.2 g is given daily in divided doses, reduced
to 600–900 mg daily in divided doses for
maintenance.

6.6   Drugs affecting bone metabolism

This section includes calcitonin and salcatonin
(section 6.6.1) and disodium etidronate (section
6.6.2).

See also plicamycin (section 8.1.2), calcium and
phosphorus compounds (sections 9.5.1.1 and
9.5.2), vitamin D preparations (section 9.6.4),
and oestrogens in postmenopausal osteoporosis
(section 6.4.1.1).

6.6.1   Calcitonin and salcatonin

Calcitonin (Calcitare®) is involved with para-
thyroid hormone in the regulation of bone turnover and hence in the maintenance of calcium
balance and homoeostasis. It is used to lower the
plasma-calcium concentration in some patients
with hypercalcaemia (notably when associated
with malignant disease). In the treatment of
severe Paget's disease of bone it is used mainly
for relief of pain but it is also effective in relieving
some of the neurological complications, for

example deafness. The prolonged use of porcine
calcitonin can lead to the production of neutralising antibodies. **Salcatonin** (Calsynar®, synthetic salmon calcitonin) is less immunogenic and
thus more suitable for long-term therapy. When
changing treatment in Paget's disease, calcitonin
80 units is equivalent to salcatonin 50 units.

CALCITONIN

Indications: Paget's   disease   of   bone;
hypercalcaemia
Cautions: see notes above; porcine calcitonin
may contain trace amounts of thyroid. Skin test
advisable in patients with history of allergy
Side-effects: nausea, vomiting, flushing, tingling
of hands, unpleasant taste, inflammatory reactions at injection site
Dose: hypercalcaemia, *by subcutaneous or intramuscular injection*, initially 4–8 units/kg daily
adjusted according to clinical and biochemical
response
Paget's disease of bone, *by subcutaneous or
intramuscular injection*, 80–160 units 3 times
weekly increased to daily in patients with bone
pain or nerve compression syndromes

PoM **Calcitare**® (Rorer)
Injection, powder for reconstitution, porcine
calcitonin. Net price 160-unit vial (with gelatin
diluent) = £11.36

SALCATONIN

Indications: Paget's disease of bone; hypercalcaemia; bone pain in neoplastic disease;
postmenopausal osteoporosis
Cautions; Side-effects: see under Calcitonin and
notes above
Dose: hypercalcaemia, *by subcutaneous or intramuscular injection*, initially up to 8 units/kg
every 6–8 hours adjusted according to clinical
and biochemical response
Paget's disease of bone, *by subcutaneous or
intramuscular injection*, 50–100 units 3 times
weekly increased to daily, in single or divided
doses, in patients with bone pain or nerve
compression syndromes, usually for 3–6 months
Bone pain in neoplastic disease, *by subcutaneous or intramuscular injection*, 200 units
every 6 hours for 48 hours
Postmenopausal osteoporosis, *by subcutaneous
or intramuscular injection*, 100 units daily with
calcium and vitamin D

PoM **Calsynar**® (Rorer)
Injection, salcatonin 100 units/ml in saline/
acetate. Net price 1-ml amp = £8.12
Injection, salcatonin 200 units/ml in saline/
acetate. Net price 2-ml vial = £29.20

6.6.2   Disodium etidronate

Disodium etidronate (Didronel®) is used mainly
in the treatment of Paget's disease of bone. It is
adsorbed onto hydroxyapatite crystals, so slowing
both their rate of growth and dissolution, and
reduces the increased rate of bone turnover

associated with the disease. The initial dose is usually 5 mg/kg daily for up to 6 months, but 10 mg/kg daily may be used for up to 3 months if more rapid suppression of bone turnover is necessary; however doses higher than this may make symptoms worse. At least 3 months should elapse before retreatment.

An injection is now available for hypercalcaemia of malignancy.

DISODIUM ETIDRONATE

Indications: see under Dose

Cautions: enterocolitis; discontinue use if fractures occur; reduce dose in renal impairment (avoid if severe)

Side-effects: nausea, diarrhoea, increase in bone pain, increased risk of fractures with high doses; transient taste loss reported

Dose: Paget's disease of bone, *by mouth*, 5 mg/kg as a single daily dose for up to 6 months; doses above 10 mg/kg daily for up to 3 months may be used with caution but doses above 20 mg/kg daily are not recommended; see also notes above

Hypercalcaemia of malignancy, *by intravenous infusion* (over at least 2 hours), 7.5 mg/kg daily for 3 days; repeat if necessary after at least 7 days; *by mouth*, on day after last intravenous dose, 20 mg/kg as a single daily dose for 30 days; max. recommended treatment period 90 days

COUNSELLING. Avoid food for at least 2 hours before and after treatment, particularly calcium-containing products

▼ PoM **Didronel**® (Norwich Eaton)
Tablets, disodium etidronate 200 mg. Net price 20 tabs = £10.46. Counselling advised, food and calcium (see above)

▼ PoM **Didronel IV**® (Norwich Eaton)
Injection, disodium etidronate 50 mg/ml. Net price 6-ml amp = £33.09

6.7 Other endocrine drugs

This section includes:
6.7.1 Bromocriptine
6.7.2 Diagnostic agents
6.7.3 Danazol
6.7.4 Trilostane

6.7.1 Bromocriptine

Bromocriptine (Parlodel®) is a stimulant of dopamine receptors in the brain; it also inhibits release of prolactin by the pituitary. Bromocriptine is used for the suppression of lactation when simpler measures fail, for the treatment of galactorrhoea and cyclical benign breast disease, and for the treatment of prolactinomas (when it reduces both plasma-prolactin concentration and tumour size). Bromocriptine also inhibits the release of growth hormone and is sometimes used in the treatment of acromegaly, the success rate is much lower than with prolactinomas.

For the use of bromocriptine in parkinsonism, see section 4.9.1.

BROMOCRIPTINE

Indications: see notes above

Cautions: monitor for pituitary enlargement, particularly during pregnancy, annual gynaecological assessment (post-menopausal, every 6 months), monitor for peptic ulceration in acromegalic patients; contraceptive advice if appropriate (oral contraceptives may increase prolactin concentrations); at high dosage caution in patients with history of psychotic disorders or with severe cardiovascular disease; alcohol may reduce tolerance. Drug interactions: see Appendix 1 (section 6.7)

Side-effects: nausea, vomiting, constipation, headache, dizziness, postural hypotension, drowsiness; *high doses*, confusion, hallucinations, dyskinesia, dry mouth, leg cramps, pleural effusions (may necessitate withdrawal of treatment), digital vasospasm; retroperitoneal fibrosis reported (monitoring required)

Dose: prevention/suppression of lactation for medical reasons, 2.5 mg on 1st day (prevention) or daily for 2–3 days (suppression); then 2.5 mg twice daily for 14 days

Hypogonadism/galactorrhoea, infertility, initially 1–1.25 mg at bedtime, increased gradually; usual dose 7.5 mg daily in divided doses, increased if necessary to a max. of 30 mg daily. Usual dose in infertility without hyperprolactinaemia, 2.5 mg twice daily

Cyclical benign breast disease and cyclical menstrual disorders (particularly breast pain), 1–1.25 mg at bedtime, increased gradually; usual dose 2.5 mg twice daily

Acromegaly, initially 1–1.25 mg at bedtime, increase gradually to 5 mg every 6 hours

Prolactinoma, initially 1–1.25 mg at bedtime; increased gradually to 5 mg every 6 hours (occasional patients may require up to 30 mg daily)

Doses should be taken with food

COUNSELLING. Hypotensive reactions may be disturbing in some patients during the first few days of treatment and particular care should be exercised when driving vehicles or operating machinery

PoM **Parlodel**® (Sandoz)
Tablets, both scored, bromocriptine (as mesylate) 1 mg, net price 20 = £2.65; 2.5 mg, 20 = £5.13. Label: 21, counselling advised, see above
Capsules, bromocriptine (as mesylate) 5 mg (blue/white), net price 20 = £10.06; 10 mg, 20 = £18.62. Label: 21, counselling advised, see above

6.7.2 Diagnostic agents for endocrine disorders

Tetracosactrin injection (section 6.5.1) is used to test adrenocortical function. Failure of the plasma cortisol concentration to rise after intramuscular administration indicates adrenocortical insufficiency.

Metyrapone (Metopirone®) is a competitive inhibitor of 11β-hydroxylation in the adrenal cortex; the resulting inhibition of cortisol production leads to an increase in ACTH production which, in turn, leads to increased synthesis and release of cortisol precursors. It may be used as a test of anterior pituitary function. For therapeutic use in Cushing's syndrome, see section 6.3.1.

Thyrotrophin-releasing hormone (TRH, **protirelin**) may be of value in difficult cases of hyperthyroidism. Failure of plasma thyrotrophin (TSH) concentration to rise after intravenous injection indicates excess circulating thyroid hormones. Impaired or absent responses also occur in some euthyroid patients with single adenoma, multinodular goitre, or endocrine exophthalmos; patients with hypopituitarism show a reduced or delayed rise.

Gonadotrophin-releasing hormone (LH-RH, **gonadorelin**) when injected intravenously in normal subjects leads to a rapid rise in plasma concentrations of both luteinising hormone (LH) and follicle-stimulating hormone (FSH). It has not proved to be very helpful, however, in distinguishing hypothalamic from pituitary lesions.

Desmopressin (section 6.5.2) is used in the differential diagnosis of diabetes insipidus. Following an intramuscular dose of 2 micrograms, restoration of the ability to concentrate urine after water deprivation confirms a diagnosis of cranial diabetes insipidus. Failure to respond occurs in nephrogenic diabetes insipidus.

The **glucose** tolerance test is used in the diagnosis of diabetes mellitus; 75 g of glucose (dextrose monohydrate) is given by mouth to the fasting patient, and plasma glucose concentrations are measured at intervals.

GONADORELIN
(LH–RH)
Indications: see preparations below
Side-effects: rarely, nausea, headache, abdominal pain, increased menstrual bleeding; irritation at injection site
Dose: see below

▼ PoM **Fertiral**® (Hoechst)
Injection, gonadorelin 500 micrograms/ml. Net price 2-ml amp = £34.30
For amenorrhoea and infertility due to abnormal release of LH–RH (endogenous gonadorelin), *by pulsatile subcutaneous infusion*, initially 10–20 micrograms over 1 minute, repeated every 90 minutes for max. of 6 months; pulsatile intravenous infusion (in association with heparin) may be required
▼ PoM **HRF**® (Wyeth)
Injection, powder for reconstitution, gonadorelin. Net price 100-microgram vial = £8.12; 500-microgram vial = £17.73 (both with diluent)
For assessment of pituitary function, *by subcutaneous or intravenous injection*, 100 micrograms; to determine the threshold of pituitary

response, initially, 25 micrograms increasing stepwise, max. 500 micrograms
PoM **Relefact LH-RH**® (Hoechst)
Injection, gonadorelin 100 micrograms/ml. Net price 1-ml amp = £9.68
For assessment of pituitary function, *by intravenous injection*, 100 micrograms
PoM **Relefact LH-RH/TRH**® (Hoechst)
Injection, gonadorelin 100 micrograms, protirelin 200 micrograms/ml. Net price 1-ml amp = £11.18.
For assessment of anterior pituitary reserve by intravenous injection, 1 ml

METYRAPONE
Indications: see under Dose
Cautions: gross hypopituitarism (risk of precipitating acute adrenal failure); many drugs interfere with estimation of steroids
Contra-indications: pregnancy, breast-feeding
Side-effects: occasional nausea, vomiting, dizziness, headache, hypotension
Dose: in the assessment of pituitary function 750 mg every 4 hours for 6 doses; CHILD 15 mg/kg (minimum 250 mg)
Management of Cushing's syndrome, range 0.25–6 g daily, tailored to cortisol production; see also section 6.3.1
Resistant oedema due to increased aldosterone secretion in cirrhosis, nephrosis, and congestive heart failure, 2.5–4.5 g daily in divided doses (with glucocorticoids)
Note. Metyrapone should only be used under specialist advice; corticosteroid replacement therapy needed with high doses

PoM **Metopirone**® (Ciba)
Capsules, metyrapone 250 mg. Net price 20 = £4.18. Label: 21

PROTIRELIN
Indications: assessment of thyroid function and thyroid stimulating hormone reserve in hypopituitarism
Cautions: severe hypopituitarism, cardiac insufficiency, bronchial asthma and obstructive airways disease, early pregnancy
Side-effects: nausea; also after rapid intravenous administration desire to micturate, flushing, dizziness, syncope, strange taste; rarely bronchospasm
Dose: by intravenous injection, adults and children 200 micrograms

PoM **TRH** (Roche)
Injection, protirelin 100 micrograms/ml. Net price 2-ml amp = £15.00

6.7.3   Danazol
Danazol (Danol®) inhibits pituitary gonadotrophin secretion, and is used in the treatment of endometriosis. It has also been used for menorrhagia and other menstrual disorders, mammary dysplasia, and gynaecomastia. It is the drug

of choice in the long-term management of hereditary angioedema.

DANAZOL

Indications: see notes above

Cautions: cardiac, hepatic, or renal impairment, epilepsy, diabetes mellitus, migraine, breast-feeding; non-hormonal contraceptive methods should be used, if appropriate. Drug interactions: see Appendix 1 (sections *2.8B, 4.8, 8*)

Contra-indications: porphyria; pregnancy, ensure that patients with amenorrhoea are not pregnant

Side-effects: nausea, dizziness, rashes, backache, flushing, skeletal muscle spasm, hair loss; mild androgenic effects including acne, oily skin, oedema, mild hirsutism, voice changes, hyper-glucagonaemia; thrombocytopenia reported

Dose: usual range 200–800 mg daily in up to 4 divided doses; in adult females all doses should start during menstruation, preferably on the first day

Endometriosis, initially 400 mg daily in 2–4 divided doses, adjusted according to response, usually for 6 months

Menorrhagia, 100–400 mg daily in 2–4 divided doses, adjusted according to response (usual dose 200 mg daily), review after 3 months

Benign breast disorders, initially 300 mg daily in divided doses, adjusted according to response, usually for 3–6 months

CHILD, precocious puberty, 100–400 mg daily according to age and response

PoM **Danol**® (Winthrop)
Capsules, pink/white, danazol 200 mg. Net price 20 = £10.98; 56-cap pack = £30.75
PoM **Danol-½**® (Winthrop)
Capsules, grey/white, danazol 100 mg. Net price 20 = £5.55

6.7.4   Trilostane

Trilostane (Modrenal®) inhibits the synthesis of mineralocorticoids and glucocorticoids by the adrenal cortex, and its use is being evaluated for Cushing's syndrome and primary hyperaldosteronism. It appears to be less effective than metyrapone (section 6.3.1) for the treatment of Cushing's syndrome.

TRILOSTANE

Indications: see notes above

Cautions: impaired liver and kidney function, monitor circulating corticosteroids and blood-electrolyte concentrations; non-hormonal contraceptive methods should be used, if appropriate. Drug interactions: see Appendix 1 (section *2.2*)

Contra-indications: pregnancy

Side-effects: rarely flushing, nausea, rhinorrhoea with high doses

Dose: 60 mg 4 times daily for at least 3 days, then adjusted according to patient's response; usual dose range 120–480 mg daily in divided doses

PoM **Modrenal**® (Sterling Research)
Capsules, pink/black, trilostane 60 mg. Net price 20 = £7.92

7: Drugs used in

OBSTETRICS, GYNAECOLOGY, and URINARY-TRACT DISORDERS

In this chapter, drugs are discussed under the following headings:

7.1 Drugs acting on smooth muscle
7.2 Treatment of vaginal and vulval conditions
7.3 Contraceptives
7.4 Drugs for urinary-tract disorders

For hormonal therapy of gynaecological disorders see sections 6.4.1 and 6.5.1.

7.1 Drugs acting on smooth muscle

This section includes prostaglandins and oxytocics (section 7.1.1) and myometrial relaxants (section 7.1.2).

Note. Because of the complexity of dosage regimens in obstetrics, in all cases detailed specialist literature should be consulted.

7.1.1 Prostaglandins and oxytocics

Myometrial stimulants are used to induce abortion or induce or augment labour and to minimise blood loss from the placental site. They include oxytocin, ergometrine, and the prostaglandins.

INDUCTION OF ABORTION. The prostaglandins **dinoprost** (Prostin F2 alpha®) and **dinoprostone** (Prostin E2®) can be used for the induction of abortion. They are contra-indicated in conditions where prolonged uterine contractions would be inappropriate.

The *intravenous route* is associated with a high incidence of side-effects and is rarely used.

Extra- or *intra-amniotic* administration of a prostaglandin is preferable for the induction of late therapeutic abortion. Extra-amniotic dinoprostone is also of value as an adjunct in 'priming' the cervix prior to suction termination. The intra-amniotic route can only be used after about 14–16 weeks gestation.

INDUCTION AND AUGMENTATION OF LABOUR. **Oxytocin** (Syntocinon®) is administered by slow intravenous infusion, preferably using an infusion pump, to induce or augment labour, often in conjunction with amniotomy. Uterine activity must be monitored and hyperstimulation avoided. Large doses of oxytocin may result in excessive fluid retention.

Prostaglandins have now been developed as vaginal tablets and vaginal gels for the induction of labour at term. The intravenous and oral routes are rarely used.

PREVENTION AND TREATMENT OF HAEMORRHAGE. Bleeding due to *incomplete abortion* can be controlled with **ergometrine** and **oxytocin** (Syntometrine®) given intravenously or intramuscularly, the dose being adjusted according to the patient's condition and blood loss. This is commonly used prior to surgical evacuation of the uterus, particularly when surgery is delayed. Oxytocin or ergometrine may be used alone but is usually less effective on the early pregnant uterus.

For the routine management of the *third stage of labour* ergometrine 500 micrograms with oxytocin 5 units (Syntometrine® 1 ml) is given by intramuscular injection with or after delivery of the shoulders. Intravenous injection is needed for the prevention of postpartum haemorrhage in *high-risk cases*, giving either ergometrine 125–250 micrograms alone *or* oxytocin 5–10 units alone after delivery of the shoulders (repeated if necessary); alternatively intravenous infusion of oxytocin 10–20 units/500 ml can be given after delivery of the shoulders, particularly when the uterus is *atonic*.

DINOPROST

Indications: see notes above
Cautions: asthma, glaucoma and raised intra-ocular pressure, grand multiparas and multiple pregnancy; excessive dosage may cause uterine rupture; see also notes above
Contra-indications: hypertonic uterine inertia, mechanical obstruction of delivery, placenta praevia, predisposition to uterine rupture, severe toxaemia, untreated pelvic infection, fetal distress
Side-effects: nausea, vomiting, diarrhoea, flushing, shivering, headache, dizziness, temporary pyrexia and raised white blood cell count; all dose-related and more common after intravenous administration; also local tissue reaction and erythema after intravenous administration
Dose: by intravenous infusion (rarely used, see notes above)
Induction of labour, fetal intra-uterine death, as a solution containing 15 micrograms/ml, 2.5 micrograms/minute for at least 30 minutes then maintained or increased; fetal intra-uterine death an initial rate of 5 micrograms/minute may be used with increases at intervals of not less than 1 hour
Therapeutic abortion, missed abortion, and hydatidiform mole, as a solution containing 50 micrograms/ml, 25 micrograms/minute for at least 30 minutes, then continued or increased to 50 micrograms/minute; should be maintained for at least 4 hours before increasing further
By slow intra-amniotic injection, therapeutic termination of pregnancy in second trimester, 40 mg (8 ml undiluted)

PoM **Prostin F2 alpha**® (Upjohn)

Intravenous injection, dinoprost 5 mg (as tro-metamol salt)/ml. For dilution and use as an infusion. Net price 1.5-ml amp = £7.47; 5-ml amp = £24.71 (Hosp. only)

Intra-amniotic injection, dinoprost 5 mg (as tro-metamol salt)/ml. Net price 4-ml amp = £19.71; 8-ml amp = £39.42 (Hosp. only)

DINOPROSTONE

Indications: Cautions; Contra-indications; Side-effects: see under Dinoprost and notes above; also avoid extra-amniotic route in cervicitis or vaginitis

Dose: by mouth, induction of labour, 500 micro-grams, followed by 0.5–1 mg (max. 1.5 mg) at hourly intervals

By intravenous infusion (rarely used, see notes above)

Induction of labour, fetal intra-uterine death, as a solution containing 1.5 micrograms/ml, 250 nanograms/minute for at least 30 minutes then maintained or increased; in fetal intra-uterine death an initial rate of 500 nanograms/minute may be used with increases at intervals of not less than 1 hour

Therapeutic abortion, missed abortion, and hydatidiform mole, as a solution containing 5 micrograms/ml, 2.5 micrograms/minute for at least 30 minutes then increased if necessary to 5 micrograms/minute; should be maintained for at least 4 hours before increasing further

By extra-amniotic instillation, therapeutic abor-tion, as a solution containing 100 micrograms/ml, 100 micrograms, followed by 100–200 micrograms every 2 hours

By vagina, induction of labour, as **gel** inserted high into posterior fornix, 1 mg, followed after 6 hours by 1–2 mg if required; max. 3 mg [gel]

By vagina, induction of labour, as **vaginal tablets** inserted high into posterior fornix, 3 mg, fol-lowed after 6–8 hours by 3 mg if labour is not established; max. 6 mg [vaginal tablets]

Note. The debris of vaginal tablets can be aspirated during birth, therefore the gel may be safer

IMPORTANT. Do not confuse dose of vaginal **gel** with that of vaginal **tablets**—not bioequivalent.

PoM **Prostin E2**® (Upjohn)

Tablets, dinoprostone 500 micrograms. Net price 10-tab pack = £14.93 (Hosp. only)

Intravenous injection, for dilution and use as an infusion, dinoprostone 1 mg/ml, net price 0.75-ml amp = £6.91; 10 mg/ml, 0.5-ml amp = £14.93 (both hosp. only)

Extra-amniotic injection, dinoprostone 10 mg/ml. Net price 0.5-ml amp (with diluent) = £14.93 (Hosp. only)

Vaginal gel, dinoprostone 400 micrograms/ml, net price 2.5 ml (1 mg) = £14.52; 800 micrograms/ml, 2.5 ml (2 mg) = £16.00

Vaginal tablets, dinoprostone 3 mg. Net price 4-vaginal tab pack = £32.52

Note. Prostin E2 Vaginal Gel and Vaginal Tablets are **not** bioequivalent

ERGOMETRINE MALEATE

Indications: active management of third stage of labour, postpartum haemorrhage

Cautions: toxaemia, cardiac disease, hyperten-sion, sepsis, multiple pregnancy

Contra-indications: 1st and 2nd stages of labour, vascular disease, impaired pulmonary, hepatic, and renal function

Side-effects: nausea, vomiting, transient hyper-tension, vasoconstriction

Dose: by mouth, 0.5–1 mg (onset about 8 minutes, duration about 1 hour)

By intramuscular injection, 200–500 micrograms (onset about 5–7 minutes, duration about 45 minutes)

By intravenous injection for emergency control of haemorrhage, 100–500 micrograms (onset about 1 minute)

See also notes above

PoM **Ergometrine Tablets**, ergometrine maleate 250 micrograms, net price 20 = £1.10; 500 micrograms, 20 = £1.45

PoM **Ergometrine Injection**, ergometrine maleate 500 micrograms/ml. Net price 1-ml amp = 18p

Combined preparation

PoM **Syntometrine**® (Sandoz)

Injection, ergometrine maleate 500 micrograms, oxytocin 5 units/ml. Net price 1-ml amp = 19p

Dose: by intramuscular injection, 1 ml; by intra-venous injection, 0.5–1 ml

GEMEPROST

Indications: softening and dilation of the cervix to facilitate transcervical operative procedures for first trimester abortion

Cautions: obstructive airways disease, cardio-vascular insufficiency, raised intra-ocular pres-sure, cervicitis or vaginitis

Side-effects: vaginal bleeding and uterine pain; nausea, vomiting, or diarrhoea; headache, mus-cle weakness, dizziness, flushing, chills, back-ache, dyspnoea, chest pain, palpitations and mild pyrexia

Dose: by vagina in pessaries, 1 mg 3 hours before surgery

▼ PoM **Cervagem**® (M&B)

Pessaries, gemeprost 1 mg. Net price 1 pessary = £18.15

OXYTOCIN

Indications: induction and augmentation of labour; management of missed or incomplete abortion; postpartum haemorrhage

Cautions: hypertension, pressor drugs (may pre-cipitate severe hypertension), multiple preg-nancy, high parity, previous Caesarean section

Contra-indications: hypertonic uterine inertia, mechanical obstruction to delivery, failed trial labour, severe toxaemia, predisposition to amniotic fluid embolism, fetal distress, and placenta praevia

Side-effects: high doses cause violent uterine contractions leading to rupture and fetal asphyxiation, arrhythmias, maternal hypertension and subarachnoid haemorrhage, water intoxication

Dose: by slow intravenous infusion, induction and augmentation of labour, as a solution containing 1 unit per litre, 1–3 milliunits per minute, adjusted according to response

Missed abortion, as a solution containing 10–20 units/500 ml given at a rate of 10–30 drops/minute, increased in strength by 10–20 units/500 ml every hour to a max. strength of 100 units/500 ml

Postpartum haemorrhage, 5–10 units/500 ml given at a rate of 15 drops/minute, adjusted according to response

PoM Syntocinon® (Sandoz)
Injection, oxytocin 1 unit/ml, net price 2-ml amp = 18p; 5 units/ml, 1-ml amp = 20p; 10 units/ml, 1-ml amp = 23p, 5-ml amp = 84p
Nasal spray—discontinued

Combined preparation—see Syntometrine

DUCTUS ARTERIOSUS

MAINTENANCE OF PATENCY
Alprostadil (prostaglandin E₁) is used to maintain patency of the ductus arteriosus in neonates with congenital heart defects, prior to corrective surgery in centres where intensive care is immediately available.

ALPROSTADIL
Indications: congenital heart defects in neonates prior to corrective surgery
Cautions: see notes above; avoid use in hyaline membrane disease, history of haemorrhage, monitor arterial pressure
Side-effects: apnoea (particularly in infants under 2 kg), flushing, bradycardia, hypotension, tachycardia, cardiac arrest, oedema, diarrhoea, fever, convulsions, disseminated intravascular coagulation, hypokalaemia; cortical proliferation of long bones, weakening of the wall of the ductus arteriosus and pulmonary artery may follow prolonged use
Dose: by intravenous infusion, initially 50–100 nanograms/kg/minute, then decreased to lowest effective dose

▼ **PoM Prostin VR®** (Upjohn)
Injection, alprostadil 500 micrograms/ml in alcohol. For dilution and use as an infusion. Net price 1-ml amp = £56.96 (Hosp. only)

CLOSURE OF DUCTUS ARTERIOSUS
Prostaglandin E₁ has the role of dilating the ductus arteriosus; indomethacin is believed to close it by inhibiting prostaglandin synthesis.

INDOMETHACIN
Indications: patent ductus arteriosus in premature infants (under specialist supervision)

Cautions: may mask symptoms of infection; may reduce renal function by 50% or more and precipitate renal insufficiency especially in infants with heart failure, sepsis, or hepatic impairment, or who are receiving nephrotoxic drugs; if urine volume reduced, discontinue until output returns to normal; may induce hyponatraemia; monitor renal function and electrolytes

Contra-indications: untreated infection, bleeding, congenital heart disease where patency of ductus arteriosus necessary for satisfactory pulmonary or systemic blood flow; thrombocytopenia, coagulation defects, necrotising enterocolitis, renal impairment

Side-effects: include haemorrhagic, renal, gastrointestinal, metabolic, and coagulation disorders; fluid retention, and exacerbation of infection

Dose: by intravenous injection, over 5–10 seconds, 3 doses at intervals of 12–24 hours, age less than 48 hours, 200 micrograms/kg then 100 micrograms/kg then 100 micrograms/kg; age 2–7 days, 200 micrograms/kg then 200 micrograms/kg then 200 micrograms/kg; age over 7 days, 200 micrograms/kg then 250 micrograms/kg then 250 micrograms/kg; solution prepared with 1–2 ml sodium chloride 0.9% or water for injections (not glucose and no preservatives)

If ductus arteriosus reopens a second course of 3 injections may be given

▼ **PoM Indocid PDA®** (Morson)
Injection, powder for reconstitution, indomethacin (as sodium trihydrate). Net price 3 × 1-mg vials = £22.50 (Hosp. only)

7.1.2   Myometrial relaxants

Beta₂-adrenoceptor stimulants (sympathomimetics) relax uterine muscle and are used in selected cases in an attempt to inhibit *premature labour*.

They should not be used unless a clear benefit is likely. Tachycardia is the commonest side-effect and may be extreme if atropine is also administered.

Drugs used in the treatment of *spasmodic dysmenorrhoea* include prostaglandin-synthetase inhibitors such as aspirin, mefenamic acid and naproxen sodium (see section 4.7.1). See sections 6.4.1.2 and 6.4.1.4 for hormone treatment.

PREMATURE LABOUR

ISOXSUPRINE HYDROCHLORIDE
Indications: premature labour
Cautions: may cause hypotension in the newborn; see notes above
Contra-indications: recent arterial haemorrhage, heart disease, premature detachment of placenta, severe anaemia, ruptured membranes, infection
Side-effects: hypotension, tachycardia, flushing, nausea, vomiting
Dose: by intravenous infusion, initially 200–300 micrograms/minute gradually increased to 500 micrograms/minute until labour is arrested; subsequently *by intramuscular injection,* 10 mg

every 3 hours for 24 hours, then every 4–6 hours for 48 hours

PoM Duvadilan® (Duphar)
Injection, isoxsuprine hydrochloride 5 mg/ml. Net price 2-ml amp = 35p

---

RITODRINE HYDROCHLORIDE

Indications: premature labour; fetal asphyxia due to hypertonic uterine action
Cautions: diabetes mellitus (monitor blood sugar during intravenous treatment), treatment with corticosteroids, anaesthetics, potassium-depleting diuretics (depresses potassium plasma concentrations); monitor blood pressure and pulse
Contra-indications: cardiac disorders, haemorrhage, hypertension, pre-eclampsia, cord compression, thyrotoxicosis, ruptured membranes, infection, treatment with monoamine-oxidase inhibitors, tricyclic antidepressants, beta-adrenoceptor blocking drugs, antihypertensives
Side-effects: nausea, vomiting, flushing, sweating, tremor; hypokalaemia, tachycardia and hypotension with high doses
Dose: by intravenous infusion, premature labour, initially 50 micrograms/minute, gradually increased to 150–350 micrograms/minute and continued for 12–48 hours after contractions have ceased; or *by intramuscular injection,* 10 mg every 3–8 hours continued for 12–48 hours after contractions have ceased; then *by mouth,* 10 mg 30 minutes before termination of intravenous infusion, repeated every 2 hours for 24 hours, followed by 10–20 mg every 4–6 hours, max. 120 mg daily
Fetal asphyxia due to hypertonic uterine action, *by intravenous infusion,* 50 micrograms/minute increased as necessary to a max. of 350 micrograms/minute, while preparations are made for delivery

PoM Yutopar® (Duphar)
Tablets, buff, scored, ritodrine hydrochloride 10 mg. Net price 20 = £4.40
Injection, ritodrine hydrochloride 10 mg/ml. Net price 5-ml amp = £2.15

SALBUTAMOL

Indications: premature labour
Cautions; Contra-indications; Side-effects: see under Ritodrine Hydrochloride
Dose: by intravenous infusion, 10 micrograms/minute gradually increased to 45 micrograms/minute until contractions have ceased, then gradually reduced; or *by intravenous or intramuscular injection,* 100–250 micrograms repeated according to patient's response; subsequently *by mouth* 4 mg every 6–8 hours

PoM Ventolin® (A&H)
Solution for intravenous infusion, salbutamol 1 mg (as sulphate)/ml. Net price 5-ml amp = £3.08
Tablets and *Injection,* see section 3.1.1.1

TERBUTALINE SULPHATE

Indications: premature labour
Cautions; Contra-indications; Side-effects: see under Ritodrine Hydrochloride
Dose: by intravenous infusion, 10 micrograms/minute (as a 0.0005% solution) for 1 hour, gradually increased to a max. of 25 micrograms/minute until contractions have ceased, then reduced; subsequently *by subcutaneous injection,* 250 micrograms every 6 hours for 3 days, and *by mouth,* 5 mg every 8 hours until 37th week of pregnancy

PoM Bricanyl® (Astra)
Injection, terbutaline sulphate 500 micrograms/ml. Net price 1-ml amp = 28p
Tablets, see section 3.1.1.1

7.2 Treatment of vaginal and vulval conditions

Topical applications to the vulva and vagina include pessaries, dusting-powders, creams, and medicated tampons. Symptoms are likely to be primarily referable to the vulva, but infections almost invariably involve the vagina also, so that external applications to the vulva at best are likely to give only symptomatic relief and will not cure infections.

Creams are usually preferable to ointments, which are not water permeable and adversely affect evaporation and dispersal of natural secretions. Aqueous medicated douches may disturb normal vaginal acidity and bacterial flora.

Topical anaesthetic agents give only symptomatic relief and may cause sensitivity reactions. They are indicated only in cases of pruritus where specific local causes have been excluded.

Systemic drugs are required in the treatment of infections, especially those which are sexually transmitted, which, whilst manifest primarily by genital tract symptoms, may also affect other tissues (see section 5.1).

  7.2.1 Topical hormones
  7.2.2 Anti-infective drugs

7.2.1 Topical hormones

When there is a lack of endogenous oestrogens (as in postmenopausal women) application of cream containing an oestrogen may be used alone or as an adjunct to other treatment in order to improve the quality of the vaginal epithelium in conditions such as menopausal vaginitis and kraurosis vulvae and increase natural resistance to infection.

Topical oestrogens are also used prior to vaginal surgery for prolapse when there is epithelial atrophy.

> Topical oestrogens should be used in the minimum effective amount and treatment discontinued as soon as possible to minimise absorption of the oestrogen.

OESTROGENS, TOPICAL

Indications: see notes above

Cautions; Contra-indications; Side-effects: see Ethinyloestradiol (section 6.4.1.1); contra-indicated in pregnancy and lactation; discontinue treatment and examine patients periodically to assess need for further treatment

PoM **Stilboestrol Pessaries,** stilboestrol 500 micrograms

Insert 2 pessaries at night for 1–2 weeks then reduced (see notes above)
Available from Penn (special order)

PoM **Hormofemin®** (Medo)

Cream, dienoestrol 0.025%. Net price 40 g with 4-g applicator = £2.19
Insert ½–1 applicatorful daily for 1–2 weeks gradually reduced to half initial dose for 1 further week; not to be repeated in less than 6 months with re-examination

PoM **Ortho Dienoestrol** (Ortho-Cilag)

Cream, dienoestrol 0.01%. Net price 78 g with applicator = £2.44
Insert 1–2 applicatorfuls daily for 1–2 weeks, then gradually reduced to 1 applicatorful 1–3 times weekly if necessary; attempts to reduce or discontinue should be made at 3–6 month intervals with re-examination

PoM **Ortho-Gynest®** (Ortho-Cilag)

Pessaries, oestriol 500 micrograms. Net price 15 pessaries = £4.94
Insert 1 pessary daily, preferably in the evening, until improvement occurs; maintenance 1 pessary twice a week; attempts to reduce or discontinue should be made at 3–6 month intervals with re-examination

▼ PoM **Ovestin®** (Organon)

Intravaginal cream, oestriol 0.1%. Net price 15 g with applicator = £3.95
Insert 1 applicatorful daily for 2–3 weeks, then reduce to twice a week (discontinue every 3 months for 4 weeks to assess need for further treatment); postmenopausal surgery, 1 applicatorful daily for 2 weeks, resuming 2 weeks after surgery

PoM **Premarin®** (Wyeth)

Vaginal cream, conjugated oestrogens 625 micrograms/g. Net price 42.5 g with calibrated applicator = £2.19
Insert 1–2 g daily, starting on 5th day of cycle, for 3 weeks, followed by 1-week interval; if therapy long term, oral progestogen for 10–12 days at end of each cycle essential

PoM **Tampovagan Stilboestrol and Lactic Acid®** (Norgine)

Pessaries, stilboestrol 500 micrograms, lactic acid 5%. Net price 10 pessaries = £5.96
Insert 2 pessaries at night for 1–2 weeks then reduce (see notes above)

7.2.2   Anti-infective drugs

Effective specific treatments are available for the common vaginal infections and the causal organism should be identified before instituting treatment.

Vaginal candidiasis is treated primarily by pessaries or cream which should be inserted high into the vagina, including the time of menstruation, using a special applicator for the cream. Candidal vulvitis is treated with cream but there is almost invariably associated vaginal infection which should also be treated.

Nystatin is a well established treatment. One or two pessaries are inserted nightly for 14 to 28 nights. It may be supplemented with cream for vulvitis and other superficial sites of infection. The imidazole drugs (clotrimazole, econazole, isoconazole, and miconazole) appear to be equally effective in shorter courses of 3 to 14 days according to the preparation used; single dose preparations are also available, which is an advantage when compliance is a problem. Tampons coated with miconazole are also available. Vaginal applications may be supplemented with cream for vulvitis and other superficial sites of infection.

Recurrence is common if the full course of treatment has not been completed and is also particularly likely if there are predisposing factors such as antibiotic therapy, oral contraceptive use, pregnancy, or diabetes mellitus. Possible reservoirs of infection may also lead to recontamination and should be treated. These include other skin sites such as the digits, nail beds, and umbilicus as well as the gut and the bladder. Also, the partner may be the source of re-infection and should be treated with the cream at the same time. Concurrent oral treatment may be necessary in resistant or recurrent infection, using **nystatin** or **miconazole** tablets (see section 5.2); for a CSM warning on oral ketoconazole, see also section 5.2. Vaginal preparations intended to restore the normal acidity (Aci-Jel®) may also prevent re-infection and permit the re-establishment of the normal vaginal flora.

Trichomonal infections commonly involve the lower urinary tract as well as the genital system and need systemic treatment with metronidazole, nimorazole, or tinidazole (see section 5.1.11) (**important:** alcohol should be avoided during treatment with these drugs).

Bacterial infections of the lower genital tract may be caused by a wide range of organisms. The treatment of gonorrhoea and syphilis is described in section 5.1, Table 1. Infections with Gram-negative organisms are particularly common in association with gynaecological operations and trauma. Metronidazole is effective against certain Gram-negative organisms, especially *Bacteroides* spp. and may be used as a prophylactic measure in gynaecological surgery.

Antibacterial creams such as Sultrin® are used in the treatment of mixed bacterial infections but are of unproven value; they are ineffective against *Candida* spp. and *Trichomonas vaginalis*.

Acyclovir preparations (see section 5.3 for systemic preparations, and section 13.10.3 for cream) may be used in the treatment of genital infection due to *herpes simplex virus*, the HSV type 2 being a major cause of genital ulceration. These preparations all have a beneficial effect on virus shedding and healing, generally giving relief from pain and other symptoms.

GENITAL ANTIFUNGAL PREPARATIONS

Indications: vaginal and vulval candidiasis
Side-effects: local irritation, possibly including burning, oedema, erythema
Administration: insert pessaries or cream high into the vagina and complete the course regardless of intervening menstruation

Canesten® (Baypharm)
Cream (topical), clotrimazole 1%. Net price 20 g = £1.82; 50 g = £4.26
    Apply to anogenital area 2–3 times daily
PoM *Vaginal cream,* clotrimazole 2%. Net price 35 g (with 5-g applicators) = £5.22
    Insert 5 g twice daily for 3 days or once nightly for 6 nights
PoM *Vaginal tablets,* clotrimazole 100 mg. Net price 6 tabs with applicator = £2.64
PoM *Vaginal tablets,* clotrimazole 200 mg. Net price 3 tabs with applicator = £2.58
    Insert 200 mg for 3 nights *or* 100 mg for 6 nights
PoM *Duopak,* clotrimazole 100-mg vaginal tablets and cream (topical) 1%. Net price 6 tabs and 20 g cream = £4.35
PoM **Canesten 1®** (Baypharm)
Vaginal tablets, clotrimazole 500 mg. Net price 1 with applicator = £2.58
    Insert 1 at night as a single dose
PoM **Canesten 10% VC®** (Baypharm)
Vaginal cream, clotrimazole 10%. Net price 5-g applicator pack = £3.43
    Insert 5 g at night as a single dose
Ecostatin® (Squibb)
Cream (topical), econazole nitrate 1%. Net price 15 g = £1.49; 30 g = £2.75
    Apply to anogenital area twice daily
PoM *Pessaries,* econazole nitrate 150 mg. Net price 3 with applicator = £3.96
    Insert 1 pessary for 3 nights
PoM *Twinpack,* econazole nitrate 150-mg pessaries and cream 1%. Net price 3 pessaries and 15 g cream = £4.98
PoM **Ecostatin-1®** (Squibb)
Pessary, econazole nitrate 150 mg. Net price 1 pessary with applicator = £4.40
    Insert 1 pessary at night as a single dose
Flagyl Compak, see section 5.1.11
PoM **Fungilin®** (Squibb)
Cream, amphotericin 3%. Net price 15 g = £1.30
    Apply to anogenital area 2–4 times daily
PoM **Gyno-Daktarin®** (Janssen)
Intravaginal cream, miconazole nitrate 2%. Net price 78 g with applicators = £4.95
    Insert 2 applicatorfuls at night for 7 nights; *topical,* apply to anogenital area twice daily
Pessaries, miconazole nitrate 100 mg. Net price 14 = £4.04
    Insert 2 pessaries for 7 nights
Tampons, coated with miconazole nitrate 100 mg. Net price 10 = £3.83
    Insert 1 tampon night and morning for 5 days
Combipack, miconazole nitrate 100-mg pessaries and cream (topical) 2%. Net price 14 pessaries and 15 g cream = £5.94

PoM **Gyno-Daktarin 1®** (Janssen)
Ovule (= vaginal capsule), miconazole nitrate 1.2 g in a fatty basis. Net price 1 ovule (with finger stall) = £3.95
    Insert 1 ovule at night as a single dose
PoM **Gyno-Pevaryl®** (Ortho-Cilag)
Cream, econazole nitrate 1%. Net price 15 g = £1.74; 30 g = £3.45
    Apply to anogenital area 2–3 times daily for 14 days
Pessaries, econazole nitrate 150 mg. Net price 3 = £3.96
    Insert 1 pessary for 3 nights
Combipack, econazole nitrate 150-mg pessaries, econazole nitrate 1% cream (to be applied to anogenital area). Net price 3 pessaries and 15 g cream = £4.98
PoM **Gyno-Pevaryl 1®** (Ortho-Cilag)
Pessary, econazole nitrate 150 mg (formulated for single-dose therapy). Net price 1 = £4.40
    Insert 1 pessary at night as a single dose
Cream and Pessary CP pack, econazole nitrate 150-mg pessary, econazole nitrate 1% cream (to be applied to anogenital area). Net price 1 pessary and 15 g cream = £5.84
PoM **Monistat®** (Ortho-Cilag)
Vaginal cream, miconazole nitrate 2%. Net price 78 g with applicator = £5.12
    Insert 1 applicatorful (approx. 5 g) at night for 14 nights; also apply to anogenital area
Pessaries, miconazole nitrate 100 mg. Net price 14 = £4.91
    Insert 100 mg at night for 14 nights
PoM **Nizoral®** (Janssen)
Cream (topical), ketoconazole 2%. Net price 15 g = £1.73
    Apply to anogenital area once or twice daily
PoM **Nyspes®** (DDSA)
Pessaries, buff, nystatin 100000 units. Net price 15 = £1.30
    Insert 1–2 pessaries for at least 14 nights
PoM **Nystan®** (Squibb)
Cream and Ointment, see section 13.10.2
Gel (topical), nystatin 100000 units/g. Net price 30 g = £2.66
    Apply to anogenital area 2–4 times daily
Vaginal cream, nystatin 100000 units/4-g application. Net price 60 g with applicator = £3.26
Pessaries, yellow, nystatin 100000 units. Net price 15 with applicator = £1.09
    Insert 1–2 applicatorfuls of cream or 1–2 pessaries at night for at least 14 nights
Triple pack, nystatin tablets 500000 units, nystatin gel 100000 units/g. Nystavescent® pessaries as below. Net price 42 tablets + 28 pessaries + 30 g gel = £8.86
    Dose: 1 tablet 3 times daily for 14 days, with gel and pessaries as above
PoM **Nystavescent®** (Squibb)
Pessaries, yellow, effervescent, nystatin 100000 units. Net price 15 with applicator = £1.55
    Insert as for Nystan® (above)

Cautionary label wordings, see inside back cover

Prices are **net**, see p. 1

Pevaryl® (Ortho-Cilag)
Cream, econazole nitrate 1%. Net price 30 g = £3.33
  Apply to anogenital area 2–3 times daily
  Lotion and *Dusting-powder*, see section 13.10.2

PoM **Pimafucin**® (Brocades)
Cream, natamycin 2%. Net price 30 g = £1.75
  Apply to anogenital area 2–3 times daily
Vaginal tablets (=pessaries), natamycin 25 mg. Net price 20 = £1.66
  Trichomonas, insert 1 pessary at night for 20 days; candidal infections, 1 pessary at night for 20 days *or* 1 pessary twice daily for 10 days

▼ PoM **Travogyn**® (Schering)
Cream (topical), isoconazole nitrate 1%. Net price 20 g = £1.88
  Apply to anogenital area twice daily
Vaginal tablets (=pessaries), isoconazole nitrate 300 mg. Net price 2 = £3.90
  Insert 2 pessaries as a single dose preferably at night

VAGINAL ANTIBACTERIAL PREPARATIONS

Indications: bacterial vaginitis and cervicitis
Side-effects: sensitivity

PoM **Sultrin**® (Ortho-Cilag)
Cream, sulphathiazole 3.42%, sulphacetamide 2.86%, sulphabenzamide 3.7%. Net price 78 g with applicator = £3.25
Vaginal tablets, sulphathiazole 172.5 mg, sulphacetamide 143.75 mg, sulphabenzamide 184 mg. Net price 20 with applicator = £2.75
  Insert 1 pessary or applicatorful of cream twice daily for 10 days, then once daily if necessary

VAGINAL ANTISEPTIC PREPARATIONS

Aci-Jel® (Ortho-Cilag)
Vaginal jelly, acetic acid 0.92% in a buffered (pH 4) basis. Net price 85 g with applicator = £2.89
  Non-specific infections, insert 1 applicatorful twice daily to restore vaginal acidity

Betadine® (Napp)
Caution: avoid in pregnancy and in breast-feeding
Side-effects: rarely sensitivity; may interfere with thyroid function tests
Pessaries, brown, povidone-iodine 200 mg. Net price 28 pessaries with applicator = £4.65
Vaginal gel, brown, povidone-iodine 10%. Net price 80 g with applicator = £2.12
  In vaginal infections insert 1 moistened pessary or 1 applicatorful (5 g) of gel twice daily for 2–4 weeks
Antiseptic Vaginal Cleansing Kit, solution, povidone-iodine 10%. For dilution before use. Net price 250 ml with measuring bottle and applicator = £2.53
  Vaginal cleansing in vaginal infections or pre-operatively, douche daily for 14 days

OTHER PREPARATIONS FOR VAGINAL INFECTIONS

▼ PoM **Gynatren**® (Cabot)
Vaccine prepared from inactivated *Lactobacillus acidophilus*. Net price 3 × 0.5-ml amp = £16.00
Dose: for recurrent trichomoniasis, by intramuscular injection, 3 doses each of 0.5 ml separated by intervals of 2 weeks

7.3   Contraceptives

The criteria by which contraceptive methods should be judged are effectiveness, acceptability, and freedom from side-effects.

Hormonal contraception is the most effective method of fertility control, short of sterilisation, but has unwanted major and minor side-effects, especially for certain groups of women.

Intra-uterine devices have a high use-effectiveness but may produce undesirable side-effects, especially menorrhagia, or be otherwise unsuitable in a significant proportion of women; their use is generally inadvisable in nulliparous women because of the increased risk of pelvic sepsis and infertility.

Barrier methods alone (condoms, diaphragms, and caps) are less effective but can be very reliable for well-motivated couples if used in conjunction with a **spermicide**. Occasionally sensitivity reactions occur.

7.3.1 Combined oral contraceptives
7.3.2 Progestogen-only contraceptives
7.3.3 Spermicidal contraceptives
7.3.4 Intra-uterine contraceptive devices

7.3.1   Combined oral contraceptives

Oral contraceptives containing an oestrogen and a progestogen are the most effective preparations for general use. The oestrogen content ranges from 20 to 50 micrograms and generally a preparation with the lowest oestrogen and progestogen content which gives good cycle control and minimal side-effects in the individual patient is chosen.

DOSAGE. The dosage regimen for *combined oral contraceptives* is usually 1 tablet daily for 21 days, followed by a 7-day interval during which menstrual bleeding occurs. If the first course is started on the 5th day of the cycle ovulation may not be inhibited during that cycle and additional contraceptive precautions should therefore be taken during the first 14 days or when changing from a high to a low oestrogen preparation. Additional contraceptive precautions are unnecessary in the first cycle if the tablets are started on the first day of the cycle as is now usually recommended.

Phased formulations more closely mimic normal endogenous cyclical hormonal activity. They are generally recommended for a day 1 start.

The tablet should be taken at approximately the same time each day. If it is delayed by longer than 12 hours, contraceptive protection may be lost.

MISSED PILL. The following advice is now recommended by family planning organisations:

'If you forget a pill, take it as soon as you remember, and the next one at your normal time. If you are 12 or more hours late with any pill (especially the first or last in the packet) the pill may not work. As soon as you remember, continue normal pill taking. However, you will not be protected for the next seven days and must either not have sex or use another method such as the sheath. IF these seven days run beyond the end of your packet, start the next packet at once when you have finished the present one, i.e. do not have a gap between packets. This will mean you may not have a period until the end of two packets but this does you no harm. Nor does it matter if you see some bleeding on tablet-taking days. If you are using everyday (ED) pills—miss out the seven inactive pills. If you are not sure which these are, ask your doctor.'

POSTCOITAL CONTRACEPTION. Combined oral contraceptives may also be given for occasional emergency use after unprotected intercourse. Two tablets of a preparation containing levonorgestrel 250 micrograms and ethinyloestradiol 50 micrograms (Eugynon 50®, Ovran®, Schering PC4®) are taken within 72 hours, and a further 2 tablets 12 hours later. The patient should always consult her doctor approximately 3 weeks after using this treatment.

SIDE-EFFECTS. Combined oral contraceptives carry a small risk of thrombo-embolic and cardiovascular complications. This increases with age, obesity, and cigarette smoking, and with predisposing conditions such as diabetes, hypertension, and familial hyperlipidaemia.

Hypertension may develop as the result of therapy but when it is due to contraceptive usage reversion to normotension occurs on cessation of treatment.

Critical factors which limit effectiveness are vomiting and diarrhoea and some antibiotics, for example ampicillin, which interfere with oestrogen absorption. Drugs which induce hepatic enzyme activity (e.g. barbiturates, phenytoin, rifampicin) also increase the risk of failure.

CHILDBIRTH. Following childbirth oral contraception can be started at any time after 3 weeks postpartum (not earlier because of the increased risk of thrombosis). Lactation may be affected by combined oral contraceptives as described under Prescribing during Breast-feeding p. 33.

SURGERY. Oestrogen-containing oral contraceptives should be discontinued (and adequate alternative contraceptive arrangements made) 4 weeks before major elective surgery and all surgery to the legs; they should normally be recommenced at the first menses occurring at least 2 weeks after the procedure. When discontinuation is not possible, e.g. after trauma or if, by oversight, a patient admitted for an elective procedure is still on an oestrogen-containing oral contraceptive, some consideration should be given to subcutaneous heparin prophylaxis. These recommendations do not apply to minor surgery with short duration of anaesthesia, e.g. laparoscopic sterilisation or tooth extraction, or to women taking oestrogen-free contraceptives.

ORAL CONTRACEPTIVES (Combined)

Indications: contraception; menstrual symptoms, see section 6.4.1.4

Cautions: see notes above; diabetes, hypertension, cardiac or renal disease, migraine, epilepsy, depression, asthma, immobilisation, contact lenses (may irritate), varicose veins; cigarette-smokers, patients over 35 years, obesity, breast-feeding. Drug interactions: see Appendix 1 (sections *2.5, 2.8, 2.8A, 3, 4.3, 6.1, 7, 8*)

Contra-indications: pregnancy; thrombosis and history of any thrombo-embolic disease, after evacuation of hydatidiform mole (until return to normal of urine and plasma gonadotrophin values); recurrent jaundice, acute and chronic liver disease, porphyria, Dubin-Johnson and Roter syndromes, hyperlipidaemia (safety not established), hyperlipidaemia, mammary or endometrial carcinoma, oestrogen-dependent tumours, severe or focal migraine, undiagnosed vaginal bleeding, history of pruritus of pregnancy or herpes gestationis, deterioration of otosclerosis

Side-effects: nausea, vomiting, headache, breast tenderness, changes in body weight, thrombosis (more common in blood groups A, B, and AB than O), changes in libido, depression, chloasma, hypertension, impairment of liver function, hepatic tumours, reduced menstrual loss, 'spotting' in early cycles, amenorrhoea; rarely photosensitivity

Dose: see notes above

Ethinyloestradiol 20 micrograms

May be less effective with less good cycle control, and regularity of pill-taking is critical; appropriate for obese patients (provided oral contraceptive use otherwise suitable).

PoM Loestrin 20® (P-D)
Tablets, blue-grey, f/c, norethisterone acetate 1 mg, ethinyloestradiol 20 micrograms. Net price 21-tab calendar pack = 81p

▼ **PoM Mercilon®** (Organon)
Tablets, desogestrel 150 micrograms, ethinyloestradiol 20 micrograms. Net price 21-tab pack = £1.69

Ethinyloestradiol 30 micrograms

Standard strength from which the initial choice is usually selected. Highly effective if the pill-free interval is not lengthened by dose omissions.

PoM Conova 30® (Gold Cross)
Tablets, f/c, ethynodiol diacetate 2 mg, ethinyloestradiol 30 micrograms. Net price 21-tab pack = 80p

PoM **Eugynon 30**® (Schering)
Tablets, s/c, levonorgestrel 250 micrograms, ethinyloestradiol 30 micrograms. Net price 21-tab pack = 69p

▼ PoM **Femodene**® (Schering)
Tablets, s/c, gestodene 75 micrograms, ethinyloestradiol 30 micrograms. Net price 21-tab pack = £1.90

PoM **Loestrin 30**® (P-D)
Tablets, green, f/c, norethisterone acetate 1.5 mg, ethinyloestradiol 30 micrograms. Net price 21-tab pack = £1.18

PoM **Marvelon**® (Organon)
Tablets, desogestrel 150 micrograms, ethinyloestradiol 30 micrograms. Net price 21-tab pack = £1.30

PoM **Microgynon 30**® (Schering)
Tablets, beige, s/c, levonorgestrel 150 micrograms, ethinyloestradiol 30 micrograms. Net price 21-tab pack = 54p

▼ PoM **Minulet**® (Wyeth)
Tablets, s/c, gestodene 75 micrograms, ethinyloestradiol 30 micrograms. Net price 3 × 21-tab pack = £5.70

PoM **Ovran 30**® (Wyeth)
Tablets, levonorgestrel 250 micrograms, ethinyloestradiol 30 micrograms. Net price 21-tab pack = 57p

PoM **Ovranette**® (Wyeth)
Tablets, levonorgestrel 150 micrograms, ethinyloestradiol 30 micrograms. Net price 21-tab pack = 62p
Dose: see above and under Ovran below

Ethinyloestradiol 35 micrograms

In common with the 30-microgram strength (above): standard strength from which the initial choice is usually selected. Highly effective if the pill-free interval is not lengthened by dose omissions.

PoM **Brevinor**® (Syntex)
Tablets, norethisterone 500 micrograms, ethinyloestradiol 35 micrograms. Net price 21-tab pack = 52p

PoM **Neocon 1/35**® (Ortho-Cilag)
Tablets, peach, norethisterone 1 mg, ethinyloestradiol 35 micrograms. Net price 21-tab calendar pack = 71p

PoM **Norimin**® (Syntex)
Tablets, yellow, norethisterone 1 mg, ethinyloestradiol 35 micrograms. Net price 21-tab calendar pack = 51p

PoM **Ovysmen**® (Ortho-Cilag)
Tablets, norethisterone 500 micrograms, ethinyloestradiol 35 micrograms. Net price 21-tab pack = 53p

---

Ethinyloestradiol 50 micrograms

Increased security but possibility of increased side-effects. Used mainly in circumstances of reduced bioavailability (e.g. during long-term use of enzyme-inducing drugs).

PoM **Eugynon 50**® (Schering)
Tablets, s/c, norgestrel 500 micrograms (≡ levonorgestrel 250 micrograms), ethinyloestradiol 50 micrograms. Net price 21-tab pack = 72p

PoM **Gynovlar 21**® (Schering)
Tablets, pink, s/c, norethisterone acetate 3 mg, ethinyloestradiol 50 micrograms. Net price 21-tab pack = 90p

PoM **Minilyn**® (Organon)
Tablets, lynoestrenol 2.5 mg, ethinyloestradiol 50 micrograms. Net price 22-tab pack = 47p
Dose: 1 tablet daily for 22 days starting on 1st day of cycle, and repeated after a 6-day interval

PoM **Minovlar**® (Schering)
Tablets, ochre, s/c, norethisterone acetate 1 mg, ethinyloestradiol 50 micrograms. Net price 21-tab pack = 90p

PoM **Minovlar ED**® (Schering)
As for Minovlar and in addition 7 white lactose tablets. Net price 28-tab pack = 90p
Dose: 1 tablet daily starting in red sector on 1st day of cycle continuing in sequence without interruption

PoM **Ovran**® (Wyeth)
Tablets, levonorgestrel 250 micrograms, ethinyloestradiol 50 micrograms. Net price 21-tab pack = 37p
Dose: contraception, spasmodic dysmenorrhoea, see above; endometriosis 1–2 tablets daily without interruption; postponement of menstruation 1 tablet daily, preferably beginning before last 5 days of cycle, increased if spotting occurs to 2 tablets daily

---

Mestranol 50 micrograms

In common with the ethinyloestradiol 50-microgram strength (above): increased security but possibility of increased side-effects. Used mainly in circumstances of reduced bioavailability (e.g. during long-term use of enzyme-inducing drugs).

PoM **Norinyl-1**® (Syntex)
Tablets, norethisterone 1 mg, mestranol 50 micrograms. Net price 21-tab pack = 50p

PoM **Ortho-Novin 1/50**® (Ortho-Cilag)
Tablets, norethisterone 1 mg, mestranol 50 micrograms. Net price 21-tab pack = 73p

---

Phased formulations

A little more complex for the user to take, but provide better cycle control (with low metabolic effect) than equivalent fixed-dose levonorgestrel or norethisterone formulations.

PoM **BiNovum**® (Ortho-Cilag)
Calendar pack, 7 white tablets, norethisterone 500 micrograms, ethinyloestradiol 35 micrograms; 14 peach tablets, norethisterone 1 mg,

---

ethinyloestradiol 35 micrograms. Net price
21 = 70p

Dose: 1 tablet daily for 21 days, starting with a
white tablet on 1st day of cycle, and repeated
after a 7-day interval

PoM **Logynon**® (Schering)

Calendar pack, all s/c, 6 light brown tablets,
levonorgestrel 50 micrograms, ethinyloestradiol 30 micrograms; 5 white tablets, levonorgestrel 75 micrograms, ethinyloestradiol 40
micrograms; 10 ochre tablets, levonorgestrel
125 micrograms, ethinyloestradiol 30 micrograms. Net price 21 = 88p

Dose: 1 tablet daily for 21 days, starting with
tablet marked 1 on 1st day of cycle, and
repeated after a 7-day interval

PoM **Logynon ED**® (Schering)

As for Logynon and in addition 7 white placebo
tablets. Net price 28-tab calendar pack = 88p

Dose: 1 tablet daily starting in red sector on 1st
day of cycle continuing in sequence without
interruption

▼ PoM **Synphase**® (Syntex)

Calendar pack, 7 white tablets, norethisterone
500 micrograms, ethinyloestradiol 35 micrograms; 9 yellow tablets, norethisterone 1 mg,
ethinyloestradiol 35 micrograms; 5 white tablets, norethisterone 500 micrograms, ethinyloestradiol 35 micrograms. Net price 21 = 88p

Dose: 1 tablet daily for 21 days, starting with
tablet marked 1 on the 5th day of the cycle, and
repeated after a 7-day interval

PoM **Trinordiol**® (Wyeth)

Calendar pack, all s/c, 6 light brown tablets,
levonorgestrel 50 micrograms, ethinyloestradiol 30 micrograms; 5 white tablets, levonorgestrel 75 micrograms, ethinyloestradiol 40
micrograms; 10 ochre tablets, levonorgestrel
125 micrograms, ethinyloestradiol 30 micrograms. Net price 21 = £1.09

Dose: 1 tablet daily for 21 days, starting with
tablet marked 1 on 1st day of cycle, and repeated after a 7-day interval

PoM **TriNovum**® (Ortho-Cilag)

Calendar pack, 7 white tablets, norethisterone
500 micrograms, ethinyloestradiol 35 micrograms; 7 light peach tablets, norethisterone 750
micrograms, ethinyloestradiol 35 micrograms;
7 peach tablets, norethisterone 1 mg, ethinyloestradiol 35 micrograms. Net price 21 =
85p

Dose: 1 tablet daily for 21 days, starting with a
white tablet on 1st day of cycle, and repeated
after a 7-day interval

Postcoital contraceptive

▼ PoM **Schering PC4**® (Schering)

Tablets, s/c, levonorgestrel 250 micrograms, ethinyloestradiol 50 micrograms. Net price 4 =
£1.40. For postcoital contraception as an
occasional emergency measure

Dose: 2 tablets as soon as possible after coitus
(up to 72 hours) then 2 tablets after 12 hours

7.3.2 Progestogen-only contraceptives

When oestrogens are contra-indicated,
progestogen-only preparations may offer a suitable alternative but have a higher failure rate
than combined preparations. They are suitable for
older patients who may be at risk from oestrogen,
heavy smokers, and those in whom oestrogens
cause severe side-effects. Menstrual irregularities
(oligomenorrhoea, menorrhagia) are more common but patients tend to revert to a more regular
cyclical menstrual pattern on long treatment. Oral
preparations are started on the 1st day of the cycle
and taken every day at the same time without a
break. Additional contraceptive precautions are
unnecessary when initiating treatment with progestogen-only contraceptives. When changing
from a combined oral contraceptive to a progestogen-only preparation treatment should start
on the day following completion of the combined
oral contraceptive course so that there is no break
in tablet taking.

The tablet should be taken at the same time
each day. If it is delayed by longer than 3 hours,
contraceptive protection may be lost. The following advice is now recommended by family
planning organisations:

'If you forget a pill, take it as soon as you remember
and carry on with the next pill at the right time. If the
pill was more than three hours overdue you are not
protected. Continue normal pill-taking but you must
also use another method, such as the sheath, for the
next 48 hours. If you have vomiting or very severe
diarrhoea the pill may not work. Continue to take it,
but you may not be protected from the first day of
vomiting or diarrhoea. Use another method, such as
the sheath, for any intercourse during the stomach upset
and for the next 48 hours.'

Medroxyprogesterone acetate (Depo-Provera®)
is a long-acting progestogen given by intramuscular injection. It is useful for short-term
interim contraception, for example, before vas-
ectomy becomes effective or after rubella
vaccination. It may also be used as a long-term
contraceptive for women who are unable to use
any other method, after counselling on the long
and short-term effects. Transient infertility and
irregular cycles may occur after discontinuation
of treatment. Heavy bleeding has been reported
in patients given medroxyprogesterone acetate in
the immediate puerperium. **Norethisterone enanthate** (Noristerat®) is a long-acting progestogen
given as an oily injection which provides contraception for 8 weeks.

Progestogen-only preparations can be administered in the early puerperium without adverse
effects; established lactation is not affected.

PROGESTOGEN-ONLY CONTRACEPTIVES

Indications: contraception

Cautions: diabetes, hypertension, heart disease,
functional ovarian cysts, malabsorption syndromes; migraine which is severe or focal or

---

has begun for first time on a combined oral contraceptive; active liver disease, recurrent cholestatic jaundice, and history of jaundice in pregnancy. Drug interactions: see under Combined Oral Contraceptives (section 7.3.1)

Contra-indications pregnancy, undiagnosed vaginal bleeding, past ectopic pregnancy, past severe arterial disease or current high risk (including any atherogenic lipid profile); liver adenoma; after evacuation of hydatidiform mole (until return to normal of urine and plasma gonadotrophin values); carcinoma of the breast and other sex hormone dependent cancers

Side-effects: menstrual irregularities (see also notes above); nausea and vomiting, headache, breast discomfort, depression, skin disorders. For other critical factors affecting contraceptive efficacy such as vomiting, diarrhoea, enzyme induction, and for comment on progestogen-only contraceptives and surgical operations, see under Combined Oral Contraceptives (section 7.3.1)

Dose: by mouth, 1 tablet daily at the same time, preferably early in the evening, starting on 1st day of cycle then continuously

Oral preparations

PoM **Femulen**® (Gold Cross)
Tablets, ethynodiol diacetate 500 micrograms. Net price 28-tab calendar pack = 94p

PoM **Micronor**® (Ortho-Cilag)
Tablets, norethisterone 350 micrograms. Net price 28-tab calendar pack = 63p

PoM **Microval**® (Wyeth)
Tablets, levonorgestrel 30 micrograms. Net price 35-tab calendar pack = £1.00

PoM **Neogest**® (Schering)
Tablets, brown, s/c, norgestrel 75 micrograms (= levonorgestrel 37.5 micrograms). Net price 35-tab calendar pack = 78p

PoM **Norgeston**® (Schering)
Tablets, s/c, levonorgestrel 30 micrograms. Net price 35-tab calendar pack = 78p

PoM **Noriday**® (Syntex)
Tablets, norethisterone 350 micrograms. Net price 28-tab calendar pack = 61p

Parenteral preparations

▼ PoM **Depo-Provera**® (Upjohn)
Injection (aqueous suspension), medroxyprogesterone acetate 50 mg/ml, net price 3-ml vial = £3.79; 150 mg/ml, 1-ml vial = £3.79
Dose: by deep intramuscular injection, 150 mg in first 5 days of cycle or first 6 weeks after parturition (delay until 6 weeks after parturition if breast-feeding); for long-term contraception, repeated every 3 months

▼ PoM **Noristerat**® (Schering)
Injection (oily), norethisterone enanthate 200 mg/ml. Net price 1-ml amp = £3.00
Dose: by deep intramuscular injection, short-term contraception, 200 mg in first 5 days of cycle or immediately after parturition (duration 8 weeks); may be repeated once after 8 weeks

(withhold breast-feeding for neonates with severe or persistent jaundice requiring medical treatment)

7.3.3 Spermicidal contraceptives

Spermicidal contraceptives are useful additional safeguards but do **not** give adequate protection if used alone; they are suitable for use in conjunction with barrier methods. They have two components: a spermicide and a vehicle which itself may have some inhibiting effect on sperm migration. They are formulated as pessaries, creams, pastes, gels, aerosol foams, and soluble films. The commonly used spermicides are all phenoxypolyethoxyethanol derivatives.

DIRECTIONS, *Creams, gels*, apply over surface and rim of diaphragm or cap within one hour of intercourse then subsequently one applicatorful; with condoms, insert 1 applicatorful before intercourse. *Pessaries*, insert 1 pessary before intercourse. *Foams*, insert 1 applicatorful before intercourse. A fresh application or an additional pessary must be inserted if intercourse is repeated or delayed by more than one hour.

C-Film® (Arun)
Film, nonoxinol '9' 67 mg in a water-soluble basis. Net price 10 films = 84p

Delfen® (Ortho-Cilag)
Cream, nonoxinol '9' 5%. Net price 70 g = £2.03
Foam, nonoxinol '9' 12.5%, pressurised aerosol unit. Net price 20 g (with applicator) = £4.18; 20 g refill = £3.33

Double Check® (FP)
Pessaries, nonoxinol '9' 6%. Net price 10 pessaries = 81p

Duracreme® (LRC)
Cream, nonoxinol '11' 2%. Net price 100-g tube = £1.61; applicator = 63p

Duragel® (LRC)
Gel, nonoxinol '11' 2%. Net price 100-g tube = £1.61; applicator = 63p

Genexol® (Rendell)
Pessaries, nonoxinols '10' and '11' 5%, in a palm kernel oil basis. Net price 12 pessaries = 95p. For use with condoms only

Gynol II® (Ortho-Cilag)
Jelly, nonoxinol '9' 2%. Net price 30 g = £1.14; 81 g = £2.26; applicator = 75p

Ortho-Creme® (Ortho-Cilag)
Cream, nonoxinol '9' 2%. Net price 70 g = £2.09; applicator = 75p

Orthoforms® (Ortho-Cilag)
Pessaries, nonoxinol '9' 5%. Net price 15 pessaries = £1.89

Ortho-Gynol® (Ortho-Cilag)
Jelly, p-di-isobutylphenoxypolyethoxyethanol 1%. Net price 81 g = £2.09; applicator = 75p

Rendells® (Rendell)
Pessaries, nonoxinols '10' & '11' 5%, in a basis containing fractionated palm kernel oil. Net price 12 pessaries = 95p. For use with condoms only

Staycept® (Syntex)
Jelly, octoxinol 1%. Net price 80 g = £1.20
Pessaries, nonoxinol '9' 6%. Net price 10 pessaries = 87p
When used with diaphragm or cap, one pessary inside device before it is placed in position and insert a second pessary before intercourse

Two's Company® (FP)
Pessaries, nonoxinol '9' 5%. Net price 10 pessaries with 10 condoms = £3.40

7.3.4 Intra-uterine contraceptive devices

The intra-uterine device (IUD) is suitable for older parous women but should be a last-resort contraceptive for young nulliparous women because of the increased risk of pelvic inflammatory disease and infertility. Inert intra-uterine devices are no longer on the UK market but may still be worn by some women.

Smaller devices have now been introduced in order to minimise side-effects; these consist of a plastic carrier wound with copper wire; some also have a central core of silver with the aim of preventing fragmentation of the copper. The recommended replacement time for these devices is from 3 to 5 years but this can be extended according to clinical judgement (especially in older women).

The timing and technique of fitting an intra-uterine device play a critical part in its subsequent performance and call for proper training and experience. Devices should not be fitted during the heavy days of the period; they are best fitted after the end of menstruation and before the calculated time of implantation.

An intra-uterine device should not be removed in mid-cycle unless an additional contraceptive was used for the previous 7 days. If removal is essential (e.g. to treat severe pelvic infection) post-coital contraception should be considered.

INTRA-UTERINE CONTRACEPTIVE DEVICES.

Indications: see notes above
Cautions: anaemia, heavy menses, history of pelvic inflammatory disease, diabetes, valvular heart disease (antibiotic cover needed), epilepsy, increased risk of expulsion if inserted before uterine involution; gynaecological examination before insertion, 3 months after, and yearly; remove if pregnancy occurs; anticoagulant therapy (avoid if possible)
Contra-indications: pregnancy, severe anaemia, very heavy menses, history of ectopic pregnancy or tubal surgery, distorted or small uterine cavity, genital malignancy, pelvic inflammatory disease, immunosuppressive therapy, *copper devices:* copper allergy, Wilson's disease, medical diathermy
Side-effects: uterine or cervical perforation, displacement, pelvic infection, heavy menses, dysmenorrhoea, allergy; *on insertion:* some

pain and bleeding; occasionally, epileptic seizure, vasovagal attack

PoM **Gravigard**® (Gold Cross)
Intra-uterine device, copper wire, surface area approx. 200 mm^2 wound on vertical stem of plastic carrier (in shape of figure 7), impregnated with barium sulphate for radio-opacity, monofilament thread attached to base of vertical stem; partially preloaded in inserter. Dimensions: transverse arm 2.6 cm, vertical stem 3.6 cm. Net price, each = £8.45
For uterine length over 6.5 cm; replacement every 3 years

NHS PoM **Mini-Gravigard**® (Gold Cross)
Intra-uterine device, as above, with dimensions: transverse arm 2.2 cm, vertical stem 2.8 cm. Net price each = £8.45
For uterine length 5.5 to 6.5 cm; replacement every 3 years

PoM **Multiload**® **Cu250** (Organon)
Intra-uterine device, copper wire, surface area approx. 250 mm^2 wound on vertical stem of plastic carrier, 3.6 cm length, with 2 down-curving flexible arms, monofilament thread attached to base of vertical stem; preloaded in inserter. Net price, each = £6.75
For uterine length over 7 cm; replacement every 3 years

PoM **Multiload**® **Cu250 Short** (Organon)
Intra-uterine device, as above, with vertical stem length 2.5 cm. Net price, each = £6.75
For uterine length 5–7 cm; replacement every 3 years

PoM **Multiload**® **Cu375** (Organon)
Intra-uterine device, as above, with copper surface area approx. 375 mm^2. Net price, each = £8.75
For uterine length over 7 cm; replacement every 5 years

PoM **Novagard**® (KabiVitrum)
Intra-uterine device, copper wire with silver core, surface area approx. 200 mm^2 wound on vertical stem of T-shaped plastic carrier, impregnated with barium sulphate for radio-opacity, monofilament thread attached to base of vertical stem; partially preloaded in inserter. Dimensions: transverse arms, vertical stem, both 3.2 cm. Net price, each = £9.00
For uterine length over 5.5 cm; replacement every 5 years

▼ PoM **Nova-T**® (Schering)
Intra-uterine device, copper wire with silver core, surface area approx. 200 mm^2 wound on vertical stem of T-shaped plastic carrier, impregnated with barium sulphate for radio-opacity, threads attached to base of vertical stem. Net price, each = £9.00
For uterine length over 6.5 cm; replacement every 5 years

PoM **Ortho Gyne-T**® (Ortho-Cilag)
Intra-uterine device, copper wire, surface area 200 mm^2, wound on vertical stem of T-shaped plastic carrier, impregnated with barium

---

sulphate for radio-opacity, 2-tail plastic thread attached to base of vertical stem. Net price each = £8.99

For uterine length over 6.5 cm; replacement every 3 years

NHS PoM **Ortho Gyne-T® 380 Slimline** (Ortho-Cilag)

Intra-uterine device, as above, with copper wire surface area 320 mm² and copper collar surface 30 mm² on distal portion of each arm. Net price each = £7.50

For uterine length over 6.5 cm; replacement every 4 years

7.4   Drugs for urinary-tract disorders

7.4.1 Drugs for urinary retention
7.4.2 Drugs for urinary frequency, enuresis, and incontinence
7.4.3 Drugs used as urinary analgesics or to alter urinary pH
7.4.4 Bladder instillations

For other drugs used in the treatment of urinary infections see chapter 5.

7.4.1   Drugs for urinary retention

Acute retention is painful and is initially treated by catheterisation. Thereafter, provided an obstructive cause is excluded, further episodes may be treated medically.

Chronic retention is painless and often long-standing. Catheterisation is unnecessary unless there is deterioration of renal function. After the cause has initially been established and treated, drugs may be required to increase detrusor muscle tone.

Parasympathomimetics produce the effects of parasympathetic nerve stimulation; they possess the muscarinic rather than the nicotinic effects of acetylcholine and improve voiding efficiency by increasing detrusor muscle contraction. In the absence of obstruction to the bladder outlet they have a limited role in the relief of urinary retention (e.g. in neurological disease or post-operatively). Generalised parasympathomimetic side-effects such as sweating, bradycardia, and intestinal colic may occur, particularly in the elderly.

Carbachol and **bethanechol** are choline esters whose actions are more prolonged than those of acetylcholine; both may relieve acute or chronic urinary retention.

Distigmine produces a similar effect by inhibiting the breakdown of acetylcholine. It may help patients with an upper motor neurone neurogenic bladder.

BETHANECHOL CHLORIDE

Indications: urinary retention (see section 1.6.2 for use in gastro-intestinal disease)
Cautions: elderly patients, asthma, cardiovascular disease, epilepsy, parkinsonism, vagotonia, hyperthyroidism
Contra-indications: intestinal or urinary obstruction, recent myocardial infarction, recent intestinal anastomosis
Side-effects: parasympathomimetic effects such as nausea, vomiting, sweating, blurred vision, bradycardia, and intestinal colic
Dose: 10–30 mg 3–4 times daily half an hour before food

PoM **Myotonine®** (Glenwood)
Tablets, both pale blue, scored, bethanechol chloride 10 mg, net price 20 = 82p; 25 mg, 20 = £1.04. Label: 22

CARBACHOL

Indications: urinary retention
Cautions; Contra-indications; Side-effects: see under Bethanechol Chloride but side-effects are more frequent
Dose: by mouth, 2 mg 3 times daily half an hour before food
By subcutaneous injection (acute symptoms, postoperative urinary retention) 250 micrograms, repeated twice if necessary at 30-minute intervals

PoM **Carbachol** (Non-proprietary)
Tablets, carbachol 2 mg. Net price 20 = 83p. Label: 22
Injection, carbachol 250 micrograms/ml. Net price 1-ml amp = 40p

DISTIGMINE BROMIDE

Indications: urinary retention due to upper motor lesions (see section 1.6.2 for use in gastro-intestinal disease)
Cautions; Contra-indications; Side-effects: see under Bethanechol Chloride; side-effects are mild but more prolonged
Dose: by mouth, 5 mg daily or on alternate days, half an hour before breakfast
By intramuscular injection, 500 micrograms 12 hours after surgery to prevent urinary retention; may be repeated every 24 hours

PoM **Ubretid®** (Rorer)
Tablets, scored, distigmine bromide 5 mg. Net price 20 = £10.86. Label: 22
Injection, distigmine bromide 500 micrograms/ml. Net price 1-ml amp = 54p

7.4.2   Drugs for urinary frequency, enuresis, and incontinence

Anticholinergic drugs such as **terodiline** and **propantheline** are used to treat *urinary frequency*; they increase bladder capacity by diminishing unstable detrusor contractions. All these drugs may cause dry mouth and blurred vision and may precipitate glaucoma. Terodiline, possessing anticholinergic and calcium antagonist properties, relaxes the detrusor muscle of the bladder and is useful in patients with urge incontinence and detrusor instability. The **tricyclic antidepressants** imipramine, amitriptyline, and nortriptyline (see section 4.3.1) are sometimes effective in the management of the unstable bladder because of their anticholinergic properties.

Nocturnal enuresis is a normal occurrence in young children but persists in as many as 5% by 10 years of age. In the absence of urinary-tract infection simple measures such as bladder training or the use of an alarm system may be successful. Drug therapy is not appropriate for children under 7 years of age and should be reserved for when alternative measures have failed. The possible side-effects and potential toxicity of these agents if taken in overdose should be borne in mind when they are prescribed.

The most widely used treatment is with tricyclics such as **amitriptyline**, **imipramine**, and less often **nortriptyline** (see section 4.3.1). They are effective, but behaviour disturbances may occur and relapse is common after withdrawal. Treatment should not normally exceed 3 months unless a full physical examination (including ECG) is given.

Desmopressin, an analogue of vasopressin, is also used for nocturnal enuresis; it should not be given for longer than 28 days.

The sympathomimetic drug **ephedrine** may also be useful.

AMITRIPTYLINE HYDROCHLORIDE
See section 4.3.1

DESMOPRESSIN
See section 6.5.2

EPHEDRINE HYDROCHLORIDE
Indications: nocturnal enuresis
Cautions; Contra-indications; Side-effects: see under Ephedrine Hydrochloride (section 3.1.1.2) and notes in section 3.10
Dose: CHILD 7–8 years 30 mg, 9–12 years 45 mg, 13–15 years 60 mg at bedtime

Preparations
See section 3.1.1.2

FLAVOXATE HYDROCHLORIDE
Indications: urinary frequency and incontinence, dysuria
Cautions; Contra-indications: see Terodiline Hydrochloride
Side-effects: anticholinergic side-effects (see Atropine Sulphate, section 1.2); see also notes above
Dose: 200 mg 3 times daily

PoM **Urispas**® (Syntex)
Tablets, s/c, flavoxate hydrochloride 100 mg. Net price 20 = 68p

IMIPRAMINE HYDROCHLORIDE
See section 4.3.1

NORTRIPTYLINE HYDROCHLORIDE
See section 4.3.1

PROPANTHELINE BROMIDE
Indications: urinary frequency and incontinence
Cautions; Contra-indications: see Terodiline Hydrochloride
Side-effects: anticholinergic side-effects (see Atropine Sulphate, section 1.2); see also notes above
Dose: 15–30 mg 2–3 times daily one hour before meals

Preparations
See section 1.2

TERODILINE HYDROCHLORIDE
Indications: urinary frequency and incontinence
Cautions: gastric retention, obstructive lesions (particularly of gastro-intestinal tract); fever, thyrotoxicosis, cardiac disease where increase in rate is undesirable, hepatic impairment; elderly. Drug interactions: see Appendix 1 (section *4.9*)
Contra-indications: urinary obstruction, bladder outflow obstruction, flaccid bladder or high residual urine, severe hepatic or biliary tract disease, glaucoma
Side-effects: anticholinergic side-effects (see under Atropine Sulphate, section 1.2); also see notes above
Dose: 12.5–25 mg twice daily (elderly patients, 12.5 mg twice daily)

▼ PoM **Terolin**® (KabiVitrum)
Tablets, f/c, terodiline hydrochloride 12.5 mg. Net price 100 = £21.50

7.4.3 Drugs used as urinary analgesics or to alter urinary pH

Potassium citrate or **sodium citrate** by their alkalinising action may relieve the discomfort of *cystitis* caused by lower urinary tract infections. A **terpene** mixture (Rowatinex®) is claimed to be of benefit in *urolithiasis* for the expulsion of calculi. Intramuscular injection of **diclofenac** (see section 10.1.1) is effective in the acute pain of *ureteric colic*, comparing favourably with pethidine; more than one injection may be required. **Lignocaine gel** is a useful topical application in *urethral pain* or to relieve the discomfort of catheterisation (see section 15.2).

Alkalinisation of urine may be undertaken with **sodium bicarbonate**, or alternatively sodium or potassium citrate. *Acidification* of urine has been undertaken with **ascorbic acid** or occasionally with ammonium chloride. Ascorbic acid is not always reliable and ammonium chloride is associated with rapid development of tolerance and a number of adverse effects, including vomiting and systemic acidosis.

For pH-modifying solutions for the maintenance of indwelling urinary catheters, see section 7.4.4.

ASCORBIC ACID

Indications: acidification of urine
Dose: by mouth, 4 g daily in divided doses

Preparations
See section 9.6.3

POTASSIUM CITRATE

Indications: relief of discomfort in mild urinary-tract infections; alkalinisation of urine
Cautions: renal impairment, cardiac disease; elderly. Drug interactions: see Appendix 1 (sections *2.2, 2.5)*
Side-effects: hyperkalaemia on prolonged high dosage, mild diuresis
Dose: cystitis, adults and children over 6 years, 3 g, well diluted with water, 3 times daily; CHILD 1–6 years 1.5 g
Alkalinisation of urine, 3–6 g with water every 6 hours

Potassium Citrate Mixture, potassium citrate 1.5 g/5 ml (see Formulary). Net price 100 ml = 31p. Label: 27
Effercitrate® (Typharm)
Tablets, effervescent, the equivalent of potassium citrate 1.5 g (13.9 mmol K$^+$), citric acid 250 mg (1 tablet ≡ 5 ml potassium citrate mixture). Net price 12 = £1.24. Label: 13

SODIUM BICARBONATE

Indications: alkalinisation of urine
Cautions; Side-effects: elderly; see also section 1.1.2
Dose: 3 g in water every 2 hours until urinary pH exceeds 7; maintenance of alkaline urine 5-10 g daily

Sodium Bicarbonate Powder. Net price 50 g = 5p. Label: 13

SODIUM CITRATE

Indications: relief of discomfort in mild urinary-tract infections
Cautions: renal impairment, cardiac disease, pregnancy, patients on a sodium-restricted diet; elderly
Side-effects: mild diuresis
Dose: see below

Urisal® (Winthrop)
Granules, yellow and white, effervescent, the equivalent of sodium citrate 4 g/sachet. Contains 41 mmol Na$^+$/sachet. Net price 9 sachets = £2.33. Label: 13
Dose: 1 sachet in a glass of water 3 times daily for max. of 3 days
Note. Although Urisal® is legally on the General Sale List it is restricted by product licence to prescription only

OTHER PREPARATIONS FOR URINARY DISORDERS

Ammonium Chloride Mixture (see Formulary). Net price 100 ml = 12p. Label: 13

Dose: 10–20 ml up to 3 times daily for the acidification of urine (but see notes above). To be taken well diluted with water
Rowatinex® (Tillotts)
Capsules, yellow, e/c, 0.1 ml of liquid of composition below. Net price 20 = £2.38. Label: 25
Dose: 1 capsule 3–4 times daily
Liquid, yellow, anethole 400 mg, borneol 1 g, camphene 1.5 g, cineole 300 mg, fenchone 400 mg, pinene 3.1 g, olive oil to 10 g. Net price 10 ml = £5.70. Label: 22, counselling advised, use of dropper
Dose: 3–5 drops 4–5 times daily before food

7.4.4 Bladder instillations

INFECTED BLADDERS. Various solutions are available as irrigations or washouts for the infected bladder.

Initial treatment is with **sterile sodium chloride solution 0.9%** (physiological saline).

Aqueous **chlorhexidine** (Hibitane®, see section 13.11) is effective against a wide range of common urinary-tract pathogens but not against most *Pseudomonas* spp. Solutions containing 1 in 5000 (0.02%) are used but they may irritate the mucosa and cause burning and haematuria (in which case they should be discontinued); solutions containing 1 in 10000 (0.01%) are usually preferred postoperatively. **Polymyxin B sulphate with neomycin** (Polybactrin®) and **colistin** (both section 5.1.7) are bactericidal to most pathogens and emergence of resistance is slow.

Noxythiolin (Noxyflex®) is also bactericidal to most pathogens with slow emergence of resistance, but initial use in the purulent infected bladder is often accompanied by an intense reaction including the passage of large clumps of fibrin. Other indications for noxythiolin include intra-peritoneal use during colonic surgery.

Bladder irrigations of **amphotericin** 100 micrograms/ml (Fungizone®, see section 5.2) may be of value in mycotic infections.

DISSOLUTION OF BLOOD CLOTS. Clot retention is usually treated by irrigation with sterile **sodium chloride** solution but sterile **sodium citrate** solution for bladder irrigation (3%) may also be helpful. **Streptokinase-streptodornase** (Varidase Topical®, see section 13.11) is an alternative.

LOCALLY ACTING CYTOTOXIC DRUGS. **Ethoglucid** (Epodyl®, see section 8.1.1) is used in the control of rapidly recurring non-invasive bladder tumours of low grade malignancy. 100 ml of a 1–2% solution is left in the bladder for as long as possible (usually 1 hour). Treatment may be given weekly for 12 weeks and then monthly for a year. It may cause dysuria and frequency.

Thiotepa (see section 8.1.1) is used for bladder tumours of low to medium grade malignancy. A solution containing 30–60 mg in 60 ml of sterile water is retained in the bladder for 2 hours. It is given weekly for 4 weeks. The concentration should be reduced if there is evidence of bone-marrow suppression.

Doxorubicin (see section 8.1.2) is used to treat recurrent superficial bladder tumours, carcinoma-in-situ, and some papillary tumours. An instillation (50 mg in 50 ml of sterile sodium chloride solution 0.9%) is retained in the bladder for one hour and treatment repeated monthly. Although systemic side-effects are few, it may cause frequency, urgency, dysuria, and occasionally reduction in bladder capacity.

INTERSTITIAL CYSTITIS. Dimethyl sulphoxide may be used for symptomatic relief in patients with interstitial cystitis (Hunner's ulcer). 50 ml of a 50% solution (Rimso-50®) is instilled into the bladder, retained for 15 minutes, and voided by the patient. Treatment is repeated at intervals of 2 weeks. Bladder spasm and hypersensitivity reactions may occur and long-term use requires ophthalmic, renal, and hepatic assessment at 6-monthly intervals.

CHLORHEXIDINE

Indications: bladder washouts, see notes above and section 13.11

See also catheter patency solutions

DIMETHYL SULPHOXIDE

Indications: bladder washouts, see notes above

PoM **Rimso-50**® (Britannia)
Bladder instillation, sterile, dimethyl sulphoxide 50%, in aqueous solution. Net price 50 ml = £19.80

NOXYTHIOLIN

Indications: see notes above
Side-effects: burning sensation on application to bladder (relieved by addition of amethocaine)
Dose: bladder instillation, 100 ml of a 2.5% solution instilled 1–2 times daily
Intraperitoneal use, 100 ml of a 2.5% solution instilled prior to closure

PoM **Noxyflex**® (Geistlich)
Solution, powder for reconstitution, noxythiolin 2.5 g, amethocaine hydrochloride 10 mg. Net price 2.5 g in 20-ml vial = £6.37; 2.5 g in 100 ml vial with transfer needle = £7.96
PoM **Noxyflex S**® (Geistlich)
Solution, powder for reconstitution, noxythiolin.

Net price 2.5 g in 20 ml vial = £6.37; 2·5 g in 100-ml vial with transfer needle = £7.96

SODIUM CHLORIDE
Indications: bladder washouts, see notes above

Note. The term 'normal saline' should not be used to describe sterile sodium chloride solution 0.9%; the term 'physiological saline' is acceptable

SODIUM CITRATE
Indications: bladder washouts, see notes above

Sterile Sodium Citrate Solution for Bladder Irrigation, sodium citrate 3%, dilute hydrochloric acid 0.2%, in purified water, freshly boiled and cooled, and sterilised

MAINTENANCE OF INDWELLING URINARY CATHETERS

The deposition which occurs in catheterised patients is usually chiefly composed of phosphate and to minimise this the catheter (if latex) should be changed at least as often as every 6 weeks. If the catheter is to be left for longer periods a silicone catheter should be used. If bladder washouts are required at frequent intervals this usually indicates that the catheter needs to be changed.

Catheter patency solutions
Uro-Tainer® (CliniMed)
 Chlorhexidine 0.02%. Net price 100-ml sachet = £1.71
 Mandelic acid 1%. Net price 100-ml sachet = £1.71
 Sodium chloride 0.9%. Net price 100-ml sachet = £1.52
 Solution R, citric acid 6%, gluconolactone 0.6%, magnesium carbonate 2.8%, disodium edetate 0.01%. Net price 100-ml sachet = £1.71
 Note. To minimise inflammation or irritation, treatment should commence with Suby G
 Suby G, citric acid 3.23%, magnesium oxide 0.38%, sodium bicarbonate 0.7%, disodium edetate 0.01%. Net price 100-ml sachet = £1.71
Uro-Tainer M® (CliniMed)
 Sodium chloride 0.9%. Net price 50- and 100-ml sachet (both) = £1.93

8: Drugs used in the treatment of

MALIGNANT DISEASE and for IMMUNOSUPPRESSION

In this chapter, drug treatment is discussed under the following headings:

8.1 Cytotoxic drugs
8.2 Drugs affecting the immune response
8.3 Sex hormones and antagonists used in malignant disease

Malignant disease may be treated by surgery, radiotherapy, and/or chemotherapy. Certain tumours are highly sensitive to chemotherapy but many are not, and inappropriate drug administration in these circumstances can only increase morbidity or mortality. Cytotoxic drugs and corticosteroids are also used as immunosuppressants. The sex hormones are used to treat certain responsive tumours.

8.1 Cytotoxic drugs

8.1.1 Alkylating drugs
8.1.2 Cytotoxic antibiotics
8.1.3 Antimetabolites
8.1.4 Vinca alkaloids and etoposide
8.1.5 Other antineoplastic drugs

Many drugs are now available which are active in malignant disease or as immunosuppressants for use in organ transplant recipients or patients with a range of medical conditions.

Great care is needed when prescribing these drugs as damage to normal tissue, which may be irreversible, is an almost invariable consequence of their use. These drugs should rarely, if ever, be used empirically in a patient with cancer, and administration should always be regarded as a clinical trial with clear objectives in mind.

In a minority of cancers, chemotherapy may be given with cure, or marked prolongation of survival, a realistic end-point. Here short-term drug-related toxicity, which may be severe, is acceptable. However, for the majority of patients, modest survival prolongation or palliation of symptoms will be the aim, and an attempt should be made to use relatively non-toxic treatments, or to consider the use of other effective modalities, e.g. radiotherapy.

Cytotoxic drugs may be used either singly, or in combination therapy. In the latter case, the initial letters of the drug names, or proprietary names, identify the regimen used and those referred to in this chapter are:

MOPP—mustine, vincristine (Oncovin®), procarbazine, and prednisolone

MVPP—mustine, vinblastine, procarbazine, and prednisolone

ABVD—doxorubicin (Adriamycin®), bleomycin, vinblastine, and dacarbazine.

Many other such combinations have been used. Drug combinations are frequently more toxic than single drugs but may have the advantage in certain tumours of enhanced response and increased survival, e.g. in Hodgkin's disease. However for some tumour types, single-agent chemotherapy remains the treatment of choice.

> Most cytotoxic drugs are teratogenic, and all may cause life-threatening toxicity; administration should, where possible, be confined to those experienced in their use.
>
> Because of the complexity of dosage regimens in the treatment of malignant disease, dose statements have been omitted from some of the drug entries in this chapter. *In all cases detailed specialist literature should be consulted.*
>
> Prescriptions should **not** be repeated except on the instructions of a specialist.

Cytotoxic drugs fall naturally into a number of classes, each with characteristic antitumour activity, sites of action, and toxicity. A knowledge of sites of metabolism and excretion is important, as impaired drug handling as a result of disease is not uncommon and may result in enhanced toxic effects. A number of side-effects are characteristic of particular agents or groups of drugs, e.g. neurotoxicity of vinca alkaloids, and details will be provided in the appropriate sections. Most toxic effects are, however, common to many of these drugs and will be briefly outlined here.

EXTRAVASATION OF INTRAVENOUS DRUGS. A number of drugs will cause severe local tissue necrosis if leakage into the extravascular compartment occurs. Recommended modes of administration must be adhered to. Infusion of vesicant drugs should be stopped immediately if local pain is experienced. Where doubt exists as to whether significant leakage has occurred, the infusion should be discontinued and the cannula resited in another vein.

NAUSEA AND VOMITING. Nausea and vomiting is a source of considerable distress to many patients receiving chemotherapy. It should be anticipated and, where possible, prevented with anti-emetic treatment tailored to the chemotherapy regimen and the response of the patient.

If first-line anti-emetics are ineffective treatment should be escalated as below. Hospital admission may be necessary.

Group 1: severe emesis unlikely
Drugs in this group include alkylating agents by mouth, intravenous fluorouracil, vinca alkaloids, and methotrexate.

Phenothiazines (e.g. prochlorperazine) or domperidone, given by mouth, when necessary, will often suffice. Premedication with these drugs is often useful before intravenous chemotherapy, treatment being continued for up to 24 hours afterwards. Both prochlorperazine and domperidone are also available as suppositories which is useful for patients who develop vomiting despite oral therapy.

For preparations and doses of anti-emetics, see section 4.6.

Group 2: moderate emesis
Drugs in this group include intravenous cyclophosphamide and doxorubicin; premedication is essential for all drugs in this group. Most patients can be treated on an out-patient basis therefore, if possible, the anti-emetics should be given by mouth.

Anti-emetics in group 1 are sufficient for some patients but it is probably preferable to start with dexamethasone 10 mg by mouth before and 6 hours after chemotherapy, or lorazepam 1 to 2 mg by mouth given similarly. Lorazepam has the advantage of causing drowsiness and amnesia, but patients cannot drive after it. Nabilone is also suitable, but may cause dysphoria.

Patients in group 1 with an unsatisfactory response can be transferred to drugs in this group.

Group 3: severe emesis
Drugs in this group include mustine, dacarbazine, and cisplatin. They commonly cause severe emesis, particularly if used in combination.

A simple well-tolerated anti-emetic regimen is dexamethasone 10 mg by mouth with lorazepam 1 to 2 mg by mouth, given before and 6 hours after chemotherapy. Out-patients should be warned not to drive. Dexamethasone and lorazepam can also be given intravenously to inpatients; the dose of lorazepam is titrated according to the patient's level of consciousness (drowsiness should be obtained with 2 to 4 mg). This regimen should be avoided in patients with chronic chest disease and care is necessary in the elderly.

Alternatively, high-dose metoclopramide can be given by intravenous infusion but it may cause dystonic reactions in younger patients (see section 4.6).

Patients in group 2 with an unsatisfactory response can be transferred to drugs in this group.

BONE-MARROW SUPPRESSION. All cytotoxic drugs except vincristine and bleomycin cause marrow depression. This commonly occurs 7 to 10 days after administration, but is delayed for certain drugs, such as carmustine, lomustine, and melphalan. Peripheral blood counts must be checked prior to each treatment, and doses should be reduced or therapy delayed if marrow recovery has not occurred. Fever occurring in a neutropenic patient (neutrophil count less than 800×10^9/litre) is an indication for immediate parenteral broad-spectrum antibiotic therapy, once appropriate bacteriological investigations have taken place.

ALOPECIA. Reversible hair loss is a common complication of these drugs, although it varies in degree between drug preparations and individual patients. No pharmacological methods of preventing this are available.

8.1.1 Alkylating drugs

Extensive experience is available with these drugs, which are among the most widely used in cancer chemotherapy. They act by damaging DNA, thus interfering with cell replication. In addition to the side-effects common to many cytotoxic drugs (section 8.1), there are two problems associated with prolonged usage. Firstly, gametogenesis is often severely affected. Almost all males will be rendered permanently sterile early in a treatment course. Females are less severely affected, though the span of reproductive life may be shortened by the onset of a premature menopause. Potency is not affected. Secondly, prolonged use of these drugs, particularly when combined with extensive irradiation, is associated with a marked increase in the incidence of acute non-lymphocytic leukaemia.

Cyclophosphamide (Endoxana®) is widely used in the treatment of chronic lymphocytic leukaemia, the lymphomas, and solid tumours. It may be given orally or intravenously and is inactive until metabolised by the liver. Acrolein, a urinary metabolite of cyclophosphamide, may cause haemorrhagic cystitis; this is a serious complication and if it occurs cyclophosphamide is not normally used again. An increased fluid intake, for example 3 to 4 litres per day after intravenous injection, will help avoid this complication. When high dose therapy is used mesna will also help prevent this complication.

Ifosfamide (Mitoxana®) is related to cyclophosphamide and is given with mesna to reduce urothelial toxicity.

Chlorambucil (Leukeran®) is a useful agent commonly used to treat chronic lymphocytic leukaemia, the indolent non-Hodgkin's lymphomas, Hodgkin's disease, and ovarian carcinoma. Side-effects, apart from marrow suppression, are uncommon, although rashes may occur.

Melphalan (Alkeran®) is used to treat myeloma and occasionally solid tumours and lymphomas. Marrow toxicity is delayed and it is usually given at intervals of 4–6 weeks.

Busulphan (Myleran®) is used almost exclusively to treat chronic myeloid leukaemia. Frequent blood counts are necessary as excessive myelosuppression may result in irreversible bone-marrow aplasia. Hyperpigmentation of the skin is a common side-effect and, rarely, progressive pulmonary fibrosis may occur.

Lomustine (CCNU®) is a lipid-soluble nitrosourea and may be given orally. It is mainly used to treat Hodgkin's disease and certain solid tumours. Marrow toxicity is delayed, and the drug is therefore given at intervals of 4 to 6 weeks. Permanent marrow damage may occur with prolonged use. Nausea and vomiting are common and moderately severe.

Carmustine (BiCNU®) is given intravenously. It has similar activity and toxicities.

Mustine is now much less commonly used. It is a very toxic drug which causes severe vomiting. The freshly prepared injection must be given into a fast-running intravenous infusion. Local extravasation causes severe tissue necrosis.

Estramustine (Estracyt®) is a stable combination of an oestrogen and mustine, designed to deliver mustine to the oestrogen receptor site of a tumour, for example prostate cancer. It is not extensively used in this country.

Treosulfan is used to treat ovarian carcinoma.

Thiotepa is usually used as an intracavitary drug for the treatment of malignant effusions or bladder cancer. It is also occasionally used to treat breast cancer, but requires parenteral administration.

Ethoglucid (Epodyl®) is used by the intracavitary route for bladder cancer.

Mitobronitol is occasionally used to treat chronic myeloid leukaemia; it is available on a named-patient basis only (as *Myelobromol*®, Sinclair).

BUSULPHAN

Indications: chronic myeloid leukaemia
Cautions; Side-effects: see section 8.1 and notes above
Dose: induction of remission, 60 micrograms/kg to max. 4 mg daily; maintenance, 0.5–2 mg daily

PoM **Myleran**® (Wellcome)
Tablets, busulphan 500 micrograms, net price 20 = £1.78; 2 mg, 20 = £2.67

CARMUSTINE

Indications: see notes above
Cautions; Side-effects: see section 8.1 and notes above; irritant to tissues

PoM **BiCNU**® (Bristol-Myers)
Injection, powder for reconstitution, carmustine. Net price 100-mg vial (with diluent) = £12.50

CHLORAMBUCIL

Indications: see notes above (for use as an immunosuppressant see section 8.2.1)
Cautions; Side-effects: see section 8.1 and notes above
Dose: used alone, usually 100–200 micrograms/kg daily for 4–8 weeks

PoM **Leukeran**® (Wellcome)
Tablets, both yellow, chlorambucil 2 mg, net price 20 = £4.30; 5 mg, 20 = £6.54

CYCLOPHOSPHAMIDE

Indications: see notes above
Cautions; Side-effects: see section 8.1 and notes above. Drug interactions: see Appendix 1 (sections 8, *15*)

PoM **Cyclophosphamide** (Farmitalia Carlo Erba)
Tablets, s/c, cyclophosphamide (anhydrous) 50 mg. Net price 20 = 76p. Label: 27

Injection, powder for preparing injections, cyclophosphamide. Net price 107-mg vial = 38p; 214-mg vial = 53p; 535-mg vial = £1.03; 1.07-g vial = £1.67

PoM **Endoxana**® (Boehringer Ingelheim)
Tablets, both compression-coated, cyclophosphamide 10 mg, net price 20 = 51p; 50 mg, 20 = £1.59. Label: 27
Injection, powder for reconstitution, cyclophosphamide. Net price 107-mg vial = 79p; 214-mg vial = £1.13; 535-mg vial = £1.97; 1.069-g vial = £3.44

ESTRAMUSTINE PHOSPHATE

Indications: prostatic carcinoma
Cautions; Contra-indications; Side-effects: see section 8.1 and under Ethinyloestradiol (section 6.4.1.1)
Dose: 0.14–1.4 g daily in divided doses (usual range 0.56–1.12 g daily)

▼ PoM **Estracyt**® (Lundbeck)
Capsules, estramustine phosphate 140 mg (as disodium salt). Net price 20 = £20.90. Label: 21, counselling advised, should not be taken with dairy products

ETHOGLUCID

Indications: non-invasive bladder carcinoma, see section 7.4.4
Side-effects: frequency of micturition, dysuria, fall in leucocyte count
Dose: by instillation, 1% solution

PoM **Epodyl**® (ICI)
Liquid, sterile ethoglucid. Plastic syringes should not be used. Net price 1-ml amp = £2.21

IFOSFAMIDE

Indications: see notes above
Cautions; Side-effects: see section 8.1 and notes under Cyclophosphamide; reduce dose in renal impairment

PoM **Mitoxana**® (Boehringer Ingelheim)
Injection, powder for reconstitution, ifosfamide. Net price 500-mg vial = £5.52; 1-g vial = £9.63; 2-g vial = £17.72 (Hosp. only)

LOMUSTINE

Indications: see notes above
Cautions; Side-effects: see section 8.1 and notes above
Dose: used alone, 120–130 mg/m² body-surface every 6–8 weeks

▼ PoM **CCNU**® (Lundbeck)
Capsules, lomustine 10 mg (blue/white), net price 20 = £9.42; 40 mg (blue), 20 = £23.69

MELPHALAN

Indications: myelomatosis
Cautions; Side-effects: see section 8.1 and notes above; reduce dose in renal impairment
Dose: by mouth, 150–300 micrograms/kg daily for 4–6 days, repeated after 4–8 weeks

---

PoM **Alkeran**® (Wellcome)
Tablets, melphalan 2 mg, net price 20 = £5.89;
5 mg, 20 = £10.42
Injection, powder for reconstitution, melphalan. Net price 100-mg vial (with solvent and
diluent) = £35.48

MUSTINE HYDROCHLORIDE

Indications: Hodgkin's disease—see notes above
Cautions; Side-effects: see section 8.1 and notes
above; also caution in handling—vesicant and
a nasal irritant

PoM **Mustine Hydrochloride** (Boots)
Injection, powder for reconstitution, mustine
hydrochloride. Net price 10-mg vial = £1.48

THIOTEPA

Indications: see notes above and section 7.4.4
Cautions; Side-effects: see section 8.1. Drug
interactions: see Appendix 1 (section *15*)

PoM **Thiotepa** (Lederle)
Injection, powder for reconstitution, thiotepa
(with sodium chloride and bicarbonate). Net
price 15-mg vial = £4.85

TREOSULFAN

Indications: see notes above
Cautions; Side-effects: see section 8.1
Dose: by mouth, courses of 1–2 g daily in 4 divided doses to provide total dose of 21–28 g over
initial 8 weeks

PoM **Treosulfan** (Leo)
Capsules, treosulfan 250 mg. Net price 20 =
£6.02. Label: 25
Injection, powder for reconstitution, treosulfan.
Net price 5 g in infusion bottle with transfer
needle = £68.76

UROTHELIAL TOXICITY

Urothelial toxicity, commonly manifest by haemorrhagic cystitis, is a problem peculiar to the use of
cyclophosphamide or ifosfamide and is caused by a
metabolite (acrolein). **Mesna** (Uromitexan®) reacts
specifically with this metabolite in the urinary tract,
preventing toxicity. Mesna is given simultaneously
with cyclophosphamide or ifosfamide, and further
doses are given orally or intravenously 4 and 8 hours
after treatment.

MESNA

Indications: see notes above
Side-effects: above max. therapeutic doses, gastro-
intestinal disturbances, fatigue, headache

▼ PoM **Uromitexan**® (Boehringer Ingelheim)
Injection, mesna 100 mg/ml. Net price 4-ml amp =
£1.18; 10-ml amp = £2.56
Note. For oral administration contents of ampoule
are taken in fruit juice

8.1.2 Cytotoxic antibiotics

Drugs within this group are widely used as anti-
cancer agents. Many act as radiomimetics and
simultaneous use of radiotherapy with these drugs
should be avoided as it may result in markedly
enhanced normal tissue toxicity.

Doxorubicin is one of the most successful and
widely used antitumour drugs, and is used to treat
the acute leukaemias, lymphomas, and a variety
of solid tumours. It is given by fast running
infusion, commonly at 21-day intervals. Local
extravasation will cause severe tissue necrosis.
Common toxic effects include nausea and
vomiting, myelosuppression, alopecia, and
mucositis. This drug is largely excreted by the
biliary tract, and an elevated bilirubin concentration is an indication for reducing the dose.
Supraventricular tachycardia related to drug
administration is an uncommon complication.
Higher cumulative doses are associated with
development of a cardiomyopathy. It is customary
to arbitrarily limit total doses to be administered
to 450–550 mg/m² body-surface area as symptomatic and potentially fatal heart failure occurs
increasingly commonly above this level. Patients
with pre-existing cardiac disease, the elderly, and
those who have received myocardial irradiation
should be treated cautiously. Cardiac monitoring,
for example by sequential radionuclide ejection
fraction measurement, may assist in safely limiting
total dosage. Evidence is available to suggest that
weekly low dose administration may be associated
with less cardiac damage.

Epirubicin (Pharmorubicin®) is closely structurally related to doxorubicin. Preliminary clinical
trials suggest that it is as effective as doxorubicin
in the treatment of breast cancer. Its principal
benefit is a reduced tendency to cause
cardiotoxicity.

Bleomycin is used to treat the lymphomas, certain solid tumours and, by the intracavitary route,
malignant effusions. It is unusual in that it causes
no marrow suppression. Dermatological toxicity
is common; increased pigmentation particularly
affecting the flexures and sclerotic
plaques may occur. Mucositis is also relatively
common and an association with Raynaud's
phenomenon is reported. Hypersensitivity reactions manifest by chills and fevers commonly
occur a few hours after drug administration and
may be prevented by simultaneous administration
of a corticosteroid, for example hydrocortisone
intravenously. The principal problem associated
with the use of bleomycin is progressive pulmonary fibrosis. This is dose related, occurring
more commonly at cumulative doses greater than
300 mg and in the elderly. Basal lung crepitations
or suspicious chest X-ray changes are an indication to stop therapy with this drug.

Actinomycin D (Cosmegen Lyovac®) is principally used to treat paediatric cancers. Its side-
effects are similar to those of doxorubicin, except
that cardiac toxicity is not a problem.

Plicamycin (mithramycin; Mithracin®) is no
longer used as a cytotoxic, but has found a useful

role in low dose in the emergency therapy of hypercalcaemia due to malignant disease (see section 9.5.1.2).

Mitomycin (Mitomycin C Kyowa®) is used to treat upper gastro-intestinal and breast cancers. It causes delayed marrow toxicity and is usually administered at 6-weekly intervals. Prolonged use may result in permanent marrow damage. It is a relatively toxic drug and may cause lung fibrosis and renal damage.

ACTINOMYCIN D
(Dactinomycin)
Indications: see notes above
Cautions; Side-effects: see section 8.1 and notes above; irritant to tissues

PoM **Cosmegen Lyovac®** (MSD)
Injection, powder for reconstitution, actinomycin D (with mannitol). Net price 500-microgram vial = £1.25

BLEOMYCIN
Indications: squamous cell carcinoma—see notes above
Cautions; Side-effects: see section 8.1 and notes above; reduce dose in renal impairment. Also caution in handling—irritant to skin

PoM **Bleomycin** (Lundbeck)
Injection, powder for reconstitution, bleomycin (as sulphate). Net price 15 mg = £13.89

DOXORUBICIN HYDROCHLORIDE
Indications: see notes above and section 7.4.4
Cautions; Side-effects: see section 8.1 and notes above; reduce dose in hepatic impairment; also caution in handling—irritant to skin and tissues

▼ PoM **Doxorubicin Rapid Dissolution** (Farmitalia Carlo Erba)
Injection, powder for reconstitution, doxorubicin hydrochloride (with lactose). Net price 10-mg vial = £9.80; 50-mg vial = £47.04
Note. This preparation has replaced Adriamycin®

EPIRUBICIN HYDROCHLORIDE
Indications: see notes above
Cautions; Side-effects: see section 8.1 and notes above; reduce dose in hepatic impairment; also irritant to tissues

▼ PoM **Pharmorubicin®** (Farmitalia Carlo Erba)
Injection, powder for reconstitution, epirubicin hydrochloride. Net price 10-mg vial = £13.72; 20-mg vial = £27.44; 50-mg vial = £67.62

MITOMYCIN
Indications: see notes above
Cautions; Side-effects: see section 8.1 and notes above; also irritant to tissues

PoM **Mitomycin C Kyowa®** (Martindale)
Injection, powder for reconstitution, mitomycin. Net price 2-mg vial = £4.40; 10-mg vial = £13.95; 20-mg vial = £27.60 (Hosp. only)

PLICAMYCIN
(Mithramycin)
Indications: see notes above
Cautions; Side-effects: see section 8.1 and notes above; irritant to tissues

PoM **Mithracin®** (Pfizer)
Injection, powder for reconstitution, plicamycin (with mannitol and sodium phosphate). Net price 2.5-mg vial = £7.51

8.1.3   Antimetabolites

Antimetabolites are incorporated into new nuclear material or combine irreversibly with vital cellular enzymes, preventing normal cellular division.

Methotrexate inhibits the enzyme dihydrofolate reductase, essential for the synthesis of purines and pyrimidines. It may be given orally, intravenously, intramuscularly, or intrathecally. High-dose methotrexate cannot generally be recommended except in clinical trials.

Methotrexate is used as maintenance therapy for childhood acute lymphoblastic leukaemia. Other uses include choriocarcinoma, non-Hodgkin lymphomas, and a number of solid tumours. Intrathecal methotrexate is used in the CNS prophylaxis of childhood acute lymphoblastic leukaemia, and as a therapy for established meningeal carcinoma or lymphoma.

Methotrexate causes myelosuppression, mucositis, and rarely pneumonitis. It is contra-indicated if significant renal impairment is present, as the kidney is its route of excretion. It should also be avoided if a significant pleural effusion or ascites are present as it tends to accumulate at these sites, and its subsequent return to the circulation will be associated with myelosuppression. For similar reasons blood counts should be carefully monitored when intrathecal methotrexate is given.

Oral or parenteral folinic acid (see below) will speed recovery from methotrexate mucositis or myelosuppression.

Cytarabine (Cytosar® etc.) acts by interfering with pyrimidine synthesis. It may be given subcutaneously, intravenously, or intrathecally. Its predominant use is in the induction of remission and maintenance therapy of acute myeloblastic leukaemia. It is a potent myelosuppressant and requires careful haematological monitoring.

Fluorouracil may be given orally but is usually given intravenously. It is used to treat a number of solid tumours, including colon and breast cancer. It may also be used topically for certain malignant skin lesions. Toxicity is unusual, but may include myelosuppression, mucositis, and rarely a cerebellar syndrome.

Mercaptopurine (Puri-Nethol®) is used almost exclusively as maintenance therapy for the acute leukaemias. The dose should be reduced if the patient is receiving concurrent allopurinol as this drug interferes with the metabolism of mercaptopurine.

Thioguanine (Lanvis®) is used orally to induce remission and for maintenance in acute myeloid leukaemia.

Azathioprine is an antimetabolite, but is commonly used as an immunosuppressant (section 8.2.1).

CYTARABINE

Indications: acute leukaemias
Cautions; Side-effects: see section 8.1 and notes above

▼ PoM **Cytarabine** (Non-proprietary)
Injection, powder for reconstitution, cytarabine. Net price 100-mg vial = £2.75; 500-mg vial = £13.33; 1-g vial = £25.86
▼ PoM **Alexan**® (Pfizer)
Injection, cytarabine 20 mg/ml. Net price 2-ml amp = £1.06; 5-ml amp = £2.65
▼ PoM **Alexan 100**® (Pfizer)
Injection, cytarabine 100 mg/ml. Net price 1-ml amp = £2.65; 10-ml amp = £26.46. For intravenous infusion
PoM **Cytosar**® (Upjohn)
Injection, powder for reconstitution, cytarabine. Net price 100-mg vial = £3.17; 500-mg vial (with diluent) = £15.45

FLUOROURACIL

Indications: see notes above
Cautions; Side-effects: see section 8.1. Drug interactions: see Appendix 1 (section 8)
Dose: by mouth, maintenance 15 mg/kg weekly; max. in one day 1 g.

PoM **Fluorouracil** (Non-proprietary)
Injection, fluorouracil (as sodium salt) 25 mg/ml. Net price 10-ml vial = £1.34; 20-ml vial = £2.60; 100-ml vial = £12.60
PoM **Fluoro-uracil** (Roche)
Capsules, blue/orange, fluorouracil 250 mg. Net price 30-cap pack = £35.38. Label: 21
Injection, fluorouracil 25 mg (as sodium salt)/ml. Net price 10-ml amp = £1.42
PoM **Efudix**® (Roche)
Cream, fluorouracil 5%. Net price 20 g = £3.75

MERCAPTOPURINE

Indications: acute leukaemias
Cautions; Side-effects: see section 8.1 and notes above; reduce dose in renal impairment. Drug interactions: see Appendix 1 (section 8)
Dose: initially 2.5 mg/kg daily

PoM **Puri-Nethol**® (Wellcome)
Tablets, fawn, scored, mercaptopurine 50 mg. Net price 20 = £8.77

METHOTREXATE

Indications: see notes above
Cautions; Side-effects: see section 8.1 and notes above; reduce dose in renal impairment; dose-related toxicity in hepatic impairment. Drug interactions: see Appendix 1 (section 8)
Dose: by mouth, leukaemia in children (maintenance), 15 mg/m^2 weekly; psoriasis, 10–25 mg weekly

PoM **Methotrexate** (Lederle)
Tablets, both yellow, scored, methotrexate 2.5 mg, net price 20 = £2.17; 10 mg also available
Injection, methotrexate 2.5 mg (as sodium salt)/ml. Net price 1-ml amp = 83p; 2-ml vial = 91p
Injection, methotrexate 25 mg (as sodium salt)/ml. Net price 1-ml vial = £1.94; 2-ml vial = £2.69; 4-ml vial = £5.14; 8-ml vial = £10.28; 20-ml vial = £25.71; 40-ml vial = £45.71; 200-ml vial = £205.71
Injection, powder for reconstitution, methotrexate (as sodium salt). Net price 500-mg vial = £32.00
PoM **Emtexate**® (Nordic)
Tablets, methotrexate 10 mg. Net price 20 = £6.62
Injection, methotrexate 2.5 mg (as sodium salt)/ml. Net price 2-ml amp = 80p
Injection, methotrexate 25 mg (as sodium salt)/ml. Net price 2-ml vial = £1.98; 10-ml vial = £8.57; 20-ml vial = £15.77; 40-ml vial = £30.58; 200-ml vial = £136.16
Injection, methotrexate 100 mg (as sodium salt)/ml. Net price 10-ml vial = £30.58; 50-ml vial = £136.16
Injection, powder for reconstitution, methotrexate (as sodium salt). Net price 500-mg vial = £16.56; 1-g vial = £30.58; 5-g vial = £136.16
PoM **Maxtrex**® (Farmitalia Carlo Erba)
Tablets, both yellow, scored, methotrexate 2.5 mg, net price 20 = £2.14; 10 mg, 20 = £9.70
Injection, methotrexate 2.5 mg (as sodium salt)/ml. Net price 2-ml vial = 56p
Injection, methotrexate 25 mg (as sodium salt)/ml. Net price 2-ml vial = £2.75; 20-ml vial = £25.00; 40-ml vial = £55.00; 200-ml vial = £212.50

THIOGUANINE

Indications: acute leukaemias
Cautions; Side-effects: see section 8.1 and notes above; reduce dose in renal impairment
Dose: initially 2–2.5 mg/kg daily

PoM **Lanvis**® (Wellcome)
Tablets, yellow, scored, thioguanine 40 mg. Net price 20 = £23.34

FOLATE RESCUE

Folinic acid is used to counteract the folate-antagonist action of methotrexate and thus speed recovery from methotrexate-induced mucositis or myelosuppression. It does not counteract the antibacterial activity of folate antagonists such as trimethoprim.

FOLINIC ACID

Indications: see notes above
Cautions: avoid simultaneous administration of methotrexate; as for Folic Acid (section 9.1.2) not indicated for pernicious anaemia or other megaloblastic anaemias where vitamin B$_{12}$ deficient
Dose: as an antidote to methotrexate (started 8–24 hours after the beginning of methotrexate

infusion), in general up to 120 mg in divided doses over 12–24 hours by intramuscular or intravenous injection or infusion, followed by 12–15 mg intramuscularly or 15 mg by mouth every 6 hours for the next 48 hours

Suspected methotrexate overdosage, immediate administration of an equal or higher dose of folinic acid

PoM **Calcium Folinate** (Non-proprietary)
Tablets, scored, folinic acid (as calcium salt) 15 mg. Net price 10-tab pack = £35.00

PoM **Calcium Leucovorin** (Lederle)
Tablets, scored, folinic acid 15 mg (as calcium salt). Net price 10-tab pack = £42.28
Injection, folinic acid 3 mg (as calcium salt)/ml. Net price 1-ml amp = £1.09
Injection, powder for reconstitution, folinic acid (as calcium salt). Net price 15-mg vial = £4.57; 30-mg vial = £8.57

PoM **Refolinon**® (Farmitalia Carlo Erba)
Tablets, yellow, scored, folinic acid 15 mg (as calcium salt). Net price 30 = £105.00
Injection, folinic acid 3 mg (as calcium salt)/ml. Net price 2-ml amp = £1·60; 10-ml amp = £6.70

PoM **Rescufolin**® (Nordic)
Tablets, folinic acid 15 mg (as calcium salt). Net price 5 tabs = £8.80
Injection, powder for reconstitution, folinic acid (as calcium salt). Net price 15-mg vial = £2.78; 50-mg vial = £9.76; also 100-mg vial

8.1.4 Vinca alkaloids and etoposide

These interfere with microtubule assembly, causing metaphase arrest. All vinca alkaloids have similar activity but vary in the predominant site of toxicity.

The vinca alkaloids are used to treat the acute leukaemias, lymphomas, and some solid tumours (e.g. breast and lung cancer). They commonly cause peripheral and autonomic neuropathy. This side-effect is most obvious with vincristine, and is manifest by peripheral paraesthesia, loss of deep tendon reflexes, and abdominal bloating and constipation. If these symptoms are severe, doses should be reduced. Significant new motor weakness is a contra-indication to further use of these drugs. Recovery of the nervous system is generally slow but complete.

Vincristine (Oncovin®) causes virtually no myelosuppression. Its use may be associated with alopecia; hyponatraemia, as a result of inappropriate ADH secretion, has been described.

Vinblastine (Velbe®) is a more myelosuppressive drug than vincristine, but causes less neurotoxicity.

Vindesine (Eldisine®) is the most recent addition to the vinca alkaloid group. It has a similar range of clinical activity, and side-effects intermediate between those of the above two drugs.

Etoposide (Vepesid®) may be given orally or intravenously, the dose when used orally being double that when given intravenously. There is limited clinical evidence to suggest that administration in divided doses over 3–5 days may be beneficial; courses may not be repeated more

frequently than at intervals of 21 days. It has useful activity in small cell carcinoma of the bronchus, the lymphomas, and testicular teratoma. Common toxic effects include alopecia, myelosuppression, nausea, and vomiting.

ETOPOSIDE

Indications: see notes above
Cautions; Contra-indications; Side-effects: see section 8.1 and notes above; irritant to tissues

PoM **Vepesid**® (Bristol-Myers)
Capsules, etoposide 50 mg, net price 20 = £113.95; 100 mg, 10-tab pack = £99.57
Injection, etoposide 20 mg/ml. To be diluted. Net price 5-ml amp = £14.58
Caution: may dissolve certain types of filter

VINBLASTINE SULPHATE

Indications: see notes above
Cautions; Side-effects: see section 8.1 and notes above; caution in handling—avoid contact with eyes; irritant to tissues

PoM **Vinblastine Injection,** powder for reconstitution, vinblastine sulphate. Net price 10-mg vial (with diluent) = £6.86

PoM **Velbe**® (Lilly)
Injection, powder for reconstitution, vinblastine sulphate. Net price 10-mg amp (with diluent) = £10.29

VINCRISTINE SULPHATE

Indications: see notes above
Cautions; Side-effects: see section 8.1 and notes above; caution in handling—avoid contact with eyes; irritant to tissues

PoM **Vincristine Injection,** powder for reconstitution, vincristine sulphate (with lactose). Net price, 1-mg vial = £3.42; 2-mg vial = £6.86; 5-mg vial = £17.14 (all with diluent)

PoM **Oncovin**® (Lilly)
Injection, powder for reconstitution, vincristine sulphate (with lactose). Net price 1-mg vial = £9.36; 2-mg vial = £18.54; 5-mg vial = £46.38 (all with diluent)
Injection, vincristine sulphate 1 mg/ml, net price 1-ml vial = £10.31; 2-ml vial = £20.40 (both with mannitol 100 mg/ml)

VINDESINE SULPHATE

Indications: see notes above
Cautions; Side-effects: see section 8.1 and notes above; caution in handling—avoid contact with eyes; irritant to tissues

PoM **Eldisine**® (Lilly)
Injection, powder for reconstitution, vindesine sulphate (with mannitol). Net price 5-mg vial (with diluent) = £51.77 (Hosp. only)

8.1.5 Other antineoplastic drugs

Amsacrine (Amsidine®) is a newly introduced drug with an action and toxic effects similar to those of doxorubicin. It is used as second-line treatment in refractory acute myeloid leukaemia. Side-effects include myelosuppression and mucositis; electrolytes should be monitored as fatal arrhythmias have occurred in association with hypokalaemia.

AMSACRINE

Indications: see notes above

Cautions; Side-effects: see section 8.1 and notes above; reduce dose in renal or hepatic impairment. Also caution in handling—irritant to skin and tissues

▼ PoM **Amsidine**® (P-D)

Concentrate for intravenous infusion, amsacrine 5 mg (as lactate)/ml, when reconstituted by mixing two solutions. Net price 1.5-ml amp with 13.5-ml vial = £30.90 (Hosp. only)

Note. Use glass infusion apparatus

Carboplatin (Paraplatin®) is a recently introduced derivative of cisplatin. Experience with this drug is still limited, but early studies suggest that it may be equipotent with cisplatin for patients with ovarian carcinoma. Nausea and vomiting are reduced in severity and nephrotoxicity, neurotoxicity, and ototoxicity are much less of a problem than with cisplatin. It is, however, more myelosuppressive than cisplatin, and for this reason should not be repeated at intervals of less than 4 weeks.

CARBOPLATIN

Indications: see notes above

Cautions; Side-effects: see section 8.1 and notes above; reduce dose in renal impairment

▼ PoM **Paraplatin**® (Bristol-Myers)

Injection, powder for reconstitution, carboplatin. Net price 150-mg vial = £68.57

Cisplatin has an alkylating action. It has useful antitumour activity in certain solid tumours including ovarian carcinoma and testicular teratoma. It is, however, a toxic drug. Common problems include severe nausea and vomiting, nephrotoxicity (pretreatment hydration recommended and the creatinine clearance should be closely monitored), myelotoxicity, ototoxicity (high tone hearing loss and tinnitus), peripheral neuropathy, and hypomagnesaemia. These toxic effects commonly necessitate dose reduction and/or drug withdrawal. It is preferable that treatment with this drug be supervised by specialists familiar with its use.

CISPLATIN

Indications: see notes above

Cautions; Side-effects: see section 8.1 and notes above; reduce dose in renal impairment. Drug interactions: see Appendix 1 (section 8)

PoM **Cisplatin** (Non-proprietary)

Injection, cisplatin 1 mg/ml. Net price 10-ml vial = £2.90; 50-ml vial = £14.00; 100-ml vial = £27.00

Injection, powder for reconstitution, cisplatin 10-mg vial, net price = £2.50; 50-mg vial = £12.10

PoM **Platosin**® (Nordic)

Injection, cisplatin 500 micrograms/ml. Net price 20-ml vial = £2.98; 100-ml vial = £12.70

Injection, powder for reconstitution, cisplatin. Net price 10-mg vial = £2.76; 25-mg vial = £6.90; 50-mg vial = £12.64

Crisantaspase is the enzyme asparaginase produced by *Erwinia chrysanthemi*. It is used almost exclusively in acute lymphoblastic leukaemia. Special precautions are necessary to reduce the risk of anaphylaxis, including skin testing (particularly if a treatment-free interval occurs); administration by the intramuscular route also minimises the risk. Other side-effects include metabolic abnormalities therefore careful monitoring is necessary and the urine is tested for glucose to exclude hyperglycaemia.

CRISANTASPASE

Indications; Cautions; Side-effects: see notes above

▼ PoM **Erwinase**® (Porton)

Injection, powder for reconstitution, crisantaspase. Net price 20 × 10000-unit vial = £460.00

Dacarbazine is not commonly used on account of its toxicity. It has been used to treat melanoma and, in combination therapy, the soft tissue sarcomas. It is also a component of a commonly used second-line combination for Hodgkin's disease (ABVD). The predominant side-effects are myelosuppression and intense nausea and vomiting.

DACARBAZINE

Indications: see notes above

Cautions; Side-effects: see section 8.1; also caution in handling—irritant to skin and tissues

PoM **DTIC-Dome** (Bayer)

Injection, powder for reconstitution, dacarbazine. Net price 100-mg vial = £4.83; 200-mg vial = £7.40

Hydroxyurea (Hydrea®) is an orally active drug used mainly in the treatment of chronic myeloid leukaemia. Myelosuppression, nausea, and skin reactions are the commonest toxic effects.

HYDROXYUREA

Indications: see notes above

Cautions; Side-effects: see section 8.1 and notes above

Dose: 20–30 mg/kg daily *or* 80 mg/kg every 3rd day

PoM **Hydrea**® (Squibb)

Capsules, pink/green, hydroxyurea 500 mg. Net price 20 = £2.39

Mitozantrone (Novantrone®) is structurally related to doxorubicin and preliminary work sug-

---

gests that it has equal activity in breast cancer; it is well tolerated apart from myelosuppression and probable dose-related cardiotoxicity.

MITOZANTRONE
Indications: see notes above
Cautions; Side-effects: see section 8.1 and notes above

▼ PoM **Novantrone®** (Lederle)
Intravenous infusion, mitozantrone 2 mg (as hydrochloride)/ml, with sodium chloride and acetate buffer. Net price 20-mg vial = £135.16; 25-mg vial = £168.95; 30-mg vial = £202.73

Procarbazine (Natulan®) is a first-line drug in Hodgkin's disease, for example in MOPP chemotherapy. It is also used to treat non-Hodgkin lymphomas and small cell carcinoma of the bronchus. It is given orally. Toxic effects include nausea, myelosuppression, and a hypersensitivity rash preventing further use of this drug. It is a mild monoamine-oxidase inhibitor and appropriate dietary advice is recommended (see section 4.3.2). Alcohol ingestion may cause a disulfiram-like reaction.

PROCARBAZINE
Indications: see notes above
Cautions; Side-effects: see section 8.1 and notes above; reduce dose in renal impairment. Drug interactions: see Appendix 1 (section 8)
Dose: initially 50 mg daily, gradually increased to 250–300 mg daily in divided doses

PoM **Natulan®** (Roche)
Capsules, ivory, procarbazine 50 mg (as hydrochloride). Net price 50-cap pack = £3.45. Label: 4

Razoxane (Razoxin®) has limited activity in the leukaemias, and is little used.

RAZOXANE
Indications: see notes above
Cautions; Side-effects: see section 8.1
Dose: 125 mg twice daily, with radiotherapy

▼ PoM **Razoxin®** (ICI)
Tablets, scored, razoxane 125 mg. Net price 20 = £16.33

8.2   Drugs affecting the immune response

8.2.1 Cytotoxic immunosuppressants
8.2.2 Corticosteroids and other immuno-
       suppressants
8.2.3 Immunostimulants
8.2.4 Interferons

8.2.1   Cytotoxic immunosuppressants

These drugs are used to suppress rejection in organ transplant recipients and are also used to treat a variety of auto-immune and collagen diseases (see section 10.1.3). They are non-specific in their action and careful monitoring of peripheral blood counts is required, with dose adjustments for marrow toxicity. Patients receiving these drugs will be prone to atypical infections, e.g. fungal infections.

Azathioprine (Imuran® etc.) is widely used for transplant recipients and is also used to treat a number of auto-immune conditions, usually when corticosteroid therapy alone has provided inadequate control. This drug is metabolised to mercaptopurine, and doses should be reduced when concurrent therapy with allopurinol is given. The predominant toxic effect is myelosuppression, although hepatic toxicity is also well recognised.

Cyclophosphamide and chlorambucil (section 8.1.1) are less commonly prescribed as immunosuppressants.

AZATHIOPRINE
Indications: see notes above
Cautions; Side-effects: see section 8.1 and notes above; also rashes. Reduce dose in severe renal impairment. Drug interactions: see Appendix 1 (section 8)
Dose: by mouth, 2–2.5 mg/kg daily.
  Chronic active hepatitis, 1–1.5 mg/kg daily
  Suppression of transplant rejection, consult specialist literature

PoM **Azamune®** (Penn)
Tablets, yellow, scored, azathioprine 50 mg. Net price 20 = £5.70
PoM **Berkaprine®** (Berk)
Tablets, yellow, scored, azathioprine 50 mg. Net price 20 = £7.02
PoM **Imuran®** (Wellcome)
Tablets, both f/c, azathioprine 25 mg (orange), net price 20 = £6.25; 50 mg (yellow), 20 = £10.42
Injection, powder for reconstitution, azathioprine (as sodium salt). Net price 50-mg vial = £13.13

8.2.2   Corticosteroids and other immunosuppressants

Prednisone and prednisolone are widely used in oncology. They have marked antitumour effect in acute lymphoblastic leukaemia, Hodgkin's disease, and the non-Hodgkin lymphomas. They are also active in hormone-sensitive breast cancer and may cause useful disease regression. Finally, they have a role in the palliation of symptomatic end-stage malignant disease when they may produce a sense of well-being.

The corticosteroids are also powerful immunosuppressants. They are used to prevent organ transplant rejection, and in high dose to treat rejection episodes. For notes on corticosteroids see section 6.3.

Antilymphocyte immunoglobulin (Pressimmune®) is obtained from immunised horses. It has mainly been used to prevent transplant rejection.

Cyclosporin (Sandimmun®) is a fungal metabolite and potent immunosuppressant which is virtually non-myelotoxic but markedly nephrotoxic. It has found particular use in the field of organ and tissue transplantation, for prevention of graft rejection following bone marrow, kidney, liver, pancreas, heart, and heart-lung transplantation, and for prophylaxis of graft-versus-host disease.

ANTILYMPHOCYTE IMMUNOGLOBULIN

Indications: see notes above
Cautions: test for hypersensitivity; acute infections
Side-effects: fever, shivering, nausea, hypotension, tachycardia; also anaphylactic reactions, urticaria, pruritus

PoM **Pressimmune**® (Hoechst)
Injection, antilymphocyte immunoglobulin (horse) 50 mg/ml. Net price 10-ml amp = £53.59 (Hosp. only)

CYCLOSPORIN

Indications: see notes above
Cautions: monitor liver and kidney function; avoid other immunosuppressants (except corticosteroids); over-suppression may increase susceptibility to infection and lymphoma; avoid during pregnancy, breast-feeding, or with systemic nephrotoxic antibiotics. Drug interactions: see Appendix 1 (section 8)
Side-effects: impairment of liver and renal function; tremor, gastro-intestinal disturbances, hypertrichosis; gum hyperplasia; hyperkalaemia; *occasionally* facial oedema, hypertension, fluid retention, and convulsions; serum creatinine, urea, bilirubin, and liver enzymes may be increased; burning sensation in hands and feet during first week of oral administration

▼ PoM **Sandimmun**® (Sandoz)
Oral solution, oily, yellow, sugar-free, cyclosporin 100 mg/ml. Net price 50 ml = £110.15
Concentrate for intravenous infusion (oily), cyclosporin 50 mg/ml. To be diluted before use. Net price 1-ml amp = £1.70; 5-ml amp = £8.09
Note. Contains polyethoxylated castor oil which has been associated with anaphylaxis

8.2.3   Immunostimulants

A suspension of inactivated *Corynebacterium parvum* organisms may be used by the intracavitary route to treat malignant effusions. Pyrexia is a common side-effect. Treatment should be avoided within 10 days of thoracotomy.

CORYNEBACTERIUM PARVUM VACCINE

Indications: see notes above
Side-effects: pyrexia, abdominal pain, nausea and vomiting

PoM **Coparvax**® (Calmic)
Injection, powder for reconstitution, *Corynebacterium parvum* (inactivated). Net price 7-mg vial = £43.56

8.2.4   Interferons

The interferons (alfa, beta, and gamma) are naturally occurring proteins with complex effects on immunity and cell function. Recently alfa interferon (formerly called lymphoblastoid interferon) has shown some antitumour effect in certain lymphomas and solid tumours. Side-effects are dose-related, but commonly include influenza-like symptoms, lethargy, and depression. Myelosuppression may also occur, particularly affecting granulocyte counts. Finally, cardiovascular problems (hypotension, hypertension, and arrhythmias) have been reported.
Drug interactions: see Appendix 1 (section 3).

▼ PoM **Intron A**® (Kirby-Warrick)
Injection, powder for reconstitution, interferon alfa-2b (rbe). Net price 3-million unit vial = £18.11; 5-million unit vial = £29.77; 10-million unit vial = £58.73; 30-million unit vial = £171.30
For use in AIDS-related Kaposi's sarcoma, hairy cell leukaemia, chronic myelogenous leukaemia, condyloma acuminata

▼ PoM **Roferon-A**® (Roche)
Injection, powder for reconstitution, interferon alfa-2a (rbe). Net price 3 million-unit vial = £16.96; 9 million-unit vial = £50.88; 18 million-unit vial = £101.77
For use in AIDS-related Kaposi's sarcoma and hairy cell leukaemia

▼ PoM **Wellferon**® (Wellcome)
Injection, interferon alfa-N1 (lns) 3 million units/ml, net price 1-ml vial = £18.20; 10 million units/ml, net price 1-ml vial = £58.95
For hairy cell leukaemia

8.3   Sex hormones and antagonists in malignant disease

8.3.1 Oestrogens
8.3.2 Progestogens
8.3.3 Androgens and anabolic steroids
8.3.4 Hormone antagonists

Hormonal manipulation has an important role in the treatment of metastatic breast, prostate, and endometrial cancer, and a more marginal role in the treatment of hypernephroma. These treatments are not curative, but may provide excellent palliation of symptoms in selected patients, sometimes for a period of years. Tumour response, and treatment toxicity should be carefully monitored and treatment changed if progression occurs or side-effects exceed benefit. More recently adjuvant hormonal treatment using tamoxifen has been used after treatment of the primary in postmenopausal patients with high-risk breast cancer.

Such treatment has consistently prolonged the period between diagnosis and the development of metastases; an effect on overall survival has not however been fully proven.

Overall, approximately 30% of patients with metastatic breast cancer respond to tamoxifen. This figure is increased to 60% in patients with oestrogen receptor positive tumours; receptor negative tumours responding in less than 10%. Tamoxifen is equivalent in effect to oophorectomy in pre-menopausal patients and it is so well tolerated that it is probably the treatment of choice in suitable patients of all ages. Whilst oophorectomy still has a therapeutic role, adrenalectomy has largely been replaced by aminoglutethimide, given together with prednisolone. Hypophysectomy is rarely used.

Patients with non-threatening metastases unresponsive to tamoxifen may still respond to a secondary hormonal treatment. Certainly, patients who initially respond to tamoxifen should receive second-line hormone treatment. No clear guidelines are available; for pre-menopausal patients oophorectomy or a progestogen may be used; for post-menopausal patients a progestogen or aminoglutethimide with corticosteroid cover may be used. Responding patients can receive further hormones at relapse, refractory patients are better treated with chemotherapy or palliative therapy.

Metastatic carcinoma of the prostate is commonly responsive to hormonal treatment designed to deprive the cancer of androgen. Treatment is probably best reserved for patients with symptomatic metastatic disease. The most simple treatment is bilateral subcapsular orchidectomy, which commonly results in responses lasting 12–18 months. Alternatively, a gonadotrophin-releasing hormone analogue (e.g. buserelin) may be given; these require parenteral administration, at least initially, and are expensive. Stilboestrol is still used; the dose should be restricted to 1–3 mg daily by mouth as higher doses are associated with unacceptable cardiovascular morbidity. Cyproterone may also be used, but it is very expensive. Second-line treatment may palliate symptoms, but rarely results in appreciable disease regression. Alternatives after orchidectomy include cyproterone or aminoglutethimide with prednisolone.

8.3.1   Oestrogens

Stilboestrol may be used in low dosage to treat symptomatic metastases from prostate cancer. It is now less commonly used in postmenopausal women with breast cancer. Toxicity is common and dose-related side-effects include nausea, fluid retention, and venous and arterial thrombosis. Impotence and gynaecomastia always occur in men, and withdrawal bleeding may be a problem in women. Hypercalcaemia and bone pain may also occur in breast cancer.

Fosfestrol (Honvan®) is activated by the enzyme acid phosphatase to produce stilboestrol. Side-effects are as for stilboestrol and, in addition,

perineal pain may complicate intravenous use in prostate cancer.

Ethinyloestradiol is the most potent oestrogen available. Unlike other oestrogens it is not metabolised in the liver. It is used in breast cancer and may be better tolerated than stilboestrol in patients suffering from nausea.

Polyestradiol (Estradurin®) is a long-acting oestrogen preparation.

ETHINYLOESTRADIOL
Indications: see notes above
Cautions; Contra-indications; Side-effects: see section 6.4.1.1 and notes above
Dose: 1–3 mg daily

Preparations
See section 6.4.1.1

FOSFESTROL TETRASODIUM
Indications: see notes above
Cautions; Contra-indications; Side-effects: see under Ethinyloestradiol (section 6.4.1.1) and notes above
Dose: by mouth, 100–200 mg 3 times daily, reducing to 100–300 mg daily
By slow intravenous injection, 552–1104 mg daily for at least 5 days; maintenance 276 mg 1–4 times weekly

PoM **Honvan**® (Boehringer Ingelheim)
Tablets, fosfestrol tetrasodium 100 mg. Net price 20 = £1.87
Injection, fosfestrol tetrasodium 55.2 mg/ml. Net price 5-ml amp = 92p

POLYESTRADIOL PHOSPHATE
Indications: prostatic carcinoma
Cautions; Contra-indications; Side-effects: see under Ethinyloestradiol (section 6.4.1.1) and notes above
Dose: by deep intramuscular injection, 80–160 mg every 4 weeks; maintenance 40–80 mg

PoM **Estradurin**® (Lundbeck)
Injection, powder for reconstitution, polyestradiol phosphate (with mepivacaine and nicotinamide). Net price 40-mg vial = £2.18; 80-mg vial = £3.51 (both with diluent)

STILBOESTROL
Indications: see notes above
Cautions; Contra-indications; Side-effects: see under Ethinyloestradiol (section 6.4.1.1) and notes above
Dose: breast cancer, 10–20 mg daily
Prostatic cancer, 1–3 mg daily

PoM **Stilboestrol Tablets,** stilboestrol 1 mg, net price 20 = 58p; 5 mg, 20 = 98p

8.3.2   Progestogens

These drugs are used largely as second- or third-line therapy in breast cancer. They are also used to treat endometrial carcinoma and hypernephroma.

Medroxyprogesterone or **megestrol** are usually used and can be given orally. High-dose or parenteral treatment cannot be recommended. Side-effects are mild but may include nausea, fluid retention, and weight gain.

GESTRONOL HEXANOATE

Indications: see notes above

Cautions; Contra-indications; Side-effects: see under Progesterone (section 6.4.1.2) and notes above

Dose: by intramuscular injection, 200–400 mg every 5–7 days

PoM **Depostat**® (Schering)

Injection (oily), gestronol hexanoate 100 mg/ml. Net price 2-ml amp = £4.28

MEDROXYPROGESTERONE ACETATE

Indications: see notes above

Cautions; Contra-indications; Side-effects: see under Progesterone (section 6.4.1.2) and notes above

Dose: by mouth, endometrial, prostatic, and renal cancer, 100–500 mg daily; breast cancer, various doses in range 0.4–1.5 g daily

By deep intramuscular injection, various doses in range 1 g daily down to 250 mg weekly

▼ PoM **Depo-Provera**® (Upjohn)

Injection, medroxyprogesterone acetate 150 mg/ml. Net price 3-ml vial = £11.35

PoM **Farlutal**® (Farmitalia Carlo Erba)

Tablets, both scored, medroxyprogesterone acetate 100 mg, net price 20 = £6.80; 250 mg, 20 = £16.00

Tablets, scored, medroxyprogesterone acetate 500 mg. Net price 20 = £31.34. Label: 27

Injection, medroxyprogesterone acetate 200 mg/ml. Net price 2.5-ml vial = £12.00; 5-ml vial = £20.00

PoM **Provera**® (Upjohn)

Tablets, medroxyprogesterone acetate 100 mg (scored), net price 20 = £8.32; 200 mg (scored), 20 = £16.47; 400 mg, 20 = £32.59

Suspension, sugar-free, medroxyprogesterone 400 mg/5 ml. Diluent purified water, freshly boiled and cooled, life of diluted suspension 28 days. Net price 100 ml = £32.59

MEGESTROL ACETATE

Indications: see notes above

Cautions; Contra-indications; Side-effects: see under Progesterone (section 6.4.1.2) and notes above

Dose: breast cancer, 160 mg daily in single or divided doses; endometrial cancer, 40–320 mg daily in divided doses

PoM **Megace**® (Bristol-Myers)

Tablets, both scored, megestrol acetate 40 mg, net price 20 = £4.98; 160 mg (off-white), 20 = £19.53

NORETHISTERONE

Indications: see notes above

Cautions; Contra-indications; Side-effects: see section 6.4.1.2 and notes above

Dose: 40 mg daily, increased to 60 mg daily if required

Preparations

See section 6.4.1.2

NORETHISTERONE ACETATE

Indications: see notes above

Cautions; Contra-indications; Side-effects: see section 6.4.1.2 and notes above

Dose: 10 mg 3 times daily, increased to 60 mg daily if required

PoM **SH 420**® (Schering)

Tablets, scored, norethisterone acetate 10 mg. Net price 20 = £4.95

8.3.3   Androgens and anabolic steroids

The androgens are given parenterally and are predominantly used as second- or third-line therapy for metastatic breast cancer.

DROSTANOLONE PROPIONATE

Indications: see notes above

Cautions; Contra-indications; Side-effects: see under Nandrolone (section 6.4.3) and notes above

Dose: by intramuscular injection, 300 mg weekly

PoM **Masteril**® (Syntex)

Injection (oily), drostanolone propionate 100 mg/ml. Net price 1-ml amp = £1.95

NANDROLONE

Indications: see notes above

Cautions; Contra-indications; Side-effects: see section 6.4.3 and notes above

Dose: by deep intramuscular injection, breast cancer, nandrolone decanoate 50 mg every 2–3 weeks; nandrolone phenylpropionate 50 mg weekly

Preparations

See section 6.4.3

8.3.4   Hormone antagonists

Tamoxifen acts as an oestrogen antagonist and blocks receptor sites in target organs. This drug, at a dose of 20 mg daily, is the hormonal treatment of choice for breast cancer in postmenopausal women with metastatic disease and is also increasingly commonly used as a first-line treatment for premenopausal women. Side-effects are unusual, but patients with bony metastases may experience an exacerbation of their pain, sometimes associated with hypercalcaemia. This reaction commonly precedes tumour response. Amenorrhoea commonly develops in premenopausal women.

Aminoglutethimide (Orimeten®) is used in postmenopausal women with breast cancer. It acts predominantly by inhibiting the conversion of androgens to oestrogens in the peripheral tissues. Corticosteroid replacement therapy is necessary (see section 6.3.1). Early toxicity is common and may include drowsiness, drug fever, and a morbilliform eruption. These side-effects generally settle spontaneously. The dose is usually increased gradually over 2 to 4 weeks. Present research suggests that this drug may be effective in rather lower dosage than currently recommended. Hepatic enzyme induction occurs, and may require modification of the doses of other drugs, e.g. oral anticoagulants and oral hypoglycaemic drugs.

Cyproterone acetate (Cyprostat®) is an antiandrogen used as a second-line therapy for metastatic prostate cancer.

Buserelin (Suprefact®) is a gonadotrophin-releasing hormone analogue which is used to treat metastatic prostate cancer. It causes an initial stimulation of luteinising hormone (LH) release by the pituitary, which in turn causes testosterone secretion by the testis; subsequently inhibition of LH release occurs, with achievement of an anorchic state.

Drugs of this type are as effective as orchidectomy or stilboestrol. Buserelin requires parenteral administration initially, then intranasal administration. During the first 1 to 2 weeks of treatment increased tumour growth may occur causing, for example, spinal cord compression. When such problems are anticipated alternative treatments (e.g. orchidectomy) or simultaneous use of an anti-androgen (e.g. cyproterone) are recommended. Other side-effects are similar to those of orchidectomy.

AMINOGLUTETHIMIDE

Indications: metastatic mammary carcinoma in postmenopausal or oophorectomised women; advanced carcinoma of prostate; Cushing's syndrome due to malignant disease
Cautions; Side-effects: see notes above. Drug interactions: see Appendix 1 (sections *2.8A*, *6.3*)
Dose: 250 mg daily for 1 week, increased once a week to 250 mg 4 times daily; given with a glucocorticoid (see notes above)

▼ PoM **Orimeten**® (Ciba)
Tablets, scored, aminoglutethimide 250 mg. Net price 20 = £6.57

BUSERELIN

Indications; Side-effects: see notes above
Dose: see below

▼ PoM **Suprefact**® (Hoechst)
Injection, buserelin 1 mg (as acetate)/ml. Net price treatment pack of 2 × 5.5-ml vial = £30.37
Dose: by subcutaneous injection, 500 micrograms every 8 hours for 7 days
Nasal spray, buserelin 100 micrograms (as acetate)/metered spray. Net price treatment pack of 4 × 10-g bottle with spray pump = £99.92
Dose: apply 1 spray into each nostril 6 times daily

CYPROTERONE ACETATE

Indications: see notes above
Cautions: hepatic disease; risk of recurrence of thrombo-embolic disease; severe depression; see also section 6.4.2
Contra-indications: none in prostate cancer; for contra-indications relating to other indications see section 6.4.2
Side-effects: see section 6.4.2
Dose: 300 mg daily in 2–3 divided doses after food

PoM **Cyprostat**® (Schering)
Tablets, scored, cyproterone acetate 50 mg. Net price 20 = £12.64. Label: 3, 21

GOSERELIN

Indications: prostate cancer
Cautions: during first month monitor patients at risk of ureteric obstruction or spinal cord compression, see notes above
Side-effects: initial increase in bone pain (due to transient increases in plasma testosterone); hot flushes, decreased libido, rashes (reversible without stopping therapy), infrequent gynaecomastia; bruising at injection site
Dose: see below

▼ PoM **Zoladex**® (ICI)
Implant, goserelin 3.6 mg (as acetate) in syringe applicator. Net price each = £114.00
Dose: by subcutaneous injection into anterior abdominal wall, 3.6 mg every 28 days (local anaesthetic if desired)

TAMOXIFEN

Indications: see notes above
Cautions: drug interactions: see Appendix 1 (section *2.8B*)
Contra-indications: pregnancy
Side-effects: hot flushes, vaginal bleeding, gastrointestinal disturbances, dizziness; rarely fluid retention, visual disturbances; see also notes
Dose: breast cancer, initially 20–40 mg daily

PoM **Tamoxifen Tablets,** tamoxifen (as citrate) 10 mg, net price 20 = £4.20; 20 mg, 20 = £6.40
PoM **Noltam**® (Lederle)
Tablets, both f/c, tamoxifen (as citrate) 10 mg, net price 20 = £4.13; 20 mg, 20 = £6.23
PoM **Nolvadex**® (ICI)
Tablets, tamoxifen 10 mg (as citrate). Net price 20 = £4.13
PoM **Nolvadex-D**® (ICI)
Tablets, tamoxifen 20 mg (as citrate). Net price 20 = £6.22
PoM **Nolvadex-Forte**® (ICI)
Tablets, scored, tamoxifen 40 mg (as citrate). Net price 20 = £14.67
PoM **Tamofen**® (Tillotts)
Tablets, off-white, scored, tamoxifen 10 mg (as citrate). Net price 20 = £4.13
PoM **Tamofen-20**® (Tillotts)
Tablets, off-white, tamoxifen 20 mg (as citrate). Net price 20 = £6.23
PoM **Tamofen-40**® (Tillotts)
Tablets, off-white, tamoxifen 40 mg (as citrate). Net price 20 = £14.67

9: Drugs affecting
NUTRITION and BLOOD

In this chapter drugs and preparations are discussed under the follwoing headings:

9.1 Anaemias and some other blood disorders

Before initiating treatment it is essential to determine which type of anaemia is present. Iron salts may be harmful and result in iron overload if given alone to patients with anaemias other than those due to iron deficiency.

9.1.1 Iron-deficiency anaemias

The only justification for iron treatment is the presence of a demonstrable iron-deficiency state. Prophylaxis is justifiable in pregnancy, menorrhagia, after subtotal or total gastrectomy, and in the management of low birth-weight infants such as premature babies, twins, and infants delivered by Caesarean section.

9.1.1.1 ORAL IRON

Iron salts should be given by mouth unless there are good reasons for using another route.

Ferrous salts show only marginal differences in efficiency of absorption of iron, but ferric salts are much less well absorbed. Haemoglobin regeneration rate is little affected by the type of salt used provided sufficient iron is given, and in most patients the time factor is not critical. Choice of preparation is thus usually decided by incidence of side-effects and cost.

The oral dose of elemental iron should be 100 to 200 mg daily; it is customary to give this as dried **ferrous sulphate**, 200 mg three times daily. If side-effects arise, dosage can be reduced or a change made to an alternative iron salt. It should be remembered, however, that an apparent improvement in tolerance on changing to another salt may be due to its lower content of elemental iron. The incidence of side-effects due to ferrous sulphate is no greater than with other iron salts when compared on the basis of equivalent amounts of elemental iron.

The following table gives the iron content of the different salts available:

Table 1: Iron Salts

Iron salt	Amount	Content of ferrous iron
Ferrous fumarate	200 mg	65 mg
Ferrous gluconate	300 mg	35 mg
Ferrous glycine sulphate	225 mg	40 mg
Ferrous succinate	100 mg	35 mg
Ferrous sulphate	300 mg	60 mg
Ferrous sulphate, dried	200 mg	60 mg

THERAPEUTIC RESPONSE. The haemoglobin concentration should rise by about 100–200 mg per 100 ml (1–2 g per litre) per day. After the haemoglobin has risen to normal, treatment should be continued for a further three months in an attempt to replenish the iron stores. Epithelial tissue changes such as atrophic glossitis and koilonychia are usually improved although the response is often slow.

COMPOUND PREPARATIONS. Some oral preparations contain ascorbic acid to aid absorption, or the iron is in the form of a chelate, which can be shown experimentally to produce a modest increase in absorption of iron. However, the therapeutic advantage is minimal and cost may be increased.

There is neither theoretical nor clinical justification for the inclusion of other therapeutically active ingredients, such as the B group of vitamins (except folic acid for pregnant women, see Iron and Folic Acid below).

SLOW-RELEASE CAPSULES AND TABLETS. These are designed to release iron gradually as the capsule or tablet passes along the gut so that a smaller amount of iron is present in the lumen at any one time. It is claimed that each dose unit contains enough iron for 24 hours, thus permitting once daily dosage.

These preparations are likely to carry the iron past the first part of the duodenum into an area of the gut where conditions for iron absorption are poor. The low incidence of side-effects may well be because of the small amounts of iron available under these conditions and so the preparations have no therapeutic advantage and should not be used.

SIDE-EFFECTS. Because iron salts are astringent, gastro-intestinal irritation may occur. Nausea and epigastric pain are dose-related but the relationship between dose and altered bowel habit (constipation or diarrhoea) is less clear.

Iron preparations taken orally may have a constipating effect in older patients, occasionally leading to faecal impaction.

FERROUS SULPHATE

Indications: iron-deficiency anaemia

Cautions: drug interactions: see Appendix 1 (sections *5.1, 9, 9, 10*)

Side-effects: large doses may produce gastro-intestinal irritation, vomiting, diarrhoea; continued administration may result in constipation

Dose: ferrous iron, therapeutic, 120–180 mg daily in divided doses; prophylactic, 60 mg daily; CHILD, therapeutic, daily in divided doses, up to 1 year 36 mg, 1–5 years 72 mg, 6–12 years 120 mg

See also under Preparations

COUNSELLING. Although iron preparations are best absorbed on an empty stomach they may be taken after food to reduce gastro-intestinal side-effects

Ferrous Sulphate (Non-proprietary)

Tablets, f/c or s/c, dried ferrous sulphate 200 mg[1](60 mg iron), net price 20 = 7p

Dose: prophylactic, 1 tablet daily; therapeutic, 1 tablet 2–3 times daily

[1]Tablets containing 300 mg (90 mg iron) also available

Paediatric mixture, ferrous sulphate 60 mg (12 mg iron)/5 ml (see Formulary). Net price 100 ml = 9p. Label: 27

Dose: therapeutic, CHILD up to 1 year, 5 ml 3 times daily; 1–5 years, 10 ml 3 times daily; 6–12 years, 15 ml 3 times daily *or* 25 ml twice daily. To be taken well diluted with water

Sustained-release preparations

Feospan® (SK&F)

Spansule® (= capsules s/r), clear/red, enclosing green and red pellets, dried ferrous sulphate 150 mg (45 mg iron). Net price 30 = 90p. Label: 25

Dose: 1–2 capsules daily; CHILD over 1 year 1 capsule daily

Ferrograd® (Abbott)

Filmtabs® (= tablets f/c), s/r, red, dried ferrous sulphate 325 mg (105 mg iron). Net price 20 = 53p. Label: 25

Dose: 1 tablet daily before food

Slow-Fe® (Ciba)

Tablets, s/r, dried ferrous sulphate 160 mg (48 mg iron). Net price 20 = 31p. Label: 25

Dose: prophylactic, 1 tablet daily; therapeutic, 2 tablets daily; CHILD over 6 years, 1 tablet daily

FERROUS FUMARATE

Indications; Cautions; Side-effects: see under Ferrous Sulphate

Dose: see under preparations below

Fersaday® (DF)

Tablets, orange, f/c, ferrous fumarate 304 mg (100 mg iron). Net price 28 = 45p

Dose: prophylactic, 1 tablet daily; therapeutic, 1 tablet twice daily

Fersamal® (DF)

Tablets, brown, ferrous fumarate 200 mg (65 mg iron). Net price 20 = 14p

Dose: 1–2 tablets 3 times daily

Syrup, brown, ferrous fumarate 140 mg (45 mg iron)/5 ml. Diluent syrup, life of diluted preparation 14 days. Net price 200 ml = £1.47

Dose: 10–20 ml twice daily; PREMATURE INFANT 0.6–2.4 ml/kg daily; CHILD up to 6 years 2.5–5 ml twice daily

Galfer® (Galen)

Capsules, red/green, ferrous fumarate 290 mg (100 mg iron). Net price 20 = 50p

Dose: 1 capsule 1–2 times daily before food

Meterfer® (Sinclair)

Tablets, blue, f/c, ferrous fumarate equivalent to 100 mg iron. Net price 20 = 34p

Dose: 1 tablet 1–2 times daily with food

Sustained-release preparations

Ferrocap® (Consolidated)

Capsules, s/r, green/orange, enclosing brown and white granules, ferrous fumarate 330 mg (110 mg iron). Net price 20 = 48p. Label: 25

Dose: 1 capsule daily

FERROUS GLUCONATE

Indications; Cautions; Side-effects: see under Ferrous Sulphate

Dose: see under preparations below

Ferrous Gluconate (Non-proprietary)

Tablets, red, s/c, ferrous gluconate 300 mg (35 mg iron). Net price 20 = 12p

Dose: prophylactic, 2 tablets daily before food; therapeutic, 4–6 tablets daily in divided doses before food; CHILD 6–12 years, prophylactic and therapeutic, 1–3 tablets daily

Fergon® (Winthrop)

Tablets, red, s/c, ferrous gluconate 300 mg (35 mg iron). Net price 20 = 39p

Dose: see above

FERROUS GLYCINE SULPHATE

Indications; Cautions; Side-effects: see under Ferrous Sulphate

Dose: see under preparations below

Plesmet® (Napp)

Syrup, ferrous glycine sulphate 141 mg (25 mg iron)/5 ml. Diluent syrup, life of diluted preparation 14 days. Net price 100 ml = 67p

Dose: 5–10 ml 3 times daily; CHILD 2–5 ml 2–3 times daily

Sustained-release preparations

Ferrocontin Continus® (Degussa)

Tablets, s/r, red, f/c, ferrous glycine sulphate 562.5 mg (100 mg iron). Net price 20 = 32p. Label: 25

Dose: 1 tablet daily

FERROUS SUCCINATE

Indications; Cautions; Side-effects: see under Ferrous Sulphate

Dose: see under preparations below

Ferromyn® (Calmic)

Elixir, brown, ferrous succinate 106 mg (37 mg iron)/5 ml. Diluent syrup, life of diluted elixir 14 days. Net price 100 ml = £2.91

Dose: 5 ml 3 times daily; CHILD up to 2 years max. 1 ml twice daily, 2–5 years 2.5 ml 3 times daily, 5–10 years 5 ml twice daily

---

POLYSACCHARIDE-IRON COMPLEX

Indications; Cautions; Side-effects: see under Ferrous Sulphate

Dose: see under preparations below

Niferex® (Tillotts)

Tablets, brown, polysaccharide-iron complex equivalent to 50 mg of iron. Net price 20 = 53p
Dose: prophylactic, 1 tablet daily; therapeutic, 2 tablets 1–2 times daily
Elixir, brown, polysaccharide-iron complex equivalent to 100 mg of iron/5 ml. Diluent water for preparations or sorbitol solution, life of diluted elixir 14 days. Net price 100 ml = £1.83; 30-ml dropper bottle for paediatric use = £1.56. Counselling advised, use of dropper
Dose: prophylactic, 2.5 ml daily; therapeutic, 5 ml daily; INFANT, 1 drop (from dropper bottle) per pound body-weight 3 times daily; CHILD 2–6 years, 2.5 ml daily, 6–12 years 5 ml daily

Niferex-150® (Tillotts)

Capsules, brown/orange, polysaccharide-iron complex equivalent to 150 mg of iron. Net price 20 = £1.80
Dose: 1–2 capsules daily

SODIUM IRONEDETATE

Indications; Cautions; Side-effects: see under Ferrous Sulphate

Dose: see under preparations below

Sytron® (P-D)

Elixir, sugar-free, sodium ironedetate 190 mg equivalent to 27.5 mg of iron/5 ml. Diluent water for preparations, life of diluted elixir 14 days. Net price 100 ml = 28p
Dose: 5 ml increasing gradually to 10 ml 3 times daily; INFANT and PREMATURE INFANT 2.5 ml twice daily following smaller initial doses; CHILD 1–5 years 2.5 ml 3 times daily, 6–12 years 5 ml 3 times daily

IRON AND FOLIC ACID

These preparations are used for the prevention of iron and folic acid deficiences in pregnancy. The prophylactic dose in pregnancy is the equivalent of approximately 100 mg of iron with folic acid 200–500 micrograms daily.

It is important to note that the small doses of folic acid contained in these preparations are inadequate for the treatment of megaloblastic anaemias.

Fefol® (SK&F)

Spansule® (= capsules s/r), clear/green, enclosing red, yellow, and white pellets, dried ferrous sulphate 150 mg (47 mg iron), folic acid 500 micrograms. Net price 30 = 90p. Label: 25
Dose: 1 capsule daily

PoM **Ferfolic SV®** (Sinclair)

Tablets, pink, s/c, ferrous gluconate 250 mg (30 mg iron), folic acid 5 mg. Net price 20 = 48p
Dose: 1 tablet 3 times daily

Ferrocap-F 350® (Consolidated)

Capsules, s/r, pink, enclosing brown, white, and yellow granules, ferrous fumarate 330 mg (110 mg iron), folic acid 350 micrograms. Net price 20 = 59p. Label: 25
Dose: 1 capsule daily

Ferrocontin Folic Continus® (Degussa)

Tablets, orange, f/c, ferrous glycine sulphate 562.5 mg (100 mg iron) for sustained release, folic acid 500 micrograms. Net price 20 = 32p. Label: 25
Dose: 1 tablet daily

Ferrograd Folic® (Abbott)

Filmtabs® (= tablets f/c), red/yellow, dried ferrous sulphate 325 mg (105 mg iron) for sustained release, folic acid 350 micrograms. Net price 20 = 54p. Label: 25
Dose: 1 tablet daily before food

Folex-350® (Rybar)

Tablets, pink, s/c, ferrous fumarate 308 mg (100 mg iron), folic acid 350 micrograms. Net price 20 = 36p
Dose: 1 tablet daily

Galfer FA® (Galen)

Capsules, red/yellow, ferrous fumarate 290 mg (100 mg iron), folic acid 350 micrograms. Net price 20 = 51p
Dose: 1 capsule daily before food

Lexpec with Iron-M® (RP Drugs)

Syrup, brown, sugar-free, ferric ammonium citrate equivalent to 80 mg iron, folic acid 500 micrograms/5 ml. Net price 125 ml = £3.50
Dose: 5–10 ml daily before food
Note. Lexpec with Iron-M® contains five times less folic acid than Lexpec with Iron®; it contains approximately the same proportion of folic acid as other iron and folic acid preparations in this list

PoM **Lexpec with Iron®** (RP Drugs)

Syrup, brown, sugar-free, ferric ammonium citrate equivalent to 80 mg iron, folic acid 2.5 mg/5 ml. Net price 125 ml = £3.70
Dose: see above
Note. Lexpec with Iron® contains five times as much folic acid as Lexpec with Iron-M®, and at least five times as much as other iron and folic acid preparations in this list

Meterfolic® (Sinclair)

Tablets, grey, f/c, ferrous fumarate equivalent to 100 mg iron, folic acid 350 micrograms. Net price 20 = 37p
Dose: 1 tablet 1–2 times daily

Pregaday® (DF)

Tablets, brown, f/c, ferrous fumarate 304 mg (100 mg iron), folic acid 350 micrograms. Net price 28 = 51p
Dose: 1 tablet 1–2 times daily

Pregnavite Forte F, see compound iron preparations

Slow-Fe Folic® (Ciba)

Tablets, s/r, ivory, f/c, dried ferrous sulphate 160 mg (50 mg iron), folic acid 400 micrograms. Net price 30-tab pack = 46p. Label: 25
Dose: 1–2 tablets daily

COMPOUND IRON PREPARATIONS

These preparations contain an iron salt and, usually, one or more vitamins or small amounts of substances intended to provide a 'mineral supplement'.

There is no justification for prescribing compound iron preparations, except for preparations of iron and folic acid for prophylactic use in pregnancy (see above).

Ferrous Sulphate Tablets, Compound, green, s/c, dried ferrous sulphate equivalent to 170 mg of $FeSO_4$, copper

sulphate 2.5 mg, manganese sulphate 2.5 mg. Net price
20 tabs = 9p
Dose: 1–2 tablets daily

NHS BC 500 with Iron® (Wyeth)
Tablets, red, f/c, ferrous fumarate 200 mg (65 mg iron)
with vitamins B group and C. Net price 20 = 94p
Dose: 1 tablet daily

NHS Fefol-Vit® (SK&F)
Spansule® (= capsules s/r), clear/white, enclosing red,
orange, yellow, and white pellets, dried ferrous sulphate
150 mg (47 mg iron) with vitamins B group and C. Net
price 20 = 83p. Label: 25
Dose: 1 capsule daily during pregnancy

Fefol Z® (SK&F)
Spansule® (= capsules s/r), blue/clear, enclosing red,
yellow, and white pellets, dried ferrous sulphate
150 mg (47 mg iron), folic acid 500 micrograms, zinc
sulphate monohydrate 61.8 mg (22.5 mg zinc). Net price
20 = £1.19. Label: 25
Dose: 1 capsule daily during pregnancy

Feospan Z® (SK&F)
Product discontinued

NHS Ferrograd C® (Abbott)
Filmtabs® (= tablets f/c), red, dried ferrous sulphate
325 mg (105 mg iron) for sustained release, ascorbic acid
500 mg (as sodium salt). Net price 20 = 71p. Label: 25
Dose: 1 tablet daily before food

NHS Fesovit® (SK&F)
Spansule® (= capsules s/r), colourless/yellow, enclosing
red, orange, and white pellets, dried ferrous sulphate
150 mg (47 mg iron) with vitamins B group and C. Net
price 20 = 57p. Label: 25
Dose: 1–2 capsules daily; CHILD over 1 year 1 capsule
daily

NHS Fesovit Z® (SK&F)
Spansule® (= capsules s/r), orange/clear, enclosing red,
orange, and white pellets, dried ferrous sulphate 150 mg
(47 mg iron), zinc sulphate monohydrate 61.8 mg
(22.5 mg zinc) with vitamins B group and C. Net price
20 = £1.25. Label: 25
Dose: 1–2 capsules daily; CHILD over 1 year 1 capsule
daily

PoM Folicin® (Paines & Byrne)
Tablets, s/c, dried ferrous sulphate 200 mg (60 mg iron),
folic acid 2.5 mg with minerals. Net price 20 = 18p
Dose: 1–2 tablets daily during pregnancy

NHS Forceval® (Unigreg)
Capsules, ferrous fumarate 30.8 mg (10 mg iron) with
vitamins A, B group, C, D, E, and minerals. Net price
20 = £1.80
Dose: 1 capsule daily
Junior capsules, red, ferrous fumarate 15.4 mg (5 mg
iron) with vitamins A, B group, C, D, E, and minerals.
Net price 30 = £2.31
Dose: CHILD over 5 years, 1 capsule daily

NHS Galfer-Vit® (Galen)
Capsules, maroon/orange, ferrous fumarate 305 mg
(100 mg iron) with vitamins B group and C. Net price
20 = 58p
Dose: 1 capsule 1–2 times daily before food

NHS Gevral® (Lederle)
Capsules, brown, ferrous fumarate 30.8 mg (10 mg iron)
with vitamins A, B group, C, D, E, and minerals. Net
price 30 = £1.78
Dose: adults and children, 1 capsule daily after food

NHS Givitol® (Galen)
Capsules, red/maroon, ferrous fumarate 305 mg (100 mg
iron) with vitamins B group and C. Net price 20 = 82p
Dose: 1 capsule daily before food

NHS Glykola® (Sinclair)
Elixir, red, ferric chloride solution 0.01 ml (500 micrograms iron), caffeine 20 mg, calcium glycerophosphate
30 mg, kola liquid extract 0.12 ml/5 ml. Net price
100 ml = 61p
Dose: 5–10 ml 3 times daily after food

NHS Irofol C® (Abbott)
Filmtabs® (= tablets, f/c), red, dried ferrous sulphate
325 mg (105 mg iron) for sustained release, folic acid
350 micrograms, ascorbic acid 500 mg (as sodium salt).
Net price 20 = 59p. Label: 25
Dose: 1 tablet daily before food during pregnancy

NHS Octovit® (SK&F)
Tablets, maroon, f/c, dried ferrous sulphate (10 mg iron)
with vitamins A, B group, C, D, E, and minerals. Net
price 14 tabs = £1.56
Dose: 1 tablet daily

NHS *Pregnavite Forte F® (Bencard)
Tablets, lilac, s/c, dried ferrous sulphate 84 mg (25.2 mg
iron), folic acid 120 micrograms, vitamin A 1333 units,
thiamine hydrochloride 500 micrograms, riboflavine 500
micrograms, nicotinamide 5 mg, pyridoxine hydrochloride 330 micrograms, ascorbic acid 13.3 mg, vitamin
D 133 units, calcium phosphate 160 mg. Net price 84-
tab pack = £1.96
* except to reduce the risk of spina bifida or anencephaly
in babies born to women who have previously given
birth to one or more babies (or aborted a fetus) with a
neural tube defect and endorsed 'S3B' ('S2B' in
Scotland)
Dose: 1 tablet 3 times daily during or after food
Note. For prophylaxis of neural tube defects in pregnancy, dosage should be started not less than 28 days
prior to conception and continue uninterrupted at least
until the date of the second missed period

NHS Tonivitan A & D® (Medo)
Syrup, green, ferric ammonium citrate 150 mg (22 mg
iron) with vitamins A, D, and minerals. Net price
125 ml = 55p
Dose: 10 ml 3 times daily; CHILD under 1 year, 2.5 ml 3
times daily, 1–10 years, 5 ml, 10–12 years, 10 ml

9.1.1.2 PARENTERAL IRON

The only valid reason for administering iron preparations parenterally is failure of oral therapy.
Such failure may be due to lack of patient co-
operation with oral treatment, gastro-intestinal
side-effects, continuing severe blood loss or
malabsorption. Provided that the oral iron preparation is taken reliably and is absorbed, then with
equivalent doses of iron the rate of haemoglobin
response is not significantly faster when the intramuscular or intravenous instead of the oral route
is used. The need for a rapid cure of the anaemia is
therefore not met by intramuscular administration
of iron.

It is customary to give a course of deep *intramuscular* injections lasting about 10 days. The
manufacturer's dosage schedules should be consulted; these usually include a supplement for
reconstitution of iron stores.

Iron dextran (Imferon®) may also be administered as a single dose by slow intravenous infusion over 6 to 8 hours provided that there is no
reaction to administration of a test dose. Although
the incidence of side-effects is low, disquieting
adverse reactions may occur, especially in allergic
subjects, and intravenous infusion is contra-indicated in asthmatic patients. Iron dextran should

only be administered *intravenously* in selected cases where proper indications exist for its use, that is, when continuing blood loss is likely to be permanent and oral prophylaxis cannot keep pace, when a patient requiring parenteral iron has a small muscle mass or a haemostatic defect contra-indicating intramuscular injection, or when psychological or social pressures make iron treatment by other means impracticable.

Preparations suitable for parenteral use contain iron either in the form of **Iron Dextran Injection**, containing a complex of ferric hydroxide with dextrans of high molecular weight, or as **Iron Sorbitol Injection** (Jectofer®), containing a complex of iron, sorbitol and citric acid. The latter preparation is **not** suitable for intravenous injection and, although the low mean molecular weight allows rapid absorption from the injection site, excretion in the saliva and substantial urinary losses from each dose also occur.

To prevent leakage along the needle track with subsequent staining of the skin, intramuscular injections should be deep for both preparations.

IRON DEXTRAN INJECTION

Contains 5% (50 mg/ml) of iron
Indications: iron deficiency anaemia (see notes above)
Cautions: risk of anaphylaxis especially in patients with history of allergy; test dose essential when given by intravenous infusion; patient should be under observation for entire period of infusion and 1 hour after; adrenaline, chlorpheniramine, and hydrocortisone should be available to control allergic reactions (see section 3.4.3)
Contra-indications: severe liver disease, acute kidney infections; intravenous infusion in asthmatic patients
Side-effects: staining of the skin if leakage along needle track occurs, transient nausea, vomiting, flushing; occasionally severe dyspnoea; rarely severe anaphylaxis (see Cautions)
Dose: see notes above and manufacturer's literature

PoM **Imferon®** (Fisons)
Injection, iron dextran injection. Net price 2-ml amp = 54p; 5-ml amp = £1.08
Intravenous infusion, iron dextran injection. Net price 20-ml amp = £4.48 (Hosp. only)

IRON SORBITOL INJECTION

Contains 5% (50 mg/ml) of iron
Indications: iron-deficiency anaemia
Cautions: oral administration of iron should be stopped at least 24 hours before giving iron sorbitol injection; administration of other injectable iron preparations should be stopped a week beforehand; urine may darken on standing
Contra-indications: liver disease, kidney disease (particularly pyelonephritis), untreated urinary-tract infections
Dose: by intramuscular injection, see notes above and manufacturer's literature

PoM **Jectofer®** (Astra)
Injection, iron sorbitol injection. Net price 2-ml amp = 47p

9.1.2 Drugs used in megaloblastic anaemias

Most megaloblastic anaemias are due to lack of either vitamin B_{12} or folate and it is essential to establish in every case which deficiency is present and the underlying cause. In emergencies, where delay might be dangerous, it is sometimes necessary to administer both substances after the bone marrow test while plasma assay results are awaited. Normally, however, appropriate treatment should be instituted only when the results of tests are available.

Vitamin B_{12} is also needed in the treatment of megaloblastosis due to prolonged nitrous oxide anaesthesia, which inactivates the vitamin, and in the rare syndrome of congenital transcobalamin II deficiency.

Vitamin B_{12} should be given prophylactically after total gastrectomy or total ileal resection (or after partial gastrectomy if a vitamin B_{12} absorption test shows vitamin B_{12} malabsorption).

Apart from dietary deficiency, all other causes of vitamin-B_{12} deficiency are attributable to malabsorption so there is little place for the use of vitamin B_{12} orally and none for vitamin B_{12} intrinsic factor complexes given by mouth.

Hydroxocobalamin has completely replaced cyanocobalamin as the form of vitamin B_{12} of choice for therapy; when vitamin B_{12} injection is prescribed hydroxocobalamin injection should be given. It is retained in the body longer than cyanocobalamin and thus for maintenance therapy need only be given at intervals of 3 months. Although a haematological response in vitamin-B_{12} deficiency may be obtained by small doses, it is customary to start treatment with 1 mg by intramuscular injection repeated 5 times at intervals of 2 to 3 days to replenish the depleted body stores. Thereafter, maintenance treatment, which is usually for life, can be instituted. There is no evidence that larger doses provide any additional benefit in vitamin-B_{12} neuropathy.

Folic acid has few indications for long-term therapy since most causes of folate deficiency are self-limiting or will yield to a short course of treatment. It should not be used in undiagnosed megaloblastic anaemia unless vitamin B_{12} is administered concurrently otherwise neuropathy may be precipitated (see above).

In folate-deficient megaloblastic anaemia (e.g. due to poor nutrition, pregnancy, or anticonvulsants), standard treatment to bring about a haematological remission and replenish body stores, is oral administration of folic acid 5 mg daily for 4 months; up to 15 mg daily may be necessary in malabsorption states.

For prophylaxis in chronic haemolytic states or in renal dialysis, it is sufficient to give folic acid 5 mg daily or even weekly, depending on the diet and the rate of haemolysis.

For prophylaxis in pregnancy the dose of folic acid is 200–500 micrograms daily (see Iron and Folic Acid, section 9.1.1.1).

There is **no** justification for prescribing multiple-ingredient vitamin preparations containing vitamin B_{12} or folic acid.

HYDROXOCOBALAMIN

Indications: Addisonian pernicious anaemia, subacute combined degeneration of the spinal cord, other causes of vitamin-B_{12} deficiency

Cautions: should not be given before diagnosis fully established but see also notes above

Dose: by intramuscular injection, initially 1 mg repeated 5 times at intervals of 2–3 days; maintenance dose 1 mg every 3 months; CHILD, dosage as for adult

PoM **Hydroxocobalamin Injection,** hydroxocobalamin 250 micrograms/ml, net price 1-ml amp = 9p; 1 mg/ml, 1-ml amp = 18p
Note. The BP directs that when vitamin B_{12} injection is prescribed or demanded hydroxocobalamin injection shall be dispensed or supplied

NHS PoM **Cobalin-H**® (Paines & Byrne)
Injection, hydroxocobalamin 1 mg/ml. Net price 1-ml amp = 18p

NHS PoM **Neo-Cytamen**® (DF)
Injection, hydroxocobalamin 250 micrograms/ ml. Net price 1-ml amp = 9p
Injection, hydroxocobalamin 1 mg/ml. Net price 1-ml amp = 18p

CYANOCOBALAMIN

Indications: see notes above

Dose: by intramuscular injection, initially 1 mg repeated 10 times at intervals of 2–3 days, maintenance 1 mg every month, but see notes above

PoM **Cyanocobalamin Injection,** cyanocobalamin 1 mg/ ml. Net price 1 ml amp = 17p
Note. The BP directs that when vitamin B_{12} injection is prescribed or demanded hydroxocobalamin injection shall be dispensed or supplied

NHS **Cytacon**® (DF)
Tablets, f/c, cyanocobalamin 50 micrograms. Net price 20 = 48p
Liquid, red, cyanocobalamin 35 micrograms/5 ml. Net price 200 ml = £1.19

NHS PoM **Cytamen**® (DF)
Injection, cyanocobalamin 1 mg/ml. Net price 1-ml amp = 17p

FOLIC ACID

Indications: see notes above

Cautions: should never be given alone in the treatment of Addisonian pernicious anaemia and other vitamin B_{12}-deficiency states because it may precipitate the onset of subacute combined degeneration of the spinal cord. Do not use in malignant disease unless megaloblastic anaemia due to folate deficiency is an important complication (some malignant tumours are folate-dependent)

Dose: initially, 5 mg daily for 4 months (see notes above); maintenance, 5 mg every 1–7 days

depending on underlying disease; CHILD up to 1 year, 500 micrograms/kg daily; over 1 year, as adult dose

PoM [1]**Folic Acid Tablets,** folic acid 5 mg, net price 20 = 6p; 100-microgram tablets also available
[1]*Note.* Can be sold to the public provided the recommended single and daily doses do not exceed 500 micrograms

PoM **Lexpec**® (RP Drugs)
Syrup, sugar-free, folic acid 2.5 mg/5 ml. Diluent sorbitol solution, life of syrup diluted to 75% up to 21 days. Net price 125 ml = £3.20

FOLINIC ACID
See section 8.1.3

9.1.3   Drugs used in hypoplastic and haemolytic anaemias

Anabolic steroids, pyridoxine hydrochloride, antilymphocyte immunoglobulin, and various corticosteroids are used in hypoplastic and haemolytic anaemias.

The place of non-androgenic **anabolic steroids** in the therapy of *aplastic anaemia* remains somewhat controversial and their effectiveness is unclear. There is a wide variation in the reported successful responses. Occasional patients, however, do seem to derive benefit. It is customary to prescribe oxymetholone in doses of the order of 2–3 mg/kg daily, and to continue therapy for at least 3 to 6 months. At these dose levels, virilising side-effects may be expected in female patients and in children. Controlled trials have shown that antilymphocyte immunoglobulin produces a response in 50% of acquired cases.

It is unlikely that dietary deprivation of **pyridoxine hydrochloride** (section 9.6.2) produces haematological effects in man. However, certain forms of *sideroblastic anaemia* respond to pharmacological doses of pyridoxine, possibly reflecting its role as a co-enzyme during haemoglobin synthesis.

Pyridoxine is indicated in both idiopathic acquired and hereditary sideroblastic anaemias. Although complete cures have not been reported, some increase in haemoglobin may occur; the dose required is usually high, up to 400 mg daily. Reversible sideroblastic anaemias respond to treatment of the underlying cause but in pregnancy, haemolytic anaemias, and alcoholism, and during antituberculous treatment, pyridoxine is also indicated.

Corticosteroids (see section 6.3) have an important place in the management of a wide variety of haematological disorders. They include conditions with an immune basis such as auto-immune haemolytic anaemias, immune thrombocytopenias and neutropenias, and major transfusion reactions. They are also used in chemotherapy schedules for all forms of lymphoreticular malignancy, lymphoid leukaemias, and paraproteinaemias, including myelomatosis. Corticosteroids are used in aplastic anaemias, where their usefulness is more debatable.

It is possible that corticosteroids in low doses may also reduce the capillary fragility which occurs in the purpuric diseases, thus lessening bleeding.

IRON OVERLOAD. Severe tissue iron overload may occur in aplastic and other refractory anaemias, mainly as the result of repeated blood transfusions. It is a particular problem in refractory anaemias with hyperplastic bone marrow, especially thalassaemia major, where excessive iron absorption from the gut and inappropriate iron therapy add to the tissue siderosis.

Venesection therapy is contra-indicated, but the long-term administration of the iron chelating compound desferrioxamine mesylate is useful. Subcutaneous infusions of desferrioxamine (0.5 to 4 g over 12 hours) are given on 5 to 7 nights each week. Desferrioxamine (up to 2 g per unit of blood) may also be given through the infusion line at the time of blood transfusion.

Iron excretion is enhanced by administration of vitamin C (section 9.6.3) in a dose of 100 to 200 mg daily; it should be given separately from food since it also enhances iron absorption.

NANDROLONE

Indications: aplastic anaemia, see notes above
Cautions; Contra-indications; Side-effects: see section 6.4.3
Dose: by deep intramuscular injection, nandrolone decanoate 50–150 mg weekly

PoM **Deca-Durabolin 100**® (Organon)
Injection (oily), nandrolone decanoate 100 mg/ml. Net price 1-ml amp = £6.68

OXYMETHOLONE

Indications: aplastic anaemia; see notes above
Cautions: cardiac and renal impairment, circulatory failure, hypertension, diabetes mellitus, epilepsy, migraine; monitor skeletal maturation in children for 6 months after treatment. Drug interactions: see Appendix 1 (sections *2.8, 2.8B*)
Contra-indications: hepatic impairment, prostatic carcinoma, pregnancy, breast-feeding
Side-effects: acne, oedema, jaundice and liver dysfunction, virilism with high doses, hypercalcaemia, menstrual irregularities; hyperglucagonaemia has also been reported with oxymetholone
Dose: aplastic anaemia, 2–3 mg/kg daily in divided doses; CHILD 2–3 mg/kg daily (less in Fanconi's anaemia)

PoM **Anapolon 50**® (Syntex)
Tablets, scored, oxymetholone 50 mg. Net price 20 = £9.86

STANOZOLOL

Indications; Cautions; Contra-indications; Side-effects: see under Oxymetholone
Dose: by deep intramuscular injection, 50 mg every 2–3 weeks

PoM **Stromba**® (Sterling Research)
Injection (aqueous suspension), stanozolol 50 mg/ml. Net price 1-ml amp = £5.93

9.1.4   Drugs used in autoimmune thrombocytopenic purpura

It is usual to commence the treatment of autoimmune (idiopathic) thrombocytopenic purpura with corticosteroids, e.g. prednisolone in the order of 1 mg/kg daily, gradually reducing the dosage over the subsequent weeks. In patients who fail to achieve a satisfactory platelet count or relapse when corticosteroid dosage is reduced or withdrawn, splenectomy is considered.

Other therapy that has been tried in refractory cases includes azathioprine (see section 8.2.1), vincristine or vinblastine (see section 8.1.4) (or vinblastine-loaded platelets), and danazol (see section 6.7.3). Intravenous immunoglobulins, e.g. Sandoglobulin® (see section 14.5), have also been used in refractory cases or where a temporary rapid rise in platelets is needed, as in pregnancy or pre-operatively. For patients with chronic severe thrombocytopenia refractory to other therapy, tranexamic acid (see section 2.11) may be given to reduce the severity of haemorrhage.

9.1.5   Prescribing in G6PD deficiency

Glucose 6-phosphate dehydrogenase (G6PD) deficiency is highly prevalent in populations originating from most parts of Africa, from most parts of Asia, from Oceania, and from Southern Europe; it can also be encountered, rarely, in any other population.

When prescribing drugs for patients who are G6PD deficient, the following three points should be kept in mind:
1. G6PD deficiency is genetically heterogeneous; different genetic variants entail different susceptibility to the haemolytic risk from drugs; thus, a drug found to be safe in some G6PD-deficient subjects may not be equally safe in others;
2. no test specifically designed to identify potential risk in G6PD-deficient subjects is currently carried out by manufacturers;
3. the risk and severity of haemolysis is almost always dose-related.

The table below should be read with these points in mind. Whenever possible, a test for G6PD deficiency should be done before prescribing a drug in the list, especially if the patient belongs to a population group in which G6PD deficiency is common.

A very small group of G6PD-deficient individuals, with chronic non-spherocytic haemolytic anaemia, have haemolysis even in the absence of an exogenous trigger. These patients must be regarded as being at high risk of severe exacerbation of haemolysis following administration of any of the drugs listed below.

Drugs with definite risk of haemolysis in most G6PD-deficient subjects

Dapsone and other sulphones (higher doses used for dermatitis herpetiformis more likely to cause problems)
Methylene blue
Nalidixic acid
Niridazole [not on UK market]
Nitrofurantoin
Pamaquin [not on UK market]
Primaquine (30 mg weekly for 8 weeks has been found to be without undue harmful effects in Afro and Asian people, see section 5.4.1)
Sulphonamides (including co-trimoxazole; some sulphonamides, e.g. sulphadiazine, have been tested and found not to be haemolytic in many G6PD-deficient subjects

Drugs with possible risk of haemolysis in some G6PD-deficient subjects

Aspirin (acceptable in a dose of at least 1 g daily in most G6PD-deficient subjects)
Chloroquine (acceptable in management of acute malaria)
Menadione, water-soluble derivatives (e.g. menadiol sodium phosphate)
Probenecid
Quinidine (acceptable in management of acute malaria when quinine unavailable)
Quinine (acceptable in management of acute malaria)

Note. Mothballs may contain naphthalene which also causes haemolysis in subjects with G6PD-deficiency.

9.2   Electrolyte and water replacement

9.2.1 Oral administration
9.2.2 Intravenous administration
9.2.3 Plasma substitutes
9.2.4 Electrolyte concentrations

9.2.1   Oral administration

9.2.1.1 Potassium salts
9.2.1.2 Sodium salts

Electrolyte preparations may be given by mouth to prevent certain electrolyte deficiencies in conditions in which it is known that these are likely to arise, or to treat established deficiencies of mild or moderate degree. Oral magnesium salts are occasionally required on a long-term basis in patients with malabsorption.

9.2.1.1   POTASSIUM SALTS

Compensation for potassium loss is especially necessary:
1. in elderly patients, since they frequently take inadequate amounts of potassium in the diet (but see below for warning on renal insufficiency);
2. in those taking digoxin or anti-arrhythmic drugs, where potassium depletion may induce arrhythmias;
3. in patients in whom secondary hyperaldosteronism occurs, e.g. renal artery stenosis, cirrhosis of the liver, the nephrotic syndrome, and severe heart failure;

4. in patients with excessive losses of potassium in the faeces, e.g. chronic diarrhoea associated with intestinal malabsorption or laxative abuse.

Measures to compensate for potassium loss may also be required during long-term administration of drugs known to induce potassium loss (e.g. corticosteroids). Potassium supplements are seldom required with the small doses of diuretics given to treat hypertension; potassium-sparing diuretics (rather than potassium supplements) are recommended with diuretics such as frusemide or the thiazides when these are given to eliminate oedema.

DOSAGE. If *prophylactic administration of potassium* is needed, doses of potassium chloride 2 to 4 g (approx. 25 to 50 mmol) daily by mouth are suitable in patients taking a normal diet. Smaller doses must be used if there is renal insufficiency (common in the elderly) otherwise there is danger of hyperkalaemia. Potassium salts cause nausea and vomiting therefore poor compliance is a major limitation to their effectiveness; where appropriate, potassium-sparing diuretics are preferable.

When there is *established potassium depletion* or when the plasma-potassium concentration is less than 3.5mmol/litre, larger doses of 10 to 15 g (approx. 135 to 200 mmol) daily of potassium chloride are required over periods of days or weeks. Potassium depletion is frequently associated with chloride depletion and with metabolic alkalosis (as in the vomiting of pyloric stenosis), and these disorders require correction.

ADMINISTRATION. Potassium salts are preferably given as a liquid preparation, rather than sustained-release tablets; the use of potassium bicarbonate should be restricted to hyperchloraemic states.

Salt substitutes. A number of salt substitutes which contain significant amounts of potassium chloride are readily available as health food products (e.g. Losalt and Ruthmol). These are not recommended in patients with renal failure as potassium intoxication may result.

POTASSIUM SALTS

Indications: potassium depletion (see notes above)
Cautions: intestinal stricture, hiatus hernia (for sustained-release preparations). Drug interactions: see Appendix 1 (sections 2.2, 2.5, 8)
Contra-indications: renal failure, plasma potassium concentrations above 5 mmol/litre
Side-effects: nausea and vomiting (severe symptoms may indicate obstruction), oesophageal or small bowel ulceration
Dose: see notes above

Potassium Tablets, Effervescent, potassium bicarbonate 500 mg, potassium acid tartrate 300 mg, each tablet providing 6.5 mmol of K$^+$. To be dissolved in water before administration. Net price 100 = £2.58p. Label: 13, 21
Note. These tablets do not contain chloride; for effervescent tablets containing potassium and chloride, see Kloref® tablets or Sando-K® tablets (below)

Kay-Cee-L® (Geistlich)
Syrup, red, sugar-free, potassium chloride 7.5% (1 mmol/ml). Do not dilute. Net price 200 ml = £1.95; 500 ml = £2.44. Label: 21

K-Contin Continus® (Napp)
Tablets, s/r, orange, f/c, potassium chloride 600 mg (8 mmol each of K$^+$ and Cl$^-$). Net price 20 = 8p. Label: 25, 27, counselling advised, swallow whole with fluid during meals while sitting or standing

Kloref® (Cox Pharmaceuticals)
Tablets, effervescent, betaine hydrochloride, potassium benzoate, bicarbonate, and chloride, equivalent to potassium chloride 500 mg (6.7 mmol each of K$^+$ and Cl$^-$). Net price 50 = £1.45. Label: 13, 21

Kloref-S® (Cox Pharmaceuticals)
Granules, effervescent, sugar-free, betaine hydrochloride, potassium bicarbonate and chloride equivalent to potassium chloride 1.5 g (20 mmol each of K$^+$ and Cl$^-$)/sachet. Net price 20 sachets = £1.72. Label: 13, 21

Leo K® (Leo)
Tablets, s/r, f/c, potassium chloride 600 mg (8 mmol each of K$^+$ and Cl$^-$). Net price 20 = 18p. Label: 25, 27, counselling advised, swallow whole with fluid during meals while sitting or standing

Nu-K® (Consolidated)
Capsules, s/r, blue, potassium chloride 600 mg (8 mmol each of K$^+$ and Cl$^-$). Net price 20 = 31p. Label: 25, 27, counselling advised, swallow whole with fluid while sitting or standing *or* open capsule and swallow enclosed granules with fluid or soft food

Sando-K® (Sandoz)
Tablets, effervescent, potassium bicarbonate and chloride equivalent to potassium 470 mg (12 mmol of K$^+$) and chloride 285 mg (8 mmol of Cl$^-$). Net price 20 = 35p. Label: 13, 21

Slow-K® (Ciba)
Tablets, s/r, orange, s/c, potassium chloride 600 mg (8 mmol each of K$^+$ and Cl$^-$). Net price 20 = 10p. Label: 25, 27, counselling advised, swallow whole with fluid during meals while sitting or standing

---

HYPERKALAEMIA

POLYSTYRENE SULPHONATE RESINS

Indications: hyperkalaemia associated with anuria or severe oliguria, and in dialysis patients
Contra-indications: avoid calcium-containing resin in hyperparathyroidism, multiple myeloma, sarcoidosis, or metastatic carcinoma; avoid sodium-containing resin in congestive heart failure and severe renal impairment
Cautions: children (impaction of resin with excessive dosage or inadequate dilution)
Side-effects: rectal ulceration following rectal administration
Dose: by mouth, 15 g 3–4 times daily in water (not fruit juice which has a high K$^+$ content)
By rectum, as an enema, 30 g in methylcellulose solution, retained for 9 hours
CHILD, any route, 0.5–1 g/kg daily

Calcium Resonium® (Winthrop)
Powder, brown, calcium polystyrene sulphonate. Net price 300 g = £38.48. Label: 13

Resonium A® (Winthrop)
Powder, buff, sodium polystyrene sulphonate. Net price 454 g = £47.45. Label: 13

9.2.1.2 SODIUM SALTS

Sodium chloride is indicated in states of sodium depletion and usually needs to be given intravenously (section 9.2.2). In chronic conditions associated with mild or moderate degrees of sodium depletion, e.g. in salt-losing renal disease, oral supplements may be sufficient.

SODIUM SALTS

Indications: sodium depletion. See also section 9.2.2 below

Sodium Chloride Tablets, sodium chloride 300 mg. Net price 20 = 18p

Slow Sodium® (Ciba)
Tablets, s/r, sodium chloride 600 mg (approx. 10 mmol each of Na$^+$ and Cl$^-$). Net price 20 = 11p. Label: 25

ORAL REHYDRATION THERAPY (ORT)

As a worldwide problem diarrhoea is by far the most important indication for fluid and electrolyte replacement. Intestinal absorption of sodium and water is enhanced by glucose, therefore replacement of fluid and electrolytes lost through diarrhoea can be achieved by administration of solutions containing sodium, potassium, and glucose.

Oral rehydration solutions should:
enhance optimally the absorption of water and electrolytes;
replace the electrolyte deficit adequately and safely;
contain an alkalising agent to counter acidosis;
be simple to use in hospital and at home;
be palatable and acceptable, especially to children;
be readily available.

It is the policy of the World Health Organization (WHO) to promote a single oral rehydration solution but use it flexibly (e.g. by giving extra water between drinks of oral rehydration solution to moderately dehydrated infants).

The WHO formulation is as follows:

Sodium Chloride	3.5 g/litre
Potassium Chloride	1.5 g/litre
Sodium Bicarbonate	2.5 g/litre
Anhydrous Glucose	20.0 g/litre

This provides

Sodium	90 mmol/litre
Potassium	20 mmol/litre
Chloride	80 mmol/litre
Bicarbonate	30 mmol/litre
Glucose	111 mmol/litre

Compared with the WHO formulation oral rehydration solutions used in the UK are low in sodium (30–50 mmol/litre) and high in glucose (approx. 200 mmol/litre). They are of benefit for mild to moderate diarrhoea, when the body's homoeostatic mechanisms are still working and will not be harmful, but they may be suboptimal in correction of fluid loss and electrolyte imbalance. In the more severe diarrhoeas the WHO formulation is marginally more effective in correcting dehydration; it carries no danger of hypernatraemia if used correctly.

ORAL REHYDRATION SALTS
(ORS)
Indications: see notes above

WHO formulation
See notes above
Note. In the BP 1988 this corresponds to Oral Rehydration Salts—Bicarbonate (Formula B); the anhydrous glucose may be replaced by Glucose BP (i.e. the monohydrate) if the sodium bicarbonate is packaged separately. In the BP 1988, Oral Rehydration Salts—Citrate (Formula C), the sodium bicarbonate in Formula B is replaced by sodium citrate 2.9 g. In the BP 1988, Oral Rehydration Salts—Formula A corresponds to Compound Sodium Chloride and Glucose Oral Powder BP 1980 (see Formulary)

Proprietary preparations
Note. After reconstitution any unused solution should be discarded no later than 1 hour after preparation unless stored in a refrigerator when it may be kept for up to 24 hours.

Dextrolyte® (Cow & Gate)
Oral solution, glucose, potassium chloride, sodium chloride, sodium lactate, providing Na+ 35 mmol, K+ 13.4 mmol, Cl−30.5 mmol, lactate 17.7 mmol, and glucose 200 mmol/litre. 100 ml (Hosp. only)

Dioralyte® (Rorer)
Effervescent tablets, sodium bicarbonate 300 mg, potassium bicarbonate 200 mg, citric acid 1.06 g, anhydrous glucose 3.6 g. Net price 10-tab pack (pineapple-flavoured or plain) = £1.20. Label: 13
Reconstitute 2 tablets with 200 ml of water (only for adults and for children over 2 years)
Note. Ten tablets when reconstituted with 1 litre of water provide Na+ 35 mmol, K+ 20 mmol, citrate 55 mmol, and glucose 200 mmol
Oral powder, sodium chloride 200 mg, potassium chloride 300 mg, sodium bicarbonate 300 mg, glucose 8 g/sachet. Net price 20 sachets (cherry- or pineapple-flavoured or plain) = £4.17. Label: 13
Reconstitute one sachet with 200 ml of water (freshly boiled and cooled for infants).
Note. Five sachets reconstituted with 1 litre of water provide Na+ 35 mmol, K+ 20 mmol, Cl− 37 mmol, HCO3− 18 mmol, and glucose 200 mmol (corresponds to Compound Sodium Chloride and Glucose Oral Powder, see Formulary)

Electrolade® (Nicholas)
Oral powder, sodium chloride 236 mg, potassium chloride 300 mg, sodium bicarbonate 500 mg, anhydrous glucose 4 g/sachet. Net price 20 sachets = £3.75. Label: 13

Reconstitute one sachet with 200 ml of water (freshly boiled and cooled for infants)
Note. Five sachets when reconstituted with 1 litre of water provide Na+ 50 mmol, K+ 20 mmol, Cl− 40 mmol, HCO3− 30 mmol, and glucose 111 mmol

Electrosol® (Macarthys)
Oral powder, sodium chloride 200 mg, potassium chloride 300 mg, sodium bicarbonate 300 mg, glucose 8 g/sachet. 24 sachets. Label: 13
Reconstitute one sachet with 200 ml of water (freshly boiled and cooled for infants).
Note. Five sachets when reconstituted with 1 litre of water provide Na+ 35 mmol, K+ 20 mmol, Cl− 37 mmol, HCO3− 18 mmol, and glucose 200 mmol corresponds to Compound Sodium Chloride and Glucose Oral Powder, see Formulary

Gluco-lyte® (Cupal)
Oral powder, sodium chloride 200 mg, potassium chloride 300 mg, sodium bicarbonate 300 mg, glucose 8 g/sachet. Net price 6 sachets = 94p. Label: 13
Reconstitute one sachet with 200 ml of water (freshly boiled and cooled for infants)
Note. Five sachets when reconstituted with 1 litre of water provide Na+ 35 mmol, K+ 20 mmol, Cl− 37 mmol, HCO3− 18 mmol, and glucose 200 mmol (corresponds to Compound Sodium Chloride and Glucose Oral Powder, see Formulary)

Paedialyte® (Abbott)
RS Rehydration Solution, sodium chloride, potassium citrate, sodium citrate, glucose, providing Na+ 75 mmol, K+ 20 mmol, Cl− 65 mmol, citrate 10 mmol, and glucose 139 mmol/litre. Net price 250-ml bottle = 95p
MS Maintenance Solution, sodium chloride, potassium citrate, sodium citrate, glucose, providing Na+ 45 mmol, K+ 20 mmol, Cl− 35 mmol, citrate 10 mmol, and glucose 139 mmol/litre. Net price 250-ml bottle = 89p

Rehidrat® (Searle)
Oral powder, sodium chloride 440 mg, potassium chloride 380 mg, sodium bicarbonate 420 mg, citric acid 440 mg, glucose 4.09 g, sucrose 8.07 g, fructose 70 mg/sachet. Net price 20 sachets (lemon and lime- or orange-flavoured) = £4.87. Label: 13
Note. Lemon and lime version stains vomit green
Reconstitute one sachet with 250 ml of water (freshly boiled and cooled for infants)
Note. Four sachets when reconstituted with one litre of water provide Na+ 50 mmol, K+ 20 mmol, Cl− 50 mmol, HCO3− 20 mmol, citrate 9 mmol, glucose 91 mmol, sucrose 94 mmol, and fructose 2 mmol

9.2.2   Intravenous administration
Solutions of electrolytes are given intravenously, to meet normal fluid and electrolyte requirements or to replenish substantial deficits or continuing losses, when the patient is nauseated or vomiting and is unable to take adequate amounts by mouth.

In an individual patient the nature and severity of the electrolyte imbalance must be assessed from the history and clinical and biochemical examination. Sodium, potassium, chloride, magnesium, phosphate, and water depletion can occur singly and in combination with or without disturbances of acid-base balance.

Isotonic solutions may be infused safely into a peripheral vein. Solutions more concentrated than plasma, for example 20% glucose are best given through an indwelling catheter positioned in a large vein.

Sodium chloride in isotonic solution provides the most important extracellular ions in near physiological concentration and is indicated in sodium depletion which may arise from such conditions as gastro-enteritis, diabetic ketoacidosis, ileus, and ascites. In a severe deficit of from 4 to 8 litres, 2 to 3 litres of isotonic sodium chloride may be given over 2 to 3 hours; thereafter infusion can usually be at a slower rate.

Excessive administration should be avoided; the jugular venous pressure should be assessed, the bases of the lungs should be examined for crepitations, and in elderly or seriously ill patients it is often helpful to monitor the right atrial (central) venous pressure.

Sodium chloride and glucose solutions are indicated when there is combined water and sodium depletion. A 1:1 mixture of isotonic sodium chloride and 5% glucose allows some of the water (free of sodium) to enter body cells which suffer most from dehydration while the sodium salt with a volume of water determined by the normal plasma Na^+ remains extracellular. Examples of combined sodium chloride and water depletion occur in persistent vomiting and hyperosmolar diabetic ketoacidosis.

Glucose solutions (5%) are mainly used to replace water deficits and should be given alone when there is no significant loss of electrolytes. Average water requirements in a healthy adult are 1.5 to 2.5 litres daily and this is needed to balance unavoidable losses of water through the skin and lungs and to provide sufficient for urinary excretion. Water depletion (dehydration) tends to occur when these losses are not matched by a comparable intake, as for example may occur in coma or dysphagia or in the aged or apathetic who may not drink water in sufficient amount on their own initiative. Water depletion also occurs in diabetic ketoacidosis; the deficit may be up to 8 litres in severe cases.

Excessive loss of water without loss of electrolytes is uncommon, occurring in fevers, hyperthyroidism, and in uncommon water-losing renal states such as diabetes insipidus or hypercalcaemia. The volume of glucose solution needed to replenish deficits varies with the severity of the disorder, but usually lies within the range of 2 to 10 litres.

Potassium chloride and sodium chloride intravenous infusion and **potassium chloride and glucose** intravenous infusion are used to correct severe hypokalaemia and depletion and when sufficient potassium cannot be taken by mouth. Potassium chloride (1.5 g in sterile ampoules) may be conveniently added to 500 ml of sodium chloride intravenous infusion or 5% glucose; the solution then contains 40mmol/litre and may be given slowly over 2 to 3 hours. Repeated measurements of plasma potassium are necessary to determine whether further infusions are required and to avoid the development of hyperkalaemia; this is especially liable to occur in renal failure.

Sodium bicarbonate is used to control severe metabolic acidosis (as in renal failure or diabetic coma). Since this condition is usually attended by sodium depletion, it is reasonable to correct this first by the administration of isotonic sodium chloride intravenous infusion, provided the kidneys are not primarily affected and the degree of acidosis is not so severe as to impair renal function. In these circumstances, isotonic sodium chloride alone is usually effective as it restores the ability of the kidneys to generate bicarbonate. In renal acidosis or in severe acidosis of any origin (for example blood pH<7.1) sodium bicarbonate (1.26%) should be infused with isotonic sodium chloride; a total volume of up to 6 litres (4 litres of sodium chloride and 2 litres of sodium bicarbonate) may be necessary in the adult. In severe shock due for example to cardiac arrest, metabolic acidosis may develop without sodium depletion; in these circumstances sodium bicarbonate is best given in a small volume of hypertonic solution, such as 200 to 300 ml of 8.4% solution intravenously; plasma pH should be monitored.

Magnesium chloride or **sulphate** is occasionally needed to correct magnesium deficiency in alcoholism or that has arisen from prolonged diarrhoea or vomiting which has been treated with parenteral fluid and nutrition without magnesium supplements; 35–50mmol of magnesium chloride (or sulphate) may be added to 1 litre of 5% glucose or other isotonic solution and given over a period of 12 to 24 hours. Repeated measurements of plasma magnesium are advisable to determine the rate and duration of the infusion. The dose should be reduced in renal failure.

Phosphate infusion is occasionally needed in circumstances similar to those that give rise to magnesium deficiency; phosphate depletion also occurs in severe diabetic ketoacidosis. A solution containing up to 50 mmol/litre can be infused in sodium chloride or glucose over 12 to 24 hours. Since potassium depletion is also commonly present the phosphate may be given as a mixture of the sodium and potassium salts.

Sodium lactate intravenous infusion is obsolete in metabolic acidosis, and carries the risk of producing lactic acidosis, particularly in seriously ill patients with poor tissue perfusion or impaired hepatic function.

GLUCOSE
(Dextrose Monohydrate)
Indications: fluid replacement (see notes above), provision of energy (section 9.3)
Side-effects: glucose injections especially if hypertonic may have a low pH and irritate the venous intima so causing thrombophlebitis
Dose: water replacement, see notes above; energy source, 1–3 litres daily of 20–50% solution

PoM **Glucose Intravenous Infusion,** glucose, usual strength 5% (50 mg/ml). 20% solution, net price 20-ml amp = £1.00; 25% solution, 25-ml

amp = £1.29; 50% solution, price 20-ml amp = 65p; 25-ml amp = £1.15; 50-ml amp = £1.92
In hospitals, 500- and 1000-ml packs, and sometimes other sizes, are available.

POTASSIUM CHLORIDE

Indications: electrolyte imbalance; see also oral potassium supplements, section 9.2.1.1
Cautions: for intravenous infusion the concentration of solution should not exceed 3.2 g (43 mmol)/litre
Side-effects: rapid injection may be toxic to heart
Dose: by slow intravenous infusion, up to 6 g (80 mmol) daily

PoM **Potassium Chloride and Glucose Intravenous Infusion,** usual strength potassium chloride 0.3% (3 g, 40 mmol each of K⁺ and Cl⁻/litre) with 5% of anhydrous glucose
In hospitals, 500- and 1000-ml packs, and sometimes other sizes, are available

PoM **Potassium Chloride and Sodium Chloride Intravenous Infusion,** usual strength potassium chloride 0.3% (3 g/litre) and sodium chloride 0.9% (9 g/litre), containing 40 mmol of K⁺, 150 mmol of Na⁺, and 190 mmol of Cl⁻/litre
In hospitals, 500- and 1000-ml packs, and sometimes other sizes, are available

PoM **Potassium Chloride, Sodium Chloride, and Glucose Intravenous Infusion,** sodium chloride 0.18% (1.8 g, 30 mmol of Na⁺/litre) with 4% of anhydrous glucose and usually sufficient potassium chloride to provide 10–40 mmol of K⁺/litre (to be specified by the prescriber)
In hospitals, 500- and 1000-ml packs, and sometimes other sizes, are available

PoM **Potassium Chloride Solution, Strong** (sterile), potassium chloride 15% (150 mg, approximately 2 mmol each of K⁺ and Cl⁻/ml). Net price 10-ml amp = 45p
IMPORTANT. Must be diluted with not less than 50 times its volume of sodium chloride intravenous infusion 0.9% or other suitable diluent and mixed well
Solutions containing 10 and 20% of potassium chloride are also available in both 5- and 10-ml ampoules.

SODIUM BICARBONATE

Indications: metabolic acidosis
Dose: by slow intravenous injection, a strong solution (up to 8.4%), or *by continuous intravenous infusion,* a weak solution (usually 1.26%), an amount appropriate to the body base deficit (see notes above)

PoM **Sodium Bicarbonate Intravenous Infusion,** usual strength sodium bicarbonate 1.26% (12.6 g, 150 mmol each of Na⁺ and HCO₃⁻/litre); various other strengths available
5% solution available in 20- and 50-ml ampoules. Net price 20-ml amp = £1.49; 50-ml amp = £2.67
In hospitals, 500- and 1000-ml packs, and sometimes other sizes, are available

SODIUM CHLORIDE

Indications: electrolyte imbalance, also section 9.2.1.2

Cautions: restrict intake in impaired renal function, cardiac failure, hypertension, peripheral and pulmonary oedema, toxaemia of pregnancy
Side-effects: administration of large doses may give rise to sodium accumulation and oedema
Dose: see notes above

PoM **Ringer's Solution for Injection,** calcium chloride (dihydrate) 322 micrograms, potassium chloride 300 micrograms, sodium chloride 8.6 mg/ml, providing the following ions (in mmol/litre), Ca²⁺ 2.2, K⁺ 4, Na⁺ 147, Cl⁻ 156
In hospitals, 500- and 1000-ml packs, and sometimes other sizes, are available

PoM **Sodium Chloride Intravenous Infusion,** usual strength sodium chloride 0.9% (9 g, 150 mmol each of Na⁺ and Cl⁻/litre), this strength being supplied when normal saline for injection is requested. Net price 2-ml amp = 23p; 5-ml amp = 30p; 10-ml amp = 34p; 20-ml amp = 62p; 50-ml amp = £1.42
In hospitals, 500- and 1000-ml packs, and sometimes other sizes, are available
Note. The term 'normal saline' should **not** be used to describe sodium chloride intravenous infusion 0.9%; the term 'physiological saline' is acceptable but it is preferable to give the composition (i.e. sodium chloride intravenous infusion 0.9%).

PoM **Sodium Chloride and Glucose Intravenous Infusion,** usual strength sodium chloride 0.18% (1.8 g, 30 mmol each of Na⁺ and Cl⁻/litre) and 4% of anhydrous glucose
In hospitals, 500- and 1000-ml packs, and sometimes other sizes are available

SODIUM LACTATE

Indications: diabetic coma, diminished alkali reserve (but see notes above)

PoM **Sodium Lactate Intravenous Infusion,** sodium lactate M/6, contains the following ions (in mmol/litre), Na⁺ 167, HCO₃⁻ (as lactate) 167
PoM **Sodium Lactate Intravenous Infusion, Compound,** (Hartmann's solution for injection), contains the following ions (in mmol/litre), Na⁺ 131, K⁺ 5, Ca²⁺ 2, HCO₃⁻ (as lactate) 29, Cl⁻ 111
In hospitals, 500- and 1000-ml packs, and sometimes other sizes, are available

PoM **Water for Injections.** Net price 1-ml amp = 11p; 2-ml amp = 11p; 5-ml amp = 16p; 20-ml amp = 47p; 50-ml amp = 94p

9.2.3   Plasma substitutes

Dextrans, **hetastarch**, and **gelatin** are macromolecular substances which are slowly metabolised; they may be used at the outset to expand and maintain blood volume in shock arising from conditions such as burns or septicaemia. They are rarely needed when shock is due to sodium and water depletion as, in these circumstances, the shock responds to water and electrolyte repletion. They should not be used to maintain plasma volume in conditions such as burns or peritonitis where there is loss of plasma protein, water and electrolytes over periods of several days or weeks. In these situations, plasma or plasma protein fractions containing large amounts of albumin should be given. These colloids should be used in haemorrhage if blood is not available as an immediate short-term measure until it is.

Dextrans may interfere with blood group cross-matching or biochemical measurements and these should be carried out before infusion is begun. Dextran 70 by intravenous infusion is used predominantly for volume expansion. Dextran 40 intravenous infusion is used in an attempt to improve peripheral blood flow in ischaemic disease of the limbs and peripheral thrombo-embolism.

Gelatin and **hetastarch** are also used for short-term volume expansion.

> **Dosage.** Because of the complex requirements relating to blood volume expansion and the primary significance of blood, plasma protein, and electrolyte replacement, detailed dose statements have been omitted. *In all cases specialist literature should be consulted.*

DEXTRAN 40 INTRAVENOUS INFUSION, Dextrans of weight average molecular weight about '40000' 10% in glucose intravenous infusion 5% or in sodium chloride intravenous infusion 0.9%
Indications: conditions associated with peripheral local slowing of the blood flow; prophylaxis of post-surgical thrombo-embolic disease
Cautions; Contra-indications; Side-effects: see under Dextran 70 Intravenous Infusion; correct dehydration before infusion and give adequate fluids during therapy; very special care in those at risk of vascular overloading
Dose: by intravenous infusion, initially 500–1000 ml; further doses are given according to the patient's condition (see notes above)

PoM **Gentran 40**® (Baxter)
Intravenous infusion, dextran 40 intravenous infusion in glucose intravenous infusion 5% or in sodium chloride intravenous infusion 0.9%. 500-ml bottle (both)
PoM **Lomodex 40**® (CP)
Intravenous infusion, dextran 40 intravenous infusion in glucose intravenous infusion 5% or in sodium chloride intravenous infusion 0.9%. Net price 500-ml bottle (both) = £5.77
PoM **Rheomacrodex**® (Pharmacia)
Intravenous infusion, dextran 40 intravenous infusion in glucose intravenous infusion 5% or in sodium chloride intravenous infusion 0.9%. Net price 500-ml bottle (both) = £6.51

DEXTRAN 70 INTRAVENOUS INFUSION, Dextrans of weight average molecular weight about '70000' 6% in glucose intravenous infusion 5% or in sodium chloride intravenous infusion 0.9%
Indications: short-term blood volume expansion; prophylaxis of post-surgical thrombo-embolic disease
Cautions: congestive heart failure, renal impairment; blood samples for cross-matching should ideally be taken before infusion

Contra-indications: severe congestive heart failure; renal failure; bleeding disorders such as thrombocytopenia and hypofibrinogenaemia
Side-effects: rarely anaphylactoid reactions
Dose: by intravenous infusion, after moderate to severe haemorrhage, 500–1000 ml rapidly initially followed by 500 ml later if necessary; severe burns, up to 3000 ml in the first few days with electrolytes (see also notes above)

PoM **Gentran 70**® (Baxter)
Intravenous infusion, dextran 70 intravenous infusion in glucose intravenous infusion 5% or in sodium chloride intravenous infusion 0.9%. 500-ml bottle (both)
PoM **Lomodex 70**® (CP)
Intravenous infusion, dextran 70 intravenous infusion in glucose intravenous infusion 5% or in sodium chloride intravenous infusion 0.9%. Net price 500-ml bottle (both) = £3.66
PoM **Macrodex**® (Pharmacia)
Intravenous infusion, dextran 70 intravenous infusion in glucose intravenous infusion 5% or in sodium chloride intravenous infusion 0.9%. Net price 500-ml bottle (both) = £4.11

DEXTRAN 110 INTRAVENOUS INFUSION, Dextrans of weight average molecular weight about '110000' 6% in glucose intravenous infusion 5% or in sodium chloride intravenous infusion 0.9%
Indications: see under Dextran 70 Intravenous Infusion
Cautions; Contra-indications; Side-effects: see under Dextran 70 Intravenous Infusion; blood samples for cross-matching should be taken before infusion
Dose: by intravenous infusion, see under Dextran 70 Intravenous Infusion

PoM **Dextraven 110**® (CP)
Intravenous infusion, dextran 110 intravenous infusion in sodium chloride intravenous infusion 0.9%. Net price 500-ml bottle = £5.77

GELATIN
Note. The gelatin is partially degraded
Indications: low blood volume
Cautions; Contra-indications; Side-effects: see under Dextran 70 Intravenous Infusion
Dose: by intravenous infusion, initially 500–1000 ml of a 3.5–4% solution (see notes above)

PoM **Gelofusine**® (Consolidated)
Intravenous infusion, succinylated gelatin (modified fluid gelatin, average molecular weight 30000) 4%, sodium chloride 0.9%. Net price 500-ml bottle = £3.16
PoM **Haemaccel**® (Hoechst)
Intravenous infusion, polygeline (degraded and modified gelatin, average molecular weight 35000) 35 g, Na$^+$145 mmol, K$^+$ 5.1 mmol, Ca^{2+} 6.25 mmol, Cl$^-$ 145 mmol/litre. Net price 500-ml bottle = £3.81

HETASTARCH

Indications: low blood volume (expansion)
Cautions; Contra-indications; Side-effects: see· under Dextran 70 Intravenous Infusion
Dose: by *intravenous infusion,* 500–1000 ml; usual max. 1500 ml daily (see notes above)

▼ PoM **Hespan**® (Du Pont)
Intravenous infusion, hetastarch 6% in sodium chloride intravenous infusion 0.9%. 500-ml Steriflex® bag

9.2.4   Electrolyte concentrations

Concentrations of electrolytes in intravenous infusion fluids are generally given in millimoles (mmol)/litre.

Table 2: Electrolyte concentrations of intravenous fluids

Intravenous infusion	Millimoles per litre				
	Na^+	K^+	HCO_3^-	Cl^-	Ca^{2+}
Normal Plasma Values	142	4.5	26	103	2.5
Citrated Plasma	150	12	—	55	—
Sodium Chloride 0.9%	150	—	—	150	—
Compound Sodium Lactate (Hartmann's)	131	5	29	111	2
Sodium Chloride 0.18% and Glucose 4%	30	—	—	30	—
Potassium Chloride 0.3% and Glucose 5%	—	40	—	40	—
Potassium Chloride 0.3% and Sodium Chloride 0.9%	150	40	—	190	—
To correct metabolic acidosis					
Sodium Bicarbonate 1.26%	150	—	150	—	—
Sodium Bicarbonate 8.4% for cardiac arrest	1000	—	1000	—	—
Sodium Lactate (M/6)	167	—	167	—	—

Table 3: Millimoles of each ion in 1 gram of salt

Electrolyte		mmol per g approx.
Ammonium chloride		18.7
Calcium chloride	Ca	6.8
(CaCl₂,2H₂O)	Cl	13.6
Potassium bicarbonate		10
Potassium chloride		13.4
Sodium bicarbonate		11.9
Sodium chloride		17.1
Sodium lactate		8.9

Faeces, vomit, or aspiration should be saved and analysed where possible if abnormal losses are

suspected; where this is impracticable the approximations in table 4 may be helpful in planning replacement therapy.

Table 4: Electrolyte content of gastro-intestinal secretions

Type of fluid	Millimoles per litre				
	H^+	Na^+	K^+	HCO_3^-	Cl^-
Gastric	40–60	20–80	5–20	—	100–150
Biliary	—	120–140	5–15	30–50	80–120
Pancreatic	—	120–140	5–15	70–110	40–80
Small bowel	—	120–140	5–15	20–40	90–130

9.3   Intravenous nutrition

When adequate feeding via the alimentary tract is not possible, nutrients may be given by intravenous infusion. This may be in addition to ordinary oral or tube feeding—**supplemental parenteral nutrition**, or may be the sole source of nutrition—**total parenteral nutrition** (TPN). Indications for this method include preparation of undernourished patients for surgery, chemotherapy, or radiation therapy; severe or prolonged disorders of the gastro-intestinal tract; major surgery, trauma, or burns; prolonged coma or refusal to eat; and some patients with renal or hepatic failure. Table 5 gives the composition of proprietary preparations available.

Protein is given as mixtures of essential and non-essential synthetic L-amino acids, which have replaced the protein hydrolysate preparations formerly used. Ideally, all essential amino acids should be included with a wide variety of non-essential ones to provide sufficient nitrogen together with electrolytes (see also section 9.2.2). However, available solutions vary in composition. Most contain amino acids alone or with a partial energy source (see Table 5) using combinations of glucose (dextrose), fructose (laevulose), sorbitol, and ethanol. Some are significantly deficient in electrolytes or particular amino acids.

Energy is provided in a ratio of 0.6 to 1.1 megajoules (150–250 kcals) per gram of protein nitrogen. Energy requirements must be met if amino acids are to be utilised for tissue maintenance. Although it has long been held that carbohydrate has a greater nitrogen-sparing effect than fat, recent studies have shown that a mixture of both energy sources, usually 30 to 50% as fat, gives better utilisation of amino acid solutions than glucose alone.

Glucose is the preferred source of carbohydrate, but if more than 180 g is given per day frequent monitoring of blood glucose is required, and insulin may be necessary. Glucose in various strengths from 10 to 50% must be infused through a central venous catheter to avoid thrombosis. Preparations are available with useful added ions and trace elements, e.g. Glucoplex®, Glucoven®.

Fructose and sorbitol have been used in an attempt to avoid the problem of hyperosmolar

Table 5: Proprietary Infusion Fluids for Parenteral Feeding

Preparation	Nitrogen g/litre	Energy kJ/litre	K⁺	Mg²⁺	Na⁺	Acet⁻	Cl⁻	Other components/litre
Aminofusin L Forte (Merck) Net price 500 ml = £10.50	15.2	1700	30	5	40	10	27.5	vitamins
Aminoplasmal L3 (Braun) Net price 500 ml = £4.70	4.82	510	25	2.5	48	59	18	acid phosphate 9 mmol, malate 7.5 mmol
Aminoplasmal L5 (Braun) Net price 500 ml = £6.10	8.03	850	25	2.5	48	59	31	acid phosphate 9 mmol, malate 7.5 mmol
Aminoplasmal L10 (Braun) Net price 500 ml = £11.60	16.06	1700	25	2.5	48	59	62	acid phosphate 9 mmol, malate 7.5 mmol
Aminoplasmal Ped (Braun) Net price 100 ml = £3.80; 250 ml = £4.60	7.4	850	25	2.5	50	27	15	
Aminoplex 5 (Geistlich) Net price 1000 ml = £10.71	5.0	4200	28	4	35	28	43	ethanol 5%, sorbitol 125 g, malic acid 1.85 g
Aminoplex 12 (Geistlich) Net price 500 ml = £10.36; 1000 ml = £17.48	12.44	1300	30	2.5	35	5	67	malic acid 4.6 g
Aminoplex 14 (Geistlich) Net price 500 ml = £10.36	13.4	1400	30		35		79	vitamins, malic acid 5.36 g
Aminoplex 24 (Geistlich) Net price 500 ml = £15.85	24.9	2600	30	2.5	35	5	67	malic acid 4.5 g
Aminoven 12 (MCP) Net price 500 ml = £8.81; 1000 ml = £14.86	12.44	1300	30	2.5	35	17.5	67	malic acid 4.6 g
Branched Chain Amino Acids (Baxter) 500-ml Viaflex® pack	4.4							
FreAmine III 8.5% (Kendall) 500 and 1000 ml	13.0	1400			10	72	<3	phosphate 10 mmol
FreAmine III 10% (Kendall) 1000 ml	15.3	1650			10	88	<2	phosphate 20 mmol
Glucoplex 1000 (Geistlich) Net price 500 ml = £2.54; 1000 ml = £2.83		4200	30	2.5	50		67	acid phosphate 18 mmol, Zn²⁺ 0.046 mmol, anhydrous glucose 240 g
Glucoplex 1600 (Geistlich) Net price 500 ml = £2.66; 1000 ml = £3.07		6700	30	2.5	50		67	acid phosphate 18 mmol, Zn²⁺ 0.046 mmol, anhydrous glucose 400 g
Glucoven 1000 (MCP) Net price 1000 ml = £2.69		4200	30	2.5	50		67	phosphate 18 mmol, zinc 0.046 mmol, anhydrous glucose 240 g
Glucoven 1600 (MCP) Net price 1000 ml = £2.91		6720	30	2.5	50		67	phosphate 18 mmol, zinc 0.046 mmol, anhydrous glucose 400 g
Intralipid 10% (KabiVitrum) Net price 100 ml = £4.35; 500 ml = £9.65		4600						fractionated soya oil 100 g, glycerol 22.5 g
Intralipid 20% (KabiVitrum) Net price 100 ml = £6.55; 500 ml = £14.40		8400						fractionated soya oil 200 g, glycerol 22.5 g
Laevuflex 20 (Geistlich) Net price 500 ml = £2.24		3400						fructose 200 g
Nephramine 5.4% (Kendall) 250 ml	6.4	840			5	44	<3	essential amino acids only
Perifusin (Merck) Net price 1000 ml = £7.20	5.0	550	30	5	40	10	9	malate 22.5 mmol
Plasma-Lyte 148 (water) (Baxter) 1000 ml		80	5	1.5	140	27	98	gluconate 23 mmol
Plasma-Lyte 148 (dextrose 5%) (Baxter) 500 ml and 1000 ml		880	5	1.5	140	27	98	gluconate 23 mmol, anhydrous glucose 50 g
Plasma-Lyte M (dextrose 5%) (Baxter) 1000 ml		800	16	1.5	40	12	40	Ca²⁺ 2.5 mmol, lactate 12 mmol, anhydrous glucose 50 g
Synthamin 9 (Baxter) Net price 500 ml = £7.15; 1000 ml = £13.25	9.1	1000	60	5	73	100	70	acid phosphate 30 mmol
Synthamin 14 (Baxter) Net price 500 ml = £10.35; 1000 ml = £18.40	14.0	1600	60	5	73	130	70	acid phosphate 30 mmol
Synthamin 14 without electrolytes (Baxter) Net price 500 ml = £10.60; 1000 ml = £18.40	14.0	1600				68	34	
Synthamin 17 (Baxter) Net price 500 ml = £13.60; 1000 ml = £24.70	16.5	1900	60	5	73	150	70	acid phosphate 30 mmol
Vamin 9 (KabiVitrum) Net price 500 ml = £6.60; 1000 ml = £11.90	9.4	1000	20	1.5	50		55	Ca²⁺ 2.5 mmol

 Prices are **net**, see p. 1

Table 5: Proprietary Infusion Fluids for Parenteral Feeding *(continued)*

Preparation	Nitrogen g/litre	Energy kJ/litre	Electrolytes mmol/litre K+	Mg²⁺	Na⁺	Acet⁻	Cl⁻	Other components/litre
Vamin 9 glucose (KabiVitrum)	9.4	2700	20	1.5	50		55	Ca²⁺ 2.5 mmol, anhydrous glucose 100 g
Net price 100 ml = £3.40; 500 ml = £7.10; 1000 ml = £12.80								
▼Vamin 14 (KabiVitrum)	13.5	1400	50	8	100	135	100	Ca²⁺ 5 mmol, SO₄²⁻ 8 mmol
Net price 500 ml = £9.55; 1000 ml = £16.95								
▼Vamin 14 (electrolyte-free) (KabiVitrum)	13.5	1400						
Net price 500 ml = £9.55; 1000 ml = £16.95								
▼Vamin 18 (electrolyte-free) (KabiVitrum)	18.0	1900						
Net price 500 ml = £12.70; 1000 ml = £22.80								
▼Vamin Infant (KabiVitrum)	9.3	1000						
Net price 100 ml = £3.80; 500 ml = £8.70								

Note. 1000 kcal = 4.1868 MJ; 1 MJ (1000 kJ) = 238.8 kcal. All entries are PoM

hyperglycaemic non-ketotic acidosis but other metabolic problems may occur, as with xylitol and ethanol which are now rarely used.

Fat emulsions have the advantages of a high energy to fluid volume ratio, neutral pH, and iso-osmolarity with plasma, and provide essential fatty acids. Available preparations are soya bean oil emulsions (Intralipid®). Several days of adaptation may be required to attain maximal utilisation. Reactions include occasional febrile episodes (usually only with 20% emulsions) and rare anaphylactic responses. Interference with biochemical measurements such as those for blood gases and calcium may occur if samples are taken before fat has been cleared. Daily checks are necessary to ensure complete clearance from the plasma. **Additives may only be mixed with fat emulsions where compatibility is known.**

Total parenteral nutrition (TPN) requires the use of a solution containing amino acids, glucose, fat, electrolytes, trace elements, and vitamins. This is now commonly provided by the pharmacy in the form of the 3-litre bag. The solution is infused through a central venous catheter inserted under full surgical precautions. Only nutritional fluids should be given by this line. Loading doses of vitamin B₁₂ and folic acid are advised and other vitamins are given parenterally twice weekly.

Before starting, the patient should be well oxygenated with a near normal circulating blood volume, renal function, and acid-base status. Appropriate biochemical tests should have been carried out beforehand and serious deficits corrected. Nutritional and electrolyte status must be monitored throughout treatment.

SUPPLEMENTARY PREPARATIONS

PoM **Addamel**® (KabiVitrum)
Solution, electrolytes and trace elements for addition to Vamin® amino acid solutions except Vamin 18 (see Table 5), Ca²⁺ 5 mmol, Mg²⁺ 1.5 mmol, Cl⁻ 13.3 mmol/10 ml; traces of Fe³⁺, Zn²⁺, Mn²⁺, Cu²⁺, F⁻, I⁻. For adult use. Net price 10-ml amp = £1.59

▼PoM **Addiphos**® (KabiVitrum)
Solution, sterile, phosphate 40 mmol, K⁺ 30 mmol, Na⁺ 30 mmol/20 ml. For addition to Vamin®

amino acid solutions (see Table 5) and glucose intravenous infusions. Net price 20-ml vial = £1.18

▼ PoM **Additrace**® (KabiVitrum)
Solution, trace elements for addition to Vamin® amino acid solutions (see Table 5); traces of Fe³⁺, Zn²⁺, Mn²⁺, Cu²⁺, Cr³⁺, Se⁴⁺, Mo⁶⁺, F⁻, I⁻. For adult use. Net price 10-ml amp = £1.79

PoM **Multibionta**® (Merck)
Solution, ascorbic acid 500 mg, dexpanthenol 25 mg, nicotinamide 100 mg, pyridoxine hydrochloride 15 mg, riboflavine sodium phosphate 10 mg, thiamine hydrochloride 50 mg, tocopheryl acetate 5 mg, vitamin A 10000 units. For addition to infusion solutions. Net price 10-ml amp = £1.47

PoM **Ped-El**® (KabiVitrum)
Solution, sterile, Ca²⁺, Cu²⁺, Fe³⁺, Mg²⁺, Mn²⁺, Zn²⁺, Cl⁻, F⁻, I⁻, P. For addition to Vamin® amino acid solutions (see Table 5). For paediatric use. Net price 20-ml vial = £1.59

PoM **Solivito N**® (KabiVitrum)
Solution, powder for reconstitution, biotin 60 micrograms, cyanocobalamin 5 micrograms, folic acid 400 micrograms, glycine 100 mg, nicotinamide 40 mg, pyridoxine hydrochloride 4.9 mg, riboflavine 3.6 mg (as sodium phosphate), sodium ascorbate 113 mg, sodium pantothenate 16.5 mg, thiamine mononitrate 3.1 mg. Dissolve in water for injections or glucose intravenous infusion for adding to glucose intravenous infusion or Intralipid; dissolve in Vitlipid N or Intralipid for adding to Intralipid only. Net price per vial = £1.80

PoM **Vitlipid N**® (KabiVitrum)
Emulsion, adult, vitamin A 330 units, ergocalciferol 20 units, dl-alpha tocopherol 1 unit, phytomenadione 15 micrograms/ml. For addition to Intralipid®. Net price 10-ml amp = £1.75
Emulsion, infant, vitamin A 230 units, ergocalciferol 40 units, dl-alpha tocopherol 0.7 unit, phytomenadione 20 micrograms/ml. For addition to Intralipid®. Net price 10-ml amp = £1.75

9.4 Oral nutrition

9.4.1 Foods for special diets
9.4.2 Enteral nutrition

9.4.1 Foods for special diets

A number of the foods listed below have been prepared to eliminate or reduce the content of a specific constituent. There are also specially formulated mixtures to substitute for foods which contain an unwanted ingredient.

ACBS. In certain clinical conditions some foods may have the characteristics of drugs and the Advisory Committee on Borderline Substances advises as to the circumstances in which such foods may be regarded as drugs and so can be prescribed in the NHS. These clinical conditions are shown with the food preparations listed below. Prescriptions for these foods issued in accordance with the advice of this committee and endorsed 'ACBS' will normally not be investigated. See Appendix 3 for a listing by clinical condition.

Corn flour and corn starch. For hypoglycaemia associated with glycogen-storage disease

Corn oil (maize oil). Net price 100 ml = 37p. For familial hypercholesterolaemia

Fructose (laevulose). Net price 500 g = £6.50. For proven glucose/galactose intolerance

Glucose for oral use (dextrose monohydrate). Net price 100 g = 10p. For glycogen storage disease and sucrose/isomaltose intolerance

Sunflower oil. Net price 100 ml = 40p. For familial hypercholesterolaemia

Aglutella® (GF Dietary Supplies)

Pasta, protein not more than 500 mg, carbohydrate 86.8 g, fat 500 mg/100 g, low Na⁺ and K⁺, gluten-free; macaroni, pasta spirals, semolina, spaghetti, spaghetti rings, tagliatelle. Net price 250 g = £2.21. For phenylketonuria; similar amino-acid abnormalities; renal failure; liver failure and liver cirrhosis; gluten-sensitive enteropathies including steatorrhoea due to gluten sensitivity, coeliac disease, and dermatitis herpetiformis

Aglutella Azeta® (GF Dietary Supplies)

Wafers, cream-filled, gluten-free, low protein, low sodium, low potassium. Net price 150 g = £3.07. For phenylketonuria; similar amino-acid abnormalities; renal failure; liver failure and liver cirrhosis

Albumaid® (Scientific Hospital Supplies)

Complete, powder, amino acids 89.4%, with vitamins, minerals, trace elements, free from carbohydrate and fat. Net price 200 g = £25.36. For malabsorption states where there is failure to hydrolyse and/or absorb protein

RVHB, powder, amino acid mixture, methionine-free. Net price 200 g = £25.12. For homocystinuria

RVHB complete, powder, amino acid mixture, methionine-free, with vitamins, minerals, and trace elements. Net price 200 g = £25.12. For homocystinuria

XP, powder, amino acids 40%, carbohydrate 50%, fat nil, phenylalanine not more than 10 mg per 100 g, with vitamins, minerals, and trace elements. Net price 200 g = £12.79. For phenylketonuria

XP Concentrate, powder, amino acids 85%, carbohydrate and fat nil, phenylalanine not more than 25 mg per 100 g, with vitamins, minerals, and trace elements. Net price 200 g = £24.43. For phenylketonuria

Alembicol D® (Alembic Products)

Fractionated coconut oil. Net price 4 kg = £35.84. For steatorrhoea associated with cystic fibrosis of the pancreas, intestinal lymphangiectasia, surgery of the intestine, chronic liver disease, liver cirrhosis, other proven malabsorption syndromes; and in a ketogenic diet in the management of epilepsy

Aminex® (Cow & Gate)

Biscuits, protein 0.9% (phenylalanine 0.021%), carbohydrate 76.1%, fat 8.4%, lactose- and sucrose-free. Net price 12 × 12.5-g biscuits = £1.14. For phenylketonuria; similar amino-acid abnormalities; liver cirrhosis; chronic renal failure; lactose with sucrose intolerance

Aminogran® (A&H)

Food Supplement, powder, containing all essential amino acids except phenylalanine, for use with mineral mixture

(see below). Net price 500 g = £43.87. For phenylketonuria

Mineral Mixture, powder, containing all appropriate minerals for use with the above food supplement and other synthetic diets. Net price 250 g = £7.43. For phenylketonuria and as a mineral supplement in synthetic diets

Aproten® (Ultrapharm)

Various products, gluten-free, low protein, low Na⁺ and K⁺. Net prices: anellini 250 g = £1.95; biscuits 180 g (36) = £2.00; crispbread 240 g = £3.58; ditalini 250 g = £1.95; flour 500 g = £1.76; rigatini 250 g = £1.95; tagliatelle 250 g = £1.95. For phenylketonuria; similar amino-acid abnormalities; renal failure; liver failure and liver cirrhosis; gluten-sensitive enteropathies including steatorrhoea due to gluten sensitivity, coeliac disease, and dermatitis herpetiformis

Bi-Aglut® (Ultrapharm)

Flour, rice flour, maize starch, with vitamins, gluten- and lactose-free. Net price 500 g = £1.95

Biscuits, starch, sugar, eggs, skimmed milk solids, flavourings, gluten-free. Net price 180 g (36) = £2.00

Cracker toast, potato starch, sugar, rice flour, soya flour, hydrogenated vegetable fat, flavourings, gluten-, lactose-, and milk-protein-free. Net price 240 g (40) = £2.58. For gluten-sensitive enteropathies including steatorrhoea due to gluten sensitivity, coeliac disease, and dermatitis herpetiformis

Calogen® (Scientific Hospital Supplies)

Emulsion, arachis oil 50% in water. Net price 1 litre = £7.23; 2 litres = £13.94. For renal failure and other conditions requiring a high-energy, low-fluid, low-electrolyte diet, disorders of amino-acid metabolism or carbohydrate absorption; in a ketogenic diet in the management of epilepsy

Caloreen® (Roussel)

Powder, water-soluble dextrins, predominantly polysaccharides containing an average of 5 glucose molecules, with less than 1.8 mmol of Na⁺ and 0.3 mmol of K⁺/100 g. Net price 250 g = £1.14; 5 kg = £19.52. For indications, see under Duocal (below).

Carobel, Instant® (Cow & Gate)

Powder, carob seed flour. Net price 150 g = £2.74. For thickening feeds in the treatment of vomiting

Casilan® (Farley)

Powder, whole protein, containing all essential amino acids, 90% with less than 0.1% Na⁺. Net price 250 g = £2.71. For biochemically proven hypoproteinaemia

Comminuted Chicken Meat (Cow & Gate)

Suspension (aqueous). Net price 110 g = 87p. For carbohydrate intolerance in association with possible or proven intolerance of milk; glucose and galactose intolerance

Dialamine® (Scientific Hospital Supplies)

Powder, essential amino acids 30%, with carbohydrate 62%, energy 1500 kJ (360 kcal)/100 g, with ascorbic acid, minerals, and trace elements. Flavour: orange. Net price 1 kg = £57.20. For oral feeding where essential amino-acid supplements are required; e.g. chronic renal failure, hypoproteinaemia, wound fistula leakage with excessive protein loss, conditions requiring a controlled nitrogen intake and haemodialysis

dp® (GF Dietary Supplies)

Biscuits, low-protein, butterscotch- or chocolate-flavoured chip cookies. Net price 170 g = £4.00. For phenylketonuria; similar amino-acid abnormalities; renal failure; liver failure and liver cirrhosis

Duocal® (Scientific Hospital Supplies)

Liquid, emulsion providing carbohydrate 23.4 g, fat 7.1 g, energy 628 kJ/100 ml. Low-electrolyte, gluten-, lactose-, and protein-free. Net price 250 ml = £1.25; 1 litre = £4.42

Powder, carbohydrate 72.7 g, fat 22.3 g, energy 1960 kJ/100 g. Low-electrolyte, gluten-, lactose-, and protein-free. Net price 100 g = £2.08. For renal failure; liver cirrhosis; disaccharide intolerance (without isomaltose intolerance), disorders of amino acid metabolism (and other similar disorders) and/or whole protein intolerance; malabsorption states and other conditions requiring a high energy, low fluid intake, whether or not sodium and/or potassium restriction is essential

Ener-G® (General Designs)

Rice bread (brown, sliced), gluten-free. Net price 400 g = £2.86. For gluten-sensitive enteropathies including steatorrhoea due to gluten sensitivity, coeliac disease, and dermatitis herpetiformis

Forceval Protein® (Unigreg)

Powder, calcium caseinate 60%, carbohydrate 30%, with vitamins and minerals, providing not less than 55% protein, not more than 1% of fat, not more than 0.12% of Na⁺. Lactose- and gluten-free. Custard, strawberry, orange, and neutral flavours. Net price 8 × 15-g sachets = £3.10; 300 g = £7.03. For biochemically proven hypoproteinaemia and as a supplement for short-bowel syndrome; intractable malabsorption; pre-operative preparation of patients who are undernourished; treatment for those with proven inflammatory bowel disease; treatment following total gastrectomy; dysphagia, where a reduced salt intake is required; bowel fistulas. Not suitable as a sole source of nutrition for infants under 1 year or for children up to about 5 years

Formula S® (Cow & Gate)

Powder, soya protein isolate, glucose syrup, vegetable oil, vitamins and minerals, providing carbohydrate 6.7%, fat 3.6%, and protein 1.8% when used as a 12.7% solution. Net price 450 g = £2.29. For milk intolerance; galactosaemia, galactokinase deficiency, and lactose intolerance

Fortical® (Cow & Gate)

Liquid, glucose polymers providing carbohydrate 61.5 g/100 ml. Low-electrolyte, protein-free. Flavours: apple, apricot, black currant, lemon, orange, and neutral. Net price 200 ml = 63p. For renal failure; liver cirrhosis, or other conditions requiring a high-energy, low-fluid, low-electrolyte diet

Galactomin® (Cow & Gate)

Formula 17, powder, protein and fat 22.3 g each, carbohydrate 50.2 g, mineral salts 3 g/100 g. Used as a 12.5% solution with additional vitamins in place of milk. Net price 400 g = £6.97. For lactose intolerance and proven galactosaemia or galactokinase deficiency

Formula 18, powder, modification of Formula 17 with reduced fat ('half-cream'—14.4%). Net price 400 g = £7.92. For indications, see under Galactomin Formula 17

Formula 19, powder, modification of Formula 17 with reduced fat (14.4%) and fructose as carbohydrate source. Net price 400 g = £14.11. For glucose plus galactose intolerance

Glutenex® (Cow & Gate)

Biscuits, free from milk products, gluten-free. Net price 250 g (pack of 18) = £1.14. For gluten-sensitive enteropathies including steatorrhoea due to gluten sensitivity, coeliac disease, and dermatitis herpetiformis

Gluten-free biscuits (Farley)

Biscuits. Net price 200 g = 79p. For indications, see under Glutenex

Gluten-free crackers (GF Dietary Supplies)

Biscuits. Net price 200 g = £1.49. For indications, see under Glutenex

Hepatic-Aid II® (Boots)

Powder, maltodextrins, sucrose, amino acids, partially hydrogenated soya oil, lecithin, mono- and diglycerides, providing amino acids 4.4%, carbohydrate 16.8%, fat 3.6% when reconstituted. Low sodium and electrolytes; mineral and vitamin supplementation is required. Flavours: chocolate, chocolate mint, custard, eggnog. Net price per packet = £7.95. For patients with chronic liver disease and/or porto-hepatic encephalopathy

Hycal® (Beecham Products)

Liquid, protein-free, low-electrolyte, glucose syrup solids 49.5%. Flavours: black currant, lemon, orange,

raspberry. Net price 171 ml = 60p. For renal failure; liver cirrhosis or other conditions requiring a high-energy, low-fluid, low-electrolyte diet

Isomil® (Abbott)

Powder, corn syrup solids, sucrose, soya protein isolate, corn oil, coconut oil, vitamins, and minerals, providing protein 1.8%, carbohydrate 6.9%, fat 4.69% when reconstituted. Lactose-free. Net price 400 g = £2.38. For milk protein intolerance and lactose intolerance; galactosaemia and galactokinase deficiency

Juvela® (GF Dietary Supplies)

Gluten-free. Bread/cake mix; net price 500 g = £3.15. Bread (sliced and unsliced); 400-g loaf = £1.35. High-fibre bread (sliced and unsliced); 400-g loaf = £1.35. Corn mix; 500 g = £3.15. Fibre mix; 500 g = £3.15. For gluten-sensitive enteropathies including steatorrhoea due to gluten sensitivity, coeliac disease, and dermatitis herpetiformis

Low Protein. Bread/cake mix; net price 500 g = £3.15. Bread (sliced and unsliced); 400-g loaf = £1.35. For phenylketonuria and similar amino-acid abnormalities; renal failure; liver failure and liver cirrhosis; gluten-sensitive enteropathies, see above

Liquigen® (Scientific Hospital Supplies)

Emulsion, medium chain triglycerides 52%. Net price 1 litre = £12.21; 2 litres = £21.96. For steatorrhoea associated with cystic fibrosis of the pancreas; intestinal lymphangiectasia, surgery of the intestine; chronic liver disease and liver cirrhosis; other proven malabsorption syndromes; ketogenic diet in the management of epilepsy; type I hyperlipoproteinaemia

Locasol New Formula® (Cow & Gate)

Powder, protein 14.6 g, carbohydrate 56.5 g, fat 26.1 g, mineral salts 1.9 g, not more than 55 mg of $Ca^{2+}/100$ g and vitamins. Used as a 13.1% solution in place of milk. Net price 450 g = £8.73. For calcium intolerance

Lofenalac® (Bristol-Myers)

Powder, glucose syrup solids, casein hydrolysate, corn oil, modified tapioca starch, vitamins, and minerals, protein 15%, carbohydrate 60%, fat 18%, phenylalanine not more than 0.1%. Gluten-, sucrose-, and lactose-free. Net price 450 g = £8.00. For phenylketonuria

Maxamaid XP® (Scientific Hospital Supplies)

Powder, essential and non-essential amino acids 30% except phenylalanine, with carbohydrates, vitamins, minerals, and trace elements. Flavour: orange. Net price 100 g = £5.23; 200 g = £10.26. For phenylketonuria

Maxamum XP® (Scientific Hospital Supplies)

Powder, essential and non-essential amino acids 47% except phenylalanine, with carbohydrates, vitamins, minerals, and trace elements. Flavoured or unflavoured. Net price 200 g = £15.80. For phenylketonuria. Not to be prescribed for children under 8 years

Maxijul® (Scientific Hospital Supplies)

Liquid, maltodextrin providing carbohydrate 50%, with potassium 0.004%, sodium 0.023%. Gluten-, lactose-, and fructose-free. Flavours: black currant, lemon and lime, orange, and neutral. Net price 200 ml = 57p

Super Soluble Powder, glucose polymer, potassium 0.004%, sodium 0.046%. Gluten-, lactose-, and fructose-free. Net price 100 g = 47p. For renal failure; liver cirrhosis; disaccharide intolerance (without isomaltose intolerance); disorders of amino-acid metabolism (and other similar disorders) and/or whole protein intolerance; malabsorption states and other conditions, including proven hypoglycaemia, requiring a high-energy, low-fluid intake

Maxijul LE® (Scientific Hospital Supplies)

Powder, modification of Maxijul with lower concentrations of sodium and potassium. Net price 100 g = 74p. For indications, see under Maxijul where sodium and/or potassium restriction is also essential

Maxipro HBV® (Scientific Hospital Supplies)

Powder, whey protein and additional amino acids 88%, with some minerals. Net price 60 g = £1.61; 1 kg =

£16.60. For biochemically proven hypoproteinaemia and as a supplement for short-bowel syndrome; intractable malabsorption; pre-operative preparation of patients who are undernourished; treatment for those with proven inflammatory bowel disease; treatment following total gastrectomy; dysphagia, where a reduced salt intake is required; bowel fistulas. Not suitable as a sole source of nutrition for infants under 1 year or for children up to about 5 years

MCT Oil® (Bristol-Myers)
Triglycerides from medium chain fatty acids. Net price 950 ml = £7.80. For steatorrhoea associated with cystic fibrosis of the pancreas; intestinal lymphangiectasia; surgery of the intestine; chronic liver disease and liver cirrhosis; other proven malabsorption syndromes; in a ketogenic diet in the management of epilepsy; in type I hyperlipoproteinaemia

MCT (1)® (Cow & Gate)
Powder, protein 25.6%, carbohydrate 40.6%, medium chain triglycerides 28%, when used as a 12.5% solution. Low in lactose and sucrose-free. Net price 400 g = £5.41. For steatorrhoea associated with cystic fibrosis of the pancreas; intestinal lymphangiectasia; chronic liver disease; surgery of the intestine in infants

Medium Chain Triglyceride (MCT) Oil® (Cow & Gate)
Triglycerides from medium chain fatty acids. Net price 1 litre = £11.87. For indications, see under MCT Oil

Metabolic Mineral Mixture® (Scientific Hospital Supplies)
Powder, essential mineral salts. Net price 100 g = £4.64. For mineral supplementation in synthetic diets

Milupa PKU 3® (Milupa)
Granules, containing essential and non-essential amino acids except phenylalanine, vitamins, minerals, and trace elements, with 3.4% sucrose. Flavour vanilla. Net price 500 g = £36.00. For phenylketonuria, not recommended for child under 8 years

Minafen® (Cow & Gate)
Powder, equivalent of 12.5% protein, carbohydrate 48%, fat 31%, not more than 0.02% of phenylalanine. For use as 12.5% solution with additional vitamins. Net price 454 g = £10.59. For phenylketonuria

MSUD Aid® (Scientific Hospital Supplies)
Powder, containing full range of amino acids except isoleucine, leucine, and valine, with vitamins, minerals, and trace elements. Net price 200 g = £25.12. For maple syrup urine disease

Nestargel® (Nestlé)
Powder, carob seed flour 96.5%, calcium lactate 3.5%. Net price 125 g = £3.46. For thickening feeds in the treatment of vomiting

Nutramigen® (Bristol-Myers)
Powder, casein hydrolysate, corn oil, corn syrup solids, glucose, vitamins, and minerals, providing protein 13%, carbohydrate 62%, fat 18%. Gluten-, sucrose-, and lactose-free. Net price 425 g = £7.00. For infants over 3 months and children with galactokinase deficiency; galactosaemia; lactose intolerance and/or sucrose intolerance; sensitivity to whole protein

PK Aid 1® (Scientific Hospital Supplies)
Powder, containing essential and non-essential amino acids except phenylalanine. Net price 200 g = £25.57. For phenylketonuria

Polial® (Ultrapharm)
Biscuits, Free from egg, milk protein, wheat starch, gluten, and lactose. Net price 200-g pack = £2.30. For gluten-sensitive enteropathies including steatorrhoea due to gluten sensitivity, coeliac disease, and dermatitis herpetiformis

Polycal® (Cow & Gate)
Powder, glucose, maltose, and polysaccharides, providing 1610 kJ (380 kcal)/100 g. Net price 400 g = £1.78; 2 kg = £7.13. For renal failure; liver cirrhosis; disaccharide intolerance (without isomaltose intolerance); disorders

of amino-acid metabolism (and other similar disorders) and/or whole protein intolerance; malabsorption states and other conditions, including proven hypoglycaemia, requiring a high-energy, low-fluid intake, whether or not sodium and/or potassium restriction is essential

Polycose® (Abbott)
Powder, glucose polymers, providing carbohydrate 94 g, energy 1600 kJ (380 kcal)/100 g. Net price 350-g can = £2.19. For renal failure; liver cirrhosis; disaccharide intolerance (without isomaltose intolerance); disorders of amino-acid metabolism (and other similar disorders) and/or whole protein intolerance; malabsorption states and other conditions, including proven hypoglycaemia, requiring a high-energy, low-fluid intake, whether or not sodium and/or potassium restriction is essential

Pregestimil® (Bristol-Myers)
Powder, glucose syrup solids, casein hydrolysate, corn oil, modified tapioca starch, medium chain triglycerides, vitamins, and minerals, providing protein 12.8%, carbohydrate 61.6%, fat 18.3%. Gluten-, sucrose-, and lactose-free. Net price 454 g = £8.01. For sucrose and/or lactose intolerance in association with whole protein intolerance, or where amino acids and peptides are indicated in conjunction with medium chain triglycerides. Also for proven malabsorption syndromes in which a reduced fat diet is indicated such as steatorrhoea associated with cystic fibrosis and surgery of the intestine; galactosaemia and galactokinase deficiency

ProMod® (Abbott)
Powder, whey protein and soya lecithin, providing protein 75.8%, carbohydrate 10.2%, fat 9.1%. Gluten-free. Net price 275-g can = £6.18. For biochemically proven hypoproteinaemia

Prosobee® (Bristol-Myers)
Liquid concentrate, prepared from soya protein isolate, soya oil, glucose syrup solids, coconut oil, L-methionine, vitamins, and minerals, providing protein 4.1%, carbohydrate 13.7%, fat 7.2%. Gluten-, sucrose-, and lactose-free. Net price 385 ml = £1.39
Powder, glucose syrup solids, soya protein isolate, corn oil, coconut oil, L-methionine, vitamins, and minerals, providing protein 15.6%, carbohydrate 51.4%, fat 27.9%. Gluten-, sucrose-, and lactose-free. Net price 400 g = £3.56. For milk intolerance; galactosaemia, galactokinase deficiency, and lactose intolerance

Protifar® (Cow & Gate)
Powder, milk proteins providing protein 88.5%. Low lactose, gluten- and sucrose-free. Net price 225 g = £3.14. For biochemically proven hypoproteinaemia

Rite-Diet® (Welfare Foods)
Gluten-free. Sweet biscuits. Net price 150 g = 79p. High-fibre crackers. 150 g = £1.10. Digestive biscuits. 150 g = 79p. Savoury biscuits. 125 g = 79p. Flour mix. 500 g = £1.32. Bread mix, 500 g (brown) = £1.45; white, 500 g = £1.29. Bread (white). 400 g = £1.35. High-fibre bread (with soya bran). 400 g = £1.35. For gluten-sensitive enteropathies including steatorrhoea due to gluten sensitivity, coeliac disease, and dermatitis herpetiformis
Low protein/gluten-free. Macaroni. Net price 250 g = £1.43. Spaghetti, shortcut. 250 g = £1.43. Rings. 250 g = £1.43. Flour mix. 400 g = £1.12p. Bread; 227 g = 96p. Bread with soya bran; 280 g = 98p. Bread (with or without salt). 227 g = 86p. White bread (with added fibre). 400 g = £1.35. Crackers. 150 g = £1.10. Sweet biscuits. 150 g = 92p. Vanilla cream wafers. 100 g = 64p. Chocolate-flavoured cream wafers, 100 g = 64p. Cream-filled biscuits (chocolate flavour). 125 g = 92p. For phenylketonuria and similar amino-acid abnormalities; renal failure; liver failure and liver cirrhosis; see also gluten-free foods above
Low sodium. Bread containing protein 8.5%, carbohydrate 53.8%, fat 5.5%, Na⁺ 0.01%, K⁺ 0.055%. Net price 227 g = 96p. For conditions in which a low-sodium diet is indicated

Tritamyl® (Procea)

Flour, self-raising (starch-based), gluten- and lactose-free. Net price 2 kg = £5.10. For gluten-sensitive entero-pathies including steatorrhoea due to gluten sensitivity, coeliac disease, and dermatitis herpetiformis

Tritamyl PK® (Procea)

Flour, self-raising (starch-based), gluten-, lactose-, and protein-free. Net price 2 kg = £3.60. For phenylketo-nuria and similar amino-acid abnormalities; renal failure; liver failure and liver cirrhosis; gluten-sensitive entero-pathies as above

Trufree® (Cantassium)

Gluten-free, wheat-free flours. For gluten-sensitive enteropathies including steatorrhoea due to gluten-sensitivity, coeliac disease, and dermatitis herpetiformis

No. 1 (formerly bread mix 420 g). Net price 1 kg = £2.70

No. 2 with rice bran (formerly bread mix with rice bran 410 g). Net price 1 kg = £3.45

No. 3 for Cantabread® (formerly Cantabread mix). Net price 1 kg = £3.60

No. 4 white. Net price 1 kg = £2.70

No. 5 brown. Net price 1 kg = £2.70

No. 6 plain (formerly Trufree plain flour). Net price 1 kg = £2.33

No. 7 self-raising (formerly Trufree self-raising flour). Net price 1 kg = £2.48

Verkade® (GF Dietary Supplies)

Biscuits, gluten-free. Net price 200 g (38) = £2.25. For gluten-sensitive enteropathies including steatorrhoea due to gluten sensitivity, coeliac disease, and dermatitis herpetiformis

Wysoy® (Wyeth)

Powder, soya protein isolate, sucrose, corn syrup solids, animal and vegetable oil, vitamins and minerals, pro-viding carbohydrate 6.9%, fat 3.6%, and protein 2.1% when reconstituted. Net price 430 g = £2.42; 860 g = £4.65. For milk intolerance, galactosaemia, galacto-kinase deficiency, and lactose intolerance

9.4.2   Enteral nutrition

The body's reserves of protein rapidly become exhausted in severely ill patients, especially during chronic illness or in those with severe burns, extensive trauma, pancreatitis, or intestinal fistula. Much can be achieved by frequent meals and by persuading the patient to take sup-plementary snacks of ordinary food between the meals.

However, extra calories, protein, other nutri-ents, and vitamins are often best given by sup-plementing ordinary meals with sip or tube feeds of one of the nutritionally complete foods.

When patients cannot feed normally at all, for example patients with severe facial injury, oeso-phageal obstruction, or coma, a diet composed solely of nutritionally complete foods must be given. This is planned by a dietitian who will take into account the protein and total energy requirement of the patient and decide on the form and relative contribution of carbohydrate and fat to the energy requirements.

There are a number of nutritionally complete foods available and their use reduces an otherwise heavy workload in hospital or in the home. Most contain protein derived from milk or soya. Some contain protein hydrolysates or free amino acids and are only appropriate for patients who have diminished ability to break down protein, as may

be the case in inflammatory bowel disease or pancreatic insufficiency.

Even when nutritionally complete feeds are being given it may be important to monitor water and electrolyte balance. Extra minerals (e.g. mag-nesium and zinc) may be needed in patients where gastro-intestinal secretions are being lost. Additional vitamins may also be needed. Regular haematological and biochemical tests may be needed particularly in the unstable patient.

Some feeds are supplemented with vitamin K; for drug interactions of vitamin K see Appendix 1 (sections *2.8, 2.8A*).

CHILDREN. Infants and young children have special requirements and in most situations liquid feeds prepared for adults are totally unsuitable and should not be given. Expert advice should be sought.

ACBS indications. Unless otherwise indicated the food preparations listed below can be prescribed on form FP10 for patients with short-bowel syndrome, intractable malabsorption, pre-operative preparation of patients who are undernourished, treatment for proven inflammatory bowel disease, treatment fol-lowing total gastrectomy, dysphagia, bowel fistulas, and anorexia nervosa.

For a listing by clinical condition, see Appendix 3. Prescriptions for these foods issued in accordance with the advice of the Advisory Committee on Bor-derline Substances and endorsed 'ACBS' will nor-mally not be investigated.

Clinifeed® (Roussel)

Complete gluten-free foods in 4 formulations. For indi-cations, see notes above. Not to be prescribed for any child under one year, unsuitable as a sole source of nutrition for young children up to 5 years of age

Clinifeed 400, protein 15 g, carbohydrate 55 g, fat 13.4 g, energy 1674 kJ (400 kcal)/375 ml, with vitamins and minerals, vanilla flavour. Fructose-free. Net price 375-ml can = £1.00

Clinifeed Favour, protein 14.1 g, carbohydrate 52.5 g, fat 12.4 g, energy 1575 kJ (375 kcal)/375 ml, with vitamins and minerals, neutral flavour. Lactose-, fruct-ose-, and sucrose-free. Net price 375-ml can = 84p (not prescribable for anorexia nervosa)

Clinifeed Iso, protein 10.5 g, carbohydrate 49 g, fat 15.4 g, energy 1575 kJ (375 kcal)/375 ml, with vitamins and minerals, vanilla flavour. Fructose-, low sucrose-, and low sodium. Net price 375-ml can = £1.12

Clinifeed Protein Rich, protein 30 g, carbohydrate 70 g, fat 11 g, energy 2092 kJ (500 kcal)/375 ml, with vitamins and minerals, vanilla flavour. Fructose-free. Net price 375-ml can = £1.12

Elemental 028® (Scientific Hospital Supplies)

Powder, amino acids 12%, carbohydrate 77.8%, fat 6.64%, energy 1673 kJ (400 kcal)/100 g with vitamins and minerals. For preparation with water before use. Net price 100-g box (orange flavoured or plain) = £3.00. For indications, see notes above (except anorexia nervosa). Not to be prescribed for any child under one year, unsuitable as a sole source of nutrition for young children up to 5 years of age

Enrich® (Abbott)

Liquid with dietary fibre, glucose syrup solids, sucrose, caseinates, corn oil, soya polysaccharides and protein isolate, vitamins, and minerals, providing protein 9.4 g, carbohydrate 38.3 g (including 5 g as dietary fibre), fat 8.8 g, energy 1090 kJ (260 kcal)/250 ml. Lactose- and gluten-free. Net price 250-ml can = £1.30. For indications, see notes above. Not to be prescribed for any child under one year, unsuitable as a sole source of nutrition for young children up to 5 years of age

Ensure® (Abbott)

Liquid, protein 3.7%, fat 3.7%, carbohydrate 14.5%, with minerals and vitamins, lactose- and gluten-free, energy 1050 kJ (253 kcal)/250 ml. Vanilla, chocolate, coffee, eggnog and nut flavours. Net price 250-ml bottle = £1.18; 250-ml can = £1.10; 946-ml bottle or can = £3.62.

Powder, same composition as Ensure liquid when reconstituted. Net price 400 g = £4.65

Neither to be prescribed for any child under one year, unsuitable as a sole source of nutrition for young children up to 5 years of age

Ensure Plus® (Abbott)

Liquid, protein 6.3%, fat 5%, carbohydrate 20%, with vitamins and minerals, lactose- and gluten-free, energy 1570 kJ (375 kcal)/250 ml. Net price 250 ml = £1.23. For indications, see notes above

Flexical® (Bristol-Myers)

Powder, corn syrup solids, hydrolysed casein, soya oil, modified tapioca starch, medium chain triglycerides, vitamins, and minerals, providing protein 9.9%, carbohydrate 67%, fat 15%. Gluten- and lactose-free. Net price 454 g = £9.36. For short-bowel syndrome, intractable malabsorption, pre-operative preparation of patients who are undernourished, and treatment following total gastrectomy, bowel fistulas, anorexia nervosa. Not to be prescribed for any child under one year, unsuitable as a sole source of nutrition for young children up to 5 years of age

Fortisip® (Cow & Gate)

Energy-plus, liquid, protein 10 g, carbohydrate 35.8 g, fat 13 g, energy 1260 kJ (300 kcal)/200 ml, with vitamins and minerals. Gluten-free and low lactose. Vanilla, banana, and orange flavours. Net price 200 ml = 62p

Standard, liquid, protein 8 g, carbohydrate 24 g, fat 8 g, energy 840 kJ (200 kcal)/200 ml, with vitamins and minerals. Gluten-free and low lactose. Net price 200 ml = 55p. Neither to be prescribed for any child under one year, unsuitable as a sole source of nutrition for young children up to 5 years of age

Fortison® (Cow & Gate)

Energy-plus, same composition as Fortisip energy-plus, providing 3150 kJ (750 kcal)/500 ml. Net price 500 ml = £1.46

Soya, liquid, protein 20 g, carbohydrate 60 g, fat 20 g, energy 2100 kJ (500 kcal)/500 ml, with vitamins and minerals. Gluten-free. Net price 500 ml = £1.45. For milk intolerance and lactose intolerance

Standard, same composition as Fortisip standard, providing 2100 kJ (500 kcal)/500 ml. Net price 500 ml = £1.33

None to be prescribed for any child under one year, unsuitable as a sole source of nutrition for young children up to 5 years of age

Fresubin® (Fresenius)

Liquid, milk and soya proteins, hydrolysed maize starch, sunflower oil, vitamins and minerals, providing protein 7.6 g, carbohydrate 27.6 g, fat 6.8 g, energy 840 kJ (200 kcal)/200 ml. Gluten-free, low lactose and cholesterol. Nut, peach, chocolate, and vanilla flavours. Net price 200-ml carton = 55p; 500-ml bottle = £1.25. For indications, see notes above. Not to be prescribed for any child under one year, unsuitable as a sole source of nutrition for young children up to 5 years of age

Fresubin Plus F® (Fresenius)

Liquid foods with dietary fibre in 2 formulations. For indications, see notes above. Not to be prescribed for any child under one year, unsuitable as a sole source of nutrition for young children up to 5 years of age

Muesli-flavour, milk protein, cereals, coconut, sunflower oil, vitamins and minerals providing protein 19.0 g, fat 17.0 g, carbohydrate 69.0 g, fibre 5.0 g, energy 2100 kJ

(500 kcal)/500 ml. Low sodium, lactose, and cholesterol. Net price 200-ml carton = 65p; 500-ml bottle = £1.50

Vegetable soup-flavour, milk protein, beef fat and protein, sunflower oil, maize starch, vitamins and minerals providing protein 19.0 g, fat 17.0 g, carbohydrate 69.0 g, fibre 3.0 g, energy 2100 kJ (500 kcal)/500 ml. Gluten-free, low sodium, lactose, and cholesterol. Net price 500-ml bottle = £1.50

Isocal® (Bristol-Myers)

Liquid, maltodextrin, soya oil, caseinate solids, medium chain triglycerides, soya protein isolate, vitamins, and minerals, providing protein 3.2%, carbohydrate 12.6%, fat 4.2%. Gluten- and lactose-free. Net price 250 ml = 60p. For indications, see notes above. Not to be prescribed for any child under one year, unsuitable as a sole source of nutrition for young children up to 5 years of age

Liquisorb® (Merck)

Liquid, milk and whey proteins and casein, maltodextrin, sucrose, soya oil, vitamins and minerals, providing protein 20 g, carbohydrate 59 g, fat 20 g, energy 2095 kJ (500 kcal)/500 ml. Gluten-free, low lactose. Banana, vanilla, chocolate, and neutral flavours. Net price 500-ml bottle = £1.30. For indications, see notes above. Not to be prescribed for any child under one year, unsuitable as a sole source of nutrition for young children up to 5 years of age

Liquisorbon MCT® (Merck)

Liquid, milk proteins, maltodextrin, sucrose, mediumchain triglycerides, vitamins and minerals, providing protein 25 g, carbohydrate 61.5 g, fat 16.5 g, energy 2095 kJ (500 kcal)/500 ml. Gluten- and fructose-free, low lactose. Chocolate, strawberry, vanilla, and neutral flavours. Net price 500 ml = £2.15. For indications see notes above. Not to be prescribed for any child under one year, unsuitable as a sole source of nutrition for young children up to 5 years of age

Nutranel® now called **Pepti-2000 LF®**

Osmolite® (Abbott)

Liquid, caseinates, soya protein isolate, hydrolysed corn starch, medium chain triglycerides, corn oil, soya oil, vitamins, and minerals, providing protein 10.5 g, carbohydrate 33.4 g, fat 8.7 g, energy 1050 kJ (250 kcal)/250 ml. Gluten- and lactose-free. Net price 250-ml can = £1.04. For indications, see notes above. Not to be prescribed for any child under one year, unsuitable as a sole source of nutrition for young children up to 5 years of age

Pepti-2000 LF® (Cow & Gate)

Powder, maltodextrin, whey protein hydrolysate, corn oil, medium chain triglycerides, vitamins and minerals, providing protein 15.8%, fat 3.9%, and carbohydrate 73.9%. Gluten-free. Net price 101 g = £1.99. For intractable malabsorption; bowel fistulas; following total gastrectomy. Not to be prescribed for any child under one year, unsuitable as a sole source of nutrition for young children up to 5 years of age

Peptisorb® (Merck)

Liquid, amino acids and peptides 3.75%, carbohydrate 18.75%, fat 1.11%, with vitamins and minerals, low lactose, and fructose- and gluten-free, energy 2100 kJ (500 kcal)/500 ml. Net price 500 ml = £4.60. For intractable malabsorption; bowel fistulas; treatment following total gastrectomy
For adults only

Peptisorbon® (Merck)

Powder, amino acids and peptides 18%, carbohydrate 70%, fat 5.3%, with vitamins and minerals, low lactose, and fructose- and gluten-free, energy 1393 kJ (333 kcal)/sachet. Net price 83.3-g sachet = £1.72. For intractable malabsorption; bowel fistulas; treatment following total gastrectomy
For adults only

Portagen® (Bristol-Myers)

Powder, corn syrup solids, medium chain triglycerides, sodium caseinate, sucrose, corn oil, vitamins, and minerals, providing protein 16.5%, carbohydrate 54%, fat 22%. Gluten- and lactose-free. Net price 454 g = £6.23. For lactose intolerance without sucrose intolerance but requiring medium chain triglycerides; malabsorption associated with cystic fibrosis of the pancreas; intestinal lymphangiectasia; surgery of the intestine; chronic liver disease and liver cirrhosis; other proven malabsorption syndromes

Reabilan® (Roussel)

Liquid, casein and whey peptides, maltodextrin, starch, medium chain triglycerides, evening primrose oil, soya oil, vitamins and minerals, providing protein 11.8 g, carbohydrate 49.3 g, fat 14.6 g, energy 1575 kJ (375 kcal)/375 ml. Gluten- and lactose-free. Net price 375 ml = £3.08. For short bowel syndrome; intractable malabsorption; pre-operative preparation of patients who are undernourished; treatment for those with inflammatory bowel disease; treatment following total gastrectomy; dysphagia; bowel fistulas. Not to be prescribed for any child under 1 year, unsuitable as a sole source of nutrition for young children up to 5 years of age

Triosorbon® (Merck)

Powder, protein 19%, carbohydrate 56%, fat 19%, with vitamins and minerals. Gluten-free. Net price 85-g sachet = £1.15. For indications, see notes above. Not to be prescribed for any child under one year, unsuitable as a sole source of nutrition for young children up to 5 years of age

PoM Vivonex® (Norwich Eaton)

Powder, amino acids 6.18 g, simple sugars 69 g, safflower oil 435 mg/80-g sachet, with added vitamins and minerals. For preparation with water before use. Net price 80-g sachet = £1.50; flavour sachets 60 × 2 g = £4.68. For short-bowel syndrome, intractable malabsorption, pre-operative preparation of patients who are under-nourished, and treatment following total gastrectomy; dysphagia due to an incurable malignancy; bowel fistulas; anorexia nervosa. Not to be prescribed for any child under one year, unsuitable as a sole source of nutrition for young children up to 5 years of age

ASSOCIATED PRODUCTS

Ketovite® (Paines & Byrne)

PoM *Tablets*, yellow, ascorbic acid 16.6 mg, riboflavine 1 mg, thiamine hydrochloride 1 mg, pyridoxine hydrochloride 330 micrograms, nicotinamide 3.3 mg, calcium pantothenate 1.16 mg, alpha tocopheryl acetate 5 mg, inositol 50 mg, biotin 170 micrograms, folic acid 250 micrograms, acetomenaphthone 500 micrograms. Net price 20 = 38p

Liquid, pink, sugar-free, vitamin A 2500 units, vitamin D 400 units, choline chloride 150 mg, cyanocobalamin 12.5 micrograms/5 ml. Diluent purified water, freshly boiled and cooled, life of diluted liquid 7 days. Net price 100 ml = £1.19

Dose: as a vitamin supplement with synthetic diets, 5 ml liquid daily and 1 tablet 3 times daily

Ruthmol® (Cantassium)

Salt substitute, potassium chloride 50%. Net price 250 g = £1.42

Supplementary Vitamin Tablets for Infants (Cow & Gate)

Tablets, ferrous sulphate 4.21 mg (850 micrograms iron), folic acid 63 micrograms, thiamine hydrochloride 250 micrograms, nicotinamide 830 micrograms, riboflavine 250 micrograms, pyridoxine hydrochloride 83 micrograms, cyanocobalamin 1 microgram, ascorbic acid 10 mg, d-α-tocopheryl acetate 1.24 mg, acetomenaphthone 125 micrograms, biotin 8 micrograms, calcium pantothenate 500 micrograms, copper 34 micrograms (as

sulphate), iodine 12 micrograms (as potassium iodate), manganese 5 micrograms (as sulphate), molybdenum 6 micrograms (as ammonium molybdate), zinc 620 micrograms (as sulphate). Contains sucrose. Net price 100 = £3.15

Note. For infants on nutritionally incomplete synthetic foods

Dose: consult manufacturer's literature

9.5   Minerals

9.5.1 Calcium
9.5.2 Phosphorus
9.5.3 Fluoride
9.5.4 Zinc

See section 9.1.1 for iron salts.

9.5.1   Calcium

9.5.1.1 Calcium supplements
9.5.1.2 Hypercalcaemia

9.5.1.1   CALCIUM SUPPLEMENTS

Calcium supplements are usually only required where dietary calcium intake is deficient. This dietary requirement varies with age and is relatively greater in childhood, pregnancy, and lactation, due to an increased demand, and in old age, due to impaired absorption. In osteoporosis a daily supplement of 800 mg (20 mmol) calcium may reduce the rate of bone loss, but larger doses have not been shown to be more effective. Patients with hypoparathyroidism rarely require calcium supplements after the early stages of stabilisation on vitamin D (section 9.6.4).

In hypocalcaemic tetany an initial intravenous injection of 10 ml (2.25 mmol) of calcium gluconate injection may be followed by the continuous infusion of about 40 ml (9 mmol) daily, but plasma calcium should be monitored. This regimen can also be used, immediately but temporarily, to reduce the toxic effects of hyperkalaemia.

In cardiac arrest 10 ml of calcium gluconate injection may be given by intravenous or intracardiac injection (see section 2.7).

CALCIUM SALTS

Indications: see notes above; calcium deficiency
Cautions: drug interactions: see Appendix 1 (section 9), parenteral calcium therapy is contra-indicated in patients receiving cardiac glycosides
Side-effects: bradycardia, arrhythmias, and irritation after intravenous injection
Dose: by mouth, daily in divided doses, as calcium gluconate or lactate, see notes above
By intramuscular or slow intravenous injection, acute hypocalcaemia, calcium gluconate 1–2 g (2.25–4.5 mmol of Ca^{2+}); avoid intramuscular route in children

Calcium Gluconate Tablets, calcium gluconate 600 mg (1.35 mmol Ca^{2+}). To be chewed before swallowing. Net price 20 = 42p. Label: 24

Calcium Gluconate Tablets, Effervescent, calcium gluconate 1 g (2.25 mmol Ca^{2+}). Net price 100 = £4.69. Label: 13
Note. Each tablet usually contains sodium 102.6 mg (4.46 mmol Na^+)
PoM **Calcium Gluconate Injection,** calcium gluconate 10%. Net price 5-ml amp = 41p; 10-ml amp = 47p
Calcium Lactate Tablets, calcium lactate 300 mg (1 mmol Ca^{2+}), net price 20 = 22p; 600 mg (2 mmol Ca^{2+}), 20 = 38p
Calcium-Sandoz® (Sandoz)
Syrup, calcium glubionate 3.27 g, calcium galactogluconate 2.17 g (325 mg calcium or 8.1 mmol Ca^{2+})/15 ml. Diluent syrup, life of diluted syrup 14 days. Net price 100 ml = 49p
PoM *Injection*, calcium glubionate equivalent to 10% of calcium gluconate (93 mg calcium or 2.32 mmol Ca^{2+}/10 ml). Net price 10-ml amp = 27p
PoM **Min-I-Jet Calcium Chloride 10%®** (IMS)
Injection, calcium chloride 100 mg/ml. Net price 10-ml disposable syringe = £2.45 and £3.10 (longer needle)
Ossopan® (Labaz)
Tablets, buff, f/c, hydroxyapatite 830 mg (4.4mmol Ca^{2+}). Net price 20 = £4.14
Oral powder, hydroxyapatite 820 mg (4.4mmol Ca^{2+})/g. Net price 50 g = £5.76
Sandocal® (Sandoz)
Tablets, effervescent, orange, calcium lactate gluconate 3.08 g, equivalent to calcium gluconate 4.5 g and provides calcium 400 mg (10 mmol Ca^{2+}), sodium 137 mg (6 mmol Na^+), potassium 176 mg (4.5 mmol K^+) and 1.1 g citric acid (1.08 g citrate ion). Net price 20 = £1.47. Label: 13
Caution: avoid in renal impairment

9.5.1.2 HYPERCALCAEMIA

The cause for hypercalcaemia should be established before treatment is started, unless the patient is seriously ill. Rehydration and the exclusion of calcium from the patient's diet are essential and on occasions are all that is necessary.

Agents such as sodium cellulose phosphate which bind calcium in the gut may be helpful, but any associated increase in plasma phosphate may be harmful. Similarly, oral and intravenous phosphate may only achieve a reduction in plasma calcium by precipitating calcium phosphate in the tissues, resulting in nephrocalcinosis and impairment of renal function.

Agents which inhibit mobilisation of calcium from the skeleton are usually required where hypercalcaemia is severe. Plicamycin (see section 8.1.2) is probably the most rapidly effective drug, but cannot be given continuously for more than a few days because of marrow toxicity. Corticosteroids (see section 6.3) and calcitonin (see section 6.6.1) may be helpful but often take several days to achieve the desired effect and may be totally ineffective even in massive dosage. Calcitonin is relatively non-toxic but expensive and a

daily dose of 200 units is usually as effective as larger doses.

Intravenous chelating agents such as trisodium edetate are rarely used although theoretically safer than intravenous phosphate if given by slow continuous infusion. They usually cause pain in the limb receiving the infusion and may cause renal damage.

Disodium etidronate (see section 6.6.2) is now indicated in hypercalcaemia of malignancy.

SODIUM CELLULOSE PHOSPHATE

Indications: hypercalcaemia, reduction of calcium absorption from food (in conjunction with low-calcium diet)
Contra-indications: congestive heart failure, renal impairment
Side-effects: occasional diarrhoea
Dose: 5 g 3 times daily with meals; CHILD 10 g daily in 3 divided doses with meals

Calcisorb® (Riker)
Sachets, sodium cellulose phosphate 5 g. Net price 10 sachets = £2.19. Label: 13, 21, counselling advised, may be sprinkled on food

TRISODIUM EDETATE

Indications: hypercalcaemia; removal of lime burns in the eye
Cautions: plasma-calcium determinations required; caution in tuberculosis
Contra-indications: impaired renal function
Side-effects: nausea, diarrhoea, cramp; in overdosage renal damage
Dose: by slow intravenous infusion, up to 70 mg/kg daily over 2–3 hours

PoM **Limclair®** (Sinclair)
Injection, trisodium edetate 200 mg/ml. Net price 5-ml amp = £2.57
For topical use in the eye, dilute 1 ml to 50 ml with sterile purified water

9.5.2 Phosphorus
9.5.2.1 Phosphate supplements
9.5.2.2 Phosphate-binding agents

9.5.2.1 PHOSPHATE SUPPLEMENTS

Oral phosphate supplements may be required in addition to vitamin D in a small minority of patients with hypophosphataemic vitamin D-resistant rickets. Diarrhoea is a common side-effect and should prompt a reduction in dosage.

Phosphate-Sandoz® (Sandoz)
Tablets, effervescent, anhydrous sodium acid phosphate 1.936 g, sodium bicarbonate 350 mg, potassium bicarbonate 315 mg, equivalent to phosphorus 500 mg (16.1 mmol P), sodium 468.8 mg (20.4 mmol Na^+), potassium 123 mg (3.1 mmol K^+). Net price 20 = 75p. Label: 13

9.5.2.2 PHOSPHATE-BINDING AGENTS

Aluminium-containing and calcium-containing antacids are used as phosphate-binding agents in the management of renal failure. They are contra-indicated in hypophosphataemia; calcium-containing phosphate-binding agents are also contra-indicated in hypercalcaemia or hypercalciuria.

ALUMINIUM HYDROXIDE
Indications: hyperphosphataemia
Cautions: hyperaluminaemia; see also notes above

Alu-Cap® (Riker)
Capsules, green/red, dried aluminium hydroxide 475 mg (low Na⁺). Net price 20 = 64p
Dose: phosphate-binding agent in renal failure, 4–20 capsules daily

CALCIUM CARBONATE
Indications: hyperphosphataemia
Cautions: see notes above
Side-effects: hypercalcaemia

Titralac® (Riker)
Tablets, calcium carbonate 420 mg, glycine 180 mg. Net price 20 = 19p
Dose: calcium supplement or phosphate-binding agent in renal failure, according to the requirements of the patient

9.5.3   Fluoride
Availability of adequate fluoride confers significant resistance to dental caries. It is now considered that the topical action of fluoride on enamel and plaque is more important than the systemic effect.

Where the natural fluoride content of the drinking water is significantly less than 1 mg per litre (one part per million) artificial fluoridation is the most economical method of supplementing fluoride intake.

Daily administration of tablets or drops is a suitable alternative, but systemic fluoride supplements should not be prescribed without prior reference to the fluoride content of the local water supply; they are not advisable when the water contains more than 700 micrograms per litre (0.7 parts per million). In addition, it is now recommended that infants should not receive fluoride supplements until the age of 6 months.

Use of dentifrices which incorporate sodium fluoride and/or monofluorophosphate is also a convenient source of fluoride.

Individuals who are either particularly caries prone or medically compromised may be given additional protection by use of fluoride rinses or by application of fluoride gels. Rinses may be used daily or weekly; daily use of a less concentrated rinse is more effective than weekly use of a more concentrated one. Gels must be applied on a regular basis under professional supervision; extreme caution is necessary to prevent the child from swallowing any excess. Less concentrated gels have recently become available for home use. Varnishes are also available and particularly valuable for young or handicapped children since they adhere to the teeth and set in the presence of moisture.

> There are arrangements for health authorities to supply fluoride tablets in the course of pre-school dental schemes, and they may also be supplied in school dental schemes.

SODIUM FLUORIDE
Note. Sodium fluoride 2.2 mg provides approx. 1 mg fluoride ion
Indications: prophylaxis of dental caries—see notes above
Contra-indications: not for areas where drinking water is fluoridated
Side-effects: occasional white flecks on teeth with recommended doses; rarely yellowish-brown discoloration if recommended doses are exceeded
Dose: CHILD, as fluoride ion:
Water content less than 300 micrograms/litre, up to 6 months, none; 6 months–2 years, 250 micrograms daily; 2–4 years, 500 micrograms daily; over 4 years, 1 mg daily
Water content between 300 and 700 micrograms/litre, up to 2 years, none; 2–4 years, 250 micrograms daily; over 4 years, 500 micrograms daily.

Tablets
COUNSELLING. Tablets should be sucked or dissolved in the mouth and taken preferably in the evening

En-De-Kay® (Stafford-Miller)
Fluotabs Additive Free, sodium fluoride 550 micrograms (250 micrograms F⁻). Net price 200-tab pack = £1.16
Fluotabs 2–4 years, natural orange-flavoured, scored, sodium fluoride 1.1 mg (500 micrograms F⁻). Net price 200-tab pack = £1.16
Fluotabs 4+ years, natural orange-flavoured, scored, sodium fluoride 2.2 mg (1 mg F⁻). Net price 200-tab pack = £1.16
Fluor-a-day® (Dental Health)
Tablets, buff, scored, sodium fluoride 2.2 mg (1 mg F⁻). Net price 200-tab pack = 98p
Fluorigard® (Hoyt)
Tablets 0.5, purple, sodium fluoride 1.1 mg (500 micrograms F⁻). Net price 120-tab pack = 84p
Tablets 1.0, sodium fluoride 2.2 mg (1 mg F⁻). Net price 120-tab pack = 84p (available in 4 colours and flavours)
Zymafluor® (Zyma)
Tablets, sodium fluoride 550 micrograms (250 micrograms F⁻), net price 400-tab pack = 75p; 2.2 mg (1 mg F⁻) (yellow-grey), 100-tab pack = 55p

---

Oral drops
Note. Fluoride supplements no longer considered necessary below 6 months of age (see notes above)
En-De-Kay® (Stafford-Miller)
Fluodrops® (= paediatric drops), sugar-free, sodium fluoride 500 micrograms (250 micrograms F⁻)/0.15 ml. Net price 60 ml = 93p
Fluorigard® (Hoyt)
Paediatric drops, sodium fluoride 275 micrograms (125 micrograms F⁻)/drop. Net price 30 ml = 90p

Mouth-washes
Rinse mouth for 1 minute and spit out
COUNSELLING. Avoid eating, drinking, or rinsing mouth for 15 minutes after use
PoM **En-De-Kay**® (Stafford-Miller)
Fluorinse (= mouth-wash), red, sodium fluoride 2%. Net price 100 ml = £1.82
For *daily* use, dilute 5 drops to 10 ml of water; for *weekly* use, dilute 20 drops to 10 ml
Fluorigard® (Hoyt)
Daily dental rinse (= mouth-wash), blue, sodium fluoride 0.05%. Net price 500 ml = £1.75
Weekly dental rinse (= mouth-wash), blue, sodium fluoride 0.2%. Net price 150 ml = £1.16

9.5.4 Zinc

Oral zinc therapy should only be given when there is good evidence of deficiency (hypoproteinaemia spuriously lowers plasma-zinc concentrations). Zinc deficiency can occur in individuals on inadequate diets, in malabsorption, with increased body loss due to trauma, burns and protein-losing conditions, and during intravenous feeding. Therapy should continue until clinical improvement occurs and be replaced by dietary measures unless there is severe malabsorption, metabolic disease, or continuing zinc loss. Side-effects of zinc salts are abdominal pain and dyspepsia. Drug interactions: see Appendix 1 (section *5.1*, *9*, *9*, *10*)
Note. Most reliable test of zinc deficiency relates to ability to taste zinc sulphate solution 0.1%; profoundly zinc-deficient patients cannot distinguish between taste of this solution and water.

ZINC SALTS
Indications; Cautions; Side-effects: see notes

▼ **Solvazinc**® (Thames)
Effervescent tablets, yellow-white, zinc sulphate 200 mg (45 mg zinc). Net price 30 = £3.00. Label: 13, 21
Dose: 1 tablet in water 1–3 times daily after food
Zincomed® (Medo)
Capsules, blue/white, zinc sulphate 220 mg. Net price 20 = 59p. Label: 21
Dose: 1 capsule 3 times daily after food
Z Span® (SK&F)
Spansule® (= capsules s/r), blue/clear, enclosing white and grey pellets, zinc sulphate monohydrate 61.8 mg (22.5 mg zinc). Net price 20 = 92p. Label: 25
Dose: adults and children over 1 year, 1–3 capsules daily as required

9.6 Vitamins

Vitamins are used for the prevention and treatment of specific deficiency states or where the diet is known to be inadequate. Their use as general 'pick-me-ups' is of unproven value and, in the case of preparations containing vitamin A or D, may actually be harmful since many patients will take more than the prescribed dose. The recent 'fad' for mega-vitamin therapy with water-soluble vitamins, such as ascorbic acid and pyridoxine, is unscientific and can also be harmful.

In the NHS, vitamins may be prescribed to prevent or treat vitamin deficiency but they are not regarded as medicines when prescribed as dietary supplements.

9.6.1 Vitamin A
9.6.2 Vitamin B group
9.6.3 Vitamin C
9.6.4 Vitamin D
9.6.5 Vitamin E
9.6.6 Vitamin K
9.6.7 Multivitamin preparations

9.6.1 Vitamin A

Deficiency of vitamin A (retinol) is rare in Britain even in disorders of fat absorption.

Massive overdose can cause rough skin, dry hair, an enlarged liver, and a raised erythrocyte sedimentation rate and raised serum calcium and serum alkaline phosphatase concentrations. Use of excessive doses should be avoided in pregnancy.

VITAMIN A
(Retinol)
Indications; Cautions; Side-effects: see notes above
Dose: by mouth, prophylactic, 4000 units daily
Treatment of deficiency, 50 000 units daily (but rare, see notes above)

PoM **Ro-A-Vit**® (Roche)
Tablets, ivory, s/c, vitamin A (retinol) 50 000 units (as acetate). Net price 20 = 36p
Injection (oily), vitamin A (retinol) 300 000 units (as palmitate)/ml. Net price 1-ml amp = 88p
Dose: deficiency, *by deep intramuscular injection*, 150 000–300 000 units monthly, increased to weekly in acute deficiency states

Preparations of vitamins A and D
Halibut-liver Oil Capsules, vitamin A 4000 units [also contains vitamin D]. Net price 20 = 16p
Vitamins A and D Capsules, vitamin A 4000 units, vitamin D 400 units. Net price 20 = 27p
NHS **Halycitrol**® (LAB)
Emulsion, vitamin A 4600 units, vitamin D 380 units/5 ml. Net price 114 ml = 86p
Dose: 5 ml daily

9.6.2 Vitamin B group

Deficiency of the B vitamins, other than deficiency of vitamin B_{12} (section 9.1.2) is rare in Britain

---

and is usually treated by preparations containing thiamine (B$_1$), riboflavine (B$_2$), and nicotinamide, which is used in preference to nicotinic acid, as it does not cause vasodilatation. Other members (or substances traditionally classified as members) of the vitamin B complex such as aminobenzoic acid, biotin, choline, inositol, and pantothenic acid or panthenol may be included in vitamin B preparations but there is no evidence of their value.

Severe deficiency states and encephalopathy, especially as seen in chronic alcoholism, are best treated by the parenteral administration of B vitamins (Pabrinex®, Parentrovite®).

As with other vitamins of the B group, pyridoxine (B$_6$) deficiency is rare, but it may occur during isoniazid therapy and is characterised by peripheral neuritis. High doses of pyridoxine are given in some metabolic disorders, such as hyperoxaluria, and it is also used in sideroblastic anaemia (section 9.1.3). Pyridoxine has been tried in a wide variety of other disorders, including the premenstrual syndrome, but there is little sound evidence to support the claims, and overdosage induces toxic effects.

THIAMINE
(Vitamin B$_1$)
Indications: see notes above
Cautions: anaphylactic shock may occasionally follow intramuscular injection
Dose: mild chronic deficiency, 10–25 mg daily; severe deficiency, 200–300 mg daily

Thiamine Hydrochloride Tablets, thiamine hydrochloride 25 mg, net price 20 = 11p; 50 mg, 20 = 18p; 100 mg, 20 = 31p; 300 mg, 20 = 51p
NHS **Benerva**® (Roche)
Tablets, thiamine hydrochloride 25 mg, net price 20 = 12p; 50 mg, 20 = 19p; 100 mg, 20 = 33p; 300 mg, 20 = 54p

Compound preparations
PoM **Vitamins B and C Injection**
Weak, for intramuscular use, ascorbic acid 500 mg, nicotinamide 160 mg, pyridoxine hydrochloride 50 mg, riboflavine 4 mg, thiamine hydrochloride 100 mg/4 ml
Strong, for intramuscular use, ascorbic acid 500 mg, nicotinamide 160 mg, pyridoxine hydrochloride 50 mg, riboflavine 4 mg, thiamine hydrochloride 250 mg/7 ml
Strong, for intravenous use, ascorbic acid 500 mg, anhydrous glucose 1 g, nicotinamide 160 mg, pyridoxine hydrochloride 50 mg, riboflavine 4 mg, thiamine hydrochloride 250 mg/ 10 ml

Available as:
PoM **Pabrinex**® (Paines & Byrne)
Intramuscular maintenance injection, vitamins B and C injection, weak, for intramuscular use. Net price 4 ml (in 2 amps) = 40p
Intramuscular high potency injection, vitamins B and C injection, strong, for intramuscular use. Net price 7 ml (in 2 amps) = 43p

Intravenous high potency injection, vitamins B and C injection, strong, for intravenous use. Net price 10 ml (in 2 amps) = 43p
PoM **Parentrovite**® (Bencard)
IMM Injection, vitamins B and C injection, weak, for intramuscular use. Net price 4 ml (in 2 amps) = 40p
IMHP Injection, vitamins B and C injection, strong, for intramuscular use. Net price 7 ml (in 2 amps) = 43p
IVHP Injection, vitamins B and C injection, strong, for intravenous use. Net price 10 ml (in 2 amps) = 43p
Oral vitamin B complex preparations, see below

RIBOFLAVINE
(Vitamin B$_2$)
Indications: see notes above

Preparations
Injections of vitamins B and C, see under Thiamine
Oral vitamin B complex preparations, see below

PYRIDOXINE HYDROCHLORIDE
(Vitamin B$_6$)
Indications: isoniazid-induced   peripheral neuritis, idiopathic sideroblastic anaemia, deficiency states
Cautions: drug interactions: see Appendix 1 (section 4.9)
Dose: deficiency states, 20–50 mg up to 3 times daily
Isoniazid neuropathy, prophylaxis 10 mg daily; therapeutic, 50 mg three times daily
Idiopathic sideroblastic anaemia, 100–400 mg daily in divided doses
Premenstrual syndrome, 50–100 mg daily (but see notes above)

Pyridoxine Tablets, pyridoxine hydrochloride 10 mg, net price 20 = 32p; 20 mg, 20 = 26p; 50 mg, 20 = 49p
NHS **Benadon**® (Roche)
Tablets, pyridoxine hydrochloride 20 mg. Net price 20 = 26p
Tablets, scored, pyridoxine hydrochloride 50 mg. Net price 20 = 52p
NHS **Complement Continus**® (Napp)
Tablets, s/r, yellow, pyridoxine hydrochloride 100 mg. Net price 28 = £1.40. Label: 25
NHS **Paxadon**® (Steinhard)
Tablets, scored, pyridoxine hydrochloride 50 mg. Net price 20 = 46p

Injections of vitamins B and C, see under Thiamine

NICOTINAMIDE
Indications: see notes above

Nicotinamide Tablets, nicotinamide 50 mg. Net price 20 = 18p
Injections of vitamins B and C, see under Thiamine
Oral vitamin B complex preparations, see below

NICOTINIC ACID
See section 2.12

FOLIC ACID
See section 9.1.2

VITAMIN B₁₂
See section 9.1.2

ORAL VITAMIN B COMPLEX PREPARATIONS

Note. Other multivitamin preparations are in section 9.6.7.

Vitamin B Tablets, Compound, nicotinamide 15 mg, riboflavine 1 mg, thiamine hydrochloride 1 mg. Net price 20 = 6p
Dose: prophylactic, 1–2 tablets daily

Vitamin B Tablets, Compound, Strong, brown, f/c or s/c, nicotinamide 20 mg, pyridoxine hydrochloride 2 mg, riboflavine 2 mg, thiamine hydrochloride 5 mg. Net price 20 = 12p
Dose: treatment of vitamin-B deficiency, 1–2 tablets 3 times daily

NHS **Aluzyme®** (Phillips Yeast)
Tablets, folic acid 14 micrograms, thiamine hydrochloride 160 micrograms, riboflavine 210 micrograms, nicotinic acid 2.5 mg, dried yeast 297 mg. Net price 20 = 3p

NHS **Becosym®** (Roche)
Tablets, brown, f/c, vitamin B tablets, compound, strong. Net price 20 = 12p
Forte tablets, brown, f/c, thiamine hydrochloride 15 mg, riboflavine 15 mg, nicotinamide 50 mg, pyridoxine hydrochloride 10 mg. Net price 20 = 40p
Syrup, orange, thiamine hydrochloride 5 mg, riboflavine 2 mg, nicotinamide 20 mg, pyridoxine hydrochloride 2 mg/5 ml. Diluent syrup, life of diluted syrup 14 days. Net price 100 ml = 85p

NHS **Benerva Compound®** (Roche)
Tablets, yellow, vitamin B tablets, compound. Net price 20 = 9p

NHS **Tonivitan B®** (Medo)
Syrup, red, thiamine hydrochloride 500 micrograms, riboflavine 400 micrograms, nicotinamide 2.5 mg, pyridoxine hydrochloride 16.5 micrograms, calcium glycerophosphate 20 mg, manganese glycerophosphate 5 mg/5 ml. Diluent syrup, life of diluted syrup 14 days. Net price 125 ml = 46p

NHS **Vigranon B®** (Wallace Mfg)
Syrup, thiamine hydrochloride 5 mg, riboflavine 2 mg, nicotinamide 20 mg, pyridoxine hydrochloride 2 mg, panthenol 3 mg/5 ml. Net price 150 ml = 94p

---

OTHER COMPOUNDS

Potassium aminobenzoate has been used in the treatment of various disorders associated with excessive fibrosis such as scleroderma but its therapeutic value is **doubtful**.

Potaba® (Glenwood)
Capsules, red/white, potassium aminobenzoate 500 mg. Net price 20 = 83p. Label: 21
Tablets, potassium aminobenzoate 500 mg. Net price 20 = 65p. Label: 21
Dose: Peyronie's disease, scleroderma, 12 g daily in divided doses after food
Envules® (= powder in sachets), potassium aminobenzoate 3 g. Net price 40 sachets = £10.01. Label: 13, 21

9.6.3 Vitamin C
(Ascorbic acid)

Vitamin C therapy is essential in scurvy, but less florid manifestations of vitamin C deficiency are commonly found, especially in the elderly. It is rarely necessary to prescribe more than 100 mg daily except early in the treatment of scurvy.

Claims that vitamin C ameliorates colds or promotes wound healing have not been proved.

ASCORBIC ACID
Indications: prevention and treatment of scurvy
Dose: prophylactic, 25–75 mg daily; therapeutic, not less than 250 mg daily in divided doses

Ascorbic Acid Tablets, ascorbic acid 25 mg, net price 20 = 5p; 50 mg, 20 = 5p; 100 mg, 20 = 22p; 200 mg, 20 = 20p; 500 mg, 20 = 49p

PoM **Ascorbic Acid Injection,** ascorbic acid 100 mg/ml. Net price 5-ml amp = 57p

NHS **Redoxon®** (Roche)
Tablets, ascorbic acid 25 mg, net price 20 = 5p; 50 mg, 20 = 5p; 200 mg, 20 = 20p; 500 mg, 20 = 49p
Tablets, effervescent, ascorbic acid 1 g. Net price 10-tab pack = 72p. Label: 13

9.6.4 Vitamin D

Note. The term Vitamin D is used for a range of compounds which possess the property of preventing or curing rickets. They include ergocalciferol (calciferol, vitamin D₂), cholecalciferol (vitamin D₃), dihydrotachysterol, alfacalcidol (1α-hydroxycholecalciferol), and calcitriol (1,25-dihydroxycholecalciferol). Calcitriol is considered to be the most active form of vitamin D, but ergocalciferol is suitable for most purposes.

Simple vitamin D *deficiency,* which is not uncommon in Asians consuming unleavened bread and in the elderly living alone, can be prevented by taking an oral supplement of only 10 micrograms (400 units) **calciferol** daily. Unfortunately there is no plain vitamin D tablet of this strength available. Some sources therefore use calcium with vitamin D tablets although the calcium in such preparations is unnecessary and better avoided.

Vitamin D deficiency caused by *intestinal malabsorption* or *chronic liver disease* usually requires pharmacological doses of up to 1 mg (40 000 units) daily.

The hypocalcaemia of hypoparathyroidism often requires doses of up to 5 mg (200 000 units) daily in order to achieve normocalcaemia and **dihydrotachysterol** may be used as an alternative.

Alfacalcidol or **calcitriol** should be prescribed for functionally *anephric* patients; these preparations offer no advantages over calciferol in the treatment of simple vitamin D deficiency and offer few advantages in most other patients where pharmacological doses of vitamin D are required.

All patients receiving pharmacological doses of vitamin D should have the plasma calcium concentration checked at intervals (initially weekly) and whenever nausea or vomiting are

---

present. Breast milk from women taking pharmacological doses of vitamin D may cause hypercalcaemia if given to an infant.

ERGOCALCIFEROL

(Calciferol, Vitamin D₂)

Indications: see notes above

Cautions: take care to ensure correct dose in infants; monitor plasma calcium in patients receiving high doses

Contra-indications: hypercalcaemia

Side-effects: symptoms of overdosage include anorexia, lassitude, nausea and vomiting, diarrhoea, weight loss, polyuria, sweating, headache, thirst, vertigo, and raised concentrations of calcium and phosphate in plasma and urine

Dose: see notes above and under preparations

Ergocalciferol and cholecalciferol

Note. There is no vitamin D tablet available of the strength suitable for treating simple deficiency (see notes above). Alternatives include vitamins capsules (see 9.6.7), preparations of vitamins A and D (see 9.6.1), and calcium with vitamin D tablets (see below).

Calciferol Tablets, High-strength, 10 000 units, BP 1980, s/c, cholecalciferol or ergocalciferol 250 micrograms. Net price 20 = 42p

Note. It is essential to include the words 'high-strength' in the prescription; these tablets are approximately one-fifth the strength of Strong Calciferol Tablets BP 1973

Calciferol Solution, cholecalciferol or ergocalciferol 75 micrograms (3000 units)/ml in oil. Net price 100 ml = £2.32

PoM **Calciferol Injection,** BP 1980, 7.5 mg (300 000 units)/ml in oil. Net price 1-ml amp = £1.30; 2-ml amp = £1.55

Ergocalciferol with calcium

Calcium with Vitamin D Tablets, calcium sodium lactate 450 mg (or calcium lactate 300 mg), calcium phosphate 150 mg, ergocalciferol 12.5 micrograms (500 units). Net price 20 = 22p. Counselling advised, crush before administration or may be chewed

NHS **Chocovite**® (Torbet)

Tablets, brown, ergocalciferol 15 micrograms (600 units), calcium gluconate 500 mg. Net price 20 = 34p

ALFACALCIDOL

(1α-Hydroxycholecalciferol)

Indications: see notes above

Cautions; Contra-indications; Side-effects: see under Ergocalciferol

Dose: see notes above and under preparations

PoM **One-alpha**® (Leo)

Capsules, alfacalcidol 250 nanograms, net price 20 = £2.20; 1 microgram (brown), 20 = £7.20

Solution, sugar-free, alfacalcidol 200 nanograms/ml. Net price 60 ml = £14.56 (with oral syringe)

Dose: ADULTS and CHILDREN over 20 kg, initially 1 microgram daily (elderly 500 nanograms), adjusted to avoid hypercalcaemia; maintenance 0.25–1 microgram daily; CHILD under 20 kg,

initially 50 nanograms/kg daily; NEONATES and premature infants 50–100 nanograms/kg daily.

Note. This solution replaces the drops which were more concentrated and required dilution

CALCITRIOL

(1,25-Dihydroxycholecalciferol)

Indications: see notes above

Cautions; Contra-indications; Side-effects: see under Ergocalciferol

Dose: see notes above and under preparations

PoM **Rocaltrol**® (Roche)

Capsules, red/white, calcitriol 250 nanograms. Net price 20 = £3.56

Capsules, red, calcitriol 500 nanograms. Net price 20 = £6.37

Dose: initially 1–2 micrograms daily, gradually increased to 2–3 micrograms daily

CHOLECALCIFEROL

(Vitamin D₃)

Indications: see notes above

Cautions; Contra-indications; Side-effects: see under Ergocalciferol

Preparations

See under Ergocalciferol

DIHYDROTACHYSTEROL

Indications: see notes above

Cautions; Contra-indications; Side-effects: see under Ergocalciferol

Dose: see notes above and under preparations

AT 10® (Sterling Research)

Oral solution, dihydrotachysterol 250 micrograms/ml. Net price 15-ml dropper bottle = £17.25

Tachyrol® (Duphar)

Tablets, scored, dihydrotachysterol 200 micrograms. Net price 20 = £2.91

Dose: initially 200 micrograms daily, adjusted according to response

9.6.5   Vitamin E

(Tocopherols)

There is little evidence that oral supplements of vitamin E are essential in adults, even where there is fat malabsorption secondary to cholestasis. In young children with congenital cholestasis, abnormally low vitamin E concentrations may be found in association with neuromuscular abnormalities, which usually respond only to the parenteral administration of vitamin E.

Vitamin E has been tried for various other conditions but there is no scientific evidence of its value. High doses have been associated with adverse effects.

ALPHA TOCOPHERYL ACETATE

Indications: see notes above

Dose: 3 to 15 mg daily

Note. The potency of alpha tocopheryl acetate (that is, *all-rac-α*-tocopheryl acetate) is about 1 unit/mg, and the potency of *d-α*-tocopheryl is about 1.36 units/mg

Vitamin E Suspension (Roche)
Oral liquid, alpha tocopheryl acetate 500 mg/ 5 ml
Ephynal® (Roche)
Tablets, alpha tocopheryl acetate 10 mg, net price 20 = 17p; 50 mg (scored), 20 = 43p; 200 mg (ivory, scored), 20 = £1.30
Vita-E® (Bioglan)
Gels (= capsules), d-α-tocopheryl acetate 75 units (yellow), net price 20 = 47p; 200 units (yellow), 20 = £1.11; 400 units (red), 20 = £1.76
Gelucaps® (= tablets), chewable, yellow, d-α-tocopheryl acetate 75 units. Net price 20 = 56p. Label: 24
Succinate tablets, yellow, d-α-tocopheryl succinate 50 units, net price 20 = 40p; 200 units, 20 = £1.19

9.6.6 Vitamin K

Vitamin K is necessary for the production of blood clotting factors and proteins necessary for the normal calcification of bone.

Because vitamin K is fat soluble, patients with *fat malabsorption*, especially if due to biliary obstruction or hepatic disease, may become deficient. For oral administration to prevent vitamin-K deficiency in malabsorption syndromes, a water-soluble preparation, **menadiol sodium phosphate** must be used; the usual dose is about 10 mg daily.

In *neonates* deficiency of vitamin K may occur because the gut is sterile and there is no synthesis of the vitamin by *Escherichia coli*. It may be treated with **phytomenadione** (vitamin K₁), 1 mg by intramuscular injection.

Oral coumarin *anticoagulants* act by interfering with vitamin K metabolism in the hepatic cells and their effects can be antagonised by giving vitamin K.

After correction of hypoprothrombinaemia, resistance to oral anticoagulants persists for up to two weeks; patients with prosthetic valves who need to continue anticoagulant therapy but who bleed, should be treated with fresh plasma to elevate the prothrombin levels and the anticoagulant dose reduced.

For the reversal of haemorrhage associated with hypoprothrombinaemia caused by overdosage of anticoagulants or of hypoprothrombinaemia due to anticoagulants, but without haemorrhage, see guidelines in section 2.8.2.

MENADIOL SODIUM PHOSPHATE

Indications; Dose: see notes above
Cautions: pregnancy. Drug interactions: see Appendix 1 (sections *2.8, 2.8A*)

Synkavit® (Roche)
Tablets, scored, menadiol sodium phosphate equivalent to 10 mg of menadiol phosphate. Net price 20 = 41p

PHYTOMENADIONE

Indications; Dose: see notes above
Cautions: intravenous injections should be given very slowly. Drug interactions: see Appendix 1 (sections *2.8, 2.8A*)

Konakion® (Roche)
Tablets, s/c, phytomenadione 10 mg. Net price 25 = £4.20. Label: 24
PoM *Injection*, phytomenadione 2 mg/ml, net price 0.5-ml amp = 22p; 10 mg/ml, 1-ml amp = 41p
Note. Contains polyethoxylated castor oil which has been associated with anaphylaxis

9.6.7 Multivitamin preparations

There are many preparations available. The proprietary preparations have no advantage over the non-proprietary preparations given separately and many are expensive.

Vitamins Capsules, ascorbic acid 15 mg, nicotinamide 7.5 mg, riboflavine 500 micrograms, thiamine hydrochloride 1 mg, vitamin A 2500 units, vitamin D 300 units. Net price 20 = 18p
Abidec® (W-L)
NHS *Capsules*, vitamins A, B group, C, and D. Net price 20 = 23p
Drops, vitamins A, B group, C, and D. Net price 2 × 25 ml (with dropper) = £1.85
NHS **Allbee with C**® (Robins)
Capsules, yellow/green, vitamins B group and C. Net price 20 = £1.00
NHS **BC 500**® (Wyeth)
Tablets, orange, f/c, vitamins B group and C. Net price 20 = 71p
NHS **Calcimax**® (Wallace Mfg)
Syrup, brown, vitamins B group, and D. Net price 150 ml = £1.11
NHS **Ce-Cobalin**® (Paines & Byrne)
Product discontinued
NHS **Concavit**® (Wallace Mfg)
Capsules, vitamins A, B group, C, D, and E. Net price 20 = 73p
Drops and *syrup*, vitamins A, B group, C, and D. Net price drops 15 ml = £1.09; syrup 150 ml = £1.28
Dalivit® (Paines & Byrne)
NHS *Capsules*, red, vitamins A, B group, C, and D. Net price 20 = 29p
Oral drops, vitamins A, B group, C, and D. Net price 15 ml = 45p
NHS *Syrup*—discontinued
NHS **Juvel**® (Bencard)
Tablets, s/c, vitamins A, B group, C, and D. Net price 20 = 46p
Elixir, vitamins A, B group, C, and D. Diluent syrup, life of diluted elixir 14 days. Net price 100 ml = 62p
NHS **Minamino**® (Consolidated)
Syrup, vitamins B group, with amino acids, extracts of liver, spleen, and gastric mucosa, and minerals. Net price 100 ml = 47p
NHS **Multivite**® (DF)
Pellets, brown, s/c, vitamin A 2500 units, thiamine hydrochloride 500 micrograms, ascorbic acid 12.5 mg, vitamin D 250 units. Net price 56-pellet pack = 98p
NHS **Orovite**® (Bencard)
Tablets, maroon, s/c, vitamins B group and C. Net price 20 = 69p
Elixir, vitamins B group and C. Diluent syrup, life of diluted elixir 14 days. Net price 100 ml = 57p
NHS **Orovite 7**® (Bencard)
Granules, orange, vitamins A, B group, C, and D. Net price 20 × 5-g sachet = £1.80. Label: 13
NHS PoM **Polyvite**® (Medo)
Capsules, red, vitamins A, B group, C, and D. Net price 20 = 48p

NHS **Surbex T**® (Abbott)
Tablets, orange, vitamins B group and C. Net price 20 = 58p

NHS PoM **Tonivitan**® (Medo)
Capsules, brown, vitamins A, B group, C, and D with dried yeast 50 mg. Net price 20 = 28p

NHS **Verdiviton**® (Squibb)
Elixir, green, vitamins B group and minerals. Net price 240 ml = £1.80

NHS **Vi-Daylin**® (Abbott)
Syrup, vitamins A, B group, C, and D. Net price 100 ml = 56p

NHS **Vitavel**® (Bencard)
Elixir, orange, sugar-free, vitamins A, B group, C, and D for reconstitution with water for preparations. Life of reconstituted product 30 days. Net price 150 ml = £1.36

9.7   Bitters and tonics

Mixtures containing simple and aromatic bitters, such as alkaline gentian mixture, are traditional remedies for loss of appetite. All depend on suggestion and there is no advantage in prescribing the many exotically coloured and flavoured products which are available.

Gentian Mixture, Acid and **Alkaline** (see Formulary). Net price 100 ml = 11p and 16p, respectively

NHS **Effico**® (Pharmax)
Tonic, green, thiamine hydrochloride 180 micrograms, nicotinamide 2.1 mg, caffeine 20.2 mg, compound gentian infusion 0.31 ml/5 ml. Net price 100 ml = 35p

NHS **Fosfor**® (Consolidated)
Syrup, pink, phosphorylcolamine 5%. Net price 100 ml = 26p

NHS **Labiton**® (LAB)
Tonic, brown, thiamine hydrochloride 375 micrograms, caffeine 3.5 mg, kola nut dried extract 3.025 mg, alcohol 1.4 ml/5 ml. Net price 100 ml = 46p

NHS **Metatone**® (W-L)
Tonic, thiamine hydrochloride 500 micrograms, calcium glycerophosphate 45.6 mg, manganese glycerophosphate 5.7 mg, potassium glycerophosphate 45.6 mg, sodium glycerophosphate 22.8 mg/5 ml. Net price 100 ml = 36p

9.8   Drugs used in metabolic disorders

This section covers drugs used in metabolic disorders and not readily classified elsewhere.

Penicillamine (see also section 10.1.3) is used in Wilson's disease (hepatolenticular degener-

ation) to aid the elimination of copper ions. For use in copper and lead poisoning, see p. 40.

Trientine is used for the treatment of Wilson's disease only, in patients intolerant of penicillamine; it is **not** an alternative to penicillamine for rheumatoid arthritis or cystinuria.

PENICILLAMINE

Indications: see Dose below
Cautions; Contra-indications; Side-effects: see section 10.1.3
Dose: Wilson's disease, 1.5–2 g daily in divided doses before food; max. 2 g daily for 1 year; maintenance 0.75–1 g daily; ELDERLY, 20 mg/kg daily in divided doses; CHILD, up to 20 mg/kg daily in divided doses, min. 500 mg daily
Chronic active hepatitis (after disease is controlled), 500 mg daily in divided doses slowly increased over 3 months; usual maintenance dose 1.25 g daily
Primary biliary cirrhosis, 250 mg daily, increasing weekly to a maintenance dose of 0.75–1 g daily in divided doses, then reduced as liver copper concentrations return to normal
Cystinuria, therapeutic, 1–3 g daily in divided doses before food, adjusted to maintain urinary cystine below 200 mg/litre. Prophylactic (maintain urinary cystine below 300 mg/litre) 0.5–1 g at bedtime; maintain adequate fluid intake (at least 3 litres daily); CHILD minimum dose to maintain urinary cystine below 200 mg/litre

Preparations: see section 10.1.3

TRIENTINE DIHYDROCHLORIDE

Indications: Wilson's disease in patients intolerant of penicillamine
Cautions: see notes above; pregnancy. Drug interactions: see Appendix 1 (section 9)
Side-effects: nausea; penicillamine-induced systemic lupus erythematosus may not resolve on transfer to trientine
Dose: 1.2–2.4 g daily in 2–4 divided doses before food

▼ PoM **Trientine Dihydrochloride Capsules,** trientine dihydrochloride 300 mg. Label: 6, 22
Available from K & K Greeff

Note. The CSM has requested that in addition to the usual CSM reporting request special records should also be kept by the pharmacist

---

10: Drugs used in the treatment of

MUSCULOSKELETAL and JOINT DISEASES

In this chapter, drug treatment is discussed under the following headings:

10.1 Drugs used in rheumatic diseases and gout
10.2 Drugs used in neuromuscular disorders
10.3 Drugs for the relief of soft-tissue inflammation

For treatment of septic arthritis see section 5.1, Table 1.

10.1 Drugs used in rheumatic diseases and gout

Most rheumatic diseases require symptomatic treatment to relieve pain and stiffness. Suitable non-steroidal anti-inflammatory drugs (NSAIDs) are described in section 10.1.1; reference should also be made to section 10.1.4 for the treatment of acute gout.

In certain circumstances corticosteroids (section 10.1.2) may be used to suppress inflammation.

Drugs are also available which may affect the disease process itself and favourably influence the outcome. For *rheumatoid arthritis* these include penicillamine, gold salts, antimalarials (chloroquine and hydroxychloroquine), immunosuppressants (azathioprine, chlorambucil, cyclophosphamide, and methotrexate), and sulphasalazine; they are sometimes known as second-line or disease-modifying antirheumatic drugs. For *psoriatic arthritis* they include gold salts, azathioprine, and methotrexate, and for *gout* they include uricosuric drugs and allopurinol.

10.1.1 Non-steroidal anti-inflammatory drugs (NSAIDs)
10.1.2 Corticosteroids and corticotrophin
10.1.2.1 Systemic corticosteroids and corticotrophin
10.1.2.2 Local corticosteroid injections
10.1.3 Drugs which suppress the disease process
10.1.4 Drugs used in the treatment of gout

Analgesic preparations and doses—see section 4.7.

10.1.1 Non-steroidal anti-inflammatory drugs (NSAIDs)

Non-steroidal anti-inflammatory drugs (NSAIDs) have two separate actions.

In *single doses* they have analgesic activity comparable to that of paracetamol (see section 4.7.1) and can therefore be taken on demand for mild or intermittent pain or as a supplement to regular treatment.

In regular *full dosage* they have both a lasting analgesic and an anti-inflammatory effect. This combination makes them particularly useful for the treatment of continuous or regular pain associated with inflammation. NSAIDs are, therefore, more appropriate than paracetamol or the narcotic analgesics ('opioids') in the inflammatory arthritides (e.g. rheumatoid arthritis) and in advanced osteoarthrosis. They may also be of benefit in the less well defined conditions of back pain and soft-tissue disorders.

Paracetamol, nefopam, and the narcotic analgesics ('opioids') have no demonstrable anti-inflammatory activity and are therefore not included in this section (see instead 4.7.1).

CAUTIONS. In general, NSAIDs should be used with caution in the elderly, and in peptic ulceration, allergic disorders (particularly salicylate hypersensitivity and asthma, see CSM warning below), pregnancy, and renal and hepatic impairment. See also Drug interactions: Appendix 1 (sections *2.1, 2.2, 2.5, 2.8C, 4.2, 4.7, 8*) and under individual entries. Dosage of anticoagulants may need to be adjusted when anti-inflammatory analgesics are used; the risk of haemorrhage is greatest with aspirin or other salicylates.

While it is preferable to avoid NSAIDs in patients with current or previous *peptic ulceration*, and to withdraw them if gastro-intestinal lesions develop, nevertheless patients with serious rheumatic diseases (e.g. rheumatoid arthritis) are usually dependent on NSAIDs for effective relief of pain and stiffness. Prophylactic administration of histamine H₂-receptor blocking drugs (cimetidine and ranitidine, see section 1.3) may permit recommencement of a NSAID without further gastro-intestinal problems.

CSM advice.
1. NSAIDs should not be given to patients with active peptic ulceration.
2. In patients with a history of peptic ulcer disease and in the elderly they should be given only after other forms of treatment have been carefully considered.
3. In all patients it is prudent to start at the bottom end of the dose range.

CSM Warning.
Any degree of worsening of asthma may be related to the ingestion of NSAIDs, either prescribed or (in the case of ibuprofen) purchased over the counter.

SIDE-EFFECTS. Side-effects are variable in severity and frequency. Gastro-intestinal discomfort, nausea, diarrhoea, and occasionally bleeding occur and may be minimised by advising that these drugs should always be taken with food or milk. Hypersensitivity reactions (particularly angioedema, asthma, and rashes), headache, dizziness, vertigo, and hearing disturbances such as tinnitus. Blood disorders have occurred. Fluid retention may occur (rarely precipitating congestive heart failure in elderly patients). Rarely, reversible acute renal failure may be provoked by NSAIDs especially in patients with pre-existing renal impairment; papillary necrosis or interstitial fibrosis associated with NSAIDs may also lead to chronic renal failure.

CHOICE OF DRUG. Differences in anti-inflammatory activity between different NSAIDs are small, but there is considerable variation in individual patient response. About 60% of patients will respond to any NSAID. Among the rest, those who do not respond to one may well respond to another. Therefore it is often necessary to try several drugs before finding one to suit a particular patient. Most NSAIDs should produce an effect within a few days. If used for analgesia alone they should be changed if no response is obtained after a week; if an anti-inflammatory action is also required they should be changed if no response is obtained after three weeks.

The main differences between NSAIDs are in the incidence and type of side-effects. Before treatment is started the prescriber should weigh efficacy against possible side-effects for each drug.

Aspirin[1] was the traditional first choice but most physicians now prefer to start treatment with other NSAIDs because they may be better tolerated and more convenient for the patient.

In regular high dosage aspirin has about the same anti-inflammatory effect as other NSAIDs. The required dose for active inflammatory joint disease is 3.6 g or more daily. There is little anti-inflammatory effect with less than 3 g daily. Gastro-intestinal side-effects such as nausea, dyspepsia, and gastro-intestinal bleeding may occur with any dosage of aspirin but anti-inflammatory doses are associated with a much higher incidence of side-effects. Gastro-intestinal side-effects may be minimised by taking the dose after food. Numerous formulations are available which improve gastric tolerance and minimise occult bleeding, including buffered, dispersible, and enteric-coated preparations.

Anti-inflammatory doses of aspirin may also cause mild chronic salicylate intoxication (salicylism) characterised by dizziness, tinnitus, and deafness; these symptoms may be controlled by reducing the dosage.

Benorylate[1] (Benoral®), an aspirin-paracetamol ester, is broken down after absorption from the gastro-intestinal tract. It need only be given twice daily and gastric tolerance is slightly better than with aspirin. As it is more slowly absorbed than paracetamol, hepatotoxicity in overdosage may be reduced. Anti-inflammatory doses are achieved with 4 to 8 g daily.

Ibuprofen is a propionic acid derivative with anti-inflammatory, analgesic, and antipyretic properties. It has fewer side-effects than other NSAID's but its anti-inflammatory properties are weaker. Doses of 1.6 to 2.4 g daily are needed for rheumatoid arthritis and it is unsuitable for conditions where inflammation is prominent such as acute gout and ankylosing spondylitis.

Other propionic acid derivatives:

Naproxen (Naprosyn® etc.) has emerged as one of the first choices as it combines good efficacy with a low incidence of side-effects and administration is only twice daily.

Fenbufen (Lederfen®) is claimed to be associated with less gastro-intestinal bleeding, but there is a high risk of rashes.

Fenoprofen (Fenopron®) is as effective as naproxen, and flurbiprofen (Froben®) may be slightly more effective. Both are associated with slightly more gastro-intestinal side-effects than ibuprofen.

Ketoprofen (Alrheumat®, Orudis®) has anti-inflammatory properties similar to ibuprofen and has more side-effects. A slow-release preparation is claimed to cause less gastro-intestinal irritation.

Tiaprofenic acid (Surgam®) is as effective as naproxen; it has more side-effects than ibuprofen.

Drugs with properties similar to those of propionic acid derivatives:

Azapropazone (Rheumox®) is similar in effect to naproxen; it has a tendency to cause rashes. Although chemically related to phenylbutazone, on present evidence azapropazone does not give rise to blood disorders. Azapropazone is also used in the treatment of gout (section 10.1.4).

Diclofenac (Voltarol® etc.) has an action similar to that of naproxen; its side-effects are also similar. Diclofenac is also available as suppositories and as a sustained-release preparation.

Diflunisal (Dolobid®) is an aspirin derivative but its clinical effect more closely resembles that of the propionic acid derivatives than that of its parent compound. Its long half-life allows twice-daily administration.

Etodolac (Lodine®) is comparable in effect to naproxen; side-effects appear to be comparable to those of ibuprofen but long-term data are awaited. It is presently only indicated for rheumatoid arthritis.

Indomethacin (Indocid® etc.) has an action equal to or superior to that of naproxen, but with a high incidence of side-effects including headaches, dizziness, and gastro-intestinal disturbances. It can also be used for acute gout.

Mefenamic acid (Ponstan®) is a related analgesic but its anti-inflammatory properties are minor and side-effects differ in that diarrhoea and occasionally haemolytic anaemia may occur which necessitate discontinuation of treatment.

Nabumetone (Relifex®) is comparable in effect to naproxen; side-effects appear to be comparable to those of ibuprofen but long-term data are awaited.

---

[1] Owing to an association with Reye's syndrome the CSM has recommended that aspirin-containing preparations should no longer be given to children under the age of 12 years, unless specifically indicated, e.g. for juvenile chronic arthritis (Still's disease).

Phenylbutazone (Butazolidin® etc.) is a potent anti-inflammatory drug but because of occasional serious side-effects its use is limited to the hospital treatment of ankylosing spondylitis. In addition to its gastric side-effects it has two rare but dangerous side-effects. It causes fluid retention and, in predisposed patients, may precipitate cardiac failure. It also causes agranulocytosis (which may occur within the first few days of treatment) and aplastic anaemia. In ankylosing spondylitis prolonged administration may be necessary but it should not be used unless other drugs have been tried and have failed.

Piroxicam (Feldene® etc.) is as effective as naproxen and has a prolonged duration of action which permits once-daily administration. It has more gastro-intestinal side-effects than ibuprofen, especially in the elderly; suppositories or dispersible tablets are available.

Sulindac (Clinoril®) is similar in tolerance to naproxen.

Tolmetin (Tolectin®) is comparable to ibuprofen.

WITHDRAWN DRUGS. Over the last few years several non-steroidal anti-inflammatory drugs have been withdrawn from the market, either by the manufacturers or on the recommendation of the CSM and licensing authorities. They include benoxaprofen (Opren®), fenclofenac (Flenac®), feprazone (Methrazone®), flufenamic acid (Meralen®), indoprofen (Flosint®), Osmosin® (sustained-release indomethacin), oxyphenbutazone (Tandacote®, Tanderil®), suprofen (Suprol®), and zomepirac (Zomax®).

In addition the CSM has recommended that the use of phenylbutazone be restricted (see notes above).

ASPIRIN AND THE SALICYLATES

ASPIRIN

Indications: pain and inflammation in rheumatic disease and other musculoskeletal disorders (including Still's disease); see also section 4.7.1

Cautions: allergic disease, severe renal or hepatic impairment, dehydration, pregnancy (particularly at term), breast-feeding, elderly patients, concurrent anticoagulant therapy. Drug interactions: see Appendix 1 (*2.1, 2.2, 2.8, 2.8E, 4.7, 4.8, 8, 10, 11*)

Contra-indications: peptic ulceration; gout; children under 12 years (except for Still's disease), association with Reye's syndrome

Side-effects: common with anti-inflammatory doses; gastro-intestinal discomfort, ulceration, bleeding, or nausea, hearing disturbances such as tinnitus (leading rarely to deafness), vertigo, mental confusion, hypersensitivity reactions (angioedema, bronchospasm and rashes); rarely oedema, myocarditis, blood disorders, particularly thrombocytopenia

Dose: 0.3–1 g every 4 hours; max. in acute conditions 8 g daily; CHILD, Still's disease, up to 80 mg/kg daily in 5–6 divided doses, increased in acute exacerbations to 130 mg/kg. Doses should be taken after food

Aspirin Tablets, aspirin 300 mg. Net price 20 = 8p. Label: 21

Aspirin Tablets, Dispersible, aspirin 300 mg. Net price 20 = 8p. Label: 13, 21

Note. From 1st December 1988 Soluble Aspirin Tablets BP will be the title of dispersible aspirin tablets which effervesce on addition of water.

Proprietary preparations
See section 4.7.1

BENORYLATE

(Aspirin-paracetamol ester)

Indications: pain and inflammation in rheumatic disease (including Still's disease) and other musculoskeletal disorders; see also section 4.7.1

Cautions; Contra-indications: see under Aspirin (above) and Paracetamol (section 4.7.1). Patients should be advised against taking analgesics containing aspirin or paracetamol

Side-effects: see under Aspirin (above) and Paracetamol (section 4.7.1). Side-effects resemble those of aspirin rather than paracetamol but tolerance is better and hepatotoxicity may be less than with paracetamol

Dose: 4–8 g daily divided into 2–3 doses; CHILD, Still's disease, initially 200 mg/kg daily, adjusted to maintain a plasma-salicylate concentration of 250 mg/litre (1.8 mmol/litre)

Benorylate (Non-proprietary)
Mixture, benorylate 2 g/5 ml. Net price 100 ml = £3.60. Label: 21, counselling advised, avoid asprin, paracetamol

Benoral® (Sterling Research)
Tablets, benorylate 750 mg. Net price 20 = £1.49. Label: 21, counselling advised, avoid aspirin, paracetamol

Granules, benorylate 2-g/sachet. Net price 10 sachets = £2.25. Label: 13, 21, counselling advised, avoid aspirin, paracetamol

Suspension, sugar-free, benorylate 2 g/5 ml. Diluent syrup, life of diluted suspension 14 days. Net price 150 ml = £5.47. Label: 21, counselling advised, avoid aspirin, paracetamol

CHOLINE MAGNESIUM TRISALICYLATE

Indications: pain and inflammation in rheumatic disease and other musculoskeletal disorders

Cautions; Contra-indications; Side-effects: see under Aspirin (above)

Dose: 0.5–1.5 g of salicylate twice daily

Trilisate® (Napp)
Tablets, orange, scored, choline magnesium trisalicylate ≡ salicylate 500 mg. Net price 20 = £1.50. Label: 12, 21

SALSALATE

Indications: pain and inflammation in mild rheumatic disease and other musculoskeletal disorders

Cautions; Contra-indications; Side-effects: see under Aspirin (above)

Dose: 0.5–1 g 3–4 times daily

PoM **Disalcid**® (Riker)
Capsules, orange/grey, salsalate 500 mg. Net price 20 = £1.15. Label: 12, 21

SODIUM SALICYLATE

Indications: pain and inflammation in rheumatic disease
Cautions; Contra-indications; Side-effects: see under Aspirin (above). Caution in patients on low-sodium diet and in congestive heart failure; avoid in acute renal disease
Dose: 0.5–2 g with food, when necessary. In acute conditions 5–10 g daily in divided doses

Sodium Salicylate Mixture, sodium salicylate 250 mg/5 ml (see Formulary). Net price 100 ml = 13p. Label: 21
Sodium Salicylate Mixture, Strong, sodium salicylate 500 mg/5 ml (see Formulary). Net price 100 ml = 12p. Label: 21

OTHER NSAIDs

IBUPROFEN

Indications: pain and mild inflammation in rheumatic disease (including Still's disease) and other musculoskeletal disorders; see also section 4.7.1
Cautions; Side-effects: see notes above. Drug interactions: see Appendix 1 (sections *2.1, 2.2, 2.5, 2.8C, 4.2, 4.7, 8*)
Dose: initially 1.2–1.8 g daily in 3–4 divided doses preferably after food; increased if necessary to max. of 2.4 g daily; maintenance dose of 0.6–1.2 g daily may be adequate; CHILD 20 mg/kg daily, children under 30 kg max. in 24 hours 500 mg

PoM **Ibuprofen** (Non-proprietary)
Tablets, f/c or s/c, ibuprofen 200 mg, net price 20 = 26p; 400 mg, 20 = 51p; 600 mg, 20 = £1.36. Label: 21
Note. Proprietary brands of ibuprofen tablets are on sale to the public
PoM **Apsifen**® (APS)
Tablets, both pink, f/c or s/c, ibuprofen 200 mg, net price 20 = 31p; 400 mg, 20 = 62p. Label: 21
Tablets, pink, f/c, ibuprofen 600 mg. Net price 20 = £1.90. Label: 21
PoM **Brufen**® (Boots)
Tablets, both magenta, s/c, ibuprofen 200 mg, net price 20 = 61p; 400 mg, 20 = £1.21. Label: 21
Tablets, magenta, f/c, ibuprofen 600 mg. Net price 20 = £1.93. Label: 21
Syrup, orange, ibuprofen 100 mg/5 ml. Diluent syrup, life of diluted syrup 14 days. Net price 100 ml = 77p. Label: 21
PoM **Ebufac**® (DDSA)
Tablets, both pink, s/c, ibuprofen 200 mg, net price 20 = 44p; 400 mg, 20 = 68p. Label: 21
PoM **Fenbid**® (SK&F)
Spansule® (= capsule s/r), maroon/pink, enclosing off-white pellets, ibuprofen 300 mg. Net price 20 = £1.19. Label: 25
Dose: 1–3 capsules every 12 hours

PoM **Ibular**® (Lagap)
Tablets, both pink, s/c, ibuprofen 200 mg, net price 20 = 32p; 400 mg, 20 = 62p. Label: 21
PoM **Lidifen**® (Berk)
Tablets, both magenta, s/c, ibuprofen 200 mg, net price 20 = 32p; 400 mg, 20 = 62p. Label: 21
PoM **Motrin**® (Upjohn)
Tablets, all f/c, ibuprofen 200 mg (red), net price 20 = 41p; 400 mg (orange), 20 = 86p; 600 mg (peach), 20 = £1.29; 800 mg (orange), 20 = £2.45. Label: 21
PoM **Paxofen**® (Steinhard)
Tablets, all pink, f/c or s/c, ibuprofen 200 mg, net price 20 = 60p; 400 mg, 20 = £1.20; 600 mg, 20 = £1.90. Label: 21

AZAPROPAZONE

Indications: pain and inflammation in rheumatic disease and other musculoskeletal disorders; gout
Cautions; Side-effects: see notes above; photosensitivity may occur. Avoid in hypersensitivity to phenylbutazone and related drugs. Drug interactions: see Appendix 1 (sections *2.1, 2.2, 2.5, 2.8B, 4.2, 4.7, 4.8, 6.1, 8*)
Dose: 1.2 g daily in 2 or 4 divided doses (elderly patients 300 mg twice daily, max. 900 mg daily)
Acute gout, initially 2.4 g in divided doses over 24 hours, then 1.8 g reducing to 1.2 g daily in divided doses
Chronic gout, 600 mg twice daily (elderly patients 300 mg twice daily, max. 900 mg daily)

PoM **Rheumox**® (Robins)
Capsules, orange, azapropazone 300 mg. Net price 20 = £3.06. Label: 21, counselling advised: in some patients direct sunlight may lead to a rash
Tablets, orange, f/c, scored, azapropazone 600 mg. Net price 20 = £5.85. Label: 21, counselling advised: in some patients direct sunlight may lead to a rash

DICLOFENAC SODIUM

Indications: pain and inflammation in rheumatic disease (including Still's disease) and other musculoskeletal disorders; acute gout
Cautions; Side-effects: see notes above. Pain may occur at the injection site; suppositories may cause irritation. Drug interactions: see Appendix 1 (sections *2.1, 2.2, 2.5, 2.8C, 4.2, 4.7, 8*)
Dose: by mouth, 75–150 mg daily in 2–3 divided doses, preferably after food
By deep intramuscular injection acute exacerbations and post-operative, 75 mg once daily (twice daily in severe cases) for max. of 2 days
Ureteric colic, 75 mg then a further 75 mg after 30 minutes if necessary
By rectum in suppositories, 100 mg, usually at night
Max. total daily dose by any route 150 mg
CHILD, Still's disease, *by mouth or by rectum,* 1–3 mg/kg daily in divided doses

---

PoM **Diclofenac Sodium** (Non-proprietary)
Tablets, both e/c, diclofenac sodium 25 mg, net price 20 = £1.62; 50 mg, 20 = £3.15. Label: 5, 25

PoM **Rhumalgan**® (Lagap)
Tablets, both orange, e/c, diclofenac sodium 25 mg, net price 20 = £1.62; 50 mg, 20 = £3.15. Label: 5, 25

PoM **Voltarol**® (Geigy)
Tablets, both e/c, diclofenac sodium 25 mg (yellow), net price 20 = £1.91; 50 mg (brown), 20 = £3.71. Label: 5, 25
Injection, diclofenac sodium 25 mg/ml. Net price 3-ml amp = 80p
Suppositories, diclofenac sodium 100 mg. Net price 10 = £3.16
Paediatric suppositories, diclofenac sodium 12.5 mg. Net price 10 = 60p

PoM **Voltarol Retard**® (Geigy)
Tablets, s/r, red, diclofenac sodium 100 mg. Net price 28 = £12.70. Label: 21, 25
Dose: 100 mg once daily preferably with food

DIFLUNISAL
Indications: pain and inflammation in rheumatic disease and other musculoskeletal disorders; see also section 4.7.1
Cautions; Side-effects: see notes above; breast-feeding. Drug interactions: see Appendix 1 (sections *2.1*, *2.2*, *2.5*, *2.8C*, *4.2*, *4.7*, *8*)
Dose: initially 1 g daily in 2 divided doses, then 0.5–1 g daily; max. 1.5 g daily
Osteoarthrosis, rheumatoid arthritis, 0.5–1 g daily as a single daily dose *or* in 2 divided doses

▼ PoM **Dolobid**® (Morson)
Tablets, both f/c, diflunisal 250 mg (peach), net price 20 = £1.80; 500 mg (orange), 20 = £3.61. Label: 21, 25, counselling advised, avoid aluminium hydroxide

ETODOLAC
Indications: acute or long-term treatment of rheumatoid arthritis only
Cautions; Side-effects: see notes above. Drug interactions: see Appendix 1 (sections *2.1*, *2.2*, *2.5*, *2.8C*, *4.2*, *4.7*, *8*)
Dose: 200 mg twice daily or 400 mg once daily; max. 600 mg daily

▼ PoM **Lodine**® (Wyeth)
Capsules, light- and dark-grey, etodolac 200 mg. Net price 20 = £5.58. Label: 21
Tablets, brown, f/c, etodolac 200 mg. Net price 20 = £5.58. Label: 21
Note. Etodolac was also formerly marketed as Ramodar®.

FENBUFEN
Indications: pain and inflammation in rheumatic disease and other musculoskeletal disorders
Cautions; Side-effects: see notes above, but high risk of rashes. Drug interactions: see Appendix 1 (sections *2.1*, *2.2*, *2.5*, *2.8C*, *4.2*, *4.7*, *8*)
Dose: 300 mg in the morning and 600 mg at bedtime *or* 450 mg twice daily

PoM **Lederfen**® (Lederle)
Capsules, dark blue, fenbufen 300 mg. Net price 21-cap pack = £4.31; 84-cap pack = £17.26. Label: 21
Tablets, both light blue, f/c, fenbufen 300 mg, net price 21-tab pack = £4.31, 84-tab pack = £17.26; 450 mg, 28-tab pack = £8.63. Label: 21

PoM **Lederfen F**® (Lederle)
Effervescent tablets, fenbufen 450 mg. Net price 14 = £5.47. Label: 13, 21

FENOPROFEN
Indications: pain and inflammation in rheumatic disease and other musculoskeletal disorders; see also section 4.7.1
Cautions; Side-effects: see notes above. Drug interactions: see Appendix 1 (sections *2.1*, *2.2*, *2.5*, *2.8C*, *4.2*, *4.7*, *8*)
Dose: 300–600 mg 3–4 times daily with food; max. 3 g daily

PoM **Fenopron 300**® (Dista)
Tablets, orange, fenoprofen 300 mg (as calcium salt). Net price 20 = £2.30. Label: 21

PoM **Fenopron 600**® (Dista)
Tablets, orange, scored, fenoprofen 600 mg (as calcium salt). Net price 20 = £4.45. Label: 21

NHS PoM **Progesic**®
See section 4.7.1

FLURBIPROFEN
Indications: pain and inflammation in rheumatic disease and other musculoskeletal disorders
Cautions; Side-effects: see notes above. On rectal administration, local irritation. Drug interactions: see Appendix 1 (sections *2.1*, *2.2*, *2.5*, *2.8C*, *4.2*, *4.7*, *8*)
Dose: by mouth or rectum 150–200 mg, daily in divided doses, increased in acute conditions to 300 mg daily

PoM **Froben**® (Boots)
Tablets, both yellow, s/c, flurbiprofen 50 mg, net price 20 = £1.77; 100 mg, 20 = £3.54. Label: 21
Suppositories, flurbiprofen 100 mg. Net price 12 = £2.90

PoM **Froben SR**® (Boots)
Capsules, s/r, yellow, enclosing white, off-white beads, flurbiprofen 200 mg. Net price 30-cap pack = £12.80. Label: 21, 25
Dose: 1 capsule daily, preferably in the evening

INDOMETHACIN
Indications: pain and moderate to severe inflammation in rheumatic disease and other acute musculoskeletal disorders; acute gout
Cautions: see notes above; dizziness may impair the ability to drive or operate machinery; breast-feeding, epilepsy, parkinsonism, psychiatric disturbances; during prolonged therapy ophthalmic and blood examinations are particularly advisable; avoid rectal administration in proctitis and haemorrhoids. Drug interactions: see Appendix 1 (sections *2.1*, *2.2*, *2.5*, *2.8C*, *4.2*, *4.7*, *8*, *10*)

Side-effects: see notes above; frequently gastro-intestinal disturbances (including diarrhoea), headache, dizziness, and light-headedness; gastro-intestinal ulceration and bleeding; rarely, drowsiness, mental confusion, insomnia, convulsions, psychiatric disturbances, depression, syncope, blood disorders (particularly thrombocytopenia), hypertension, hyperglycaemia, blurred vision, corneal deposits, peripheral neuropathy. On rectal administration pruritus, discomfort, bleeding

Dose: by mouth, 50–200 mg daily in divided doses, with food

By rectum in suppositories, 100 mg at night and in the morning if required

Combined oral and rectal treatment, max. total daily dose 150–200 mg

PoM Indomethacin (Non-proprietary)
Capsules, indomethacin 25 mg, net price 20 = 18p; 50 mg, 20 = 55p. Label: 21
Suppositories, indomethacin 100 mg. Net price 10 = £1.83

▼ **PoM Flexin Continus®** (Napp)
Tablets, s/r yellow, scored, indomethacin 75 mg. Net price 28 = £10.47. Label: 21, 25
Dose: 1 tablet once or twice daily

PoM Imbrilon® (Berk)
Capsules, both yellow, indomethacin 25 mg, net price 20 = 63p; 50 mg, 20 = £1.25. Label: 21
Suppositories, indomethacin 100 mg. Net price 10 = £1.33

PoM Indocid® (Morson)
Capsules, indomethacin 25 mg, net price 20 = 99p; 50 mg, 20 = £1.78. Label: 21
Suspension, sugar-free, indomethacin 25 mg/5 ml. Do not dilute. Net price 100 ml = £1.56. Label: 21
Suppositories, indomethacin 100 mg. Net price 10 = £2.43

PoM Indocid-R® (Morson)
Capsules, s/r, ivory/clear, enclosing white and blue pellets, indomethacin 75 mg. Net price 20 = £5.71. Label: 21, 25
Dose: 1–2 capsules daily

PoM Indoflex® (Unimed)
Capsules, indomethacin 25 mg. Net price 20 = 62p. Label: 21

PoM Indolar SR® (Lagap)
Capsules, s/r, blue/clear, enclosing white pellets, indomethacin 75 mg. Net price 20 = £4.02. Label: 21, 25
Dose: 1 capsule 1–2 times daily

PoM Indomod® (Pharmacia)
Capsules, both s/r, orange/brown, enclosing e/c pellets, indomethacin 25 mg, net price 20 = £2.33; 75 mg, 20 = £7.00. Label: 25

PoM Mobilan® (Galen)
Capsules, both purple/blue, indomethacin 25 mg, net price 20 = 62p; 50 mg, 20 = £1.22. Label: 21

PoM Rheumacin LA® (CP)
Capsules, s/r, yellow/maroon, enclosing off-white pellets, indomethacin 75 mg. Net price 20 = £2.84. Label: 21, 25
Dose: 1–2 capsules daily

PoM Slo-Indo® (Generics)
Capsules, s/r, red/yellow enclosing off-white pellets, indomethacin 75 mg. Net price 20 = £4.47. Label: 21, 25
Dose: 1–2 capsules daily

Indocid PDA: see section 7.1.1

KETOPROFEN

Indications: pain and mild inflammation in rheumatic disease and other musculoskeletal disorders; dysmenorrhoea

Cautions; Side-effects: see notes above; suppositories may cause irritation. Drug interactions: see Appendix 1 (sections *2.1, 2.2, 2.5, 2.8C, 4.2, 4.7, 8*)

Dose: by mouth, 100–200 mg daily in 2–4 divided doses with food

By rectum in suppositories, 100 mg at bedtime

Combined oral and rectal treatment, max. total daily dose 200 mg

PoM Alrheumat® (Bayer)
Capsules, off-white, ketoprofen 50 mg. Net price 20 = £1.22. Label: 21

PoM Orudis® (M&B)
Capsules, ketoprofen 50 mg (green/purple), net price 20 = £1.29; 100 mg (pink), 20 = £2.58. Label: 21
Suppositories, ketoprofen 100 mg. Net price 7 = £2.32

PoM Oruvail® (M&B)
Capsules, both s/r, enclosing white pellets, ketoprofen 100 mg (pink/purple), net price 20 = £4.88; 200 mg (pink/white), 28-tab pack = £14.40. Label: 21, 25
Dose: 100–200 mg once daily with food

MEFENAMIC ACID

Indications: mild to moderate pain in rheumatoid arthritis (including Still's disease), osteoarthrosis, and related conditions; see also section 4.7.1

Cautions: see notes above; blood tests required during long-term treatment. Drug interactions: see Appendix 1 (sections *2.1, 2.2, 2.5, 2.8C, 4.2, 4.7, 8*)

Side-effects: see notes above; drowsiness; withdraw treatment in diarrhoea, hypersensitivity, bronchospasm, rashes, cholestatic jaundice, thrombocytopenia, haemolytic anaemia; convulsions in overdosage

Dose: 500 mg 3 times daily preferably after food; CHILD over 6 months, 25 mg/kg daily in divided doses for not longer than 7 days, except in Still's disease

PoM Mefenamic Acid (Non-proprietary)
Capsules, mefenamic acid 250 mg. Net price 20 = 89p. Label: 21

PoM Ponstan® (P-D)
Capsules, ivory/blue, mefenamic acid 250 mg. Net price 20 = £1.26. Label: 21
Tablets forte, yellow, f/c, mefenamic acid 500 mg. Net price 20 = £2.47. Label: 21

Paediatric suspension, mefenamic acid 50 mg/5 ml. Diluent syrup, life of diluted suspension 14 days. Net price 125 ml = £3.21. Label: 21
PoM **Ponstan Dispersible**® (P-D)
Dispersible tablets, blue, mefenamic acid 250 mg. Net price 20 = £1.53. Label: 13, 21

NABUMETONE
Indications: osteoarthrosis and rheumatoid arthritis
Cautions; Side-effects: see notes above. Drug interactions: see Appendix 1 (sections *2.1, 2.2, 2.5, 2.8C, 4.2,* 4.7, *8*)
Dose: 1 g at night, in severe conditions 0.5–1 g in morning as well; elderly 0.5–1 g daily

▼ PoM **Relifex**® (Bencard)
Tablets, red, f/c, nabumetone 500 mg. Net price 56-tab pack = £15.68. Label: 21, 25

NAPROXEN
Indications: pain and inflammation in rheumatic disease (including Still's disease) and other musculoskeletal disorders; acute gout; see also Naproxen Sodium, section 4.7.1
Cautions; Side-effects: see notes above. Drug interactions: see Appendix 1 (sections *2.1, 2.2, 2.5, 2.8C, 4.2,* 4.7, *8*)
Dose: by mouth in rheumatic disease, 0.5–1 g daily in 2 divided doses; CHILD (over 5 years), Still's disease, 10 mg/kg daily in 2 divided doses
Acute musculoskeletal disorders, 500 mg initially, then 250 mg every 6–8 hours as required
Acute gout, 750 mg initially, then 250 mg every 8 hours until attack has passed
By rectum in suppositories, 500 mg at bedtime; if necessary 500 mg in morning as well

PoM **Naproxen** (Non-proprietary)
Tablets, naproxen 250 mg, net price 20 = £1.62; 500 mg, 20 = £3.24. Label: 21
PoM **Laraflex**® (Lagap)
Tablets, both scored, naproxen 250 mg, net price 20 = £1.60; 500 mg, 20 = £3.19. Label: 21
PoM **Naprosyn**® (Syntex)
Tablets, both yellow, scored, naproxen 250 mg, net price 20 = £2.43; 500 mg, 60-tab pack = £14.57. Label: 21
Suspension, yellow, naproxen 125 mg/5 ml. Diluent water for preparations or equal quantities of syrup and water for preparations, life of diluted suspension 14 days. Net price 100 ml = £1.65. Label: 21
Granules, naproxen 500 mg/sachet. Net price 60 sachets = £19.47. Label: 13, 21
Suppositories, naproxen 500 mg. Net price 10 = £2.96
Synflex: see section 4.7.1

PHENYLBUTAZONE
Indications: ankylosing spondylitis (in hospital)
Cautions: blood counts before and during treatment if for more than 7 days; elderly patients (reduce dose); breast-feeding; withdraw treat-

ment if acute pulmonary syndrome including fever and dyspnoea occurs; see also notes above. Drug interactions: see Appendix 1 (sections *2.1, 2.2, 2.5, 2.8B, 4.2,* 4.7, *4.8, 6.1, 6.2, 8, 10*)
Contra-indications: cardiovascular disease, renal and hepatic impairment; pregnancy; history of peptic ulceration, gastro-intestinal haemorrhage, or blood disorders; thyroid disease; children under 14
Side-effects: see notes above; parotitis, stomatitis, goitre, pancreatitis, hepatitis, nephritis, visual disturbances; rarely leucopenia, thrombocytopenia, agranulocytosis, aplastic anaemia, erythema multiforme, toxic epidermal necrolysis
Dose: 200 mg 2–3 times daily, with milk or antacids if necessary, or after food, usually for 2 days, then reduced to effective minimum, usually 100 mg 2–3 times daily
Not for children under 14 years

PoM **Butacote**® (Geigy)
Tablets, both violet, e/c, s/c, phenylbutazone 100 mg, net price 20 = 37p; 200 mg, 20 = 78p. Label: 5, 21, 25
PoM **Butazolidin**® (Geigy)
Tablets, both s/c, phenylbutazone 100 mg (red), net price 20 = 26p; 200 mg, 20 = 52p. Label: 21
PoM **Butazone**® (DDSA)
Tablets, both s/c, phenylbutazone 100 mg (red), net price 20 = 6p; 200 mg, 20 = 9p. Label: 21

PIROXICAM
Indications: pain and inflammation in rheumatic disease (including Still's disease) and other musculoskeletal disorders; acute gout
Cautions: see notes above. Drug interactions: see Appendix 1 (sections *2.1, 2.2, 2.5, 2.8C, 4.2,* 4.7, *8*)
Side-effects: see notes above
Dose: initially 20 mg daily, maintenance 10–30 mg daily, in single or divided doses
CHILD (over 6 years), Still's disease, less than 15 kg, 5 mg daily; 16–25 kg, 10 mg; 26–45 kg, 15 mg; over 46 kg, 20 mg
Acute musculoskeletal disorders, 40 mg daily in single or divided doses for 2 days, then 20 mg daily for 7–14 days
Acute gout, 40 mg initially, then 40 mg daily in single or divided doses for 4–6 days

PoM **Piroxicam** (Non-proprietary)
Capsules, piroxicam 10 mg, net price 20 = £2.85; 20 mg, 20 = £5.70. Label: 21
PoM **Feldene**® (Pfizer)
Capsules, piroxicam 10 mg (maroon/blue), net price 60 = £9.50; 20 mg (maroon), 30 = £9.50. Label: 21
Dispersible tablets, piroxicam 10 mg (scored), net price 60 = £10.45; 20 mg, 30 = £10.45. Label: 13, 21
Suppositories, piroxicam 20 mg. Net price 10 = £5.20
PoM **Larapam**® (Lagap)
Capsules, piroxicam 10 mg (blue/white), net price 20 = £2.55; 20 mg (blue), 20 = £5.10. Label: 21

SULINDAC

Indications: pain and inflammation in rheumatic disease and other musculoskeletal disorders; acute gout

Cautions; Side-effects: see notes above. Drug interactions: see Appendix 1 (sections *2.1*, *2.2*, *2.5*, *2.8C*, *4.2*, *4.7*, *8*)

Dose: 200 mg twice daily with food (may be reduced according to response); max. 400 mg daily; acute gout should respond within 7 days; limit treatment of peri-articular disorders to 7–10 days

PoM **Clinoril**® (MSD)
Tablets, both yellow, scored, sulindac 100 mg, net price 20 = £2.24; 200 mg, 20 = £4.11. Label: 21

TIAPROFENIC ACID

Indications: pain and inflammation in rheumatic disease and other musculoskeletal disorders

Cautions; Side-effects: see notes above. Drug interactions: see Appendix 1 (sections *2.1*, *2.2*, *2.5*, *2.8C*, *4.2*, *4.7*, *8*)

Dose: 600 mg daily in 2–3 divided doses

PoM **Surgam**® (Roussel)
Tablets, tiaprofenic acid 200 mg, net price 20 = £3.28; 300 mg, 20 = £5.15. Label: 21
Granules, off-white, tiaprofenic acid 300 mg/sachet. Net price 20 sachets = £5.15. Label: 13, 21

▼ PoM **Surgam SA**® (Roussel)
Capsules, s/r, maroon/pink enclosing white pellets, tiaprofenic acid 300 mg. Net price 56-cap pack = £14.41. Label: 21, 25
Dose: 2 capsules at night

TOLMETIN

Indications: pain and inflammation in rheumatic disease and other musculoskeletal disorders

Cautions; Side-effects: see notes above. Drug interactions: see Appendix 1 (sections *2.1*, *2.2*, *2.5*, *2.8C*, *4.2*, *4.7*, *8*)

Dose: initially 400 mg 3 times daily preferably with food, adjusted according to response to 0.8–1.6 g daily in 2–4 divided doses

PoM **Tolectin DS**® (Ortho-Cilag)
Capsules, ivory/blue, tolmetin 400 mg (as sodium salt). Net price 20 = £3.56. Label: 21

10.1.2   Corticosteroids and corticotrophin

Drugs in this group have been divided into systemic corticosteroids and corticotrophin (section 10.1.2.1) and local corticosteroid injections (section 10.1.2.2).

10.1.2.1   SYSTEMIC CORTICOSTEROIDS AND CORTICOTROPHIN

The general actions and uses of the corticosteroids are described in section 6.3. Treatment with corticosteroids in rheumatic diseases should be reserved for specific indications, e.g. when other anti-inflammatory drugs unsuccessful.

In severe, possibly life-threatening, situations a high initial dose of corticosteroid is given to induce remission and the dose then gradually reduced to the lowest maintenance dose that will control the disease or, if possible, discontinued altogether. A major problem is that relapse may occur as dosage reduction is made, particularly if this is carried out too rapidly. The tendency is therefore to increase and maintain dosage and consequently the patient becomes dependent on corticosteroids. For this reason pulse doses of corticosteroids (e.g. methylprednisolone 1 g intravenously or methylprednisolone 320 mg intravenously on three consecutive days) is under consideration.

Prednisolone is used for most purposes; it has the advantage over the more potent corticosteroids (see section 6.3.2) of permitting finer dosage adjustments. To minimise side-effects the maintenance dose of prednisolone should be kept as low as possible, usually 7.5 mg daily and seldom exceeding 10 mg daily.

Corticosteroids should preferably be **avoided** in children as they prevent growth by suppressing the hypothalamic-pituitary-adrenal axis, and corticotrophin (see section 6.5.1) may be used instead. However, alternate day treatment with prednisolone may be preferred to injections of corticotrophin after the initial treatment has controlled disease activity.

Polymyalgia rheumatica and *temporal (giant cell) arteritis* are always treated with corticosteroids. The usual initial dose of prednisolone in polymyalgia rheumatica is 10 to 15 mg daily and in temporal arteritis 40 to 60 mg daily (the higher dose being used if visual symptoms occur). Treatment should be continued until remission occurs and doses then gradually reduced. Relapse is common if therapy is stopped within 3 years but most patients can discontinue treatment after approximately 3 to 6 years after which recurrences become rare.

Polyarteritis nodosa and *polymyositis* are usually treated with corticosteroids. An initial dose of 60 mg of prednisolone daily is often used and reduced to a maintenance dose of 10 to 15 mg daily.

Systemic lupus erythematosus is treated with corticosteroids when necessary using a similar dosage regimen to that for polyarteritis nodosa and polymyositis (above). Patients with pleurisy pericarditis, or other systemic manifestations will respond to corticosteroids. It may then be possible to reduce the dosage; alternate-day treatment is sometimes adequate, and the drug may be gradually withdrawn. In some mild cases corticosteroid treatment may be stopped after a few months Many mild cases of systemic lupus erythematosus do not require corticosteroid treatment. Alternative treatment with anti-inflammatory analgesics and possibly chloroquine, should be considered.

Since effective doses of systemic corticosteroids may cause Cushing's syndrome these drugs should **not** be used to suppress symptoms of *rheumatoid arthritis* unless alternative anti-inflammatory drug and drugs which may affect the disease process (section 10.1.3) have proved unsuccessful, with increasing disability due to the inflammatory process. The smallest effective dose should be used and increased if necessary, but should not exceed the equivalent of prednisolone 7.5 to 10 mg daily. Attempts should always be made gradually to reduce the dose. Corticosteroids in low dosage may be useful in the elderly patient, and similar nocturnal doses may relieve morning stiffness.

Ankylosing spondylitis should not be treated with long-term corticosteroids; rarely, pulse doses may be needed and may be useful in extremely active disease that does not respond to conventional treatment. Corticotrophin may rarely be required in patients with *acute gout* who do not respond to the usual drugs (section 10.1.4).

10.1.2.2 LOCAL CORTICOSTEROID INJECTIONS

Corticosteroids are injected locally for an anti-inflammatory effect. In inflammatory conditions of the joints, particularly in rheumatoid arthritis, they are given by *intra-articular injection* to relieve pain, increase mobility, and reduce deformity in one or a few joints. Full aseptic precautions are essential. Infected areas should be avoided. An almost insoluble, long-acting compound such as triamcinolone hexacetonide is preferred for intra-articular injection.

Smaller amounts of corticosteroids may also be injected directly into soft tissues for the relief of inflammation in conditions such as *tennis* or *golfer's elbow* or *compression neuropathies*. In *tendinitis*, injections should be made into the tendon sheath and not directly into the tendon. A soluble, short-acting compound such as prednisolone sodium phosphate or betamethasone is preferred for injection into the carpal tunnel.

Cortisone acetate is **not** effective for local injection and hydrocortisone acetate or one of the synthetic analogues such as triamcinolone hexacetonide is generally used. The risk of necrosis and muscle wasting may be slightly increased with triamcinolone.

Corticosteroid injections are also injected into soft tissues for the treatment of skin lesions (see section 13.4).

DEXAMETHASONE SODIUM PHOSPHATE

Indications: local inflammation of joints and soft tissues

Cautions; Contra-indications; Side-effects: see notes above and section 6.3.3

Dose: by intra-articular, intralesional, or soft-tissue injection, dexamethasone 0.4–4 mg, according to size of joint or amount of soft-tissue, at intervals of 3–21 days according to response

Note. 1.3 mg dexamethasone sodium phosphate ≡ 1.2 mg dexamethasone phosphate ≡ 1 mg dexamethasone

PoM **Decadron**® (MSD)

Injection, dexamethasone phosphate 4 mg/ml (as sodium salt) (≡ 3.33 mg/ml dexamethasone). Net price 2-ml vial = £1.76

PoM **Oradexon**® (Organon)

Injection, dexamethasone 4 mg/ml (as sodium phosphate), net price 1-ml amp = 83p; 2-ml vial = £1.27

HYDROCORTISONE ACETATE

Indications: local inflammation of joints and soft tissues

Cautions; Contra-indications; Side-effects: see notes above and section 6.3.3

Dose: by intra-articular, intrasynovial, or soft-tissue injection, 5–50 mg, according to joint size or amount of soft tissue; not more than 3 joints should be treated on any one day

PoM **Hydrocortisone Acetate Injection** (aqueous suspension), hydrocortisone acetate 25 mg/ml. Net price 1-ml amp = 36p

PoM **Hydrocortistab**® (Boots)

Injection (aqueous suspension), hydrocortisone acetate 25 mg/ml. Net price 1-ml vial = 80p

METHYLPREDNISOLONE ACETATE

Indications: local inflammation of joints and soft-tissues

Cautions; Contra-indications; Side-effects: see notes above and section 6.3.3

Dose: by intra-articular, intrasynovial, intra-lesional, or soft-tissue injection, 4–80 mg, according to joint size or amount of soft tissue, repeated every 1–5 weeks according to the response

PoM **Depo-Medrone**® (Upjohn)

Injection (aqueous suspension), methyl-prednisolone acetate 40 mg/ml. Net price 1-ml vial = £2.59; 2-ml vial or syringe = £4.65; 5-ml vial = £10.40

PoM **Depo-Medrone with Lidocaine**® (Upjohn)

Injection (aqueous suspension), methyl-prednisolone acetate 40 mg, lignocaine hydrochloride 10 mg/ml. For injection into joints, bursae, or tendon sheaths. Net price 2-ml vial = £4.65

PREDNISOLONE ACETATE

Indications: local inflammation of joints and soft tissues

Cautions; Contra-indications; Side-effects: see notes above and section 6.3.3

Dose: by intra-articular, intrasynovial, or soft-tissue injection, 5–25 mg according to joint size or amount of soft tissue; not more than 3 joints should be treated on any one day

PoM **Deltastab**® (Boots)

Injection (aqueous suspension), prednisolone acetate 25 mg/ml. Net price 5-ml vial = 90p

PREDNISOLONE SODIUM PHOSPHATE

Indications: local inflammation of joints and soft tissues

Cautions; Contra-indications; Side-effects: see notes above and section 6.3.3

Dose: by intra-articular, intrasynovial, intra-lesional, or soft-tissue injection, prednisolone 1.6–24 mg, according to joint size or amount of soft tissue, at intervals of 3–21 days according to response

PoM **Codelsol®** (MSD)
Injection, prednisolone 16 mg/ml (as prednisolone sodium phosphate). Net price 2-ml vial = £1.39

TRIAMCINOLONE ACETONIDE

Indications: local inflammation of joints and soft tissues

Cautions; Contra-indications; Side-effects: see notes above and section 6.3.3

Dose: by intra-articular injection, 2.5–40 mg according to joint size, to a max. of 80 mg in multiple injections

By intralesional injection, 2–3 mg; max. 30 mg (5 mg at any one site). Doses are repeated every 1–2 weeks according to the response

PoM **Adcortyl Intra-articular / Intradermal®** (Squibb)
Injection (aqueous suspension), triamcinolone acetonide 10 mg/ml. Net price 1-ml amp = £1.02; 5-ml vial = £4.14

PoM **Kenalog Intra-articular / Intramuscular®** (Squibb)
Injection (aqueous suspension), triamcinolone acetonide 40 mg/ml. Net price 1-ml vial = £1.70

TRIAMCINOLONE HEXACETONIDE

Indications: local inflammation of joints and soft tissues

Cautions; Contra-indications; Side-effects: see notes above and section 6.3.3

Dose: by intra-articular, intrasynovial, or soft-tissue injection, 2–30 mg, according to joint size or amount of soft tissue, repeated at intervals of not less than 3–4 weeks according to the response

By intracutaneous injection of a suspension containing not more than 5 mg/ml, up to 500 micrograms/square inch of affected skin

PoM **Lederspan®** (Lederle)
Injection (aqueous suspension), triamcinolone hexacetonide 5 mg/ml. For intralesional or sublesional injection. Net price 5-ml vial = £2.54

Injection (aqueous suspension), triamcinolone hexacetonide 20 mg/ml. For intra-articular or intrasynovial injection. Net price 1-ml vial = £2.21; 5-ml vial = £8.61

10.1.3 Drugs which may affect the rheumatic disease process

Certain drugs such as gold, penicillamine, hydroxychloroquine, chloroquine, immunosuppressants, and sulphasalazine may affect the disease process in *rheumatoid arthritis,* as may

gold and immunosuppressants in *psoriatic arthritis.* They differ from the NSAIDs in a number of ways. They do not produce an immediate therapeutic effect but reach a full response after 4 to 6 months of treatment. They may improve not only the symptoms and signs of inflammatory joint disease but also extra-articular manifestations such as vasculitis. They reduce the erythrocyte sedimentation rate and sometimes the titre of rheumatoid factor. Some (e.g. the immunosuppressants) may retard erosive damage as judged radiologically.

These drugs are used in rheumatoid arthritis where treatment with NSAIDs has been unsuccessful, so that there is evidence of disease progression including continuing active joint inflammation and worsening radiological changes. Since, in the first few months, the course of rheumatoid arthritis is unpredictable, it is usual to delay treatment for about 6 months depending on the progress of the disease, but treatment should be initiated before joint damage becomes irreversible.

Penicillamine and immunosuppressants are also sometimes used in rheumatoid arthritis where there are troublesome extra-articular features such as vasculitis, and in patients who are taking excessive doses of corticosteroids. Where the response is satisfactory there is often a striking reduction in requirements of both corticosteroids and other drugs. Gold, penicillamine, and related drugs may also be used to treat *juvenile chronic arthritis* (Still's disease) when indications are similar.

Gold and penicillamine are effective in palindromic rheumatism and chloroquine is sometimes used to treat *systemic* and *discoid lupus erythematosus.*

GOLD

Gold may be given by intramuscular injection as sodium aurothiomalate or by mouth as auranofin.

Sodium aurothiomalate must be given by deep intramuscular injection and the area gently massaged. Test doses of 10 and 20 mg should be given at weekly intervals to test the patient's tolerance; thereafter doses of 50 mg are given at weekly intervals until remission occurs or a total of 1 g has been given. Benefit is not to be expected until about 500 mg has been given. The interval between injections is then gradually increased to 2 and then to 4 weeks. If relapse occurs dosage may be immediately increased to 50 mg weekly and only once control has been obtained should a reduction in dosage again be instituted. It is important to avoid complete relapse since second courses of gold are not usually effective. Treatment should be continued indefinitely subject to tolerance.

Auranofin is given by mouth as 3 mg tablets, initially in a dose of 6 mg daily which may be increased to 9 mg daily after 3 to 6 months in the absence of response. If there is no response after 9 months treatment should be discontinued.

Gold therapy should be discontinued in the presence of blood disorders or proteinuria (associated with immune complex nephritis) which is repeatedly above 300 mg/litre without other cause (such as urinary-tract infection). Urine tests and full blood counts (including total and differential white cell and platelet counts) must therefore be performed before each intra-muscular injection; in the case of oral treatment the urine and blood tests should be carried out monthly. Rashes with pruritus often occur after 2 to 6 months of intramuscular treatment and may necessitate discontinuation of treatment; the most common side-effect of oral therapy, diarrhoea with or without nausea or abdominal pain, may respond to temporary reduction in dosage.

SODIUM AUROTHIOMALATE

Indications: active progressive rheumatoid arthritis, Still's disease

Cautions: see notes above; patients should report pruritus, metallic taste, fever, sore throat or tongue, buccal ulceration, purpura, epistaxis, bleeding gums, bruising, menorrhagia, diarrhoea; renal and hepatic impairment, elderly, breast-feeding, history of urticaria, eczema, colitis, drugs which cause blood disorders; annual chest x-ray

Contra-indications: severe renal and hepatic disease (see notes above); history of blood disorders or bone marrow aplasia, exfoliative dermatitis, systemic lupus erythematosus, necrotising enterocolitis, pulmonary fibrosis; pregnancy

Side-effects: severe reactions (occasionally fatal) in up to 5% of patients; mouth ulcers, skin reactions, oedema, proteinuria, blood disorders (sometimes sudden and fatal); rarely colitis, peripheral neuritis, pulmonary fibrosis, hepatotoxicity with cholestatic jaundice

Dose: administered on expert advice, ADULT, see notes above; CHILD, *by deep intramuscular injection,* slowly increased to the following maximum weekly doses: under 20 kg 10 mg, 20–50 kg 20 mg, over 50 kg 30 mg

PoM **Myocrisin**® (M&B)
Injection 5 mg, sodium aurothiomalate 10 mg/ml. Net price 0.5-ml amp = 86p
Injection 10 mg, sodium aurothiomalate 20 mg/ml. Net price 0.5-ml amp = £1.11
Injection 20 mg, sodium aurothiomalate 40 mg/ml. Net price 0.5-ml amp = £1.62
Injection 50 mg, sodium aurothiomalate 100 mg/ml. Net price 0.5-ml amp = £3.14

AURANOFIN

Indications: active progressive rheumatoid arthritis when NSAIDs inadequate alone

Cautions; Contra-indications: see under Sodium Aurothiomalate

Side-effects: diarrhoea most common; see also under Sodium Aurothiomalate

Dose: 6 mg daily (initially in 2 divided doses then if tolerated as single dose), if response

inadequate after 6 months, increase to 9 mg daily (in 3 divided doses), discontinue if no response after a further 3 months

▼ PoM **Ridaura**® (Bridge)
Tablets, pale yellow, f/c, auranofin 3 mg. Net price 60-tab pack = £28.00. Label: 21

PENICILLAMINE

Penicillamine has a similar action to gold, and more patients are able to continue treatment than with gold but side-effects occur frequently. An initial dose of 125 to 250 mg daily before food is given for 1 month, increased by this amount every 4 to 12 weeks until remission occurs. Penicillamine should be discontinued if there is no improvement within 1 year. The usual maintenance dose is 500 to 750 mg daily, but up to 1.5 g may rarely be required.

Patients should be warned not to expect improvement for at least 6 to 12 weeks after treatment is initiated. If remission has been sustained for 6 months, reduction of dosage by 125 to 250 mg every 12 weeks may be attempted.

Blood counts, including platelets, and urine examinations should be carried out every 1 or 2 weeks for the first 2 months then every 4 weeks to detect blood disorders and proteinuria. A reduction in platelet count indicates that treatment with penicillamine should be stopped, subsequently re-introduced at a lower dosage level and then, if possible, gradually increased. Proteinuria, associated with immune complex nephritis, occurs in up to 30% of patients, but may resolve despite continuation of treatment; treatment may be continued provided that renal function tests remain normal, oedema is absent, and the 24-hour urinary excretion of protein does not exceed 2 g.

Nausea may occur but is not usually a problem provided that penicillamine is taken before food or on retiring and that low initial doses are used and only gradually increased. Loss of taste may occur about 6 weeks after treatment is started but usually returns 6 weeks later irrespective of whether or not treatment is discontinued; mineral supplements are not recommended. Rashes are a common side-effect. Those which occur in the first few months of treatment disappear when the drug is stopped and treatment may then be re-introduced at a lower dose level and gradually increased. Late rashes are more resistant and often necessitate discontinuation of treatment.

PENICILLAMINE

Indications: severe active or progressive rheumatoid arthritis, Still's disease. For use in Wilson's disease, see section 9.8

For use in copper and lead poisoning, see Emergency Treatment of Poisoning

Cautions: see notes above; renal impairment, pregnancy, and portal hypertension; avoid concurrent gold, chloroquine, hydroxychloroquine, or immunosuppressive treatment. Drug interactions: see Appendix 1 (section 10)

Contra-indications: lupus erythematosus
Side-effects: hypersensitivity reactions (may necessitate discontinuation of treatment); nausea, anorexia, taste loss, mouth ulcers, muscle weakness, skin reactions (see notes above), oedema, proteinuria, agranulocytosis or severe thrombocytopenia (sometimes fatal); rarely myasthenia, febrile reactions, lupus erythematosus
Dose: rheumatoid arthritis, administered on expert advice, ADULT, see notes above; CHILD initial dose, 50 mg daily before food for 1 month, increased at 4-week intervals to a maintenance dose of 15–20 mg/kg daily

PoM **Distamine**® (Dista)
Tablets, all f/c, penicillamine 50 mg (scored), net price 20 = £1.26; 125 mg, 20 = £2.52; 250 mg, 20 = £4.34. Label: 6, 22

PoM **Pendramine**® (Degussa)
Tablets, both scored, f/c, penicillamine 125 mg, net price 20 = £1.79; 250 mg, 20 = £3.09. Label: 6, 22

ANTIMALARIALS

Chloroquine and **hydroxychloroquine** have a similar action to, and are better tolerated than, gold or penicillamine but their use is limited by their ocular toxicity. However, retinopathy is rare provided the doses given below are not exceeded. Nevertheless, all patients should have a full ophthalmic examination before starting treatment and then subsequently at intervals of 3 to 6 months. Ocular toxicity is also reduced if the drug is not given continuously for longer than 2 years and some physicians advise their patients to stop treatment for 2 months of each year.

These drugs should not be used for psoriatic arthritis and are best **avoided** in elderly patients as it is difficult to distinguish ageing changes from drug-induced retinopathy.

They are also used in systemic lupus erythematosus (section 10.1.2.1).

CHLOROQUINE
Indications: active rheumatoid arthritis, systemic and discoid lupus erythematosus
Cautions: renal and hepatic impairment, pregnancy, porphyria, psoriasis, neurological disorders, severe gastro-intestinal disorders, glucose 6-phosphate dehydrogenase deficiency; elderly patients, children; regular ophthalmic examinations required (see notes above). Drug interactions: see Appendix 1 (sections 10, *10*)
Contra-indications: pre-existing maculoretinopathy concurrent therapy with hepatotoxic drugs or sodium aurothiomalate
Side-effects: gastro-intestinal disturbances, headache, visual disturbances, irreversible retinal damage, corneal opacities, depigmentation or loss of hair, skin reactions (sometimes severe—may necessitate discontinuation of treatment), hearing disturbances such as tinnitus, leading rarely to deafness; rarely neuromyopathy,

myopathy, psychiatric disturbances, photosensitisation, and blood disorders (usually thrombocytopenia)
Dose: administered on expert advice, chloroquine 150 mg daily preferably after food; CHILD, 3 mg/kg daily
Note. 150 mg chloroquine ≡ 200 mg chloroquine sulphate ≡ 250 mg chloroquine phosphate (approx.)

Preparations
See section 5.4.1

HYDROXYCHLOROQUINE SULPHATE
Indications: active rheumatoid arthritis (including Still's disease), systemic and discoid lupus erythematosus
Cautions; Contra-indications; Side-effects: see under Chloroquine and notes (above)
Dose: administered on expert advice, initially 400 mg daily in divided doses; maintenance 200–400 mg daily; max. 6.5 mg/kg daily; CHILD, up to 6.5 mg/kg daily (dosage form not suitable for children under 3 years)

PoM **Plaquenil**® (Sterling Research)
Tablets, orange, s/c, hydroxychloroquine sulphate 200 mg. Net price 20 = £6.29. Label: 5

IMMUNOSUPPRESSANTS

When used in *rheumatoid arthritis* **immunosuppressants** have a similar action to gold and are useful alternatives in cases that have failed to respond to gold, penicillamine, chloroquine, or hydroxychloroquine.

Azathioprine (see section 8.2.1) is usually chosen and is given in a dose of 1.5 to 2.5 mg per kilogram body-weight daily in divided doses. Blood counts should be carried out every 4 weeks to detect possible neutropenia and/or thrombocytopenia which is usually resolved by reducing the dose. Nausea, vomiting, and diarrhoea may occur, usually starting early during the course of treatment, and may necessitate withdrawal of the drug. Herpes zoster infection may also occur during treatment.

Chlorambucil (see section 8.1.1) is another immunosuppressant which is used in rheumatoid arthritis; a dose of 100 to 200 micrograms/kg daily is usually given initially; most patients require between 2.5 and 7.5 mg daily. Regular blood counts including platelets should be carried out. **Cyclophosphamide** is more toxic but may be used at a dose of 1 to 1.5 mg/kg daily for rheumatoid arthritis with severe systemic manifestations.

Immunosuppressants are also used in the management of severe cases of *systemic lupus erythematosus* and other connective tissue disorders. They are often given in conjunction with corticosteroids for patients with severe or progressive renal disease though the evidence for their benefit is doubtful. They may be used in cases of *polymyositis* which are resistant to corticosteroids. They are used for their corticosteroid-sparing effect in patients whose corticosteroid requirements are excessive. **Azathioprine** is usually used but **chlorambucil** is an alternative and **methotrexate** (see section 8.1.3) has been used in polymyositis and rheumatoid arthritis.

Azathioprine and methotrexate are used in the treatment of *psoriatic arthropathy* for severe or progressive cases which are not controlled with anti-inflammatory drugs. There is an impression that **azathioprine** is the more effective for psoriatic arthritis and that **methotrexate** is the more effective for skin manifestations. Methotrexate is usually given in a dose of 10–25 mg weekly by mouth. Regular blood counts should be carried out.

SULPHASALAZINE

Sulphasalazine was initially introduced for the treatment of rheumatoid arthritis. Recently, it has again attracted attention and evidence is accumulating that it has a beneficial effect in suppressing the inflammatory activity of rheumatoid arthritis. Side-effects include rashes, gastro-intestinal intolerance and, especially in patients with rheumatoid arthritis, occasional leucopenia, neutropenia, and thrombocytopenia. These haematological abnormalities occur usually in the first 3 to 6 months of treatment and are reversible on cessation of treatment. Close monitoring of full blood counts is necessary throughout treatment and especially during the first 12 weeks.

SULPHASALAZINE

Indications: active rheumatoid arthritis
Cautions; Contra-indications; Side-effects: see section 1.5
Dose: by mouth, administered on expert advice, as enteric-coated tablets, initially 500 mg daily, increased by 500 mg at intervals of 1 week to a max. of 2–3 g daily in divided doses

PoM **Salazopyrin EN-tabs**® (Pharmacia)
Tablets, e/c, yellow, f/c, sulphasalazine 500 mg. Net price 125-tab pack = £11.94. Label: 5, 14, 25

10.1.4 Drugs used in the treatment of gout

It is important to distinguish drugs used for the treatment of acute attacks of gout from those used in the long-term control of the disease. The latter exacerbate and prolong the acute manifestations if started during an attack.

ACUTE ATTACKS

Acute attacks of gout are usually treated with high doses of **anti-inflammatory analgesics** such as azapropazone, diclofenac, indomethacin, naproxen, piroxicam, and sulindac (section 10.1.1). Colchicine is an alternative. Aspirin is contra-indicated in gout. Allopurinol and uricosurics are not effective in treating an acute attack and may prolong it indefinitely if started during the acute episode.

Indomethacin is often chosen in acute attacks. High doses are usually well tolerated for short periods (50 to 100 mg repeated after a few hours if necessary and followed by reducing doses every 6 hours as the patient improves). If courses of treatment last for less than one week side-effects are unusual despite the high doses used.

Colchicine is probably as effective as indomethacin but its use is limited by its toxicity.

In resistant cases of acute gout **corticotrophin** (see section 6.5.1) is very effective and is given in a dose of 80 units by intramuscular injection repeated after a day or two if necessary.

COLCHICINE

Indications: acute gout, short-term prophylaxis during initial therapy with allopurinol and uricosuric drugs
Cautions: elderly and debilitated patients, cardiac or gastro-intestinal disease, renal impairment, pregnancy and breast-feeding
Side-effects: most common are nausea, vomiting, and abdominal pain; excessive doses may also cause profuse diarrhoea, gastro-intestinal haemorrhage, rashes, and renal damage. Rarely peripheral neuritis, alopecia, and with prolonged treatment blood disorders
Dose: 1 mg initially, followed by 500 micrograms every 2–3 hours until relief of pain is obtained or vomiting or diarrhoea occurs, or until a total dose of 10 mg has been reached. The course should not be repeated within 3 days
Prevention of attacks during initial treatment with allopurinol or uricosuric drugs, 500 micrograms 2–3 times daily

PoM **Colchicine Tablets,** colchicine 250 micrograms, net price 20 = 42p; 500 micrograms, 20 = 50p

INTERVAL TREATMENT

For long-term ('interval') control of gout the formation of uric acid from purines may be reduced with the **xanthine-oxidase inhibitor** allopurinol, or the **uricosuric drugs** probenecid or sulphinpyrazone may be used to increase the excretion of uric acid in the urine. Treatment should be continued indefinitely once the decision has been made to prevent further attacks of gout by correcting the hyperuricaemia. These drugs should never be started during an acute attack. The initiation of treatment may precipitate an acute attack therefore colchicine or an anti-inflammatory analgesic should be used as a prophylactic for the first few months of treatment until the hyperuricaemia has been corrected.

Allopurinol (Zyloric® etc.) is a convenient well tolerated drug which is now widely used. It is especially useful in patients with renal impairment or urate stones where uricosuric drugs cannot be used. It is usually given once daily, as the active metabolite of allopurinol has a long half-life, but doses over 300 mg daily should be divided. Allopurinol treatment should not be started until an acute attack of gout has completely subsided, as further attacks may be precipitated. It is well tolerated in most patients but may occasionally cause rashes.

The uricosuric drugs include **probenecid** (Benemid®) and **sulphinpyrazone** (Anturan®). They can be used instead of allopurinol, or in conjunction with it in cases that are resistant to treatment.

If an acute attack develops in a patient taking allopurinol or a uricosuric the treatment should continue at the same dosage while the acute attack is treated in its own right.

Azapropazone (section 10.1.1) also has a uricosuric effect and may be useful in the long-term treatment of chronic gout.

Salicylates antagonise the uricosuric drugs; they do not antagonise allopurinol but are nevertheless contra-indicated in gout.

Crystallisation of urate in the urine may occur with the uricosuric drugs and it is important to ensure that there is an adequate urine output especially in the first few weeks of treatment. As an additional precaution the urine may be rendered alkaline.

The anti-inflammatory analgesics are described in section 10.1.1.

ALLOPURINOL

Indications: gout prophylaxis, hyperuricaemia

Cautions: administer prophylactic colchicine or anti-inflammatory analgesic for about 1 month during initial therapy; ensure adequate fluid intake (2 litres/day); render urine alkaline if uric acid overload is high; hepatic disease; reduce dose in renal impairment (dosage adjustment necessary during dialysis). In neoplastic conditions treatment with allopurinol (if required) should be commenced before cytotoxic drugs are given. Drug interactions: see Appendix 1 (sections *2.8C, 8*)

Contra-indications: as a treatment for acute gout (but continue if attack develops when already receiving allopurinol, and treat attack separately, see notes above)

Side-effects: rashes, sometimes with fever (withdraw therapy; if rash mild re-introduce cautiously but discontinue immediately if recurrence); gastro-intestinal disorders. Rarely malaise, headache, vertigo, drowsiness, taste disturbances, hypertension, symptomless xanthine deposits in muscle, alopecia, hepatotoxicity

Dose: initially 100 mg daily as a single dose, after food, gradually increased over 1–3 weeks according to the plasma or urinary uric acid concentration, to about 300 mg daily; usual maintenance dose 200–600 mg, rarely 900 mg daily, divided into doses of not more than 300 mg; CHILD (in neoplastic conditions, enzyme disorders) 10–20 mg/kg daily

PoM **Allopurinol** (Non-proprietary)
Tablets, allopurinol 100 mg, net price 20 = 50p; 300 mg, 20 = £1.71. Label: 8, 21, 27

PoM **Aloral**® (Lagap)
Tablets, both scored, allopurinol 100 mg, net price 20 = 50p; 300 mg, 20 = £1.68. Label: 8, 21, 27

PoM **Aluline**® (Steinhard)
Tablets, both scored, allopurinol 100 mg, net price 20 = £2.52; 300 mg, 28-tab pack = £8.48. Label: 8, 21, 27

PoM **Caplenal**® (Berk)
Tablets, both scored, allopurinol 100 mg, net price 20 = £2.17; 300 mg, 28-tab pack = £7.53. Label: 8, 21, 27

PoM **Cosuric**® (DDSA)
Tablets, allopurinol 100 mg, net price 20 = £2.12; 300 mg, 20 = £4.40. Label: 8, 21, 27

PoM **Hamarin**® (Nicholas)
Tablets, both scored, allopurinol 100 mg, net price 20 = £1.65; 300 mg, 20 = £4.96. Label: 8, 21, 27

PoM **Zyloric**® (Calmic)
Tablets, allopurinol 100 mg, net price 20 = £3.55; 300 mg, 30-tab pack = £13.62. Label: 8, 21, 27

PROBENECID

Indications: gout prophylaxis, hyperuricaemia; reduction of tubular excretion of penicillins and certain cephalosporins

Cautions: during initial gout therapy administer prophylactic colchicine or other appropriate therapy, ensure adequate fluid intake (about 2 litres daily), render urine alkaline if uric acid overload is high; peptic ulceration, renal impairment; transient false-positive Benedict's test. Drug interactions: see Appendix 1 (sections *4.7, 5.1, 5.3, 8*, 10, *10*)

Contra-indications: concurrent salicylate therapy, history of blood disorders, nephrolithiasis, acute gout attack and 3 weeks after

Side-effects: infrequent; occasionally nausea and vomiting, urinary frequency, headache, flushing, dizziness, rashes; rarely hypersensitivity, nephrotic syndrome, hepatic necrosis, aplastic anaemia

Dose: uricosuric therapy, initially 250 mg twice daily after food, increased after a week to 500 mg twice daily then up to 2 g daily in 2–4 divided doses according to plasma-uric acid concentration and reduced for maintenance Penicillin and cephalosporin therapy, 2 g daily in divided doses; CHILD over 2 years initially 25 mg/kg (700 mg/m²) daily, then 10 mg/kg (300 mg/m²) every 6 hours; over 50 kg, adult dose. Single-dose treatment, 1 g at the same time as oral penicillin or cephalosporin or 30 minutes before an intramuscular injection

PoM **Benemid**® (MSD)
Tablets, scored, probenecid 500 mg. Net price 20 = 55p. Label: 12, 21, 27

SULPHINPYRAZONE

Indications: gout prophylaxis, hyperuricaemia

Cautions; Contra-indications: see under Probenecid. Regular blood counts are advisable. Avoid in hypersensitivity to phenylbutazone and related drugs. Drug interactions: see Appendix 1 (sections *2.8B*, *3*, *4.8*, *6.1*, 10)

Side-effects: gastro-intestinal disorders, occasionally hypersensitivity reactions; rarely blood disorders

Dose: initially 100–200 mg daily with food (or milk) increasing over 2–3 weeks to 600 mg daily, continued until serum uric acid concentration normal then reduced for maintenance

---

PoM **Anturan**® (Geigy)

Tablets, both yellow, s/c, sulphinpyrazone 100 mg, net price 20 = 78p; 200 mg, 28-tab pack = £2.17. Label: 12, 21

10.2 Drugs used in neuromuscular disorders

Drugs in this section have been divided into those which enhance neuromuscular transmission (section 10.2.1) and skeletal muscle relaxants (section 10.2.2).

10.2.1 Drugs which enhance neuromuscular transmission

Anticholinesterase drugs are used to enhance neuromuscular transmission in voluntary and involuntary muscle in conditions such as *myasthenia gravis*. They prolong the action of acetylcholine by inhibiting the action of the enzyme acetylcholinesterase. Excessive dosage of these drugs may impair neuromuscular transmission and precipitate 'cholinergic crises' by causing a depolarising block. This may be difficult to distinguish from a worsening myasthenic state.

Side-effects of anticholinesterases are due to their parasympathomimetic action. Muscarinic effects include increased sweating, salivary, and gastric secretion, also increased gastro-intestinal and uterine motility, and bradycardia. These effects are antagonised by atropine.

Edrophonium (Tensilon®) has a very brief action and is therefore used only for the diagnosis of myasthenia gravis. A single test-dose will cause a dramatic but transient improvement in muscle power in patients with the disease (if respiration already impaired, *only* in conjunction with someone skilled at intubation).

It can also be used to determine whether a patient with myasthenia is receiving inadequate or excessive treatment with cholinergic drugs; if treatment is excessive an injection of edrophonium would either have no effect or intensify symptoms (if respiration already impaired, *only* in conjunction with or someone skilled at intubation).

Neostigmine (Prostigmin®) produces a therapeutic effect for up to 4 hours. Its pronounced muscarinic action is a disadvantage, and simultaneous administration of an anticholinergic drug such as atropine or propantheline may be required to prevent colic, excessive salivation, or diarrhoea. In severe disease neostigmine may be

given every 2 hours. The maximum that most patients can tolerate is 180 mg daily.

Pyridostigmine (Mestinon®) is less powerful and slower in action than neostigmine but it has a longer duration of action. It is sometimes preferred in patients whose muscles are weak on wakening. It has a comparatively mild gastro-intestinal effect but an anticholinergic drug may still be required. Pyridostigmine would therefore appear to have some advantages over neostigmine in the treatment of myasthenia gravis. It is inadvisable to exceed a daily dose of 720 mg.

Distigmine (Ubretid®) has the most protracted action but the danger of a 'cholinergic crisis' caused by accumulation of the drug is greater than with shorter-acting drugs. **Physostigmine** is now mainly used as a miotic (see section 11.6).

Corticosteroids (see section 6.3) are established as treatment for myasthenia gravis where *thymectomy* is inadvisable or to reduce the risk of surgery beforehand. The initial dose may be high (up to 100 mg **prednisolone** daily) but most advise starting with a smaller dose (20 mg prednisolone daily) and gradually increasing it. There is grave risk of exacerbation of the myasthenia during the initial stages of therapy, particularly in the first 2–3 weeks, therefore inpatient supervision is essential. Improvement usually begins after about 2 weeks on the high-dose regimen. In some patients a prolonged remission may be induced, but often patients need a maintenance dose of 25–40 mg of prednisolone daily; alternate-day therapy is popular. Patients who need a corticosteroid may benefit from the addition of **azathioprine** which may allow a reduction in corticosteroid dosage.

Plasmapheresis produces a striking but temporary remission in myasthenia gravis in many patients and is indicated where severe disease is unresponsive to other forms of treatment.

Neostigmine and edrophonium are also used to reverse the actions of the non-depolarising muscle relaxants (see section 15.1.6).

DISTIGMINE BROMIDE

Indications: myasthenia gravis

Cautions; Contra-indications; Side-effects: see under Neostigmine

Dose: initially 5 mg daily half an hour before breakfast, increased at intervals of 3–4 days if necessary to a max. of 20 mg daily; CHILD up to 10 mg daily according to age

---

PoM **Ubretid**® (Berk)

Tablets, scored, distigmine bromide 5 mg. Net price 20 = £10.86. Label: 22

EDROPHONIUM CHLORIDE

Indications: diagnosis of myasthenia gravis, detection of underdosage or overdosage with cholinergic drugs (see notes above)

Cautions; Contra-indications; Side-effects: see under Neostigmine; great caution in respiratory distress

---

Dose: diagnosis of myasthenia gravis, *by intravenous injection*, 2 mg followed after 30 seconds (if no adverse reaction has occurred) by 8 mg; in adults without suitable veins, *by intramuscular injection*, 10 mg

Detection of overdosage or underdosage of cholinergic drugs, *by intravenous injection*, 2 mg one hour after the last dose of cholinergic drug

PoM **Tensilon®** (Roche)
Injection, edrophonium chloride 10 mg/ml. Net price 1-ml amp = 27p

NEOSTIGMINE

Indications: myasthenia gravis
Cautions: asthma, bradycardia, recent myocardial infarction, epilepsy, hypotension, parkinsonism, vagotonia, pregnancy. Atropine or other antidote to muscarinic effects may be necessary (particularly when neostigmine is given by injection), but it should not be given routinely as it may mask signs of overdosage. Drug interactions: see Appendix 1 (sections *10*, *15*)
Contra-indications: intestinal or urinary obstruction
Side-effects: nausea, vomiting, increased salivation, diarrhoea, abdominal cramps (more marked with higher doses). Signs of overdosage are increased gastro-intestinal discomfort, bronchial secretions, and sweating, involuntary defaecation and micturition, miosis, nystagmus, bradycardia, hypotension, agitation, excessive dreaming, and weakness eventually leading to fasciculation and paralysis
Dose: by mouth, neostigmine bromide 15–30 mg at suitable intervals throughout day, total daily dose 75–300 mg (but see also notes above); NEONATE 1–5 mg every 4 hours, half an hour before feeds; CHILD up to 6 years initially 7.5 mg, 6–12 years initially 15 mg, usual total daily dose 15–90 mg
By subcutaneous or intramuscular injection, neostigmine methylsulphate 1–2.5 mg at suitable intervals throughout day (usual total daily dose 5–20 mg); NEONATE 50–250 micrograms every 4 hours; CHILD 200–500 micrograms as required

PoM **Prostigmin®** (Roche)
Tablets, scored, neostigmine bromide 15 mg. Net price 20 = 53p
Injection, neostigmine methylsulphate 500 micrograms/ml, net price 1-ml amp = 16p; 2.5 mg/ml, 1-ml amp = 16p

PYRIDOSTIGMINE BROMIDE

Indications: myasthenia gravis
Cautions; Contra-indications; Side-effects: see under Neostigmine; weaker muscarinic action
Dose: by mouth, 30–120 mg at suitable intervals throughout day, total daily dose 0.3–1.2 g (but see also notes above); NEONATE 5–10 mg every 4 hours, ½–1 hour before feeds; CHILD up to 6 years initially 30 mg, 6–12 years initially 60 mg, usual total daily dose 30–360 mg

PoM **Mestinon®** (Roche)
Tablets, scored, pyridostigmine bromide 60 mg. Net price 20 = £1.01

10.2.2   Skeletal muscle relaxants

Drugs described in this section are used for the relief of muscle spasm or spasticity. They act principally on the central nervous system with the exception of dantrolene which has a peripheral site of action. They differ in action from the muscle relaxants used in anaesthesia (see section 15.1.5) which block transmission of impulses at the neuromuscular junction.

The underlying cause of spasticity should be treated and any aggravating factors (e.g. pressure sores, infection) remedied. Skeletal muscle relaxants are effective in most forms of spasticity except the rare alpha variety. The major disadvantage of treatment with these drugs is that reduction in muscle tone can cause a loss of splinting action of the spastic leg and trunk muscles and sometimes lead to an increase in disability.

Diazepam may be tried in the first instance. Sedation and, occasionally, extensor hypotonus are disadvantages associated with its use. Other benzodiazepines also have muscle-relaxant properties. Muscle-relaxant doses of benzodiazepines are similar to anxiolytic doses (see section 4.1.2).

Baclofen (Lioresal®) has a clinical effect similar to that of diazepam; it inhibits transmission at spinal level and also depresses the central nervous system. The dose should be increased slowly to avoid sedation and hypotonia.

Dantrolene (Dantrium®) acts directly on skeletal muscle and produces fewer central adverse effects making it a drug of choice. As with baclofen the dose should be increased slowly.

Quinine salts (see section 5.4.1) 200 to 300 mg at bedtime are effective in relieving nocturnal leg cramps. They are toxic in overdosage and accidental fatalities have occurred in children.

DIAZEPAM

Indications: muscle spasm of varied aetiology; tetanus
Cautions; Side-effects: see section 4.1.2; also hypotonia; special precautions for intravenous injection (see section 4.8.2)
Dose: by mouth, 2–15 mg daily in divided doses, increased if necessary in spastic conditions to 60 mg daily according to response
Spasticity with minimal brain damage, CHILD 2–40 mg daily in divided doses
By intramuscular or slow intravenous injection, in acute muscle spasm, 10 mg repeated if necessary after 4 hours; CHILD, 100–200 micrograms/kg, repeated if necessary
Tetanus, *by intravenous injection,* 100–300 micrograms/kg repeated every 1–4 hours; *by intravenous infusion,* 3–10 mg/kg over 24 hours, adjusted according to response

Preparations
See section 4.1.2

BACLOFEN

Indications: muscle spasm in spastic conditions
Cautions: psychiatric illness, cerebrovascular disease, elderly patients; reduce dose in renal impairment, epilepsy; avoid abrupt withdrawal
Side-effects: nausea, vomiting, drowsiness, confusion, fatigue, muscle hypotonia, hypotension
Dose: 5 mg 3 times daily, preferably after food, gradually increased; max. 100 mg daily; CHILD up to 8 years 5–10 mg daily in 3–4 divided doses, gradually increased to a max. of 40 mg daily; over 8 years 10 mg daily in divided doses, gradually increased to a max. of 60 mg daily

PoM **Baclofen** (Non-proprietary)
Tablets, baclofen 10 mg. Net price 20 = £2.60. Label: 2, 8
PoM **Lioresal**® (Ciba)
Tablets, scored, baclofen 10 mg. Net price 20 = £2.60. Label: 2, 8
Liquid, sugar-free, baclofen 5 mg/5 ml. Diluent purified water, freshly boiled and cooled, life of diluted liquid 14 days. Net price 300 ml = £6.84. Label: 2, 8

DANTROLENE SODIUM

Indications: muscle spasm in spastic conditions
Cautions: impaired cardiac, pulmonary, and hepatic function; test liver function before and 6 weeks after initiating therapy. Therapeutic effect may take a few weeks to develop but if treatment is ineffective it should be discontinued after 4–6 weeks. Patients should not drive or operate machinery until therapy is stabilised. Avoid in children or when spasticity is useful, for example, locomotion. May enhance effects of CNS depressants
Side-effects: transient drowsiness, dizziness, weakness, malaise, fatigue, diarrhoea (reduce dose if necessary), occasionally urinary or musculoskeletal disturbances, rashes, and, rarely, jaundice
Dose: initially 25 mg daily, gradually increased over 7 weeks to a max. of 100 mg 4 times daily

PoM **Dantrium**® (Norwich Eaton)
Capsules, both orange/brown, dantrolene sodium 25 mg, net price 20 = £3.11; 100 mg, 20 = £10.88. Label: 2
Injection—see section 15.1.8

OTHER MUSCLE RELAXANTS

The clinical efficacy of carisoprodol, chlormezanone and meprobamate (see section 4.1.2), methocarbamol, and orphenadrine as muscle relaxants is **not** well established although they are often included in compound analgesic preparations.

CARISOPRODOL

Indications: muscle spasm (see notes above)
Cautions; Side-effects: see under Meprobamate, section 4.1.2. Drowsiness is common
Dose: 350 mg 3–4 times daily

PoM **Carisoma**® (Pharmax)
Tablets, carisoprodol 125 mg, net price 20 = 38p; 350 mg, 20 = 42p. Label: 2

METHOCARBAMOL

Indications: muscle spasm, usually in muscle injury (see notes above)
Cautions: may cause drowsiness, enhance action of CNS depressants, and increase effects of alcohol; persons affected should not drive or operate machinery. Avoid injection in renal impairment
Contra-indications: coma or pre-coma, brain damage, epilepsy, tachycardia, glaucoma, prostatic hypertrophy, bladder-neck obstruction
Side-effects: lassitude, light-headedness, dizziness, restlessness, anxiety, confusion, drowsiness, nausea, allergic rash or angioedema, convulsions
Dose: by mouth, 1.5 g 4 times daily
By slow intravenous injection or by infusion, 1–3 g; max. 3 g daily for 3 days

PoM **Robaxin 750**® (Robins)
Tablets, scored, methocarbamol 750 mg. Net price 20 = £2.24. Label: 2
Injection, methocarbamol 100 mg/ml in aqueous macrogol '300'. Net price 10-ml amp = £1.32
Robaxisal Forte—see section 4.7.1.1

ORPHENADRINE CITRATE

Indications: muscle spasm, usually in muscle injury (but see notes above)
Cautions; Contra-indications: see under Benzhexol, section 4.9.2. Avoid in children
Side-effects: dry mouth and other anticholinergic side-effects; see also Orphenadrine Hydrochloride, section 4.9.2
Dose: by mouth, 200–300 mg daily in 2 divided doses; reduce dose in elderly (preferably avoid)
By intramuscular or by slow intravenous injection (over 5 minutes), 60 mg repeated after 12 hours if necessary

PoM **Norflex**® (Riker)
Tablets, s/r, orphenadrine citrate 100 mg. Net price 20 = 91p. Label: 25
Injection, orphenadrine citrate 30 mg/ml. Net price 2-ml amp = 60p
Norgesic—see section 4.7.1.1

10.3 Drugs for the relief of soft-tissue inflammation

10.3.1 Enzymes

The enzymes in this section have fibrinolytic or proteolytic activity. Their therapeutic effectiveness is **doubtful**. They are claimed to relieve inflammation, bruising, swelling, and other soft-tissue trauma by removing coagulated blood, exudate, and necrotic tissue. They include **bromelains**, **chymotrypsin**, and **trypsin**. Some are also used to facilitate expectoration by liquefaction of bronchial secretions. See section 2.10 for streptokinase and urokinase, which also have fibrinolytic activity, and section 13.13 for desloughing agents used in ulcer treatment.

BROMELAINS

Indications: adjunctive treatment of soft tissue inflammation and oedema

Cautions: disturbances of blood-clotting mechanism; severe hepatic or renal impairment; avoid in pineapple sensitivity
Side-effects: nausea, vomiting, rashes

Ananase Forte® (Fisons)
Tablets, orange, e/c, bromelains 100 000 Rorer units. Net price 20 = £1.87. Label: 5, 25
Dose: 1 tablet 4 times daily

CHYMOTRYPSIN
Indications: adjunctive treatment of soft-tissue inflammation and oedema
Cautions: anticoagulant therapy; test for sensitivity before intramuscular injection
Side-effects: nausea, vomiting, diarrhoea, rarely severe hypersensitivity, rash

PoM **Chymar®** (Rorer)
Injection, powder for reconstitution, alpha-chymotrypsin 5000 Armour units. Net price vial (with diluent) = £1.32
Dose: by intramuscular injection, 5000 Armour units 1–3 times daily
Chymoral® (Rorer)
Tablets, red, e/c, trypsin, alpha-chymotrypsin, providing 50 000 Armour units. Net price 20 = £1.90. Label: 5, 22, 25
Tablets forte, pink, e/c, twice strength of Chymoral Tablets. Net price 20 = £3.18. Label: 5, 22, 25
Dose: 100000 Armour units 4 times daily, half an hour before food

HYPODERMOCLYSIS

Hyaluronidase (Hyalase®) is used to render the tissues more easily permeable to injected fluids, e.g. for introduction of fluids by subcutaneous infusion (termed hypodermoclysis).

HYALURONIDASE
Indications: enhance permeation of subcutaneous or intramuscular injections; promote resorption of excess fluids and blood
Contra-indications: intravenous route, bites or stings, infection or malignancy at site
Dose: to enhance tissue permeability, *by subcutaneous or intramuscular injection*, usually 1500 units, either mixed with the injection fluid or injected into the site before injection is administered
By subcutaneous infusion, 1500 units administered before 500–1000 ml infusion fluid

PoM **Hyalase®** (CP)
Injection, powder for reconstitution, hyaluronidase (ovine). Net price 1500-unit amp = £1.98

10.3.2   Rubefacients and other topical antirheumatics

Rubefacients act by counter-irritation. Pain, whether superficial or deep-seated, is relieved by any method which itself produces irritation of the

skin, for example, heat or mustard oil. There is little evidence that the blood supply to the viscera is improved by stimulation of the skin.

Counter-irritation is comforting in painful lesions of the muscles, tendons, and joints, and in non-articular rheumatism. An unnecessarily large number of substances have been, and still are, used as counter-irritants. They probably all act through the same essential mechanism and differ mainly in intensity and duration of action.

Aerosol sprays containing volatile compounds relieve pain by chilling the affected area.

There is no satisfactory evidence that preparations of adrenaline or aspirin, applied topically are of value in the relief of deep-seated pain.

Liniments and **ointments** should be applied with gentle massage 2–3 times daily avoiding broken or inflamed skin.

Adrenaline Cream (Drug Tariff Formula), adrenaline solution (1 in 1000) 20 ml, chlorocresol 100 mg, emulsifying ointment 30 g, dilute hydrochloric acid 0.04 ml, sodium metabisulphite 40 mg/100 g, in purified water, freshly boiled and cooled. Contains adrenaline 1 in 5000. Net price 50 g = 31p
Kaolin Poultice, heavy kaolin 52.7%, thymol 0.05%, boric acid 4.5%, peppermint oil 0.05%, methyl salicylate 0.2%, glycerol 42.5%. Net price 200 g = £1.18
Warm and apply directly or between layers of muslin; avoid application of overheated poultice
Kaolin Poultice K/L Pack® (K/L)
Kaolin poultice. Net price 4 × 100-g pouches = £3.16
Methyl Salicylate Liniment, methyl salicylate 25% (see Formulary). Net price 100 ml = 50p
Methyl Salicylate Ointment, methyl salicylate 50%, white beeswax 25%, hydrous wool fat 25%. Net price 100 g = 95p
Turpentine Liniment, turpentine oil 65%, camphor 5%, soft soap 7.5%, water 22.5%. Net price 100 ml = 37p
White Liniment, turpentine oil 25%, ammonium chloride 1.25%, dilute ammonia solution 4.5%, oleic acid 8.5%, water 62.5%. Net price 100 ml = 22p
Algesal® (Duphar)
Cream, diethylamine salicylate 10%. Net price 50 g = 75p
Algipan® (Wyeth)
Cream, methyl nicotinate 1%, capsicum oleoresin 0.1%, glycol salicylate 10%. Net price 40 g = 60p
Spray application, methyl nicotinate 1.5%, glycol salicylate 10%. Net price 120-ml aerosol spray = 86p
Aradolene® (Fisons)
Cream, diethylamine salicylate 5%, 'capsicin water-soluble' 0.4%, menthol 2.5%, rectified camphor oil 1.4% in a lanolin basis. Net price 40 g = 67p
Aspellin® (Fisons)
Liniment, ammonium salicylate 1%, camphor 0.6%, menthol 1.4%, ethyl and methyl salicylate 0.54%. Net price 100 ml = 52p; 500 ml = £2.60; 150-ml spray can = 96p
Balmosa® (Pharmax)
Cream, camphor 4%, capsicum oleoresin 0.035%, menthol 2%, methyl salicylate 4%. Net price 20 g = 36p; 40 g = 47p
Bayolin® (Bayer)
Cream, benzyl nicotinate 2.5%, glycol salicylate 10%, heparinoid 50 units/g. Net price 35 g = 70p
Bengué's Balsam® (Bengué)
Ointment, menthol 20%, methyl salicylate 20% in a lanolin basis. Net price 25 g = 59p
Bengué's Balsam SG® (Bengué)
Cream, menthol 10%, methyl salicylate 15% in a vanishing cream basis. Net price 25 g = 59p

---

Cremalgin® (Rorer)
Balm (= cream), capsicin 0.1%, glycol salicylate 10%, methyl nicotinate 1%. Net price 30 g = 44p
Difflam® (Riker)
Cream, benzydamine hydrochloride 3%. Net price 50 g = £3.77; 100 g = £7.13
Dubam® (Norma)
Spray application, glycol salicylate 5%, methyl nicotinate 1.6%, methyl salicylate 1%, ethyl salicylate 4%. Net price 113-g aerosol spray = £2.16
Finalgon® (Boehringer Ingelheim)
Ointment, butoxyethyl nicotinate 2.5%, vanillylnonanamide 0.4%. Net price 20 g (with applicator) = 27p

Intralgin® (Riker)
Gel, benzocaine 2%, salicylamide 5% in an alcoholic vehicle. Net price 50 g = 51p
PoM **Movelat®** (Panpharma)
Cream, corticosteroids 0.02% (as adrenocortical extract), heparinoid 0.2%, salicylic acid 2%. Net price 100 g = £3.90
Gel, ingredients as for cream but in a colourless alcoholic basis. Net price 100 g = £3.90
Transvasin® (R&C)
Cream, benzocaine 2%, ethyl nicotinate 2%, hexyl nicotinate 2%, tetrahydrofurfuryl salicylate 14%. Net price 30 g = 41p

11: Drugs acting on the

EYE

In this chapter, drug treatment is discussed under the following headings:

11.1 Administration of drugs to the eye
11.2 Control of microbial contamination
11.3 Anti-infective preparations
11.4 Corticosteroids and other anti-inflammatory preparations
11.5 Mydriatics and cycloplegics
11.6 Treatment of glaucoma
11.7 Local anaesthetics
11.8 Miscellaneous ophthalmic preparations
11.9 Contact lenses

The entries in this chapter generally relate only to local eye treatment. Systemic indications and side-effects of many of the drugs are given elsewhere (see index).

11.1 Administration of drugs to the eye

EYE-DROPS AND EYE OINTMENTS. When administered in the form of eye-drops, drugs penetrate the eyeball, probably through the cornea. However, systemic effects, which are usually undesirable, may well arise from absorption of drugs into the general circulation via conjunctival vessels or from the nasal mucosa after the excess of the preparation has drained down through the tear ducts. For example, timolol (a beta-blocker), administered as eye-drops may induce bronchospasm or bradycardia in susceptible individuals. Generally it is inadvisable for patients to continue to wear hydrophilic (soft) contact lenses when receiving eye-drops.

Eye ointments are often applied to lid margins for blepharitis. They may also be used in the conjunctival sac for other conditions especially where a prolonged action is required.

When two different preparations in the form of eye-drops are required at the same time of day, for example pilocarpine and timolol in glaucoma, dilution and overflow may occur when one immediately follows the other. The patient should therefore leave an interval of a few minutes. At night, an eye ointment for the second drug will reduce the problem.

For warnings relating to eye-drops and contact lenses, see section 11.9.

EYE LOTIONS. These are solutions for the irrigation of the conjuctival sac. They act mechanically to flush out irritants or foreign bodies as a first-aid treatment. **Sodium Chloride Eye Lotion** (section 11.8.2) is usually used. However, the lotion, which is sterile, should be used once only from a previously unopened container for first aid, while for treatment it should be used for no longer than 24 hours after the container is first opened. Single-application containers of the lotion are available.

In emergency, tap water drawn freshly from the main (not stored water) will suffice.

OTHER PREPARATIONS. Subconjunctival injection may be used to administer anti-infective drugs, mydriatics, or corticosteroids for conditions not responding to topical therapy. The drug diffuses through the sclera to the anterior and posterior chambers and vitreous humour in higher concentration than can be achieved by absorption from eye-drops. However, because the dose-volume is limited (usually not more than 1 ml), this route is suitable only for drugs which are readily soluble.

Drugs such as antibiotics and corticosteroids may be administered systemically to treat an eye condition.

Suitable plastic devices which gradually release a specified amount of drug over a period of, say, 1 week are also used (e.g. Ocuserts®).

11.2 Control of microbial contamination

Preparations for the eye should be sterile when issued. For routine domiciliary use they are supplied in multiple-application containers for individual use. They contain a suitable preservative and provided that contamination is avoided they may be used for about one month after which a new container should be opened (if treatment is to be continued) and the old one discarded.

In eye surgery it is wise to use single-application containers. Preparations used during intra-ocular procedures and others that may penetrate into the anterior chamber must be isotonic and without preservatives and buffered if necessary to a neutral pH. Large volume intravenous infusion preparations are not suitable for this purpose. For all surgical procedures, a previously unopened container is used for each patient.

11.3 Anti-infective preparations

11.3.1 Topical preparations
11.3.2 Systemic preparations

11.3.1 Topical preparations

ADMINISTRATION. Lachrymation quickly dilutes or eliminates aqueous solutions. Ideally, therefore, eye-drops should be non-irritant and instilled very frequently (at least every 2 hours) to treat acute infection or inflammation.

A useful addition for night-time use is an eye ointment because of its longer action. It will also soften crusts which cause the lids and eye lashes to adhere together when the patient is asleep. A small quantity of eye ointment is applied to the eye or lid margin as appropriate.

ANTIBACTERIAL PREPARATIONS. When prescribing antibiotics, in general, it is preferable to use topically in the eye antibiotics that are seldom or never used for systemic infections. However, the possibility of systemic absorption (section 11.1) must be taken into consideration. Examples of antibiotics with a wide spectrum of activity are **chloramphenicol**, **framycetin**, **gentamicin**, and **neomycin**. **Gentamicin** and **tobramycin** are effective for treating infections due to *Pseudomonas aeruginosa*. **Sulphacetamide** should no longer be used topically to treat eye infections, since it is rarely of any value.

Propamidine isethionate eye-drops (Brolene®) are suitable for the treament of *blepharitis* and acute and chronic *conjunctivitis*. The use of **mercuric oxide** eye ointment, even for short periods, is **not** recommended.

ANTIBACTERIAL/CORTICOSTEROID PREPARATIONS. Many antibiotic preparations also incorporate a corticosteroid but such mixtures should **not** be used unless a patient is under close specialist supervision (section 11.4). A 'red eye' is sometimes caused by the herpes simplex virus which produces a dendritic ulcer. This may be difficult to diagnose. Treatment with corticosteroids with or without antibiotics will aggravate the condition with a significant chance of loss of vision or even loss of the eye.

ANTIVIRAL PREPARATIONS. Herpes simplex infections producing, for example, dendritic corneal ulcer can be treated with **idoxuridine**. Alternatively **vidarabine** (Vira-A®) may be used. **Acyclovir** (Zovirax®) is a new drug that is activated within herpes-infected cells.

TRACHOMA. For mass antitrachoma treatment, the World Health Organization recommends **tetracycline hydrochloride** eye ointment (Achromycin®) applied to both eyes twice daily for 5 days in each month for 6 months. Chlortetracycline eye ointment (Aureomycin®) may also be used but chloramphenicol is not as effective.

For active trachoma in the individual, one or both of the following are effective. (i) For adults, orally administered sulphonamides for 2 weeks or the long-acting sulphadimethoxine (no longer on UK market) 1 g initially followed by 500 mg daily for 10 days (see section 5.1.8). For children, erythromycin should be used (see section 5.1.5). (ii) Tetracycline eye ointment three times daily for 6 weeks.

ACYCLOVIR
Indications: local treatment of herpes simplex infections
Apply 5 times daily

▼ PoM **Zovirax**® (Wellcome)
Eye ointment, acyclovir 3%. Net price 4.5 g = £7.37

CHLORAMPHENICOL
Indications: local treatment of infections (see notes above)
Apply eye-drops or eye ointment every 3 hours or more frequently if required

PoM **Chloramphenicol Eye-drops,** chloramphenicol 0.5%. Net price 10 ml = 66p
PoM **Chloromycetin**® (P-D)
Ophthalmic ointment (= eye ointment), chloramphenicol 1%. Net price 4 g = 64p
Redidrops (= eye-drops), chloramphenicol 0.5%. Net price 5 ml = £1.10; 10 ml = £1.18
PoM **Minims Chloramphenicol** (S&N Pharm.)
Eye-drops, chloramphenicol 0.5%. Net price 20 × 0.5 ml = £4.15
PoM **Opulets Chloramphenicol**® (Alcon)
Eye-drops, chloramphenicol 0.5%. Net price 20 × 0.5 ml = £3.54
PoM **Sno Phenicol**® (S&N Pharm.)
Eye-drops, chloramphenicol 0.5%, in a viscous vehicle. Net price 10 ml = 93p

CHLORTETRACYCLINE
Indications: local treatment of infections, including trachoma (see notes above)
Apply eye ointment every 2 hours (acute infections)

PoM **Aureomycin**® (Lederle)
Ophthalmic ointment (= eye ointment), chlortetracycline hydrochloride 1%. Net price 3.5 g = 94p

FRAMYCETIN SULPHATE
Indications: local treatment of infections (see notes above)
Apply eye-drops or eye ointment 3–4 times daily

PoM **Framycetin Sulphate Eye-drops,** framycetin sulphate 0.5%. Net price 5 ml = £1.27; 8 ml = £2.54
PoM **Framycetin Sulphate Eye Ointment,** framycetin sulphate 0.5%. Net price 3.5 g = 61p; 5 g = 61p
PoM **Framygen**® (Fisons)
Drops (for ear or eye), framycetin sulphate 0.5%. Net price 5 ml = £1.27
Eye ointment, framycetin sulphate 0.5%. Net price 3.5 g = 61p
PoM **Soframycin**® (Roussel)
Eye-drops, framycetin sulphate 0.5%. Net price 8 ml = £2.70
Eye ointment, framycetin sulphate 0.5%. Net price 5 g = £1.09
Ophthalmic powder, framycetin sulphate (sterile) for preparing subconjunctival injections. Net price 500-mg vial = £3.85

GENTAMICIN
Indications: local treatment of infection (see notes above)
Apply eye-drops 3–6 times daily, eye ointment 2–4 times daily

PoM Cidomycin® (Roussel)
Drops (for ear or eye), gentamicin 0.3% (as sulphate). Net price 8 ml = £1.34
Eye ointment, gentamicin 0.3% (as sulphate). Net price 3 g = £1.21

PoM Garamycin® (Kirby-Warrick)
Drops (for ear or eye), gentamicin 0.3% (as sulphate). Net price 10 ml = £1.79

PoM Genticin® (Nicholas)
Eye-drops, gentamicin 0.3% (as sulphate). Net price 10 ml = £1.79
Eye ointment, gentamicin 0.3% (as sulphate). Net price 3 g = £1.30

PoM Minims Gentamicin (S&N Pharm.)
Eye-drops, gentamicin 0.3% (as sulphate). Net price 20 × 0.5 ml = £4.72

IDOXURIDINE

Indications: local treatment of herpes simplex infections
  Apply eye-drops every hour during the day and every 2 hours at night; eye ointment every 4 hours

PoM Idoxene® (Spodefell)
Eye ointment, idoxuridine 0.5%. Net price 3 g = 95p

PoM Kerecid® (Allergan)
Eye-drops, idoxuridine 0.1%, polyvinyl alcohol (Liquifilm®) 1.4%. Net price 15 ml = £3.35
Dose, as above *or* 1 drop every minute for 5 minutes, schedule repeated every 4 hours day and night
Eye ointment, idoxuridine 0.5%. Net price 4 g = £3.68

PoM Ophthalmadine® (Sas)
Eye-drops, idoxuridine 0.1%. Net price 10 ml = £1.05
Eye ointment, idoxuridine 0.5%. Net price 3 g = £1.05

NEOMYCIN SULPHATE

Indications: local treatment of infections (see notes above)
  Apply eye-drops or eye ointment 3–4 times daily

PoM Neomycin Sulphate Eye-drops, neomycin sulphate 0.5%. Net price 10 ml = £1.53

PoM Graneodin® (Squibb)
Ophthalmic ointment (= eye ointment), gramicidin 0.025%, neomycin sulphate 0.25%. Net price 3.6 g = 61p
  Apply 3–4 times daily

PoM Minims Neomycin Sulphate (S&N Pharm.)
Eye-drops, neomycin sulphate 0.5%. Net price 20 × 0.5 ml = £4.72

PoM Myciguent® (Upjohn)
Eye ointment, neomycin sulphate 0.5%. Net price 3.9 g = 68p

PoM Neosporin® (Calmic)
Eye-drops, gramicidin 25 units, neomycin sulphate 1700 units, polymyxin B sulphate 5000 units/ml. Net price 5 ml = £3.19
  Apply 2–4 times daily or more frequently if required

POLYMYXIN B SULPHATE

Indications: local treatment of infections (see notes above)

PoM Polyfax® (Calmic)
Eye ointment, polymyxin B sulphate 10 000 units, bacitracin zinc 500 units/g. Net price 4 g = £1.94
  Apply twice daily

PoM Polytrim® (Wellcome)
Eye-drops, trimethoprim 0.1%, polymyxin ▶ sulphate 10 000 units/ml. Net price 5 ml = £2.5.
  Apply 4 times daily
▼ *Eye ointment*, trimethoprim 0.5%, polymyxin B sulphate 10000 units/g. Net price 4 g = £2.5.
  Apply 3–4 times daily

PROPAMIDINE ISETHIONATE

Indications: local treatment of infections (see notes above)

Brolene® (M&B)
Eye-drops, propamidine isethionate 0.1%. Net price 10 ml = £1.13
  Apply 4 times daily

SULPHACETAMIDE SODIUM

Indications: not recommended, see notes above
  Apply eye-drops every 2–6 hours, eye ointment 2–4 times daily or at night

PoM Sulphacetamide Eye-drops, sulphacetamide sodium 10%, net price 10 ml = £1.42; 30%, 10 ml = £1.45
Note. When Weak Sulphacetamide Eye-drops are prescribed a 10% solution is supplied; when Strong Sulphacetamide Eye-drops are prescribed a 30% solution is supplied

PoM Albucid® (Nicholas)
Eye-drops, sulphacetamide sodium 10%, net price 10 ml = 85p; 20%, 10 ml = 87p; 30%, 10 ml = 89p
Eye ointment, greasy basis, sulphacetamide sodium 2.5%, 4 g = 57p; 6%, 4 g = 60p
Eye ointment, water-miscible basis, sulphacetamide sodium 10%. Net price 4 g = 63p

PoM Minims Sulphacetamide Sodium (S&N Pharm.)
Eye-drops, sulphacetamide sodium 10%. Net price 20 × 0.5 ml = £4.72

PoM Ocusol® (Boots)
Eye-drops, sulphacetamide sodium 5%, zinc sulphate 0.1%. Net price 10 ml = 90p

TETRACYCLINE HYDROCHLORIDE

Indications: local treatment of infections, including trachoma (see notes above)
  Apply eye-drops 2–4 times daily or eye ointment every 2 hours (acute infections)

PoM Achromycin® (Lederle)
Ophthalmic oil suspension (= eye-drops), tetracycline hydrochloride 1%, in sesame oil vehicle. Net price 6 ml = £1.85
Ointment (for ear or eye), tetracycline hydrochloride 1%. Net price 3.5 g = 70p

TOBRAMYCIN

Indications: local treatment of infections (see notes above)
  Apply eye-drops every 2–4 hours depending on severity

PoM **Tobralex®** (Alcon)
Eye-drops, tobramycin 0.3%. Net price 5 ml =
£1.43

VIDARABINE

Indications: local treatment of Herpes simplex
infections
Apply 5 times daily

PoM **Vira-A®** (P-D)
Eye ointment, vidarabine 3%. Net price 3.5 g =
£6.42

FUNGAL INFECTIONS OF THE EYE

Fungal infections of the cornea are rare but tend
to occur after agricultural injuries, especially in
hot and humid climates. Orbital mycosis is rare,
and when it occurs is usually due to direct spread
of infection from the paranasal sinuses. Increasing
age, debility, or immunosuppression by drugs,
for example, following renal transplantation, may
encourage fungal proliferation in many parts of
the body. The spread of infection via the blood-
stream occasionally produces a metastatic
endophthalmitis.

A wide range of fungi are capable of producing
ocular mycosis and may be identified by appropriate laboratory procedures.

Antifungal preparations for the eye are not
generally available. Treatment will normally be
carried out at specialist centres, but requests for
information about supplies of preparations not
available commercially should be addressed to the
District Pharmaceutical Officer (or equivalent in
Scotland or Northern Ireland) or to Moorfields
Eye Hospital, City Road, London EC1V 2PD
(01-253 3411).

11.3.2 Systemic preparations

In severe infections, systemic treatment is given
in addition to topical therapy as, for example,
in gonococcal conjunctivitis in the newborn and
infective endophthalmitis. The blood-aqueous
barrier usually breaks down in the latter case
allowing intra-ocular penetration of systemically
administered drugs. Subconjunctival injection of
a suitable drug may also help to achieve a high
intra-ocular concentration.

Pyrimethamine (see section 5.4.1) administered
systemically is appropriate for treatment of toxoplasma choroidoretinitis; clindamycin and sulphadiazine are other possibilities.

Other drugs suitable for the systemic treatment
of eye infections are included in chapter 5.

11.4 Corticosteroids and other anti-inflammatory preparations

Corticosteroids administered topically, by subconjunctival injection, and systemically have an
important place in treating uveitis and scleritis;

they are also used to reduce post-operative
inflammation following eye operations.

Topical corticosteroids should normally only be
used under expert supervision; they should not be
prescribed for undiagnosed 'red eye'. There are
two main dangers from topical corticosteroids.
First is enhancement of herpetic corneal disease,
due to misdiagnosis already referred to (section
11.3.1), when the corticosteroid is administered
in eye-drops. Second, again arising from the use
of eye-drop formulations, a 'steroid glaucoma'
may be produced, after a few weeks treatment, in
patients predisposed to chronic simple glaucoma,
especially with dexamethasone and prednisolone.

Systemic corticosteroids can usefully be given
on an alternate-day basis to minimise side-effects.
The risk of producing glaucoma is not great, but
'steroid cataract' is a very high risk (75%) if more
than 15 mg of prednisolone or equivalent is given
daily for several years. The longer the duration,
the greater is the risk. A dose of less then 10 mg
per day is usually safe.

Oxyphenbutazone eye ointment (Tanderil®)
does not have the disadvantages of corticosteroids
and has been used in the treatment of episcleritis.

Topical preparations of **antihistamines** such as
eye-drops containing antazoline sulphate (with
xylometazoline hydrochloride as Otrivine-Anti-
stin®) may be used for short-term treatment of
allergic conjunctivitis.

Sodium cromoglycate eye-drops (Opticrom®)
may be useful for vernal catarrh and other allergic
forms of conjunctivitis.

ANTAZOLINE

Indications: allergic conjunctivitis

Otrivine-Antistin® (Zyma)
Eye-drops, antazoline sulphate 0.5%, xylometa-
zoline hydrochloride 0.05%. Net price 10 ml =
92p
Apply 2–3 times daily
PoM **Vasocon A®** (CooperVision)
Eye-drops, antazoline phosphate 0.5%,
naphazoline hydrochloride 0.05%. Net price
10 ml = £2.19
Apply every 3–4 hours

BETAMETHASONE

Indications: local treatment of inflammation
Cautions; Side-effects: see notes above
Apply eye-drops every 1–2 hours or eye oint-
ment 2–4 times daily

PoM **Betnesol®** (Glaxo)
Drops (for ear, eye, or nose), betamethasone
sodium phosphate 0.1%. Net price 5 ml = 80p;
10 ml = £1.31
Eye ointment, betamethasone sodium phosphate
0.1%. Net price 3 g = 56p
PoM **Betnesol-N®** (Glaxo)
Drops (for ear, eye, or nose), see section 12.1.1
Eye ointment, betamethasone sodium phosphate 0.1%,
neomycin sulphate 0.5%. Net price 3 g = 64p

PoM **Vista-Methasone®** (Daniel)
Drops (for ear, eye, or nose), betamethasone sodium phosphate 0.1%. Net price 5 ml = 60p; 10 ml = 95p
PoM **Vista-Methasone N®** (Daniel)
Drops (for ear, eye, or nose), see section 12.1.1

CLOBETASONE BUTYRATE
Indications: local treatment of inflammation
Cautions; Side-effects: see notes above; reduced tendency to raise intra-ocular pressure
Apply eye-drops every 1–6 hours

PoM **Eumovate®** (Glaxo)
Eye-drops, clobetasone butyrate 0.1%. Net price 5 ml = £1.46; 10 ml = £2.70
PoM **Eumovate-N®** (Glaxo)
Eye-drops, clobetasone butyrate 0.1%, neomycin sulphate 0.5%. Net price 5 ml = £1.46; 10 ml = £2.70

DEXAMETHASONE
Indications: local treatment of inflammation
Cautions; Side-effects: see notes above
Apply eye-drops every 1–4 hours

PoM **Maxidex®** (Alcon)
Eye-drops, dexamethasone 0.1%, hypromellose 0.5%. Net price 5 ml = £1.53; 10 ml = £3.03
PoM **Maxitrol®** (Alcon)
Eye-drops, dexamethasone 0.1%, hypromellose 0.5%, neomycin 0.35% (as sulphate), polymyxin B sulphate 6000 units/ml. Net price 5 ml = £1.81
Eye ointment, dexamethasone 0.1%, neomycin 0.35% (as sulphate), polymyxin B sulphate 6000 units/g. Net price 3.5 g = £1.56
PoM **Sofradex®** (Roussel)
Ointment (for ear or eyelid), see section 12.1.1

FLUOROMETHOLONE
Indications: local treatment of inflammation
Cautions; Side-effects: see notes above; reduced tendency to raise intra-ocular pressure
Apply eye-drops every 1–4 hours

PoM **FML®** (Allergan)
Ophthalmic suspension (= eye-drops), fluorometholone 0.1%, polyvinyl alcohol (Liquifilm®) 1.4%. Net price 5 ml = £1.78; 10 ml = £2.83
▼ PoM **FML-Neo®** (Allergan)
Eye-drops, fluorometholone 0.1%, neomycin sulphate 0.5%, polyvinyl alcohol (Liquifilm®) 1.4%. Net price 5 ml = £1.90

HYDROCORTISONE ACETATE
Indications: local treatment of inflammation
Cautions; Side-effects: see notes above

PoM **Hydrocortisone** (Non-proprietary)
Eye-drops, hydrocortisone acetate 1%. Net price 10 ml = £1.70
PoM **Chloromycetin Hydrocortisone®** (P-D)
Eye ointment, chloramphenicol 1%, hydrocortisone acetate 0.5%. Net price 4 g = 70p
PoM **Cortucid®** (Nicholas)
Eye drop cream (= eye ointment), hydrocortisone acetate 0.5%, sulphacetamide sodium 10%. Net price 3 g = 81p

PoM **Framycort®** (Fisons)
Drops (for ear or eye), framycetin sulphate 0.5%, hydrocortisone acetate 0.5%. Net price 5 ml = £2.21
Eye ointment, framycetin sulphate 0.5%, hydrocortisone acetate 0.5%. Net price 3.5 g = £1.17
PoM **Neo-Cortef®** (Upjohn)
Drops and *ointment* (for ear or eye), see section 12.1.

OXYPHENBUTAZONE
Indications: local treatment of inflammation
Apply eye ointment 2–5 times daily

PoM **Tanderil®** (Zyma)
Eye ointment, oxyphenbutazone 10%. Net price 5 g = 63p
PoM **Tanderil Chloramphenicol®** (Zyma)
Eye ointment, chloramphenicol 1%, oxyphenbutazone 10%. Net price 5 g = £1.02

PREDNISOLONE
Indications: local treatment of inflammation
Cautions; Side-effects: see notes above
Apply eye-drops every 1–2 hours

PoM **Minims Prednisolone** (S&N Pharm.)
Eye-drops, prednisolone sodium phosphate 0.5%. Net price 20 × 0.5 ml = £4.72
▼ PoM **Pred Forte®** (Allergan)
Eye-drops, prednisolone acetate 1%. Net price 5 ml = £1.55; 10 ml = £3.09
Apply 2–4 times daily
PoM **Predsol®** (Glaxo)
Drops (for ear or eye), prednisolone sodium phosphate 0.5%. Net price 5 ml = 80p; 10 ml = £1.31
PoM **Predsol-N®** (Glaxo)
Drops (for ear or eye), see section 12.1.1

SODIUM CROMOGLYCATE
Indications: allergic conjunctivitis
Apply eye-drops 4 times daily; eye ointment apply 2–3 times daily

PoM **Opticrom®** (Fisons)
Eye-drops, sodium cromoglycate 2%. Net price 13.5 ml = £5.59
Eye ointment, sodium cromoglycate 4%. Net price 5 g = £5.99

11.5 Mydriatics and cycloplegics

The two properties of dilatation of the pupil and paralysis of the ciliary muscle are usually possessed equally by anticholinergic drugs applied topically but they vary in potency. Short-acting, relatively weak mydriatics which paralyse the sphincter pupillae are used by the ophthalmologist to allow a better view of the fundus of the eye. The relative potencies and durations of action of the principal drugs, in ascending order, are tropicamide (3 hours), cyclopentolate, hyoscine and homatropine (all 24 hours), and atropine (6 days or longer).

Cyclopentolate 1% or **atropine** are preferable for producing cycloplegia for refraction in young

hildren. Atropine 1% (in ointment form) is pre-
erred for children under 5 years of age. Atropine
s also used for the treatment of iridocyclitis
nainly to prevent posterior synechiae, often with
phenylephrine 10% eye-drops (2.5% in children
nd those with cardiac disease). Phenylephrine
nay interact with systemically administered
nonoamine-oxidase inhibitors.

Contact dermatitis is not uncommon with all of
he above mydriatic drugs, especially atropine,
and toxic systemic reactions to this drug may occur
n the very young and the very old.

Mydriasis may precipitate acute closed-angle
'congestive') glaucoma in a few patients, usually
aged over 60 years, who are predisposed to the
condition because of a small eyeball with a shallow
anterior chamber and small diameter cornea. A
amily history is significant. Mydriatics should
be avoided in such patients. Patients should be
warned to be cautious in driving after mydriasis.

ANTICHOLINERGICS

ATROPINE SULPHATE
Indications: refraction procedures in young children; see also notes above
Cautions: action persistent, may precipitate glaucoma; see also notes above

PoM **Atropine Eye-drops,** atropine sulphate 1%.
Net price 10 ml = 66p
PoM **Atropine Eye Ointment,** atropine sulphate
1%. Net price 3 g = 60p
PoM **Isopto Atropine**® (Alcon)
Eye-drops, atropine sulphate 1%, hypromellose
0.5%. Net price 5 ml = £1.02
PoM **Minims Atropine Sulphate** (S&N Pharm.)
Eye-drops, atropine sulphate 1%. Net price
20 × 0.5 ml = £4.15
PoM **Opulets Atropine Sulphate**® (Alcon)
Eye-drops, atropine 1%. Net price 20 × 0.5 ml =
£3.54

CYCLOPENTOLATE HYDROCHLORIDE
Indications: see notes above
Cautions: patients with raised intra-ocular
pressure; see notes above

PoM **Minims Cyclopentolate Hydrochloride**
(S&N Pharm.)
Eye-drops, cyclopentolate hydrochloride 0.5 and
1%. Net price 20 × 0.5 ml (both) = £4.15
PoM **Mydrilate**® (Boehringer Ingelheim)
Eye-drops, cyclopentolate hydrochloride 0.5%,
net price 5 ml = 67p; 1%, 5 ml = 90p
PoM **Opulets Cyclopentolate Hydrochloride**®
(Alcon)
Eye-drops, cyclopentolate hydrochloride 1%.
Net price 20 × 0.5 ml = £3.54

HOMATROPINE HYDROBROMIDE
Indications; Cautions: see notes above

PoM **Homatropine Eye-drops,** homatropine
hydrobromide 1%, net price 10 ml = £1.66; 2%,
10 ml = £1.76

PoM **Minims Homatropine Hydrobromide** (S&N
Pharm.)
Eye-drops, homatropine hydrobromide 2%. Net
price 20 × 0.5 ml = £4.72

HYOSCINE HYDROBROMIDE
Indications; Cautions: see notes above

PoM **Hyoscine Eye-drops,** usual strength hyoscine
hydrobromide 0.25%. Net price 10 ml = 83p

LACHESINE CHLORIDE
Indications: see notes above; useful in patients
hypersensitive to other mydriatics
Cautions: see notes above

Lachesine Eye-drops, lachesine chloride 1%.
Net price 10 ml = £3.60

TROPICAMIDE
Indications; Cautions: see notes above

PoM **Minims Tropicamide** (S&N Pharm.)
Eye-drops, tropicamide 0.5 and 1%. Net price
20 × 0.5 ml (both) = £4.72
PoM **Mydriacyl**® (Alcon)
Eye-drops, tropicamide 0.5%, net price 5 ml =
£1.39; 1%, 5 ml = £1.72

SYMPATHOMIMETICS

ADRENALINE
See section 11.6

PHENYLEPHRINE HYDROCHLORIDE
Indications; Cautions: see notes above

Phenylephrine Eye-drops, phenylephrine
hydrochloride 10%. Net price 10 ml = £1.73
Minims Phenylephrine Hydrochloride (S&N
Pharm.)
Eye-drops, phenylephrine hydrochloride 2.5%,
net price 20 × 0.5 ml = £4.72; 10%,
20 × 0.5 ml = £4.72
See also under Hypromellose (section 11.8.1)

11.6 Treatment of glaucoma

An abnormally high intra-ocular pressure, glaucoma, may result in blindness associated with
pressure-excavation of the optic disk ('glau-
comatous cupping'). In virtually all cases, rise in
pressure is due to reduced outflow of aqueous
humour, the inflow remaining constant.

Glaucoma is treated by the application of eye-
drops containing miotics, adrenaline (and guanethidine), or beta-blockers. Acetazolamide and
dichlorphenamide are given by mouth and, in
emergency or before surgery, mannitol may be
given by intravenous infusion.

Probably the commonest condition is *chronic
simple glaucoma* where the obstruction is in the
trabecular meshwork. It is commonly first treated

with a topical beta-blocker and other drugs added as necessary to control the intra-ocular pressure e.g. adrenaline or pilocarpine.

If supplementary topical treatment is required after *iridectomy* or a drainage operation in either open-angle or closed-angle glaucoma, a beta-blocker is preferred to pilocarpine. This is because of the risk that posterior synechiae will be formed as a result of the miotic effect of pilocarpine, especially in closed-angle glaucoma. It is then also advantageous to utilise the mydriatic side-effect of adrenaline.

MIOTICS

The small pupil is an unfortunate side-effect of these drugs (except when **pilocarpine** is used temporarily while patients await operation for *closed-angle glaucoma*). The key factor is the opening up of the inefficient drainage channels in the trabecular meshwork resulting from contraction or spasm of the ciliary muscle. This unfortunately also produces accommodation spasm that may result in blurring of vision and browache, which is especially disadvantageous in patients under 40 years of age. Pilocarpine has a duration of action of 3 to 4 hours. **Physostigmine** is more potent; it is still used with pilocarpine but is not usually used alone. **Carbachol** is sometimes used to lower intra-ocular pressure, usually in conjunction with other miotics such as physostigmine. In severe cases **ecothiopate iodide** (Phospholine Iodide®) produces a more prolonged potent effect but the risk of cataract and other side-effects has to be weighed against the benefit.

CARBACHOL

Indications: see notes above
Apply eye-drops 3 times daily

PoM **Isopto Carbachol**® (Alcon)
Eye-drops, carbachol 3%, hypromellose 1%. Net price 10 ml = £1.80

DEMECARIUM BROMIDE

Indications: glaucoma
Apply eye-drops 1–2 times daily

PoM **Tosmilen**® (Sinclair)
Eye-drops, demecarium bromide 0.25% (named-patient basis only)

ECOTHIOPATE IODIDE

Indications; Side-effects: see notes above
Cautions: drug interactions: see Appendix 1 (section *15*)
Apply eye-drops 1–2 times daily

PoM **Phospholine Iodide**® (Wyeth)
Eye-drops, ecothiopate iodide (when reconstituted) 0.03%, net price 5 ml = £1.82; 0.06%, 5 ml = £2.07; 0.125%, 5 ml = £2.28; 0.25%, 5 ml = £2.64

PHYSOSTIGMINE SULPHATE

Indications; Side-effects: see notes above
Apply eye-drops 2–6 times daily

PoM **Physostigmine** (Non-proprietary)
Eye-drops, physostigmine sulphate 0.25 an 0.5%. Net price 10 ml (both) = £1.89

PoM **Physostigmine and Pilocarpine** (Nor proprietary)
Eye-drops, physostigmine sulphate 0.25%, pilo carpine hydrochloride 2%. Net price 10 ml = £1.28
Eye-drops, physostigmine sulphate 0.25%, pilo carpine hydrochloride 4%. Net price 10 ml = £1.87
Eye-drops, physostigmine sulphate 0.5%, pilo carpine hydrochloride 4%. Net price 10 ml = £1.87

PILOCARPINE

Indications; Side-effects: see notes above
Apply eye-drops 3–6 times daily

Pilocarpine hydrochloride
PoM **Pilocarpine** (Non-proprietary)
Eye-drops, pilocarpine hydrochloride 0.5 an 1%, net price 10 ml = £1.10; 2%, 10 ml = £1.19; 3%, 10 ml = £1.35; 4%, 10 ml = £1.50
PoM **Isopto Carpine**® (Alcon)
Eye-drops, all with hypromellose 0.5%; pilo carpine hydrochloride 0.5%, net price 10 ml = 75p; 1%, 10 ml = 83p; 2%, 10 ml = 92p; 3% 10 ml = 99p; 4%, 10 ml = £1.07
PoM **Opulets Pilocarpine**® (Alcon)
Eye-drops, pilocarpine hydrochloride 1, 2, an 4%. Net price 20 × 0.5 ml (all) = £3.54
PoM **Sno Pilo**® (S&N Pharm.)
Eye-drops, in a viscous vehicle, pilocarpin hydrochloride 1%, net price 10 ml = 90p; 2% 10 ml = 98p; 4%, 10 ml = £1.17

Pilocarpine nitrate
PoM **Minims Pilocarpine Nitrate** (S&N Pharm.
Eye-drops, pilocarpine nitrate 1, 2, and 4%. Ne price 20 × 0.5 ml (all) = £4.15

Sustained-release (as base)
▼ PoM **Ocusert**® (M&B)
Pilo-20 ocular insert, s/r, pilocarpine 20 micr grams released per hour for 1 week. Net pri per insert = £2.79. Counselling advise method of use
Pilo-40 ocular insert, s/r, pilocarpine 40 micr grams released per hour for 1 week. Net pri per insert = £3.20. Counselling advise method of use

ADRENALINE/GUANETHIDINE

Adrenaline probably acts both by reducing th rate of production of aqueous humour and b increasing the outflow through the trabecula meshwork. It is contra-indicated in closed-ang glaucoma because it is a mydriatic, unless an ir dectomy has been carried out. Side-effects includ

---

severe smarting and redness of the eye; adrenaline should be used with caution in patients with heart disease.

Dipivefrine (Propine®) is an ester and prodrug of adrenaline. It is stated to pass more rapidly through the cornea and is then converted to the active form.

Guanethidine (Ganda®, Ismelin®) enhances and prolongs the effects of adrenaline. It is also used alone and produces an initial mydriasis together with an increased aqueous outflow followed by a miosis and reduced aqueous secretion. Prolonged use, particularly of the higher strengths may result in conjunctival fibrosis with secondary corneal changes; the conjunctiva and cornea should be examined at least every six months.

ADRENALINE
Indications; Contra-indications: see notes above
  Apply eye-drops 1–2 times daily

PoM **Epifrin®** (Allergan)
Eye-drops, adrenaline 1% (as hydrochloride). Net price 10 ml = £1.95
Eppy® (S&N Pharm.)
Eye-drops, adrenaline 1%. Net price 7.5 ml = £3.26
Isopto Epinal® (Alcon)
Eye-drops, adrenaline 1% (as borate complex) and hypromellose 0.5%. Net price 7.5 ml = £1.62
PoM **Simplene®** (S&N Pharm.)
Eye-drops, adrenaline, in a viscous vehicle, 0.5%, net price 7.5 ml = £2.79; 1%, 7.5 ml = £3.06

DIPIVEFRINE HYDROCHLORIDE
Indications; Contra-indications: see notes above
  Apply 1 drop twice daily

▼ PoM **Propine®** (Allergan)
Eye-drops, dipivefrine hydrochloride 0.1%. Net price 10 ml = £4.65

GUANETHIDINE MONOSULPHATE
Indications: see notes above
  Apply eye-drops 1–2 times daily
Cautions: see notes above

▼ PoM **Ganda®** (S&N Pharm.)
Eye-drops '1 + 0.2', guanethidine monosulphate 1%, adrenaline 0.2% in a viscous vehicle. Net price 7.5 ml = £3.87
Eye-drops '3 + 0.5', guanethidine monosulphate 3%, adrenaline 0.5% in a viscous vehicle. Net price 7.5 ml = £5.06
PoM **Ismelin®** (Zyma)
Eye-drops, guanethidine monosulphate 5%. Net price 5 ml = £1.87

BETA-BLOCKERS

Topical application of a beta-blocker to the eye reduces intra-ocular pressure effectively in chronic simple glaucoma, probably by reducing the rate of production of aqueous humour. Administration by mouth also reduces intra-ocular pressure but this route is not used (see comment under Systemic Drugs).

Beta-blockers used as eye-drops include **timolol maleate** (Timoptol®) and, more recently, **betaxolol hydrochloride** (Betoptic®), **carteolol hydrochloride** (Teoptic®), and **metipranolol** (Glauline®).

SIDE-EFFECTS. Systemic absorption may follow topical application, therefore beta-blocker eye-drops are contra-indicated in patients with asthma or a history of obstructive airways disease; betaxolol and possibly carteolol are least likely to be hazardous but nevertheless should not be used.

> **CSM advice.** The CSM has advised that beta-blockers, even those with apparent cardio-selectivity, should not be used in patients with asthma or a history of obstructive airways disease, unless no alternative treatment is available. In such cases the risk of inducing bronchospasm should be appreciated and appropriate precautions taken.

Eye-drops containing a beta-blocker are also contra-indicated in patients with bradycardia, heart block, or heart failure.

Local side-effects of eye-drops containing a beta-blocker include transitory dry eyes and allergic blepharoconjunctivitis.

DRUG INTERACTIONS. Administration may give rise notably to an interaction with drugs such as verapamil. See Appendix 1 (sections *2.3*, 2.4, *2.5*, *2.7*, *4.2*, *6.1*, *10*, *15*).

BETAXOLOL HYDROCHLORIDE
Indications; Cautions; Contra-indications; Side-effects: see notes above
  Apply eye-drops twice daily

▼ PoM **Betoptic®** (Alcon)
Eye-drops, betaxolol 0.5% (as hydrochloride). Net price 5 ml = £5.30

CARTEOLOL HYDROCHLORIDE
Indications; Cautions; Contra-indications; Side-effects: see notes above
  Apply eye-drops twice daily

▼ PoM **Teoptic®** (Dispersa)
Eye-drops, carteolol hydrochloride 1%, net price 5 ml = £5.05; 2%, 5 ml = £5.67

METIPRANOLOL
Indications; Cautions; Contra-indications; Side-effects: see notes above
  Apply eye-drops twice daily

▼ PoM **Glauline®** (S&N Pharm.)
Eye-drops, metipranolol 0.1%, net price 5 ml = £3.73; 0.3%, 5 ml = £4.45; 0.6%, 5 ml = £4.94

▼ PoM **Minims Metipranolol** (S&N Pharm.)
Eye-drops, metipranolol 0.1%, net price
20 × 0.5 ml = £8.50; 0.3%, 20 × 0.5 ml =
£9.90; 0.6%, 20 × 0.5 ml = £10.90

TIMOLOL MALEATE

*Indications; Cautions; Contra-indications; Side-
effects:* see notes above
Apply eye-drops twice daily

PoM **Timoptol**® (MSD)
Eye-drops, in Ocumeter® metered-dose unit,
timolol (as maleate) 0.25%, net price 5 ml =
£5.18; 0.5%, 5 ml = £5.82

SYSTEMIC DRUGS

The side-effects of beta-blockers are probably sufficient to prevent their being prescribed by the
ophthalmologist for administration by mouth.
Hence **acetazolamide** (Diamox®) will retain a
significant place in treatment. It inhibits carbonic
anhydrase, thus reducing the bicarbonate in aqueous humour and the water secreted with it,
resulting in a fall in the intra-ocular pressure.
Dichlorphenamide (Daranide®) has a similar but
more prolonged action. Both these drugs have a
moderate incidence of side-effects, giving rise,
especially in the elderly, to paraesthesia, hypokalaemia, lack of appetite, drowsiness and
depression. Intravenous hypertonic **mannitol**, or
glycerol by mouth, are useful short-term ocular
hypotensive drugs. Acetazolamide by intramuscular or preferably intravenous injection is
also useful in the pre-operative treatment of
closed-angle glaucoma.

ACETAZOLAMIDE

Indications; Side-effects: see notes above
Cautions: avoid in renal impairment. Drug interactions: see Appendix 1 (sections *2.2, 2.3, 4.2,*
11)
Dose: by mouth or by intravenous injection, 0.25–
1 g daily in divided doses
By intramuscular injection, as for intravenous
injection but preferably avoided because of
alkaline pH

PoM **Acetazolamide** (Non-proprietary)
Tablets, acetazolamide 250 mg. Net price 20 =
30p. Label: 3
PoM **Diamox**® (Lederle)
Sustets® (= capsules s/r), orange, acetazol-
amide 500 mg. Net price 20 = £5.49. Label: 3,
25
Dose: 1 capsule twice daily
Tablets, acetazolamide 250 mg. Net price 20 =
£1.96. Label: 3
Sodium Parenteral (= injection), powder for
reconstitution, acetazolamide (as sodium salt).
Net price 500-mg vial = £15.14

DICHLORPHENAMIDE

Indications; Side-effects: see notes above

Dose: initially 100–200 mg, then 100 mg every
12 hours, adjusted according to the patient's
response

PoM **Daranide**® (MSD)
Tablets, yellow, scored, dichlorphenamide
50 mg. Net price 20 = 79p

11.7   Local anaesthetics

Oxybuprocaine and amethocaine are probably
the most widely used topical local anaesthetics.
Proxymetacaine (Ophthaine®) causes less initial
stinging and is useful for children. Cocaine, by
potentiating noradrenaline, produces useful vasoconstriction, but is now much less used in surgery.
Oxybuprocaine or a combined preparation of lignocaine and fluorescein is used for tonometry.
Lignocaine, with or without adrenaline, is injected
into the eyelids for minor surgery, while a retro-
bulbar injection may be used for major eye
surgery.

AMETHOCAINE HYDROCHLORIDE

Indications: local anaesthetic

PoM **Amethocaine Eye-drops,** amethocaine
hydrochloride 0.5%, net price, 10 ml = £1.65;
1%, 10 ml = £1.46
PoM **Minims Amethocaine Hydrochloride**
(S&N Pharm.)
Eye-drops, amethocaine hydrochloride 0.5 and
1%. Net price 20 × 0.5 ml (both) = £4.72

COCAINE HYDROCHLORIDE

Indications: local anaesthetic

CD **Cocaine Eye-drops,** cocaine hydrochloride
4%. Net price 10 ml = £2.65
CD **Cocaine and Homatropine Eye-drops,**
cocaine hydrochloride 2%, homatropine hydrobromide 2%.

LIGNOCAINE HYDROCHLORIDE

Indications: local anaesthetic

PoM **Minims Lignocaine and Fluorescein**
(S&N Pharm.)
Eye-drops, lignocaine hydrochloride 4%, fluorescein sodium 0.25%. Net price 20 × 0.5 ml =
£5.68

OXYBUPROCAINE HYDROCHLORIDE

Indications: local anaesthetic

PoM **Minims Benoxinate (Oxybuprocaine)
Hydrochloride** (S&N Pharm.)
Eye-drops, oxybuprocaine hydrochloride 0.4%.
Net price 20 × 0.5 ml = £4.15
PoM **Opulets Benoxinate (Oxybuprocaine)
Hydrochloride**® (Alcon)
Eye-drops, oxybuprocaine hydrochloride 0.4%.
Net price 20 × 0.5 ml = £3.54

PROXYMETACAINE HYDROCHLORIDE

Indications: local anaesthetic

PoM **Ophthaine**® (Squibb)
Eye-drops, proxymetacaine hydrochloride 0.5%. Net price 15 ml = £3.90

11.8 Miscellaneous ophthalmic preparations

11.8.1 Preparations for tear deficiency
11.8.2 Other preparations

11.8.1 Preparations for tear deficiency

Chronically sore eyes associated with reduced tear secretion, usually in cases of rheumatoid arthritis (Sjögren's syndrome), often respond to hypromellose eye-drops and mucolytic agents.

ACETYLCYSTEINE

Indications: tear deficiency, mucolytic
Apply eye-drops 3–4 times daily

PoM **Ilube**® (DF)
Eye-drops, acetylcysteine 5%, hypromellose 0.35%. Net price 15 ml = £4.96

HYPROMELLOSE

Indications: tear deficiency

Hypromellose Eye-drops, hypromellose '4000' (or '4500' or '5000') 0.3%. Net price 10 ml = 74p
BJ6 (Macarthys; Thornton & Ross)
Eye-drops, hypromellose 0.25%. Net price 10 ml = 73p and 75p, respectively
Isopto Alkaline® (Alcon)
Eye-drops, hypromellose 1%. Net price 10 ml = £1.02
Isopto Plain® (Alcon)
Eye-drops, hypromellose 0.5%. Net price 10 ml = 87p
Tears Naturale® (Alcon)
Eye-drops, dextran '70' 0.1%, hypromellose 0.3%. Net price 15 ml = £1.72

With phenylephrine
Isopto Frin® (Alcon)
Eye-drops, phenylephrine hydrochloride 0.12%, hypromellose 0.5%. Net price 10 ml = £1.17

LIQUID PARAFFIN

Indications: tear deficiency

Lacri-Lube® (Allergan)
Eye ointment, liquid paraffin. Net price 3.5 g = £1.76

POLYVINYL ALCOHOL

Indications: tear deficiency

Hypotears® (CooperVision)
Eye-drops, macrogol '8000' 2%, polyvinyl alcohol 1%. Net price 10 ml = £1.71

Liquifilm Tears® (Allergan)
Eye-drops, polyvinyl alcohol 1.4%. Net price 15 ml = £1.33
Sno Tears® (S&N Pharm.)
Eye-drops, polyvinyl alcohol 1.4%. Net price 10 ml = 88p

11.8.2 Other preparations

Zinc sulphate is a traditional astringent which has been used in eye-drops for treatment of excessive lachrymation. Zinc sulphate and adrenaline eye-drops should not be used because not only is there considerable doubt as to efficacy but there is a risk in using adrenaline in patients predisposed to closed-angle glaucoma.

Simple eye ointment is a bland sterile preparation which may be used to soften crusts in blepharitis or as a bland lubricant at night.

Sodium chloride eye lotion has already been mentioned (section 11.1).

Thymoxamine is used to reverse the mydriasis produced by phenylephrine.

Fluorescein sodium and **rose bengal** are used in diagnostic procedures and for locating damaged areas of the cornea due to injury or disease. Rose bengal is much more efficient for the diagnosis of conjunctival epithelial damage.

Certain eye-drops, e.g. benzylpenicillin, colistin, desferrioxamine, and trisodium edetate, may be prepared aseptically from material supplied for injection.

ACETYLCHOLINE CHLORIDE

Indications: cataract surgery, penetrating keratoplasty, iridectomy, and other anterior segment surgery requiring rapid miosis

PoM **Miochol**® (CooperVision)
Solution for intra-ocular irrigation, acetylcholine chloride 1%, mannitol 3% when reconstituted. 2 ml

CASTOR OIL

Indications: emollient and lubricant used in removal of foreign bodies

Minims Castor Oil (S&N Pharm.)
Eye-drops, castor oil. Net price 20 × 0.5 ml = £4.72

CHYMOTRYPSIN

Indications: zonulolysis in intracapsular cataract extraction

PoM **Zonulysin**® (Henleys)
Injection, powder for reconstitution, alphachymotrypsin 300 USP units (≡ 1.5 microkatals). Net price per vial (with diluent) = £3.42

PARAFFIN, YELLOW, SOFT

Indications: see notes above

Simple Eye Ointment, liquid paraffin 10%, wool fat 10%, in yellow soft paraffin. Net price 3 g = 90p

---

SODIUM CHLORIDE

Indications: irrigation, including first-aid removal of harmful substances

Sodium Chloride Eye Lotion, sodium chloride 0.9%. Net price 200 ml = £1.35

Balanced Salt Solution

Solution (sterile), sodium chloride 0.64%, sodium acetate 0.39%, sodium citrate 0.17%, calcium chloride 0.048%, magnesium chloride 0.03%, potassium chloride 0.075%. Available from Alcon (15 ml and 30 ml) and from CooperVision (15 ml)

Minims Sodium Chloride (S&N Pharm.)

Eye-drops, sodium chloride 0.9%. Net price 20 × 0.5 ml = £4.15

Normasol Undine® (Seton Prebbles)

Solution (sterile), sodium chloride 0.9%. Net price 10 × 20-ml disposable containers = £2.00

Opulets Sodium Chloride® (Alcon)

Eye-drops, sodium chloride 0.9%. Net price 20 × 0.5 ml = £3.54

SODIUM HYALURONATE

(a visco-elastic polymer normally present in the aqueous and vitreous humour)

Indications: used during surgical procedures on the eye

Side-effects: occasional hypersensitivity (avian origin)

PoM **Healonid**® (Pharmacia)

Injection, sodium hyaluronate 10 mg/ml in disposable syringes, net price 0.5 ml = £39.35, 0.75 ml = £59.00

THYMOXAMINE HYDROCHLORIDE

Indications: see notes above

Side-effects: minimal conjunctival hyperaemia for a few hours; rarely transient ptosis

Apply one drop as required

▼ PoM **Minims Thymoxamine Hydrochloride** (S&N Pharm.)

Eye-drops, thymoxamine hydrochloride 0.5%. Net price 20 × 0.5 ml = £4.72

ZINC SULPHATE

Indications; Cautions: see notes above

Zinc Sulphate Eye-drops, zinc sulphate 0.25%. Net price 10 ml = £1.63

Zinc Sulphate and Adrenaline Eye-drops, zinc sulphate 0.25%, adrenaline acid tartrate 0.09% (equivalent to 1 in 2000 adrenaline). Net price 10 ml = £1.63

DIAGNOSTIC PREPARATIONS

FLUORESCEIN SODIUM

Indications: detection of lesions and foreign bodies, but see notes above

Minims Fluorescein Sodium (S&N Pharm.)

Eye-drops, fluorescein sodium 1 or 2%. Net price 20 × 0.5 ml (both) = £4.15

Opulets Fluorescein Sodium® (Alcon)

Eye-drops, fluorescein sodium 1%. Net price 20 × 0.5 ml = £3.54

ROSE BENGAL

Indications: detection of lesions and foreign bodies

Minims Rose Bengal (S&N Pharm.)

Eye-drops, rose bengal 1%. Net price 20 × 0.5 ml = £4.72

11.9   Contact lenses

Many patients wear these lenses and special care is required in prescribing eye preparations for them. Unless medically indicated the lenses should not be worn during treatment. If the patient is wearing hard lenses the use of eye-drops containing anti-inflammatory drugs over long periods of time is to be deprecated. Some drugs can spoil hydrophilic soft lenses. Therefore unless eye-drops are specifically indicated as safe to use with hydrophilic contact lenses, the lenses should be removed before instillation and not worn during the period of treatment.

Hydrophilic plastic used for many soft contact lenses will selectively bind certain preservatives and could then be a source of irritation. Thiomersal is usually satisfactory. Chlorhexidine acetate is satisfactory in some cases, while phenylmercuric acetate or nitrate is usually satisfactory but is not recommended for long-term treatment. Benzalkonium chloride is unsuitable in all cases.

Sodium chloride solution 0.9% (sterile) can be used to store soft hydrophilic lenses provided that the case, lenses, and solution are regularly subjected to a heat treatment to reduce microbial contamination (such as 80°C for 40 minutes).

12: Drugs used in the treatment of diseases of the
EAR, NOSE, and OROPHARYNX

In this chapter, drug treatment is discussed under the following headings:

12.1 Drugs acting on the ear
12.2 Drugs acting on the nose
12.3 Drugs acting on the oropharynx

12.1 Drugs acting on the ear

12.1.1 Otitis externa
12.1.2 Otitis media
12.1.3 Removal of ear wax

For treatment of labyrinthine disorders see section 4.6.

12.1.1 Otitis externa

Otitis externa is an eczematous reaction of the meatal skin. It is important to exclude an underlying chronic otitis media before treatment is commenced. Many cases recover after thorough cleansing of the meatus by suction, dry mopping, or gentle syringing. The main problem in resistant cases is the difficulty in applying lotions and ointments satisfactorily to the relatively inaccessible affected skin. The most effective method is to introduce a ribbon gauze dressing soaked in an **astringent** such as **aluminium acetate**, or anti-inflammatory **corticosteroid** solution. When this is not practical, the ear should be gently cleaned with a probe covered in cotton wool and the patient encouraged to lie with the affected ear uppermost for ten minutes after the canal has been filled with a liberal quantity of the appropriate solution.

If infection is present, a topical anti-infective which is not used systemically (such as **framycetin**, **neomycin**, or **clioquinol**) may be used, but for only about a week as excessive use may result in fungal infections. These may be difficult to treat and require expert advice. Sensitivity to the anti-infective or solvent may occur and resistance to antibacterials is a possibility with prolonged use. Chloramphenicol ear-drops contain propylene glycol and cause sensitivity in about 10% of patients. An eye ointment of chloramphenicol may be used. Solutions containing an anti-infective and a corticosteroid (such as Locorten-Vioform®) are used for treating cases where infection is present with inflammation and eczema. The CSM has warned that when otitis externa is treated topically with preparations containing chlorhexidine, aminoglycosides (e.g. neomycin, framycetin), or polymyxins in patients who have a perforation of the tympanic membrane, there is an increased risk of drug-induced deafness. It is therefore important to ensure that there is no perforation in such patients before prescription of these preparations.

An acute infection may cause severe pain and a systemic antibiotic and a simple analgesic are required. When a resistant staphylococcal infection (a boil) is present in the external auditory meatus, **flucloxacillin** is the drug of choice (see section 5.1.1.2). Ampicillin or phenoxymethylpenicillin are used for other infections (see sections 5.1, Table 1).

The skin of the pinna adjacent to the ear canal is often affected by eczema, and topical corticosteroid creams and ointments (see section 13.4) are then required and should be applied five or six times daily. Prolonged use should be avoided.

Ear-drops or **ointment** should be applied using 3–4 drops of a liquid preparation or a similar quantity of ointment, warmed if necessary, inserted into the affected ear. If discharge is profuse, ear-drops applied directly may be washed away; in these circumstances the ear canal should be carefully cleaned and a quarter-inch gauze wick impregnated with the ear-drops should be introduced into it.

ASTRINGENT PREPARATIONS

ALUMINIUM ACETATE
Indications: inflammation in otitis externa

Aluminium Acetate Ear-drops (13%) consists of aluminium acetate solution, BP.
Insert into the meatus or apply on a gauze wick which should be kept saturated with the ear-drops
Available from Macarthys and Penn (special order)
Aluminium Acetate Ear-drops (8%), prepared by diluting 8 parts of aluminium acetate solution, BP, with 5 parts of purified water, freshly boiled and cooled. It must be freshly prepared.
Directions as above

ANTI-INFLAMMATORY PREPARATIONS

BETAMETHASONE SODIUM PHOSPHATE
Indications: eczematous inflammation in otitis externa
Cautions: avoid prolonged use
Contra-indications: untreated infection

PoM **Betnesol**® (Glaxo)
Drops (for ear, eye, or nose), betamethasone sodium phosphate 0.1%. Net price 5 ml = 80p; 10 ml = £1.31
Apply every 2–3 hours; reduce frequency of application when relief is obtained
PoM **Vista-Methasone**® (Daniel)
Drops (for ear, eye, or nose), betamethasone sodium phosphate 0.1%. Net price 5 ml = 60p; 10 ml = 95p
Apply every 3–4 hours; reduce frequency of application when relief is obtained

---

Cautionary label wordings, see inside back cover

Prices are **net**, see p. 1

PREDNISOLONE SODIUM PHOSPHATE

Indications: eczematous inflammation in otitis externa
Cautions: avoid prolonged use
Contra-indications: untreated infection

PoM **Predsol**® (Glaxo)
Drops (for ear or eye), prednisolone sodium phosphate 0.5%. Net price 5 ml = 80p; 10 ml = £1.31
Apply every 2–3 hours; reduce frequency of application when relief is obtained

ANTI-INFECTIVE PREPARATIONS

CHLORAMPHENICOL

Indications: bacterial infection in otitis externa
Cautions: avoid prolonged use (see notes above)
Side-effects: high incidence of sensitivity reactions to vehicle
Apply 2–3 times daily

PoM **Chloramphenicol Ear-drops 5%** and **10%,** chloramphenicol in propylene glycol. Net price 10 ml (5%) = £1.75; 10 ml (10%) = 70p

CLIOQUINOL

Indications: mild bacterial or fungal infections in otitis externa
Cautions: avoid prolonged use; see also notes above
Side-effects: local sensitivity; stains skin and clothing

PoM **Locorten-Vioform**® (Zyma)
Ear-drops, clioquinol 1%, flumethasone pivalate 0.02%. Net price 7.5 ml = £1.05
Apply 2–3 drops twice daily

CLOTRIMAZOLE

Indications: fungal infection in otitis externa
Side-effects: occasional skin irritation or sensitivity

Canesten® (Baypharm)
Solution, clotrimazole 1% in polyethylene glycol. Net price 20 ml = £2.38
Apply 2–3 times daily continuing for at least 14 days after disappearance of infection

FRAMYCETIN SULPHATE

Indications: bacterial infection in otitis externa
Cautions: avoid prolonged use; perforated eardrum; see also notes above
Side-effects: local sensitivity; ototoxicity (see notes above)
Apply 3–4 times daily

PoM **Framycort**® (Fisons)
Drops (for ear or eye), framycetin sulphate 0.5%, hydrocortisone acetate 0.5%. Net price 5 ml = £2.21
PoM **Framygen**® (Fisons)
Drops (for ear or eye), framycetin sulphate 0.5%. Net price 5 ml = £1.27

GENTAMICIN

Indications; Cautions; Side-effects: see under Framycetin Sulphate
Apply 3–4 times daily and at night

PoM **Gentamicin Ear-drops,** gentamicin 0.3% (as sulphate). Net price 10 ml = £1.79
PoM **Cidomycin**® (Roussel)
Drops (for ear or eye), gentamicin 0.3% (as sulphate). Net price 8 ml = £1.34
PoM **Garamycin**® (Kirby-Warrick)
Drops (for ear or eye), gentamicin 0.3% (as sulphate). Net price 10 ml = £1.79
PoM **Genticin**® (Nicholas)
Drops (for ear or eye), gentamicin 0.3% (as sulphate). Net price 10 ml = £1.79
PoM **Gentisone HC**® (Nicholas)
Ear-drops, gentamicin 0.3% (as sulphate), hydrocortisone acetate 1%. Net price 10 ml = £2.94

NEOMYCIN SULPHATE

Indications; Cautions; Side-effects: see under Framycetin Sulphate
Apply ear-drops every 2–3 hours; ear ointment 2–4 times daily. Reduce frequency of application when relief is obtained

PoM **Betnesol-N**® (Glaxo)
Drops (for ear, eye, or nose), betamethasone sodium phosphate 0.1%, neomycin sulphate 0.5%. Net price 5 ml = 87p; 10 ml = £1.35
PoM **Neo-Cortef**® (Upjohn)
Drops (for ear or eye), hydrocortisone acetate 1.5%, neomycin sulphate 0.5%. Net price 5 ml = £3.07
Ointment (for ear or eye), hydrocortisone acetate 1.5%, neomycin sulphate 0.5%. Net price 3.9 g = £2.21
PoM **Predsol-N**® (Glaxo)
Drops (for ear or eye), neomycin sulphate 0.5%, prednisolone sodium phosphate 0.5%. Net price 5 ml = 77p; 10 ml = £1.20
PoM **Vista-Methasone N**® (Daniel)
Drops (for ear, eye, or nose), betamethasone sodium phosphate 0.1%, neomycin sulphate 0.5%. Net price 5 ml = 65p; 10 ml = £1.05

TETRACYCLINE HYDROCHLORIDE

Indications: susceptible bacterial infection in otitis externa
Cautions: avoid prolonged use
Side-effects: local sensitivity; stains skin and clothing
Apply every 2 hours

PoM **Achromycin**® (Lederle)
Ointment (for ear or eye), tetracycline hydrochloride 1%. Net price 3.5 g = 70p

COMPOUND ANTI-INFECTIVE PREPARATIONS

PoM **Audicort**® (Lederle)
Ear-drops, neomycin 0.35%, undecenoic acid 0.7% (as neomycin undecenoate), triamcinolone acetonide 0.1%, benzocaine 5%. Net price 10 ml = £5.85
Apply 3–4 times daily

PoM **Otosporin**® (Calmic)
Ear-drops, hydrocortisone 1%, neomycin sulphate 0.439%, polymyxin B sulphate 0.119%. Net price 5 ml = £3.65; 10 ml = £6.24
Apply 3–4 times daily

PoM **Sofradex**® (Roussel)
Ear-drops, dexamethasone sodium metasulphobenzoate 0.05%, framycetin sulphate 0.5%, gramicidin 0.005%. Net price 8 ml = £4.00
Apply 3–4 times daily
Ointment (for ear or eyelid), dexamethasone 0.05%, framycetin sulphate 0.5%, gramicidin 0.005%. Net price 5 g = £3.31
Apply 2–3 times daily and at bedtime

PoM **Soframycin**® (Roussel)
Cream, framycetin sulphate 1.5%, gramicidin 0.005% in a water-miscible basis. Net price 15 g = £1.56
Ointment, ingredients as for cream, but in a greasy basis. Net price 15 g = £1.56
Apply 1–3 times daily

PoM **Terra-Cortril**® (Pfizer)
Ear suspension (= ear-drops), hydrocortisone acetate 1.5%, oxytetracycline 0.5% (as hydrochloride), polymyxin B sulphate 0.119%. Net price 5 ml = 68p
Apply 3 times daily

PoM **Tri-Adcortyl Otic**® (Squibb)
Ear ointment, gramicidin 0.025%, neomycin 0.25% (as sulphate), nystatin 3.33%, triamcinolone acetonide 0.1% in Plastibase®. Net price 10 g = £1.58
Apply 2–4 times daily

OTHER AURAL PREPARATIONS

Choline salicylate and phenazone are mild analgesics but are of doubtful value when applied topically. There is no place for the use of local anaesthetics in ear-drops.

Audax® (Napp)
Ear-drops, choline salicylate 20%, glycerol 10%. Net price 8 ml = £1.15

Auralgicin® (Fisons)
Ear-drops, benzocaine 1.4%, chlorbutol 1%, ephedrine hydrochloride 1%, phenazone 5.5%, potassium hydroxyquinoline sulphate 0.1% in glycerol. Net price 12.5 ml = £1.28

Auraltone® (Fisons)
Ear-drops, benzocaine 1%, phenazone 5% in glycerol. Net price 15 ml = 77p

12.1.2 Otitis media

Acute otitis media is the commonest cause of severe pain in small children and recurrent attacks, especially in infants, are particularly distressing. Sero-mucinous otitis media ('glue ear') is present in about 10% of the child population and in 90% of children with cleft palates. Chronic otitis media is thought to be a legacy from untreated or resistant cases of sero-mucinous otitis media.

ACUTE OTITIS MEDIA. Local treatment is ineffective and there is no place for drops containing a local anaesthetic. Many attacks are viral in origin and need only treatment with a **simple analgesic** such as paracetamol for pain. Severe attacks of bacterial origin should be treated with **systemic antibiotics**. Identification of the infecting organism by bacterial examination of the discharge, if present, is helpful in selecting the appropriate treatment (see section 5.1, Table 1). Again, simple analgesics such as paracetamol are used to relieve pain. In recurrent acute otitis media a daily dose of a prophylactic antibiotic (co-trimoxazole or erythromycin) during the winter months can be tried.

SERO-MUCINOUS OTITIS MEDIA ('GLUE EAR'). This condition should be referred to hospital because of the risk of permanent damage to middle ear function and impaired language development.

CHRONIC OTITIS MEDIA. The organisms recovered from patients with chronic otitis media are often opportunists living in the debris, keratin, and necrotic bone present in the middle ear and mastoid. Thorough cleansing with an aural suction tube may completely control infection of many years duration. Acute exacerbations of chronic infection may require systemic antibiotics (see section 5.1, Table 1). A swab should be taken to determine the organism present and its antibiotic sensitivity. Unfortunately the culture often produces *Pseudomonas aeruginosa* and *Proteus* spp, sensitive only to parenteral antibiotics. Local debridement of the meatal and middle ear contents may then be followed by topical treatment with ribbon gauze dressings as for otitis externa (section 12.1.1). This is particularly true with infections in mastoid cavities when dusting powders can also be tried.

12.1.3 Removal of ear wax

Wax is a normal bodily secretion which provides a protective film on the meatal skin and need only be removed if it causes deafness or interferes with a proper view of the eardrum. It may be removed by syringing with warm water. If necessary, wax can be softened before syringing with topical solutions, the most effective of which is **sodium bicarbonate ear-drops**. Other simple remedies are **olive oil** and **almond oil**. The patient should lie with the affected ear uppermost for 5 to 10 minutes after a generous amount of the solution has been introduced into the ear. Some proprietary preparations containing organic solvents can cause irritation of the meatal skin, and in most cases the simple remedies which are indicated above are just as effective and less likely to cause irritation. **Docusate sodium** is an ingredient in a number of proprietary preparations.

Almond Oil (warm before use). Net price 10 ml = 8p

Olive Oil (warm before use). Net price 10 ml = 6p

Sodium Bicarbonate Ear-drops (see Formulary). Net price 10 ml = 2p

Audinorm® (Carlton)
Ear-drops, docusate sodium 5%, glycerol 10%. Net price 12 ml = 30p

Cerumol® (LAB)
Ear-drops, chlorbutol 5%, paradichlorobenzene 2%, turpentine oil 10%. Net price 11 ml = 79p

Dioctyl® (Medo)
Ear-drops, docusate sodium 5% in macrogol. Net price
7 ml = 57p
Exterol® (Dermal)
Ear-drops, urea-hydrogen peroxide complex 5% in
glycerol. Net price 12 ml = £2.14
Molcer® (Wallace Mfg)
Ear-drops, docusate sodium 5%. Net price 15 ml = 76p
Soliwax® (Martindale)
Ear capsules (= ear-drops), docusate sodium 5% in oil,
red, single-application capsules. Net price 10 = 67p
Waxsol® (Norgine)
Ear-drops, docusate sodium 0.5%. Net price 10 ml = 86p

12.2   Drugs acting on the nose

Rhinitis is often self-limiting and sinusitis is best
treated with antibiotics (see section 5.1, Table 1).
There are few indications for the use of sprays
and drops except in allergic rhinitis where topical
preparations of corticosteroids or sodium cromoglycate have much to offer. Most other preparations contain sympathomimetic drugs which
may damage the nasal cilia and their prolonged
use causes mucosal oedema and severe nasal
obstruction (rhinitis medicamentosa). Symptomatic relief in chronic nasal obstruction may be
obtained with **systemic nasal decongestants** (see
section 3.10). Douching the nose with salt and
water is **not** recommended.

12.2.1 Drugs used in nasal allergy
12.2.2 Topical nasal decongestants
12.2.3 Anti-infective nasal preparations

12.2.1   Drugs used in nasal allergy

Mild cases are controlled by **oral antihistamines**
and **systemic nasal decongestants** (see sections
3.4.1 and 3.10). Many patients with severe symptoms can now expect relief from topical preparations of **corticosteroids** or **sodium
cromoglycate**. Treatment should begin 2 to 3
weeks before the hay fever season commences
and may have to be continued for months or even
years in some patients. No significant side-effects
have been reported. Very disabling symptoms
occasionally justify the use of **systemic corticosteroids** for short periods (see section 6.3), for
example in students taking important examinations. They may also be used at the beginning of
a course of treatment with a corticosteroid spray
to relieve severe mucosal oedema and allow the
spray to penetrate the nasal cavity.

For reference to injections of **allergen extracts**
see section 3.4.2.

BECLOMETHASONE DIPROPIONATE

Indications: allergic and vasomotor rhinitis
Cautions: untreated nasal infection, prolonged
use in children, previous treatment with corticosteroids by mouth
Side-effects: sneezing after administration
Adults and children over 6 years, apply 100
micrograms (2 puffs) into each nostril twice
daily or 50 micrograms (1 puff) 3–4 times daily;
max. 8 puffs daily

PoM Beconase® (A&H)
Nasal aerosol, beclomethasone dipropionate 50
micrograms/metered inhalation. Net price 200-
dose unit with nasal adaptor = £5.01
PoM Beconase Aqueous® (A&H)
Nasal spray, beclomethasone dipropionate
50 micrograms/metered spray. Net price 200-
dose unit with nasal applicator = £5.01

BETAMETHASONE SODIUM PHOSPHATE

Indications; Cautions; Side-effects: see under
Beclomethasone Dipropionate
Apply 2–3 drops into each nostril 2–3 times
daily

PoM Betnesol® (Glaxo)
Drops (for ear, eye, or nose), betamethasone
sodium phosphate 0.1%. Net price 5 ml = 80p;
10 ml = £1.31
PoM Vista-Methasone® (Daniel)
Drops (for ear, eye, or nose), betamethasone
sodium phosphate 0.1%. Net price 5 ml = 60p;
10 ml = 95p

BUDESONIDE

Indications: allergic and vasomotor rhinitis
Cautions: see under Beclomethasone Dipropionate; also patients with pulmonary
tuberculosis
Side-effects: see under Beclomethasone
Dipropionate
Apply 100 micrograms (2 puffs) into each nostril twice daily, reducing to 50 micrograms (1
puff) twice daily

PoM Rhinocort® (Astra)
Nasal aerosol, budesonide 50 micrograms/
metered inhalation, 200-dose unit with nasal
adaptor. Net price complete unit = £5.66

FLUNISOLIDE

Indications; Cautions; Side-effects: see under
Beclomethasone Dipropionate
Apply 50 micrograms (2 sprays) into each nostril 2–3 times daily; CHILD over 5 years 25 micrograms (1 spray) into each nostril 3 times daily,
reduced for maintenance

PoM Syntaris® (Syntex)
Nasal spray, flunisolide 25 micrograms/0.1 ml
metered spray. Net price 24 ml with pump and
applicator = £4.87

SODIUM CROMOGLYCATE

Indications: prophylaxis of allergic rhinitis (see
notes above)
Side-effects: local irritation, particularly during
initial treatment with insufflations; rarely transient bronchospasm

Rynacrom® (Fisons)
Nasal insufflation, cartridges, pink, sodium cromoglycate 10 mg for use with insufflator. Net
price 20 cartridges = 78p; insufflator = £1.66
Adults and children, insufflate 10 mg into each
nostril up to 4 times daily

Nasal drops, sodium cromoglycate 2%. Net price 15 ml = £4.31

Adults and children, instil 2 drops into each nostril 6 times daily

Nasal spray, sodium cromoglycate 2% (2.6 mg/squeeze). Net price 26 ml with pump = £5.36

Adults and children, apply 1 squeeze into each nostril 4–6 times daily

Rynacrom Compound® (Fisons)

Nasal spray, sodium cromoglycate 2% (2.6 mg/metered spray) and xylometazoline hydrochloride 0.025% (32.5 micrograms/metered spray). Net price 26 ml with pump = £5.94

Apply 1 spray into each nostril 4 times daily

12.2.2 Topical nasal decongestants

The nasal mucosa is sensitive to changes in the atmospheric temperature and humidity and these alone may cause slight nasal congestion. The nose and nasal sinuses produce a litre of mucus in twenty-four hours and much of this finds its way silently into the stomach via the nasopharynx. Slight changes in the nasal airway, accompanied by an awareness of mucus passing along the nasopharynx causes some patients to be inaccurately diagnosed as suffering from chronic sinusitis. These symptoms are particularly noticeable in the later stages of the common cold for which there is no effective treatment at the moment; the temptation to use nasal drops should be resisted. **Sodium chloride** 0.9% given as nasal drops may relieve nasal congestion by helping to liquefy mucous secretions.

Symptomatic relief from the nasal congestion associated with vasomotor rhinitis, nasal polypi, and the common cold can be obtained by the short-term use of decongestant nasal drops and sprays. These all contain sympathomimetic drugs which exert their effect by vasoconstriction of the mucosal blood vessels which in turn reduces the thickness of the nasal mucosa. They are of limited value as they can give rise to a rebound phenomenon as their effects wear off, due to a secondary vasodilatation with a subsequent temporary increase in nasal congestion. This in turn tempts the further use of the decongestant, leading to a vicious circle of events. **Ephedrine nasal drops** is the safest sympathomimetic preparation and can give relief for several hours. The more potent sympathomimetic drugs oxymetazoline, phenylephrine, and xylometazoline are more likely to cause a rebound effect. **All** of these preparations may cause a hypertensive crisis if used during treatment with a monoamine-oxidase inhibitor.

Steam inhalations are useful in the treatment of symptoms of acute infective conditions, and the use of compounds containing volatile substances such as menthol and eucalyptus may encourage their use (see section 3.8). There is no evidence that nasal preparations containing antihistamines and anti-infective agents have any therapeutic effect.

Systemic nasal decongestants—see section 3.10.

EPHEDRINE HYDROCHLORIDE

Indications: nasal congestion

Cautions: avoid excessive use; caution in infants under 3 months (no good evidence of value—if irritation occurs might narrow nasal passage). Drug interactions: see Appendix 1 (section *4.3*)

Side-effects: local irritation; after excessive use tolerance with diminished effect, rebound congestion

Instil 1–2 drops (see below) into each nostril when required

Ephedrine Nasal Drops, ephedrine hydrochloride 0.5% (see Formulary). Net price 10 ml = 3p

Note. Ephedrine Nasal Drops 1% also available; if no strength specified 0.5% should be supplied

OXYMETAZOLINE HYDROCHLORIDE

Indications: nasal congestion

Cautions; Side-effects: see under Ephedrine

NHS **Afrazine®** (Kirby-Warrick)

Nasal drops, oxymetazoline hydrochloride 0.05%. Net price 15 ml = 70p

Instil 2–3 drops into each nostril every 12 hours when required

Paediatric nasal drops, oxymetazoline hydrochloride 0.025%. Net price 15 ml = 67p

CHILD up to 5 years instil 2–3 drops into each nostril every 12 hours when required

Nasal spray, oxymetazoline hydrochloride 0.05%. Net price 15 ml = 70p

Apply 2–3 times to each nostril every 12 hours when required

PHENYLEPHRINE HYDROCHLORIDE

Indications: nasal congestion

Cautions; Side-effects: see under Ephedrine

NHS **Neophryn®** (Winthrop)

Nasal drops, phenylephrine hydrochloride 0.25%. Net price 15 ml = 69p

Instil 2–3 drops in each nostril every 3–4 hours if necessary; CHILD 1–2 drops

Nasal spray, phenylephrine hydrochloride 0.5%. Net price 15 ml = 85p

2 applications to each nostril every 3–4 hours if necessary

XYLOMETAZOLINE HYDROCHLORIDE

Indications: nasal congestion

Cautions; Side-effects: see under Ephedrine

Xylometazoline Nasal Drops, xylometazoline hydrochloride 0.1%, net price 10 ml = 55p

Instil 2–3 drops into each nostril every 8–12 hours when required

Xylometazoline Nasal Drops, Paediatric xylometazoline hydrochloride 0.05%, net price 10 ml = 55p

CHILD instil 1–2 drops into each nostril 1–2 times daily when required

Note. The brand name NHS Otrivine® (Ciba Consumer) relates to xylometazoline nasal drops 0.1%, paediatric nasal drops 0.05%, and nasal spray 0.1%.

COMPOUND NASAL DECONGESTANT PREPARATIONS

NHS **Hayphryn**® (Winthrop)
Nasal spray, phenylephrine hydrochloride 0.5%, thenyldiamine hydrochloride 0.1%. Net price 15 ml = 91p
NHS **Otrivine-Antistin**® (Ciba Consumer)
Nasal drops and *spray*, antazoline sulphate 0.5%, xylometazoline hydrochloride 0.05%. Net price 10 ml (both) = 60p

12.2.3   Anti-infective nasal preparations

There is **no** evidence that topical anti-infective nasal preparations have any therapeutic value.
Systemic treatment of sinusitis—see section 5.1, Table 1.

PoM **Betnesol-N**® (Glaxo)
Drops (for ear, eye, or nose), section 12.1.1
PoM **Dexa-Rhinaspray**® (Boehringer Ingelheim)
Nasal inhalation, dexamethasone 21-isonicotinate 20 micrograms, neomycin sulphate 100 micrograms, tramazoline hydrochloride 120 micrograms/metered inhalation. Net price 125-dose unit = £1.79
PoM **Locabiotal**® (Servier)
Nasal inhalation, fusafungine 125 micrograms/metered inhalation. Net price 200-dose unit = £1.59
PoM **Vibrocil**® (Zyma)
Nasal drops, dimethindene maleate 0.025%, neomycin sulphate 0.35%, phenylephrine 0.25%. Net price 15 ml = 52p
Nasal gel, dimethindene maleate 0.025%, neomycin sulphate 0.35%, phenylephrine 0.25%. Net price 12 g = 52p
Nasal spray, dimethindene maleate 0.025%, neomycin sulphate 0.35%, phenylephrine 0.25%. Net price 10 ml = 52p
PoM **Vista-Methasone N**® (Daniel)
Drops (for ear, eye, or nose), section 12.1.1

NASAL STAPHYLOCOCCI

Elimination of organisms such as staphylococci from the nasal vestibule can be achieved by the use of a cream containing **chlorhexidine and neomycin** (Naseptin®), but re-colonisation frequently occurs. Coagulase-positive staphylococci can be obtained from the noses of 40% of the population.

▼ PoM **Bactroban**® **Nasal** (Beecham)
Nasal ointment, mupirocin 2% in white soft paraffin basis. Net price 3 g = £5.15
Apply 2–3 times daily to the inner surface of each nostril
PoM **Naseptin**® (ICI)
Cream, chlorhexidine hydrochloride 0.1%, neomycin sulphate 0.5%. Do not dilute. Net price 5 g = 28p
For treatment of staphylococcal infections apply to nostrils 4 times daily for 10 days; for preventing nasal carriage of staphylococci apply to nostrils twice daily

12.3   Drugs acting on the oropharynx

12.3.1   Drugs used in aphthous ulcers
12.3.2   Oropharyngeal anti-infective drugs
12.3.3   Antiseptic lozenges and sprays
12.3.4   Mouth-washes, gargles, and dentifrices

12.3.1   Drugs used in aphthous ulcers

Recurrent single or multiple aphthous ulcers are often a nuisance and occasionally are extremely painful. Local treatment aims at protecting the ulcerated area and at relieving pain or reducing inflammation.

A **carmellose gelatin** paste (Orabase®) or powder (Orahesive®) has a mechanical protective effect; it is difficult to apply effectively to some parts of the mouth.

Corticosteroids in lozenges (Corlan®) or in paste (Adcortyl in Orabase®) are the most effective particularly if used in the 'prodromal' phase.

Carbenoxolone gel may be of value; **tetracycline** rinsed in the mouth may also be of value.

Choline salicylate dental gel may relieve the pain of minor aphthous ulcers; excessive application or confinement under a denture irritates the mucosa and can itself cause ulceration. Relief obtained in teething may merely be due to pressure of application (comparable with biting a teething ring); excessive use may give rise to salicylate poisoning.

Benzydamine (Difflam®) is used as an analgesic mouth-wash or spray for oral ulceration and other painful conditions.

Local anaesthetics as in benzocaine lozenges also provide pain relief but may cause sensitisation. Care must be taken not to produce anaesthesia before meals as this might lead to choking.

Secondary bacterial infection may be a feature of any mucosal ulceration and can delay healing. Use of a **chlorhexidine** mouth-wash (section 12.3.4) is often beneficial and may accelerate healing of recurrent aphthae.

Local application of **silver nitrate** or **alum** is not recommended; it causes tissue damage and delays healing.

BENZYDAMINE HYDROCHLORIDE
Indications: painful inflammatory conditions of oropharynx
Side-effects: occasional numbness or stinging

Difflam® (Riker)
Oral rinse, green, benzydamine hydrochloride 0.15%. Net price 200 ml = £2.43
Rinse or gargle, using 15 ml, diluted if necessary, every 1½–3 hours as required, usually for not more than 7 days; not suitable for children under 12
Spray, benzydamine hydrochloride 0.15%. Net price 30-ml unit = £3.23
4–8 puffs onto affected area every 1½–3 hours; CHILD 6–12 years 4 puffs every 1½–3 hours

---

CARBENOXOLONE SODIUM

Indications: mild oral and perioral lesions

Bioral Gel® (Winthrop)
Gel, carbenoxolone sodium 2% in adhesive basis. Net price 5 g = £1.37
Apply after meals and at bedtime

▼ PoM **Bioplex**® (Thames)
Mouth-wash granules, carbenoxolone sodium 1%. Net price 24 × 2-g sachets = £9.60
For mouth ulcers, rinse with 2 g in 30–50 ml of warm water 3 times daily and at bedtime

CARMELLOSE SODIUM

Indications: mechanical protection of oral and perioral lesions

Orabase® (Squibb)
Oral paste, carmellose sodium 16.58%, pectin 16.58%, gelatin 16.58%, in Plastibase®. Net price 30 g = £1.18; 100 g = £2.60
Apply a thin layer when necessary after meals

Orahesive® (Squibb)
Powder, carmellose sodium, pectin, gelatin, equal parts. Net price 25 g = £1.30
Sprinkle on the affected area

CORTICOSTEROIDS

Indications: oral and perioral lesions
Contra-indications: untreated oral infection

PoM **Adcortyl in Orabase**® (Squibb)
Oral paste, triamcinolone acetonide 0.1% in adhesive basis. Net price 10 g = £1.10
Apply a thin layer 2–4 times daily

PoM **Corlan**® (Glaxo)
Pellets (= lozenges), hydrocortisone 2.5 mg (as sodium succinate). Net price 20 lozenges = £1.40
One lozenge 4 times daily, allowed to dissolve slowly in the mouth in contact with the ulcer; if ulcers recur rapidly treatment may be continued for a period at reduced dosage

LOCAL ANAESTHETICS

Indications: relief of pain in oral lesions
Cautions: avoid prolonged use; hypersensitivity may occur

Benzocaine Lozenges, benzocaine 10 mg. Net price 20 lozenges = 52p
Dissolve one slowly in the mouth when necessary
Note. It is essential not to confuse these with compound benzocaine lozenges which contain ten times the amount of benzocaine

Dequacaine® (Farley)
Lozenges, amber, benzocaine 10 mg, dequalinium chloride 250 micrograms. Net price 24 lozenges = 73p
Dissolve 1 lozenge slowly in the mouth when necessary; max. 8 lozenges daily

Medilave® (Martindale)
Gel, benzocaine 1%, cetylpyridinium chloride 0.01%. Net price 10 g = 55p
Adults and children over 6 months, apply a thin layer 3–4 times daily

Oral-B® (Oral-B)
Oral gel, lignocaine 0.6%, cetylpyridinium chloride 0.02%, cineole 0.1%, menthol 0.06%. Net price 15 g = 49p
Apply every 3 hours when required

For endoscopy or laryngoscopy

Benzocaine Lozenges, Compound, benzocaine 100 mg, menthol 3 mg. Net price 20 lozenges = 48p
Dissolve one slowly in the mouth when necessary
Note. It is essential not to confuse these with benzocaine lozenges which contain one-tenth the amount of benzocaine

SALICYLATES

Indications: mild oral and perioral lesions
Cautions: frequent application, especially in children, may give rise to salicylate poisoning
Note. The recent CSM warning on aspirin and Reye's syndrome does not apply to non-aspirin salicylates or to topical preparations such as teething gels

Choline Salicylate Dental Gel (formerly Choline Salicylate Dental Paste), choline salicylate 8.7% in a suitable water-miscible basis.
Apply every 3–4 hours with gentle massage before food and at bedtime

Bonjela® (R&C)
Oral gel, sugar-free, choline salicylate dental gel containing choline salicylate 8.7%. Net price 10 g = 65p

Pyralvex® (Norgine)
Oral paint, brown, anthraquinone glycosides 5%, salicylic acid 1%. Net price 10 ml with brush = £1.15
Apply 3–4 times daily

Teejel® (Napp)
Oral gel, choline salicylate dental gel containing choline salicylate 8.7%. Net price 10 g = 52p

TETRACYCLINE

Indications: severe recurrent aphthous ulceration; oral herpes (section 12.3.2)
Side-effects: fungal superinfection

PoM **Tetracycline Mixture**[1], consists of tetracycline hydrochloride 125 mg (as tetracycline)/5 ml
10 ml to be held in the mouth for 2–3 minutes 3 times daily for not longer than 3 days followed by a break of at least 3 days before treatment is recommended (to avoid oral thrush); it should preferably not be swallowed

Note. Tetracycline stains teeth; avoid in children under 12 years of age
1. Available as Achromycin® Syrup (see section 5.1.3); alternatively the contents of a 250-mg capsule can be stirred in a small amount of water and used in the same way as the mixture—this ensures a sugar-free version

12.3.2   Oropharyngeal anti-infective drugs

The commonest cause of a sore throat is a viral infection which does not benefit from anti-infective treatment. Streptococcal sore throats require systemic **penicillin** therapy (see section 5.1.1). Acute ulcerative (Vincent's) gingivitis responds to systemic **metronidazole** 200 mg 3 times daily for 3 days (see section 5.1.11) or **nimorazole** 500 mg twice daily for 2 days (see section 5.4.3).

Candida albicans may cause thrush and other forms of stomatitis which are sometimes a sequel to the use of broad-spectrum antibiotics or antineoplastics; withdrawing the causative drug may lead to rapid resolution. Otherwise, **nystatin**, **amphotericin**, or **miconazole** may be effective; **polynoxylin** and **dequalinium** are less effective. **Crystal violet** paint (see section 13.11) is no longer recommended for application to mucous membranes.

Herpes infections in the mouth, if they require treatment, may respond to **tetracycline** rinsed in the mouth (see above). Systemic **acyclovir** may be required for recurrent or resistant infections (see section 5.3); acyclovir cream is indicated for herpes labialis (see section 13.10.3). Idoxuridine 0.1% Paint has been superseded by more effective preparations.

AMPHOTERICIN

Indications: oral and perioral fungal infections

PoM **Fungilin**® (Squibb)
Lozenges, yellow, amphotericin 10 mg. Net price 20 lozenges = £1.20. Label: 9, 24, counselling advised, after food
Dissolve 1 lozenge slowly in the mouth 4 times daily, may require 10–15 days' treatment; increase to 8 daily if infection severe
Suspension, yellow, sugar-free, amphotericin 100 mg/ml. Net price 12 ml with pipette = £2.10. Label: 9, counselling advised, use of pipette, hold in mouth, after food
Place 1 ml in the mouth after food and retain near lesions 4 times daily for 14 days

DEQUALINIUM CHLORIDE

Indications: mild oral fungal infections

Dequadin® (Farley)
Lozenges, orange, dequalinium chloride 250 micrograms. Net price 20 lozenges = 37p
Dissolve 1 lozenge slowly in the mouth when required
Labosept® (LAB)
Pastilles, red, dequalinium chloride 250 micrograms. Net price 20 pastilles = 50p
Suck 1 pastille slowly when required

MICONAZOLE

Indications: oral fungal infections
Cautions: pregnancy. Drug interactions: see Appendix 1 (sections *2.8B*, *4.8*, *6.1*)

Daktarin® (Janssen)
Oral gel, sugar-free, miconazole 25 mg/ml. Net price 40 g = £2.50. Label: 9, counselling advised, hold in mouth, after food
Place 5–10 ml in the mouth after food and retain near lesions before swallowing, 4 times daily; CHILD up to 2 years 2.5 ml twice daily, 2–6 years 5 ml twice daily, over 6 years 5 ml 4 times daily
Localised lesions, smear affected area with clean finger; a 15-g tube (net price £1.17) also available
Tablets—see section 5.2

NATAMYCIN

Indications: oral fungal infections

PoM **Pimafucin**® (Brocades)
Oral suspension, off-white, sugar-free, natamycin 10 mg/ml. Net price 5-ml dropper bottle = 67p. Label: 9, counselling advised, use of pipette, hold in mouth
Place 10 drops in the mouth after food and retain near lesions; INFANTS 4 drops

NYSTATIN

Indications: oral and perioral fungal infections

PoM **Nystatin Mixture,** nystatin 100 000 units/ml. Do not dilute. Net price 30 ml = £2.32. Label: 9, counselling advised, use of pipette, hold in mouth, after food
Place 1 ml in the mouth after food and retain near lesions 4 times daily, continued for 48 hours after lesions have resolved
PoM **Nystan**® (Squibb)
Pastilles, yellow/brown, nystatin 100 000 units. Net price 28 pastilles = £3.95. Label: 9, 24, counselling advised, after food
Suck 1 pastille slowly, 4 times daily after food
Suspension, yellow, nystatin 100 000 units/ml. Net price 30 ml with pipette = £2.27. Label: 9, counselling advised, use of pipette, hold in mouth, after food
Suspension, gluten-, lactose-, and sugar-free, nystatin 100 000 units/ml when reconstituted with water for preparations. Measure with pipette. Net price 24 ml with pipette = £1.67. Label: 9, counselling advised, use of pipette
PoM **Nystatin-Dome**® (Lagap)
Suspension, yellow, nystatin 100 000 units/ml. Net price 30 ml with 1-ml spoon = £2.36. Label: 9, counselling advised, use of 1-ml spoon, hold in mouth, after food

POLYNOXYLIN

Indications: mild oral fungal infections

Anaflex® (Geistlich)
Lozenges, polynoxylin 30 mg. Net price 50 lozenges = £3.00. Label: 9,24, counselling advised, after food
Suck 1 lozenge slowly 6–10 times daily

TETRACYCLINE
Section 12.3.1

12.3.3 Antiseptic lozenges and sprays

There is no convincing evidence that antiseptic lozenges and sprays have a beneficial action and they sometimes irritate and cause sore tongue and sore lips. Some of these preparations also contain local anaesthetics which relieve pain but may cause sensitisation.

Benzalkonium Lozenges, benzalkonium chloride 500 micrograms. Net price 20 lozenges = 48p

AAA® (Rorer)
Mouth and throat spray, benzocaine 1.5%, cetalkonium chloride 0.0413%. Net price 60-dose unit = £2.19

Bradosol® (Ciba)
Lozenges, domiphen bromide 500 micrograms. Net price 24 lozenges = 53p

Eludril® (Concept)
Aerosol spray, amethocaine hydrochloride 0.015%, chlorhexidine gluconate 0.05%. Net price 55 ml = £1.37

PoM **Locabiotal**® (Servier)
Aerosol spray, fusafungine 125 micrograms/metered inhalation. Net price 200-dose unit with nasal and oral adaptor = £1.59

Merocaine® (Merrell)
Lozenges, green, benzocaine 10 mg, cetylpyridinium chloride 1.4 mg. Net price 24 lozenges = 70p

Merocets® (Merrell)
Lozenges, yellow, cetylpyridinium chloride 0.066%. Net price 24 lozenges = 61p

Oralcer® (Vitabiotics)
Lozenges, green, ascorbic acid 6 mg, clioquinol 35 mg. Net price 20 lozenges = 50p

Tyrozets® (MSD)
Lozenges, pink, benzocaine 5 mg, tyrothricin 1 mg. Net price 24 lozenges = 59p

12.3.4 Mouth-washes, gargles, and dentifrices

Mouth-washes have a mechanical cleansing action and freshen the mouth. Warm **compound sodium chloride mouth-wash** or **compound thymol glycerin** is as useful as any.

Hydrogen peroxide mouth-wash has a mechanical cleansing effect due to frothing when in contact with oral debris. **Sodium perborate** (Bocasan®) is similar in effect to hydrogen peroxide.

There is recent evidence that **chlorhexidine** has a specific effect in inhibiting the formation of plaque on teeth. A chlorhexidine mouth-wash may be useful as an adjunct to other oral hygiene measures in cases of oral infection or when tooth-brushing is not possible.

There is no convincing evidence that gargles are effective.

Artificial saliva (see Formulary) may be indicated for dry mouth. Proprietary preparations are available (see next page).

CETYLPYRIDINIUM CHLORIDE
Indications: oral hygiene

Merocet® (Merrell)
Solution (= mouth-wash or gargle), yellow, cetylpyridinium chloride 0.05%. Net price 200 ml = 84p
To be used undiluted or diluted with an equal volume of warm water

CHLORHEXIDINE GLUCONATE
Indications: oral hygiene; inhibition of plaque formation
Side-effects: idiosyncratic mucosal irritation; reversible brown staining of teeth

Corsodyl® (ICI)
Dental gel, chlorhexidine gluconate 1%. Net price 50 g = 69p
Brush on the teeth once or twice daily
Mouth-wash, chlorhexidine gluconate 0.2% (original or mint-flavoured). Net price 300 ml = £1.05
Rinse the mouth with 10 ml for about 1 minute twice daily

Eludril® (Concept)
Mouth-wash, red, chlorhexidine gluconate 0.1%, chlorbutol 0.1%, chloroform 0.5%. Net price 90 ml = 67p; 250 ml = £1.38; 500 ml = £2.75
Use 10 ml in half a tumblerful of warm water 3–4 times daily

HEXETIDINE
Indications: oral hygiene

Oraldene® (W-L)
Mouth-wash or *gargle*, red, hexetidine 0.1%. Net price 100 ml = 48p
Use 15 ml undiluted 2–3 times daily

HYDROGEN PEROXIDE
Indications: oral hygiene, see notes above

Hydrogen Peroxide Mouth-wash, consists of hydrogen peroxide solution (6% ≡ approx. 20 volume). Net price 100 ml = 20p
Rinse the mouth for 2–3 minutes with 15 ml in half a tumblerful of warm water 2–3 times daily

PHENOL
Indications: oral hygiene

Phenol Gargle, phenol glycerin 5% (see Formulary). Net price 100 ml = 5p
To be diluted with an equal volume of warm water

Chloraseptic® (Richardson Vicks)
Throat spray or *gargle*, green, phenol and sodium phenolate (total phenol 1.4%), menthol, thymol, and glycerol. Net price 115 ml with spray = £1.40; 150 ml = £1.42
Use every 2 hours if necessary, undiluted as a throat spray, undiluted or diluted with an equal volume of water as a mouth-wash or gargle

---

POVIDONE-IODINE

Indications: oral hygiene
Cautions: pregnancy; breast-feeding
Side-effects: idiosyncratic mucosal irritation and hypersensitivity reactions

Betadine® (Napp)
Mouth-wash or *gargle*, amber, povidone-iodine 1%. Net price 250 ml = 75p
To be used undiluted or diluted with an equal volume of warm water every 2–4 hours if necessary

SODIUM CHLORIDE

Indications: oral hygiene, see notes above

Sodium Chloride Mouth-wash, Compound, sodium chloride 1.5% (see Formulary). Net price 100 ml = 5p
To be diluted with an equal volume of warm water

SODIUM PERBORATE

Indications: oral hygiene, see notes above
Cautions: avoid prolonged use (over 1 month) because of possible borate poisoning

Bocasan® (Oral-B)
Mouth-wash, sodium perborate 70%. Net price 8 × 1.7-g sachets = 43p
Use 1 sachet in 30 ml of water

THYMOL

Indications: oral hygiene, see notes above

Mouth-wash Solution-tablets, consist of tablets which may contain antimicrobial, colouring, and flavouring agents in a suitable soluble effervescent basis to make a mouth-wash suitable for dental purposes. Net price 20 solution-tablets = 26p
Dissolve 1 tablet in a tumblerful of warm water
Thymol Glycerin, Compound, glycerol 10%, thymol 0.05% with colouring and flavouring. Net price 100 ml = 15p
To be used undiluted or diluted with 3 volumes of warm water

OTHER PREPARATIONS FOR OROPHARYNGEAL USE

Glandosane® (Fresenius)
Aerosol spray, carmellose sodium 500 mg, sorbitol 1.5 g, potassium chloride 60 mg, sodium chloride 42.2 mg, magnesium chloride 2.6 mg, calcium chloride 7.3 mg, and dipotassium hydrogen phosphate 17.1 mg/50 g. Net price 50-ml unit (neutral or flavoured) = £3.00
Spray onto oral and pharyngeal mucosa as required to provide artificial saliva
Saliva Orthana® (Nycomed)
Aerosol spray, gastric mucin (porcine) 3.5%, with preservatives and flavouring agents. Net price 50-ml spray bottle = £3.75; 450-ml refill bottle = £25.10
Dry mouth, spray 2–3 times onto oral and pharyngeal mucosa, when required

---

13: Drugs acting on the

SKIN

The skin is particularly amenable to treatment by local application as there is intimate contact between the drug and the target tissue with a minimum of systemic effects. However, when a substance is used topically there may be difficulty in regulating the total quantity applied to the area concerned and lack of patient compliance may be a problem.

In this chapter, drug treatment is discussed under the following headings:

13.1 Vehicles and diluents
13.2 Emollient and barrier preparations
13.3 Local anaesthetic and antipruritic preparations
13.4 Topical corticosteroids
13.5 Preparations for psoriasis and eczema
13.6 Preparations for acne
13.7 Preparations for warts and calluses
13.8 Sunscreens and camouflaging preparations
13.9 Scalp preparations
13.10 Anti-infective skin preparations
13.11 Skin disinfecting and cleansing agents
13.12 Antiperspirants
13.13 Wound management products
13.14 Topical preparations for circulatory disorders

13.1 Vehicles and diluents

VEHICLE. Both the vehicle and the active ingredients are important in the treatment of skin conditions and it is being increasingly recognised that the vehicle alone may have a greater therapeutic value than a mere placebo effect. The vehicle affects the degree of hydration of the skin, has a mild anti-inflammatory effect, and aids the penetration of active drug in the preparation.

Additives. The following additives in topical preparations may be associated with sensitisation, particularly of eczematous skin. Where available, details of whether they are contained in preparations listed in the BNF are given after the preparation entry.

Most commonly	Less commonly	Rarely[1]
Wool fat and related substances	Benzyl alcohol	Beeswax
Chlorocresol	Butylated hydroxyanisole	Edetic acid (EDTA)
Ethylenediamine	Butylated hydroxytoluene	Isopropyl palmitate
Fragrances	Hydroxybenzoates (parabens)	
	Polysorbates	
	Propylene glycol	
	Sorbic acid	

[1] Non-dermatologists can reasonably disregard the substances in this category

The vehicle, the indication for which the drug is prescribed, solubility, cosmetic and general acceptability to the patient, and the safety and stability of the final preparation should all be considered.

DILUTION. Because of the complexity of many formulations, dilution is undesirable except where a particular diluent is known to be suitable. Suitable diluents for individual preparations are given in the relevant entries. Inappropriate diluents may impair the activity or stability of the preparation, even though no physical change is apparent. Diluted creams are generally given a life of 2 weeks.

QUANTITY. Suitable quantities of dermatological preparations to be prescribed for specific areas of the body are given below.

The following recommendations do not apply to corticosteroid preparations which should be applied sparingly. Corticosteroid creams and ointments are available in various pack sizes, commonly 15 g or 30 g, while corticosteroid lotions are usually packed in 20- or 100-ml sizes.

	Creams and Ointments	Lotions
Face	5 to 15 g	100 ml
Both hands	25 to 50 g	200 ml
Scalp	50 to 100 g	200 ml
Both arms or both legs	100 to 200 g	200 ml
Body	200 g	500 ml
Groins and genitalia	15 to 25 g	100 ml
Dusting-powders	50 to 100 g	
Paints	10 to 25 ml	

These amounts are usually suitable for 2 to 4 weeks.

CHOICE OF VEHICLE

The vehicle may take the form of a cream, ointment, lotion, paste, dusting-powder, application, collodion, liniment, or paint basis. The properties of the various forms are described below but it should be noted that there are some vehicles having intermediate properties, for example ointments with some properties of a cream.

CREAMS are either water-miscible and readily washed off, or oily and not so easily washed off. They contain a preservative to minimise microbial growth. Generally, creams are cosmetically more acceptable to the patient as they are less greasy than ointments and easier to apply.

Aqueous Cream, emulsifying ointment 30%, phenoxyethanol 1%, in freshly boiled and cooled purified water. Net price 100 g = 27p
Buffered Cream, emulsifying ointment 30%, citric acid monohydrate 0.5%, sodium phosphate

2.5%, chlorocresol 0.1%, in freshly boiled and cooled purified water. Net price 100 g = 37p

Cetomacrogol Cream, *Formula A*, cetomacrogol emulsifying ointment 30%, chlorocresol 0.1%, in freshly boiled and cooled purified water. Net price 100 g = £2.94

Formula B, cetomacrogol emulsifying ointment 30%, propyl hydroxybenzoate 0.08%, methyl hydroxybenzoate 0.15%, benzyl alcohol 1.5%, in freshly boiled and cooled purified water. Net price 100 g = £1.60

Diprobase® (Kirby-Warrick)

Cream, cetomacrogol 2.25%, cetostearyl alcohol 7.2%, liquid paraffin 6%, white soft paraffin 15%, water-miscible basis used for Diprosone® cream. Net price 50 g = £1.60
Additives: chlorocresol

Lipobase® (Brocades)

Cream, fatty cream basis used for Locoid Lipocream®. Net price 50 g = £2.05
Additives: hydroxybenzoates (parabens)

Locobase® (Brocades)

Cream, water-miscible basis used for Locoid® cream. Net price 100 g = £2.70
Additives: hydroxybenzoates (parabens)

Ultrabase® (Schering)

Cream, water-miscible, containing liquid paraffin and white soft paraffin. Net price 50 g = £1.05; 500 g = £5.70
Additives: hydroxybenzoates (parabens), disodium edetate, fragrance

OINTMENTS are greasy preparations which are normally anhydrous and insoluble in water, and are more occlusive than creams. The most commonly used ointment bases consist of soft paraffin or a combination of soft paraffin with liquid paraffin and hard paraffin. Some modern ointment bases have both hydrophilic and lipophilic properties; they may have occlusive properties on the skin surface, encourage hydration, and be miscible with water. They often have a mild anti-inflammatory effect. Water-soluble ointments contain macrogols which are freely soluble in water and are therefore readily washed off. They have a limited but useful application in circumstances where ready removal is desirable. Ointments are particularly suitable for chronic, dry lesions. Contact sensitivity to wool fat (lanolin) and wool alcohols may occur and ointments containing these substances must be avoided in sensitised patients.

Cetomacrogol Emulsifying Ointment, cetomacrogol emulsifying wax 30%, liquid paraffin 20%, white soft paraffin 50%. Net price 100 g = 35p

Emulsifying Ointment, emulsifying wax 30%, white soft paraffin 50%, liquid paraffin 20%. Net price 100 g = 30p

Hydrous Ointment (oily cream), dried magnesium sulphate 0.5%, phenoxyethanol 1%, water for preparations 48.5%, in wool alcohols ointment. Net price 100 g = 37p

Hydrous Wool Fat, wool fat 70% in freshly boiled and cooled purified water. Net price 100 g = 69p

Hydrous Wool Fat Ointment, hydrous wool fat 50%, yellow soft paraffin 50%. Net price 100 g = 68p

Macrogol Ointment, macrogol '4000' 35%, macrogol '300' 65%

Paraffin, white soft (white petroleum jelly). Net price 100 g = 35p

Paraffin, yellow soft (yellow petroleum jelly). Net price 100 g = 35p

Paraffin Ointment, (see Formulary). Net price 100 g = 41p

Simple Ointment, cetostearyl alcohol 5%, hard paraffin 5%, wool fat 5%, in yellow or white soft paraffin. Net price 100 g = 37p

Wool Alcohols Ointment, wool alcohols 6%, yellow or white soft paraffin 10%, hard paraffin 24%, in liquid paraffin. Net price 100 g = 97p

Diprobase® (Kirby-Warrick)

Ointment, liquid paraffin 5%, white soft paraffin 95%, basis used for Diprosone® ointment. Net price 50 g = £1.60
Additives: none as listed in table above

Locobase® (Brocades)

Ointment, basis for Locoid® ointment. Net price 100 g = £2.70
Additives: none as listed in table above

Unguentum Merck® (Merck)

Cream (hydrophilic and lipophilic), cetostearyl alcohol 9%, glyceryl monostearate 3%, saturated neutral oil 2%, liquid paraffin 3%, white soft paraffin 32%, propylene glycol 5%, polysorbate '40' 8%, silicic acid 0.1%, sorbic acid 0.2%. Net price 50 g = £1.63; 100 g = £3.21; 200 ml = £6.35; 500 g = £9.80; 900 g = £12.42

LOTIONS are usually aqueous solutions or suspensions which cool diffusely inflamed unbroken skin. They cool by evaporation and should be reapplied frequently. Volatile solvents increase the cooling effect but are liable to cause stinging. Lotions are also used to apply drugs to the skin and may be preferred to ointments or creams when it is intended to apply a thin layer of the preparation over a large or hairy area.

SHAKE LOTIONS (such as calamine lotion) containing insoluble powders are applied to less acute, scabbed, dry lesions. In addition to cooling they leave a deposit of inert powder on the skin surface.

PASTES are stiff preparations containing a high proportion of finely powdered solids such as zinc oxide and starch. The standard example is **Compound Zinc Paste** to which other active ingredients may be added (e.g. dithranol). Pastes are used for circumscribed lesions such as those which occur in lichen simplex, chronic eczema, or psoriasis. They are less occlusive than ointments and can be used to protect sub-acute, lichenified, or excoriated skin.

Zinc Paste, Compound, zinc oxide 25%, starch 25%, white soft paraffin 50%. Net price 25 g = 8p

APPLICATIONS are usually viscous solutions, emulsions, or suspensions for application to the skin.

COLLODIONS are painted on the skin and allowed to dry to leave a flexible film over the site of application. Flexible collodion may be used to seal minor cuts and wounds. Collodions may also be used to provide a means of holding a dissolved drug in contact with the skin for a long period, e.g. salicylic acid collodion (section 13.7).

Collodion, Flexible, castor oil 2.5%, colophony 2.5% in a collodion basis, prepared by dissolving pyroxylin (10%) in a mixture of 3 volumes of ether and 1 volume of alcohol (90%). Net price 10 ml = 10p. Label: 15
Caution: highly flammable

LINIMENTS are liquid preparations which are intended for external application and may contain substances possessing analgesic, rubefacient, soothing, or stimulating properties.

For preparations see section 10.3.2.

PAINTS are liquid preparations intended for application with a brush to the skin or mucous surfaces.

13.2 Emollient and barrier preparations

13.2.1 Emollients and barrier creams
13.2.2 Emollient bath additives
13.2.3 Dusting-powders

13.2.1 Emollients and barrier creams

Emollients soothe, smooth and hydrate the skin and are indicated for all dry scaling disorders (such as ichthyosis). Their effects are short-lived and they should be applied frequently even after improvement occurs. They are useful in dry eczematous disorders, and to a lesser extent in psoriasis (section 13.5). Simple preparations such as **aqueous cream** are often as effective as the more complex proprietary formulations; sprays offer little advantage but, in general, the choice depends on patient preference. Some ingredients may cause sensitisation, notably hydrous wool fat (lanolin) or antibacterials and this should be suspected if an eczematous reaction occurs at the site of application.

Camphor, menthol, and phenol have a mild antipruritic effect when used in emollient preparations. Calamine and zinc oxide may also be included as they slightly enhance therapeutic efficacy; they are particularly useful in dry eczema. Zinc and titanium preparations have mild astringent properties. Thickening agents such as talc and kaolin may also be included. Preparations containing antibacterial drugs should be avoided unless infection is present (section 13.10).

Urea is employed as a hydrating agent. It is used in scaling conditions and may be useful in elderly patients and infantile eczemas. It is often used with other topical agents such as corticosteroids to enhance penetration.

Barrier creams often contain water-repellent substances such as **dimethicone** or other silicones. They are used to give protection against irritation or repeated hydration (napkin rash, areas around stomata, sore areas in the elderly, bedsores, etc.). Whatever is applied is no substitute for adequate nursing care, and it is doubtful if these water-repellent creams are any more effective than the traditional compound zinc ointments.

Napkin rash is usually a local dermatitis. The first line of treatment is to ensure that napkins are changed frequently, and that tightly fitting rubber pants are avoided. The rash may clear when left exposed to the air and an emollient, or preparations containing calamine and emollients, may be helpful. See also section 13.4.

For preparations used in stoma care, see section 1.8.1.

Aqueous Cream—section 13.1
Dimethicone Cream, dimethicone '350' 10%, cetostearyl alcohol 5%, cetrimide 0.5%, chlorocresol 0.1%, liquid paraffin 40%, freshly boiled and cooled purified water 44.4%. Net price 50 g = 26p
Hydrous Ointment—section 13.1
Titanium Dioxide Paste, titanium dioxide 20%, chlorocresol 0.1%, red ferric oxide 2%, glycerol 15%, light kaolin 10%, zinc oxide 25%, in water for preparations. For napkin and urinary rash and as a sunscreen
Zinc Cream, zinc oxide 32%, arachis oil 32%, calcium hydroxide 0.045%, oleic acid 0.5%, wool fat 8%, in freshly boiled and cooled purified water. Net price 50 g = 36p. For napkin and urinary rash and eczematous conditions
Zinc Ointment, zinc oxide 15%, in simple ointment. Net price 25 g = 16p. For napkin and urinary rash and eczematous conditions
Zinc and Castor Oil Ointment, zinc oxide 7.5%, castor oil 50%, arachis oil 30.5%, white beeswax 10%, cetostearyl alcohol 2%. Net price 25 g = 13p. For napkin and urinary rash
Alcoderm® (Alcon)
Cream, water-miscible, containing carbomer, cetyl alcohol, liquid paraffin, polysorbate 60, sodium lauryl sulphate, stearyl alcohol, triethanolamine. Net price 60 g = £1.43
Additives: isopropyl palmitate, hydroxybenzoates (parabens)
Lotion, water-miscible, ingredients as above. Net price 120 ml = £1.54
Additives: hydroxybenzoates (parabens)
▼ **Conotrane®** (Boehringer Ingelheim)
Cream, benzalkonium chloride 0.1%, dimethicone '350' 22%. Net price 50 g = 59p; 450 g = £3.28
Additives: fragrance
Diprobase—section 13.1
E45® (Crookes Products)
Cream, light liquid paraffin 11.6%, white soft paraffin 14.5%, wool fat 1%, with methyl hydroxybenzoate, self-emulsifying monostearin, stearic acid, triethanolamine. Net price 50 g = 71p; 125 g = £1.43; 500 g = £2.93

Eczederm® (Quinoderm Ltd)
Cream, calamine 20.88%, arachis oil 12.5%, in an emollient basis. Net price 25 g = 92p; 50 g = £1.58; 500 g = £8.45
Additives: fragrance

Emulsiderm® (Dermal)
Liquid emulsion (= lotion), liquid paraffin 25%, isopropyl myristate 25%, benzalkonium chloride 0.5%. Net price 250 ml (with 10-ml measure) = £2.82; 1 litre = £11.30
Additives: polysorbate 60

Hewletts Cream® (Astra)
Cream, hydrous wool fat 4%, zinc oxide 8%. Net price 35 g = 45p; 400 g = £2.52

Humiderm® (BritCair)
Cream, pyrrolidone carboxylic acid 5% (as sodium salt). Net price 60 g = £3.20
Additives: hydroxybenzoates (parabens), propylene glycol

Kamillosan® (Norgine)
Ointment, extract of chamomile 10%, volatile oil of chamomile 0.5%. Net price 5 g = 57p (hosp. only); 24 g = £1.31. For napkin rash, cracked nipples and chapped hands
Additives: beeswax, hydroxybenzoates (parabens), wool fat

Keri® (Bristol-Myers)
Lotion, mineral oil 16%, with lanolin oil. Net price 190-ml pump pack = £3.65; 380-ml pump pack = £5.96
Additives: hydroxybenzoates (parabens), propylene glycol, fragrance

Lacticare® (Stiefel)
Lotion, lactic acid 5%, sodium pyrrolidone carboxylate 2.5%, in an emulsion basis. Net price 150 ml = £3.19
Additives: isopropyl palmitate, fragrance

Locobase—section 13.1

Massé Breast Cream® (Ortho-Cilag)
Cream (water-miscible), containing arachis oil, cetyl alcohol, glycerol, glyceryl monostearate, wool fat, polysorbate 60, potassium hydroxide, sorbitan monostearate, stearic acid. Net price 28 g = 66p. For pre- and postnatal nipple care
Additives: hydroxybenzoates (parabens)

Metanium® (Bengué)
Ointment, titanium dioxide 20%, titanium peroxide 5%, titanium salicylate 3%, titanium tannate 0.1%, in a silicone basis. Net price 25 g = 52p. For napkin rash and related disorders
Additives: none as listed in section 13.1

Morhulin® (Napp)
Ointment, cod-liver oil 11.4%, zinc oxide 38%, in a basis containing wool fat and paraffin. Net price 50 g = 49p; 350 g = £2.90. For minor wounds, varicose ulcers, and pressure sores

Morsep® (Napp)
Cream, cetrimide 0.5%, ergocalciferol 10 units/g, vitamin A 70 units/g. Net price 40 g = 43p; 300 g = £2.22. For urinary rash
Additives: wool fat derivative, fragrance

Natuderm® (Burgess)
Cream (hydrophilic and lipophilic), free fatty acids 5%, glycerides 15.5%, glycerol 3.7%, phospholipids 0.2%, polysorbate '60' 1.1%, sorbitan monostearate 1%, squalane 0.5%, squalene 3.3%, free sterols 0.8%, sterol esters 1.3%, α-tocopherol 0.003%, waxes 7%, butyl-

ated hydroxyanisole 0.003%. Net price 40 g = £1.02; 100 g = £2.08; 450 g = £8.19

Noratex® (Norton)
Cream, cod-liver oil 2.15%, light kaolin 3.5%, talc 7.4%, wool fat 1.075%, zinc oxide 21.8%. Net price 500 g = £2.50. For napkin and urinary rash and pressure sores

Oilatum® (Stiefel)
Cream, arachis oil 21%, povidone (polyvinylpyrrolidone) 1%, in a water-miscible basis. Net price 40 g = £1.79; 80 g = £2.78
Additives: fragrance

Rikospray Balsam® (Riker)
Spray application, benzoin 12.5%, prepared storax 2.5% (pressurised aerosol pack). Net price 150-g unit = £2.31. For application to skin under adhesive plasters, in ileostomy and colostomy care, bedsores, cracked nipples and skin fissures
Additives: information not disclosed for BNF

Rikospray Silicone® (Riker)
Spray application, aldioxa 0.5%, cetylpyridinium chloride 0.02%, in a water-repellent basis containing dimethicone 1000. Net price 200-g pressurised aerosol pack = £2.45. For urinary rash, pressure sores, and colostomy care
Additives: information not disclosed for BNF

Siopel® (Care)
Barrier cream, dimethicone '1000' 10%, cetrimide 0.3%. Net price 50 g = 35p; 500 g = £1.80. For dermatoses, colostomy and ileostomy care, urinary rash, and related conditions
Additives: information not disclosed for BNF

Sprilon® (Pharmacia)
Spray application, dimethicone 0.6%, zinc oxide 7.2%, in a basis containing wool fat, wool alcohols, cetyl alcohol, dextran, white soft paraffin, liquid paraffin, propellants. Net price 200-g pressurised aerosol unit = £2.82. For urinary rash, pressure sores, and colostomy and ileostomy

Sudocrem® (Tosara)
Cream, benzyl alcohol 0.39%, benzyl benzoate 1.01%, benzyl cinnamate 0.15%, wool fat 4%, zinc oxide 15.25%. Net price 25 g = 15p; 60 g = 50p; 125 g = 82p; 250 g = £1.49; 400 g = £2.17. For napkin rash and pressure sores
Additives: beeswax (synthetic), butylated hydroxyanisole, propylene glycol, fragrance

Thovaline® (Ilon)
Ointment, cod-liver oil 1.5%, light kaolin 2.5%, talc 3.3%, wool fat 2.5%, zinc oxide 19.8%. Net price 15 g = 36p; 40 g = 42p; 50 g = 55p; 90 g = 85p; 125 g = £1.15; 500 g = £2.80. For napkin and urinary rash and pressure sores
Additives: fragrance
Spray application, ingredients as for ointment in pressurised aerosol pack. Net price 142 g = £1.95

Ultrabase—section 13.1

Unguentum Merck—section 13.1

Vasogen® (Pharmax)
Barrier cream, dimethicone 20%, calamine 1.5%, zinc oxide 7.5%. Net price 50 g = 57p; 100 g = 97p. For napkin and urinary rash, pressure sores, and pruritus ani
Additives: hydroxybenzoates (parabens), wool fat

Vita-E® (Bioglan)
Ointment, d-α-tocopheryl acetate 30 units/g in yellow soft paraffin. Net price 50 g = £1.51. For pressure sores and related conditions
Additives: none as listed in section 13.1

Preparations containing urea
Aquadrate® (Norwich Eaton)
Cream, urea 10% in a powder-in-cream basis. Net price 30 g = £1.63; 100 g = £4.91
Additives: none as listed in section 13.1
Apply sparingly and rub into area when required
Calmurid® (Pharmacia)
Cream, urea 10%, lactic acid 5%, in a water-miscible basis. Diluent aqueous cream, life of diluted cream 14 days. Net price 50 g = £1.76; 100 g = £3.49; 400-g dispenser = £12.50
Additives: none as listed in section 13.1
Apply a thick layer for 3–5 minutes, massage into area, and remove excess, usually twice daily. Use half-strength cream for 1 week if stinging occurs with undiluted preparation
Nutraplus® (Alcon)
Cream, urea 10% in a water-miscible basis. Net price 60 g = £2.01
Additives: hydroxybenzoates (parabens), propylene glycol
Apply 2–3 times daily

13.2.2 Emollient bath additives

For bath additives containing tar, see section 13.5 and for antiseptic bath additives, see section 13.11.

Alpha Keri Bath® (Bristol-Myers)
Bath oil, liquid paraffin 91.7%, oil-soluble fraction of wool fat 3%. Net price 240 ml = £3.54; 480 ml = £6.59
Additives: fragrance
Aveeno Oilated® (Dendron)
Bath additive, oat (protein fraction) 41%, liquid paraffin 35%. Net price 6 × 30-g sachets = £2.28
Additives: none as listed in section 13.1
Add 1 sachet/bath
¹Aveeno Regular® (Dendron)
Bath additive, oat (protein fraction). Net price 6 × 50-g sachets = £2.28
Additives: none as listed in section 13.1
Add 1 sachet/bath
¹Formerly Aveeno Colloidal
Balneum® (Merck)
Bath oil, soya oil 84.75%. Net price 225 ml = £2.70; 500 ml = £6.00; 1 litre = £12.00
Additives: butylated hydroxytoluene, propylene glycol, fragrance
Add 20 ml/bath
Balneum with Tar—section 13.5
Emulsiderm —section 13.2.1
Add 20–30 ml/bath and soak for 5–10 minutes
Hydromol Emollient® (Quinoderm Ltd)
Bath additive, isopropyl myristate 13%, light liquid paraffin 37.8%. Net price 150 ml = £1.28; 350 ml = £2.98
Additives: fragrance

Oilatum Emollient® (Stiefel)
Bath additive (emulsion), acetylated wool alcohols 5%, liquid paraffin 63.7%. Net price 150 ml = £1.12; 350 ml = £2.62
Additives: isopropyl palmitate, fragrance
Add 5–15 ml/bath and soak for 10–20 minutes

13.2.3 Dusting-powders

Dusting-powders are used in folds where friction may occur between opposing skin surfaces. They should not be applied in areas that are very moist as they tend to cake and abrade the skin. **Talc** acts as a lubricant powder but does not absorb moisture whereas **starch** is less lubricant but absorbs water. Other inert powders such as kaolin or zinc oxide may also be used in the formulation of dusting-powders.

See also section 13.11 for antiseptic dusting-powders.

Talc Dusting-powder, starch 10% in sterilised purified talc. Net price 100 g = 25p
Zinc, Starch and Talc Dusting-powder, zinc oxide 25%, starch 25%, sterilised purified talc 50%. Net price 50 g = 14p
ZeaSORB® (Stiefel)
Dusting-powder, aldioxa 0.2%, chloroxylenol 0.5%, pulverised maize core 45%. Net price 50 g = £2.15
Additives: fragrance

13.3 Local anaesthetic and antipruritic preparations

Pruritus may be caused by systemic disease (such as drug hypersensitivity, obstructive jaundice, endocrine disease, and certain malignant diseases) as well as by skin disease (e.g. psoriasis, eczema, urticaria, and scabies). Where possible the underlying causes should be treated.

There is no really effective antipruritic. **Calamine** preparations are widely prescribed. **Emollient** preparations (section 13.2.1) may also be of value. **Oral antihistamines** (section 3.4.1) should be used in allergic rashes.

Some topical antihistamines and local anaesthetics may cause sensitisation. Topical antihistamines are only marginally effective. Insect bites and stings, though often treated with such preparations, are best treated with calamine preparations or emollients.

Crotamiton (Eurax®) shows little evidence of greater effectiveness than calamine in the relief of pruritus.

For preparations used in pruritus ani, see section 1.7.1.

CALAMINE
Indications: pruritus

Calamine Application, Compound, calamine 10%, zinc oxide 5%, zinc stearate 2.5%, wool fat 2.5%, yellow soft paraffin 25%, liquid paraffin 55%. Net price 50 g = 20p

Calamine Cream, Aqueous, calamine 4%, zinc oxide 3%, arachis oil 30%, emulsifying wax 6%, freshly boiled and cooled purified water 57%. Net price 50 g = 26p

Calamine Lotion, calamine 15%, zinc oxide 5%, glycerol 5%, bentonite 3%, sodium citrate 0.5%, liquefied phenol 0.5%, in freshly boiled and cooled purified water. Net price 200 ml = 70p

Calamine Lotion, Oily, calamine 5%, arachis oil 50%, oleic acid 0.5%, wool fat 1%, in calcium hydroxide solution. Net price 200 ml = 80p

Calamine Ointment, calamine 15%, in white soft paraffin. Net price 25 g = 9p

Eczederm—section 13.2.1

CROTAMITON

Indications: pruritus
Cautions: avoid use near eyes
Contra-indications: acute exudative dermatoses

Eurax® (Ciba Consumer)
Lotion, crotamiton 10%. Net price 150 ml = £1.72
Additives: propylene glycol
Cream, crotamiton 10%. Net price 30 g = 80p; 100 g = £1.56
Additives: beeswax, hydroxybenzoates (parabens)

LOCAL ANAESTHETICS

Indications: relief of local pain, see notes above. See section 15.2 for use in surface anaesthesia
Cautions: may cause hypersensitivity

Note. Topical local anaesthetic preparations may be absorbed, especially through mucosal surfaces, therefore excessive application should be avoided, particularly in infants and children.

Anethaine® (Evans)
Cream, amethocaine hydrochloride 1%, in a water-miscible basis. Net price 25 g = 73p
Additives: fragrance

Solarcaine® (Plough)
Cream, benzocaine 1%, triclosan 0.2%. Net price 25 ml = 94p
Additives: benzyl alcohol, disodium edetate
Lotion, benzocaine 0.5%, triclosan 0.2%. Net price 75 ml = £1.38
Additives: disodium edetate, hydroxybenzoates (parabens)
Spray (= application), benzocaine 5%, triclosan 0.1%, pressurised aerosol unit. Net price 100 g = £1.82
Additives: propylene glycol

Xylocaine® (Astra)
Ointment, lignocaine 5% in a water-miscible basis. Net price 15 g = 83p
Additives: none as listed in section 13.1
For other Xylocaine® preparations, see section 15.2

TOPICAL ANTIHISTAMINES

Indications: pruritus, urticaria, see notes above
Cautions: may cause hypersensitivity; avoid in eczema; photosensitivity (diphenhydramine and promethazine)

Anthical® (Fisons)
Cream, mepyramine maleate 1.5%, zinc oxide 15%, in a vanishing-cream basis. Net price 25 g = 96p
Additives: hydroxybenzoates (parabens)
Apply 3–4 times daily for up to 3 days

Anthisan® (Fisons)
Cream, mepyramine maleate 2%. Net price 25 g = 90p
Additives: hydroxybenzoates (parabens), fragrance
Apply 2–3 times daily for up to 3 days

Caladryl® (W-L)
Cream, diphenhydramine hydrochloride 1%, calamine 8%, camphor 0.1%, in a water-miscible basis. Net price 42 g = 98p
Additives: hydroxybenzoates (parabens), polysorbate 60, propylene glycol
Lotion, ingredients as for cream. Net price 125 ml = 99p
Additives: fragrance
Apply 3–4 times daily for up to 3 days

R.B.C.® (Rybar)
Cream, antazoline hydrochloride 1.8%, calamine 8%, camphor 0.1%, cetrimide 0.5%. Net price 25 g = 98p
Additives: propylene glycol
Apply when required for up to 3 days

13.4   Topical corticosteroids

Topical corticosteroids are used for the treatment of inflammatory conditions of the skin other than those due to an infection, in particular the eczematous disorders. Corticosteroids suppress various components of the inflammatory reaction while in use; they are in no sense curative, and when treatment is discontinued a rebound exacerbation of the condition may occur. They are indicated for the relief of symptoms and for the suppression of signs of the disorder when potentially less harmful measures are ineffective.

Corticosteroids are of no value in the treatment of urticaria and are **contra-indicated** in rosacea and in ulcerative conditions as they worsen the condition. They should not be used indiscriminately in pruritus.

CHOICE OF PREPARATION. The preparation containing the **least potent** drug at the **lowest strength** which is effective is the one of choice, but extemporaneous dilution should be avoided whenever possible.

Topical corticosteroid preparations are divided into four groups in respect of potency. In ascending order these are:

	Potency	Examples
IV	Mild	Hydrocortisone 1%
III	Moderately potent	Clobetasone butyrate 0.05% (Eumovate®)
II	Potent	Betamethasone 0.1% (as valerate) (Betnovate®); hydrocortisone butyrate (Locoid®)
I	Very potent	Clobetasol propionate 0.05% (Dermovate®)

Intradermal corticosteroid injections (see section 10.1.2.2) are more effective than the very potent topical corticosteroid preparations and they should be reserved for severe cases where there are localised lesions and topical treatment has failed. Their effects last for several weeks.

SIDE-EFFECTS. Unlike groups I and II, groups III and IV are rarely associated with side-effects. The more potent the preparation the more care is required, as absorption through the skin can cause severe pituitary-adrenal-axis suppression and hypercorticism (see section 6.3.3), both of which depend on the area of the body treated and the duration of the treatment. It must also be remembered that absorption is greatest from areas of thin skin, raw surfaces, and intertriginous areas, and is increased by occlusion.

Local side-effects from the use of corticosteroids topically include:

(a) spread and worsening of untreated infection;
(b) thinning of the skin which may be restored over a period of time although the original structure may never return;
(c) irreversible striae atrophicae;
(d) increased hair growth;
(e) perioral dermatitis, an inflammatory papular disorder on the face of young women;
(f) acne at the site of application in some patients;
(g) mild depigmentation and vellus hair.

CHOICE OF FORMULATION. Water-miscible creams are particularly suitable for treating moist or weeping lesions whereas ointments are generally chosen for use on dry, lichenified or scaly lesions or where a more occlusive effect is required. Lotions may be useful when minimal application to a large area is required. Occlusive polythene dressings may be used to increase the effect, but also increase the risk of side-effects. The inclusion of urea increases the penetration of the corticosteroid.

USE IN CHILDREN. Children, especially babies, are particularly susceptible to side-effects. The more potent corticosteroids should be **avoided** in paediatric treatment or if necessary used with great care for short periods; a mild corticosteroid such as hydrocortisone is useful for treating napkin rash and infantile eczemas. Napkins and plastic pants may however act as an occlusive dressing and increase absorption.

COMPOUND PREPARATIONS. The advantages of including other substances with corticosteroids in topical preparations are debatable. The commonest ones are the **antibacterials**.

LABELS. The application of excessive quantities of external corticosteroid preparations can result in undesirable local and systemic side-effects (see above). Accordingly, label 28 (To be applied sparingly) should be used with all external corticosteroid preparations.

HYDROCORTISONE

Indications: mild inflammatory skin disorders
Cautions: see notes above; also avoid prolonged use in infants and children, and on the face
Contra-indications: untreated bacterial, fungal, or viral skin lesions
Side-effects: see notes above
Administration: apply sparingly 2–4 times daily, reducing strength and frequency as condition responds

---

Over-the-counter sales. Proprietary brands of hydrocortisone cream (0.1 and 1%) and ointment (1%) are on sale to the public for treatment of allergic contact dermatitis, irritant dermatitis, and insect bite reactions only
Cautions: not for children under 10 years or in pregnancy, without medical advice
Contra-indications: eyes/face, anogenital region, broken or infected skin (including cold sores, acne, and athlete's foot)
Administration: apply sparingly over small area 1–2 times daily for max. of 1 week
Labelling must state. If the condition is not improved, consult your doctor.

Creams

PoM **Hydrocortisone Cream,** hydrocortisone in a suitable basis. When hydrocortisone cream is prescribed and no strength is stated, the 1% strength should be supplied. Net price, 0.1%, 30 g = 16p;   0.5%,   15 g = 36p;   30 g = 59p; 50 g = 97p;   100 g = £1.94;   1%,   15 g = 46p; 30 g = 90p; 50 g = £1.61;   100 g = £2.90; 2.5%, 15 g = 71p. Potency IV

PoM **Cobadex**® (Cox Pharmaceuticals)
Cream, hydrocortisone 0.5 or 1%, dimethicone '350' 20%, in a water-miscible basis, net price 20 g   (0.5%) = £1.17;   20 g   (1%) = £1.68. Potency IV
Additives: hydroxybenzoates (parabens), polysorbate 80, propylene glycol

PoM **Dioderm**® (Dermal)
Cream, hydrocortisone 0.1%, in a water-miscible basis. Net price 30 g = £2.14. Potency IV
Additives: propylene glycol

PoM **Efcortelan**® (Glaxo)
Cream, hydrocortisone in a water-miscible basis. Diluent cetomacrogol cream (formula A), life of diluted cream 14 days. Net price 0.5%, 15 g = 30p; 1%, 15 g = 37p, 50 g = 99p; 2.5%, 15 g = 83p. Potency IV
Additives: chlorocresol

PoM **Hydrocortistab**® (Boots)
Cream, hydrocortisone acetate 1%, in a water-miscible basis. Net price 15 g = 30p. Potency IV
Additives: chlorocresol

PoM **Hydrocortisyl**® (Roussel)
Cream, hydrocortisone 1%, in a water-miscible basis. Net price 15 g = 51p. Potency IV
Additives: chlorocresol

Ointments

PoM **Hydrocortisone Ointment,** hydrocortisone, in white soft paraffin or a mixture of this with liquid paraffin, with or without wool fat. When hydrocortisone ointment is prescribed and no strength is stated, the 1% strength should be supplied. Net price 15 g (0.5%) = 36p; 15 g (1%) = 47p; 30 g (1%) = 92p; 100 g (1%) = £3.00. Potency IV

PoM **Efcortelan**® (Glaxo)
Ointment, hydrocortisone in a paraffin basis. Diluent white soft paraffin, life of diluted ointment 14 days. Net price 0.5%, 15 g = 30p; 1%, 15 g = 37p,   50 g = 99p;   2.5%,   15 g = 83p. Potency IV
Additives: none as listed in section 13.1

PoM **Hydrocortistab**® (Boots)
Ointment, hydrocortisone 1%, in an anhydrous greasy basis. Net price 15 g = 30p. Potency IV
Additives: none as listed in section 13.1

PoM **Hydrocortisyl**® (Roussel)
Ointment, hydrocortisone 1%, in an anhydrous greasy basis. Net price 15 g = 51p. Potency IV
Additives: wool fat

Lotions
PoM **Efcortelan**® (Glaxo)
Lotion, hydrocortisone 1%, in a water-miscible basis. Do not dilute. Net price 20 ml = 44p. Potency IV
Additives: hydroxybenzoates (parabens)

Dressings
Cortacream® *see* Hydrocortisone and Silicone Bandage, section 13.13.1

Compound preparations
Note. For compound preparations with coal tar, see section 13.5

PoM **Alphaderm**® (Norwich Eaton)
Cream, hydrocortisone 1%, urea 10%, in a powder-in-cream basis. Net price 30 g = £2.42; 100 g = £7.51. Potency III
Additives: none as listed in section 13.1
Apply sparingly twice daily

PoM **Calmurid HC**® (Pharmacia)
Cream, hydrocortisone 1%, urea 10%, lactic acid 5%, in a water-miscible basis. Diluent aqueous cream, life of diluted cream 14 days. Net price 30 g = £2.33; 100 g = £6.75. Potency III
Additives: none as listed in section 13.1
Apply sparingly twice daily. Use half-strength cream for 1 week if stinging occurs with undiluted preparation

PoM **Eczederm with Hydrocortisone**® (Quinoderm Ltd)
Cream, hydrocortisone 0.5%, calamine 20.88%, starch 2.09%. Net price 25 g = £1.06. Potency IV
Additives: fragrance
Apply sparingly up to 3 times daily

PoM **Epifoam**® (Stafford-Miller)
Foam (= application), hydrocortisone acetate 1%, pramoxine hydrochloride 1%, in a mucoadherent basis (pressurised aerosol pack). Net price 12-g unit (approx. 20 applications of 5 ml) = £2.81. Potency IV
Additives: information not disclosed for BNF
For perineal trauma including post-episiotomy pain and dermatoses
Apply on a pad 3–4 times daily

PoM **Eurax-Hydrocortisone**® (Zyma)
Cream, hydrocortisone 0.25%, crotamiton 10%. Net price 30 g = 93p. Potency IV
Additives: hydroxybenzoates (parabens), propylene glycol
Apply sparingly 2–3 times daily

▼ PoM **Sential**® (Pharmacia)
Cream, hydrocortisone 0.5%, urea 4%, sodium chloride 4%, in a water-miscible basis. Net price 30 g = £2.40; 100 g = £7.25. Potency IV
Additives: sorbic acid
Apply sparingly twice daily

With antimicrobials
PoM **Hydrocortisone and Neomycin Cream**, hydrocortisone 0.5%, neomycin sulphate 0.5%, in a water-miscible basis. Net price 15 g = 65p. Potency IV
Apply sparingly 2–3 times daily

PoM **Barquinol HC**® (Fisons)
Cream, hydrocortisone acetate 0.5%, clioquinol 3%. Net price 15 g = 58p. Potency IV
Additives: hydroxybenzoates (parabens), wool fat
Apply sparingly 2–3 times daily
Caution: stains clothing

PoM **Canesten HC**® (Baypharm)
Cream, hydrocortisone 1%, clotrimazole 1%. Net price 30 g = £3.18. Potency IV
Additives: benzyl alcohol
Apply sparingly twice daily

PoM **Daktacort**® (Janssen)
Cream, hydrocortisone 1%, miconazole nitrate 2%, in a water-miscible basis. Net price 30 g = £2.82. Potency IV
Additives: butylated hydroxyanisole, disodium edetate
Ointment, hydrocortisone 1%, miconazole nitrate 2%, in a greasy basis. Net price 30 g = £3.10. Potency IV
Additives: none as listed in section 13.1
Apply sparingly 2–3 times daily

▼ PoM **Econacort**® (Squibb)
Cream, hydrocortisone 1%, econazole nitrate 1%. Net price 30 g = £2.85. Potency IV
Additives: butylated hydroxyanisole
Apply sparingly twice daily

PoM **Framycort**® (Fisons)
Ointment, hydrocortisone acetate 0.5%, framycetin sulphate 0.5%. Net price 15 g = £1.82. Potency IV
Additives: none as listed in section 13.1
Apply sparingly 2–3 times daily

PoM **Fucidin H**® (Leo)
Cream, hydrocortisone acetate 1%, fusidic acid 2%. Net price 15 g = £3.00; 30 g = £5.17. Potency IV
Additives: butylated hydroxyanisole, potassium sorbate
Gel, hydrocortisone acetate 1%, fusidic acid 2%, in a water-miscible basis. Net price 15 g = £2.91; 30 g = £5.06. Potency IV
Additives: hydroxybenzoates (parabens), polysorbate 80
Ointment, hydrocortisone acetate 1%, sodium fusidate 2%. Net price 15 g = £2.70; 30 g = £4.68. Potency IV
Additives: wool fat
Apply sparingly 3–4 times daily

PoM **Genticin HC**® (Nicholas)
Cream, hydrocortisone acetate 1%, gentamicin 0.3% (as sulphate), in a water-miscible basis. Net price 15 g = £1.86. Potency IV
Additives: hydroxybenzoates (parabens), polysorbates, propylene glycol
Ointment, ingredients as for cream but greasy basis. Net price 15 g = £1.86. Potency IV
Additives: hydroxybenzoates (parabens), polysorbates, propylene glycol
Apply sparingly 3–4 times daily

PoM **Gregoderm**® (Unigreg)
Ointment, hydrocortisone 1%, neomycin sulphate 0.4%, nystatin 100 000 units/g, polymyxin B sulphate 7250 units/g. Net price 4 g = 78p; 15 g = £1.70. Potency IV
Additives: none as listed in section 13.1
Apply sparingly 2–3 times daily

PoM **Hydroderm**® (MSD)
Ointment, hydrocortisone 1%, neomycin sulphate 0.5%, bacitracin zinc 1000 units/g, in an emollient basis. Net price 15 g = 81p. Potency IV
Additives: beeswax, wool fat
Apply sparingly 2–3 times daily

PoM **Nystaform-HC**® (Bayer)
Cream, hydrocortisone 0.5%, nystatin 100 000 units/g, chlorhexidine hydrochloride 1%, in a water-miscible basis. Net price 15 g = £1.73; 30 g = £2.73. Potency IV
Additives: benzyl alcohol, polysorbate 60
Ointment, hydrocortisone 1%, nystatin 100 000 units/g, chlorhexidine acetate 1%, in a water-repellent basis. Net price 30 g = £2.73. Potency IV
Additives: none as listed in section 13.1
Apply sparingly 2–3 times daily

PoM **Quinocort**® (Quinoderm Ltd)
Cream, hydrocortisone 1%, potassium hydroxyquinoline sulphate 0.5% in a vanishing cream basis. Net price 30 g = £2.29. Potency IV
Additives: edetic acid (EDTA)
Apply sparingly 2–3 times daily

PoM **Terra-Cortril**® (Pfizer)
Topical ointment, hydrocortisone 1%, oxytetracycline 3% (as hydrochloride), in a paraffin basis. Net price 15 g = £1.01; 30 g = £1.82. Potency IV
Additives: none as listed in section 13.1
Apply sparingly 2–4 times daily
Spray application, hydrocortisone 50 mg, oxytetracycline 150 mg (as hydrochloride), 30-ml pressurised aerosol unit, net price = £1.44; double these amounts in 60-ml unit, net price = £2.50. Potency IV
Additives: none as listed in section 13.1
Spray area sparingly 2–4 times daily

PoM **Terra-Cortril Nystatin**® (Pfizer)
Cream, hydrocortisone 1%, nystatin 100 000 units/g, oxytetracycline 3% (as calcium salt). Net price 30 g = £1.76. Potency IV
Additives: hydroxybenzoates (parabens), polysorbate, propylene glycol, fragrance
Apply sparingly 2–4 times daily

PoM **Timodine**® (R&C)
Cream, hydrocortisone 0.5%, nystatin 100 000 units/g, benzalkonium chloride solution 0.2%, dimethicone '350' 10%. Net price 30 g = £2.38. Potency IV
Additives: butylated hydroxyanisole, hydroxybenzoates (parabens), sorbic acid
Apply sparingly 3 times daily (napkin rash, after each change)

PoM **Vioform-Hydrocortisone**® (Zyma)
Cream, hydrocortisone 1%, clioquinol 3%. Net price 30 g = £1.57. Potency IV
Ointment, hydrocortisone 1%, clioquinol 3%. Net price 30 g = £1.57. Potency IV
Apply sparingly 1–3 times daily
Caution: stains clothing

HYDROCORTISONE BUTYRATE

Indications: severe inflammatory skin disorders such as eczema in patients unresponsive to less potent corticosteroids

Cautions; Contra-indications; Side-effects: see under Hydrocortisone and notes above
Administration: apply sparingly 2–4 times daily, reducing frequency as condition responds

PoM **Locoid**® (Brocades)
Cream, hydrocortisone butyrate 0.1%, in a water-miscible basis. Diluent Locobase® cream, life of diluted cream 14 days. Net price 30 g = £2.38; 100 g = £7.29. Potency II
Additives: hydroxybenzoates (parabens)
Lipocream, hydrocortisone butyrate 0.1% in a fatty cream basis. Diluent Lipobase® cream, life of diluted cream 14 days. Net price 30 g = £2.38; 100 g = £7.29. Potency II
Additives: hydroxybenzoates (parabens)
Ointment, hydrocortisone butyrate 0.1%, in an anhydrous greasy basis. Diluent Locobase® ointment, life of diluted ointment 14 days. Net price 30 g = £2.27; 100 g = £6.95. Potency II
Additives: none as listed in section 13.1
Scalp lotion, hydrocortisone butyrate 0.1%, in an aqueous isopropyl alcohol basis. Net price 30 ml = £3.20; 100 ml = £9.81. Potency II
Additives: none as listed in section 13.1
Apply 1–2 times daily, reducing frequency as condition responds
Caution: flammable

With antimicrobials
PoM **Locoid C**® (Brocades)
Cream, hydrocortisone butyrate 0.1%, chlorquinaldol 3%. Net price 30 g = £2.97. Potency II
Additives: none as listed in section 13.1
Ointment, ingredients as for cream, in a greasy basis. Net price 30 g = £2.97. Potency II
Additives: none as listed in section 13.1
Apply sparingly 2–4 times daily. Max. 60 g for up to 14 days

ALCLOMETASONE DIPROPIONATE

Indications: inflammatory skin disorders such as eczema
Cautions; Contra-indications; Side-effects: see under Hydrocortisone and notes above
Administration: apply sparingly 2–3 times daily, reducing frequency as condition responds

▼ PoM **Modrasone**® (Kirby-Warrick)
Cream, alclometasone dipropionate 0.05%. Net price 15 g = £1.70; 50 g = £4.80. Potency IV
Additives: chlorocresol, propylene glycol
Ointment, alclometasone dipropionate 0.05%. Net price 15 g = £1.70; 50 g = £4.80. Potency IV
Additives: beeswax

BECLOMETHASONE DIPROPIONATE

Indications: severe inflammatory skin disorders such as eczema in patients unresponsive to less potent corticosteroids
Cautions; Contra-indications; Side-effects: see under Hydrocortisone and notes above
Administration: apply sparingly twice daily, reducing strength and frequency as condition responds. Under occlusion, max. 2 g daily of 0.5% preparation

PoM **Propaderm**® (A&H)

Cream, beclomethasone dipropionate 0.025%. Diluent cetomacrogol cream (formula A), life of diluted cream 14 days. Net price 15 g = 79p; 50 g = £2.06. Potency II
Additives: chlorocresol

Ointment, beclomethasone dipropionate 0.025%. Diluent white soft paraffin, life of diluted ointment 14 days. Net price 15 g = 79p; 50 g = £2.06. Potency II
Additives: propylene glycol

With antibacterials
PoM **Propaderm-A**® (A&H)

Ointment, beclomethasone dipropionate 0.025%, chlortetracycline hydrochloride 3%. Diluent white soft paraffin, life of diluted ointment 14 days. Net price 15 g = 89p; 50 g = £2.23. Potency II
Additives: none as listed in section 13.1

Initially apply sparingly twice daily

Caution: stains clothing

BETAMETHASONE ESTERS

Indications: severe inflammatory skin disorders such as eczema in patients unresponsive to less potent corticosteroids

Cautions; Contra-indications; Side-effects: see under Hydrocortisone and notes above. Application of more than 100 g per week of 0.1% preparation is likely to cause adrenal suppression

Administration: apply sparingly 2–3 times daily, reducing strength and frequency as condition responds

PoM **Betnovate**® (Glaxo)

Cream, betamethasone 0.1% (as valerate), in a water-miscible basis. Diluent cetomacrogol cream (formula A), life of diluted cream 14 days. Net price 15 g = 78p; 30 g = £1.40; 100 g = £3.95. Potency II
Additives: chlorocresol

Ointment, betamethasone 0.1% (as valerate), in an anhydrous paraffin basis. Diluent white soft paraffin or a mixture of this with liquid paraffin, life of diluted ointment 14 days. Net price 15 g = 78p; 30 g = £1.40; 100 g = £3.95. Potency II
Additives: none as listed in section 13.1

Lotion, betamethasone 0.1% (as valerate). Do not dilute. Net price 20 ml = 95p. Potency II
Additives: hydroxybenzoates (parabens)

Scalp application, betamethasone 0.1% (as valerate), in a thickened alcoholic basis. Net price 30 ml = £1.74; 100 ml = £5.18. Potency II
Additives: none as listed in section 13.1

Apply sparingly 1–2 times daily, reducing frequency as condition responds

Caution: flammable

PoM **Betnovate-RD**® (Glaxo)

Cream, betamethasone 0.025% (as valerate) in a water-miscible basis (1 in 4 dilution of Betnovate cream). Net price 100 g = £3.26. Potency III
Additives: chlorocresol

Ointment, betamethasone 0.025% (as valerate) in an anhydrous paraffin basis (1 in 4 dilution of Betnovate ointment). Net price 100 g = £3.26. Potency III
Additives: none as listed in section 13.1

▼ PoM **Diprosalic**® (Kirby-Warrick)

Ointment, betamethasone 0.05% (as dipropionate), salicylic acid 3%. Net price 30 g = £2.95; 100 g = £8.25. Potency II
Additives: none as listed in section 13.1

[1]*Scalp application*, betamethasone 0.05% (as dipropionate), salicylic acid 2%, in an alcoholic basis. Net price 30 ml = £3.95; 100 ml = £9.95. Potency II
Additives: disodium edetate

Apply sparingly 1–2 times daily
[1] formerly Diprosalic lotion

▼ PoM **Diprosone**® (Kirby-Warrick)

Cream, betamethasone 0.05% (as dipropionate), in a water-miscible basis. Diluent Diprobase® cream, life of diluted cream 14 days. Net price 30 g = £2.34; 100 g = £6.66. Potency II
Additives: chlorocresol

Duopack, Diprosone cream 30 g with Diprobase cream 100 g. Net price = £4.92

Ointment, betamethasone 0.05% (as dipropionate). Diluent Diprobase® ointment, life of diluted ointment 14 days. Net price 30 g = £2.34; 100 g = £6.66. Potency II
Additives: none as listed in section 13.1

Apply sparingly once or twice daily

Duopack, Diprosone ointment 30 g with Diprobase ointment 100 g. Net price = £4.92

[2]*Lotion*, betamethasone 0.05% (as dipropionate), in a thickened alcoholic basis. Net price 30 ml = £2.94; 100 ml = £8.45. Potency II
Additives: none as listed in section 13.1

Apply twice daily, reducing as condition responds
[2] formerly Diprosalic scalp applicaton

With antimicrobials
PoM **Betnovate-C**® (Glaxo)

Cream, betamethasone 0.1% (as valerate), clioquinol 3%, in a water-miscible basis. Diluent cetomacrogol cream (formula A), life of diluted cream 14 days. Net price 15 g = 94p; 30 g = £1.72. Potency II
Additives: chlorocresol

Ointment, betamethasone 0.1% (as valerate), clioquinol 3%, in a paraffin basis. Diluent white soft paraffin or a mixture of this with liquid paraffin, life of diluted ointment 14 days. Net price 15 g = 94p; 30 g = £1.72. Potency II
Additives: none as listed in section 13.1

Apply sparingly 2–3 times daily

Caution: stains clothing

PoM **Betnovate-N**® (Glaxo)

Cream, betamethasone 0.1% (as valerate), neomycin sulphate 0.5%, in a water-miscible basis. Diluent cetomacrogol cream (formula A), life of diluted cream 14 days. Net price 15 g = 94p; 30 g = £1.72; 100 g = £4.77. Potency II
Additives: chlorocresol

Ointment, betamethasone 0.1% (as valerate), neomycin sulphate 0.5%, in a paraffin basis.

Diluent white soft paraffin or a mixture of this with liquid paraffin, life of diluted ointment 14 days. Net price 15 g = 94p; 30 g = £1.72; 100 g = £4.77. Potency II
Additives: none as listed in section 13.1

Apply sparingly 2–3 times daily

PoM **Fucibet**® (Leo)

Cream, betamethasone 0.1% (as valerate), fusidic acid 2%, in a water-miscible basis. Net price 15 g = £3.49; 30 g = £5.89. Potency II
Additives: chlorocresol

Apply sparingly 2–3 times daily

▼ PoM **Lotriderm**® (Kirby-Warrick)

Cream, betamethasone 0.05% (as dipropionate), clotrimazole 1%. Net price 15 g = £3.49. Potency II
Additives: benzyl alcohol, propylene glycol

Apply sparingly twice daily

CLOBETASOL PROPIONATE

Indications: short-term treatment only of severe exacerbations in inflammatory skin disorders such as discoid lupus erythematosus in patients unresponsive to less potent corticosteroids

Cautions; Contra-indications; Side-effects: see under Hydrocortisone and notes above. Not more than 50 g of 0.05% preparation should be applied per week

Administration: apply sparingly 1–2 times daily for up to 4 weeks, reducing frequency as condition responds

PoM **Dermovate**® (Glaxo)

Cream, clobetasol propionate 0.05%, in a water-miscible basis. Diluents cetomacrogol cream (formula A), aqueous cream, or buffered cream, life of diluted cream 14 days. Net price 25 g = £2.13; 100 g = £7.52. Potency I
Additives: beeswax (or beeswax substitute), chlorocresol, propylene glycol

Ointment, clobetasol propionate 0.05%, in an anhydrous paraffin basis. Diluents white soft paraffin or a mixture of this with liquid paraffin, life of diluted ointment 14 days. Net price 25 g = £2.13; 100 g = £7.52. Potency I
Additives: propylene glycol

Scalp application, clobetasol propionate 0.05%, in a thickened alcoholic basis. Net price 25 ml = £2.79; 100 ml = £9.91. Potency I
Caution: flammable
Additives: none as listed in section 13.1

With antimicrobials
PoM **Dermovate-NN**® (Glaxo)

Cream, clobetasol propionate 0.05%, neomycin sulphate 0.5%, nystatin 100 000 units/g. Net price 25 g = £2.23. Potency I
Additives: beeswax substitute

Ointment, ingredients as for cream, in a paraffin basis. Diluent white soft paraffin, life of diluted ointment 14 days. Net price 25 g = £2.23. Potency I
Additives: none as listed in section 13.1

Apply sparingly once or twice daily, for up to 4 weeks reducing as condition responds

CLOBETASONE BUTYRATE

Indications: inflammatory skin disorders in patients unresponsive to less potent corticosteroids

Cautions; Contra-indications; Side-effects: see under Hydrocortisone and notes above

Administration: apply sparingly up to 4 times daily, reducing frequency as condition responds

PoM **Eumovate**® (Glaxo)

Cream, clobetasone butyrate 0.05%, in a water-miscible basis. Net price 25 g = £1.47; 100 g = £5.16. Potency III
Additives: beeswax substitute, chlorocresol

Ointment, clobetasone butyrate 0.05%, in an anhydrous paraffin basis. Net price 25 g = £1.47; 100 g = £5.16. Potency III
Additives: none as listed in section 13.1

With antimicrobials
PoM **Trimovate**® (Glaxo)

Cream, clobetasone butyrate 0.05%, oxytetracycline 3% (as calcium salt), nystatin 100 000 units/g, in a water-miscible basis. Net price 25 g = £2.61. Potency III
Additives: chlorocresol

Ointment, clobetasone butyrate 0.05%, chlortetracycline hydrochloride 3%, nystatin 100 000 units/g, in a paraffin basis. Net price 25 g = £2.61. Potency III
Additives: none as listed in section 13.1

Apply sparingly up to 4 times daily
Caution: stains clothing

DESONIDE

Indications: severe inflammatory skin disorders such as eczema in patients unresponsive to less potent corticosteroids

Cautions; Contra-indications; Side-effects: see under Hydrocortisone and notes above

Administration: apply sparingly 2–3 times daily reducing frequency as condition responds

PoM **Tridesilon**® (Lagap)

Cream, desonide 0.05%, in a water-miscible basis. Diluents cetomacrogol cream (formula A or B) or aqueous cream, life of diluted cream up to 3 months. Net price 15 g = £1.73; 30 g = £2.99. Potency II
Additives: beeswax, hydroxybenzoates (parabens)

DESOXYMETHASONE

Indications: acute inflammatory, allergic, and chronic skin disorders

Cautions; Contra-indications; Side-effects: see under Hydrocortisone and notes above

Administration: apply sparingly 2–3 times daily reducing frequency as condition responds

▼ PoM **Stiedex**® (Stiefel)

Oily cream, desoxymethasone 0.25%, in an oily basis. Diluent oily cream, life of diluted cream 14 days. Net price 30 g = £3.43. Potency II
Additives: wool fat

LP Oily cream, desoxymethasone 0.05%, in an oily basis. Diluent oily cream, life of diluted cream 14 days. Net price 30 g = £2.86. Potency III
Additives: edetic acid (EDTA), wool fat

With antibacterials
▼ PoM **Stiedex LPN**® (Stiefel)
Oily cream, desoxymethasone 0.05%, neomycin (as sulphate) 0.5%, in an oily basis. Net price 15 g = £2.17. Potency III
Additives: edetic acid (EDTA), wool fat
Apply sparingly 2–3 times daily

DIFLUCORTOLONE VALERATE

Indications: severe inflammatory skin disorders such as eczema in patients unresponsive to less potent corticosteroids; high strength preparations (0.3%), short term treatment of severe exacerbations
Cautions; Contra-indications; Side-effects: see under Hydrocortisone and notes above. Not more than 50 g of 0.3% preparation should be applied per week
Administration: apply sparingly 2–3 times daily for up to 4 weeks (0.1% preparations) or 2 weeks (0.3% preparations), reducing strength and frequency as condition responds

PoM **Nerisone**® (Schering)
Cream, diflucortolone valerate 0.1%, in a water-miscible basis. Diluent aqueous cream or Ultrabase®, life of diluted cream 14 days. Net price 30 g = £2.56. Potency II
Additives: disodium edetate, hydroxybenzoates (parabens)
Oily cream, diflucortolone valerate 0.1%, in a water-in-oil basis. Diluent hydrous ointment (oily cream), life of diluted cream 14 days. Net price 30 g = £2.56. Potency II
Additives: none as listed in section 13.1
Ointment, diflucortolone valerate 0.1%, in an anhydrous basis. Diluent white soft paraffin, life of diluted ointment 14 days. Net price 30 g = £2.56. Potency II
Additives: none as listed in section 13.1

PoM **Nerisone Forte**® (Schering)
Oily cream, diflucortolone valerate 0.3%, in a water-in-oil basis. Diluent hydrous ointment (oily cream), life of diluted cream 14 days. Net price 15 g = £2.09. Potency I
Additives: none as listed in section 13.1
Ointment, diflucortolone valerate 0.3% in an anhydrous fatty basis. Diluent white soft paraffin, life of diluted ointment 14 days. Net price 15 g = £2.09. Potency I
Additives: none as listed in section 13.1

PoM **Temetex**® (Roche)
Cream, diflucortolone valerate 0.1%, in a water-miscible basis. Net price 30 g = £2.33. Potency II
Additives: disodium edetate, hydroxybenzoates (parabens)
Fatty ointment, diflucortolone valerate 0.1%, in an anhydrous basis. Net price 30 g = £2.33. Potency II
Additives: none as listed in section 13.1
Ointment, diflucortolone valerate 0.1%, in a water-in-oil cream basis. Diluent white soft paraffin, life of diluted ointment 14 days. Net price 30 g = £2.33. Potency II
Additives: beeswax

FLUCLOROLONE ACETONIDE

Indications: severe inflammatory skin disorders such as eczema in patients unresponsive to less potent corticosteroids

Cautions; Contra-indications; Side-effects: see under Hydrocortisone and notes above
Administration: apply sparingly twice daily, reducing frequency as condition responds

PoM **Topilar**® (Syntex)
Cream, fluclorolone acetonide 0.025%, in a non-aqueous, water-miscible basis. Net price 30 g = £1.48; 100 g = £4.02. Potency II
Additives: propylene glycol
Ointment, fluclorolone acetonide 0.025%, in an ointment basis. Diluent white soft paraffin, life of diluted ointment 14 days. Net price 30 g = £1.48; 100 g = £4.02. Potency II
Additives: propylene glycol, wool fat

FLUOCINOLONE ACETONIDE

Indications: inflammatory skin disorders such as eczema, 0.0025–0.01% preparations in milder conditions, 0.025% preparations in severe conditions
Cautions; Contra-indications; Side-effects: see under Hydrocortisone and notes above
Administration: apply sparingly 2–3 times daily, reducing strength and frequency as condition responds

PoM **Synalar**® (ICI)
Cream, fluocinolone acetonide 0.025%, in a water-miscible basis. Diluent cetomacrogol cream (formula B), life of diluted cream 14 days. Net price 15 g = 69p; 30 g = £1.24; 50 g = £1.87. Potency II
Additives: propylene glycol
Gel, fluocinolone acetonide 0.025%, in a water-miscible basis. Net price 30 g = £1.32. For use on scalp and other hairy areas. Potency II
Additives: hydroxybenzoates (parabens), propylene glycol
Ointment, fluocinolone acetonide 0.025%, in a greasy basis. Diluents white or yellow soft paraffin or eye ointment basis, life of diluted ointment 14 days. Net price 15 g = 69p; 30 g = £1.24; 50 g = £1.87. Potency II
Additives: propylene glycol, wool fat

PoM **Synalar 1 in 4 Dilution**® (ICI)
Cream, fluocinolone acetonide 0.00625% in a water-miscible basis. Net price 50 g = £1.42. Potency III
Additives: propylene glycol
Ointment, fluocinolone acetonide 0.00625% in a greasy basis. Net price 50 g = £1.67. Potency III
Additives: propylene glycol, wool fat

PoM **Synalar 1 in 10 Dilution**® (ICI)
Cream, fluocinolone acetonide 0.0025% in a water-miscible basis. Net price 50 g = £1.35. Potency IV
Additives: propylene glycol

With antibacterials
PoM **Synalar C**® (ICI)
Cream, fluocinolone acetonide 0.025%, clioquinol 3%, in a water-miscible basis. Diluent cetomacrogol cream (formula B), life of diluted cream 14 days. Net price 15 g = 85p. Potency II
Additives: hydroxybenzoates (parabens), propylene glycol

Ointment, ingredients as for cream, in a greasy basis. Diluents white or yellow soft paraffin or eye ointment basis, life of diluted ointment 14 days. Net price 15 g = 85p. Potency II
Additives: propylene glycol, wool fat
Apply sparingly 2–3 times daily
Caution: stains clothing

PoM **Synalar N**® (ICI)
Cream, fluocinolone acetonide 0.025%, neomycin sulphate 0.5%, in a water-miscible basis. Diluent as above. Net price 15 g = 74p; 30 g = £1.29. Potency II
Additives: hydroxybenzoates (parabens), propylene glycol
Ointment, ingredients as for cream, in a greasy basis. Diluents as above. Net price 15 g = 74p; 30 g = £1.29. Potency II
Additives: propylene glycol, wool fat
Apply sparingly 2–3 times daily

FLUOCINONIDE

Indications: severe inflammatory skin disorders such as eczema in patients unresponsive to less potent corticosteroids
Cautions; Contra-indications; Side-effects: see under Hydrocortisone and notes above
Administration: apply sparingly 3–4 times daily, reducing frequency as condition responds

PoM **Metosyn**® (Stuart)
FAPG cream, fluocinonide 0.05%, in a non-aqueous water-miscible basis. Net price 25 g = 96p; 100 g = £3.64. Potency II
Additives: propylene glycol
Ointment, fluocinonide 0.05%, in a paraffin basis. Diluent white soft paraffin, life of diluted ointment 14 days. Net price 25 g = 96p; 100 g = £3.64. Potency II
Additives: propylene glycol, wool fat
Scalp lotion, fluocinonide 0.05% in a propylene glycol-alcohol basis. Net price 30 ml (with applicator) = £2.30. Potency II
Additives: propylene glycol
Apply 1–2 times daily, reducing frequency as condition responds
Caution: flammable

FLUOCORTOLONE

Indications: 0.25% preparations—severe inflammatory skin disorders such as eczema in patients unresponsive to less potent corticosteroids; 0.1% preparations—milder inflammatory skin disorders
Cautions; Contra-indications; Side-effects: see under Hydrocortisone and notes above
Administration: apply sparingly 2–3 times daily, reducing strength and frequency as condition responds

PoM **Ultradil Plain**® (Schering)
Cream, fluocortolone hexanoate 0.1%, fluocortolone pivalate 0.1%, in a water-miscible basis. Diluent aqueous cream or Ultrabase®, life of diluted cream 14 days. Net price 50 g = £2.86; 100 g = £5.41. Potency III
Additives: disodium edetate, hydroxybenzoates (parabens), fragrance

Ointment, fluocortolone hexanoate 0.1%, fluocortolone pivalate 0.1%, in a water-in-oil emulsion basis. Diluent hydrous ointment (oily cream), life of diluted ointment 14 days. Net price 50 g = £2.86; 100 g = £5.41. Potency III
Additives: wool fat, fragrance

PoM **Ultralanum Plain**® (Schering)
Cream, fluocortolone hexanoate 0.25%, fluocortolone pivalate 0.25%, in a water-miscible basis. Diluent aqueous cream or Ultrabase®, life of diluted cream 14 days. Net price 30 g = £3.06; 50 g = £4.65. Potency III
Additives: disodium edetate, hydroxybenzoates (parabens), fragrance
Ointment, fluocortolone 0.25%, fluocortolone pivalate 0.25%, in a water-in-oil emulsion basis. Diluent as for Ultradil Plain ointment. Net price 30 g = £3.06; 50 g = £4.65. Potency III
Additives: wool fat, fragrance

FLURANDRENOLONE

Indications: 0.05%   preparations—severe inflammatory skin disorders such as eczema in patients unresponsive to less potent corticosteroids;   0.0125%   preparations—milder inflammatory skin disorders
Cautions; Contra-indications; Side-effects: see under Hydrocortisone and notes above
Administration: apply sparingly 2–3 times daily, reducing strength and frequency as condition responds

PoM **Haelan**® (Dista)
Cream, flurandrenolone 0.0125%, in a water-miscible basis. Diluent aqueous cream, life of diluted cream 14 days. Net price 60 g = £3.96. Potency III
Additives: propylene glycol
Ointment, flurandrenolone 0.0125%, in an anhydrous greasy basis. Diluent white soft paraffin. Net price 60 g = £3.96. Potency III
Additives: beeswax, polysorbate

PoM **Haelan-X**® (Dista)
Cream, flurandrenolone 0.05%, in a water-miscible basis. Diluent as above. Net price 15 g = £1.92. Potency III
Additives: propylene glycol
Ointment, flurandrenolone 0.05%, in an anhydrous greasy basis. Diluent as above. Net price 15 g = £1.92. Potency III
Additives: beeswax, polysorbate

With antibacterials
PoM **Haelan-C**® (Dista)
Cream, flurandrenolone 0.0125%, clioquinol 3%. Diluent aqueous cream, life of diluted cream 14 days. Net price 30 g = £2.69. Potency III
Additives: hydroxybenzoates (parabens), sodium edetate
Ointment, flurandrenolone 0.0125%, clioquinol 3%. Diluent white soft paraffin, life of diluted ointment 14 days. Net price 30 g = £2.69. Potency III
Additives: none as listed in section 13.1
Apply sparingly 2–3 times daily
Caution: stains clothing

HALCINONIDE

Indications: severe inflammatory skin disorders such as eczema in patients unresponsive to less potent corticosteroids

Cautions; Contra-indications; Side-effects: see under Hydrocortisone and notes above

Administration: apply sparingly 2–3 times daily, reducing frequency as condition responds

PoM **Halciderm Topical**® (Squibb)
Cream, halcinonide 0.1%, in a water-miscible basis. Net price 30 g = £3.40. Potency I
Additives: propylene glycol

METHYLPREDNISOLONE ACETATE

Indications: see notes above
Cautions; Contra-indications; Side-effects: see under Hydrocortisone

PoM **Neo-Medrone**® (Upjohn)
Cream, methylprednisolone acetate 0.25%, neomycin sulphate 0.5%. Net price 15 g = £1.44. Potency IV
Additives: information not disclosed for BNF
Apply sparingly 1–3 times daily

TRIAMCINOLONE ACETONIDE

Indications: severe inflammatory skin disorders such as eczema in patients unresponsive to less potent corticosteroids

Cautions; Contra-indications; Side-effects: see under Hydrocortisone and notes above

Administration: apply sparingly 2–4 times daily, reducing frequency as condition responds

PoM **Adcortyl**® (Squibb)
Cream, triamcinolone acetonide 0.1%, in a water-miscible basis. Diluents cetomacrogol cream (formula B), or aqueous cream provided that chlorocresol content is increased to 0.2%, life of diluted cream 14 days. Net price 30 g = £1.98. Potency II
Additives: benzyl alcohol, propylene glycol
Ointment, triamcinolone acetonide 0.1%, in an anhydrous greasy basis. Diluent white soft paraffin. Net price 30 g = £1.98. Potency II
Additives: none as listed in section 13.1

PoM **Ledercort**® (Lederle)
Cream, triamcinolone acetonide 0.1%, in water-miscible basis. Diluent aqueous cream, life of diluted cream 4 weeks. Net price 15 g = £1.72; 250 g = £25.90. Potency II
Additives: hydroxybenzoates (parabens), polysorbate 80
Ointment, triamcinolone acetonide 0.1%, in an anhydrous greasy basis. Diluent 1 part wool fat, 9 parts white soft paraffin. Net price 15 g = £1.72; 250 g = £25.90. Potency II
Additives: hydroxybenzoates (parabens), wool fat

With antimicrobials
PoM **Adcortyl with Graneodin**® (Squibb)
Cream, triamcinolone acetonide 0.1%, gramicidin 0.025%, neomycin 0.25% (as sulphate), in a vanishing-cream basis. Do not dilute. Net price 15 g = £1.80. Potency II
Additives: benzyl alcohol, propylene glycol

Ointment, ingredients as for cream, in an ointment basis. Do not dilute. Net price 15 g = £1.80. Potency II
Additives: none as listed in section 13.1
Apply sparingly 2–4 times daily

PoM **Aureocort**® (Lederle)
Cream, triamcinolone acetonide 0.1%, chlortetracycline hydrochloride 3% (as chlortetracycline), in a water-miscible basis. Do not dilute. Net price 15 g = £2.77. Potency II
Additives: chlorocresol
Ointment, triamcinolone acetonide 0.1%, chlortetracycline hydrochloride 3%, in an anhydrous greasy basis containing wool fat and white soft paraffin. Do not dilute. Net price 15 g = £2.77. Potency II
Additives: hydroxybenzoates (parabens), wool fat
Caution: stains clothing
Apply sparingly 2–3 times daily

PoM **Nystadermal**® (Squibb)
Cream, triamcinolone acetonide 0.1%, nystatin 100 000 units/g. Net price 15 g = £2.27. Potency II
Additives: benzyl alcohol, propylene glycol, fragrance
Apply sparingly 2–4 times daily on moist weeping lesions

PoM **Tri-Adcortyl**® (Squibb)
Cream, triamcinolone acetonide 0.1%, gramicidin 0.025%, neomycin 0.25% (as sulphate), nystatin 100 000 units/g. Net price 15 g = £1.72; 30 g = £3.23. Potency II
Additives: benzyl alcohol, ethylenediamine, propylene glycol, fragrance
Ointment, ingredients as for cream, in an ointment basis. Net price 15 g = £1.72; 30 g = £3.23. Potency II
Additives: none as listed in section 13.1
Apply sparingly 2–4 times daily

13.5 Preparations for psoriasis and eczema

Eczema ('dermatitis') is due to a particular type of epidermal inflammation and is caused by a wide variety of factors; where possible the causative factors should be established and removed (see also hyposensitisation, section 3.4.2). In many cases no underlying factor can be identified (atopic eczema).

Dry, fissured, scaly lesions are treated with bland **emollients** (section 13.2.1) which are often all that is necessary to allay irritation and permit healing. Preparations containing zinc oxide and calamine are sometimes useful; zinc may have a weak anti-eczematous action. **Topical corticosteroids** are described in section 13.4. Perfumes and perfumed soaps should be **avoided** and preparations such as **emulsifying ointment** used as soap substitutes and in the bath. **Keratolytics** such as salicylic acid, followed by ichthammol or coal tar (see below) are used in chronic eczematous conditions where there is marked thickening of the skin and pronounced scaling.

Weeping eczemas may be treated with corticosteroids; they are, however, commonly secondarily infected. Wet dressings of **potassium**

---

permanganate (0.01%) (section 13.11) are applied. If a large area is involved, potassium permanganate baths are taken. When necessary **topical antibacterials** are used (section 13.10.1) but those which are not given systemically should be chosen.

Psoriasis is characterised by epidermal thickening and scaling. It has less tendency to heal spontaneously than eczema. For mild conditions, treatment, other than reassurance and an emollient, may be unnecessary. In more troublesome cases, local application of **salicylic acid**, **coal tar**, or **dithranol** may have a beneficial effect. Topical and systemic corticosteroids should be avoided or given under specialist supervision because, although they may be effective, subsequent treatment becomes more difficult, as tachyphylaxis may occur and they may induce or precipitate severe pustular psoriasis (see also section 6.3.3). In resistant cases an antimetabolite, usually methotrexate (see section 8.1.3), may be used for its antimitotic activity but this must always be done under hospital supervision and the dose adjusted according to severity of the condition and in accordance with haematological and biochemical measurements; the usual dose is 15 to 25 mg of methotrexate weekly, usually by mouth.

Salicylic acid may be used in all hyperkeratotic and scaling conditions to enhance the rate of loss of surface scale. Preparations containing salicylic acid 2% are used initially and then gradually increased to concentrations of 3 to 6%. Side-effects are few but include allergic contact sensitivity, or, when large areas are treated, salicylism (see section 10.1.1).

Ichthammol has a milder action than coal tar and is useful in the less acute forms of eczema. It can be applied conveniently to flexures of the limbs as **zinc paste and ichthammol bandage** (section 13.13.1).

Coal tar is more active than salicylic acid and has antipruritic and keratolytic properties. It is used in psoriasis and eczema. Coal tar has superseded wood tar as it is more active. The formulation and strength chosen depends on patient acceptability and severity of the condition; the 'thicker' the patch of eczema or psoriasis the stronger the concentration of coal tar required. **Coal tar paste** or **zinc and coal tar paste** are generally suitable for most cases but are limited by their unpleasant appearance and smell and they may not be used on the face. Some of the newer preparations are less unsightly and may be preferred. Preparations such as Carbo-Dome® are suitable for treating the face. **Zinc paste and coal tar bandage** (section 13.13.1) is useful for treating the limbs. **Tar** shampoos are described in section 13.9. When lesions are extensive coal tar baths are useful. Combinations of coal tar with zinc or salicylic acid have no advantage over the simpler preparations. Preparations containing hydrocortisone and coal tar are useful in eczemas.

Dithranol is used in psoriasis and is the most potent topical preparation available for this condition. The preparation is applied carefully to the lesion, covered with a dressing, and left for one hour. Traditionally applications have been left on the skin overnight but this has now been shown to be unnecessary as short contact applications of 30 to 60 minutes are equally effective. Usual concentrations are 0.1–2% although in individual patients 5% or more may be used. Dithranol must be used with caution as it can cause quite severe skin irritation. For this reason it must be applied only to the lesions and it is customary to start with low concentrations and gradually build up to the maximum concentration which produces a therapeutic effect without irritation. Hands should be washed thoroughly after use. Some patients are intolerant to dithranol in low concentrations and it is important to recognise them early in treatment. Fair skin is more sensitive than dark skin. Proprietary preparations such as Dithrocream® are most commonly used as they may cause less staining and irritation than dithranol paste. Dithranol and urea combinations (Psoradrate®) may improve skin texture by rehydration. **Dithranol triacetate** (Exolan®) has no advantage over traditional preparations.

Ingram's method of applying dithranol is a frequent method used in hospitals. The patient soaks in a warm bath containing coal tar solution 1 in 800 and after drying is exposed to ultraviolet radiation B (UVB) to produce a slight erythema. **Dithranol paste** is applied to the lesions and the normal skin protected by applying talc and stockinette dressings. The procedure is repeated daily.

PUVA, photochemotherapy using psoralens with long-wave ultraviolet irradiation (UVA), is an effective method of treating some patients with psoriasis. Special lamps are required, and a psoralen, generally methoxsalen (available on named-patient basis only) is given by mouth about 2 hours beforehand, to sensitise the skin to the effects of irradiation. A course of PUVA may last 4 to 6 weeks and requires a variable number of treatments. Treatment is only available in specialist centres; it has to be carefully regulated, owing to the short-term hazard of severe burning and the long-term hazards of cataract formation, accelerated ageing, and the development of skin cancer.

Etretinate (Tigason®) is a newly introduced drug given by mouth for the treatment of severe resistant or complicated psoriasis and some of the congenital disorders of keratinisation including Darier's disease (keratosis follicularis). It should be prescribed only by consultant dermatologists or under hospital supervision. It is a retinoid compound with marked effects on keratinising epithelia. A therapeutic effect occurs after 2 to 4 weeks with maximum benefit after 4 to 6 weeks. Etretinate should be administered continuously because it treats only manifestations not the ultimate causes of these diseases, but treatment should be limited to a period of 6 to 9 months with a 3- to 4-month rest period before repeating treatment, as experience with this drug is limited. Most patients suffer from dryness and cracking of the lips. Other side-effects include mild transient alopecia, occasional generalised pruritus, paronychia, and nose bleeds. There is a tendency for the plasma lipids to rise in some patients. Etretinate is teratogenic and must be **avoided** in pregnancy. Contraceptive measures must be taken during treatment by women who may become pregnant and for one year after a course of the drug.

Bufexamac (Parfenac®) is used in mild inflammatory skin conditions.

COAL TAR

Indications: chronic eczema and psoriasis
Cautions: avoid broken or inflamed skin
Side-effects: skin irritation and acne-like eruptions, photosensitivity; stains skin, hair, and fabric
Administration: apply 1–3 times daily starting with low-strength preparations

Ointments and similar preparations
Calamine and Coal Tar Ointment (see Formulary). Net price 25 g = 11p
Coal Tar and Salicylic Acid Ointment (see Formulary). Net price 25 g = 14p
Coal Tar Paint, coal tar 10%, in acetone. Net price 25 ml = 14p. Label: 15
Caution: highly flammable
Coal Tar Paste, strong coal tar solution 7.5%, in compound zinc paste. Net price 25 g = 15p
Zinc and Coal Tar Paste, zinc oxide 6%, coal tar 6%, emulsifying wax 5%, starch 38%, yellow soft paraffin 45%. Net price 25 g = 17p
Alphosyl® (Stafford-Miller)
Cream, coal tar extract 5%, allantoin 2%, in a vanishing-cream basis. Net price 75 g = £1.56.
Additives: information not disclosed for BNF
For application to skin particularly intertriginous areas
Lotion, coal tar extract 5%, allantoin 2%. Net price 250 ml = £2.28. For application to skin or scalp
Additives: information not disclosed for BNF
Apply liberally 2–4 times daily
Carbo-Dome® (Lagap)
Cream, coal tar solution 10%, in a water-miscible basis. Net price 30 g = £1.48; 100 g = £4.47
Additives: beeswax, hydroxybenzoates (parabens)
Apply 2–3 times daily
Clinitar® (S&N Pharm.)
Cream, coal tar extract 1%. Net price 60 g = £3.00
Additives: information not disclosed for BNF
Gel, coal tar extract 2.5%. Net price 40 g = £2.85
Additives: information not disclosed for BNF
Apply 1–2 times daily
Gelcosal® (Quinoderm Ltd)
Gel, strong coal tar solution 5%, pine tar 5%, salicylic acid 2% in a water-miscible basis. Net price 50 g = £2.54. Apply twice daily
Additives: none as listed in section 13.1
Gelcotar® (Quinoderm Ltd)
Gel, strong coal tar solution 5%, pine tar 5%, in a water-miscible basis. Net price 50 g = £2.31; 500 g = £11.95. Apply twice daily
Additives: none as listed in section 13.1
Liquid, see section 13.9

Meditar® (Brocades)
Application, coal tar 5% in a wax stick. Net price 20 g = £2.46
Additives: beeswax, butylated hydroxytoluene
Apply 1–2 times daily
Pragmatar® (Bioglan)
Ointment, cetyl alcohol-coal tar distillate 4%, salicylic acid 3%, sulphur (precipitated) 3%, in a water-miscible basis. Net price 25 g = £1.29; 100 g = £4.79
Additives: fragrance
Apply sparingly daily; for scalp apply weekly to clean hair or in severe cases daily. Dilute with a few drops of water before application to infants
Psoriderm® (Dermal)
Cream, coal tar 6%, lecithin 0.4%. Net price 225 ml = £2.83
Additives: hydroxybenzoates (parabens), isopropyl palmitate, propylene glycol
Apply 1–2 times daily
PsoriGel® (Alcon)
Gel, coal tar solution USP 7.5% in an alcoholic emollient basis. Net price 90 g = £2.82
Additives: propylene glycol
Apply 1–2 times daily

Impregnated dressings
Zinc Paste and Coal Tar Bandage (Coltapaste®, Tarband®), see section 13.13.1

Bath preparations
Coal Tar Solution, coal tar 20%, polysorbate '80' 5%, in alcohol. Net price 100 ml = 62p
Use 100 ml in a bath
Note. This is Coal Tar Solution BP; Strong Coal Tar Solution BP contains coal tar 40%
Balneum with Tar® (Merck)
Bath oil, coal tar distillate 30%, soya oil 55%. Net price 225 ml = £3.72
Additives: none as listed in section 13.1
Use 1 measure (20 ml) in bath
Polytar Emollient® (Stiefel)
Bath additive, coal tar solution 2.5%, arachis oil extract of coal tar 7.5%, tar 7.5%, cade oil 7.5%, liquid paraffin 35%. Net price 350 ml = £4.20. ACBS: for psoriasis, eczema, atopic and pruritic dermatoses
Additives: isopropyl palmitate
Use 2–4 capfuls in bath and soak for 20 minutes
Psoriderm® (Dermal)
Bath emulsion, coal tar 40%. Net price 200 ml = £2.44
Additives: polysorbate 20
Use 30 ml in a bath and soak for 5 minutes

Shampoo preparations
Section 13.9
Coal tar and corticosteroid preparations
PoM **Alphosyl HC®** (Stafford-Miller)
Cream, coal tar extract 5%, hydrocortisone 0.5%, allantoin 2%, in a vanishing-cream basis. Net price 30 g = £1.70; 45 g = £2.41. Potency IV
Additives: information not disclosed for BNF
Apply sparingly 2–4 times daily

PoM **Carbo-Cort**® (Lagap)
Cream, coal tar solution 3%, hydrocortisone 0.25%, in a water-miscible basis. Price 30 g = £2.71. Potency IV
Additives: beeswax, hydroxybenzoates (parabens)
Apply sparingly 2–3 times daily

PoM **Tarcortin**® (Stafford-Miller)
Cream, coal tar extract 5%, hydrocortisone 0.5%, in a vanishing-cream basis. Net price 30 g = £1.21; 45 g = £1.55. Potency IV
Additives: information not disclosed for BNF
Apply sparingly 2–4 times daily

BUFEXAMAC

Indications: mild inflammatory skin disorders
Side-effects: skin irritation
Administration: apply sparingly 2–3 times daily

PoM **Parfenac**® (Lederle)
Cream, bufexamac 5%, in a water-miscible basis. Do not dilute. Net price 30 g = £2.16
Additives: hydroxybenzoates (parabens)

DITHRANOL

Indications: subacute and chronic psoriasis, see notes above
Cautions: avoid use near eyes
Contra-indications: hypersensitivity; acute psoriasis
Side-effects: local burning sensation and irritation; stains skin, hair, and fabrics
Administration: see notes above

****Dithranol Ointment**, dithranol, in yellow soft paraffin; usual strengths 0.1–2%. Part of basis may be replaced by hard paraffin if a stiffer preparation is required. Net price 25 g = 11p. Label: 28
*PoM if dithranol content more than 1%, otherwise P
Dithranol Paste, dithranol in zinc and salicylic acid (Lassar's) paste. Usual strengths 0.1% ('weak dithranol paste') and 1% ('strong dithranol paste') of dithranol. Net price 0.1%, 25 g = 18p; 1%, 25 g = 42p. Label: 28

PoM **Anthranol 0.4**® (Stiefel)
Ointment, dithranol 0.4%. Net price 50 g = £3.50. Label: 28. For application to skin or scalp
Additives: none as listed in section 13.1; contains salicylic acid 0.4% as an antioxidant

PoM **Anthranol 1.0**® (Stiefel)
Ointment, dithranol 1%. Net price 50 g = £4.25. Label: 28. For short contact application to skin or scalp
Additives: none as listed in section 13.1; contains salicylic acid 0.5% as an antioxidant

PoM **Anthranol 2.0**® (Stiefel)
Ointment, dithranol 2%. Net price 50 g = £6.00. Label: 28. For short contact application to skin or scalp
Additives: none as listed in section 13.1; contains salicylic acid 0.5% as an antioxidant

Antraderm Mild® (Brocades)
Application, dithranol 0.5% in a wax stick. Net price 20 ml = £5.48. Label: 28. For sensitive skins
Additives: beeswax, butylated hydroxytoluene

PoM **Antraderm**® (Brocades)
Application, dithranol 1% in a wax stick. Net price 20 ml = £6.13. Label: 28
Additives: beeswax, butylated hydroxytoluene

PoM **Antraderm Forte**® (Brocades)
Application, dithranol 2% in a wax stick. Net price 20 ml = £6.78. Label: 28
Additives: beeswax, butylated hydroxytoluene

Dithrocream® (Dermal)
Cream, dithranol in a water-miscible basis, 0.1%, net price 50 g = £3.13; 0.25%, 50 g = £3.37; 0.5% (Forte), 50 g = £3.78; 1% (HP), 50 g = £4.38; 2%, 50 g = £6.25. Label: 28. For application to skin or scalp
Additives: chlorocresol

Dithrolan® (Dermal)
Ointment, dithranol 0.5%, salicylic acid 0.5%. Diluent yellow soft paraffin, life of diluted ointment 14 days. Net price 90 g = £4.52. Label: 28
Additives: none as listed in section 13.1

Psoradrate® (Norwich Eaton)
Cream, dithranol in a powder-in-cream basis containing urea. 0.1%, net price 30 g = £2.54, 100 g = £7.59; 0.2%, 30 g = £2.81, 100 g = £8.72; 0.4%, 100 g = £10.03. Label: 28
Additives: polysorbate 40

Psorin® (Thames)
Ointment, dithranol 0.11%, crude coal tar 1%, salicylic acid 1.6%, in an emollient basis. Net price 25 g = £2.79; 50 g = £5.30; 100 g = £10.50. Label: 28
Additives: beeswax, wool fat

DITHRANOL TRIACETATE

Indications; Cautions; Contra-indications; Side-effects; Administration: see under Dithranol and notes above

Exolan® (Dermal)
Cream, dithranol triacetate 1% in a water-miscible basis. Net price 50 g = £2.76. Label: 28
Additives: chlorocresol
Apply daily to skin and scalp

ETRETINATE

Indications: severe extensive psoriasis resistant to other forms of therapy; palmo-plantar pustular psoriasis; severe congenital ichthyosis; severe Darier's disease (keratosis follicularis)
Cautions: monitor hepatic function and plasma lipids (especially in hypertriglyceridaemia) at start, 1 month after initiating treatment, and then at intervals of 3 months; exclude pregnancy before starting; patients should avoid pregnancy at least 1 month before, during, and for at least 1 year after treatment, should avoid concomitant high doses of vitamin A, and should not donate blood during or for 1 year after stopping therapy (teratogenic risk); investigate atypical musculoskeletal symptoms and avoid long-term use in children (skeletal hyperostosis and extra-osseous calcification)
Contra-indications: hepatic and renal impairment; pregnancy and breast-feeding
Side-effects: (mainly dose-related) dryness of mucous membranes (sometimes erosion), of skin (sometimes scaling, thinning, erythema,

and pruritus), and of conjunctiva (sometimes conjunctivitis); palmar and plantar exfoliation, epistaxis, and epidermal fragility reported, also paronychia; reversible alopecia; myalgia and arthralgia; occasional nausea, headache, malaise, drowsiness and sweating; benign intracranial hypertension reported; raised liver enzymes, rarely jaundice and hepatitis; raised triglycerides

Dose: administered in accordance with expert advice, adults and children, initially up to 750 micrograms/kg daily in divided doses for 2–4 weeks, increased to 1 mg/kg daily if necessary (max. daily dose 75 mg), then reduced to 500 micrograms/kg daily for a further 6–8 weeks, then intermittently as necessary; usual maintenance dose 250–500 micrograms/kg daily (see also notes above)

▼ PoM **Tigason**® (Roche)
Capsules, etretinate 10 mg (yellow), net price 20 = £6.94; 25 mg (orange/yellow), 20 = £14.98 (hosp. only). Label: 10, patient information card, 21

ICHTHAMMOL

Indications: chronic eczema
Side-effects: skin irritation and sensitisation
Administration: apply 1–3 times daily

Ichthammol Ointment, ichthammol 10%, yellow soft paraffin 45%, wool fat 45%. Net price 25 g = 17p
Zinc and Ichthammol Cream, ichthammol 5%, cetostearyl alcohol 3%, wool fat 10%, in zinc cream. Net price 100 g = 48p
Zinc Paste and Ichthammol Bandage (Ichthopaste®, Icthaband®), see section 13.13.1

SALICYLIC ACID

Indications: hyperkeratoses
Cautions: see notes above; avoid broken or inflamed skin
Side-effects: sensitivity, excessive drying, irritation, systemic effects after prolonged use (see section 10.1.1)

Salicylic Acid Collodion —section 13.7
Salicylic Acid Ointment, salicylic acid 2%, in wool alcohols ointment. Net price 25 g = 18p
Apply twice daily
Zinc and Salicylic Acid Paste (Lassar's Paste), zinc oxide 24%, salicylic acid 2%, starch 24%, white soft paraffin 50%. Net price 25 g = 15p
Apply twice daily
Keralyt® (Bristol-Myers)
Gel, salicylic acid 6%. Net price 55 g = £2.44
  Additives: propylene glycol
Apply to hydrated skin, cover with an occlusive dressing, preferably overnight, and remove by washing; wash hands thoroughly after use

---

13.6   Preparations for acne

TOPICAL TREATMENT. Most topical preparations are intended for removing follicular plugs and reducing skin flora. The skin is cleansed regularly with detergent solutions, for example cetrimide solution (section 13.11). Abrasive agents may also be used but their effectiveness is uncertain.

Cleansing is followed by application of **antiseptics** and **keratolytics**. Preparations usually contain benzoyl peroxide, potassium hydroxyquinoline sulphate, sulphur, salicylic acid, or tretinoin. Many of these irritate the skin but it is doubtful if a therapeutic effect can be obtained without some degree of irritation, which subsides with continued treatment. Topical application of **tretinoin** (Retin-A®) has been shown to be useful in treating acne but patients should be warned that some redness and skin peeling may occur after application for several days. Tretinoin is a vitamin A derivative.

Thick greasy preparations are generally **contraindicated** in acne. Topical antimicrobials are also used but their value is uncertain and they may cause sensitisation, particularly with neomycin. They may also cause resistant strains to appear in the skin flora. Preparations containing resorcinol should be avoided as prolonged application may interfere with thyroid function.

Topical **corticosteroids** should **not** be used in acne.

SYSTEMIC TREATMENT. Systemic antibacterial treatment is useful. **Tetracycline** (see section 5.1.3), **erythromycin** (see section 5.1.5), and occasionally other antibacterials are used. The usual dosage regimen for tetracycline and erythromycin, taken before meals, is 250 mg 3 times daily for 1–4 weeks and then reduced to twice daily until improvement occurs. Maximum improvement usually occurs after three or four months but in resistant cases treatment may need to be continued for two or more years. As there have been some reports of pseudomembranous colitis with tetracycline, caution is necessary in long-term administration.

Cyproterone acetate with **ethinyloestradiol** (Dianette®) contains an anti-androgen and is used to treat women with severe acne refractory to prolonged oral antibacterial therapy. Improvement of acne probably occurs because of decreased sebum secretion which is under androgen control. Some women with mild to moderate idiopathic hirsutism may also benefit as hair growth is also androgen-dependent (see also section 6.4.2). Dianette® may also be used as an oral contraceptive but should be reserved for women who are being treated for androgen-dependent skin conditions. It is contra-indicated in pregnancy and in patients with a predisposition to thrombosis.

Isotretinoin (Roaccutane®) has recently been introduced for the systemic treatment of severe cystic and conglobate acne. It should only be given after the usual treatments have proved ineffective and then only under the guidance of experts familiar with its actions and side-effects. It is given in doses of 500 micrograms/kg/day for 12–16 weeks but doses may be adjusted if necessary after 4 weeks. Repeat courses should not normally be given. An exacerbation is common some 2–4 weeks after starting treatment but usually subsides after a few weeks.

Side-effects include dry lips, sore eyes, nose bleeds, mild transient hair loss, and joint pains. Plasma lipids and liver function should be checked by investigation monthly as there is a tendency for the plasma lipids to rise in some patients. The drug is teratogenic and must **not** be given to women who are pregnant or those who may become pregnant unless there is concomitant effective contraception and then only after detailed explanation by the physician. The contraceptive measures must continue for at least one month after ceasing treatment with the drug.

TOPICAL ACNE PREPARATIONS

ABRASIVE AGENTS
Indications: cleansing in acne vulgaris
Cautions: avoid contact with eyes; discontinue use temporarily if skin becomes irritated
Contra-indications: superficial venules, telangiectasia

Brasivol® (Stiefel)
Paste No. 1, aluminium oxide 38.09% in fine particles, in a soap-detergent basis. Net price 70 g = £2.49
Additives: fragrance
Paste No. 2, aluminium oxide 52.2% in medium particles, in a soap-detergent basis. Net price 85 g = £2.49
Additives: fragrance
Paste No. 3, aluminium oxide 65.2% in coarse particles, in a soap-detergent basis. Net price 100 g = £2.49
Additives: fragrance
Use instead of soap 1–3 times daily, starting with fine grade and progressing to coarser grades if required

Ionax Scrub® (Alcon)
Gel, polyethylene granules 21.9%, benzalkonium chloride 0.25% in a foaming aqueous alcoholic basis. Net price 60 g = £1.19. ACBS: for control and hygiene of acne and cleansing of the skin prior to acne treatment
Additives: propylene glycol
Use instead of soap 1–2 times daily

ANTIBIOTICS
Indications: acne vulgaris

▼ PoM **Dalacin T**® (Upjohn)
Topical solution, clindamycin (as phosphate) 1%, in an aqueous alcoholic basis. Net price 30 ml (with applicator) = £5.50
Additives: propylene glycol
Apply to clean skin twice daily for up to 12 weeks

▼ PoM **Topicycline**® (Norwich Eaton)
Solution, powder for reconstitution, tetracycline hydrochloride, 4-epitetracycline hydrochloride, providing tetracycline hydrochloride 2.2 mg/ml when reconstituted with solvent containing n-decyl methyl sulphoxide and citric acid in 40% alcohol. Net price (with solvent) = £7.90
Additives: none as listed in section 13.1
Apply to clean skin twice daily

BENZOYL PEROXIDE
Indications: acne vulgaris
Cautions: avoid contact with eyes, mouth, and mucous membranes; may bleach fabrics
Contra-indications: acne rosacea
Side-effects: skin irritation
Administration: apply 1–2 times daily to clean skin, starting treatment with lower-strength preparations

Acetoxyl 2.5® (Stiefel)
Gel, benzoyl peroxide 2.5%, in an aqueous-acetone-gel basis. Net price 40 g = £1.59
Additives: propylene glycol

Acetoxyl 5® (Stiefel)
Gel, benzoyl peroxide 5%, in an aqueous-acetone-gel basis. Net price 40 g = £1.76
Additives: propylene glycol

Acnegel® (Kirby-Warrick)
Gel, benzoyl peroxide 5%, in an aqueous alcoholic basis. Net price 50 g = £2.17
Additives: none as listed in section 13.1
Forte gel, benzoyl peroxide 10%, in an aqueous alcoholic basis. Net price 50 g = £2.38
Additives: none as listed in section 13.1

Acnidazil® (Janssen)
Cream, benzoyl peroxide 5%, miconazole nitrate 2%. Net price 15 g = £1.74; 20 g = £2.31
Additives: polysorbate 20, propylene glycol

Benoxyl 5® (Stiefel)
Cream, benzoyl peroxide 5%, in a non-greasy basis. Net price 40 g = £1.29
Additives: isopropyl palmitate, propylene glycol
Lotion, benzoyl peroxide 5%, in a non-greasy basis. Net price 30 ml = £1.03
Additives: isopropyl palmitate, propylene glycol

Benoxyl 5 with Sulphur® (Stiefel)
Cream, benzoyl peroxide 5%, sulphur 2%, in a water-miscible basis. Net price 40 g = £1.39
Additives: isopropyl palmitate, propylene glycol
Apply once daily. Use if tolerance develops to Benoxyl 5® but before progressing to Benoxyl 10®

Benoxyl 10® (Stiefel)
Lotion, benzoyl peroxide 10%, in a water-miscible basis. Net price 30 ml = £1.09
Additives: isopropyl palmitate, propylene glycol

Benoxyl 10 with Sulphur® (Stiefel)
Cream, benzoyl peroxide 10%, sulphur 5%, in a water-miscible basis. Net price 40 g = £1.49
Additives: isopropyl palmitate, propylene glycol

Benzagel 5® (Bioglan)
Gel, benzoyl peroxide 5%. Net price 40 g = £1.89
Additives: fragrance

Benzagel 10® (Bioglan)
Gel, benzoyl peroxide 10%. Net price 40 g = £2.05
Additives: fragrance

Nericur® (Schering)
Gel 5, benzoyl peroxide 5%, in an aqueous gel basis. Net price 30 g = £1.45
Additives: propylene glycol
Gel 10, benzoyl peroxide 10%, in an aqueous gel basis. Net price 30 g = £1.60
Additives: propylene glycol

Panoxyl 2.5® (Stiefel)
Aquagel (= aqueous gel), benzoyl peroxide 2.5%. Net price 40 g = £1.72
Additives: propylene glycol

Panoxyl 5® (Stiefel)

Gel, benzoyl peroxide 5%, in an aqueous alcoholic basis. Net price 40 g = £1.44
Additives: fragrance

Aquagel (= aqueous gel), benzoyl peroxide 5%. Net price 40 g = £1.92
Additives: propylene glycol

Panoxyl 10® (Stiefel)

Gel, benzoyl peroxide 10%, in an aqueous alcoholic basis. Net price 40 g = £1.63
Additives: fragrance

Aquagel (= aqueous gel), benzoyl peroxide 10%. Net price 40 g = £2.12
Additives: propylene glycol

Wash, benzoyl peroxide 10%, in a detergent basis. Net price 150 ml = £3.50
Additives: none as listed in section 13.1

Quinoderm® (Quinoderm Ltd)

Cream, benzoyl peroxide 10%, potassium hydroxyquinoline sulphate 0.5%, in an astringent vanishing-cream basis. Net price 25 g = 94p; 50 g = £1.56
Additives: edetic acid (EDTA)

Cream 5, benzoyl peroxide 5%, potassium hydroxyquinoline sulphate 0.5%, in an astringent vanishing-cream basis. Net price 50 g = £1.41
Additives: edetic acid (EDTA)

Lotio-gel 5%, benzoyl peroxide 5%, potassium hydroxyquinoline sulphate 0.5%, in an astringent creamy basis. Net price 30 ml = £1.22
Additives: edetic acid (EDTA)

Lotio-gel 10%, benzoyl peroxide 10%, potassium hydroxyquinoline sulphate 0.5%, in an astringent creamy basis. Net price 30 ml = £1.31
Additives: edetic acid (EDTA)

Apply 1–3 times daily

Theraderm 5® (Bristol-Myers)

Gel, benzoyl peroxide 5% in a water-miscible basis. Net price 56 g = £2.02
Additives: disodium edetate

Theraderm 10® (Bristol-Myers)

Gel, benzoyl peroxide 10% in a water-miscible basis. Net price 56 g = £2.11
Additives: disodium edetate

SULPHUR

Indications: acne vulgaris

Cautions: avoid contact with eyes, mouth, and mucous membranes

Side-effects: skin irritation

Administration: apply to clean skin 1–2 times daily

Resorcinol and Sulphur Paste, resorcinol 5%, precipitated sulphur 5%, emulsifying ointment 50%, zinc oxide 40%. Net price 25 g = 11p

Salicylic Acid and Sulphur Cream, salicylic acid 2%, precipitated sulphur 2%, in aqueous cream. Net price 50 g = 18p

Salicylic Acid and Sulphur Ointment, salicylic acid 3%, precipitated sulphur 3%, in hydrous ointment (oily cream). Net price 25 g = 21p

Sulphur Lotion, Compound, precipitated sulphur 4% (see Formulary). Net price 100 ml = 18p

Sulphur Ointment, precipitated sulphur 10%, in simple ointment. Net price 25 g = 9p

Dome-Acne® (Lagap)

Cream, resorcinol monoacetate 3%, colloidal sulphur 4%, in a non-greasy basis. Net price 30 g = £1.53
Additives: propylene glycol

Lotion, ingredients as for cream. Net price 50 ml = £1.92
Additives: polysorbate, propylene glycol

Eskamel® (SK&F)

Cream, resorcinol 2%, sulphur 8%, in a non-greasy flesh-coloured basis. Net price 25 g = 60p
Additives: propylene glycol, fragrance

TRETINOIN

Indications: acne vulgaris

Cautions: avoid contact with eyes, mouth, and mucous membranes; do not use simultaneously with other peeling agents (can be alternated every 12 hours with benzoyl peroxide); do not use with ultra-violet lamps

Contra-indications: eczema, broken skin

Side-effects: irritation, erythema, peeling, with excressive use; changes in pigmentation, photosensitivity

Administration: apply to clean skin 1–2 times daily

PoM **Retin-A**® (Ortho-Cilag)

Cream, tretinoin 0.025%, net price 60 g = £5.65; 0.05%, 60 g = £5.65. For dry or fair skin
Additives: butylated hydroxytoluene, sorbic acid

Gel, tretinoin 0.025%. Net price 60 g = £5.65. For severe acne, initial treatment, or dark and oily skins
Additives: butylated hydroxytoluene

Lotion, tretinoin 0.025%. Net price 80 ml = £5.65. For application to large areas such as the back
Additives: butylated hydroxytoluene

CORTICOSTEROIDS

Indications: see notes above

Cautions; Contra-indications; Side-effects: section 13.4 and notes above

Administration: apply to clean skin 1–2 times daily but see notes above

PoM **Actinac**® (Roussel)

Lotion (powder for reconstitution), chloramphenicol 1.25%, hydrocortisone acetate 1.25%, allantoin 0.75%, butoxyethyl nicotinate 0.75%, precipitated sulphur 10%, when reconstituted with solvent. Discard after 21 days. Net price 2 × 5-g bottles powder with 2 × 16-ml bottles solvent = £7.27. Potency IV
Additives: fragrance

PoM **Medrone**® (Upjohn)

Acne lotion, methylprednisolone acetate 0.25%, aluminium chlorhydroxide complex 10%, sulphur (colloidal) 5%. Net price 25 ml = £2.26; 75 ml = £6.07. Potency IV
Additives: information not disclosed for BNF

PoM **Neo-Medrone**® (Upjohn)

Acne lotion, methylprednisolone acetate 0.25%, neomycin sulphate 0.25%, aluminium chlorhydroxide complex 10%, sulphur 5%. Net price 50 ml = £4.80; 75 ml = £6.43. Potency IV
Additives: information not disclosed for BNF

PoM **Quinoderm with Hydrocortisone**® (Quinoderm Ltd)

Cream, hydrocortisone 1%, benzoyl peroxide 10%, potassium hydroxyquinoline sulphate 0.5%, in an astringent vanishing-cream basis. Net price 30 g = £1.61. Potency IV
Additives: edetic acid (EDTA)

ORAL PREPARATIONS

CYPROTERONE ACETATE

Indications: see notes above
Cautions; Contra-indications; Side-effects: see under Combined Oral Contraceptives (section 7.3.1)

▼ PoM **Dianette**® (Schering)
Tablets, beige, s/c, cyproterone acetate 2 mg, ethinyloestradiol 35 micrograms. Net price 21-tab pack = £4.40
Dose: 1 tablet daily for 21 days starting on 5th day of menstrual cycle and repeated after a 7-day interval, usually for several months

ISOTRETINOIN

Indications; Cautions; Side-effects: see notes above
Contra-indications: pregnancy; renal or hepatic impairment
Dose: 500 micrograms/kg daily after food for the first 4 weeks, adjusted if necessary to 100–200 micrograms/kg daily (sensitive patients), or 1 mg/kg daily (unresponsive patients) for a further 8–12 weeks

▼ PoM **Roaccutane**® (Roche)
Capsules, isotretinoin 5 mg (red/white), net price 20 = £6.81; 20 mg (red-violet/white), 20 = £19.64 (Hosp. only). Label: 10, patient information card, 21

13.7 Preparations for warts and calluses

The least destructive method possible should be chosen to treat these lesions as they are self-limiting and all viral warts including those on the soles of the feet (verrucas) eventually disappear spontaneously. The preparations used are keratolytics which slowly remove the hyperkeratotic layers and destroy the underlying epidermis. Salicylic acid and podophyllin preparations are useful but can cause considerable irritation of the treated area, and podophyllin treatment may be painful. **Salicylic acid** collodion and proprietary preparations are suitable for removal of warts and calluses.

Podophyllin preparations may also be useful. Podophyllum resin made into a paint, in concentrations of between 5 and 20% is employed for the treatment of anogenital warts. The paint should be allowed to stay on the treated area for not longer than 6 hours and then washed off. Care should be taken to avoid splashing the surrounding skin during application; it must be covered with soft paraffin as a protection. Where there are a large number of warts only a few should be treated at any one time as severe toxicity caused by absorption of podophyllin has been reported. It should also be avoided in pregnancy. **Posalfilin**® is suitable for treating plantar warts.

Preparations containing formaldehyde, glutaraldehyde, and bromine are also available but their effects are unpredictable. Formaldehyde preparations may irritate and sensitise the skin.

Ointments and liquid preparations are applied to the wart or callus, avoiding contact with surrounding skin, and covered with a plaster. Dead skin may be removed at intervals by rubbing with a pumice stone.

SALICYLIC ACID

Indications: removal of warts and hard skin
Cautions: avoid normal skin and application to large areas; application to the face and anogenital region is contra-indicated for most salicylic acid preparations

Salicylic Acid Adhesive Plaster 20% or 40%. Net price 10 plasters 75 mm × 45 mm = £1.40 (20%); £1.70 (40%)
Salicylic Acid Collodion, salicylic acid 12%, in flexible collodion. Net price 5 ml = 5p. Label: 15
Apply daily or on alternate days
Cuplex® (S&N Pharm.)
Gel, salicylic acid 11%, lactic acid 4%, copper acetate (= Cu^{2+} 0.0011%), in a collodion basis. Net price 5 g = £2.01. For plantar and mosaic warts, corns, and calluses
Additives: information not disclosed for BNF
Apply twice daily
Duofilm® (Stiefel)
Paint, salicylic acid 16.7%, lactic acid 16.7%, in flexible collodion. Net price 15 ml (with applicator) = £1.95. For plantar and mosaic warts
Additives: none as listed in section 13.1
Apply daily
Salactol® (Dermal)
Paint, salicylic acid 16.7%, lactic acid 16.7%, in flexible collodion. Net price 10 ml (with applicator) = £1.61. For warts, particularly plantar warts
Additives: none as listed in section 13.1
Apply daily
Verrugon® (Pickles)
Ointment, salicylic acid 50% in a paraffin basis. Net price 6 g = 94p
Additives: wool fat derivative
Apply daily

BROMINE COMPLEXES

Indications: warts, particularly plantar warts
Cautions: avoid normal skin

Callusolve® (Dermal)
Paint, benzalkonium chloride-bromine adduct 25%. Net price 10 ml (with applicator) = £1.96. For warts, particularly plantar and mosaic warts
Additives: none as listed in section 13.1
Apply daily

FORMALDEHYDE

Indications: warts, particularly plantar warts
Cautions: avoid normal skin

Veracur® (Typharm)
Gel, formaldehyde solution 1.5% in a water-miscible gel basis. Net price 15 g = 90p
Additives: none as listed in section 13.1
Apply twice daily

GLUTARALDEHYDE

Indications: warts, particularly plantar warts
Cautions: avoid normal skin; stains skin brown

Glutarol® (Dermal)
Solution (= application), glutaraldehyde 10%. Net price 10 ml (with applicator) = £1.85
Additives: none as listed in section 13.1
Apply twice daily

Verucasep® (Galen)
Gel, glutaraldehyde 10%. Net price 15 g = £1.86
Additives: none as listed in section 13.1
Apply twice daily

PODOPHYLLUM RESIN

Indications: anogenital and plantar warts
Cautions: avoid normal skin
Contra-indications: pregnancy; facial warts
Side-effects: may cause pain on application
Administration: see notes above

PoM **Podophyllin Paint, Compound,** podophyllum resin 15% (see Formulary). Net price 25 ml = 66p. Label: 15, counselling advised, application, see notes above. For warts, including anogenital warts
Apply daily to plantar warts, weekly to anogenital warts

PoM **Posalfilin®** (Norgine)
Ointment, podophyllum resin 20%, salicylic acid 25%. Net price 10 g = £2.38. For plantar warts
Additives: wool fat
Apply 2–3 times weekly

13.8 Sunscreens and camouflaging preparations

13.8.1 Sunscreening preparations
13.8.2 Camouflaging preparations

13.8.1 Sunscreening preparations

Ultraviolet radiation may be harmful in certain diseases, for example lupus erythematosus, photosensitive dermatitis, and rosacea. Protection may also be required in patients who have developed signs of chronic solar damage in the skin. Certain individuals are naturally sensitive to the sun's rays, while others are sensitised by systemic drugs, for example, demeclocycline, chlorpromazine, and nalidixic acid.

There are two types of preparation which protect the skin from ultraviolet radiation. One type merely places an opaque, reflectant barrier between the sun's rays and the skin; an example is titanium dioxide paste (section 13.2.1). This is thick and greasy and not very acceptable to the patient. The second type listed below is more useful. It contains substances that absorb the erythema-producing portions of the ultraviolet spectrum, for example **aminobenzoic acid** and **padimate O** (Spectraban®).

For maximum benefit these preparations must be applied frequently. Because they filter out only a proportion of harmful rays, burning may still occur in intense sunlight and patients with light-sensitive skin should spend as little time as possible exposed to sunlight. The sun protection factor (SPF, usually indicated in the preparation title) provides some guidance on the degree of protection offered. This indicates the multiples of protection against burning provided, compared to unprotected skin; for example, an SPF of 8 should enable a patient to remain 8 times longer in the sun without burning. Unfortunately no preparation of this type exists which completely blocks the range of sunlight responsible for some photosensitive reactions, particularly the porphyrias and drug-induced photosensitivity, although the reflectant sunscreens do give moderate protection.

Some of the sunscreens, particularly aminobenzoates, may rarely cause photosensitivity reactions. Sunscreen preparations containing bergamot oil (which contains 5-methoxypsoralen) occasionally cause photosensitisation with subsequent pigmentation; these are suspected of increasing the incidence of skin cancers, but this is not established.

BORDERLINE SUBSTANCES. The preparations marked 'ACBS' are regarded as drugs when prescribed for skin protection against ultraviolet radiation in photodermatoses, including those resulting from radiotherapy. Prescriptions issued in accordance with this advice and endorsed 'ACBS' will normally not be investigated. See Appendix 3 for listing by clinical condition.

Aminobenzoic Acid Lotion, aminobenzoic acid 5 g, glycerol 20 ml, industrial methylated spirit 60 ml, purified water, freshly boiled and cooled, to 100 ml
Apply undiluted and allow to dry before exposure; repeat every 2 hours if necessary
Caution: stains clothing

Coppertone Supershade 15® (Scholl)
Lotion, padimate-O 7%, oxybenzone 3%. Net price 125 ml = £4.95. ACBS
Additives: benzyl alcohol, wool fat, fragrance

Coppertone Ultrashade 23® (Scholl)
Lotion, ethylhexyl *p*-methoxycinnamate 7.5%, oxybenzone 3%, padimate-O 2.5%. Net price 150 ml = £5.95. ACBS
Additives: benzyl alcohol, disodium edetate, hydroxybenzoate (parabens), wool fat, fragrance

Piz Buin® (Colson & Kay)
NHS *Creme No. 6*, 2-ethylhexyl *p*-methoxycinnamate 4.1%, oxybenzone 1.3%. Net price 50 ml = £2.47
Additives: information not disclosed for BNF

NHS *Creme No. 8*, 2-ethylhexyl *p*-methoxycinnamate 4.8%, oxybenzone 1.7%. Net price 50 ml = £2.47
Additives: information not disclosed for BNF

Creme No. 12, 2-ethylhexyl *p*-methoxycinnamate 4.8%, oxybenzone 2.2%, zinc oxide 4.5%, talc 4.5%. Net price 30 ml = £2.44. ACBS
Additives: information not disclosed for BNF

NHS *Lipstick*, factor 8, 2-ethylhexyl *p*-methoxycinnamate 4.8%, oxybenzone 1.7%. Net price 5-g stick = £1.22
Additives: information not disclosed for BNF

RoC Total Sunblock® (RoC)
Cream 15 A + B, colourless or tinted, ethylhexyl *p*-methoxycinnamate 7%, zinc oxide. Net price 50 ml = £3.05.
Additives: beeswax, hydroxybenzoates (parabens)

Apply every 2 hours or more frequently

Spectraban® (Stiefel)
4 Lotion, padimate-O 3.2%, in an alcoholic basis. Net price 150 ml = £2.24. ACBS
Additives: fragrance

15 Lotion, aminobenzoic acid 5%, padimate-O 3.2%, in an alcoholic basis. Net price 150 ml = £2.49. ACBS
Additives: fragrance

Apply once daily; renew after bathing or excessive sweating

Caution: flammable; stains clothing

13.8.2 Camouflaging preparations

Disfigurement of the skin can be very distressing to patients and have a marked psychological effect. In skilled hands, or with experience, these preparations can be very effective in concealing scars, areas of discoloration, and birthmarks.

BORDERLINE SUBSTANCES. The preparations marked 'ACBS' are regarded as drugs when prescribed for postoperative scars and other deformities and as adjunctive therapy in the relief of emotional disturbances due to mutilating skin disease. Prescriptions issued in accordance with this advice and endorsed 'ACBS' will normally not be investigated. See Appendix 3 for listing by clinical condition.

Boots Covering Cream® (Boots)
Cream (4 shades). 20 g. ACBS
Additives: hydroxybenzoates (parabens)

Covermark® (Stiefel)
Additives: beeswax, hydroxybenzoates (parabens), fragrance
Cream rouge (3 shades). Net price 4.5 g = £2.96. ACBS
Spotstick—discontinued
Grey toner (= cream). Net price 8 g = £2.96. ACBS
Masking cream (covering cream, 10 shades). Net price 25 g = £4.35. ACBS
Shading cream. Net price 4.5 g = £2.96. ACBS
Finishing powder. Net price 50 g = £2.62; 250 g = £9.37. ACBS

Dermacolor® (Fox)
Camouflage creme, 30 shades. Net price 30 g = £5.33. ACBS
Additives: information not disclosed for BNF
Fixing powder, 5 shades. Net price 75 g = £4.23. ACBS
Additives: information not disclosed for BNF

Keromask® (Innoxa)
Masking cream, 2 shades. Net price 15 ml = £1.75. ACBS
Additives: butylated hydroxyanisole, hydroxybenzoates (parabens), wool fat
Finishing powder. Net price 25 g = £1.88. ACBS
Additives: none as listed in section 13.1

Veil® (Blake)
Cover cream, 16 shades. Net price 19 g = £2.03; 44 g = £2.90; 70 g = £4.06. ACBS
Additives: hydroxybenzoates (parabens), wool fat derivative

13.9 Scalp preparations

SHAMPOOS. Dandruff (*pityriasis capitis*) is excessive non-inflammatory scaling of the scalp, and often increases at puberty. The treatment of choice is the frequent use of a mild detergent shampoo generally once or twice weekly; this will rid the scalp of scale but should not be expected to have a therapeutic effect in itself. Shampoos containing antimicrobial agents such as **pyrithione zinc** have beneficial effects but are not prescribable in the general medical service. Shampoos containing **tar** extracts, for example Polytar®, may be useful and they are also used in psoriasis, both as adjunctive treatment and for the removal of pastes etc. Shampoos containing **selenium sulphide** are of no more value than the other shampoos and should not be used within 48 hours of applying hair colouring or permanent waving preparations.

APPLICATIONS. When shampoos are insufficient, preparations such as **salicylic acid and sulphur cream** (section 13.6) may be useful. For the more severe conditions, weak **corticosteroid** gels and lotions (section 13.4), applied to the scalp may be helpful.

Cradle cap in infants may be treated with **olive oil** or **arachis oil** applications before shampooing.

See also section 13.5 (psoriasis and eczema), section 13.10.4 (lice), and section 13.10.2 (ringworm).

BORDERLINE SUBSTANCES. The preparations marked 'ACBS' are regarded as drugs when prescribed in accordance with the advice of the Advisory Committee on Borderline Substances for the clinical conditions listed. Prescriptions issued in accordance with this advice and endorsed 'ACBS' will normally not be investigated. See Appendix 3 for listing by clinical condition.

Shampoos
  Use once or twice weekly

Cetrimide Solution —section 13.11

Alphosyl® (Stafford-Miller)
Application PC, allantoin 0.2%, refined coal tar extract 5%, in a shampoo basis. Net price 60 g = 48p. ACBS: for psoriasis and other scaly disorders of the scalp
Additives: information not disclosed for BNF

Baltar® (Merck)

Shampoo, coal tar distillate 1.5% in soap-free basis. Net price 225 ml = £2.63; 500 ml = £4.60
Additives: fragrance

Betadine® (Napp)

Scalp and skin cleanser—section 13.11

Shampoo solution, povidone-iodine 4%, in a surfactant solution. Net price 250 ml = £1.58. ACBS: for seborrhoeic scalp conditions associated with excessive dandruff, pruritic scaling, seborrhoeic dermatitis, pityriasis capitis, infected lesions of the scalp, pyodermas (recurrent furunculosis, infective folliculitis, impetigo)
Additives: wool fat, fragrance

Calmurid® (Pharmacia)

Solution, urea 20%, lactic acid 5%, in an aqueous vehicle. Net price 125 ml = £4.10
Additives: polysorbate 20

Apply twice daily to scalp

Capitol® (Dermal)

Gel (= shampoo application), benzalkonium chloride 0.5%. Net price 120 g = £2.29. ACBS: for pityriasis capitis and seborrhoeic dermatitis of the scalp
Additives: none as listed in section 13.1

Ceanel Concentrate® (Quinoderm Ltd)

Shampoo, cetrimide 10%, undecenoic acid 1%, phenethyl alcohol 7.5%. Net price 50 ml = 68p; 150 ml = £2.04; 500 ml = £6.80. ACBS: for psoriasis or seborrhoeic conditions
Additives: fragrance

Cetavlon PC® (Care)

Solution (= shampoo application), cetrimide 17.5%. Net price 125 ml = 53p. ACBS: for seborrhoea capitis and seborrhoeic dermatitis
Additives: information not disclosed for BNF

Clinitar® (S&N Pharm.)

Shampoo solution, coal tar extract 2%. Net price 60 g = £2.24
Additives: information not disclosed for BNF

Gelcotar® (Quinoderm Ltd)

Liquid, strong coal tar solution 1.25%, cade oil 0.5%, in a shampoo basis. Net price 150 ml = 99p; 350 ml = £2.31. ACBS: for psoriasis of the scalp, seborrhoeic dermatitis, and dandruff
Additives: fragrance

Gel, see section 13.5

Genisol® (Fisons)

Liquid (= shampoo application), prepared coal tar 2% (as purified coal tar fractions), sodium sulphosuccinated undecylenic monoalkylolamide 1%. Net price 58 ml = 90p; 250 ml = £2.60; 600 ml = £6.24. ACBS: for psoriasis, eczema, and scaling of the scalp (psoriasis, dandruff, or eczema)
Additives: fragrance

Ionil T® (Alcon)

Shampoo application, benzalkonium chloride 0.2%, coal tar solution 5%, salicylic acid 2% in an alcoholic basis. Net price 240 ml = £1.71. ACBS: for seborrhoeic dermatitis of the scalp
Additives: tetrasodium edetate

Lenium® (Winthrop)

Cream (= shampoo application), selenium sulphide 2.5%. Net price 9 g sachet = 15p; 42 g = 60p; 100 g = £1.15
Additives: fragrance

Polytar® (Stiefel)

Liquid (= shampoo application), arachis oil extract of crude coal tar 0.3%, cade oil 0.3%, coal tar solution 0.1%, oleyl alcohol 1%, tar 0.3%. Net price 65 ml = 40p; 150 ml = 93p; 350 ml = £2.17. ACBS: for psoriasis, eczema, and scaling of the scalp (psoriasis, dandruff, and eczema)
Additives: polysorbate 80, fragrance

Polytar Plus® (Stiefel)

Liquid (= shampoo application), ingredients as above with hydrolysed animal protein 3%. Net price 150 ml = £1.75; 350 ml = £3.29. ACBS: for scalp disorders such as scaling (psoriasis, dandruff, eczema), pruritus, and in the removal of pastes and pomades used in the treatment of psoriasis
Additives: fragrance

Pragmatar—section 13.5

Psoriderm® (Dermal)

Scalp lotion (= shampoo), coal tar 2.5%, lecithin 0.3%. Net price 250 ml = £4.98
Additives: disodium edetate

Selsun® (Abbott)

Shampoo application, selenium sulphide 2.5%. Net price 50 ml = 51p; 100 ml = £1.02; 150 ml = £1.53
Additives: fragrance

Synogist® (Townendale)

Shampoo solution, sodium sulphosuccinated undecylenic monoalkylolamide 2%. Net price 200 ml = £12.98
Additives: hydroxybenzoates (parabens)

T/Gel® (Neutrogena)

Shampoo, coal tar extract 2%. Net price 125 ml = £1.80. ACBS: for psoriasis, eczema, and scaling of the scalp (psoriasis, dandruff, and eczema)
Additives: hydroxybenzoates (parabens), tetrasodium edetate, fragrance

Applications

Apply once or twice daily

Arachis Oil. Net price 50 ml = 23p
Olive Oil. Net price 50 ml = 29p
Salicylic Acid and Sulphur Cream—section 13.6
Salicylic Acid Lotion, salicylic acid 2% (see Formulary). Net price 100 ml = 16p. Label: 15
Caution: highly flammable

13.10 Anti-infective skin preparations

13.10.1 Antibacterial preparations
13.10.2 Antifungal preparations
13.10.3 Antiviral preparations
13.10.4 Parasiticidal preparations
13.10.5 Preparations for minor skin infections

13.10.1 Antibacterial preparations

13.10.1.1 Antibacterial preparations only used topically
13.10.1.2 Antibacterial preparations also used systemically

For many skin infections such as erysipelas and cellulitis systemic antibacterial treatment is the method of choice because the infection is too deeply sited for adequate penetration of topical preparations. For details of suitable treatment see section 5.1, Table 1. Impetigo may be treated by local application with **chlortetracycline** (Aureomycin®) or, if there is systemic toxicity, with oral **flucloxacillin** (see section 5.1, Table 1). Mild antiseptic solutions such as **sodium hypochlorite** or **povidone-iodine** (section 13.11) are used to remove crusts and exudate.

Although there are a great many antibacterial drugs presented in topical preparations they are potentially hazardous and frequently their use is not necessary if adequate hygienic measures can be taken. Moreover not all skin conditions that are oozing, crusted, or characterised by pustules are actually infected.

To minimise the development of resistant organisms it is advisable to limit the choice of drugs applied topically to those not used systemically. Unfortunately some of these drugs, for example neomycin, may cause sensitisation and, if large areas of skin are being treated, ototoxicity may be a hazard, particularly in children and the elderly. Resistant organisms are more common in hospitals, and whenever possible swabs for examination should be taken before beginning treatment.

Mupirocin (Bactroban®) is not related to any other antibiotic in use, and cross resistance with other antibiotics has not been demonstrated. Its antibacterial spectrum is appropriate for skin infections and percutaneous absorption is low, thus making it suitable for topical use.

Mafenide (Sulfamylon®) and **silver sulphadiazine** (Flamazine®) are useful in the treatment of infected burns.

13.10.1.1 ANTIBACTERIAL PREPARATIONS ONLY USED TOPICALLY

COLISTIN SULPHATE
Indications: Gram-negative skin infections
Side-effects: transient irritation

PoM **Colomycin**® (Pharmax)
Powder, sterile, for making topical preparations (usually 1%), colistin sulphate. Net price 1 g vial = £18.60

FRAMYCETIN SULPHATE
Indications; Cautions; Side-effects: see under Neomycin Sulphate
Administration: apply 3 times daily

PoM **Framygen**® (Fisons)
Cream, framycetin sulphate 0.5%, in a water-miscible basis. Net price 15 g = £1.65
Additives: hydroxybenzoates (parabens)

PoM **Soframycin**® (Roussel)
Cream, framycetin sulphate 1.5%, gramicidin 0.005%, in a vanishing-cream basis. Net price 15 g = £1.56
Additives: hydroxybenzoates (parabens)
Ointment, ingredients as for cream, in a wool fat and paraffin basis. Net price 15 g = £1.56
Additives: wool fat
Sterile powder for preparing topical solutions, framycetin sulphate. Net price 500-mg vial = £3.85
Sofra-Tulle *see* Framycetin Sulphate Gauze Dressing, section 13.13.6

MAFENIDE
Indications: skin infections, particularly pseudomonal infection of second- and third-degree burns
Cautions: pulmonary dysfunction
Contra-indications: sensitivity to sulphonamides
Side-effects: allergic reactions including rashes, metabolic acidosis

PoM **Sulfamylon**® (Winthrop)
Cream, mafenide 8.5% (as acetate), in a water-miscible basis. Net price 500 g = £39.19
Additives: disodium edetate, hydroxybenzoates (parabens)
Apply liberally 1–2 times daily with sterile applicator

MUPIROCIN
(Pseudomonic Acid)
Indications: bacterial skin infections
Cautions: see below
Administration: apply up to 3 times daily for up to 10 days

▼ PoM **Bactroban**® (Beecham)
Ointment, mupirocin 2%, in a water-miscible macrogol basis. Net price 15 g = £3.55
Additives: none as listed in section 13.1
Note. Contains macrogol therefore caution in renal impairment; may sting
Nasal ointment, see section 12.2.3

NEOMYCIN SULPHATE
Indications: skin infections
Cautions: see notes above; large open wounds, sensitivity to other aminoglycosides
Side-effects: local hypersensitivity reactions
Administration: apply 3 times daily

Creams and ointments
PoM **Neomycin Cream,** neomycin sulphate 0.5%, cetomacrogol emulsifying ointment 30%, chlorocresol 0.1%, disodium edetate 0.01%, freshly boiled and cooled purified water 69.39%. Net price 15 g = 43p
PoM **Cicatrin**® (Calmic)
Cream, neomycin sulphate 0.5%, bacitracin zinc 250 units/g, cysteine 0.2%, glycine 1%, threonine 0.1%. Net price 15 g = £3.69; 30 g = £6.70
Additives: wool fat derivative
Apply 3 times daily; max. 60 g daily for 3 weeks

PoM **Graneodin**® (Squibb)
Ointment, neomycin sulphate 0.25%, gramicidin
0.025%. Net price 15 g = 88p
Additives: none as listed in section 13.1
Apply 3 times daily

PoM **Myciguent**® (Upjohn)
Ointment, neomycin sulphate 0.5%, in an anhy-
drous greasy basis. Net price 28.4 g = £1.25
Additives: information not disclosed for BNF

Powders and sprays

PoM **Cicatrin**® (Calmic)
Dusting-powder, neomycin sulphate 0.5%, bacitracin zinc 250 units/g, cysteine 0.2%, glycine
1%, threonine 0.1%. Net price 15 g = £3.97;
50 g = £10.04. Max. 50 g daily for 4 weeks
Powder spray, neomycin sulphate 2%, bacitracin
zinc 1250 units/g, cysteine 1.2%, glycine 6%;
pressurised aerosol unit. Net price 3 g = £9.57.
Max. 3 g daily for 12 weeks

PoM **Polybactrin**® (Calmic)
Powder spray, neomycin sulphate 495 000 units,
bacitracin zinc 37 500 units, polymyxin B
sulphate 150 000 units/pressurised aerosol unit.
Net price per unit (115 ml) = £14.52. Max. 1
unit daily for 7 days
Additives: none as listed in section 13.1

PoM **Tribiotic**® (Riker)
Spray application, neomycin sulphate
500 000 units, bacitracin zinc 10 000 units, polymyxin B sulphate 150 000 units/pressurised
aerosol unit. Net price per unit (110 g) = £5.72.
Max. 1 unit daily for 7 days
Additives: information not disclosed for BNF

NITROFURAZONE
Indications: superficial skin infections
Side-effects: local hypersensitivity reactions
Administration: apply 3 or more times daily

PoM **Furacin**® (Norwich Eaton)
Soluble ointment, nitrofurazone 0.2%, in a water-miscible macrogol basis. Net price 25 g =
£1.20
Additives: none as listed in section 13.1
Note. Contains macrogol therefore caution in renal
impairment

POLYMYXIN B SULPHATE
Indications; skin infections
Cautions: see notes above; large open wounds
Side-effects: local hypersensitivity reactions

PoM **Polyfax**® (Calmic)
Ointment, polymyxin B sulphate 10 000 units,
bacitracin zinc 500 units/g, in a paraffin basis.
Net price 20 g = £5.04
Additives: none as listed in section 13.1
Apply 3 times daily

SILVER SULPHADIAZINE
Indications: skin infection, particularly Gram-
negative infections such as pseudomonal infections in second- and third-degree burns,
infected leg ulcers, and pressure sores
Cautions: hepatic and renal impairment

Contra-indications: sensitivity to sulphonamides
Side-effects: rarely allergic reactions including
rashes

PoM **Flamazine**® (S&N Pharm.)
Cream, silver sulphadiazine 1%, in a water-soluble basis. Net price 50 g = £3.65; 250 g =
£9.65; 500 g = £17.10
Additives: information not disclosed for BNF
In burns apply daily with sterile applicator; in
leg ulcers apply at least 3 times a week

13.10.1.2   ANTIBACTERIAL PREPARATIONS ALSO USED SYSTEMICALLY

CHLORTETRACYCLINE HYDROCHLORIDE
Indications: susceptible skin infections; impetigo,
see section 5.1, Table 1
Cautions: see notes above; overgrowth with non-
susceptible organisms may occur; stains
clothing
Side-effects: rarely local hypersensitivity
reactions
Administration: apply 3 times daily

PoM **Aureomycin**® (Lederle)
Cream, chlortetracycline hydrochloride 3% (as
chlortetracycline), in a water-miscible basis.
Net price 30 g = £1.82
Additives: chlorocresol
Ointment, chlortetracycline hydrochloride 3%,
in a greasy basis. Diluent wool fat 10% in white
soft paraffin, life of diluted ointment 14 days.
Net price 30 g = £1.82
Additives: hydroxybenzoates (parabens), wool fat

FUSIDIC ACID
Indications: staphylococcal skin infections and
abscesses
Cautions: see notes above; avoid contact with
eyes
Side-effects: rarely local hypersensitivity
reactions
Administration: apply 3 times daily

PoM **Fucidin**® (Leo)
Cream, fusidic acid 2%. Net price 15 g = £2.67;
30 g = £4.51
Additives: butylated hydroxyanisole, polysorbates, pot-
assium sorbate
Gel, fusidic acid 2%, in a water-miscible basis.
Net price 15 g = £2.54; 30 g = £4.40
Additives: hydroxybenzoates (parabens), polysorbate 80
Caviject gel, fusidic acid 2%, in a single-dose
unit (7 g) fitted with elongated nozzle. For treat-
ment of abscesses. Net price 1 unit = £1.49
Inject once only into curetted abscess and apply
dressing
Ointment, sodium fusidate 2%, in an anhydrous
greasy basis. Net price 15 g = £2.40; 30 g =
£4.07
Additives: wool fat
Fucidin Intertulle *see* Sodium Fusidate Gauze
Dressing Sterile, section 13.13.6

GENTAMICIN

Indications: skin infections
Cautions: see notes above; large open wounds, sensitivity to other aminoglycosides
Administration: apply 3 times daily

PoM **Cidomycin Topical**® (Roussel)
Cream, gentamicin 0.3% (as sulphate), in a water-miscible basis. Do not dilute. Net price 15 g = £1.59; 30 g = £3.09
Additives: hydroxybenzoates (parabens), propylene glycol
Ointment, gentamicin 0.3% (as sulphate), in a paraffin basis. Do not dilute. Net price 15 g = £1.59; 30 g = £3.09
Additives: none as listed in section 13.1

PoM **Genticin**® (Nicholas)
Cream, gentamicin 0.3% (as sulphate), in a water-miscible basis. Net price 15 g = £1.37; 100 g = £9.15
Additives: hydroxybenzoates (parabens)
Ointment, gentamicin 0.3% (as sulphate), in an anhydrous greasy basis. Net price 15 g = £1.37; 100 g = £9.15
Additives: hydroxybenzoates (parabens)

TETRACYCLINE HYDROCHLORIDE

Indications; Cautions; Side-effects: see under Chlortetracycline Hydrochloride

PoM **Achromycin Topical**® (Lederle)
Ointment, tetracycline hydrochloride 3%, in a wool fat and paraffin basis. Net price 30 g = £1.48
Additives: hydroxybenzoates (parabens), wool fat
Apply 3 times daily

13.10.2 Antifungal preparations

Ideally skin scrapings should be examined to confirm diagnosis before treatment is begun. Widespread or intractable fungal infections are treated systemically (see section 5.2). Most localised infections are treated with the topical preparations described below.

Nail ringworm (tinea unguium) and scalp ringworm (*T. capitis*) are best treated systemically (see section 5.2). Most other ringworm infections, including tinea pedis, may be adequately treated with topical preparations. The imidazoles **clotrimazole** (Canesten®), **econazole** (Ecostatin®, Pevaryl®), and **miconazole** (Daktarin®, Dermonistat®) are all effective and commonly used. **Sulconazole** (Exelderm®) is a recently introduced imidazole with similar properties. Combinations of imidazoles and weak corticosteroids may be of use in the treatment of some eczematous disorders and, in the first few days only, of a severely inflamed patch of ringworm. **Compound benzoic acid ointment** (Whitfield's ointment) is also quite effective but cosmetically less acceptable than the proprietary preparations. It is generally used to treat patches of ringworm (tinea) on the trunk, limbs, palms, or soles. The **undecenoates** and **tolnaftate** are less effective in treating ringworm infections.

Candidal skin infections may also be treated by topical application with the broad-spectrum antifungals, clotrimazole, econazole, and miconazole. **Amphotericin** (Fungilin®) and **nystatin** preparations are also equally as effective in candidiasis although they are ineffective against infections due to dermatophyte fungi (tinea).

Lotions are generally chosen for application to large and hairy areas. Ointments are best avoided on moist surfaces because of their occlusive properties. Dusting-powders have no place in the treatment of fungal infections, except for toiletry or cosmetic purposes, as they are therapeutically ineffective and may cause skin irritation.

AMPHOTERICIN

Indications: skin infections due to *Candida* spp.
Administration: apply 2–4 times daily

PoM **Fungilin**® (Squibb)
Cream, amphotericin 3%, in a water-miscible basis. Do not dilute. Net price 15 g = £1.30
Additives: benzyl alcohol, propylene glycol
Ointment, amphotericin 3%, in Plastibase®. Do not dilute. Net price 15 g = £1.30
Additives: none as listed in section 13.1

BENZOIC ACID

Indications: ringworm (tinea)

Benzoic Acid Ointment, Compound (Whitfield's ointment), benzoic acid 6%, salicylic acid 3%, in emulsifying ointment. Net price 25 g = 14p
Apply twice daily

BENZOYL PEROXIDE

Indications: fungal skin infections, particularly tinea pedis

Quinoped® (Quinoderm Ltd)
Cream, benzoyl peroxide 5%, potassium hydroxyquinoline sulphate 0.5%, in an astringent basis. Net price 25 g = 80p.
Additives: edetic acid (EDTA)
Apply twice daily

CLOTRIMAZOLE

Indications: fungal skin infections
Side-effects: occasional skin irritation or sensitivity
Administration: apply 2–3 times daily continuing for 14 days after lesions have healed

Canesten® (Baypharm)
Cream, clotrimazole 1%, in a water-miscible basis. Net price 20 g = £1.82; 50 g = £4.26
Additives: benzyl alcohol, polysorbate 60
Solution, clotrimazole 1% in macrogol 400. Net price 20 ml = £2.38. For hairy areas
Additives: none as listed in section 13.1
Spray, clotrimazole 1%, in 30% isopropyl alcohol. Net price 40-ml atomiser = £5.12. For large or hairy areas
Additives: propylene glycol
Caution: flammable
Dusting-powder, clotrimazole 1%. Net price 30 g = £1.56
Additives: none as listed in section 13.1

ECONAZOLE NITRATE

Indications; Side-effects: see under Clotrimazole
Administration: apply 2–3 times daily continuing for 14 days after lesions have healed; nail infections, apply daily under occlusive dressing

Ecostatin® (Squibb)
Cream, econazole nitrate 1%, in a water-miscible basis. Net price 15 g = £1.49; 30 g = £2.75
Additives: butylated hydroxyanisole, fragrance
Lotion, econazole nitrate 1%. Net price 30 ml = £2.75
Additives: butylated hydroxyanisole, fragrance
Spray solution, econazole nitrate 1% in an alcoholic solution. Net price 150 g = £3.48
Additives: propylene glycol, fragrance
Dusting-powder, econazole nitrate 1% in a talc basis. Net price 30 g = £2.90
Additives: fragrance
Spray-powder, econazole nitrate 1% in a talc basis. Net price 200-g unit = £2.64
Additives: fragrance

Pevaryl® (Ortho-Cilag)
Cream, econazole nitrate 1% in a water-miscible basis. Net price 30 g = £3.33
Additives: butylated hydroxyanisole, fragrance
Lotion, econazole nitrate 1% in a water-miscible basis. Net price 30 ml = £3.33
Additives: butylated hydroxyanisole, fragrance
Spray-powder, econazole nitrate 1%. Net price 200-g pressurised aerosol unit (20 g powder) = £3.33
Additives: fragrance

KETOCONAZOLE

Indications; Side-effects: see under Clotrimazole
Administration: apply 1–2 times daily, continuing for a few days after lesions have healed

▼ PoM **Nizoral**® (Janssen)
Cream, ketoconazole 2% in a water-miscible basis. Net price 15 g = £1.73
Additives: polysorbates, propylene glycol

MICONAZOLE NITRATE

Indications; Side-effects: see under Clotrimazole
Administration: apply twice daily continuing for 10 days after lesions have healed; nail infections, apply daily under occlusive dressing

Daktarin® (Janssen)
Cream, miconazole nitrate 2%, in a water-miscible basis. Net price 30 g = £2.07
Additives: butylated hydroxyanisole
Dusting-powder, miconazole nitrate 2%. Net price 20 g = £1.17
Spray powder, miconazole nitrate 0.16%, in an aerosol basis. Net price 100 g = £1.17
Additives: none as listed in section 13.1
Twin pack, 1 × 30 g pack of cream miconazole nitrate 2%, with 1 × 30 g dusting-powder miconazole nitrate 2%. Net price (complete pack) = £3.80

Dermonistat® (Ortho-Cilag)
Cream, miconazole nitrate 2%, in a water-miscible basis. Net price 30 g = £2.60
Additives: butylated hydroxyanisole

NATAMYCIN

Indications: skin infections due to *Candida* spp.
Administration: apply 2–3 times daily

PoM **Pimafucin**® (Brocades)
Cream, natamycin 2%, in a water-miscible basis. Net price 30 g = £1.75
Additives: hydroxybenzoates (parabens)

NITROPHENOL

Indications: fungal skin infections, particularly tinea

Phortinea® (Philip Harris)
Paint, 4-nitrophenol 2% in an alcoholic basis. Net price 10 ml (with applicator) = 75p
Additives: information not disclosed for BNF
Apply twice daily

NYSTATIN

Indications: skin infections due to *Candida* spp.
Administration: apply 2–4 times daily, continuing for 7 days after lesions have healed

PoM **Multilind**® (Squibb)
Ointment, nystatin 100000 units/g, zinc oxide 20% in an emollient basis. Net price 50 g = £3.45. For superinfection, particularly in napkin rash
Additives: fragrance

PoM **Nystaform**® (Bayer)
Cream, nystatin 100000 units/g, chlorhexidine hydrochloride 1%. Net price 30 g = £2.69
Additives: benzyl alcohol, polysorbate 60
Ointment, nystatin 100000 units/g, chlorhexidine acetate 1%, in a water-repellent basis. Net price 30 g = £2.69
Additives: none as listed in section 13.1

PoM **Nystan**® (Squibb)
Cream, nystatin 100000 units/g, in a water-miscible basis. Net price 15 g = £1.55; 30 g = £2.66
Additives: benzyl alcohol, propylene glycol, fragrance
Gel, nystatin 100000 units/g. Net price 30 g = £2.66
Additives: chlorocresol, fragrance
Ointment, nystatin 100000 units/g, in Plastibase®. Net price 15 g = £1.09; 30 g = £2.14
Additives: none as listed in section 13.1
Dusting-powder, nystatin 100000 units/g. Net price 15 g = £1.09
Additives: none as listed in section 13.1

PoM **Tinaderm-M**® (Kirby-Warrick)
Cream, nystatin 100000 units/g, tolnaftate 1%, in a water-miscible basis. Net price 20 g = £1.83. For *Candida* infections and tinea
Additives: butylated hydroxytoluene, hydroxybenzoates (parabens), fragrance
Apply 2–3 times daily

SALICYLIC ACID

Indications: fungal skin infections, particularly tinea
Side-effects: hypersensitivity reactions

Phytex® (Pharmax)

Paint, salicylic acid 1.46% (total combined), tannic acid 4.89% and boric acid 3.12% (as borotannic complex), in a vehicle containing alcohol and ethyl acetate. Net price 25 ml (with brush) = £1.33. For fungal nail infections (onychomycosis)
Additives: none as listed in section 13.1
Apply twice daily
Caution: flammable; avoid in pregnancy and children under 5 years

Phytocil® (Fisons)

Cream, salicylic acid 1.5%, 2-*p*-chlorophenoxyethanol 1%, menthol 1%, 1-phenoxypropan-2-ol 2%. Net price 25 g = 49p. For tinea pedis, tinea cruris, and tinea circinata
Additives: none as listed in section 13.1
Apply 2–3 times daily

SULCONAZOLE NITRATE

Indications; Side-effects: see under Clotrimazole
Cautions: avoid contact with eyes (lens changes in *animals* after high oral doses)
Administration: apply 1–2 times daily continuing for 2–3 weeks after lesions have healed

▼ PoM **Exelderm®** (ICI)

Cream, sulconazole nitrate 1%, in a water-miscible basis. Net price 30 g = £3.25
Additives: information not disclosed for BNF

TIOCONAZOLE

Indications: fungal nail infections
Side-effects: local irritation, usually during first week of treatment; discontinue if sensitivity reaction develops
Administration: apply to nails and surrounding skin twice daily for up to 6 months (may be extended to 12 months)

▼ PoM **Trosyl®** (Pfizer)

Nail solution, tioconazole 28%. Net price 12 ml (with applicator brush) = £25.00
Additives: none as listed in section 13.1

TOLNAFTATE

Indications: skin infections, particularly tinea pedis
Side-effects: rarely hypersensitivity

Timoped® (R&C)

Cream, tolnaftate 1%, triclosan 0.25%. Net price 30 g = £3.10
Additives: none as listed in section 13.1
Apply twice daily

UNDECENOATES

Indications: skin infections, particularly tinea pedis

Monphytol® (LAB)

Paint, undecenoic acid 5% (as methyl and propyl esters), boric acid 2%, salicylic acid 31% (free and as methyl ester), chlorbutol 3%. Net price 18 ml (with brush) = 89p. For fungal (particularly nail) infections
Additives: fragrance
Apply 4 times daily

Mycota® (Crookes Products)

Cream, zinc undecenoate 20%, undecenoic acid 5%. Net price 25 g = 51p
Additives: fragrance

Dusting-powder, zinc undecenoate 20%, undecenoic acid 2%. Net price 70 g = 87p
Additives: fragrance

Spray application, undecenoic acid 2.5%, dichlorophen 0.25% (pressurised aerosol pack). Net price 110 g = 87p
Additives: none as listed in section 13.1
Apply 1–2 times daily

Phytocil® (Fisons)

Dusting-powder, zinc undecenoate 5.8%, 2-*p*-chlorophenoxyethanol 1%, 1-phenoxypropan-2-ol 2%. Net price 50 g = 68p. For use with cream
Additives: none as listed in section 13.1

Tineafax® (Wellcome)

Ointment, zinc undecenoate 8%, zinc naphthenate solution 8%, in a water-miscible basis. Net price 25 g = 47p
Additives: chlorocresol
Apply 1–2 times daily

Dusting-powder, zinc undecenoate 10%. Net price 50-g puffer pack = 73p
Additives: none as listed in section 13.1

13.10.3 Antiviral preparations

Idoxuridine solution (5% in dimethyl sulphoxide) is used for severe herpetic infections of the skin. Herpes simplex seems to respond well to frequent applications if started early and continued for 3 to 4 days, but may be less successful if delayed after 7 days. Evidence of its value in herpes zoster infections is conflicting.

Acyclovir (Zovirax®) cream is indicated for the treatment of initial and recurrent labial and genital herpes simplex infections; treatment should begin as early as possible. Systemic treatment is necessary for buccal or vaginal infections; herpes zoster (shingles) also requires systemic treatment (see section 5.3).

ACYCLOVIR

Indications: see notes above
Side-effects: transient stinging or burning on application; occasionally erythema or drying of the skin
Application: apply to lesions every 4 hours (5 times daily) for 5 days

▼ PoM **Zovirax®** (Wellcome)

Cream, acyclovir 5% in an aqueous cream basis. Net price 2 g = £5.78; 10 g = £17.42
Additives: propylene glycol
Eye ointment, see section 11.3.1

IDOXURIDINE IN DIMETHYL SULPHOXIDE

Indications: see notes above
Cautions: avoid contact with the eyes, mucous membranes, and textiles; pregnancy, breast-feeding
Side-effects: stinging on application, changes in taste; overuse may cause maceration
Administration: apply 5% solution to lesions 4 times daily for 3–4 days; in severe zoster (shingles) apply 40% solution over affected area daily for 4 days
Note. Not to be used in the mouth

PoM **Herpid**® (Boehringer Ingelheim)
Application, idoxuridine 5% in dimethyl
sulphoxide. Net price 5 ml (with brush) = £7.04
Additives: none as listed in section 13.1

PoM **Iduridin**® (Ferring)
Application, idoxuridine 5% in dimethyl
sulphoxide. Net price 5 ml (with applicator) =
£4.90
Additives: none as listed in section 13.1

Application, idoxuridine 40% in dimethyl
sulphoxide. Net price 5 ml (with applicator) =
£19.00; 20 ml with dropper = £39.00
Additives: none as listed in section 13.1

13.10.4   Parasiticidal preparations

SCABIES. Applications of benzyl benzoate,
lindane, or monosulfiram are all effective. The
preparations are traditionally applied after a hot
bath although there is no controlled study to confirm or otherwise the efficacy of the practice.
Lotions are usually preferred to creams as they
give better coverage.

Benzyl benzoate and **lindane** are widely used.
All members of an affected household are treated
over the whole body, omitting the head and neck.
Benzyl benzoate is irritant to the skin; applications for infants should be suitably diluted, and
less irritant preparations such as lindane or monosulfiram may be preferred for treating children.

Monosulfiram (Tetmosol®) is particularly useful for treating scabies in children. Patients should
avoid alcohol as a disulfiram-like reaction may
occur.

The role of malathion in scabies is uncertain.

The itch of scabies persists long after the infes-
tation has been eliminated and antipruritic treatment may be required. Application of **crotamiton**
(Eurax®) is useful in controlling itching after
treatment with more effective acaricides.

PEDICULOSIS. **Malathion** and **carbaryl** have now
become the treatment of choice for pediculosis
(lice). **Lindane** is no longer recommended for
head lice because of the emergence of resistant
strains. Lotions should be used in preference to
shampoos, which are not in contact with the hair
for long enough to be fully effective. A contact
time of 12 hours is usually recommended. On the
basis of *in vitro* tests some sources have suggested
that a 2-hour contact period may be sufficient, but
more information is required before this can be
regarded as proven.

BORDERLINE SUBSTANCES. The preparations
marked 'ACBS' are regarded as drugs when
prescribed in accordance with the advice of the
Advisory Committee on Borderline Substances
for the clinical conditions listed. Prescriptions
issued in accordance with this advice and endorsed
'ACBS' will normally not be investigated. See
Appendix 3 for listing by clinical condition.

BENZYL BENZOATE

Indications: scabies, pediculosis
Cautions: children (see notes above), avoid contact with the eyes

Side-effects: slight skin irritation, transient burning sensation, occasionally rashes

Administration: scabies—apply 25% application
over the whole body, omitting the head and
neck. The application should be repeated without bathing on the following day and washed
off 24 hours later. The application should be
diluted with 1 volume of water for children or
3 volumes for infants
Pediculosis—apply 25% application to affected
area for 24 hours, remove by washing; in severe
cases repeat 2–3 times

Benzyl Benzoate Application, benzyl benzoate
25%, emulsifying wax 2%, in purified water,
freshly boiled and cooled. Net price 150 ml =
52p

Ascabiol® (M&B)
Application, benzyl benzoate 25% in an emul-
sion basis. Net price 200 ml = £1.52
Additives: fragrance

CARBARYL

Indications: pediculosis
Cautions: avoid contact with eyes
Administration: lotion—apply to dry hair and rub
into the hair and scalp or affected areas, allow
to dry, comb, and remove by washing 12 hours
later (see also notes above); repeat procedure
if necessary after 7–9 days; shampoo—leave on
hair for 5 minutes, rinse, allow to dry, comb,
repeat twice at intervals of 3 days

Carylderm® (Napp)
Lotion, carbaryl 0.5%, in an alcoholic basis. Net
price 55 ml = 87p
Additives: none as listed in section 13.1
Caution: flammable
Shampoo, carbaryl 1%. Net price 100 ml = £1.15
Additives: wool fat derivative, fragrance

Clinicide® (De Witt)
Lotion, carbaryl 0.5% in an aqueous basis con-
taining 10% alcohol. Net price 50 ml = 78p
Additives: none as listed in section 13.1

Derbac® (International Labs)
Shampoo solution, carbaryl 0.5% in a shampoo
basis. Net price 75 ml = 81p
Additives: hydroxybenzoates (parabens), fragrance

Suleo-C® (International Labs)
Lotion, carbaryl 0.5%, in an alcoholic basis. Net
price 55 ml = 81p; 210 ml = £1.68
Additives: fragrance
Caution: flammable
Shampoo solution, carbaryl 0.5% in a shampoo
basis. Net price 75 ml = 81p
Additives: fragrance

CROTAMITON

Indications: scabies, pruritus
Cautions; Contra-indications: section 13.3
Administration: scabies—apply over the whole
body omitting the head and neck, after a hot
bath, and remove by washing on the following
day. The application may be repeated 24 hours
later but a bath should not be taken until the
following day

Preparations
Section 13.3

LINDANE

Indications: pediculosis, scabies (see notes above)

Cautions: avoid contact with eyes

Side-effects: rarely skin irritation

Administration: pediculosis—rub 0.1–2% application into hair and scalp or affected area, allow to dry, and remove by washing after 24 hours (kills parasites within a few days); shampoos, leave on hair for 5 minutes, rinse, allow to dry, comb, repeat once after 7 days

Scabies—apply 1% lotion or cream over whole body, omitting the head and neck, and wash off after 24 hours. Repeat after 1–3 days

Lindane Application, lindane 100 mg, emulsifying wax 4 g, lavender oil 1 ml, xylene (of commerce) 15 ml/100 ml, in purified water, freshly boiled and cooled. For pediculosis

Lorexane® (Care)

Cream, lindane 1%, in a water-miscible basis. Net price 50 g = 28p. For scabies and pediculosis
Additives: information not disclosed for BNF

Shampoo, lindane 2% in a detergent basis, for pediculosis. Net price 30 g = 29p
Additives: information not disclosed for BNF

Quellada® (Stafford-Miller)

Lotion, lindane 1%, in a lotion basis. Net price 100 ml = 42p; 500 ml = £2.10. For scabies
Additives: information not disclosed for BNF

Application PC, lindane 1%, in a shampoo basis. Net price 100 ml = 51p; 500 ml = £2.55. For pediculosis
Additives: information not disclosed for BNF

MALATHION

Indications: pediculosis, scabies

Cautions: avoid contact with eyes. Do not use more than once a week for 3 weeks at a time

Administration: pediculosis—rub 0.5% lotion into dry hair, scalp, and affected area, comb, allow to dry, remove by washing after 12 hours (see also notes above), repeat if necessary after 7–9 days; apply 1% shampoo to hair for 5 minutes, rinse, comb, repeat if necessary after 7–9 days

Scabies—apply 0.5% preparation over whole body, omitting the head and neck, and wash off after 24 hours, but see notes above

Derbac-M® (International Labs)

Liquid, malathion 0.5% in an aqueous basis. Net price 55 ml = 81p; 200 ml = £2.03
Additives: hydroxybenzoates (parabens), fragrance

Prioderm® (Napp)

Lotion, malathion 0.5%, in an alcoholic basis. Net price 55 ml = 87p
Additives: fragrance
Caution: flammable

Cream shampoo, malathion 1%. Net price 40 g = 87p
Additives: disodium edetate, hydroxybenzoates (parabens), propylene glycol, wool fat derivative, fragrance

Suleo-M® (International Labs)

Lotion, malathion 0.5%, in an alcoholic basis. Net price 55 ml = 81p; 210 ml = £1.68
Additives: fragrance
Caution: flammable

MONOSULFIRAM

Indications: scabies, particularly in children

Cautions: avoid contact with eyes. Drug interactions: see Appendix 1 (section 13)

Side-effects: rarely hypersensitivity

Administration: apply diluted solution over whole body omitting head and neck. Repeat if necessary for 2–3 consecutive nights

Tetmosol® (ICI)

Solution, monosulfiram 25%, in industrial methylated spirit. Dilute with 2–3 parts of water before use. Net price 100 ml = £1.00. Label: 4. ACBS: for control of scabies
Additives: information not disclosed for BNF
Caution: flammable

13.10.5 Preparations for minor skin infections

Some of the preparations listed are used in minor burns, and abrasions. They are applied as necessary. Preparations containing camphor, hydrargaphen, and sulphonamides should be **avoided**. Preparations such as magnesium sulphate paste are also listed but are now rarely used to treat carbuncles and boils as these are best treated with antibiotics (see section 5.1.1.2).

Flexible collodion (section 13.1) may be used to seal minor cuts and wounds.

Sprays and paints for minor infections are described in section 13.11.

Cetrimide Cream, cetrimide 0.5% in a suitable water-miscible basis such as cetostearyl alcohol 5%, liquid paraffin 50% in freshly boiled and cooled purified water. Net price 50 g = 14p

Chlorhexidine Cream, chlorhexidine gluconate solution usually 5% (= chlorhexidine gluconate 1%), cetomacrogol emulsifying wax 25%, liquid paraffin 10%, in purified water, freshly boiled and cooled

Proflavine Cream, proflavine hemisulphate 0.1%, yellow beeswax 2.5%, chlorocresol 0.1%, liquid paraffin 67.3%, freshly boiled and cooled purified water 25%, wool fat 5%. Net price 100 ml = 32p
Caution: stains clothing

Anaflex® (Geistlich)

Aerosol spray (= application), polynoxylin 2% with talc, in a pressurised aerosol unit. Net price 100 g = £2.85
Additives: none as listed in section 13.1

Cream, polynoxylin 10%, in a water-miscible basis. Net price 50 g = £2.35
Additives: fragrance

Dusting-powder, polynoxylin 10% in a talc basis. Net price 30 g = £2.65
Additives: none as listed in section 13.1

Paste, polynoxylin 10%. For application to moist areas. Net price 20 g = £1.20
Additives: none as listed in section 13.1

Bactrian® (Loveridge)

Cream, cetrimide 1%. Net price 45 g = 39p
Additives: information not disclosed for BNF

Betadine® (Napp)

Ointment, povidone-iodine 10%, in a water-miscible basis. Net price 80 g = £1.85
Additives: none as listed in section 13.1

Brulidine® (Fisons)

Cream, dibromopropamidine isethionate 0.15%, in a water-miscible basis. Net price 25 g = 63p
Additives: hydroxybenzoates (parabens), fragrance

Cetavlex® (Care)

Cream, cetrimide 0.5%, in a water-miscible basis. Net price 50 g = 41p; 500 g = £2.75
Additives: information not disclosed for BNF

Dermalex® (Dermalex)

Skin lotion, allantoin 0.25%, hexachlorophane 0.5%, squalane 3% in an emulsion basis. Net price 100 ml = £2.05; 250 ml = £5.35. For prevention of pressure sores and prevention and treatment of urinary rash. Avoid in children under 2 years
Additives: information not disclosed for BNF

Drapolene® (Calmic)

Cream, benzalkonium chloride 0.01%, cetrimide 0.2% in a water-miscible basis. Net price 55 g = 52p; 100 g = 81p. For urinary rash and minor wounds
Additives: chlorocresol, wool fat

Hibitane® (ICI)

Antiseptic cream, chlorhexidine gluconate solution 5% (1% chlorhexidine gluconate), in a water-miscible basis. Net price 50 g = 30p
Additives: information not disclosed for BNF

PoM **Miol (Formula M1)**® (BritCair)

Cream, alcloxa 1%, calcium chloride 0.2%, camphor 4%, chlorphenesin 0.1%, magnesium chloride 1.5%, sodium chloride 2.1% in a water-miscible basis. Net price 30 g = £2.08
Additives: none as listed in section 13.1

Lotion, alcloxa 1%, calcium chloride 0.17%, camphor 1%, magnesium chloride 1.42%, sodium chloride 1.98%. Net price 100 ml = £2.40
Additives: none as listed in section 13.1

Ponoxylan® (Rorer)

Gel, polynoxylin 10%. Net price 25 g = 87p
Additives: fragrance

Preparations for boils

Magnesium Sulphate Paste, dried magnesium sulphate 38%, phenol 0.5%, in anhydrous glycerol. Net price 25 g = 19p
Apply under dressing

Ilonium® (Ilon)

Ointment, colophony 15.6%, phenol 0.1%, turpentine oil 8%, venice turpentine 8.1%, thymol 0.03%. Net price 30 g = 56p; 100 g = £1.30
Additives: beeswax, wool fat, fragrance

Secaderm—section 13.14

13.11   Skin disinfecting and cleansing agents

The choice of *cleansing agent* is an important factor in treating skin conditions. For example, scaling disorders are best treated with **emulsifying ointment** (section 13.1) or other cleansers that do not irritate the skin; when treating ulcerated areas, a less irritant solution such as **dilute sodium hypochlorite** or **hydrogen peroxide** may be preferred; weeping eczemas may be treated with an astringent preparation (section 13.5 and below) such as **potassium permanganate solution**.

Sodium chloride solution 0.9% is suitable for general cleansing of skin and wounds. Useful *disinfectants* for skin cleansing include **cetrimide** (which has useful detergent properties), **chlorhexidine, potassium permanganate solution** 1 in 8000 and **dilute sodium hypochlorite** solution. Some patients may find these irritant and the more recent preparations, such as **povidone-iodine,** which are less irritant, may be preferred. Topical preparations of **hexachlorophane** should be used with caution in neonates and should **not** be used on large raw surfaces.

Disinfectant solutions may be prescribed for the treatment of skin conditions, but they are not regarded as drugs when used for general hygienic purposes. See Appendix 3, borderline substances. They are commonly used for cleansing of wounds and ulcers, skin cleansing in acne (section 13.6), adjunctive treatment of infected skin conditions, and skin preparation before surgery. Patients have suffered severe burns, however, when diathermy has been preceded by application of alcoholic skin disinfectants.

Astringent preparations, such as aluminium acetate lotion and potassium permanganate solution are useful for treating eczematous reactions and suppurating wounds. They may assist in sealing an exuding surface as they precipitate protein. Silver nitrate lotion is now rarely used as it stains the skin black and may cause toxic effects if used for prolonged periods.

BORDERLINE SUBSTANCES. The preparations marked 'ACBS' are regarded as drugs when prescribed in accordance with the advice of the Advisory Committee on Borderline Substances for the clinical conditions listed. Prescriptions issued in accordance with this advice and endorsed 'ACBS' will normally not be investigated. See Appendix 3 for listing by clinical condition.

DISINFECTING AND CLEANSING AGENTS

ALCOHOL

Indications: skin preparation before injection
Cautions: flammable; avoid broken skin

Industrial Methylated Spirit. Net price 100 ml = 14p. Label: 15

Surgical Spirit. Net price 100 ml = 16p. Label: 15

ALUMINIUM ACETATE

Indications: suppurating and exudative eczematous reactions and wounds

Aluminium Acetate Lotion, aluminium acetate approx. 0.65%, in water (see Formulary). To be used undiluted as a wet dressing
Note. Aluminium acetate solution (13%) for the preparation of aluminium acetate lotion (0.65%) is available from Macarthys, Penn, etc. on special order

BENZALKONIUM CHLORIDE

Indications: skin disinfection such as pre-operative skin preparation, obstetrics, wound cleansing and bladder irrigation
Cautions: avoid contact with eyes

Benzalkonium Chloride Solution, benzalkonium chloride 50%. Net price 50 ml = 32p. To be used diluted 1 in 500 to 1 in 10000

Roccal® (Winthrop)
Solution, blue, benzalkonium chloride 1%. Net price 250 ml = £1.05; 500 ml = £2.10. To be used diluted 1 in 10 to 1 in 200
Additives: fragrance

Roccal Concentrate 10X® (Winthrop)
Concentrate, blue, benzalkonium chloride 10%. Net price 2.25 litres = £25.88. For preparation of Roccal Solution with freshly boiled and cooled purified water
Additives: fragrance

CETRIMIDE
Indications: skin disinfection; soap or shampoo substitute in acne, skin infections and seborrhoea of the scalp
Cautions: avoid contact with eyes; avoid use in body cavities
Side-effects: skin irritation and occasionally sensitisation

Cetrimide Solution, yellow, cetrimide 1% in purified water freshly boiled and cooled. Net price 100 ml = 5p. To be used undiluted

Cetrimide Solution Strong, yellow, cetrimide 20 to 40%, with alcohol (95%) 7.5%, tartrazine 0.0075%. It may be perfumed. Used for preparation of cetrimide solutions. Net price 100 ml = 52p (20%); 78p (40%). To be diluted before use

Cetavlon® (ICI)
Solution, corresponds to Cetrimide Solution Strong (40%). For preparation of cetrimide solutions. Net price 100 ml = 24p. For pre-operative scrubbing, skin cleansing and disinfection use as a 1% solution; for shampooing in seborrhoeic conditions use as a 1–3% solution; for cleansing in wounds and burns use as a 0.1% solution

CHLORHEXIDINE
Indications: skin disinfection such as pre-operative skin preparation, obstetrics and wound cleansing; bladder irrigation (see also section 7.4.4)
Cautions: bladder irrigations of concentrated solutions may cause haematuria
Side-effects: sensitivity may occur, avoid contact with mucous membranes and meninges
Administration: chlorhexidine acetate or gluconate, body cavity and bladder irrigation 0.01–0.02%, urethral disinfection and catheter lubrication 0.05% (in glycerol), pre-operative skin preparation 0.5% (in alcohol 70%); chlorhexidine hydrochloride 1% as a dusting-powder or cream
Note. See section 7.4.4 for a comment that solutions containing chlorhexidine 0.01% are usually preferred for postoperative bladder instillation

Chlorhexidine Dusting-powder, chlorhexidine hydrochloride 0.5%.
Note. A sterile dusting-powder containing chlorhexidine acetate 1% (CX Antiseptic Dusting Powder) is now available from Bio-Medical, net price 15 g = £2.00

Bacticlens® (S&N)
Solution (sterile), pink, chlorhexidine gluconate 0.05%. Net price 50 × 25-ml sachet = £4.45; 25 × 100-ml sachet = £5.35. To be used undiluted for skin disinfection
Additives: none as listed in section 13.1

Cetriclens® (S&N)
Solution (sterile), yellow, chlorhexidine gluconate 0.015%, cetrimide 0.15%. Net price 50 × 25-ml sachet = £2.88; 25 × 100-ml sachet = £4.09. To be used undiluted for skin disinfection and wound cleansing
Additives: none as listed in section 13.1
Forte solution (sterile), yellow, chlorhexidine gluconate 0.05%, cetrimide 0.5%. Net price 25 × 100-ml sachet = £5.27. To be used undiluted for cleansing physically contaminated wounds
Additives: none as listed in section 13.1

Chlorasept® (Baxter)
2000 Solution (sterile), pink, chlorhexidine acetate 0.05%. Net price 20 × 25-ml sachet = £1.50; 10 × 100-ml sachet = £1.70; 250, 500, and 1000 ml packs also available. For general disinfection and wound cleansing
Additives: none as listed in section 13.1

Cyteal® (Concept)
Antiseptic skin cleanser, yellow, chlorhexidine gluconate 0.5%, chlorocresol 0.3%, hexamidine isethionate 0.1%. Net price 500 ml = 70p. For pre-operative scrubbing use undiluted; for cleansing infections use undiluted or diluted 1 in 10 and apply twice daily; for wound and ulcer cleansing dilute 1 in 10 and use daily

Dispray 1 Quick Prep® (Stuart)
Aerosol application, chlorhexidine gluconate solution 2.5% (≡ 0.5% chlorhexidine gluconate), in alcohol 70%, pressurised aerosol unit. Net price 400-ml unit = £1.01. For skin disinfection before injections or operations
Caution: flammable

Hibidil® (ICI)
Solution (sterile), pink, chlorhexidine gluconate solution 0.25% (≡ chlorhexidine gluconate 0.05%) in sterile aqueous solution. Net price 25 × 25-ml sachets = £2.00; 6 × 100-ml sachets = £1.15; 1000 ml also available. To be used undiluted for skin disinfection in wounds, burns and obstetrics

Hibiscrub® (ICI)
Cleansing solution, red, chlorhexidine gluconate solution 20% (≡4% chlorhexidine gluconate), perfumed, in a surfactant solution. Net price 250 ml = 65p; 500 ml = £1.30. Use instead of soap as pre-operative scrub or disinfectant wash for hands and skin

Hibisol® (ICI)
Solution, blue, chlorhexidine gluconate solution 2.5% (≡0.5% chlorhexidine gluconate), in isopropyl alcohol 70% with emollients. Net price 250 ml = 47p; 500 ml = 94p. To be used undiluted for hand and skin disinfection

Hibitane® (ICI)
Chlorhexidine acetate powder. 50 g. For preparation of chlorhexidine solutions

Hibitane 5% Concentrate® (ICI)
Solution, red, chlorhexidine gluconate solution 25% ($\equiv$ 5% chlorhexidine gluconate), in a perfumed aqueous solution. Net price 50 × 10-ml sachet = £3.05; 500 ml = £1.18. To be used diluted 1 in 10 (0.5%) with alcohol 70% for pre-operative skin preparation, or 1 in 100 (0.05%) with water for general skin disinfection

Hibitane Gluconate 20%® (ICI)
Solution, chlorhexidine gluconate 20% in an aqueous solution. Net price 500 ml = £4.25. To be used diluted as above in body cavity and bladder irrigation, urethral disinfection and catheter lubrication

Hibitane Obstetric® (ICI)
Cream, chlorhexidine gluconate solution 5% ($\equiv$ 1% chlorhexidine gluconate), in a pourable water-miscible basis. Net price 250 ml = 91p. For use in obstetrics as a vaginal lubricant and for application to the vulva and perineum during labour

pHiso-MED® (Winthrop)
Solution, chlorhexidine gluconate 4% in an emulsion basis. Net price 150 ml = £4.54. For use as a soap or shampoo substitute in acne and seborrhoeic conditions; for bathing mothers and babies in maternity units (as 1 in 10 dilution) to prevent cross-infection and for pre-operative hand and skin preparation
Additives: benzyl alcohol, wool fat derivative

Rotersept® (Roterpharma)
Spray application, chlorhexidine gluconate 0.2% in a pressurised aerosol unit. Net price 284-g unit = £1.99. For prevention and treatment of sore cracked nipples

Savloclens® (ICI)
Solution (sterile), yellow, chlorhexidine gluconate solution 0.25% ($\equiv$ chlorhexidine gluconate 0.05%), cetrimide 0.5% = a dilution of 1 in 30 of Savlon Hospital Concentrate. Net price 100-ml sachet = 20p. To be used undiluted in general skin disinfection and wound cleansing

Savlodil® (ICI)
Solution (sterile), yellow, chlorhexidine gluconate solution 0.075% ($\equiv$ chlorhexidine gluconate 0.015%), cetrimide 0.15% (sterile). Net price 25 × 25-ml sachets = £1.29; 6 × 100-ml sachets = 88p; 1000 ml also available. To be used undiluted for general skin disinfection and wound cleansing

Savlon Hospital Concentrate® (ICI)
Solution, orange, chlorhexidine gluconate solution 7.5% ($\equiv$ chlorhexidine gluconate 1.5%), cetrimide 15%. Net price 50 × 10-ml sachets = £1.98; 25 × 25-ml sachets = £1.74; 1 litre = £1.60. To be used diluted 1 in 100 (1%) to 1 in 30 with water for skin disinfection and wound cleansing, and diluted 1 in 30 in alcohol 70% for pre-operative skin preparation

Tisept® (Seton Prebbles)
Solution (sterile), yellow, chlorhexidine gluconate 0.015%, cetrimide 0.15%. Net price

25 × 25-ml sachet = £1.45; 6 × 100-ml sachet = 90p; 500 ml = 66p; 1000 ml = 70p. To be used undiluted for general skin disinfection and wound cleansing
Additives: none as listed in section 13.1

Travasept 30® (Baxter)
Solution (sterile), yellow, chlorhexidine acetate 0.05%, cetrimide 0.5%. Net price 100 ml = 73p; 250 ml = 69p; 500 ml = 74p; 1000 ml = 79p; 25- and 100-ml sachets also available. To be used undiluted for skin cleansing and disinfection of wounds
Additives: none as listed in section 13.1

Travasept 100® (Baxter)
Solution (sterile), yellow, chlorhexidine acetate 0.015%, cetrimide 0.15%. Net price 20 × 25-ml sachet = £1.04; 10 × 100-ml sachet = £1.45; 100 ml = 73p; 500 ml = 74p; 1000 ml = 79p. To be used undiluted in skin disinfection such as wound cleansing and obstetrics
Additives: none as listed in section 13.1

Unisept® (Seton Prebbles)
Solution (sterile), pink, chlorhexidine gluconate 0.05%. Net price 25 × 25-ml sachet = £2.10; 6 × 100-ml sachet = £1.20; 500 ml = 66p; 1000 ml = 70p. To be used undiluted for general skin disinfection and wound cleansing
Additives: none as listed in section 13.1

CHLORINATED SOLUTIONS

Indications: skin disinfection particularly wound and ulcer cleansing
Cautions: bleaches fabric; solutions may be irritant

Chlorinated Lime and Boric Acid Solution (Eusol), chlorinated lime 1.25%, boric acid 1.25%, in water for preparations. Contains not less than 0.25% available chlorine. It must be freshly prepared. To be used undiluted for skin disinfection, particularly in wound and ulcer cleansing when it may be applied as a wet dressing

Chlorinated Soda Solution, Surgical (Dakin's Solution), boric acid, chlorinated lime, sodium carbonate, sufficient of each to provide a solution containing 0.5% of available chlorine in water. Net price 500 ml = 56p. To be used undiluted for cleansing wounds and ulcers. Surrounding tissues should be protected with petroleum jelly during application as solutions are irritant

Sodium Hypochlorite Solution, Strong, contains not less than 8% available chlorine. To be diluted before use

Sodium Hypochlorite Solution, Dilute, contains about 1% available chlorine. For general disinfection. Only diluted solutions containing up to 0.5% available chlorine are suitable for use on the skin and in wounds

▼ **Chlorasol®** (Seton Prebbles)
Solution (sterile), sodium hypochlorite, containing 0.3–0.4% available chlorine. Net price 25 × 25-ml sachets = £2.75
Additives: none as listed in section 13.1

CHLOROXYLENOL

Indications: skin disinfection
Cautions: may irritate skin and cause sensitisation

Chloroxylenol Solution, chloroxylenol 5%, alcohol about 20%, terpineol 10% in a detergent solution. Net price 100 ml = 25p. To be used as 1 in 20 dilution (5%)
Dettol® (R&C)
Lotion—discontinued

CRYSTAL VIOLET

Indications: see below
Cautions: stains clothes and skin
Side-effects: mucosal ulcerations

Crystal Violet Paint, crystal violet 0.5%, in water for preparations. To be used undiluted
Note. DHSS has restricted use to topical application on unbroken skin only; no longer recommended for application to mucous membranes or open wounds

HEXACHLOROPHANE

Indications: see under preparations (below)
Contra-indications: avoid use on badly burned or excoriated skin; pregnancy; children under 2 years except on medical advice
Side-effects: sensitivity; rarely photosensitivity

PoM **Ster-Zac DC Skin Cleanser®** (Hough)
Cream, hexachlorophane 3%. Net price 100 ml = 63p. Use 3–5 ml instead of soap as pre-operative scrub for hands
Additives: information not disclosed for BNF
Ster-Zac Powder® (Hough)
Dusting-powder, hexachlorophane 0.33%, zinc oxide 3%, talc 88.67%, starch 8% (sterile). Net price 30 g = 58p
Additives: information not disclosed for BNF
Prevention of neonatal staphylococcal sepsis, after ligature of cord sprinkle on perineum, groin, front of abdomen, and axillas; after cutting cord and spraying with plastic dressing, powder stump and adjacent skin; after every napkin change powder stump, adjacent skin, perineum, groin, axillas, buttocks, and front of abdomen; continue until stump drops away and wound healed
Adjunct for treatment of recurrent furunculosis, powder daily area of skin normally subject to furunculosis

HYDROGEN PEROXIDE

Indications: skin disinfection, particularly cleansing and deodorising wounds and ulcers
Cautions: bleaches fabric; solutions above 6% should be diluted before application to the skin

Hydrogen Peroxide Solution 27% (about 90 vols). Dilute before use. Net price 100 ml = 38p
Hydrogen Peroxide Solution 6% (20 vols). Net price 100 ml = 20p
Hydrogen Peroxide Solution 3% (10 vols). Net price 100 ml = 9p
Hioxyl see Desloughing Agents (below)

IODINE COMPOUNDS

Indications: skin disinfection; surfactant solutions—soap or shampoo substitute in acne, skin infections, and seborrhoea of the scalp
Cautions: pregnancy, breast-feeding
Side-effects: rarely sensitivity; may interfere with thyroid function tests

Weak Iodine Solution (Iodine Tincture), iodine 2.5%, potassium iodide 2.5%, purified water 2.5%, in alcohol (90%). Net price 10 ml = 4p. To be used undiluted in minor skin wounds; stains skin and clothes and causes considerable pain
Betadine® (Napp)
Antiseptic spray, povidone-iodine 5%, in a pressurised aerosol unit. Net price 200-ml unit = £2.79. For use in skin disinfection, particularly minor wounds and infections
Additives: none as listed in section 13.1
Antiseptic paint, povidone-iodine 10% in an alcoholic solution. Net price 8 ml (with applicator brush) = 63p. Apply undiluted to minor wounds and infections, twice daily
Additives: none as listed in section 13.1
Alcoholic solution, povidone-iodine 10%. Net price 500 ml = £1.12. To be applied undiluted in pre- and post-operative skin disinfection
Additives: none as listed in section 13.1
Antiseptic solution, povidone-iodine 10% in aqueous solution. Net price 500 ml = 98p. To be applied undiluted in pre- and post-operative skin disinfection
Additives: none as listed in section 13.1
Dry powder spray, povidone-iodine 2.5% in a pressurised aerosol unit. Net price 150-g unit = £2.15. For skin disinfection, particularly minor wounds and infections
Scalp and skin cleanser solution, povidone-iodine 7.5%, in a surfactant basis. Net price 250 ml = £1.88. ACBS: for infective conditions of the skin. Retain on scalp for 5 minutes before rinsing
Skin cleanser solution, povidone-iodine 4%, in a surfactant basis. Net price 250 ml = £1.58. ACBS: for infective conditions of the skin. Retain on skin for 5 minutes before rinsing
Surgical scrub, povidone-iodine 7.5%, in a non-ionic surfactant basis. Net price 500 ml = 88p. To be used as a pre-operative scrub for hands and skin
Additives: wool fat derivative
Disadine DP® (Stuart)
Dry powder spray (= application), povidone-iodine 0.5%, in a pressurised aerosol unit. Net price 150-g unit = £1.99. For skin disinfection, particularly wounds, surgery, and bedsores
Additives: information not disclosed for BNF
Videne® (Riker)
Disinfectant solution, red-brown, povidone-iodine 10% (≡ 1% available iodine), in an aqueous solution. Net price 500 ml = 96p. (hosp. only)
Additives: none as listed in section 13.1
Apply undiluted in skin disinfection and pre-operative skin preparation
Disinfectant tincture, red-brown, povidone-iodine 10% (≡ 1% available iodine), in industrial methylated spirit. Net price 500 ml = £1.16

(hosp. only). Apply undiluted in pre-operative skin disinfection, particularly orthopaedic surgery
Additives: none as listed in section 13.1
Caution: flammable
Dusting-powder, povidone-iodine 5%. Net price 15 g = £2.60. For minor wounds and infections
Surgical scrub, red-brown, povidone-iodine 7.5% (≡ 0.75% available iodine), in a detergent basis. Net price 500 ml = 88p. To be used as a pre-operative scrub for hands and skin and disinfecting site of incision before surgery
Additives: none as listed in section 13.1

POTASSIUM PERMANGANATE

Indications: cleansing and deodorising suppurating eczematous reactions and wounds
Cautions: irritant to mucous membranes; stains skin and clothing
Administration: wet dressings or baths, approx. 0.01% solution (10 g/bath)

Potassium Permanganate Solution, potassium permanganate 0.1% in water (see Formulary). Net price 500 ml = 1p
Permitabs® (Bioglan)
Tablets, for preparation of topical solution, potassium permanganate 400 mg. Net price 100 = £2.00
1 tablet dissolved in 4 litres of water provides a 0.01% solution

SILVER NITRATE

Indications: suppurating lesions (short-term)
Cautions: see notes above

Silver Nitrate Lotion, silver nitrate 0.5%, in water (see Formulary). Do not use if precipitate is present. Net price 50 ml = 24p. To be used undiluted

SODIUM CHLORIDE

Indications: see notes above

Normasol® (Seton Prebbles)
Solution (sterile), sodium chloride 0.9%. Net price   25 × 25-ml   sachet = £2.20;   6 × 100-ml sachet = £1.75. To be used undiluted for topical irrigation of burns, wounds, and eyes
Additives: none as listed in section 13.1
See also section 11.8.2
Topiclens® (S&N)
Solution (sterile), sodium chloride 0.9%. Net price 50 × 25-ml sachet = £4.62; 25 × 100-ml sachet = £7.37. To be used undiluted for irrigating eyes and wounds
Additives: none as listed in section 13.1

SOFT SOAP

Indications: removal of adherent crusts

Soap Spirit, soft soap 65% in alcohol (90%). Net price 100 ml = 44p

TRICLOSAN

Indications: skin disinfection
Cautions: avoid contact with eyes

Manusept® (Hough)
Antibacterial hand rub, blue, triclosan 0.5%, isopropyl alcohol 70%. Net price 250 ml = 96p; 500 ml = £1.47. For disinfection and pre-operative hand preparation
Additives: information not disclosed for BNF
Ster-Zac Bath Concentrate® (Hough)
Solution, triclosan 2%. Net price 28.5 ml = 38p; 500 ml = £3.65. ACBS: for staphyloccal skin infections. For prevention of cross-infection use 1 sachet/bath
Additives: information not disclosed for BNF

ZINC SULPHATE

Indications: indolent ulcers

Zinc Sulphate Lotion (Lotio Rubra), zinc sulphate 1%, with amaranth, in water (see Formulary). Net price 200 ml = 2p. Apply undiluted as a wet dressing

DESLOUGHING AGENTS

Desloughing agents for ulcers are second-line treatment and the underlying causes should be treated. The main beneficial effect is removal of slough and clot and the ablation of local infection. Preparations which absorb or help promote the removal of exudate may also help (section 13.13.8). It should be noted that substances applied to an open area are easily absorbed and perilesional skin is easily sensitised. Gravitational dermatitis may be due to neomycin or lanolin sensitivity. Enzyme preparations such as streptokinase-streptodornase (Varidase®) or alternatively dextranomer (Debrisan®, section 13.13.9) are designed for sloughing ulcers and may help.

Usually all that is required is washing with an antiseptic solution such as dilute sodium hypochlorite solution, cetrimide, or potassium permanganate and covering the lesion with an adequate dressing.

Aserbine® (Bencard)
Cream, benzoic acid 0.024%, hexachlorophane 0.015%, malic acid 0.36%, propylene glycol 1.7%, salicylic acid 0.006%. Net price 100 g = 96p
Additives: chlorocresol, hydroxybenzoates (parabens), propylene glycol
Solution, benzoic acid 0.15%, malic acid 2.25%, propylene glycol 40%, salicylic acid 0.0375%. Net price 500 ml = £1.46
Additives: propylene glycol, fragrance
PoM **Benoxyl 20**® (Stiefel)
Lotion, benzoyl peroxide 20%. For cutaneous ulcers. Net price 100 ml = £3.46
Additives: isopropyl palmitate, propylene glycol
Apply 8–12 hourly as wet dressing; protect perilesional skin
Hioxyl® (Quinoderm Ltd)
Cream, hydrogen peroxide (stabilised) 1.5%. Net price 25 g = £1.43; 100 g = £4.46. For leg ulcers and pressure sores
Additives: none as listed in section 13.1
Apply when necessary and if necessary cover with a dressing

PoM **Iodosorb**® (Perstorp)
Powder, cadexomer iodine (modified starch gel microbeads containing 0.9% iodine). Net price 3-g sachet = £1.56. For venous leg ulcers and pressure sores
Sprinkle 3mm on wound surface and renew daily

Malatex® (Norton)
Cream, benzoic acid 0.024%, malic acid 0.36%, propylene glycol 1.7%, salicylic acid 0.006%. Net price 100 g = 77p; 125 g = 95p
Solution, benzoic acid 0.15%, malic acid 2.25%, propylene glycol 40%, salicylic acid 0.0375%. Net price 500 ml = £1.16

Variclene® (Dermal)
Gel, brilliant green 0.5%, lactic acid 0.5%, in an aqueous basis. Net price 50 g = £4.58. For venous and other skin ulcers
Additives: none as listed in section 13.1
Apply to cleaned and dried lesion with a sterile applicator avoiding surrounding skin; in severe ulceration apply on dressing and repeat as required at intervals of not more than 7 days

PoM **Varidase Topical**® (Lederle)
Powder, streptokinase 100 000 units, streptodornase 25 000 units. For preparing solutions for topical use. Net price per vial = £6.69
Additives: none as listed in section 13.1
Apply as wet dressing usually 1–2 times daily
Also used to dissolve clots in the bladder or urinary catheters

SOAP SUBSTITUTES

See also above; section 13.2.2 (emollient bath additives) and section 13.6 (acne)

Emulsifying ointment—section 13.1

13.12 Antiperspirants

Aluminium chloride and hydroxychloride are potent antiperspirants used in the treatment of severe hyperhidrosis.

Dusting-powders are described in section 13.2.3.

ALUMINIUM CHLORIDE

Indications: hyperhidrosis
Cautions: avoid contact with eyes; do not shave axilla or use depilatories within 12 hours of use
Side-effects: skin irritation—may be less with hydroxychloride
Administration: apply at night to dry skin, wash off on following morning, initially daily then reduce frequency as condition improves—do not bathe immediately before use

PoM **Anhydrol Forte**® (Dermal)
Solution (= application), aluminium chloride hexahydrate 20%. Net price 10-ml bottle with roll-on applicator = £2.66
Additives: none as listed in section 13.1
Caution: flammable

PoM **Driclor**® (Stiefel)
Application, aluminium chloride hexahydrate 20% in an alcoholic basis. Net price 60-ml bottle with roll-on applicator = £2.82
Additives: none as listed in section 13.1
Caution: flammable

Hyperdrol® (BritCair)
Cream, aluminium hydroxychloride 19%. Net price 60 g = £2.48
Additives: hydroxybenzoates (parabens), propylene glycol
Gel, aluminium hydroxychloride 19%. Net price 60-g roll-on applicator = £3.00
Additives: none as listed in section 13.1

13.13 Wound management products

13.13.1 Bandages
13.13.2 Surgical adhesive tapes
13.13.3 Adhesive dressings
13.13.4 Surgical absorbents
13.13.5 Wound dressing pads
13.13.6 Tulle dressings
13.13.7 Semipermeable adhesive film
13.13.8 Gel and colloid dressings
13.13.9 Foam dressings

13.13.1 Bandages

RETENTION BANDAGES

Non-stretch fabric retention bandages
Open-wove Bandage, BP (types 1, 2 and 3). Cotton cloth, plain weave, warp of cotton, weft of cotton, viscose, or combination, one continuous length. Type 1, 5 m (all): 2.5 cm, net price = 20p; 5 cm = 32p; 7.5 cm = 46p; 10 cm = 59p (most suppliers) 5 m × 5 cm supplied when size not stated
Uses: protection and retention of absorbent dressings; support for minor strains, sprains; securing splints
Note. Type 1 bandage formerly described as Open-Wove Bandage BPC 1973; Type 2 formerly described as 'medium quality'; Type 3 formerly described as 'hospital quality'
Triangular Calico Bandage, BP. Unbleached calico rt. angle triangle. 90 cm × 90 cm × 1.27 m, net price = 70p (most suppliers)
Uses: sling
NHS **Domette Bandage**, BP. Fabric, plain weave, cotton warp and wool weft (hospital quality also available, all cotton). 5 m (all): 5 cm, net price = 54p; 7.5 cm = 81p; 10 cm = £1.08; 15 cm = £1.61 (Robert Bailey, Vernon-Carus)
Uses: protection and support where warmth required
Multiple Pack Dressing No. 1 (Drug Tariff). Contains absorbent cotton, absorbent cotton gauze type 13 light (sterile), open-wove bandages (banded). Net price per pack = £2.05
Multiple Pack Dressing No. 2 (Drug Tariff). As for No. 1 (above) but with larger quantities of cotton and cotton gauze and two sizes of bandages. Net price per pack = £3.34

Stretch fabric retention bandages
Cotton Conforming Bandage, BP. Cotton fabric, plain weave, treated to impart some elasticity to warp and weft. 3.5 m (all):
type A, 5 cm, net price = 37p; 7.5 cm = 48p; 10 cm = 59p; 15 cm = 79p (S&N—*Crinx*®)
type B, 5 cm = 35p; 7.5 cm = 46p; 10 cm = 56p; 15 cm = 76p (J&J—*Kling*®)
Uses: retention of dressings in difficult positions (e.g. over joints)

Polyamide and Cellulose Contour Bandage, BP (formerly Nylon and Viscose Stretch Bandage). Fabric, plain weave, warp of polyamide filament, weft of cotton or viscose, fast edges, one continuous length. 4 m stretched (all): Cuxson Gerrard—*Slinky®* (net price 5 cm = 29p, 7.5 cm = 40p, 10 cm = 49p, 15 cm = 68p); Robinsons—*Stayform®* (5 cm = 20p, 7.5 cm = 26p, 10 cm = 30p, 15 cm = 49p)
Uses: retention of dressings

NHS **Tubular Gauze Bandage, Seamless.** Unbleached cotton yarn, positioned with applicators. 20 m roll (all): 00, net price = £1.45; 01 = £1.59; 12 = £2.20; 34 = £3.11; 56 = £4.35; 78 = £5.05; T1 = £6.90; T2 = £8.90 (Seton—*Tubegauz®*)
Uses: retention of dressings on limbs, abdomen, trunk

Elasticated Surgical Tubular Stockinette, BP. Knitted fabric, elasticated threads of rubber-cored polyamide or polyester with cotton or cotton and viscose yarn, tubular. Lengths 50 cm and 1 m, various widths 6.25 cm–12 cm, net price = 45p–£1.21 (Lastonet—*Lastogrip®*; Salt—*Rediform®*; S&N—*Tensogrip®*; Seton—*Tubigrip®*)
Uses: retention of dressings on limbs, abdomen, trunk

Foam Padded Elasticated Surgical Tubular Stockinette (Drug Tariff). Fabric as for Elasticated Surgical Tubular Stockinette with polyurethane foam lining. Heel or elbow, small, net price = £1.47; medium = £1.59, large = £1.71; sacral, small, medium, and large (all) = £7.55 (Seton—*Tubipad®*)
Uses: relief of pressure and elimination of friction in relevant areas; porosity of foam lining allows normal water loss from skin surface

Elastic Net Surgical Tubular Stockinette (Drug Tariff). Lightweight elastic open-work net tubular fabric.
type A: arm/leg, 40 cm × 1.8 cm (size C), net price = 32p; thigh/head, 60 cm × 2.5 cm (size E) = 58p; trunk (adult), 60 cm × 4.5 cm (size F) = 85p; trunk (OS adult) 60 cm × 5.4 cm (size G) = £1.14 (Lenton—*Netelast®*)
type B: withdrawn
type C: arm/leg, 40 cm × 1.8 cm (size C) = 25p; thigh/head, 60 cm × 2.7 cm (size E) = 48p; trunk (adult), 60 cm × 5.5 cm (size F) = 67p; trunk (OS adult) 60 cm × 6 cm (size G) = 85p (Macarthys—*Macrofix®*)
Drug Tariff requires size and type to be specified by prescriber
Uses: retention of dressings, particularly on awkward sites

Cotton Surgical Tubular Stockinette, BP. Knitted fabric, cotton yarn, tubular. 1 m × 2.5 cm, net price = 16p; 5 cm = 25p; 7.5 cm = 32p; 6 m × 10 cm = £2.19 (J&J, Seton)
Uses: 1 m lengths, basis (with wadding) for Plaster of Paris bandages etc.; 6 m length, compression bandage

Ribbed Cotton and Viscose Surgical Tubular Stockinette, BP. Knitted fabric of 1:1 ribbed structure, singles yarn spun from blend of two-thirds cotton and one third viscose fibres, tubular. Length 5 m (all):
type A (lightweight): arm/leg (child), arm (adult) 5 cm, net price = £1.32; arm (OS adult), leg (adult) 7.5 cm = £1.72; leg (OS adult) 10 cm = £2.27; trunk (child) 15 cm = £3.28; trunk (adult) 20 cm = £3.78; trunk (OS adult) 25 cm = £4.53 (Seton)
type B (heavyweight): sizes and prices as for type A (Sallis—*Eesiban®*)
Drug Tariff specifies various combinations of sizes to provide sufficient material for part or full body coverage
Uses: protective dressings with tar-based and other non-steroid ointments

SUPPORT AND COMPRESSION BANDAGES

Non-adhesive woven extensible bandages

Crepe Bandage, BP. Fabric, plain weave, warp of wool threads and crepe-twisted cotton threads; weft of cotton threads; stretch bandage. 4.5 m stretched (all): 5 cm, net

price = 54p; 7.5 cm = 74p; 10 cm = £1.01; 15 cm = £1.44 (most suppliers)
Uses: light support system for strains, sprains, compression over paste bandages for varicose veins

Cotton Crepe Bandage, BP. Fabric, plain weave, warp of crepe-twisted cotton threads, weft of cotton and/or viscose threads; stretch bandage. 4.5 m stretched (both): 7.5 cm, net price = £1.66; 10 cm = £2.15; other sizes NHS (most suppliers)
Uses: light support system for strains, sprains, compression over paste bandages for varicose ulcers

NHS **Cotton Stretch Bandage**, BP. Fabric, plain weave, warp of crepe-twisted cotton threads, weft of cotton threads; stretch bandage, lighter than cotton crepe. 4.5 m stretched (all): 5 cm, net price = 30p; 7.5 cm = 41p; 10 cm = 54p; 15 cm = 76p (most suppliers)
Uses: light support system for strains, sprains, compression over paste bandages for varicose veins

Cotton Suspensory Bandage (Drug Tariff). Type 1: cotton net bag with draw tapes and webbing waistband; net price small, medium, and large (all) = 94p, extra large = 98p. Type 2: cotton net bag with elastic edge and webbing waistband; small = 98p, medium = £1.02, large = £1.06, extra large = £1.10. Type 3: cotton net bag with elastic edge and webbing waistband with elastic insertion; small, medium, and large (all) = £1.12; extra large = £1.16
Type supplied to be endorsed
Uses: support of scrotum

NHS **Cotton and Rubber Elastic Bandage**, BP. Fabric, plain weave, warp of combined cotton and rubber threads, weft of cotton threads (S&N)
Uses: provision of high compression and medium support

Heavy Cotton and Rubber Elastic Bandage, BP. Heavy version of above with one end folded as foot loop; fastener also supplied. 1.8 m unstretched × 7.5 cm, net price = £7.17 (Marlow, Seton, S&N—*Elastoweb®*).
Uses: provision of high even compression over large surface

Elastic Web Bandage, BP. (also termed Blue Line Webbing). Characteristic fabric woven ribbon fashion, warp threads of cotton and rubber with mid-line threads coloured blue, weft threads of cotton or combined cotton and viscose; may be dyed skin colour; with or without foot loop. 7.5 cm, net price = 54p; 10 cm = 75p; with foot loop 7.5 cm each = £2.77 (Marlow, Seton)
Uses: provision of support and high compression over large surface

Elastic Web Bandage without Foot Loop (also termed Red Line Webbing) (Scott-Curwen). Characteristic fabric woven ribbon fashion, warp threads of cotton and rubber with mid-line threads coloured red, weft threads of cotton or combined cotton and viscose. 7.5 cm × 2.75 m (2.5 m approx. unstretched), net price = £1.76; 7.5 cm × 3.75 m (3.5 m approx. unstretched) = £2.28
Uses: provision of support and high compression over large surfaces

Adhesive woven extensible bandages

Titanium Dioxide Elastic Adhesive Bandage, BP. (Drug Tariff title: Porous Flexible Adhesive Bandage). Woven fabric, elastic in warp (crepe-twisted cotton threads), weft of cotton and/or viscose threads, spread with adhesive mass containing titanium dioxide but free from rubber and zinc oxide. 4.5 m stretched × 7.5 cm, net price = £2.75 (Scholl—*Poroplast®*)
Uses: compression for chronic leg ulcers; continuous pressure and support in patients hypersensitive to rubber and zinc oxide

Elastic Adhesive Bandage, BP. Woven fabric, elastic in warp (crepe-twisted cotton threads), weft of cotton and/or viscose threads spread with adhesive mass containing zinc oxide. 4.5 m stretched (all): 5 cm, net price = £1.95; 7.5 cm = £2.84; 10 cm = £3.78 (S&N—*Elastoplast*

Bandage®). 7.5 cm width supplied when size not stated

NHS Half-spread Elastic Adhesive Bandage, BP. Fabric as for elastic adhesive bandage but only partially spread with adhesive. (S&N)

Uses: compression for leg ulcers; compression and support for fractured ribs, clavicles, swollen/sprained joints

NHS Ventilated Elastic Adhesive Bandage, BP. Fabric as for elastic adhesive bandage but adhesive spread such that there are regular strips of unspread fabric along length. (S&N)

Uses: compression for leg ulcers; compression and support for fractured ribs, clavicles, swollen/sprained joints

NHS Extension Plaster, BP. Woven fabric, elastic in weft, spread with adhesive mass containing zinc oxide, warp threads cotton and/or viscose, weft threads crepe-twisted cotton. (S&N)

Uses: support of light strains, joints and limbs removed from plaster casts, fractured ribs; traction bandaging

NHS Cohesive extensible bandages.
These elastic bandages adhere to themselves and not to the patient's skin, which prevents slipping during use. 2.25 m (both): 5 cm, net price = £1.30; 10 cm = £2.25; 4.5 m (all): 5 cm, net price = £1.32; 7.5 cm = £1.66; 10 cm = £1.94; 15 cm = £2.80 (Boots, 3M—*Coban®*, J&J—*Secure®*, Seton, Steriseal—*Cohepress®*)

Uses: support of sprained joints

MEDICATED BANDAGES

Hydrocortisone and Silicone Bandage (Drug Tariff). Cotton fabric, plain weave, impregnated with suitable cream containing hydrocortisone acetate 1%. Requires additional bandaging. Net price 2 m × 7.5 cm = £4.63. Potency IV. (S&N—*Cortacream®*, *additives:* sorbic acid)

Zinc Paste Bandage, BP. Cotton fabric, plain weave, impregnated with suitable paste containing zinc oxide; requires additional bandaging. Net price 6 m × 7.5 cm = £1.79 (Seton—*Zincaband®*, *additives:* hydroxybenzoates); £1.85 (S&N—*Viscopaste PB7®*, *additives:* hydroxybenzoates)

Zinc Paste and Calamine Bandage (Drug Tariff). Cotton fabric, plain weave, impregnated with suitable paste containing calamine and zinc oxide; requires additional bandaging. Net price 6 m × 7.5 cm = £1.79 (Seton—*Calaband®*, *additives:* hydroxybenzoates)

Zinc Paste, Calamine, and Clioquinol Bandage, BP. Cotton fabric, plain weave, impregnated with suitable paste containing calamine, clioquinol, and zinc oxide; requires additional bandaging. Net price 6 m × 7.5 cm = £1.79 (Seton—*Quinaband®*, *additives:* hydroxybenzoates)

Zinc Paste and Coal Tar Bandage, BP. Cotton fabric, plain weave, impregnated with a suitable paste containing coal tar and zinc oxide; requires additional bandaging. Net price 6 m × 7.5 cm = £1.89 (Seton—*Tarband®*, *additives:* hydroxybenzoates; S&N—*Coltapaste®*, *additives:* wool fat)

Uses: see section 13.5

Zinc Paste and Ichthammol Bandage, BP. Cotton fabric, plain weave, impregnated with suitable paste containing ichthammol and zinc oxide; requires additional bandaging. Net price 6 m × 7.5 cm = £1.86 (Seton—*Icthaband®*, *additives:* hydroxybenzoates; S&N—*Ichthopaste®*, *additives:* none as listed in section 13.1)

Uses: see section 13.5

13.13.2 Surgical adhesive tapes

PERMEABLE SURGICAL ADHESIVE TAPES

Zinc Oxide Surgical Adhesive Tape, BP. (Zinc Oxide Plaster). Fabric, plain weave, warp and weft of cotton and/or viscose, spread with an adhesive containing zinc oxide. 1.25 cm, net price 1 m = 18p; 3 m = 35p, 5 m = 50p; 2.5 cm, 1 m = 25p; 3 m = 53p; 5 m = 72p; 5 cm × 5 m = £1.22; 7.5 cm × 5 m = £1.73 (most suppliers)

Drug Tariff specifies 1 m × 2.5 cm supplied when size not stated

Uses: securing dressings and immobilising small areas

Permeable Woven Surgical Synthetic Adhesive Tape, BP. Non-extensible closely woven fabric, spread with a polymeric adhesive. 5 m (all): 1.25 cm, net price = 43p; 2.5 cm = 67p; 5 cm = £1.23 (J&J—*Dermicel®*)

Uses: securing dressings

For patients with skin reaction to other plasters and strapping, requiring use for long periods

Elastic Surgical Adhesive Tape, BP (Elastic Adhesive Plaster). Woven fabric, elastic in warp (crepe-twisted cotton threads), weft of cotton and/or viscose threads, spread with adhesive mass containing zinc oxide. 1.5 m stretched × 2.5 cm, net price = 41p; 4.5 m stretched × 2.5 cm = 80p (Robinsons—*Flexoplast®*; S&N—*Elastoplast®*)

Uses: securing dressings

For 5 cm width, see Elastic Adhesive Bandage, section 13.13.1

Permeable Non-woven Surgical Synthetic Adhesive Tape, BP. Backing of paper-based or non-woven textile material spread with a polymeric adhesive mass. 5 m (all): Associated Hospital Supply—*Scanpor®* (net price 1.25 cm = 34p, 2.5 cm = 54p, 5 cm = 96p); J&J—*Dermilite®* (1.25 cm = 40p, 2.5 cm = 60p, 5 cm = £1.13); 3M—*Micropore®* (1.25 cm = 43p, 2.5 cm = 67p, 5 cm = £1.19); S&N—*Hypal 2®* (1.25 cm = 40p, 2.5 cm = 62p, 5 cm = £1.13)

Where no brand stated by prescriber, net price of tape supplied not to exceed 34p (1.25 cm), 54p (2.5 cm), 96p (5 cm)

Uses: securing dressings; skin closures for small incisions

For patients with skin reaction to other plasters and strapping, requiring use for long periods

NHS Permeable Plastic Surgical Adhesive Tape, BP. Extensible perforated plastic film spread with an adhesive mass; permeable to air and water (most suppliers)

Uses: securing dressings and appliances; covering sites of infection; allows immersion in water without loss of adhesion

SEMIPERMEABLE SURGICAL ADHESIVE TAPES

NHS Semipermeable Waterproof Plastic Surgical Adhesive Tape, BP. Extensible water-impermeable, air and water-vapour permeable plastic film spread with an adhesive mass. (3M; J&J; S&N)

Uses: covering dressings and appliances where free passage of air and water-vapour but exclusion of water required; covering possible sites of infection; preparation of waterproof, microporous plastic wound dressings

OCCLUSIVE SURGICAL ADHESIVE TAPES

Impermeable Plastic Surgical Adhesive Tape, BP. Extensible water-impermeable plastic film spread with an adhesive mass. 2.5 cm × 1 m, net price = 34p; 3 m = 69p; 5 m = £1.04; 5 cm × 5 m = £1.34; 7.5 cm × 5 m = £1.92 (Robinsons; Seton; S&N)

Uses: securing dressings; covering site of infection where exclusion of air, water, and water vapour is required

Impermeable Plastic Surgical Synthetic Adhesive Tape, BP. Extensible water-impermeable plastic film spread with a polymeric adhesive mass. 5 m (both): net price, 2.5 cm = 99p; 5 cm = £1.88 (3M—*Blenderm®*)

Uses: isolating wounds from external environment; covering sites where total exclusion of water and water vapour required; securing dressings and appliances

13.13.3 Adhesive dressings

(also termed Island dressings)

PERMEABLE ADHESIVE DRESSINGS

NHS **Elastic Adhesive Dressing**, BP. Wound dressing or dressing strip, pad attached to piece of extension plaster, leaving suitable adhesive margin; both pad and margin covered with suitable protector; pad may be dyed yellow and may be impregnated with suitable antiseptic (see below); extension plaster may be perforated or ventilated (most suppliers)

Uses: general purpose wound dressing
Note. Permitted antiseptics are aminacrine hydrochloride, chlorhexidine hydrochloride (both 0.07–0.13%), chlorhexidine gluconate (0.11–0.20%); domiphen bromide (0.05–0.25%)

NHS **Permeable Plastic Wound Dressing**, BP. Consisting of an absorbent pad, which may be dyed and impregnated with a suitable antiseptic (see under Elastic Adhesive Dressing), attached to a piece of permeable plastic surgical adhesive tape, to leave a suitable adhesive margin; both pad and margin covered with suitable protector (most suppliers)

Uses: general purpose wound dressing, permeable to air and water

SEMIPERMEABLE ADHESIVE DRESSINGS

Semipermeable Waterproof Plastic Wound Dressing, BP. Consists of absorbent pad, may be dyed and impregnated with suitable antiseptic (see under Elastic Adhesive Dressing), attached to piece of semipermeable waterproof surgical adhesive tape, to leave suitable adhesive margin; both pad and margin covered with suitable protector. 8.5 cm × 6 cm, net price = 21p (S&N—*Airstrip®*)

Uses: general purpose waterproof wound dressing, permeable to air and water vapour

OCCLUSIVE ADHESIVE DRESSINGS

NHS **Impermeable Plastic Wound Dressing**, BP. Consists of absorbent pad, may be dyed and impregnated with suitable antiseptic (see under Elastic Adhesive Dressing), attached to piece of impermeable plastic surgical adhesive tape, to leave suitable adhesive margin; both pad and margin covered with suitable protector (most suppliers)

Uses: protective covering for wounds requiring an occlusive dressing

13.13.4 Surgical absorbents

Absorbent Cotton, BP. Carded cotton fibres of not less than 10 mm average staple length, available in rolls and balls. 25 g, net price = 36p; 100 g = 80p; 500 g = £2.85 (most suppliers). 25-g pack to be supplied when weight not stated

Uses: cleansing and swabbing wounds, pre-operative skin preparation, application of medicaments; supplementary absorbent pad to absorb excess wound exudate

Absorbent Cotton, Hospital Quality. As for absorbent cotton but lower quality materials, shorter staple length etc. 100 g, net price = 59p; 500 g = £1.88 (most suppliers) Drug Tariff specifies to be supplied only where specifically ordered

Uses: suitable only as general purpose absorbent, for swabbing, and routine cleansing of incontinent patients; not for wound cleansing

Gauze and Cotton Tissue, BP. Consists of absorbent cotton enclosed in absorbent cotton gauze type 12 or absorbent cotton and viscose gauze type 2. 500 g, net price = £3.79 (most suppliers)

Uses: absorbent and protective pad, as burns dressing on non-adherent layer

Gauze and Cotton Tissue (Drug Tariff). Similar to above. 500 g, net price = £2.90 (most suppliers) Drug Tariff specifies to be supplied only where specifically ordered

Uses: absorbent and protective pad, as burns dressing on non-adherent layer

Absorbent Lint, BPC. Cotton cloth of plain weave with nap raised on one side from warp yarns. 25 g, net price = 50p; 100 g = £1.49; 500 g = £6.40 (most suppliers). 25-g pack supplied where no quantity stated

Uses: external absorbent protective dressing

Absorbent Cotton Gauze, BP. Cotton fabric of plain weave, in rolls and as swabs (see below), usually Type 13 light, sterile. 90 cm (all) × 1 m, net price = 59p; 3 m = £1.24; 5 m = £1.91; 10 m = £3.73 (most suppliers). 1-m packet supplied when no size stated

Uses: pre-operative preparation, for cleansing and swabbing
Note. Drug Tariff also includes unsterilised absorbent cotton gauze, 25 m roll, net price = £8.55

Cellulose Wadding, BP. Delignified wood pulp bleached white, in multiple laminate form. 500 g, net price = £1.49 (most suppliers, including Robinsons—*Cellosene®*)

Uses: absorbing large volumes of fluid

Gauze and Cellulose Wadding Tissue, BP. Consists of thick layer of cellulose wadding enclosed in absorbent cotton gauze type 12 or absorbent cotton and viscose gauze type 2. 500 g, net price = £1.88 (most suppliers)

Uses: absorbing large volumes of fluid

NHS **Absorbent Muslin**, BP. Fabric of plain weave, warp threads of cotton, weft threads of cotton and/or viscose (most suppliers)

Uses: wet dressing, soaked in 0.9% sterile sodium chloride solution

NHS **Absorbent Cotton Ribbon Gauze**, BP. Cotton fabric of plain weave in ribbon form with fast selvedge edges (most suppliers)

Uses: post-surgery cavity packing for sinus, dental, throat cavities etc.

Absorbent Cotton and Viscose Ribbon Gauze, BP. Woven fabric in ribbon form with fast selvedge edges, warp threads of cotton, weft threads of viscose or combined cotton and viscose yarn, sterile. 5 m (both) × 1.25 cm, net price = 43p; 2.5 cm = 47p (most suppliers)

Uses: post-surgery cavity packing for sinus, dental, throat cavities etc.

Gauze Swab, BP. Consists of absorbent cotton gauze type 13 light or absorbent cotton and viscose gauze type 1 folded into squares or rectangles of 8-ply with no cut edges exposed. Sterile, 7.5 cm square, net price 5-pad packet = 21p; non-sterile, 100-pad packet = £3.58 (most suppliers)

Filmated Gauze Swab, BP. As for Gauze Swab, but with thin layer of Absorbent Cotton enclosed within. Non sterile, 10 cm × 10 cm, net price 100-pad packet = £4.47 (Vernon-Carus—*Cotfil®*)

Uses: general swabbing and cleansing

Non-woven Swab (Drug Tariff). Consists of non-woven viscose fabric folded 4-ply; alternative to gauze swabs type 13 light. Sterile, 7.5 cm square, net price 5-pad packet = 19p; non-sterile, 10 cm square, 100-pad packet = £2.49 (J&J—*Sofnet II®*)

Uses: general purpose swabbing and cleansing; absorbs more quickly than gauze

Non-woven Filmated Swab (Drug Tariff). Film of viscose fibres enclosed within non-woven viscose fabric folded 8-ply. 10 cm square, net price 100-pad packet = £3.32 (J&J—*Regal®*)

Uses: general purpose swabbing and cleansing

13.13.5 Wound dressing pads

Perforated Film Absorbent Dressing, BP. Low-adherence dressing consisting of 3 layers; wound-facing layer film of poly-(ethylene terephthalate) perforated in reg

---

ular pattern; absorbent middle layer of type 1 consists of non-woven bleached cotton and viscose fibres or mixture of these with polyacrylonitrile fibres; in type 2 (NHS) middle layer consists of bleached cotton fibres; backing layer of type 1 is apertured non-woven cellulose material; in type 2, the backing layer is identical with wound-facing layer. Type 1, 5 cm × 5 cm, net price, each = 7p; 10 cm × 10 cm = 15p; 20 × 10 cm = 28p (S&N—*Melolin*® (type 1); Kendall—*Telfa*® (type 2)). 5 cm size supplied where size not stated

Uses: dressing for post-operative and low exudate wounds; low adherence property and low absorption capacity

Knitted Viscose Primary Dressing, BP. (Drug Tariff title: Sterile Knitted Viscose Dressing). Warp knitted fabric manufactured from a bright viscose monofilament. 9.5 cm × 9.5 cm (both): type 1, net price = 20p; type 2 = 15p (J&J—*N-A Dressing*® (type 1); S&N—*Tricotex*® (type 2))

Uses: low adherence wound contact layer for use on ulcerative and other granulating wounds with superimposed absorbent pad

Sterile Dressing Pack (Drug Tariff specification 10). Contains gauze and cotton tissue pad, gauze swabs, absorbent cotton balls, absorbent paper towel, water repellent inner wrapper. Net price per pack = 48p

Sterile Dressing Pack with Non-woven Pads (Drug Tariff specification 35). Contains non-woven fabric covered dressing pad (*Surgipad*®), non-woven fabric swabs (*Sofnet II*®), absorbent cotton wool balls, absorbent paper towel, water repellent inner wrapper. Net price per pack = 49p

NHS* **Surgipad**®. Absorbent pad of absorbent cotton and viscose in sleeve of non-woven viscose fabric (J&J)

Uses: for heavily exuding wounds requiring frequent dressing changes

* Except in Sterile Dressing Pack with Non-woven Pads (see above)

NHS **Perfron**®. Absorbent pad consisting of alternate layers of absorbent cotton and crepe cellulose tissue, in sleeve of non-woven viscose fabric with coating of polypropylene (J&J)

Uses: low adherence pad for heavily exuding wounds; laminate structure delays strike through

NHS **Melolite**®. Absorbent fabric pad covered on both sides by polyethylene net (S&N)

Uses: primary dressing over clean sutured wounds, lacerations, and abrasions

NHS **Mesorb**®. Cellulose wadding pad with gauze wound contact layer and non-woven water repellent backing (Molnlycke)

Uses: post-operative dressing for heavily exuding wounds

NHS **Ete**®. Wound pad of rayon wadding with rayon silk wound contact layer stitched in chequered pattern (Molnlycke)

Uses: leg wounds, decubitus ulcers, minor burns, donor sites

NHS **Release II**®. Two layered knitted construction of bright viscose in non-woven, non-adherent sleeve. Pack of 100 (all): 5 cm × 5 cm, net price = £4.56; 10 cm × 10 cm = £10.53; 10 cm × 20 cm = £17.34 (J&J)

Uses: high absorbency, low adherence wound contact dressing

Charcoal cloth dressings

NHS **Actisorb**®. Woven fabric of activated charcoal sealed within spun-bonded porous nylon sleeve. Net price (each) 10.5 cm × 10.5 cm = £1.41; 19 cm × 10.5 cm = £2.73 (J&J)

NHS **Actisorb Plus**®. Knitted fabric of activated charcoal, with one-way stretch, with silver residues, within spun-bonded nylon sleeve. Net price (each) 10.5 cm × 10.5 cm = £1.32; 19 cm × 10.5 cm = £2.56 (J&J)

NHS **Carbonet**®. Activated charcoal dressing. 10 cm × 10 cm, net price, each = £1.39; 10 cm × 20 cm = £2.71 (S&N)

NHS **Carbosorb**®. Outer cover of non-woven polyester-nylon fabric, activated charcoal cloth layer bonded to outer cover and semipermeable polyurethane film contact layer (Seton)

NHS **Lyofoam C**®. Lyofoam sheet with layer of activated charcoal cloth and additional outer envelope of polyurethane foam. 10 cm × 10 cm, net price, each = 88p; 15 cm × 20 cm = £1.97 (Ultra)

Uses: to deodorise discharging, infected, malodorous wounds and ulcers

13.13.6 Tulle dressings

Non-medicated tulle dressings

Paraffin Gauze Dressing, BP. Fabric of leno weave, weft and warp threads of cotton and/or viscose yarn, impregnated with white or yellow soft paraffin; sterile. 10 cm × 10 cm, net price, each = 20p; pack of 10 pieces = £1.42 (most suppliers including J&J—*Paratulle*®; S&N—*Jelonet*®)

Uses: treatment of abrasions, burns, and other injuries of skin, and ulcerative conditions; post-operatively as penial and vaginal dressing and for sinus packing; heavier loading for skin graft transfer

Medicated tulle dressings

Chlorhexidine Acetate Gauze Dressing, BP. Fabric of leno weave, weft and warp threads of cotton and/or viscose yarn, impregnated with ointment containing chlorhexidine acetate; sterile. 5 cm × 5 cm, net price = 15p; 10 cm × 10 cm = 31p (J&J—*Serotulle*®; Roussel—*Clorhexitulle*®; S&N—*Bactigras*®)

PoM **Framycetin Sulphate Gauze Dressing**, BP. Fabric of leno weave, weft and warp threads of cotton, impregnated with ointment containing framycetin sulphate 1% in white soft paraffin containing 10% wool fat; sterile. 10 cm × 10 cm, net price = 24p (Roussel—*Sofra-Tulle*®)

PoM **Sodium Fusidate Gauze Dressing Sterile** (Drug Tariff). Leno weave cotton gauze impregnated with ointment containing sodium fusidate 2% in white soft paraffin and wool fat. 10 cm × 10 cm, net price = 22p (Leo—*Fucidin Intertulle*®)

Povidone-Iodine Fabric Dressing. Woven rayon dressing impregnated with povidone iodine ointment 10%. 5 cm × 5 cm, net price, each = 14p; 9.5 cm × 9.5 cm = 26p (J&J—*Inadine*®)

Uses: wound contact layer for abrasions and superficial burns; max. 4 dressings at same time

13.13.7 Semipermeable adhesive film

Semipermeable Adhesive Film, BP. Sterile, extensible, waterproof, water vapour-permeable polyurethane film coated with synthetic adhesive mass; transparent. Supplied in single-use pieces. Type 1: 10 cm × 10 cm, net price = 88p (S&N—*Opsite*®), Type 2: 10 cm × 12 cm, net price = 84p (3M—*Tegaderm*®). Type 3: 10.2 cm × 12.7 cm, net price = 82p (J&J—*Bioclusive*®)

Uses: post-operative dressing, donor sites, IV sites, superficial decubitus ulcers, amputation stumps, stoma care; protective cover to prevent skin breakdown

NHS **Transite Film Dressing**®. Primary exudate transfer film composed of two layers which allow excess exudate to pass to secondary absorbent dressing through fine slits which narrow again when exudation decreases. Pack of 10 (all): 10 cm × 10 cm, net price = 89p; 15 cm × 20 cm = £1.41; 30 cm × 40 cm = £2.67 (S&N)

Uses: donor sites; partial and full thickness burns

13.13.8 Gel and colloid dressings

Occlusive or semi-occlusive dressings which adhere to dry skin and interact with moisture in the wound to form a gel; may remain on a wound for up to 7 days.

NHS **Bard Absorption Dressing**®. A dry polysaccharide derivative in flake form which is mixed with water and applied directly into the wound. 60-g pack
Uses: treatment of wounds and ulcers.

NHS **Biofilm**®. Dressing with non-woven fibre backing; also in powder form for direct application into wound: 10 cm × 10 cm, net price 10 = £16.50; 20 cm × 20 cm, 5 = £28.50; powder, 10 sachets = £18.20 (CliniMed)

NHS **Comfeel Ulcus**®. Soft elastic pad consisting of carmellose sodium particles embedded in adhesive mass; smooth outer layer and polyurethane film backing; available as sheets, powder in plastic blister units and paste in tubes for direct application into the wound: 10 cm × 10 cm, net price 10 = £18.00; 15 cm × 15 cm, 5 = £19.10; 20 cm × 20 cm, 5 = £30.90; powder 6 g, 10 = £23.60; paste 50 g, each = £3.49 (Coloplast)

Debrisan®. Spherical beads of dextranomer packed in plastic castors, single-use sachets, paste or NHS pads. Beads sprinkled onto cleansed wound and covered with a suitable non-woven, adhesive, semi-occlusive covering, or sterile dressing. Alternatively paste or pad is applied and covered in similar manner. Beads, net price 4-g sachet = £1.99, 60 g = £29.75; paste in sachets, 4 × 10 g = £20.40; pads, 7 × 3 g = £19.88 (Pharmacia)
Uses: debriding agent to remove necrotic tissue

NHS **Dermiflex**®. Hydrocolloid dressing bonded to PVC foam 10.2 cm × 10.2 cm, net price, each = £1.95 (J&J)

NHS **Geliperm**®. Gel sheets, dry and wet forms; tubed granulated gel. Dry, 11 cm × 25 cm, net price, 6 sheets = £51.23; granulate, 20 g, 6 tubes = £20.82, 50 g, 6 tubes = £52.04. Wet, 10 cm × 10 cm, net price, 20 sheets = £39.00, 12 cm × 13 cm, 6 sheets = £25.62; 12 cm × 26 cm, 6 sheets = £51.23 (Geistlich)
Uses: wound and ulcer dressing, burns, donor sites

Granuflex®. Hydrocolloid wound contact layer bonded to plastic foam layer, with outer impermeable plastic film. 10 cm × 10 cm, net price each = £1.66; other sizes (NHS), 15 cm × 20 cm, 3 = £14.21, 20 cm × 20 cm, 3 = £17.58, 15 cm × 15 cm with adhesive foam border, 5 = £18.90; also Granuflex Paste (NHS), net price 30 g = £2.61 (Squibb Surgicare)
Uses: chronic ulcers, pressure sores, open wounds, debridement of wounds; powders and pastes used with sheet dressings to fill deep or heavily exuding wounds

Kaltostat®. (Drug Tariff title: Calcium Alginate Dressing, type 2). Calcium alginate fibre, flat non-woven pads, 5 cm × 5 cm, net price, each = 35p; other sizes (NHS), 7.5 cm × 12 cm, 50 = £41.50; 10 cm × 20 cm, 25 = £43.25; 15 cm × 25 cm, 25 = £79.50; wound packing, 2 g, 25 = £25.75 (BritCair)
Uses: haemostatic

NHS **Scherisorb**® **Gel.** A ready-mixed hydrogel containing Graft T® starch copolymer applied directly into the wound. 25-g sachet, net price 10 sachets = £15.10 (S&N)

Sorbsan® (Drug Tariff title: Calcium Alginate Dressing, type 1). Calcium alginate fibre, highly absorbent, flat non-woven pads, 5 cm × 5 cm, net price, each = 77p; other sizes (NHS) 10 cm × 10 cm, 10 = £19.50; 10 cm × 20 cm, 5 = £16.25; surgical packing 30 cm, 5 = £19.50; ribbon, 40 cm (+12.5-cm probe), 5 = £12.50 (Steriseal)
Uses: heavily to moderately exuding wounds

Varihesive®. Wafers containing gelatin 20%, pectin 20%, polyisobutylene 40%, carmellose sodium 20%. 10 cm × 10 cm, net price 5 dressings = £7.13 (Squibb Surgicare)
Uses: wound dressing for leg ulcers

NHS **Vigilon**®. Semi-permeable hydrogel sheets on a polyethylene mesh support. Sterile, 3 in × 6 in, net price 10 = £31.50, 4 in × 4 in, 10 = £31.50; non-sterile, 4 in × 4 in, 10 = £22.00, 13 in × 24 in, 2 = £38.80 (Seton)

13.13.9　Foam dressings

NHS **Polyurethane Foam Dressing**, BP. Absorbent foam dressing of low adherence; sterile. 7.5 cm × 7.5 cm, net price, 25 = £10.62; 10 cm × 10 cm, 25 = £12.58; 10 cm × 17.5 cm, 25 = £22.66; 15 cm × 20 cm, 20 = £23.16; 10 cm × 25 cm, 35 = £43.55; 25 cm × 30 cm, each = £2.80 (Ultra—*Lyofoam*®)
Uses: treatment of burns, decubitus ulcers, donor sites, granulating wounds

NHS **Allevyn**®. Hydrophilic polyurethane dressing; foam sheets with trilaminate structure, non-adherent wound contact layer, foam based central layer, bacteria and waterproof outer layer. 10 cm × 10 cm, each = £3.34 (S&N)
Uses: treatment of heavily exuding wounds, specifically venous leg ulcers

NHS **Silicone Foam Cavity Wound Dressing**, BP. Soft slightly absorbent wound dressing of low adherence prepared from fluid silicone elastomer base and tin (II) 2-ethylhexanoate by mixing thoroughly for 15 seconds immediately before use and allowing to expand to about 4 times its volume within the wound. Foam dressing, 20 g, net price = £5.10; 500 g = £83.43; foam sheeting, 10 cm × 15 cm, 10 = £44.20; 15 cm × 30 cm, 10 = £132.20; gel sheeting, 12 cm × 15 cm, 10 = £77.50 (Dow Corning—*Silastic*®)
Uses: in the managment of open granulating wounds such as pressure sores, abdominal wall breakdown, pilonidal sinus excision

13.14　Topical preparations for circulatory disorders

These preparations are used to improve circulation in conditions such as bruising, superficial thrombophlebitis, chilblains and varicose veins but are of little value. Chilblains are best managed by avoidance of exposure to cold; neither systemic nor topical vasodilator therapy is recommended. Sclerotherapy of varicose veins is described in section 2.13.

Rubefacients are described in section 10.3.2.

Akrotherm® (Napp)
Cream, acetylcholine chloride 0.2%, histamine 0.034%, cholesterol 1%. For chilblains. Net price 40 g = 87p
Additives: wool fat derivative, fragrance
Apply 3–4 times daily

Hirudoid® (Panpharma)
Cream, heparinoid 0.3% in a vanishing-cream basis. Net price 40 g = £1.90
Additives: hydroxybenzoates (parabens)
Gel, heparinoid 0.3%. Net price 40 g = £1.90
Additives: propylene glycol, fragrance
Apply up to 4 times daily in superficial soft-tissue injuries and varicose conditions

Lasonil® (Bayer)
Ointment, heparinoid 50 units, hyaluronidase 150 units/g. Net price 14 g = 38p; 40 g = £1.08
Additives: wool fat derivative
Apply 2–5 times daily in superficial tissue injuries and varicose conditions

Pernomol® (LAB)
Paint, camphor 10%, chlorbutol 2%, phenol 0.95%, soap spirit 34%, tannic acid 2.2%. For chilblains. Net price 2.5 ml (with applicator) = 65p
Additives: none as listed in section 13.1
Apply 3–4 times daily

Secaderm® (Radiol)
Salve (= ointment), colophony 26%, melaleuca oil 5.6%, phenol 2.4%, terebene 5.25%, turpentine oil 6%. For boils and chilblains. Net price 15 g = 63p
Additives: beeswax
Apply 1–2 times daily and cover with dressing

14: Immunological products and
VACCINES

In this chapter, immunisation is discussed under the following headings:

14.1 Active immunity
14.2 Passive immunity
14.3 Storage and use
14.4 Vaccines and antisera
14.5 Immunoglobulins
14.6 Vaccination programmes
14.7 International travel

14.1 Active immunity

Vaccines are designed to produce specific protection against a given disease. They may consist of

1. an attenuated form of an infective agent, as in the vaccines which are used against virus diseases such as rubella and measles, or BCG used against tuberculosis,
2. inactivated preparations of the virus (e.g. influenza vaccine) or bacteria (e.g. typhoid vaccine), or
3. extracts of or detoxified exotoxins produced by a micro-organism, e.g. tetanus vaccine.

Vaccines stimulate the production of protective antibodies and other components of the immune mechanism.

In the case of vaccines consisting of **living** agents, immunisation is generally achieved with a single dose, but 3 doses are required in the case of oral poliomyelitis vaccine. Live virus multiplies in the body and usually produces a durable immunity but not always as long as that of the natural infection. When two live virus vaccines are required (and are not available as a combined preparation) they should be given either simultaneously at different sites or with an interval of at least 3 weeks.

Inactivated vaccines usually require a primary series of doses of vaccine to produce an adequate antibody response and in most cases reinforcing or 'booster' injections are required. The duration of immunity following the use of inactivated vaccines varies from months to many years.

The health departments of the UK have issued a memorandum, *Immunisation against Infectious Disease* which describes the vaccines, immunoglobulins, and antisera in routine use in the UK; suggested schemes for immunisation in childhood are included and advice is given on storage, technique, and record keeping.

Immunisation against Infectious Disease can be obtained from:
DHSS Health Publications Unit
No. 2 Site
Manchester Road
Heywood
Lancs OL10 2PZ
Note. A new edition was published during 1988.

SIDE-EFFECTS. Some vaccines (e.g. poliomyelitis vaccines) produce very few reactions, while others (e.g. measles and rubella vaccines) may produce a very mild form of the disease. Some of the inactivated vaccines may produce mild discomfort at the site of injection and mild fever and malaise. Occasionally there are more serious untoward reactions and these should always be reported in the usual way to the CSM.

CONTRA-INDICATIONS. Most vaccines have some basic contra-indication to their use, and the manufacturer's leaflet should always be consulted. In general, vaccination should be postponed if a febrile illness or any active infection is present or suspected.

Some viral vaccines contain small quantities of antibiotics used in their production, such as neomycin or polymyxin or both. Vaccines may need to be withheld from individuals who are known to be sensitive to the antibiotic which it contains.

Live virus vaccines should never be routinely administered to pregnant women because of possible harm to the fetus. They should not be given to individuals with impaired immune responsiveness, whether occurring naturally or as a result of radiotherapy or treatment with corticosteroids or other immunosuppressive drugs. They should not be given to those suffering from malignant conditions or other tumours of the reticulo-endothelial system.

VACCINES AND AIDS. The DHSS has advised that HIV-positive subjects with or without symptoms can receive the following live vaccines as appropriate:
measles[1], mumps, polio[2], rubella;
and the following inactivated vaccines:
cholera, diphtheria, hepatitis B, pertussis, polio[2], tetanus, typhoid.
HIV-positive subjects should **not** receive:
BCG, yellow fever[3]

1. Consideration should be given to use of normal immunoglobulin after exposure to measles.
2. Virus may be excreted for longer periods than in normal subjects; contacts should be warned of this and of need for washing hands after changing a vaccinated infant's nappies; HIV-positive contacts are at greater risk than normal contacts.
   For HIV-positive symptomatic subjects inactivated polio vaccine can be used at discretion of clinician.
3. Insufficient evidence for advice on yellow fever in asymptomatic subjects.
Note. The above advice differs from that for other immunocompromised patients.

14.2 Passive immunity

Immunity with immediate protection against certain infective organisms can be obtained by injecting preparations made from the plasma of immune individuals with adequate levels of antibody to

Prices are **net**, see p. 1

the disease for which protection is sought. This passive immunity lasts only a few weeks; where necessary passive immunisation can be repeated.

Antibodies of human origin are usually termed *immunoglobulins*. The term *antiserum* is applied to material prepared in animals. Because of serum sickness and other allergic-type reactions that may follow injections of antisera, this therapy has been replaced wherever possible by the use of immunoglobulins. Reactions are theoretically possible after injection of human immunoglobulins but reports of such reactions are very rare.

14.3   Storage and use

Care must be taken to store all vaccines and other immunological products under the conditions recommended in the manufacturer's leaflet, otherwise the preparation may become denatured and totally ineffective. **Refrigerated storage** is usually necessary; many vaccines need to be stored at 2–8°C and not allowed to freeze. Opened multidose vials which have not been fully used should be discarded within one hour if no preservative is present (most live virus vaccines) or within 3 hours or at the end of a session (when vaccines containing a preservative are used but also including oral poliomyelitis vaccine).

Particular attention must be paid to the instructions on the use of diluents and ampoules of vaccine should always be adequately shaken before use to ensure uniformity of the material to be injected.

Note. The DHSS has advised against the use of jet guns for vaccination owing to the risk of transmitting bloodborne infections, such as AIDS.

14.4   Vaccines and antisera

AVAILABILITY OF VACCINES AND OTHER IMMUNOLOGICAL PRODUCTS. Anthrax, rabies (human diploid cell), smallpox (freeze-dried), and yellow fever vaccines, botulism antitoxin, and snake and scorpion venom antitoxins are available from local designated holding centres. Details of current arrangements with names, addresses, and telephone numbers of holding centres are given in:
The Health Service Supply Purchasing Guide, section D pp. 1101–1199
and
The Pharmaceutical Supplies Bulletin, volume 8, no. 5, Oct. 1985, 63/85

Enquiries for vaccines not available commercially can also be made to
DHSS
Room 423
14 Russell Square
London WC1B 5EP
telephone 01-636-6811 extn 3117/3236.
In Scotland information about availability of vaccines can be obtained from the Chief Administrative Pharmaceutical Officer of the local Health Board. In Wales enquiries should be directed to the Welsh Office, Cathays Park, Cardiff CF1 3NQ, telephone 0222 825111, extn 4658

and in Northern Ireland to the Department of Health and Social Services, Dundonald House, Belfast BT4 3FS, telephone 0232 63939 extn 2841.

For further details of availability, see under individual vaccines.

ANTHRAX VACCINE

An inactivated bacterial vaccine is available for anyone subject to heavy exposure to anthrax, such as those exposed to infected hides and carcasses and to imported bonemeal, fishmeal, and feeding stuffs. The vaccine is prepared from a culture of *Bacillus anthracis* and, following the primary course of injections, reinforcing doses should be given at about yearly intervals.

PoM Anthrax Vaccine
Dose: initial course 3 doses of 0.5 ml by intramuscular or deep subcutaneous injection at intervals of 3 weeks followed by a 4th dose after an interval of 6 months
Reinforcing doses: 0.5 ml annually
Available from local designated centres

BCG VACCINES

BCG (Bacillus Calmette-Guérin) is a live attenuated strain derived from bovine *Mycobacterium tuberculosis* which stimulates the development of hypersensitivity to *M. tuberculosis*. BCG vaccine should be given intradermally by operators skilled in the technique (see below); the percutaneous vaccine is **not** recommended.

After about 1 week a small swelling appears at the injection site which progresses to a papule or to a benign ulcer about 10 mm in diameter after 3 weeks and heals in 6–12 weeks. A dry dressing may be used if the ulcer discharges, but the air should **not** be excluded. The CSM has reported that serious reactions with BCG are uncommon and most often consist of prolonged ulceration or subcutaneous abscess formation due to faulty injection technique.

BCG is recommended for the following groups if negative for tuberculoprotein hypersensitivity:
contacts of those with active respiratory tuberculosis (children of immigrants in whose communities there is a high incidence of tubereulosis may be regarded as contacts—newborn infants need not be tested for sensitivity but should be vaccinated without delay);
children between their tenth and fourteenth birthdays (see schedule, section 14.6);
students (including those in teacher training colleges).
Apart from newborn infants any person being considered for BCG vaccination is first given a skin test for hypersensitivity to tuberculoprotein.
See section 14.1 for contra-indications.

PoM Bacillus Calmette-Guérin Vaccine. BCG
Vaccine, Dried Tub/Vac/BCG. A freeze-dried preparation of live bacteria of a strain derived from the bacillus of Calmette and Guérin.
Dose: 0.1 ml (infants under 3 months 0.05 ml) by intradermal injection
Available from District Health Authorities (also from Evans)

INTRADERMAL INJECTION TECHNIQUE. After swabbing with spirit and allowing to dry, skin is stretched between thumb and forefinger and needle inserted (bevel upwards) for about 2 mm into superficial layers of dermis (almost parallel with surface). Needle should be short with short bevel (can usually be seen through epidermis during insertion). Raised blanched bleb showing tips of hair follicles is sign of correct injection; 7 mm bleb ≡ 0.1 ml injection; if considerable resistance not felt, needle is removed and reinserted before giving more vaccine.

Injection site is at insertion of deltoid muscle (sites higher on arm more likely to lead to keloid formation); tip of shoulder should be avoided; in girls, for cosmetic reasons, upper and lateral surface of thigh may be preferred.

PoM **Bacillus Calmette-Guérin Vaccine, Isoniazid-Resistant.** A freeze-dried preparation of live bacteria of an isoniazid-resistant strain derived from the bacillus of Calmette and Guérin.

Dose: 0.1 ml (infants under 3 months 0.05 ml) by intradermal injection; for active immunisation of tuberculosis contacts receiving prophylactic treatment with isoniazid.

Available from Evans

PoM Bacillus Calmette-Guérin Vaccine, Percutaneous Tub/Vac/BCG(Perc). A preparation of live bacteria of a strain derived from the bacillus of Calmette and Guérin.

Dose: 0.02 ml by percutaneous administration but not recommended, see notes above.

Available from Evans

DIAGNOSTIC AGENTS. In the *Mantoux test* the initial diagnostic dose is 1 unit of tuberculin PPD in 0.1 ml by intradermal (intracutaneous) injection and in subsequent tests 10 and finally 100 units in 0.1 ml may be given. For routine pre-BCG skin-testing the 10-unit dose of tuberculin PPD is used. In the *Heaf test* (multiple puncture) a solution containing 100 000 units in 1 ml is used. For the *Tine, Imotest,* and other similar tests a special device impregnated with tuberculin is used.

PoM **Tuberculin PPD.** Prepared from the heat-treated products of growth and lysis of the appropriate species of mycobacterium, and containing 100 000 units/ml. Net price 1-ml amp = £4.47. Also available diluted 1 in 100 (1000 units/ml), 1 in 1000 (100 units/ml), and 1 in 10000 (10 units/ml). Net price 1 ml (all) = £1.69
Available from District Health Authorities

BOTULISM ANTITOXIN

A trivalent botulism antitoxin is available for the post-exposure prophylaxis of botulism and for the treatment of persons thought to be suffering from botulism. It specifically neutralises the toxins produced by *Clostridium botulinum* types A, B, and E. It is not effective against infantile botulism as the toxin (type A) is seldom, if ever, found in the blood in this type of infection.

Hypersensitivity reactions are a problem. It is essential to read the contra-indications, warnings, and details of sensitivity tests on the package insert. Prior to treatment checks should be made regarding previous administration of any antitoxin and history of any allergic condition, e.g. asthma,

hay fever, etc. All patients should be tested for sensitivity (diluting the antitoxin if history of allergy).

▼ PoM **Botulism Antitoxin.** A preparation containing the specific antitoxic globulins that have the power of neutralising the toxins formed by types A, B, and E of *Clostridium botulinum*.
Note. The BP title Botulinum Antitoxin is not used because the preparation currently available has a higher phenol content (0.45% against 0.25%).
Dose: prophylaxis, 20 ml by intramuscular injection as soon as possible after exposure; treatment, 20 ml by slow intravenous infusion followed by 10 ml 12 hours later if necessary, and further doses at intervals of 12–24 hours.
Available from designated holding centres

CHOLERA VACCINE

Cholera vaccine contains Inaba and Ogawa subtypes of *Vibrio cholerae*, Serovar O1. Although a certificate of vaccination (see p. 414) is still required for entry to some countries, it is now recognised that while cholera vaccine may provide some individual protection for about 6 months it cannot control the spread of the disease. Reinforcing injections are recommended every 6 months for those living in endemic areas.

Patients who travel in a country where cholera exists should be warned that attention to the hygiene of food and water is still essential, even after vaccination.

PoM **Cholera Vaccine** Cho/Vac. Net price 1.5-ml amp = £3.50; 10-ml vial = £5.57
Dose: first dose, as specified on the label, usually 0.5 ml by deep subcutaneous or intramuscular injection; second dose, after at least a week and preferably 4 weeks, 1 ml; CHILD 1–5 years 0.1 ml, second dose 0.3 ml, 5–10 years 0.3 ml, second dose 0.5 ml
Note. To minimise adverse local reactions, second and subsequent doses may be given intradermally in a volume of 0.2 ml (0.1 ml at two separate sites) when the subcutaneous dose is more than 0.5 ml, and 0.1 ml when the subcutaneous dose is 0.5 ml or less. Some countries, however, may be unwilling to accept travellers who have not received the subcutaneous dose.
Available from Wellcome

DIPHTHERIA VACCINES

Protection against diphtheria is essentially due to the presence in the blood stream of antitoxin, the production of which is stimulated by vaccines prepared from the toxin of *Corynebacterium diphtheriae*. These are more effective if adsorbed onto a mineral carrier, and adsorbed diphtheria vaccines are generally used for the routine immunisation of babies and given in the form of a triple vaccine, **adsorbed diphtheria, tetanus, and pertussis vaccine**. A dose of poliomyelitis vaccine, live (oral) is generally given at the time of each of the doses of the triple vaccine (see schedule, section 14.6). Adsorbed diphtheria and tetanus vaccine is used in place of the triple vaccine when it is decided not to immunise against whooping-cough.

A reinforcing dose of adsorbed diphtheria and tetanus vaccine is recommended at the age of school entry. This should preferably be given after an interval of at least 3 years from the last dose of the basic course.

Further reinforcing doses of diphtheria vaccine are not recommended as a routine except in the case of those who work in units where there is a potentially high risk of infection such as those employed in infectious disease units or microbiology laboratories. A dilute vaccine, adsorbed diphtheria vaccine for adults, is available for this purpose; the small quantity of diphtheria toxoid present in the preparation is sufficient to recall immunity in individuals previously immunised against diphtheria but whose immunity may have diminished with time. It is insufficient to cause the reactions that may occur when diphtheria vaccine of conventional formulation is used in adults, and may be given without prior Schick testing.

Diphtheria antitoxin is used for passive immunisation; it is prepared in horses therefore reactions are common after administration.

It is now only used in suspected cases of diphtheria (without waiting for bacteriological confirmation); tests for hypersensitivity should be first carried out.

It is no longer used for prophylaxis because of the risk of hypersensitivity; unimmunised contacts should be promptly investigated and given erythromycin prophylaxis (see section 5.1, table 2) and vaccine (see below).

Combined vaccines
With tetanus and pertussis (triple vaccine)
PoM **Adsorbed Diphtheria, Tetanus, and Pertussis Vaccine** DTPer/Vac/Ads. Prepared from diphtheria formol toxoid, tetanus formol toxoid, and pertussis vaccine with a mineral carrier (aluminium hydroxide).
Dose: primary immunisation of children, 0.5 ml by intramuscular or deep subcutaneous injection at 3 months followed by second dose after 6–8 weeks and third dose after 4–6 months (see schedule, section 14.6)
Available as **Trivax-AD®** (Wellcome). Net price 0.5-ml amp = 89p; 5-ml vial = £4.73
PoM **Diphtheria, Tetanus, and Pertussis Vaccine** DTPer/Vac. A mixture of diphtheria formol toxoid, tetanus formol toxoid, and pertussis vaccine. The adsorbed vaccine is preferred
Available as **Trivax**(®) (Wellcome). Net price 0.5-ml amp = 89p; 5-ml vial = £4.73

With tetanus only
PoM **Adsorbed Diphtheria and Tetanus Vaccine** DT/Vac/Ads. Prepared from diphtheria formol toxoid and tetanus formol toxoid with a mineral carrier (aluminium hydroxide).
Dose: primary immunisation of children omitting pertussis component, 0.5 ml by intramuscular or deep subcutaneous injection at 3 months followed by second dose after 6–8 weeks and third dose after 4–6 months (see schedule, section 14.6); reinforcement at school entry, 0.5 ml (see schedule, section 14.6)

Available from Wellcome (net price 0.5-ml amp = 77p; 5-ml vial = £3.34) and from Evans (net price 0.5-ml amp = 75p; 5-ml vial = £2.62)
PoM **Diphtheria and Tetanus Vaccine** DT/Vac/FT. A mixture of diphtheria formol toxoid and tetanus formol toxoid. The adsorbed vaccine is preferred
Available from Wellcome. Net price 5-ml vial = £3.34

Monovalent vaccines
PoM **Diphtheria Vaccine, Adsorbed** Dip/Vac/Ads. Prepared from diphtheria formol toxoid with a mineral carrier (aluminium hydroxide). Net price 0.5-ml amp = 75p
Note. Used only for contacts of a diphtheria case or carrier; immunised children under 10 years are given one dose of 0.5 ml, unimmunised children under 10 years are given three doses of 0.5 ml with an interval of 6–8 weeks between first and second doses and 4–6 months between second and third; adults and children over 10 years are given diphtheria vaccine for adults, adsorbed (see below).
Available from Wellcome

Dilute vaccine for adults
PoM **Diphtheria Vaccine for Adults, Adsorbed.** Dip/Vac/Ads for Adults. Net price 0.5-ml amp = £3.00
Dose: primary immunisation in patients over 10 years without prior Schick testing, three doses each of 0.5 ml by intramuscular or deep subcutaneous injection separated by intervals of 1 month; reinforcement, 0.5 ml
Note. Unimmunised adults and children over 10 years who are contacts of a diphtheria case or carrier are given the primary immunisation course; immunised adults and children over 10 years are given the reinforcement dose.
Available from distributor (Regent)

Antisera
PoM **Diphtheria Antitoxin** Dip/Ser.
Dose: prophylactic 500 to 2000 units by intramuscular injection (but no longer used, see notes above); therapeutic 10 000 to 30 000 units increased to 40 000 to 100 000 units in severe cases; doses of up to 30 000 units should be given intramuscularly but for those over 40 000 units a portion is given intramuscularly followed by the bulk of the dose intravenously after an interval of ½–2 hours
Note. Children require the same dose as adults, depending on the severity of the case.
Available from distributor (Regent) or stocks may be held by hospital pharmacies

HEPATITIS B VACCINE

Hepatitis B vaccine is an alum-adsorbed, inactivated hepatitis B virus surface antigen (HBsAg) vaccine. It is prepared from the plasma of human carriers or made biosynthetically using recombinant DNA technology. The vaccine is used in individuals at high risk of contracting hepatitis B.

In the UK high-risk groups include health care personnel and patients in units where there is a high incidence of hepatitis B or a direct risk of contact with contaminated human blood, and also certain family contacts of carriers. Similar persons in indirect contact with a source of infection and at a lower risk would be considered a lower priority group. Another group for whom vaccination is recommended is infants born to hepatitis B carriers or HBsAg-positive mothers, particularly if they are e antigen-positive or are without anti-e antibody. Active immunisation combined with hepatitis B immunoglobulin is started immediately after delivery.

It should be borne in mind that immunisation takes up to 6 months to confer adequate protection; the duration of immunity is thought to last for 3 to 5 years.

More detailed guidance is given in DHSS circular CMO(82)13/CNO(82)11. Vaccination does not eliminate the need for commonsense precautions for avoiding the risk of infection from known carriers by the routes of infection which have been clearly established, see DHSS circular CMO(84)11/CNO(84)7. Accidental inoculation of hepatitis B virus-infected blood into a wound, incision, needle-prick, or abrasion may lead to infection, whereas it is unlikely that indirect exposure to a carrier will do so.

Specific antihepatitis B virus immunoglobulin ('HBIG') is available for use with the vaccine in those accidentally infected and in infants (section 14.5).

PoM **H-B-Vax**® (MSD)
A suspension of hepatitis B surface antigen 20 micrograms/ml adsorbed onto alum. Net price 0.5-ml vial = £9.05; 1-ml vial = £12.07
Dose: by intramuscular injection (see note below), 3 doses of 1 ml, the second 1 month and the third 6 months after the first dose; CHILD birth to 10 years 3 doses of 0.5 ml; INFANTS born to HBsAg-positive mothers, 3 doses of 0.5 ml, first dose at birth with antihepatitis B immunoglobulin injection
Dialysis and immunocompromised patients, 3 doses of 2 ml (as two 1-ml doses at different sites)

▼ PoM **Engerix B**® (SK&F)
A suspension of hepatitis B surface antigen (prepared from yeast cells by recombinant DNA technique) 20 micrograms/ml adsorbed onto aluminium hydroxide. Net price 1-ml vial = £10.50
Dose: Adults and children, by intramuscular injection (see note below), 3 doses of 1 ml, the second 1 month and the third 6 months after the first dose; more rapid (e.g. for travellers), third dose 2 months after first dose with booster at 12 months; INFANTS born to HBsAg-positive mothers, 3 doses of 1 ml, first dose at birth with antihepatitis B immunoglobulin injection
Note. The deltoid muscle is the preferred site of injection in adults; the anterolateral thigh is the preferred site in infants and children. The paediatric doses for H-B-Vax and for Engerix B differ.

INFLUENZA VACCINES
While most viruses are antigenically stable, the influenza viruses A and B (especially A) are constantly altering their antigenic structure as indi-

cated by changes in the haemagglutinins (H) and neuraminidases (N) on the surface of the viruses. It is essential that influenza vaccines in use contain the H and N components of the prevalent strain or strains. Every year the World Health Organization recommends which strains should be included; the number of doses depends on the differences between the H and N components of the prevalent strains.

The recommended strains are grown in the allantoic cavity of chick embryos (therefore **contra-indicated** in those hypersensitive to eggs or feathers).

Since influenza vaccines will not control epidemics they are recommended only for persons at high risk, e.g. those with chronic disease of the cardiovascular, respiratory, renal, and endocrine systems, and those living in closed institutions where opportunites for contact and spread are great; the elderly in the above groups may be particularly vulnerable. In non-pandemic years immunisation is not recommended for Health Service staff, except for those at high risk.

Purified surface-antigen vaccines should be used in children aged 4–13 years (two doses with an interval of 4–6 weeks are recommended for primary vaccination of these high-risk groups); older children and adults may be vaccinated with surface-antigen or split virion vaccine.

PoM **Fluvirin**® (Servier)
Inactivated influenza vaccine, surface antigen. Net price 0.5-ml syringe = £4.50
Dose: 0.5 ml by deep subcutaneous or intramuscular injection

PoM **Influvac Sub-unit**® (Duphar)
Inactivated influenza vaccine, surface antigen. Net price 0.5-ml amp or syringe = £4.55; 5-ml vial = £41.45; 25-ml vial = £176.43
Dose: 0.5 ml by deep subcutaneous or intramuscular injection

PoM **MFV-Ject**® (Merieux)
Inactivated influenza vaccine (split virion vaccine). Net price 0.5-ml syringe = £4.52
Dose: 0.5 ml by deep subcutaneous or intramuscular injection

MEASLES VACCINE
Note. From 1st October 1988 Measles, Mumps, and Rubella Vaccine (Live) will replace Measles Vaccine for all eligible children. Single antigen measles vaccine will not be given routinely after this date; single antigen rubella vaccine **will** still be used for girls between their tenth and fourteenth birthdays and non-immune women.

Measles vaccine consists of a live attenuated strain of measles virus grown in chick-embryo fibroblast-tissue cultures (since it contains virtually no residual egg protein it is contra-indicated only in those known to suffer from severe hypersensitivity to egg protein with a history of the anaphylactoid type). It should be offered to all unprotected children from the second year of life and may be expected to produce a durable immunity (**important:** see note above).

Administration of measles vaccine to children may be associated with a mild measles-like syndrome with a measles-like rash and pyrexia which come on about a week after the injection of the vaccine. Much less commonly, convulsions and, very rarely, encephalitis have been reported as being associated with measles vaccines. Convulsions in babies are relatively common and may occur by chance following any immunisation procedure; they are certainly much less frequently associated with measles vaccine than with other conditions leading to febrile episodes.

Serious neurological complications following measles vaccine are extremely rare, perhaps of the order of 1 in 87 000 vaccinees and probably about 12–20 times less common than such complications associated with natural infections of measles, but it is difficult to get exact figures because of variable criteria of what is diagnosed as a serious neurological condition. Subacute sclerosing panencephalitis follows natural measles infection at a rate of approximately 5 to 10 cases for every million children who have developed measles. This condition may be associated with live measles vaccine at a rate of 0.5–1.0 case per million doses of vaccine distributed, and so it appears that measles vaccination to some extent protects against subacute sclerosing panencephalitis.

Measles vaccine may also be used in the control of outbreaks and should be offered to unprotected school and playstreet contacts within 3 days of exposure to infection (**important:** see note above).

Because of the generally poor uptake of measles vaccine in the second year of life, it would seem wise to offer the vaccine also to unprotected children at entry to playgroup, nursery, or primary school. Again it would seem sensible to offer vaccine to any child entering secondary school who has not had either a natural infection or a previous dose of vaccine.

Children with a personal history of convulsions, or whose parents or siblings (first-degree relatives) have a history of idiopathic epilepsy should be given suitable prophylactic treatment against febrile convulsions (see section 4.8.3) but simultaneous administration of specially diluted normal immunoglobulin is no longer recommended.

Children with partially or totally impaired immune responsiveness should not receive live vaccines (for advice on AIDS see p. 403). If they have been exposed to measles infection they should be given normal immunoglobulin (section 14.5).

For further contra-indications to live vaccines, see section 14.1

▼ PoM **Attenuvax**® (Morson)
Measles vaccine, live, Enders' Edmonston strain. Net price single-dose vial (with diluent) = £1.32
Dose: 0.5 ml by deep subcutaneous injection
PoM **Mevilin-L**® (Evans)
Measles vaccine, live, Schwarz strain. Net price single-dose vial (with diluent) = £1.32
Dose: 0.5 ml by deep subcutaneous or intramuscular injection

PoM **Rimevax**® (SK&F)
Measles vaccine, live, Schwarz strain. Net price single-dose vial (with diluent) = £1.31
Dose: 0.5 ml by deep subcutaneous or intramuscular injection

Combined vaccines
With mumps and rubella
See note above

MUMPS VACCINE

Mumps vaccine consists of a live attenuated strain of virus grown in chick-embryo tissue culture.
See section 14.1 for contra-indications.

PoM **Mumpsvax**® (Morson)
Mumps vaccine (Jeryl Lynn strain). Net price single-dose vial (with diluent) = £4.00
Dose: adults and children over 1 year, 0.5 ml by subcutaneous injection

Combined vaccines
With measles and rubella
See under Measles Vaccine

PERTUSSIS VACCINE
(Whooping-cough vaccine)
Pertussis vaccine is usually given combined with diphtheria and tetanus vaccine starting after the third month of life (see schedule, section 14.6) but may also be given as a monovalent vaccine.

Pertussis-containing vaccines may give rise to local reactions at the site of injection, mild pyrexia, and irritability. With some vaccines available in the early 1960s persistent screaming and collapse were reported but these reactions are rarely observed with the vaccines now available.

Convulsions and encephalopathy have been reported as rare complications, but such conditions may arise from other causes and be falsely attributed to the vaccine. The best estimate of risk to an apparently normal infant of suffering a severe neurological reaction after pertussis vaccine is about 1 in 100 000 injections; most of these reactions are prolonged febrile convulsions from which there is usually recovery without consequence. Neurological complications after whooping cough itself are considerably more common than after the vaccine.

As with any other elective immunisation procedure it is advisable to postpone vaccination if the child is suffering from any acute febrile illness, particularly if it is respiratory, until fully recovered. Minor infections without fever or systemic upset are not regarded as contra-indications. Vaccination should not be carried out in children who have:

a history of any severe local or general reaction, *including a neurological reaction*, to a preceding dose; or
a history of cerebral irritation or damage in the neonatal period, or who have suffered from fits or convulsions.

There are certain groups of children in whom whooping-cough vaccination is not absolutely contra-indicated but who require special consideration as to its advisability. These are:

children whose parents or siblings have a history of idiopathic epilepsy;
children with developmental delay thought to be due to a neurological defect; and
children with neurological disease.

For these groups the risk of vaccination may be higher than in normal children but the effects of whooping-cough may be more severe, so that the benefits of vaccination would also be greater. The balance of risk and benefit should be assessed with special care in each individual case.

Allergy is not a contra-indication to pertussis vaccine.

PoM Pertussis Vaccine Per/Vac. A sterile suspension of killed *Bordetella pertussis*. Net price 0.5-ml amp = 89p

Dose: primary immunisation if pertussis component has been omitted from earlier vaccinations, three doses each of 0.5 ml by intramuscular or deep subcutaneous injection, separated by intervals of 1 month (see section 14.6)

Available from Wellcome

Combined vaccines, see under Diphtheria Vaccines

PNEUMOCOCCAL VACCINE

A polyvalent pneumococcal vaccine is available for the immunisation of persons for whom the risk of contracting pneumococcal pneumonia is unusually high, for example patients who have had a splenectomy. It is effective in a single dose if the types of pneumonia in the community are reflected in the polysaccharides contained in the vaccine. Studies with other pneumococcal vaccines suggest that protection may last for 5 years. Revaccination should not be carried out because of the risk of adverse reactions. The vaccine should not be given to children under 2 years, in pregnancy, or when there is infection. It should be used with caution in cardiovascular or respiratory disease. Hypersensitivity reactions may occur.

PoM Pneumovax® (Morson)
Polysaccharide from each of 23 capsular types of pneumococcus
Dose: 0.5 ml by subcutaneous or intramuscular injection

POLIOMYELITIS VACCINE

There are two types of poliomyelitis vaccine, namely poliomyelitis vaccine, inactivated, and poliomyelitis vaccine, live (oral). The oral vaccine, consisting of a mixture of attenuated strains of virus types 1, 2, and 3 is at present generally used in the UK.

INITIAL COURSE. **Poliomyelitis vaccine, live (oral)** is given on 3 occasions, usually at the same time as routine immunisation against diphtheria, tetanus, and pertussis (see schedule, section 14.6).

The initial course of 3 doses should also be given to all unimmunised adults.

REINFORCEMENT. A reinforcing dose of oral poliomyelitis vaccine is recommended at school entry at which time children should also receive a reinforcing dose of diphtheria and tetanus vaccine. Oral poliomyelitis vaccine is also recommended at school leaving.

Vaccine-associated poliomyelitis and poliomyelitis in contacts or vaccinees are both rare, occurring about once in one to five million vaccinated persons. However, the contacts of a recently vaccinated baby should be advised of the necessity for personal hygiene, particularly of the need to wash their hands after changing the baby's napkins.

Contra-indications to the use of oral poliomyelitis vaccine include diarrhoea and immunodeficiency disorders (or household contacts of patients with immunodeficiency disorders). See section 14.1 for further contra-indications.

Poliomyelitis vaccine (inactivated) may be used for those in whom poliomyelitis vaccine (oral) is contra-indicated because of pregnancy or immunosuppressive disorders (for advice on AIDS see p. 403).

TRAVELLERS. Travellers to areas other than Australia, New Zealand, Europe, and North America should be given a full course of oral poliomyelitis vaccine if they have not been immunised in the past. Those who have not received immunisation within the last 10 years should be given a booster dose of oral poliomyelitis vaccine.

PoM Poliomyelitis Vaccine, Inactivated Pol/Vac (Inact). An inactivated suspension of suitable strains of poliomyelitis virus, types 1, 2, and 3. *Dose:* 0.5 ml or as stated on the label by deep subcutaneous or intramuscular injection; for primary immunisation 3 doses are required (see schedule, section 14.6)

Available from DHSS, Room 220, 14 Russell Square, London WC1B 5EP, telephone 01-636 6811, extn 3117/3236 *and* Scottish Home and Health Department, telephone 031-552 6255, extn 2162

Note. Should be ordered one dose at a time and only when required for use. Some brands currently available have a dose volume of 1 ml and a recommended dosage schedule of 4 doses for primary immunisation.

PoM Poliomyelitis Vaccine, Live (Oral) Pol/Vac (Oral)[1]. A suspension of suitable live attenuated strains of poliomyelitis virus, types 1, 2, and 3. Available in single-dose and 10-dose containers *Dose:* 3 drops from a multidose container or the total contents of a single-dose container; for primary immunisation 3 doses are required (see schedule, section 14.6)

Available from District Health Authorities (also from SK&F and Wellcome)

1. BP 1988 permits code OPV for vaccine in single doses provided it also appears on pack.

RABIES VACCINE

A human diploid cell **rabies vaccine** is now in use. It should be offered prophylactically to those at high risk—those working in quarantine stations, animal handlers, veterinary surgeons, and field workers who may be exposed to bites of wild animals. A detailed list is given in Health Circular HC(77)29. For *prophylactic* use the vaccine produces a good antibody response when given in a 2-dose schedule with an interval of one month between doses and a reinforcing dose after an interval of 6–12 months with further reinforcing doses every 1–3 years when required. Studies have shown that when this vaccine is administered into the gluteal region there is a poor response.

For *post-exposure treatment* of previously unvaccinated patients a course of injections should be started as soon as possible after exposure (days 0, 3, 7, 14, 30, and 90). The course may be discontinued if it is proved that the patient was not at risk. There are no known contra-indications to this diploid cell vaccine and its use should be considered whenever a patient has been attacked by an animal in a country where rabies is endemic, even if there is no direct evidence of rabies in the attacking animal. Antirabies immunoglobulin (section 14.5) should also be given.

Staff in attendance on a patient who is highly suspected of, or known to be suffering from, rabies should be offered vaccination. Four intradermal doses of 0.1 ml of human diploid cell vaccine (Merieux) given on the same day at different sites has been suggested for this purpose.

Advice on post-exposure vaccination and treatment of rabies is available from the Duty Medical Officer, Central Public Health Laboratory, Colindale Avenue, Colindale, London NW9 5HT, telephone 01-200 4400.

▼ PoM **Merieux Inactivated Rabies Vaccine®** (Merieux)

Freeze-dried human diploid cell rabies vaccine prepared from Wistar strain PM/WI 38 1503-3M. Single-dose vial with syringe containing diluent

Dose: prophylactic, 1 ml by deep subcutaneous injection, followed by a second dose after 1 month and a third after 6–12 months; also further reinforcing doses every 1–3 years depending on the risk of infection

Post-exposure, 1 ml on the first, third, seventh and fourteenth day and after 1 and 3 months

Staff in attendance, see notes above

Also available from local designated centres (special workers and post-exposure treatment)

RUBELLA VACCINE

The selective policy of protecting women of child-bearing age from the risks of rubella (German measles) in pregnancy has been extended to a policy of eliminating the circulation of rubella among young children. The existing rubella vaccination policy will therefore be reinforced by the mass vaccination of children of both sexes, using a combined measles, mumps, and rubella vaccine (see under Measles Vaccine).

Rubella vaccine is still recommended for pre-pubertal girls between their tenth and fourteenth birthdays and for seronegative women of child-bearing age (see schedule, section 14.6) as well as those who might put pregnant women at risk of infection (e.g. nurses and doctors in obstetric units).

Rubella vaccination should be avoided in early pregnancy, and women of child-bearing age should be advised not to become pregnant within 1 month of vaccination. However, despite active surveillance in the UK, the USA, and Germany, no case of congenital rubella syndrome has been reported following inadvertent vaccination shortly before or during pregnancy. There is thus no evidence that the vaccine is teratogenic, and termination of pregnancy following inadvertant vaccination should not be routinely recommended; potential parents should be given this information before making a decision about termination. For short-term interim contraception at the time of vaccination a long-acting progestagen injection (section 7.3.2) may be suitable.

Vaccine may conveniently be offered to previously unvaccinated and seronegative post-partum women. Again they must avoid pregnancy for 1 month. Immunising susceptible post-partum women a few days after delivery is important as far as the overall reduction of congenital abnormalities in the UK is concerned, for about 60% of these abnormalities occur in the babies of multiparous women.

Susceptible pregnant women who are exposed to rubella and who do not want therapeutic abortion may be offered normal immunoglobulin injection (section 14.5).

See section 14.1 for further contra-indications.

PoM **Rubella Vaccine, Live** Rub/Vac (Live). A freeze-dried suspension of a suitable live attenuated strain of rubella virus grown in suitable cell cultures.

Dose: 0.5 ml by deep subcutaneous injection (see schedule, section 14.6 and notes above)

Available as

PoM **Almevax®** (Wellcome)

Rubella vaccine, live, prepared from Wistar RA 27/3 strain propagated in human diploid cells. Net price single-dose amp with diluent = £2.38; 10-dose vial with diluent = £19.76

▼ PoM **Ervevax®** (SK&F)

Rubella vaccine, live, prepared from Wistar RA 27/3 strain propagated in human diploid cells. Net price single-dose vial = £2.30; 10-dose vial = £19.10 (both with diluent)

▼ PoM **Meruvax II®** (Morson)

Rubella vaccine, live, prepared from Wistar RA27/3 strain propagated in human diploid cells. Net price single-dose vial with diluent = £1.80

Combined vaccines
With measles and mumps
  See under Measles Vaccine

SMALLPOX VACCINE

Smallpox vaccination is no longer required routinely in the UK and other countries because global eradication of smallpox has now been achieved. The vaccine is offered to a small number of doctors and other health workers who may be called upon to deal with suspected cases of smallpox. Otherwise the only requirement for smallpox vaccination is for a few workers in institutions dealing with pox viruses. There is no requirement for smallpox vaccination of travellers.

Contra-indications to elective smallpox vaccine were pregnancy, babies under 1 year, illness at the time of vaccination, eczema in the vaccinees or in members of their households, and impaired immune responsiveness.

PoM**Smallpox Vaccine** Var/Vac. Consists of a suspension of live vaccinia virus grown in the skin of living animals, supplied in freeze-dried form with diluent

Dose: 0.05 ml by multiple pressure inoculation or through a single linear scratch not more than 2–3 mm long

Available free of charge from Virus Reference Laboratory, Central Public Health Laboratory, Colindale (01-200 4400, extn. 3207)

TETANUS VACCINES

(Tetanus toxoids)

Tetanus vaccines stimulate the production of the protective antitoxin. In general, adsorption on aluminium hydroxide, aluminium phosphate, or calcium phosphate improves antigenicity. Adsorbed tetanus vaccine is offered routinely to babies in combination with adsorbed diphtheria vaccine (DT/Vac/Ads) and more usually also combined with killed *Bordetella pertussis* organisms as a triple vaccine, adsorbed diphtheria, tetanus, and pertussis vaccine (DT Per/Vac/Ads), see schedule, section 14.6.

Of the monovalent tetanus vaccines adsorbed tetanus vaccine is again preferred to the plain vaccine. Adsorbed vaccine must not be given intradermally (intracutaneously).

In children, the triple vaccine not only gives protection against tetanus in childhood but also gives the basic immunity for subsequent reinforcing doses of tetanus vaccine at school entry and at school leaving and also when a potentially tetanus-contaminated injury has been received. Normally, tetanus vaccine should not be given unless more than 5 years have elapsed since the last reinforcing dose because of the possibility that hypersensitivity reactions may develop.

Active immunisation is important for persons in older age groups who may never have had a routine or complete course of immunisation when younger. In these persons a course of adsorbed tetanus vaccine may be given. Very rarely, tetanus has developed after abdominal surgery; patients awaiting elective surgery should be asked about tetanus immunisation and immunised if necessary.

For serious, potentially contaminated wounds antitetanus immunoglobulin injection (section

14.5) should be selectively used in addition to wound toilet, adsorbed tetanus vaccine, and benzylpenicillin or another appropriate antibiotic.

Monovalent vaccines

PoM**Adsorbed Tetanus Vaccine** Tet/Vac/Ads. Prepared from tetanus formol toxoid with a mineral carrier (aluminium hydroxide). Net price 0.5-ml amp = 59p; 5-ml vial = £3.21

Dose: 0.5 ml or as stated on the label, by intramuscular or deep subcutaneous injection followed after 6–8 weeks by a second dose and after a further 4–6 months by a third

Available from Evans and Wellcome. 0.5-ml amp and 5-ml vial

Available from Merieux (as **Tetavax®**). Net price 0.5-ml amp = 55p; 0.5-ml single-dose syringe = £1.20; 5-ml vial = £2.80

PoM**Tetanus Vaccine** Tet/Vac/FT. Tetanus formol toxoid. 0.5-ml amp and 5-ml vial

Dose: as for Adsorbed Tetanus Vaccine which is preferred (see notes above)

Available from Wellcome

Combined vaccines, see under Diphtheria Vaccines

TUBERCULOSIS VACCINES

see BCG Vaccines

TYPHOID VACCINE

Typhoid vaccination is no substitute for personal precautions in avoiding typhoid fever in countries where the disease is endemic; green salads and uncooked vegetables should be avoided and only fruits which can be peeled should be eaten. Only suitable bottled water, or water that has been boiled, or treated with sterilising tablets should be used for drinking purposes.

Typhoid vaccine (monovalent typhoid vaccine) is used. Local reactions, which consist of swelling, pain, and tenderness, appear about 2–3 hours after the subcutaneous or intramuscular injection of the vaccine. Systemic reactions which consist of fever, malaise, and headache may also occur and usually last for about 48 hours after injection. If severe reactions are experienced after the first dose intradermal (intracutaneous) injection may be preferred for the second dose, as these reactions are virtually absent when this route is used. Normally, 2 doses should be given at 4–6 weeks interval for primary immunisation, with reinforcing doses about every 3 years on continued exposure.

PoM**Typhoid Vaccine** Typhoid/Vac. A suspension of killed *Salmonella typhi* organisms. Net price 1.5-ml vial = £3.19

Dose: 0.5 ml by deep subcutaneous or intramuscular injection; CHILD 1–10 years 0.25 ml

Second dose after 4–6 weeks, 0.5 ml (or 0.1 ml by intradermal injection); CHILD 1–10 years 0.25 ml (or 0.1 ml by intradermal injection)

Available from Wellcome

TYPHUS VACCINE

The vaccine consists of formalin-inactivated *Rickettsia prowazekii* grown in the yolk sac of embryonated hens' eggs and is effective against louse-borne typhus. This vaccine is not necessary for travellers visiting countries where the disease is endemic if they will be staying in urban accommodation but it could be of value for those living in close personal contact with the indigenous population of such areas. The vaccine is no longer distributed in the United Kingdom but may be obtained on a named patient basis from the Commonwealth Serum Laboratories, Parkville 3052, Victoria, Australia.

WHOOPING-COUGH VACCINES

see Pertussis Vaccines

YELLOW FEVER VACCINE

Yellow fever vaccine consists of a live attenuated yellow fever virus (17D strain) grown in developing chick embryos. It should not be given to children under 9 months of age since there is a small risk of encephalitis. The vaccine should not be given during pregnancy or to those with impaired immune responsiveness, or who are sensitive to eggs. See section 14.1 for further contra-indications. Reactions are few. The immunity which probably lasts for life is officially accepted for 10 years starting from 10 days after primary vaccination and for a further 10 years immediately after revaccination.

PoM **Yellow Fever Vaccine, Live** Yel/Vac. A suspension of chick embryo proteins containing attenuated 17D strain virus
Dose: the volume indicated on the label by subcutaneous injection
Available (only to designated Yellow Fever Vaccination centres) as
PoM **Arilvax®** (Wellcome)
Freeze-dried yellow fever vaccine, live. 1-, 5-, and 10-dose vials (with diluent)

14.5   Immunoglobulins

Injection of immunoglobulins produces immediate protection. Foreign immunoglobulins (antisera) are frequently associated with hypersensitivity; this has led to virtual abandonment of animal antisera for passive protection and human immunoglobulins have taken their place.

There are essentially two types of human immunoglobulin preparation: human **normal immunoglobulin** and **specific immunoglobulins**.

AVAILABILITY. Normal immunoglobulin and the specific immunoglobulins are available from the Public Health Laboratory Service laboratories and Regional Blood Transfusion Centres in England and Wales with the exception of antitetanus immunoglobulin which is distributed through Regional Blood Transfusion Centres to hospital pharmacies or blood transfusion departments and is also available to general medical practitioners. Antirabies immunoglobulin is available from the Central Public Health Laboratory, London.

In Scotland all immunoglobulins are available from the Blood Transfusion Service. Antitetanus immunoglobulin is distributed by the Blood Transfusion Service to hospitals and general medical practitioners on demand.

Normal immunoglobulin injection and antitetanus immunoglobulin injection are also available commercially.

For further details of availability see under individual immunoglobulins.

NORMAL IMMUNOGLOBULIN

(Gamma Globulin)

Human **normal immunoglobulin injection** ('HNIG') is prepared from pools of at least 1000 donations of human plasma, available in liquid form or as a freeze-dried preparation for reconstitution. It is administered by intramuscular injection for the protection of susceptible contacts against hepatitis A virus (infective hepatitis), measles and, to a lesser extent, rubella.

Live virus vaccine should not normally be given until 3 months after a dose of normal immunoglobulin. Normal immunoglobulin should not be given for at least 2 weeks after a live virus vaccine, except in special circumstances (see below and section 14.7).

There are no suitable techniques available for growing **hepatitis A** (infective hepatitis) virus in quantities which would make vaccine preparation possible. Control depends on good hygiene and many studies have also shown the value of normal immunoglobulin in the prevention and control of outbreaks of this disease. It is recommended for controlling infection in contacts in closed institutions and also, under certain conditions, in school and home contacts and for travellers going to areas where the disease is highly endemic. The usual prophylactic dose by intramuscular injection for adults and children is 0.02–0.04 ml/kg. This usually gives immunological protection for 3 months; for longer periods of exposure or in areas of high endemicity, the dose is 0.06–0.12 ml/kg, repeated every 4–6 months on continued exposure.

Normal immunoglobulin may be used to modify or prevent **measles** in the few babies in whom an attack of measles must be avoided and in children in whom live measles vaccine is contra-indicated.

Normal immunoglobulin may lessen the likelihood of infection and fetal damage in pregnant women exposed to **rubella** for whom therapeutic abortion is unacceptable. The usual dose is 20 ml (two doses of 5–10 ml separated by a few days). For routine prophylaxis, see Rubella Vaccine.

For intramuscular use
PoM **Human Normal Immunoglobulin** (BPL)
Human normal immunoglobulin injection. 1.7-ml amp (250 mg); 5-ml amp (750 mg)

PoM **Gammabulin**® (Immuno)

Human normal immunoglobulin injection. Net price 2-ml vial = £3.20; 5-ml vial = £6.50; 10-ml vial = £11.00; 320-mg vial with 2 ml water for injections = £3.50

PoM **Kabiglobulin**® (KabiVitrum)

Human normal immunoglobulin injection 16%. Net price 2-ml amp = £3.40; 5-ml amp = £8.20

REPLACEMENT THERAPY

Special forms for intravenous administration are available for replacement therapy for patients with congenital agammaglobulinaemia and hypogammaglobulinaemia and for the treatment of idiopathic thrombocytopenic purpura.

▼ PoM **Gamimune-N**® (Cutter)

Human normal immunoglobin injection 5% in maltose 10% for intravenous infusion. Net price 10-ml vial = £7.80; 50-ml vial = £39.00; 100-ml vial = £75.00

▼ PoM **Intraglobin**® (Biotest)

Human normal immunoglobulin injection. Powder for reconstitution for intravenous use. Net price 250 mg = £4.00; 500 mg = £7.80; 2.5 g = £38.00 (all with solvent)

▼ PoM **Sandoglobulin**® (Sandoz)

Human normal immunoglobulin injection. Net price 1-, 3- and 6-g bottle with 33, 100, and 200 ml sodium chloride intravenous infusion 0.9% = £19.50, £46.80, and £93.60, respectively. Transfer needle and giving set with 3- and 6-g packs

SPECIFIC IMMUNOGLOBULINS

Specific immunoglobulins are prepared by pooling the blood of convalescent patients or of immunised donors who have recently been specifically boosted.

Although a hepatitis B vaccine is now available for those at high risk of infection, specific **anti-hepatitis B virus immunoglobulin** ('HBIG') is available for use in association with the vaccine for the prevention of infection in laboratory and other personnel who have accidentally become contaminated with hepatitis B virus, and in babies born to mothers who have become infected with this virus in pregnancy.

Following exposure to a rabid animal, specific **antirabies immunoglobulin**, if possible of human origin, should be injected at the site of the bite and also given intramuscularly. Rabies vaccine should also be given.

Antitetanus immunoglobulin of human origin ('HTIG') should be used selectively in addition to wound toilet, vaccine, and benzylpenicillin (or another appropriate antibiotic) for the more seriously contaminated wounds; it is rarely required for those with an established immunity in whom protection may be achieved by a reinforcing dose of vaccine if considered advisable. The administration of antitetanus immunoglobulin should be considered for patients not known to have received active immunisation (a) whose wound was sustained more than 6 hours before treatment was received and (b) with puncture wounds or wounds potentially heavily contaminated with tetanus spores, septic, or with much devitalised tissue. A dose of adsorbed tetanus vaccine should be given at the same time as the antitetanus immunoglobulin and the course of vaccine subsequently completed.

Other specific immunoglobulins include antivaricella/zoster immunoglobulin ('ZIG'), antiherpes simplex immunoglobulin and are in limited supply. Others are under study, but their availability and evaluation requires the cooperation of general practitioners to provide blood from patients who are convalescent from these and other specific viral infections in order to prepare specific immunoglobulin preparations.

PoM **Anti-HBs Immunoglobulin (Specific) Injection** See notes above

Available from the Central Public Health Laboratory (also from BPL)

PoM **Antirabies Immunoglobulin Injection.** Used for protection of persons who have been bitten by rabid animals or otherwise exposed to infection (see notes above)

Dose: 20 units/kg by intramuscular injection and infiltration around wounds

Available from the Central Public Health Laboratory (also from BPL)

PoM **Antitetanus Immunoglobulin Injection** Used for the protection of unimmunised persons when there is a specific risk of tetanus

Dose: by intramuscular injection, prophylactic 250 units, increased to 500 units if more than 24 hours have elapsed or there is risk of heavy contamination

Therapeutic, 30–300 units/kg (multiple sites)

Available from BPL and Wellcome (as Humotet®; net price 1-ml vial = £15.73)

PoM **Antivaccinia Immunoglobulin Injection.** Used to treat patients with generalised vaccinia or with localised vaccinial infection that endangers the eye (see notes above)

Available from Central Public Health Laboratories (also from BPL)

PoM **Anti-Varicella-Zoster Immunoglobulin Injection.** Used for protection of immuno-suppressed persons and neonates at risk.

Available from the Central Public Health Laboratory (also from BPL)

ANTI-D (Rh$_0$) IMMUNOGLOBULIN

Anti-D immunoglobulin is available to prevent a rhesus-negative mother from forming antibodies to fetal rhesus-positive cells which may pass into the maternal circulation during childbirth or abortion. It must be injected within 72 hours of the birth or abortion. The objective is to protect any further child from the hazard of haemolytic disease.

PoM **Anti-D (Rh₀) Immunoglobulin Injection.** See notes above

Dose: for rhesus-negative women, 500 units by intramuscular injection following birth of rhesus-positive infant; 250 units if before 20 weeks gestation; after transfusion, up to 5000 units

Note. Rubella vaccine may be administered in the post-partum period simultaneously with anti-D (Rh₀) immunoglobulin injection providing separate syringes are used and the products are administered into contralateral limbs. A blood test should be done not sooner than 8 weeks later to ensure that rubella antibodies have been produced. If blood transfusion was necessary vaccination should be delayed for 3 months.

Available from the Central Public Health Laboratory (also from BPL)

14.7   International travel

Note. For advice on malaria chemoprophylaxis, see section 5.4.1.

No particular immunisation is required for travellers to the United States, Europe, Australia, or New Zealand. In Non-European areas surrounding the Mediterranean, in Africa, the Middle East, Asia, and South America, certain special precautions are required.

Typhoid vaccine is indicated for travellers to those countries where typhoid is endemic but is no substitute for personal precautions. Green salads and uncooked vegetables should be avoided and only fruits which can be peeled should be eaten. Only suitable bottled water, or water that has been boiled, or treated with sterilising tablets should be used for drinking purposes. This advice also applies to cholera and other diarrhoeal diseases (including travellers' diarrhoea).

Long-term travellers to areas that have a high incidence of **poliomyelitis** or **tuberculosis** should be immunised with the appropriate vaccine; in the case of poliomyelitis previously vaccinated adults may be given a reinforcing dose of oral poliomyelitis vaccine. BCG vaccination is recommended for travellers proposing to stay for longer than one month in Asia, Africa, or Central and South America; it should preferably be given three months or more before departure.

Overland travellers to Asia and Africa and others at high risk may be given **normal immunoglobulin injection** (section 14.5) for protection against hepatitis A. It is preferable to complete active immunisation and wait 4 weeks before administering the immunoglobulin. An interval of 2 weeks is acceptable provided the immunoglobulin is given just before departure. If time is short, it can be given with any vaccine (including polio).

Although **cholera vaccine** is no substitute for personal hygiene it has some protective value for about 6 months in preventing individual infections. Some countries require evidence of vaccination, which can be provided in the form of a Certificate of Cholera Vaccination available from the DHSS. Stamped certificates supplied to general medical practitioners by Family Practitioner Committees (in Scotland by Health Boards) do not require to be authenticated by health authorities.

International Certificates of vaccination against **yellow fever** (section 14.4) are still required for travel to much of Africa and South America.

Meningococcal vaccine is recommended for travellers to the Sudan, Ethiopia, and Chad owing to an outbreak of group A meningococcal meningitis in these countries. The vaccine is available from Merieux and from SK&F on a named-patient basis.

The DHSS has issued two leaflets, *Before You Go* (SA 40) and *While You're Away* (SA 41) which can be obtained from travel agents or by telephoning 0800 555 777 (24-hour service); bulk copies may be ordered from:

DHSS Leaflets Unit
PO Box 21
Stanmore
Middx HA7 1AY

Before You Go provides details of vaccination requirements or recommendations country-by-country; further advice may be obtained from the DHSS memorandum, *Immunisation against Infectious Disease* (for details, see p. 403).

Vaccination requirements change from time to time, and information on the current requirements for any particular country may be obtained from the

DHSS,
Alexander Fleming House
London SE1 6BY
telephone 01-407 5522

Scottish Home and Health Department
St. Andrew's House
Edinburgh EH1 3DE
telephone 031-556 8501

Welsh Office
Cathays Park,
Cardiff CF1 3NQ
telephone Cardiff 825111

Department of Health and Social Services
Dundonald House
Upper Newtownards Road
Belfast BT4 3FS
telephone 0232 63939;

or from the embassy or legation of the appropriate country.

14.6 Vaccination programmes

The full details of the schedule set out below can be obtained from the DHSS memorandum *Immunisation Against Infectious Disease* (see section 14.1). The principal points are as follows:
1. The *basic course* is as set out below.
2. An *alternative basic course* which completes the protection against pertussis at an earlier age can be considered in the event of a whooping-cough epidemic. Three doses are given at monthly intervals commencing at 3 months of age; a booster dose of adsorbed diphtheria and tetanus vaccine is necessary at 12–18 months of age to

achieve a satisfactory level of immunity against diphtheria and tetanus.
3. There is no contra-indication to administration of pertussis vaccine to unimmunised older children in order to protect infants and siblings.

If the pertussis component has been omitted from earlier vaccinations 3 doses of pertussis vaccine can be given at monthly intervals to provide protection.

Where the basic course against diphtheria and tetanus is incomplete triple vaccine may be used to begin or complete the course against whooping-cough so that the infant is not given more injections than necessary.

Age	Vaccine	Interval	Notes
During the first year of life	DTPer/Vac/Ads *and* Pol/Vac (Oral) (1st dose)		The first doses should be given at 3 months of age. If pertussis vaccine is contra-indicated or the parents decline, DT/Vac/Ads should be given
	DTPer/Vac/Ads *and* Pol/Vac (Oral) (2nd dose)	Preferably after an interval of 6–8 weeks	
	DTPer/Vac/Ads *and* Pol/Vac (Oral) (3rd dose)	Preferably after an interval of 4–6 months	
During the second year of life	Meas/Vac (Live)		From 1st October 1988 replaced by Meas/Mump/Rub Vac (live)
At school entry or entry to nursery school	DT/Vac/Ads *and* Pol/Vac (Oral)	Preferable to allow an interval of at least 3 years after completing basic course	
Between 10th and 14th birthdays	BCG	Leave an interval of not less than 3 weeks between BCG and rubella vaccination	For tuberculin-negative children. For tuberculin-negative contacts at any age
Between 10th and 14th birthdays (girls only)	Rub/Vac (Live)		All girls of this age should be offered rubella vaccine regardless of a past history of an attack of rubella or administration of Meas/Mump/Rub Vac
On leaving school or before employment or entering further education	Pol/Vac (Oral) *or* Pol/Vac (Inact); *and* Tet/Vac/Ads		
Adult life	Pol/Vac (Oral) *or* Pol/Vac (Inact) if previously unvaccinated	3 doses at intervals of 4 weeks	No adult should remain unimmunised; reinforcing doses for travellers to countries where polio endemic and for health care workers in possible contact with polio
	Rub/Vac (Live) for susceptible women of child-bearing age		Women of child-bearing age should be tested for rubella antibodies and if sero-negative offered rubella vaccination. Pregnancy must be excluded and patient warned not to become pregnant for 1 month after
	Tet/Vac/Ads if previously unvaccinated	For previously unvaccinated adults: 2 doses at an interval of 6–8 weeks followed by a third dose 6 months later	

Note. Poliomyelitis vaccine, live (oral) is usually issued in 10-dose containers (although single-dose containers are also available). The vaccine should be stored unopened at 4° but once the containers are opened the vaccine may lose its potency however it is stored. For this reason any vaccine remaining in the containers at the end of an immunisation session should be discarded. There is particular need to conserve supplies of vaccines, which in any case are expensive. As far as possible immunisation sessions should therefore be arranged to avoid undue wastage of vaccines, although it is recognised that it will not always be possible to muster those to be vaccinated in groups of 10. The practicability of dispensing vaccines in smaller doses is being considered.

15: Drugs used in

ANAESTHESIA

This chapter describes briefly drugs used in anaesthesia in minor and major surgery. The reader is referred to other sources for more detailed information on techniques of anaesthesia. This chapter is divided into two sections: general anaesthesia (15.1) and local anaesthesia (15.2).

15.1 General anaesthesia

15.1.1	Intravenous anaesthetics
15.1.2	Inhalational anaesthetics
15.1.3	Anticholinergic premedication drugs
15.1.4	Sedative and analgesic peri-operative drugs
15.1.4.1	Opioid analgesics
15.1.4.2	Anxiolytics and neuroleptics
15.1.5	Muscle relaxants
15.1.6	Anticholinesterases used in surgery
15.1.7	Antagonists for central and respiratory depression
15.1.8	Antagonists for malignant hyperthermia

Note. The drugs in section 15.1 should be used only by experienced personnel and in premises where adequate resuscitative equipment is available.

MODERN ANAESTHETIC TECHNIQUE. It is now common practice to administer several drugs with different actions to produce a state of surgical anaesthesia with minimal risk of toxic effects. An intravenous agent is frequently used for induction, followed by maintenance with inhalational anaesthetics, perhaps supplemented by other drugs administered intravenously. Specific drugs are often used to produce muscular relaxation. Many of the agents used interfere with the reflex maintenance of spontaneous respiration and intermittent positive pressure ventilation by manual or mechanical means is commonly employed.

For certain procedures controlled hypotension may be required. Labetalol (see section 2.4), sodium nitroprusside (see section 2.5.1), and trimetaphan camsylate (see section 2.5.6) are used.

Beta-blockers (see section 2.4) may be used to control arrhythmias during anaesthesia.

Anaesthetists must know whether a patient is taking or has been taking corticosteroids as adrenal suppression may result in a failure to secrete cortisol (endogenous hydrocortisone) in response to surgical stress, usually evidenced by falls in arterial pressure during anaesthesia or in the immediate postoperative period.

For drug interactions of general anaesthetics, see Appendix 1 (section 15).

GAS CYLINDERS

Each gas cylinder bears a label with the name of the gas contained in the cylinder. The name or chemical symbol of the gas is stencilled in paint on the shoulder of the cylinder; the letters are not less than 9 mm high on cylinders up to and including 80 mm diameter, not less than 12 mm high on cylinders over 80 mm and up to and including 105 mm diameter, and 19 mm high on cylinders above 105 mm diameter. The name or chemical symbol of the gas is also clearly and indelibly stamped on the cylinder valve. The colours applied to the valve end of the cylinder extend down the cylinder to the shoulder; in the case of mixed gases the colours for the individual gases are applied in four segments, two for each colour. See table below.

Gas cylinders should be stored in a cool well-ventilated room, free from materials of a flammable nature.

No lubricant of any description should be used.

Name of gas	Symbol	Colour of cylinder body	Colour of valve end where different from body
Oxygen	O_2	Black	White
Nitrous oxide	N_2O	Blue	—
Cyclopropane	C_3H_6	Orange	—
Carbon dioxide	CO_2	Grey	—
Ethylene	C_2H_4	Violet	—
Helium	He	Brown	—
Nitrogen	N_2	Grey	Black
Oxygen and carbon dioxide mixture	$O_2 + CO_2$	Black	White and Grey
Oxygen and helium mixture	$O_2 + He$	Black	White and Brown
Oxygen and nitrous oxide mixture	$O_2 + N_2O$	Blue	Blue and White
Air (medical)	AIR	Grey	White and Black

British Standard 1319:1976; Medical gas cylinders, valves and yoke connections. The colours used for gas cylinders comply with specifications in British Standards 4800 and 5252.

15.1.1   Intravenous anaesthetics

Intravenous anaesthesics may be used alone to produce anaesthesia for short surgical procedures but are more commonly used for induction only. Intravenous anaesthetics are potent drugs which nearly all produce their effect in one arm-brain circulation time and can cause apnoea and hypotension, and so adequate resuscitative facilities **must** be available. Large doses should be avoided in obstetrics, as the drug may cross the placental barrier. The drugs are **contra-indicated** in any dose in patients in whom the anaesthetist is not confident to maintain the airway, for example if there are tumours in the pharynx or larynx. Extreme care is required in surgery of the mouth, pharynx, or larynx and patients with acute cardiovascular failure (shock) or fixed cardiac output. Patients with a full stomach present a hazard during induction since there is a danger of silent regurgitation.

Individual requirements vary considerably and the recommended dosage is only a guide. Smaller dosage is indicated in ill, shocked, or debilitated patients, while robust individuals may require more. The estimated dosage should be injected over 20 seconds and a further 20 to 30 seconds allowed to assess the effect before a supplementary dose is given. For tracheal intubation, induction should be followed by inhalational anaesthesia or by a neuromuscular blocking drug.

Thiopentone sodium (Intraval®) is the most widely used intravenous anaesthetic, but has no analgesic properties. Induction is generally smooth and rapid, but owing to the potency of the drug, overdosage with cardiorespiratory depression may occur. Aqueous solutions are unstable, particularly when exposed to air. The solution is alkaline and therefore irritant on misplaced injection outside the vein, while arterial injection is particularly dangerous. The usual strength used is 2.5% solution in water for injections.

Awakening from a moderate dose of thiopentone is rapid due to redistribution of the drug in the whole body tissues. Metabolism is, however, slow and some sedative effects may persist for up to 24 hours during which time the subject is particularly susceptible to the effects of alcohol. Repeated doses have a cumulative effect.

Methohexitone sodium (Brietal Sodium®) is less irritant to tissues than thiopentone; it is usually used in 1% solution. Recovery is marginally more rapid than in the case of thiopentone. Induction is less smooth with an incidence of hiccup, tremor, involuntary movements, and pain on injection.

Both thiopentone and methohexitone are **contra-indicated** in porphyria.

Etomidate (Hypnomidate®) is an induction agent associated with rapid recovery without hangover effect. It causes less hypotension than other agents. There is a high incidence of extraneous muscle movement and pain on injection. These effects can be minimised by premedication with a narcotic analgesic and use of larger veins. There is evidence that repeated doses of etomidate have an undesirable suppressant effect on adrenocortical function.

Propofol (Diprivan®) is associated with rapid recovery without hangover effect. There is sometimes pain on intravenous injection, but significant extraneous muscle movements do not occur.

Ketamine (Ketalar®) can be given by the intravenous or the intramuscular route, and has good analgesic properties when used in sub-anaesthetic dosage. The maximum effect occurs in more than one arm-brain circulation time. Muscle tone is increased and the airway is usually well maintained. There is cardiovascular stimulation and arterial pressure may rise with tachycardia. The main disadvantage is the high incidence of hallucinations and other transient psychotic sequelae, though it is believed that these are much less significant in children. The incidence can be reduced when agents such as droperidol or diazepam are also used. It is contra-indicated in patients with hypertension or in those with a history of mental illness. It is used mainly for paediatric anaesthesia, particularly when repeated administrations are required. Recovery is relatively slow.

TOTAL INTRAVENOUS ANAESTHESIA. This is a technique in which major surgery is carried out with all anaesthetic drugs being given intravenously. Respiration is controlled, the lungs being inflated with oxygen-enriched air. Muscle relaxant drugs are used to provide relaxation and prevent reflex muscle movements. The main problem to be overcome is the assessment of depth of anaesthesia in the paralysed ventilated patient.

THIOPENTONE SODIUM

Indications: induction of general anaesthesia; anaesthesia of short duration in minor surgical procedures

Cautions; Contra-indications; Side-effects: see notes above. Drug interactions: see Appendix 1 (section 15)

Dose: by intravenous injection, in fit premedicated adults, initially 100–150 mg (4–6 ml of 2.5% solution) over 10–15 seconds, repeated if necessary according to the patient's response after 20–30 seconds; *or* up to 4 mg/kg; CHILD, induction 4–8 mg/kg

By continuous intravenous infusion, as a 0.2–0.4% solution, according to the patient's response

PoM **Add-A-Med Thiopentone Sodium®** (IMS)
Injection, thiopentone sodium 2.5 g with 100 ml diluent to provide a 2.5% solution, net price per unit = £8.06; 5 g with 200 ml diluent to provide a 2.5% solution, net price per unit = £16.13

PoM **Intraval Sodium®** (M&B)
Injection 2.5%, powder for reconstitution, thiopentone sodium. Net price 500-mg amp = £1.49; 2.5-g vial = £4.10
Injection 5%, powder for reconstitution, thiopentone sodium. Net price 1-g amp = £1.79

Cautionary label wordings, see inside back cover Prices are **net**, see p. 1

PoM **Min-i-Mix Thiopentone Sodium**® (IMS)

Injection, thiopentone sodium 500 mg with diluent to provide a 2.5% solution on reconstitution. Net price per unit = £4.19

ETOMIDATE

Indications: induction of anaesthesia
Cautions; Side-effects: see notes above
Dose: by slow intravenous injection, 300 micrograms/kg; high-risk patients, 100 micrograms/kg/minute until anaesthetised (about 3 minutes)

PoM **Hypnomidate**® (Janssen)

Injection, etomidate 2 mg/ml in propylene glycol 35%. Net price 10-ml amp = £1.05

Concentrate injection, etomidate 125 mg (as hydrochloride)/ml. To be diluted before use. Net price 1-ml amp = £3.55

Note. Use only glass syringes, avoid contact with plastics

KETAMINE

Indications: induction and maintenance of anaesthesia
Cautions; Side-effects: see notes above
Dose: by slow intravenous injection, 1–2 mg/kg over 60 seconds, repeated according to the patient's response
By deep intramuscular injection, 4–10 mg/kg, repeated according to the patient's response

PoM **Ketalar**® (P-D)

Injection, ketamine 10 mg (as hydrochloride)/ml. Net price 20-ml vial = £3.42

Injection, ketamine 50 mg (as hydrochloride)/ml. Net price 10-ml vial = £6.90

Injection, ketamine 100 mg (as hydrochloride)/ml. Net price 5-ml vial = £6.33

METHOHEXITONE SODIUM

Indications: induction and maintenance of anaesthesia for short procedures; with other agents for more prolonged anaesthesia
Cautions; Side-effects: see notes above
Dose: by slow intravenous injection, usually as a 1% solution, 50–120 mg according to the patient's response at rate of 10 mg in 5 seconds; maintenance, 20–40 mg (2–4 ml of 1% solution) every 4–7 minutes; CHILD, induction approx. 1 mg/kg

PoM **Brietal Sodium**® (Lilly)

Injection, powder for reconstitution, methohexitone sodium. Net price 100 mg in 10-ml vial = 77p

Injection, powder for reconstitution, methohexitone sodium. Net price 500 mg in 50-ml vial = £2.00

Injection, powder for reconstitution, methohexitone sodium. Net price 2.5 g in 250-ml vial = £7.46

PROPOFOL

Indications: induction and maintenance of general anaesthesia
Cautions; Side-effects: see notes above
Dose: induction, *by intravenous injection*, 2–2.5 mg/kg; maintenance, *by intravenous infusion*, 100–200 micrograms/kg/minute

▼ PoM **Diprivan**® (ICI)

Injection (emulsion), propofol 10 mg/ml. 20-ml amp

15.1.2   Inhalational anaesthetics

Inhalational agents may be gases or volatile liquids. They can be used both for induction and maintenance of anaesthesia and may be used following induction with an intravenous agent (section 15.1.1).

Gaseous agents require suitable equipment for storage and administration. They may be supplied via hospital pipelines or from metal cylinders. In clinical use it is necessary to monitor flow rate. Volatile agents are usually administered using calibrated vaporisers, using air, oxygen, or nitrous oxide–oxygen mixtures as the carrier gas.

To prevent hypoxia gaseous agents must be given with adequate concentrations of oxygen.

Nitrous oxide is used for induction and maintenance of anaesthesia and, in sub-anaesthetic concentrations, for analgesia in a variety of situations. For anaesthesia it is commonly used in a concentration of 50 to 70% in oxygen as part of a balanced technique in association with other inhalational or intravenous agents. Nitrous oxide is unsatisfactory as a sole agent owing to lack of potency, but is useful as part of a sequence of drugs since it allows a significant reduction of dosage of other agents.

A mixture of nitrous oxide and oxygen containing 50% of each gas (Entonox®) is used to produce analgesia without loss of consciousness. Self-administration using a demand valve is popular and may be appropriate in obstetric practice, for changing painful dressings, as an aid to postoperative physiotherapy, and in emergency ambulances.

Nitrous oxide may have a deleterious effect if used in patients with an air-containing closed space since nitrous oxide diffuses into such a space with a resulting build up of pressure. This effect may be dangerous in the presence of a pneumothorax which may enlarge to compromise respiration. Exposure of patients to nitrous oxide for prolonged periods, either by continuous or intermittent administration, may result in megaloblastic anaemia due to interference with the action of vitamin B_{12}. For the same reason, exposure of anaesthetists and theatre staff to nitrous oxide should be minimised. Depression of white cell formation may also occur.

Halothane (Fluothane®) is a widely used volatile agent. Its advantages are that it is a potent agent, induction is smooth, the vapour is non-irritant, pleasant to inhale, and seldom induces coughing or breath-holding. The incidence of postoperative vomiting is low.

It is used for induction and maintenance of anaesthesia in major surgery with oxygen or nitrous oxide–oxygen mixtures. Concentrations of 2 to 4% may be used for induction, and 0.5 to 2% for maintenance.

Halothane causes cardiorespiratory depression and because of its potency is administered from calibrated vaporisers. Respiratory depression results in elevation of arterial carbon dioxide tension and perhaps ventricular dysrhythmias. Intermittent positive-pressure ventilation must be carried out with care as myocardial depression may follow increase in blood concentrations. Halothane depresses the cardiac muscle fibres and may cause bradycardia. The result is diminished cardiac output and fall of arterial pressure. There is also peripheral vasodilatation. Adrenaline infiltrations should be used with care as ventricular dysrhythmias may result.

Halothane produces moderate muscle relaxation, but this may be inadequate for major abdominal surgery and specific muscle relaxants are then used.

In a publication on findings confirming that *severe hepatotoxicity* can follow halothane anaesthesia the CSM has reported that this occurs more frequently after repeated exposures to halothane and has a high mortality. The risk of severe hepatotoxicity appears to be increased by repeated exposures within a short time interval, but even after a long interval (sometimes of several years) susceptible patients have been reported to develop jaundice. Since there is no reliable way of identifying susceptible patients the CSM recommends the following precautions prior to use of halothane:
1. a careful anaesthetic history should be taken to determine previous exposure and previous reactions to halothane;
2. repeated exposure to halothane within a period of at least 3 months should be avoided unless there are overriding clinical circumstances;
3. a history of unexplained jaundice or pyrexia in a patient following exposure to halothane is an absolute contra-indication to its future use in that patient.

Cyclopropane is a potent gas which may be used for induction and maintenance. It forms explosive mixtures with air and oxygen and is used in a closed-circuit system. Muscle relaxation is produced and muscle relaxant drugs are potentiated. Respiration is depressed but arterial blood pressure is usually well maintained. It is a useful induction agent in paediatric and obstetric practice but has lost popularity as a maintenance agent in major surgery because of its explosive properties. For major surgery it is best used in association with intermittent positive-pressure ventilation or the respiratory depressant action may result in elevation of arterial carbon dioxide tension with resultant ventricular dysrhythmias. Adrenaline infiltration should be avoided because of the danger of dysrhythmias. Recovery is rapid, though associated with postoperative vomiting and restlessness.

Trichloroethylene (Trilene®) is a weak anaesthetic agent and poor muscle relaxant, but a potent analgesic. In analgesic concentrations it can be used to supplement nitrous oxide–oxygen anaesthesia in major surgery. In a concentration of 0.35 to 1% it is without serious side-effects and its use is associated with cardiovascular stability. Arterial blood pressure does not change and ventricular dysrhythmias are rare if arterial carbon dioxide tension is not allowed to rise. It is inadvisable to administer adrenaline. Respiratory rate increases during trichloroethylene supplemented anaesthesia, but this can be controlled by judicious administration of narcotic analgesic drugs. Trichloroethylene can be used in low concentration to prevent awareness during nitrous oxide–oxygen anaesthesia with muscle relaxants.

Trichloroethylene is unsuitable as the sole agent for induction, the best results being obtained as a supplement to nitrous oxide–oxygen following premedication with narcotic analgesics and induction with an intravenous agent. Recovery is relatively slow and there is some postoperative vomiting. Administration should therefore be discontinued before the close of the operation.

Enflurane (Ethrane®) is a volatile anaesthetic agent similar to halothane, but it is less potent, about twice the concentration being necessary for induction and maintenance. Administration from a calibrated vaporiser is recommended.

Enflurane is a powerful cardiorespiratory depressant. Shallow respiration is likely to result in a rise of arterial carbon dioxide tension, but ventricular dysrhythmias are uncommon and it is probably safe to use adrenaline infiltrations. Myocardial depression may result in a fall in cardiac output and arterial hypotension.

Enflurane is usually given to supplement nitrous oxide–oxygen mixtures in concentrations of 1 to 3%. It is likely that enflurane does not cause liver dysfunction, possibly because only a small fraction of the drug is metabolised. The drug is often used in preference to halothane when repeated anaesthesia is required.

Isoflurane is an isomer of enflurane. It has a potency intermediate between that of halothane and enflurane, and even less of an inhaled dose is metabolised than with enflurane. Heart rhythm is generally stable during isoflurane anaesthesia, but heart-rate may rise, particularly in younger patients. Systemic arterial pressure may fall, due to a decrease in systemic vascular resistance and with less decrease in cardiac output than occurs with halothane. Respiration is depressed. Muscle relaxation is produced and muscle relaxant drugs potentiated.

Anaesthetic ether (diethyl ether) is a potent anaesthetic agent, but is no longer on the UK market. The vapour forms flammable and explosive mixtures with oxygen. Both induction and recovery from anaesthesia are slow, and there is a high incidence of nausea and vomiting. Cardiac rhythm is stable and adrenaline infiltration may be allowed. Arterial blood pressure is well maintained.

CYCLOPROPANE

Indications; Cautions; Side-effects: see notes above

Dose: using a suitable closed-circuit anaesthetic apparatus, for light *anaesthesia* 7–10% in oxygen, for moderate to deep anaesthesia 20–30%

ENFLURANE

Indications; Cautions; Side-effects: see notes above

Dose: using a specifically calibrated vaporiser, *induction*, increased gradually from 1% to 5% in air, oxygen, or nitrous oxide–oxygen, according to the patient's response

Maintenance, 1–3%

Ethrane® (Abbott)
Enflurane. 250 ml

HALOTHANE

Indications; Cautions; Side-effects: see notes above

Dose: using a suitable vaporiser, *induction*, increased gradually to 2–4% in oxygen or nitrous oxide–oxygen; CHILD 1.5–2%

Maintenance, 0.5–2%

Halothane (M&B)
Net price 250 ml = £10.49
Fluothane® (ICI)
Halothane. 250 ml. Net price 250 ml = £10.49

ISOFLURANE

Indications; Cautions; Side-effects: see notes above

Dose: using a specifically calibrated vaporiser, *induction*, increased gradually from 0.5% to 3%, in oxygen or nitrous oxide–oxygen

Maintenance, 1–2.5%

Forane® (Abbott)
Isoflurane. Net price 100 ml = £33.50

NITROUS OXIDE

Indications; Cautions; Side-effects: see notes above

Dose: using a suitable anaesthetic apparatus, a mixture with 20–30% oxygen for *induction* and *maintenance* of light anaesthesia

Analgesic, as a mixture with 50% oxygen, according to the patient's needs

TRICHLOROETHYLENE

Indications; Cautions; Side-effects: see notes above; must not be used with soda lime in closed circuits

Dose: maintenance of light anaesthesia, 0.5–1% as a supplement to nitrous oxide and oxygen

Analgesic, 0.35–0.5% using a suitable vaporiser

Trilene® (ICI)
Trichloroethylene. Net price 500 ml = £2.17

15.1.3   Anticholinergic premedication drugs

Anticholinergic premedication agents, usually atropine, hyoscine (scopolamine), or glycopyrronium (Robinul®), are used to dry bronchial and salivary secretions which are increased by intubation and the inhalational anaesthetics. They are also used to prevent excessive bradycardia and hypotension caused by halothane, cyclopropane, suxamethonium, and neostigmine. In some patients, especially the elderly, hyoscine may cause the central anticholinergic syndrome (excitement, ataxia, hallucinations, behavioural abnormalities, and drowsiness).

Atropine is the most commonly used. Intravenous administration immediately before anaesthesia or intramuscular injection (which should be given 30–60 minutes before the operation) is satisfactory.

Hyoscine is also an effective drying agent and provides a degree of amnesia. It produces less tachycardia than atropine.

Glycopyrronium bromide produces good drying of salivary secretions. When given intravenously it produces less tachycardia than atropine.

Phenothiazine derivatives have too little activity to be effective drying agents when used alone.

ATROPINE SULPHATE

Indications: drying secretions, reversal of excessive bradycardia; with neostigmine for reversal of competitive neuromuscular block

Cautions: cardiovascular disease

Side-effects: tachycardia; see also section 1.2

Dose: premedication, *by intravenous injection*, 300–600 micrograms immediately before induction of anaesthesia, and in incremental doses of 100 micrograms for the treatment of bradycardia

By intramuscular injection, 300–600 micrograms 30–60 minutes before induction; CHILD 20 micrograms/kg

For control of muscarinic side-effects of neostigmine in reversal of competitive neuromuscular block, *by intravenous injection*, 0.6–1.2 mg

PoM **Atropine** (Non-proprietary)
Tablets, atropine sulphate 600 micrograms. Net price 20 = £1.00
Injection, atropine sulphate 600 micrograms. Net price 1-ml amp = 30p
Note. Other strengths also available
Morphine and Atropine Injection—see under Morphine Salts (section 15.1.4.1)

GLYCOPYRRONIUM BROMIDE

Indications; Cautions; Side-effects: see under Atropine Sulphate

Dose: premedication, *by intramuscular or intravenous injection*, 200–400 micrograms, *or* 4–5 micrograms/kg to a max. of 400 micrograms; CHILD, *by intramuscular or intravenous injection*, 4–8 micrograms/kg to a max. of 200 micrograms; intra-operative use, *by intravenous injection*, as for premedication

For control of muscarinic side-effects of neostigmine in reversal of competitive neuromuscular block, *by intravenous injection*, 10–15 micrograms/kg with 50 micrograms/kg neostigmine; CHILD, 10 micrograms/kg with 50 micrograms/kg neostigmine

PoM **Robinul®** (Robins)
Injection, glycopyrronium bromide 200 micrograms/ml. Net price 1-ml amp = 59p; 3-ml amp = 99p
Robinul-Neostigmine —see section 15.1.6

HYOSCINE HYDROBROMIDE
(Scopolamine Hydrobromide)
Indications: drying secretions, amnesia
Cautions: see under Atropine Sulphate; may slow heart; avoid in the elderly (see notes above)
Dose: premedication, *by subcutaneous or intramuscular injection*, 200–600 micrograms 30–60 minutes before induction of anaesthesia, usually with papaveretum; CHILD 15 micrograms/kg

PoM **Hyoscine Injection,** hyoscine hydrobromide 400 micrograms/ml, net price 1-ml amp = 74p; 600 micrograms/ml, 1-ml amp = 74p
PoM **Papaveretum and Hyoscine Injection,** see under Papaveretum (section 15.1.4.1)

15.1.4 Sedative and analgesic peri-operative drugs

These drugs are given to allay the apprehension of the patient in the pre-operative period (including the night before operation), to relieve pain and discomfort when present, and to augment the action of subsequent anaesthetic agents. A number of the drugs used also provide some degree of pre-operative amnesia. The choice will vary with the individual patient, the nature of the operative procedure, the anaesthetic to be used and other prevailing circumstances such as outpatients, obstetrics, recovery facilities etc. The choice would also vary in elective and emergency operations.

For many procedures, particularly minor operations, premedication is omitted completely and in these circumstances antisialogogues will usually be given intraveneously, either with or just before the induction agent.

The most common premedicants are still the **opioid analgesics**, e.g. morphine, papaveretum, and pethidine given intramuscularly about an hour before operation, usually combined with an antisialogogue. Sometimes they are combined with a phenothiazine or droperidol. The main side-effects are respiratory depression, cardiovascular depression, and nausea and vomiting. The principal advantages are that opioid analgesics provide analgesia persisting into the operative period giving a reduced chance of awareness during anaesthesia with full doses of muscle relaxants.

Oral premedication is increasing in popularity using **benzodiazepines** such as diazepam, lorazepam, and temazepam. Trimeprazine is still used in children, although many anaesthetists prefer the same drugs that are used in adults, given on a weight basis. Atropine or hyoscine is often given orally to children, but may be given intravenously immediately before induction.

Diazepam is used to produce light sedation with amnesia. The 'sleep' dose shows too great an individual variation to recommend it for induction of anaesthesia, and while this variation exists with regard to its sedative effect, it is probably less marked with lower doses and of little clinical significance. It is particularly valuable in sub-anaesthetic doses to produce light sedation for unpleasant procedures or for operations under local anaesthesia, including dentistry; sub-anaesthetic doses allow retention of the pharyngeal reflexes while a local block is performed, and the resultant amnesia is such that the patient is unlikely to have any unpleasant memories of the procedure. Diazepam can also be used in a similar manner for endoscopy, with or without an opioid analgesic.

Preparations of diazepam in organic solvents (Valium®) are painful on intravenous injection and followed by a high incidence of venous thrombosis which may not be noticed until a week after the injection. They are also painful on intramuscular injection, and absorption from the injection site is erratic. An emulsion preparation of diazepam (Diazemuls®) is less irritant on intravenous injection and is followed by a negligible incidence of venous thrombosis, but it should not be given intramuscularly. Diazepam is also available as a rectal solution (Stesolid®).

Diazepam and related drugs are of particular value for sedation of patients in an intensive care unit, particularly those on ventilators. It can be given 4–6 hourly but dosage should be gradually reduced after some days to prevent delay in recovery, which can be caused by a build up of its metabolite. Since it has no analgesic action it is often given in conjunction with small doses of opiates.

Diazepam may on occasions cause marked respiratory depression and facilities for treatment of this are essential. Dental patients who are sitting in one position for a long time may develop hypotonia after diazepam and they should be warned about this possibility. Outpatients should be advised that this is a long-acting drug, and that a second period of drowsiness can occur 4–6 hours after its administration.

By virtue of its physical characteristics, diazepam can accumulate in the fetus and, particularly after the mother has been given large doses, babies can be born in a depressed state, with hypotonia and a tendency to develop hypothermia.

Temazepam has a shorter action and relatively more rapid onset than diazepam. Used orally in a dose of 10–30 mg as a premedicant, 45 to 60 minutes prior to surgery, anxiolytic and sedative effects are produced which continue for one and a half hours. After this period patients are usually fully alert but there may be residual drowsiness. It has proved useful as a premedicant in inpatient and day-case surgery.

Lorazepam produces more prolonged sedation than diazepam. In addition amnesia is commonplace. It is particularly useful when used as a premedicant the night prior to major surgery; sound sleep is assured when an oral dose of 1 to 5 mg is given. A further, smaller, dose the following morning will be required if any delay in the commencement of surgery is anticipated. Alternatively the first dose may be given in the early morning of the day of operation.

Midazolam (Hypnovel®) is a water-soluble benzodiazepine which is used in a similar manner to diazepam. Recovery is faster than with diazepam. The incidence of side-effects is low but the CSM has received reports of respiratory depression (sometimes associated with severe hypotension) following intravenous administration. A preparation containing 2 mg per ml has been made available to ensure easier titration of dosage.

Chlormethiazole has been used as an intravenous infusion to maintain sleep during surgery carried out under regional analgesia, including extradural block. It has no analgesic effect, little cardiac and respiratory depression, and may be used in elderly patients.

PREMEDICATION IN CHILDREN. Oral or rectal administration is preferred to injections where possible but is not altogether satisfactory. Oral **trimeprazine** is still used but when given alone it may cause postoperative restlessness when pain is present. An alternative is **diazepam**. Some anaesthetists prefer the use of adult regimens, with dosage on a weight basis. (For guidelines on dose calculation in children, see Prescribing for Children.)

INTRA-OPERATIVE ANALGESIA. Many of the conventional opioid analgesics are used to supplement general anaesthesia, usually in combination with nitrous oxide–oxygen and a muscle relaxant. Pethidine was the first to be used for this purpose but other drugs now available include alfentanil, fentanyl, levorphanol, meptazinol, nalbuphine, and phenoperidine. The longer-acting drugs morphine and papaveretum, although equally effective for this purpose, are not commonly used because of the problems of respiratory depression in the postoperative period.

Small doses of opioids given immediately before or with thiopentone will reduce the induction dose of the barbiturate and this is a popular technique in poor-risk patients. **Alfentanil** (Rapifen®) and **fentanyl** (Sublimaze®) are particularly useful in this respect because of their short duration of action although there may be some cumulation with large doses. Alfentanil may be employed as a continuous infusion during long procedures.

Repeated doses of intra-operative analgesics should be given with care, since not only may the respiratory depression persist into the postoperative period but it may become apparent for the first time postoperatively when the patient is away from immediate nursing attention. The specific opioid antagonist, naloxone, will immediately reverse this respiratory depression but the dose may have to be repeated. In clinical doses it will also reverse most of the analgesia. An alternative and equally acceptable approach is to use the specific respiratory stimulant, doxapram, which can be given in an infusion and which will not affect the opioid analgesia. The use of intra-operative opioids should be borne in mind when prescribing postoperative analgesics. In many instances they will delay the need for the first dose but caution is necessary since there may be some residual respiratory depression potentiated by the postoperative analgesic.

Fentanyl may produce severe respiratory depression, especially in patients with decreased respiratory function or when other respiratory depressant drugs have been given. Respiratory depression may be treated by artificial ventilation or be reversed by naloxone or doxapram. Alfentanil may also cause severe respiratory depression, especially when other respiratory depressant drugs have already been given; this may be reversed with naloxone.

Meptazinol (Meptid®) can be used for analgesia during or after operation. It is associated with nausea and vomiting, but is claimed to have a reduced incidence of respiratory depression.

For further notes on analgesics see section 4.7.

15.1.4.1 OPIOID ANALGESICS

ALFENTANIL
Indications: analgesia especially during short operative procedure and outpatient surgery; enhancement of anaesthesia
Cautions; Side-effects: see under Fentanyl and notes above
Dose: by intravenous injection, spontaneous respiration, adults, initially up to 500 micrograms over 30 seconds; supplemental, 250 micrograms
With assisted ventilation, adults and children, initially 30–50 micrograms/kg; supplemental, 15 micrograms/kg
By intravenous infusion, with assisted ventilation, adults and children, initially 50–100 micrograms/kg over 10 minutes *or* as a bolus, followed by maintenance of 0.5–1 micrograms/kg/minute

▼ **CD Rapifen®** (Janssen)
Injection, alfentanil 500 micrograms (as hydrochloride)/ml. Net price 2-ml amp = 74p; 10-ml amp = £3.39
Paediatric injection, alfentanil 100 micrograms (as hydrochloride)/ml. Net price 5-ml amp = 46p

FENTANYL

Indications: analgesia during operation, neuroleptanalgesia, enhancement of anaesthesia; respiratory depressant in assisted respiration

Cautions: chronic respiratory disease, myasthenia gravis; reduce dose in elderly, hypothyroidism, chronic liver disease; obstetric use may cause respiratory depression in neonate; see also notes above. Drug interactions: see section 4.7.2

Side-effects: respiratory depression, transient hypotension, bradycardia, nausea and vomiting

Dose: by intravenous injection, with spontaneous respiration, 50–200 micrograms, then 50 micrograms as required; CHILD 3–5 micrograms/kg
With assisted ventilation, 300–500 micrograms; CHILD 15 micrograms/kg

CD **Fentanyl Citrate** (Non-proprietary)
Injection, fentanyl 50 micrograms (as citrate)/ml, net price 2-ml amp = 45p; 10-ml amp = £2.05
CD **Sublimaze**® (Janssen)
Injection, fentanyl 50 micrograms (as citrate)/ml. Net price 2-ml amp = 45p; 10-ml amp = £2.05
CD **Thalamonal**® (Janssen)
Injection, fentanyl 50 micrograms (as citrate), droperidol 2.5 mg/ml. Net price 2-ml amp = 76p
Dose: premedication, by intramuscular injection 1–2 ml; induction, by intravenous injection 6–8 ml; CHILD, by intramuscular injection 0.4–1.5 ml

LEVORPHANOL TARTRATE

Indications: analgesia during operation; enhancement of anaesthesia

Cautions; Contra-indications; Side-effects: see section 4.7.2 and notes above

Dose: by subcutaneous, intramuscular, or intravenous injection, 250–500 micrograms, repeated to a max. of 1.5–2 mg

CD **Dromoran**® (Roche)
Injection, levorphanol tartrate 2 mg/ml. Net price 1-ml amp = 25p

MEPTAZINOL

Indications: analgesia during and after operation
Cautions; Contra-indications; Side-effects: see section 4.7.2 and notes above

Dose: by mouth, 200 mg every 3–6 hours as required
By intramuscular injection, 75–100 mg, repeated every 2–4 hours as required
By slow intravenous injection, 50–100 mg, repeated as above

▼ PoM **Meptid**® (Wyeth)
Tablets, orange, f/c, meptazinol 200 mg. Net price 20 = £2.85. Label: 2
Injection, meptazinol 100 mg (as hydrochloride)/ml. Net price 1-ml amp = 79p

MORPHINE SALTS

Indications: analgesia during and after operation; enhancement of anaesthesia; pre-operative sedation

Cautions; Contra-indications; Side-effects: see section 4.7.2 and notes above

Dose: by subcutaneous or intramuscular injection, up to 10 mg 1–1½ hours before operation; CHILD, *by intramuscular injection,* 150 micrograms/kg. See also section 4.7.2 for analgesia

CD **Morphine Sulphate Injection,** morphine sulphate, 10, 15 and 30 mg/ml. Net price 1- and 2-ml amp (all) = 35–62p
CD **Morphine and Atropine Injection,** morphine sulphate 10 mg, atropine sulphate 600 micrograms/ml. Net price 1-ml amp = 35p
Dose: by subcutaneous injection, 0.5–1 ml

NALBUPHINE HYDROCHLORIDE

Indications: peri-operative analgesia
Cautions; Contra-indications; Side-effects: see section 4.7.2 and notes above; also caution in ambulant patients (impairment of mental and physical ability)

Dose: by subcutaneous, intramuscular, or intravenous injection, 10–20 mg, adjusted according to response

▼ PoM **Nubain**® (Du Pont)
Injection, nalbuphine hydrochloride 10 mg/ml. Net price 1-ml amp = 75p; 2-ml amp = £1.16

PAPAVERETUM

The hydrochlorides of alkaloids of opium, containing the equivalent of anhydrous morphine 47.5–52.5%, anhydrous codeine 2.5–5%, noscapine 16–22%, and papaverine 2.5–7%

Indications: analgesia during and after operation; enhancement of anaesthetics; pre-operative sedation

Cautions; Contra-indications; Side-effects: see section 4.7.2 and notes above

Dose: acute pain, *by subcutaneous or intramuscular injection,* 20 mg repeated every 4 hours if necessary (10 mg for lighter patients); CHILD up to 1 month 150 micrograms/kg, 1–12 months 200 micrograms/kg, 1–12 years 200–300 micrograms/kg

By slow intravenous injection, ¼–½ corresponding subcutaneous or intramuscular dose

Pre-operative sedation, *by subcutaneous or intramuscular injection,* 10–20 mg 45–60 minutes before anaesthesia; CHILD single doses as above

Note: Papaveretum 20 mg is approximately equivalent to morphine 12.5 mg

CD **Papaveretum Injection,** papaveretum 10 mg/ml, net price 1-ml amp = 27p; 20 mg/ml, 1-ml amp = 31p
CD **Papaveretum and Hyoscine Injection,** papaveretum 20 mg, hyoscine hydrobromide 400 micrograms/ml. Net price 1-ml amp = 30p
Dose: by subcutaneous or intramuscular injection, 1 ml
CD **Omnopon**® (Roche)
Injection, papaveretum 20 mg/ml. Net price 1-ml amp = 13p
Paediatric injection, papaveretum 10 mg/ml. Net price 1-ml amp = 13p

---

Cautionary label wordings, see inside back cover

Prices are **net**, see p. 1

CD Omnopon-Scopolamine® (Roche)
Injection, papaveretum 20 mg, hyoscine hydrobromide 400 micrograms/ml. Net price 1-ml
amp = 14p
Dose: by subcutaneous or intramuscular injection, 1 ml

PETHIDINE HYDROCHLORIDE

Indications: peri-operative analgesia, enhancement of anaesthesia, for basal narcosis with
phenothiazines
Cautions; Contra-indications; Side-effects: see section 4.7.2 and notes above
Dose: premedication, *by intramuscular injection*,
50–100 mg 1 hour before operation; CHILD
1–2 mg/kg
Adjunct to nitrous oxide–oxygen, *by
intravenous injection*, 10–25 mg repeated when
required

CD Pethidine Injection, pethidine hydrochloride
50 mg/ml, net price 1-ml amp = 11p; 2-ml amp =
14p; 10 mg/ml, 5-ml amp = 45p; 10-ml amp =
49p

CD Pamergan P100® (Martindale)
Injection, pethidine hydrochloride 50 mg, promethazine hydrochloride 25 mg/ml. Net price
2-ml amp = 35p
Dose: 2 ml by intramuscular injection or,
diluted to 10 ml, by intravenous injection, 1–1½
hours before operation; CHILD, by intramuscular injection, 8–12 years 0.75 ml, 13–16
years 1 ml

PHENOPERIDINE HYDROCHLORIDE

Indications: analgesia during operation, neuroleptanalgesia, enhancement of anaesthetics;
respiratory depressant in prolonged assisted
respiration
Cautions; Contra-indications; Side-effects: see
under Pethidine Hydrochloride and Fentanyl.
Doses above 1 mg cause respiratory depression
and require assisted ventilation (effects may be
terminated with naloxone or doxapram)
Dose: by intravenous injection, with spontaneous
respiration, 0.5–1 mg, then 500 micrograms
every 40–60 minutes as required; CHILD 30–50
micrograms/kg
With assisted ventilation, 2–5 mg, then 1 mg as
required; CHILD 100–150 micrograms/kg

CD Operidine® (Janssen)
Injection, phenoperidine hydrochloride 1 mg/
ml. Net price 2-ml amp = 64p; 10-ml amp =
£3.35

15.1.4.2 ANXIOLYTICS AND NEUROLEPTICS

CHLORMETHIAZOLE EDISYLATE

Indications: sedative during regional anaesthesia
Cautions; Side-effects: see section 4.8.2
Contra-indications: acute pulmonary insuf-
ficiency

Dose: by intravenous infusion, 25 ml (200 mg)/
minute for 1–2 minutes; maintenance 1–4 ml
(8–32 mg)/minute

PoM Heminevrin® (Astra)
Intravenous infusion 0.8%, chlormethiazole
edisylate 8 mg/ml. Net price 500-ml bottle =
£5.25

CHLORPROMAZINE HYDROCHLORIDE

Indications: see under Dose
Cautions; Contra-indications; Side-effects: see
section 4.2.1
Dose: induction of hypothermia (to prevent
shivering), *by deep intramuscular injection*, 25–
50 mg every 6–8 hours; CHILD 1–12 years,
initially   0.5–1 mg/kg,   maintenance
500 micrograms/kg every 4–6 hours

PoM Largactil® (M&B)
Injection, chlorpromazine hydrochloride 25 mg/
ml. Net price 2-ml amp = 27p

DIAZEPAM

Indications: premedication; sedation with
amnesia, and in conjunction with local
anaesthesia
Cautions; Side-effects: see notes above and section 4.1.2
Dose: by mouth, 5 mg at night, 5 mg on waking,
and 5 mg 2 hours before minor or dental surgery
By slow intravenous injection, 10–20 mg over 2–
4 minutes as sedative cover for minor surgical
and medical procedures; premedication 100–
200 micrograms/kg
By rectum in solution, adults and children over
3 years 10 mg; CHILD 1–3 years and elderly
patients 5 mg

Oral and rectal preparations: see section 4.1.2

Parenteral preparations
PoM Diazemuls® (KabiVitrum)
Injection (emulsion), diazepam 5 mg/ml. For
intravenous injection or infusion. See Appendix
2. Net price 2-ml amp = 44p
PoM Stesolid® (CP)
Injection, diazepam 5 mg/ml. See Appendix 2.
Net price 2-ml amp = 25p
PoM Valium® (Roche)
Injection, diazepam 5 mg/ml. See Appendix 2.
Net price 2-ml amp = 26p

DROPERIDOL

Indications: anti-emetic, pre-operative sedation;
neuroleptanalgesia
Cautions; Contra-indications; Side-effects: see
notes above and section 4.2.1
Dose: premedication, *by intramuscular injection,*
up to 10 mg 60 minutes before operation; CHILD
200–500 micrograms/kg
Neuroleptanalgesia, *by intravenous injection,*
5–15 mg at induction with a narcotic analgesic;
CHILD 200–300 micrograms/kg

PoM **Droleptan**® (Janssen)
Injection, droperidol 5 mg/ml. Net price 2-ml
amp = 70p
Thalamonal®—see under Fentanyl (section
15.1.4.1)

LORAZEPAM

Indications: sedation with amnesia; as premedication
Cautions; Side-effects: see under Diazepam
Dose: by mouth, 1–3 mg at night *or* 1–5 mg 2–6
hours before surgery
By slow intravenous injection, preferably diluted
with an equal volume of sodium chloride intravenous infusion 0.9% or water for injections,
50 micrograms/kg
By intramuscular injection, diluted as above, 50
micrograms/kg 1–1½ hours before operation

Oral preparations: see section 4.1.2

Parenteral preparations
PoM **Ativan**® (Wyeth)
▼ *Injection*, lorazepam 4 mg/ml in solvent. Net
price 1-ml amp = 40p

MIDAZOLAM

Indications: sedation with amnesia, and in conjunction with local anaesthesia; premedication,
induction
Cautions; Side-effects: see under Diazepam; see
notes above for CSM warning. Drug interactions: see Appendix 1 (section 4.1)
Dose: sedation, *by slow intravenous injection*, 70
microgram/kg until patient becomes drowsy;
usual dose range 2.5 to 7.5 mg (2.5 mg in elderly
patients)
Premedication, *by intramuscular injection*,
70–100 micrograms/kg 30–60 minutes before
surgery; usual dose 5 mg (2.5 mg in elderly
patients)
Induction, *by slow intravenous injection*, 200–
300 micrograms/kg (elderly patients, 100–200
micrograms/kg)

▼ PoM **Hypnovel**® (Roche)
Injection, midazolam 2 mg (as hydrochloride)/
ml. Net price 5-ml amp = 83p
Injection, midazolam 5 mg (as hydrochloride)/
ml. Net price 2-ml amp = 70p

PERPHENAZINE

Indications: anti-emetic, pre-operative sedation
Cautions; Contra-indications; Side-effects: see
section 4.2.1
Dose: premedication, *by intramuscular injection*,
5 mg 1 hour before operation

PoM **Fentazin**® (A&H)
Injection, perphenazine 5 mg/ml. Net price 1-ml
amp = 15p

PROMETHAZINE HYDROCHLORIDE

Indications: anti-emetic, pre-operative sedative
and anticholinergic agent
Cautions; Side-effects: see section 4.6 and notes
above
Dose: premedication, *by mouth,* CHILD 1–5 years
15–20 mg, 6–10 years 20–25 mg
By deep intramuscular injection, 25–50 mg 1 hour
before operation; CHILD 5–10 years, 6.25–
12.5 mg

Preparations
See section 3.4.1

TEMAZEPAM

Indications: premedication before minor
surgery; anxiety before investigatory
procedures
Cautions; Side-effects: see under Diazepam
Dose: see notes above

Preparations
See section 4.1.1

TRIMEPRAZINE TARTRATE

Indications: pre-operative sedation, anti-emetic
Cautions: avoid alcohol. See also notes above
and section 3.4.1
Side-effects: drowsiness, dryness of the mouth,
allergic skin reactions
Dose: premedication, 3–4.5 mg/kg 1–2 hours
before operation; CHILD 2–7 years 2–4 mg/kg

Preparations
See section 3.4.1

15.1.5 Muscle relaxants

Muscle relaxants used in anaesthesia are also
known as **neuromuscular blocking drugs** or
myoneural blocking drugs. By specific blockade
of the neuromuscular junction they enable light
levels of anaesthesia to be employed with
adequate relaxation of the muscles of the abdomen and diaphragm. They also relax the vocal
cords and allow the passage of a tracheal tube.
Their action differs from the muscle relaxants
acting on the spinal cord or brain which are used
in musculoskeletal disorders (see section 10.2.2).

Patients who have received a muscle relaxant
should **always** have their respiration assisted or
controlled until the drug has been inactivated
or antagonised (section 15.1.6). As depolarising
relaxants may cause painful muscle spasm they
should be given after induction of anaesthesia.

NON-DEPOLARISING MUSCLE
RELAXANTS

Drugs of this group (also known as competitive
muscle relaxants) cause blockade by competing
with acetylcholine at the receptor site at the
neuromuscular junction. These drugs are best
suited to the production of paralysis of long duration. They have a slower, less complete action than
the depolarising muscle relaxants and should be
avoided in myasthenia gravis.

These drugs may be used during surgical operations and for patients receiving long-term ventilation in intensive care units, when larger total doses will be appropriate.

The action of the competitive muscle relaxants may be reversed with anticholinesterases such as neostigmine (section 15.1.6).

Tubocurarine may be regarded as the standard non-depolarising muscle relaxant but in recent years its use has declined. It starts to act between 3–5 minutes and lasts for about 30 minutes after injection. It may cause an erythematous rash on the chest and neck and this is probably due to histamine release. Onset of blockade may be associated with hypotension and this, though transient, may be important in poor-risk patients.

Pancuronium (Pavulon®) has the advantages of a quicker onset of action and of not causing significant histamine release or significant changes in blood pressure; there is no evidence that it causes ganglionic blockade.

Gallamine (Flaxedil®) has a more rapid onset of action and recovery than tubocurarine or pancuronium. It causes undesirable tachycardia by its vagolytic action. It should be avoided in patients with severe renal disease as it is excreted via the kidneys.

Alcuronium (Alloferin®) appears to have no significant advantages over tubocurarine or pancuronium. Its duration of action is similar to tubocurarine.

Atracurium (Tracrium®) has a duration of action of 15 to 35 minutes. Histamine release may occur. The drug is without vagolytic or sympatholytic properties. It has an advantage over other non-depolarising muscle relaxants in patients with renal or hepatic impairment, as it is degraded by non-enzymatic Hofmann elimination, which is independent of liver and kidney function. It is non-cumulative on repeated dosage. Its action is reversed by neostigmine. Duration of action may be prolonged in hypothermia.

Vecuronium (Norcuron®) is a recently introduced muscle relaxant with a duration of action of 20 to 30 minutes. Large doses may have a cumulative effect. The drug does not cause histamine release, sympathetic blockade, or vagolytic effects.

ALCURONIUM CHLORIDE

Indications: non-depolarising muscle relaxant of medium duration
Cautions; Side-effects: see notes above. Reduce dose in renal impairment. Drug interactions: see Appendix 1 (section 15)
Dose: by intravenous injection, initially 200–250 micrograms/kg, then incremental doses of one-sixth to one-quarter of the initial dose, as required; CHILD, 125–200 micrograms/kg

PoM **Alloferin**® (Roche)
Injection, alcuronium chloride 5 mg/ml. Net price 2-ml amp = 58p

ATRACURIUM BESYLATE

Indications: non-depolarising muscle relaxant of medium duration
Cautions: see notes above; inactivated by thiopentone and other alkaline solutions. Drug interactions: see Appendix 1 (section 15)
Side-effects: see notes above
Dose: by intravenous injection, initially 300–600 micrograms/kg, then 100–200 micrograms/kg repeated as required
By intravenous infusion, 5–10 micrograms/kg/ minute (300–600 micrograms/kg/hour)

▼ PoM **Tracrium**® (Calmic)
Injection, atracurium besylate 10 mg/ml. Net price 2.5-ml amp = £1.43; 5-ml amp = £2.75

GALLAMINE TRIETHIODIDE

Indications: non-depolarising muscle relaxant of medium duration
Cautions; Side-effects: see notes above. Drug interactions: see Appendix 1 (section 15)
Dose: by intravenous injection, 80–120 mg, then 20–40 mg as required; CHILD, 1.5 mg/kg

PoM **Flaxedil**® (M&B)
Injection, gallamine triethiodide 40 mg/ml. Net price 2-ml amp = 44p

PANCURONIUM BROMIDE

Indications: non-depolarising muscle relaxant of medium duration
Cautions; Side-effects: see notes above; caution where tachycardia could be dangerous. Reduce dose in obesity and in renal impairment. Drug interactions: see Appendix 1 (section 15)
Dose: by intravenous injection, initially for intubation 50–100 micrograms/kg then 10–20 micrograms/kg as required; CHILD initially 60–100 micrograms/kg, then 10–20 micrograms/ kg, neonate 30–40 micrograms/kg initially then 10–20 micrograms/kg
Intensive care, *by intravenous injection*, 60 micrograms/kg every 1–1½ hours; *by intramuscular injection*, 30–60 micrograms every 1–2 hours

PoM **Pavulon**® (Organon-Teknika)
Injection, pancuronium bromide 2 mg/ml. Net price 2-ml amp = 67p

TUBOCURARINE CHLORIDE

Indications: non-depolarising muscle relaxant of medium to long duration
Cautions; Side-effects: see notes above. Reduce dose in renal impairment. Drug interactions: see Appendix 1 (section 15)
Dose: by intravenous injection, 20–45 mg according to circumstances; CHILD, average initial dose of between 300–500 micrograms/kg

PoM **Jexin**® (DF)
Injection, tubocurarine chloride 10 mg/ml. Net price 1.5-ml amp = 71p

PoM **Tubarine Miscible**® (Calmic)
Injection, tubocurarine chloride 10 mg/ml. Net price 1.5-ml amp = £1.28

VECURONIUM BROMIDE

Indications: non-depolarising muscle relaxant of short to medium duration

Cautions; Side-effects: see notes above. Drug interactions: see Appendix 1 (section 15)

Dose: by intravenous injection, initially 80–100 micrograms/kg, then 30–50 micrograms/kg as required; CHILD, as adult dose (onset more rapid)

By intravenous infusion, 50–80 micrograms/kg/ hour

PoM **Norcuron**® (Organon-Teknika)
Injection, powder for reconstitution, vecuronium bromide. Net price 10-mg vial = £3.12 (with water for injections)

DEPOLARISING MUSCLE RELAXANTS

Suxamethonium is the only commonly used drug of this group. With a 5-minute duration of action it is the ideal agent for passage of a tracheal tube but may be used in repeated dosage for longer procedures.

It acts by mimicking the action of acetylcholine at the neuromuscular junction but causes blockade. Depolarisation is prolonged since disengagement from the receptor site and subsequent breakdown is slower than for acetylcholine.

It produces rapid, complete, and predictable paralysis, and recovery is spontaneous. Unlike the non-depolarising muscle relaxants its action cannot be reversed and clinical application is therefore limited.

Paralysis is usually preceded by muscle fasciculation. There is a transient rise in plasma potassium and creatine phosphokinase and there may be muscle pains postoperatively. Suxamethonium is **contra-indicated** in severe liver disease and in burned patients. Premedication with atropine is desirable.

Prolonged muscle paralysis may occur in patients with low or atypical plasma pseudocholinesterase enzymes. Prolonged paralysis may also occur in **dual block,** which occurs after repeated doses of suxamethonium have been used and is caused by the development of a non-depolarising block following the primary depolarising block. Artificial ventilation should be continued until muscle function is restored. Dual block is diagnosed by giving a short-acting anticholinesterase such as edrophonium; if an improvement occurs the block is treated with neostigmine (section 15.1.6).

SUXAMETHONIUM CHLORIDE

Indications: depolarising muscle relaxant of short duration

Cautions; Side-effects: see notes above. Drug interactions: see Appendix 1 (section 15)

Dose: by intravenous injection, 20–100 mg, according to the patient's needs. CHILD, initially 1–1.5 mg/kg, then ⅓rd of the initial dose

By intravenous infusion, as a 0.1% solution, 2–5 mg/minute (2–5 ml/minute)

PoM **Anectine**® (Calmic)
Injection, suxamethonium chloride 50 mg/ml. Net price 2-ml amp = 50p
PoM **Scoline**® (DF)
Injection, suxamethonium chloride 50 mg/ml. Net price 2-ml amp = 31p

15.1.6 Anticholinesterases used in surgery

Anticholinesterase drugs reverse the effects of the non-depolarising (competitive) muscle relaxant drugs such as tubocurarine but they prolong the action of the depolarising muscle relaxant drug suxamethonium.

Edrophonium (Tensilon®) has a transient action and is used to diagnose dual block caused by suxamethonium (section 15.1.5).

Neostigmine has a longer duration of action than edrophonium. It is the specific drug for reversal of non-depolarising (competitive) blockade. It acts within one minute of intravenous injection and lasts for 20 to 30 minutes; a second dose may then be necessary. A suitable dose is 1 mg per 20 kg body-weight. It is also used in the treatment of dual block.

Atropine or **glycopyrronium** (section 15.1.3) should be given before or with neostigmine in order to prevent bradycardia, excessive salivation, or other muscarinic actions of neostigmine. Suitable doses are 0.6 to 1.2 mg of atropine sulphate or 600 micrograms of glycopyrronium intravenously.

For drugs used in myasthenia gravis see section 10.2.1.

EDROPHONIUM CHLORIDE

Indications: brief reversal of non-depolarising neuromuscular blockade; diagnosis of dual block (section 15.1.5)

Cautions; Side-effects: see section 10.2.1 and notes above. Atropine should also be given

Dose: reversal of blockade, *by intravenous injection,* 10 mg (after or with atropine sulphate 0.6–1.2 mg), repeated at intervals of 10 minutes according to the patient's response

Diagnosis of dual block, *by intravenous injection,* 10 mg (with atropine)

PoM **Tensilon**® (Roche)
Injection, edrophonium chloride 10 mg/ml. Net price 1-ml amp = 27p

NEOSTIGMINE METHYLSULPHATE

Indications: reversal of non-depolarising neuromuscular blockade

Cautions; Side-effects: see section 10.2.1 and notes above. Atropine should also be given

Dose: by intravenous injection, 1–5 mg *or* 1 mg/20 kg, after or with atropine sulphate 0.6–1.2 mg

PoM **Prostigmin**® (Roche)
Injection, neostigmine methylsulphate 500 micrograms/ml, net price 1-ml amp = 16p; 2.5 mg/ml, 1-ml amp = 16p

PoM **Robinul-Neostigmine**® (Robins)
Injection, neostigmine methylsulphate 2.5 mg, glycopyrronium bromide 500 micrograms/ml. Net price 1-ml amp = 99p
Dose: by intravenous injection over 10–30 seconds, 1–2 ml *or* 0.02 ml/kg

15.1.7   Antagonists for central and respiratory depression

Opioid antagonists, usually **naloxone** (Narcan®), are used at the end of an operation to reverse respiratory depression caused by opioid analgesics. Unless the dosage is carefully adjusted, analgesia may also be reversed. For respiratory stimulants see section 3.5. **Doxapram** is a respiratory stimulant which does not reverse the other effects of opioid analgesics.

Flumazenil is a newly introduced benzodiazepine antagonist for the reversal of the central sedative effects of benzodiazepines in anaesthetic and similar procedures.

DOXAPRAM HYDROCHLORIDE

Indications: postoperative respiratory depression
Cautions; Contra-indications: see section 3.5
Side-effects: see section 3.5
Dose: by intravenous injection, 1–1.5 mg/kg repeated if necessary after 1 hour
By intravenous infusion, 2–3 mg/minute

PoM **Dopram**® (Robins)
Injection, doxapram hydrochloride 20 mg/ml. Net price 5-ml amp = £2.00
Intravenous infusion: see section 3.5

FLUMAZENIL

Indications: reversal of sedative effects of benzodiazepines in anaesthetic, intensive care, and diagnostic procedures
Cautions: short-acting (repeat doses may be necessary); benzodiazepine effects may persist for at least 24 hours; benzodiazepine dependence; ensure neuromuscular blockade cleared before giving; avoid rapid injection in high-risk or anxious patients and following major surgery; hepatic impairment
Contra-indications: epileptics who have received prolonged benzodiazepine therapy
Side-effects: nausea, vomiting, and flushing; if wakening too rapid, agitation, anxiety, and fear; transient increase in blood-pressure and heart-rate in intensive care patients; very rarely convulsions (particularly in epileptics)
Dose: by slow intravenous injection, 200 micrograms over 15 seconds, then 100 micrograms at 60-second intervals if required; usual dose range, 300–600 micrograms; max. total dose 1 mg (2 mg in intensive care); question aetiology if no response to repeated doses
By intravenous infusion, if drowsiness recurs after injection, 100–400 micrograms/hour, adjusted according to level of arousal

▼ PoM **Anexate**® (Roche)
Injection, flumazenil 100 micrograms/ml. Net price 5-ml amp = £16.32

NALOXONE HYDROCHLORIDE

Indications: reversal of opioid-induced respiratory depression
Cautions: see under Emergency Treatment of Poisoning
Dose: by intravenous injection, 100–200 micrograms (1.5–3 micrograms/kg); if response inadequate, increments of 100 micrograms every 2 minutes; further doses *by intramuscular injection* after 1–2 hours if required
Neonate, *by subcutaneous, intramuscular, or intravenous injection,* 10 micrograms/kg, repeated every 2 to 3 minutes *or* 200 micrograms (60 micrograms/kg) *by intramuscular injection* as a single dose at birth

PoM **Naloxone Hydrochloride** (Non-proprietary)
Injection, naloxone hydrochloride 20 micrograms/ml. Net price 2-ml amp = £3.57
Injection, naloxone hydrochloride 400 micrograms/ml—see under Emergency Treatment of Poisoning
Narcan®—see under Emergency Treatment of Poisoning
PoM **Narcan Neonatal**® (Du Pont)
Injection, naloxone hydrochloride 20 micrograms/ml. Net price 2-ml amp = £3.57

15.1.8   Antagonists for malignant hyperthermia

Dantrolene (Dantrium®) is used in the prophylaxis and treatment of malignant hyperthermia which is a rare but lethal complication of anaesthesia. It is characterised by a rapid rise in temperature, increasing muscle rigidity, tachycardia, and acidosis and can be triggered off by several agents including halothane and suxamethonium. Dantrolene acts on skeletal muscle by interfering with calcium efflux in the muscle cell and stopping the contractile process. The oral preparation (see section 10.2.2) has been advocated for prophylactic use in malignant hyperthermia in susceptible individuals. The recommended dose is 5 mg/kg given in the 24 hours prior to surgery. Known trigger agents should be avoided during anaesthesia.

DANTROLENE SODIUM

Indications: malignant hyperthermia
Cautions: avoid extravasation
Dose: by rapid intravenous injection, 1 mg/kg, repeated at 5–10 minute intervals as required to a cumulative max. of 10 mg/kg

PoM **Dantrium Intravenous**® (Norwich Eaton)
Injection, powder for reconstitution, dantrolene sodium, with mannitol. Net price 20-mg vial = £22.52 (hosp. only)

15.2   Local anaesthesia

The use of local anaesthetics by injection or by application to mucous membranes to produce local analgesia is discussed in this section.

The following sections also include information on local anaesthetics acting on the sites shown:

1.7 Colon and rectum
11.7 Eye
12.3 Oropharynx
13.3 Skin

USE OF LOCAL ANAESTHETICS

Local anaesthetic drugs act by causing a reversible block to conduction along nerve fibres. The smaller the nerve fibre the more sensitive it is so that a differential block may occur where the smaller fibres carrying pain sensation and automatic impulses are blocked, sparing coarse touch and movement. The drugs used vary widely in their potency, toxicity, duration of action, stability, solubility in water, and ability to penetrate mucous membranes. These variations determine their suitability for surface infiltration, regional, epidural, and spinal anaesthesia.

ADMINISTRATION. In estimating the safe dosage of these drugs it is important to take account of the rate at which they are absorbed and excreted as well as their potency. The patient's age, weight, physique, and clinical condition, the degree of vascularity of the area to which the drug is to be applied, and the duration of administration are other factors which must be taken into account.

Local anaesthetics do not rely on the circulation to transport them to their sites of action, but uptake into the general circulation is important in terminating their action. Following most regional anaesthetic procedures, maximum arterial plasma concentrations of anaesthetic develop within about 10 to 25 minutes, so careful surveillance for toxic effects is necessary during the first 30 minutes after injection.

TOXICITY. Toxic effects associated with the local anaesthetics are usually a result of excessively high plasma concentrations. The main effects are excitation of the central nervous system (nervousness, nausea, and convulsions) followed by depression. Less commonly the cardiovascular system is depressed. Hypersensitivity reactions occur mainly with the ester-type local anaesthetics such as amethocaine, benzocaine, cocaine, and procaine; reactions are less frequent with the amide types such as lignocaine, bupivacaine, and prilocaine.

USE OF VASOCONSTRICTORS. Toxicity may occur with repeated dosages due to accumulation of the drug, and reducing doses should therefore be given. Toxic effects may also occur if the injection is too rapid. Local anaesthetics should not be injected into inflamed or infected tissues nor should they be applied to the traumatised urethra.

Under these conditions the drug may be so rapidly absorbed that a systemic rather than a local reaction is produced.

Most local anaesthetics, with the exception of cocaine, cause dilatation of blood vessels. The addition of a vasoconstrictor such as adrenaline diminishes local blood flow, slows the rate of absorption of the local anaesthetic, and prolongs its local effect. Care is necessary when using adrenaline for this purpose because, in excess, it may produce ischaemic necrosis.

Adrenaline should not be added to injections used in digits and appendages. When adrenaline is included in an injection of lignocaine or procaine the final concentration should be 1 in 200000. In dental surgery, up to 1 in 80000 of adrenaline is used with local anaesthetics. There is no justification for using higher concentrations.

The total dose of adrenaline should not exceed 500 micrograms and it is essential not to exceed a concentration of 1 in 200000 if more than 50 ml of the mixture is to be injected. For drug interactions, see Appendix 1 (section 2.7).

LOCAL ANAESTHETIC DRUGS

Lignocaine is the most widely used local anaesthetic drug. It acts more rapidly and is more stable than most other local anaesthetics. It is effectively absorbed from mucous membranes and is a useful surface anaesthetic in concentrations of 2 to 4%. Except for surface anaesthesia, solutions should not usually exceed 1% in strength. The duration of the block (with adrenaline) is about 1½ hours. Concentrations of 1.5% are used for extradural block, and for spinal anaesthesia a 5% solution in glucose intravenous infusion is used as a hyperbaric solution.

The great advantage of bupivacaine (Marcain®) over other local anaesthetics is its duration of action of up to 8 hours when used for nerve blocks. It has a slow onset of action, taking up to 30 minutes for full effect. It is often used in lumbar epidural blockade and is particularly suitable for continuous epidural analgesia in labour; it then has a 2- to 3-hour duration of action. The maximum dose is 2 mg/kg in any 4-hour period. It is also used for spinal anaesthesia.

Prilocaine (Citanest®) is a local anaesthetic of low toxicity which is similar to lignocaine. It can be used for infiltration, regional nerve block, and spinal anaesthesia and regional intravenous analgesia. The maximum adult dose is 400 mg, or 600 mg if adrenaline or felypressin is added. If used in high doses, methaemoglobinaemia may occur which can be treated with intravenous methylene blue 1% injection using a dose of 75–100 mg.

Amethocaine is an effective local anaesthetic for topical application. It is rapidly absorbed from mucous membranes and should never be applied to inflamed, traumatised, or highly vascular surfaces. It should never be used to provide anaesthesia for bronchoscopy or cystoscopy, as lignocaine is a safer alternative. It is used in ophthalmology (see section 11.7) and in skin preparations (see section 13.3). Hypersensitivity to amethocaine has been reported.

Benzocaine is a local anaesthetic of low potency and toxicity. Its only use is in surface anaesthesia for the relief of pain and irritation in the oropharynx (see section 12.3.1).

Cocaine readily penetrates mucous membranes and is an effective surface anaesthetic but it has now been replaced by less toxic alternatives. It potentiates the action of adrenaline and possesses vasoconstrictor and mydriatic properties and should therefore **not** be used with adrenaline. It should **never** be given by injection because of its toxicity and doses not exceeding 3 mg/kg should be applied to mucous membranes. It stimulates the central nervous system and is a drug of addiction. Concentrations of 4 to 20% (50–200 mg/ml) are applied to the nose, throat, and larynx. For the use of cocaine in ophthalmology see section 11.7.

Procaine is now seldom used. It is as potent an anaesthetic as lignocaine but has a shorter duration of action. It provides less intense analgesia because it has less tendency to spread through the tissues. It is poorly absorbed from mucous membranes and is of no value as a surface anaesthetic. When used for infiltration or regional anaesthesia, adrenaline 1 in 200000 is generally added. Its metabolite para-amino-benzoic acid inhibits the action of the sulphonamides.

LIGNOCAINE HYDROCHLORIDE

Indications: see under Dose; also dental anaesthesia

Cautions: epilepsy, hepatic impairment, impaired cardiac conduction, bradycardia. Reduce dose in elderly or debilitated patients. Resuscitative equipment should be available. See section 2.3.3 for effects on heart

Contra-indications: hypovolaemia, complete heart block. Do not use solutions containing adrenaline for anaesthesia in appendages

Side-effects: hypotension, bradycardia, cardiac arrest. CNS effects include agitation, euphoria, respiratory depression, convulsions. See also notes above

Dose: adjusted according to the site of operation and response of the patient

By injection, max. dose 200 mg, or 500 mg with solutions which also contain adrenaline. Max. dose of adrenaline 500 micrograms

Infiltration anaesthesia, 0.25–0.5%, with adrenaline 1 in 200000, using 2–50 ml of a 0.5% solution in minor surgery and up to 60 ml in more extensive surgery

Nerve blocks, with adrenaline 1 in 200000, 1% to a max. of 50 ml, 2% to a max. of 25 ml

Epidural and caudal block, with adrenaline 1 in 200000, 1% to a max. of 50 ml, 2% to a max. of 25 ml

Surface anaesthesia, usual strengths 2–4%. Mouth, throat, and upper gastro-intestinal tract, max. 200 mg

Lignocaine hydrochloride injections

PoM **Min-I-Jet Lignocaine Hydrochloride with Adrenaline**® (IMS)

Injection, lignocaine hydrochloride 5 mg/ml, adrenaline 1 in 200000 (500 micrograms/ 100 ml). Net price 5-ml disposable syringe = £2.10

PoM **Xylocaine**® (Astra)

Injection 0.5%, anhydrous lignocaine hydrochloride 5 mg/ml. Net price 10-ml amp = 12p; 20 ml vial = 67p; 50-ml vial = 93p

Injection 0.5% with adrenaline 1 in 200000, anhydrous lignocaine hydrochloride 5 mg/ml, adrenaline 1 in 200000. Net price 50-ml vial = 95p

Injection 1%, anhydrous lignocaine hydrochloride 10 mg/ml. Net price 2-ml amp = 5p; 10-ml amp = 12p; 20-ml vial = 69p; 50-ml vial = 95p

Injection 1% with adrenaline 1 in 200000, anhydrous lignocaine hydrochloride 10 mg/ml, adrenaline 1 in 200000. Net price 10-ml amp = 14p; 20-ml vial = 71p; 50-ml vial = 97p

Injection 1.5%, for epidural use, anhydrous lignocaine hydrochloride 15 mg/ml. Net price 25-ml amp = £1.21

Injection 2%, anhydrous lignocaine hydrochloride 20 mg/ml. Net price 5-ml amp = 8p; 20-ml vial = 73p; 50-ml vial = £1.00

Injection 2% with adrenaline 1 in 200000, anhydrous lignocaine hydrochloride 20 mg/ml, adrenaline 1 in 200000. Net price 20-ml vial = 75p; 50-ml vial = £1.02

Lignocaine injections for dental use

A large variety of lignocaine injections, plain or with adrenaline or noradrenaline, is also available in dental cartridges under the names **Lidocaton, Lignostab, Neo-Lidocaton, Xylocaine,** and **Xylotox.**

Lignocaine for surface anaesthesia

PoM **Emla**® (Astra)

Drug Tariff cream, lignocaine 2.5%, prilocaine 2.5%. Net price 10 × 5-g tube = £17.00

Surgical pack cream, lignocaine 2.5%, prilocaine 2.5%. Net price 30-g tube (with spatula) = £10.25

NHS *Hospital pack cream,* lignocaine 2.5%, prilocaine 2.5%. Net price 10 × 5-g tube with 25 occlusive dressings = £19.50

Anaesthesia before venepuncture, apply a thick layer for 1–2 hours under an occlusive dressing

PoM **Instillagel**® (CliniMed)

Gel, lignocaine hydrochloride 2%, chlorhexidine gluconate solution 0.25%, in a sterile lubricant basis in disposable syringe. Net price 6-ml syringe = 85p; 11-ml syringe = 95p

Dose: 6–11 ml into urethra

Xylocaine® (Astra)

Antiseptic gel, lignocaine hydrochloride 2%, chlorhexidine gluconate solution 0.25% in a sterile lubricant water-miscible basis. Net price 20 g = £1.09

Gel, anhydrous lignocaine hydrochloride 2%, in a sterile lubricant water-miscible basis. Net price 20 g = 78p; 20-g single-use syringe (Accordion®) = £1.00

Ointment, lignocaine 5% in a water-miscible basis. Net price 15 g = 83p

Spray (= aerosol spray), lignocaine 10% (100 mg/g) with cetylpyridinium chloride 0.01% in a metered spray container supplying 10 mg lignocaine/dose; 800 spray doses per container. With sterilisable spray nozzles. Net price 80-g bottle = £4.67

Topical 4%, anhydrous lignocaine hydrochloride 40 mg/ml. Net price 30-ml bottle = £1.24

Dose: bronchoscopy, 2–3 ml with suitable spray; biopsy in mouth, 3–4 ml with suitable spray *or* swab (with adrenaline if necessary); max. 5 ml

Xylocaine Viscous® (Astra)

Oral solution 2%, anhydrous lignocaine hydrochloride 20 mg/ml, for surface anaesthesia of the upper digestive tract. Net price 125 ml = £1.53

Dose: after tonsillectomy, 5 ml rinsed in mouth and swallowed slowly; max. 6 doses in 24 hours; min. 4 hours between doses; no food for 3 hours after dose

Introduction of instruments into stomach, 15 ml

Severe hiccup, 10 ml swallowed quickly in one gulp; max 3 doses in 24 hours

BUPIVACAINE HYDROCHLORIDE

Indications: see under Dose

Cautions; Contra-indications; Side-effects: see under Lignocaine Hydrochloride and notes above; myocardial depression may be more severe and more resistant to treatment; contraindicated in intravenous regional anaesthesia

Dose: adjusted according to the site of operation and response of the patient

Local infiltration, 0.25% (up to 60 ml)

Peripheral nerve block, 0.25% (max. 60 ml), 0.5% (max. 30 ml)

Epidural block,

Surgery, *lumbar*, 0.5–0.75% (max. 20 ml of either)

caudal, 0.5% (max. 30 ml)

Labour, *lumbar*, 0.25–0.5% (max. 12 ml of either)

caudal, 0.25% (max. 30 ml), 0.5% (max. 20 ml)

Note. 0.75% contra-indicated for epidural use in obstetrics.

▼ PoM **Marcain Heavy®** (Astra)

Injection, bupivacaine hydrochloride 5 mg, glucose 80 mg/ml. Net price 4-ml amp = £1.00

Dose: spinal anaesthesia, 2–4 ml

PoM **Marcain Plain®** (Astra)

Injection 0.25%, bupivacaine hydrochloride 2.5 mg/ml. Net price 10-ml amp = £1.13

Injection 0.5%, bupivacaine hydrochloride 5 mg/ml. Net price 10-ml amp = £1.30

Injection 0.75%, bupivacaine hydrochloride 7.5 mg/ml. Net price 10-ml amp = £1.95

PoM **Marcain with Adrenaline®** (Astra)

Injection 0.25%, bupivacaine hydrochloride 2.5 mg/ml, adrenaline 1 in 200000. Net price 10-ml amp = £1.27

Injection 0.5%, bupivacaine hydrochloride 5 mg/ml, adrenaline 1 in 200000. Net price 10-ml amp = £1.43

PRILOCAINE HYDROCHLORIDE

Indications: see under Dose; also dental anaesthesia

Cautions; Contra-indications; Side-effects: see under Lignocaine Hydrochloride and notes above

Dose: adjusted according to the site of operation and response of patient, to a max. of 400 mg used alone, or 600 mg if used with adrenaline or felypressin

PoM **Citanest®** (Astra)

Injection 0.5%, prilocaine hydrochloride 5 mg/ml. Net price 20-ml multidose vial = 73p; 50-ml multidose vial = £1.02; 50-ml single dose vial = £1.30

Injection 1%, prilocaine hydrochloride 10 mg/ml. Net price 20-ml vial = 75p; 50-ml vial = £1.06

PoM **Citanest with Octapressin®** (Astra)

Injection 3%, prilocaine hydrochloride 30 mg/ml, felypressin 0.03 unit/ml. Net price 2-ml cartridge and self-aspirating cartridge (both) = 11p

PROCAINE HYDROCHLORIDE

Indications: local anaesthesia by infiltration and regional routes

Cautions; Side-effects: see notes above

Dose: adjusted according to the site of operation and the patient's response

By injection, up to 1 g (200 ml of 0.5% solution or 100 ml of 1%) with adrenaline 1 in 200000

PoM **Procaine Injection**, procaine hydrochloride 2% (20 mg/ml) in sodium chloride intravenous infusion. Net price 2-ml amp = 35p; 1% in 2-ml amp also available

Appendix 1: Drug Interactions

Two or more drugs given at the same time may exert their effects independently or may interact. The interaction may be potentiation or antagonism of one drug by another, or occasionally some other effect. Adverse drug interactions should be reported to the CSM as for other adverse drug reactions.

Drug interactions may be **pharmacodynamic** or **pharmacokinetic**.

Pharmacodynamic interactions

These are interactions between drugs which have similar or antagonistic pharmacological effects or side-effects. They may be due to competition at receptor sites, or occur between drugs acting on the same physiological system. They are usually predictable from a knowledge of the pharmacology of the interacting drugs and, in general, interactions demonstrated with one drug are likely to occur with related drugs. They occur to a greater or lesser extent in most patients who receive the interacting drugs.

Pharmacokinetic interactions

These occur when one drug alters the absorption, distribution, metabolism, or excretion of another, thus increasing or reducing the amount of drug available to produce its pharmacological effects. They are not easily predicted and many of them affect only a small proportion of patients taking the combination of drugs. Pharmacokinetic interactions occurring with one drug cannot be assumed to occur with related drugs unless their pharmacokinetic properties are known to be similar.

Pharmacokinetic interactions are of several types:

AFFECTING ABSORPTION. The rate of absorption or the total amount absorbed can both be altered by drug interactions. Delayed absorption is rarely of clinical importance unless high peak plasma concentrations are required (e.g. when giving an analgesic). Reduction in the total amount absorbed, however, may result in ineffective therapy.

DUE TO CHANGES IN PROTEIN BINDING. To a variable extent most drugs are loosely bound to plasma proteins. Protein-binding sites are non-specific and one drug can displace another thereby increasing its proportion free to diffuse from plasma to its site of action. This only produces a detectable increase in effect if it is an extensively bound drug (more than 90%) that is not widely distributed throughout the body. Even so displacement rarely produces more than transient potentiation because this increased concentration of free drug results in an increased rate of elimination.

Displacement from protein binding plays a part in the potentiation of warfarin by phenylbutazone, sulphonamides, and tolbutamide but the importance of these interactions is due mainly to the fact that warfarin metabolism is also inhibited.

AFFECTING METABOLISM. Many drugs are metabolised in the liver. Induction of the hepatic microsomal enzyme system by one drug can gradually increase the rate of metabolism of another, resulting in lower plasma concentrations and a reduced effect. On withdrawal of the inducer plasma concentrations increase and toxicity may occur. Barbiturates, dichloralphenazone, griseofulvin, most antiepileptics, and rifampicin are the most important enzyme inducers in man. Drugs affected include warfarin and the oral contraceptives.

Conversely when one drug inhibits the metabolism of another higher plasma concentrations are produced, rapidly resulting in an increased effect with risk of toxicity. Some drugs which potentiate warfarin and phenytoin do so by this mechanism.

AFFECTING RENAL EXCRETION. Drugs are eliminated through the kidney both by glomerular filtration and by active tubular secretion. Competition occurs between those which share active transport mechanisms in the proximal tubule. Thus probenecid delays the excretion of many drugs including penicillins, some cephalosporins, indomethacin, and dapsone; aspirin may increase the toxicity of methotrexate by a similar mechanism.

Relative importance of interactions

Many drug interactions are harmless and many of those which are potentially harmful only occur in a small proportion of patients; moreover, the severity of an interaction varies from one patient to another. Drugs with a small therapeutic ratio (e.g. phenytoin) and those which require careful control of dosage (e.g. anticoagulants, antihypertensives, and antidiabetics) are most often involved.

Patients at increased risk from drug interactions include the elderly and those with impaired renal or liver function.

The following table contains section numbers which correspond with those used in the chapters these also appear in the monographs:
roman type indicates
'drug affected' (column 1)
italic type indicates
'drug interacting' (column 2).
EXAMPLE. The reference given in the paragraph headed 'cautions' under Latamoxef Disodium reads 'Drug interactions: see Appendix 1 (sections 2.8B, 5.1)'. In Appendix 1, under 2.8B, in column 2 is the information that latamoxef (drug interacting) potentiates the action of warfarin (drug affected); under 5.1 in column 1 is the information that latamoxef (drug affected) taken with alcohol (drug interacting) produces an 'Antabuse reaction.

Table of Drug Interactions

Drug affected	Drug interacting	Effect
1: Gastro-intestinal system		
Carbenoxolone	Amiloride, spironolactone	Inhibition of ulcer healing
Cimetidine	Rifampicin	Reduced plasma concentrations of cimetidine
Domperidone, metoclopramide—see section 4.6		
Sucralfate	Antacids, cimetidine, ranitidine	Sucralfate works best in acid medium. Avoid combined use
2: Cardiovascular system		
2.1 Digoxin and other cardiac glycosides	Anti-inflammatory analgesics	May exacerbate heart failure, reduce GFR, and increase plasma-digoxin concentrations
	Carbenoxolone; diuretics—acetazolamide, bumetanide, ethacrynic acid, frusemide, piretanide, thiazides	Increased toxicity if hypokalaemia occurs
	Cholestyramine, colestipol	Reduced absorption
	Aminoglutethimide, phenobarbitone, phenytoin, rifampicin	Inhibition (digitoxin only)
Digoxin	Amiodarone, quinidine, quinine (e.g. for cramp)	Potentiation. Halve maintenance dose of digoxin
	Calcium salts	Large intravenous doses can precipitate arrhythmias
	Diltiazem, erythromycin, nicardipine, spironolactone, verapamil	Potentiation may occur
2.2 Diuretics	Anti-inflammatory analgesics such as indomethacin; carbenoxolone, corticosteroids, corticotrophin; oestrogens	Antagonism
Bumetanide, Frusemide, Piretanide, Thiazides	Acetazolamide, carbenoxolone, corticosteroids, corticotrophin	Hypokalaemia
Indapamide	Carbenoxolone; diuretics—bumetanide, frusemide, piretanide, thiazides, xipamide	Hypokalaemia
Metolazone	Frusemide	Profound diuresis can occur
Potassium-sparing diuretics	Captopril, enalapril, indomethacin (and possibly other NSAIDs), potassium supplements, trilostane	Hyperkalaemia
Potassium-sparing diuretics with thiazides	Chlorpropamide	Increased risk of hyponatraemia
Spironolactone	Aspirin, indomethacin	Antagonism of diuretic effect
Thiazides	Cholestyramine	Reduced absorption. Give at least 2 hours apart

Drug affected	Drug interacting	Effect
Triamterene	Indomethacin	Occasional reports of decreased renal function
2.3 Anti-arrhythmic drugs	Any combinations of 2 or more	Increased myocardial depression
Amiodarone	Diltiazem, verapamil	Increased risk of bradycardia and myocardial depression
Amiodarone, Disopyramide, Flecainide, Quinidine	Diuretics—bumetanide, ethacrynic acid, frusemide, piretanide, thiazides	Toxicity increased by hypokalaemia
Disopyramide	Anticholinergic drugs (e.g. antispasmodics, antiparkinsonian drugs)	Increased anticholinergic side-effects
Disopyramide, Flecainide, Quinidine	Amiodarone	Increased risk of ventricular arrhythmias
Disopyramide, Quinidine	Phenobarbitone, phenytoin, primidone, rifampicin	Reduced plasma concentrations
Flecainide, Mexiletine, Quinidine	Acetazolamide, antacids	Reduced excretion in alkaline urine may occasionally increase plasma concentrations
Flecainide, Procainamide, Quinidine	Amiodarone, cimetidine	Increased plasma concentrations
Lignocaine	Cimetidine, propranolol	Increased risk of lignocaine toxicity
Lignocaine, Mexiletine, Tocainide	Diuretics—bumetanide, ethacrynic acid, frusemide, piretanide, thiazides	Antagonised by hypokalaemia
Mexiletine	Atropine, opioid analgesics	Delayed absorption
	Phenytoin, rifampicin	Reduced plasma concentrations
Quinidine	Verapamil	Increased plasma concentrations; extreme hypotension may occur
2.4 Beta-blockers	Adrenaline	Severe hypertension, especially with non-selective beta-blockers
	Amphetamines, phenylephrine, phenylpropanolamine, and other sympathomimetic amines	Severe hypertension reported rarely
	Diltiazem	Increased risk of bradycardia and AV block
	Ergotamine	Increased peripheral vasoconstriction
	Lignocaine and similar anti-arrhythmic drugs	Increased risk of myocardial depression and bradycardia

Drug affected	Drug interacting	Effect
2.4 Beta-blockers (continued)	Nifedipine	Severe hypotension and heart failure occasionally in susceptible patients
	Prenylamine	Increased myocardial depression
Labetalol	Cimetidine	Increased plasma concentration of labetalol
Propranolol	Cimetidine	Increased plasma concentration of propranolol
	Rifampicin	Reduced plasma concentration of propranolol
Sotalol	Diuretics— bumetanide, ethacrynic acid, frusemide, piretanide, thiazides	Risk of ventricular arrhythmias increased by hypokalaemia
2.5 Antihypertensive drugs	Anti-inflammatory analgesics such as indomethacin; carbenoxolone, corticosteroids, corticotrophin; oestrogens, oral contraceptives	Reduced effect
	Alcohol, antidepressants, anxiolytics, hypnotics, phenothiazines; diethylpropion, fenfluramine; levodopa; vasodilators such as nitrates, nifedipine; verapamil	Potentiation
Bethanidine, Debrisoquine, Guanethidine	Sympathomimetic amines (including some common cold remedies); mazindol, pizotifen; tricyclic antidepressants	Antagonism
Captopril, Enalapril	Diuretics	Potentiation. Extreme hypotension can occur
	Indomethacin (and possibly other non-steroidal anti-inflammatory drugs), potassium supplements, potassium-sparing diuretics	Hyperkalaemia
Clonidine	Beta-blockers, tricyclic antidepressants	Increased risk of clonidine withdrawal hypertension
	Tricyclic antidepressants	Antagonism
Metirosine, Reserpine	Haloperidol, metoclopramide, phenothiazines	Increased risk of extrapyramidal effects
Prazosin, Terazosin	Beta-blockers, diuretics	Potentiation of initial hypotensive effect
2.6 Vasodilators Diltiazem, Nicardipine, Nifedipine	Cimetidine	Increased plasma concentrations
Glyceryl trinitrate	Anticholinergic drugs, e.g. disopyramide, tricyclic antidepressants	Loss of effect due to failure to dissolve under tongue

Drug affected	Drug interacting	Effect
Lidoflazine, Prenylamine	Diuretics—bumetanide, ethacrynic acid, frusemide, piretanide, thiazides	Risk of ventricular arrhythmias increased by hypokalaemia
Verapamil	Beta-blockers	Asystole, hypotension, heart failure
	Rifampicin	Reduced plasma concentrations
2.7 Vasoconstrictors Adrenaline, Noradrenaline	Tricyclic antidepressants	Potentiation (*note:* local anaesthetics with adrenaline appear to be safe)
	Beta-blockers	Potentiation of hypertensive effect
2.8 Anticoagulants Heparin	Aspirin, dipyridamole	Potentiation
Phenindione	Oral contraceptives, vitamin K (*note:* present in some enteral feeds)	Inhibition
	Anabolic steroids (e.g. oxymetholone, stanozolol), aspirin, bezafibrate, cholestyramine, clofibrate, dipyridamole, gemfibrozil, neomycin, thyroxine	Potentiation
Warfarin and nicoumalone	A: aminoglutethimide, barbiturates, carbamazepine, dichloralphenazone, griseofulvin, oral contraceptives, primidone, rifampicin, vitamin K (*note:* present in some enteral feeds)	Inhibition
	B: alcohol, amiodarone, anabolic steroids (e.g. oxymetholone, stanozolol), azapropazone, aztreonam, bezafibrate, cephamandole, chloramphenicol, cimetidine, clofibrate, co-trimoxazole, danazol, dextrothyroxine, disulfiram, erythromycin, gemfibrozil, ketoconazole, latamoxef, metronidazole, miconazole, phenylbutazone, sulphinpyrazone, sulphonamides, tamoxifen, thyroxine	Potentiation
	Broad-spectrum antibiotics	Studies have failed to demonstrate interaction between oral antibiotics and warfarin, but common experience in anticoagulant clinics is that prothrombin times can be prolonged by few seconds following course of broad-spectrum antibiotic e.g. ampicillin

Drug affected	Drug interacting	Effect
Warfarin and nicoumalone (*continued*)	C: allopurinol; diflunisal, flurbiprofen, mefenamic acid, piroxicam, sulindac and possibly other anti-inflammatory analgesics; chloral hydrate, cholestyramine, dextropropoxyphene, fluvoxamine, nalidixic acid, neomycin, quinidine, Rowachol®, tetracyclines	Potentiation may occur
	D: phenytoin	Both potentiation and inhibition reported
	E: aspirin, dipyridamole	Increased risk of bleeding due to anti-platelet effect

3: Respiratory system

Theophylline	Cimetidine, ciprofloxacin, erythromycin, interferons, oral contraceptives, propranolol, viloxazine	Potentiation (propranolol should also be avoided on pharmacological grounds)
	Aminoglutethimide, barbiturates, carbamazepine, phenytoin, rifampicin, sulphinpyrazone	Plasma concentrations of theophylline may be reduced

4: Central nervous system

4.1 Hypnotics and anxiolytics

	Alcohol, antidepressants, antihistamines, opioid analgesics, phenothiazines	Potentiation
Alprazolam, Chlordiazepoxide, Chlormethiazole, Clobazam, Diazepam, Flurazepam, Midazolam, Nitrazepam, Triazolam	Cimetidine	Increased plasma concentrations
Chlordiazepoxide, Diazepam	Disulfiram	Potentiation because of decreased hepatic metabolism

4.2 Antipsychotic drugs

Chlorpromazine	Antacids	Reduced absorption
	Propranolol	Increased plasma concentrations of chlorpromazine
Haloperidol	Carbamazepine, rifampicin	Reduced plasma concentrations of haloperidol
	Indomethacin	Severe drowsiness has been reported
Haloperidol, Phenothiazines	Metoclopramide, tetrabenazine	Increased risk of extrapyramidal effects
Lithium	Diuretics, sodium depletion	Potentiation due to reduced lithium clearance. Loop diuretics are safer than thiazides
	Acetazolamide, sodium bicarbonate, theophylline	Increased lithium excretion

Drug affected	Drug interacting	Effect
Lithium (*continued*)	Amiloride	Antagonism of lithium-induced polyuria without reduced lithium clearance
	Carbamazepine, diltiazem, methyldopa, phenytoin, verapamil	Neurotoxicity may occur without increased plasma concentrations
	Diclofenac, ibuprofen, indomethacin, mefenamic acid, naproxen (and possibly other NSAIDs) phenylbutazone, piroxicam	Potentiation
	Enalapril	Plasma lithium concentration may be increased
	Haloperidol, metoclopramide, phenothiazines	Increased risk of extrapyramidal effects and possibly of neurotoxicity
Phenothiazines	Anticholinergic drugs such as procyclidine	Reduced plasma concentrations of phenothiazines
4.3 Antidepressants *Monoamine-oxidase inhibitors* N.B. Interactions can occur up to 2 weeks after stopping MAOI. Interactions can occur with many tyramine-containing foods and drinks (including alcoholic and dealcoholised beverages).	Sympathomimetics such as amphetamines, common cold remedies, diethylpropion, ephedrine, phenylephrine; fenfluramine, isometheptene, levodopa, pemoline	Hypertensive crisis
	Fluvoxamine	Potentiation of CNS effects and toxicity possible
	Oxypertine, pethidine (and possibly other opioid analgesics), reserpine, tetrabenazine, tricyclic antidepressants	CNS excitation, hypertension
	Tryptophan	CNS excitation. Confusional states. Reduce dose of tryptophan
Tricyclic antidepressants	Alcohol	Potentiation of sedative effect
	Antiepileptics, barbiturates	Reduced plasma concentrations of tricyclic antidepressants
	Oral contraceptives	Reduced effect but side-effects may be increased due to higher plasma concentrations
	Phenothiazines	Increased side-effects
	Disulfiram	Increased plasma concentrations. Increased 'Antabuse' effect with alcohol and amitriptyline

Drug affected	Drug interacting	Effect
Amitriptyline, Desipramine, Doxepin, Imipramine, Nortriptyline	Cimetidine	Increased plasma concentrations
4.6 Drugs used in nausea		
Betahistine	Antihistamines	Antagonism
Domperidone, Metoclopramide	Anticholinergic drugs such as atropine, benzhexol, propantheline; opioid analgesics	Antagonism—they have opposing effects on gastro-intestinal activity
4.7 Analgesics		
Anti-inflammatory analgesics	Diuretics, captopril, enalapril	Increased risk of renal failure
Aspirin	Antacids (large doses)	Reduce plasma concentrations by hastening renal excretion of aspirin
	Corticosteroids	Reduced plasma concentrations of aspirin
	Metoclopramide	Potentiation
Diflunisal	Antacids	Reduced absorption
Ergotamine	Erythromycin	Ergotism has been reported
Indomethacin, Ketoprofen, Naproxen	Probenecid	Increased plasma concentrations
Methadone	Rifampicin	Reduced effect due to increased metabolism
Paracetamol	Cholestyramine	Reduced absorption
	Metoclopramide	Potentiation
Pethidine	Cimetidine	Increased plasma concentrations
4.8 Antiepileptics	Antidepressants, phenothiazines	Antagonism
Carbamazepine	Cimetidine, danazol, dextropropoxyphene, diltiazem, erythromycin, isoniazid, verapamil, viloxazine	Potentiation
Clonazepam	Carbamazepine, phenobarbitone, phenytoin	Reduced effect due to increased metabolism
Ethosuximide	Carbamazepine	Reduced plasma concentrations of ethosuximide
	Isoniazid	Increased plasma concentrations and increased toxicity of ethosuximide
	Sodium valproate	Increased plasma concentrations of ethosuximide
Phenobarbitone, Primidone	Phenytoin, sodium valproate	Increased sedation

Drug affected	Drug interacting	Effect
Phenytoin	Amiodarone, azapropazone, chloramphenicol, cimetidine, co-trimoxazole, diazepam, disulfiram, influenza vaccine, isoniazid, ketoconazole, metronidazole, miconazole, phenylbutazone, sulphinpyrazone, viloxazine	Potentiation
	Aspirin, sodium valproate	Transient potentiation
	Folic acid	Occasionally reduces plasma concentration of phenytoin
	Rifampicin	Reduced plasma concentration of phenytoin
	Sucralfate	Reduced absorption of phenytoin
Sodium valproate	Carbamazepine, phenobarbitone, phenytoin, primidone	Reduced plasma concentrations of valproate
4.9 Drugs for parkinsonism	Haloperidol, phenothiazines; methyldopa, metirosine, metoclopramide, reserpine, tetrabenazine	These have extra-pyramidal side-effects
Anticholinergic antiparkinsonian drugs such as benzhexol etc.	Amantadine, antidepressants, antihistamines, disopyramide, phenothiazines, terodiline	Increased anticholinergic side-effects, dry mouth, urine retention, confusion etc.
Levodopa	Chlordiazepoxide, diazepam, lorazepam, and possibly other benzodiazepines	Antagonism—occasionally
	Metoclopramide	Increased plasma concentrations of levodopa
	Pyridoxine	Antagonism (does not occur if dopa decarboxylase inhibitor also given)

5: Infections
5.1 Antibacterial drugs
Aminoglycosides

Gentamicin etc.	Ethacrynic acid, frusemide, piretanide, vancomycin	Increased ototoxicity
Cephalothin, and possibly other cephalosporins	Ethacrynic acid, frusemide, piretanide; gentamicin, vancomycin	Increased nephrotoxicity
Cephamandole, Latamoxef	Alcohol	'Antabuse' reaction
Chloramphenicol	Phenobarbitone, rifampicin	Reduced plasma concentrations
Ciprofloxacin	Antacids	Reduced absorption
Dapsone	Probenecid	Reduced excretion—increased side-effects
Lincomycin	Kaolin mixtures	Reduced absorption

Drug affected	Drug interacting	Effect
Metronidazole	Alcohol	'Antabuse' reaction
	Cimetidine	Increased plasma concentrations
	Disulfiram	Psychotic reactions
	Phenobarbitone	Reduced effect
Nalidixic acid	Probenecid	Reduced excretion—increased side-effects
Nitrofurantoin	Probenecid	Reduced excretion—increased side-effects
Penicillins		
Phenoxymethylpenicillin	Guar gum, neomycin	Reduced absorption
Pivampicillin	Antacids	Reduced absorption
Rifampicin	Antacids	Reduced absorption
Tetracyclines	Antacids, oral iron, sucralfate, zinc sulphate	Reduced absorption
	Dairy products (not doxycycline and minocycline)	Reduced absorption
Doxycycline	Barbiturates, carbamazepine, phenytoin	Reduced plasma concentrations
Vancomycin	Cholestyramine	Antagonism
5.2 Antifungal drugs		
Griseofulvin	Phenobarbitone	Antagonism
Ketoconazole	Antacids, anticholinergic drugs, cimetidine, ranitidine	Decreased absorption
	Phenytoin, rifampicin	Reduced plasma concentration of ketoconazole
5.3 Antiviral drugs		
Acyclovir	Probenecid	Reduced excretion and increased plasma concentrations
Zidovudine	Other nephrotoxic or myelosuppressive drugs	Increased risk of toxicity
	Probenecid	Increased plasma concentrations
5.4 Antimalarials		
Chloroquine	Antacids	Reduced absorption
Quinine	Cimetidine	Increased plasma concentration of quinine

6: Endocrine system

6.1 Antidiabetic drugs

(oral and insulin)	Alcohol; beta-blockers; monoamine-oxidase inhibitors	Potentiation
	Bezafibrate, clofibrate	May improve glucose tolerance and have an additive effect
	Corticosteroids, corticotrophin; diazoxide; bumetanide, frusemide, thiazides; oral contraceptives	Antagonism
	Lithium	May occasionally impair glucose tolerance

Drug affected	Drug interacting	Effect
Metformin	Alcohol	Increased risk of lactic acidosis
	Cimetidine	Increased plasma concentrations of metformin
Sulphonylureas—Chlorpropamide, Tolbutamide etc.	Azapropazone, chloramphenicol, clofibrate, co-trimoxazole, miconazole, phenylbutazone, sulphinpyrazone	Potentiation
	Nifedipine	May occasionally impair glucose tolerance
Chlorpropamide	Alcohol	Flushing in susceptible patients
Chlorpropamide, Glymidine, Tolbutamide, and possibly other sulphonylureas	Rifampicin	Reduced effect
6.2 Thyroxine	Cholestyramine	Reduced absorption
	Phenylbutazone	False low total plasma-thyroxine concentration
	Carbamazepine, phenytoin	Increased thyroxine metabolism and may increase thyroxine requirements in primary hypothyroidism
6.3 Corticosteroids, Corticotrophin	Carbenoxolone; diuretics—bumetanide, ethacrynic acid, frusemide, piretanide, thiazides	Increased potassium loss
Cortisone, Dexamethasone, Hydrocortisone, Prednisolone, Prednisone	Barbiturates, carbamazepine, phenytoin, primidone, rifampicin	Reduced effect
Dexamethasone	Aminoglutethimide	Reduced effect
6.7 Bromocriptine	Antipsychotic drugs, domperidone, metoclopramide	Antagonism of hypoprolactinaemic effect

7: Obstetrics, gynaecology, and urinary-tract disorders

Oral contraceptives	Barbiturates, carbamazepine, dichloralphenazone, griseofulvin, phenytoin, primidone, rifampicin	Reduced effect
Combined oral contraceptives only	Oral antibiotics such as ampicillin, tetracycline	Reduced effect—risk probably small

8: Malignant disease and immunosuppression

Azathioprine, Mercaptopurine	Allopurinol	Potentiation—increased toxicity
Cisplatin	Aminoglycosides	Increased risk of nephrotoxicity and possibly ototoxicity
Cyclophosphamide	Allopurinol	Bone-marrow toxicity may be increased

Drug affected	Drug interacting	Effect
Cyclosporin	Captopril, enalapril, potassium supplements, potassium-sparing diuretics	Increased risk of hyperkalaemia
	Danazol, diltiazem, erythromycin, ketoconazole, nicardipine, progestogens, verapamil	Increased plasma concentrations of cyclosporin
	Nephrotoxic drugs, e.g. aminoglycosides, amphotericin	Increased risk of nephrotoxicity
	Phenobarbitone, phenytoin, rifampicin	Reduced plasma concentration of cyclosporin
Fluorouracil	Cimetidine	Increased plasma concentrations
Methotrexate	Aspirin, azapropazone, indomethacin, ketoprofen, phenylbutazone (and probably other NSAIDs), probenecid	Delayed excretion— increased toxicity
	Antiepileptics; co-trimoxazole, pyrimethamine, trimethoprim	Increased anti-folate effect
Procarbazine	Alcohol	'Antabuse' reaction

9: Nutrition and blood

Calcium salts	Thiazides	Increased risk of hypercalcaemia
Oral iron	Magnesium trisilicate; tetracyclines; trientine; zinc salts	Reduced absorption
Zinc salts	Oral iron	Reduced absorption

10: Musculoskeletal and joint diseases

Anti-inflammatory analgesics, see section 4.7

Chloroquine, Hydroxychloroquine	Antacids	Reduced absorption
Neostigmine, Pyridostigmine	Aminoglycosides, chloroquine, clindamycin, lincomycin, lithium, propranolol, quinidine	Antagonism and deterioration in myasthenia gravis
Penicillamine	Antacids, oral iron, zinc sulphate	Reduced absorption
Phenylbutazone	Cholestyramine	Reduced absorption
Probenecid, Sulphinpyrazone	Aspirin	Inhibition
	Pyrazinamide	Antagonism

11: Eye

Acetazolamide	Aspirin	Reduced excretion of acetazolamide and risk of toxicity

Beta-blocker eye-drops *see* section 2.4

13: Skin

Monosulfiram	Alcohol	'Antabuse' reaction

15: Anaesthesia

General anaesthetics	Antihypertensive drugs; beta-blockers; chlorpromazine	Potentiation of hypotensive effect
	Adrenaline, isoprenaline, levodopa	Arrhythmias with halothane, cyclopropane, trichloroethylene

Drug affected	Drug interacting	Effect
General anaesthetics (*continued*)		
	Verapamil	Potentiation of hypotensive effect and AV delay
Thiopentone	Sulphonamides	Potentiation
Muscle relaxants	Colistin, polymyxin B; lithium, propranolol, quinidine	Potentiation
Competitive neuromuscular blocking drugs such as Tubocurarine	Aminoglycosides, clindamycin, lincomycin; magnesium salts, verapamil	Potentiation
Depolarising neuromuscular blocking drugs such as Suxamethonium	Cyclophosphamide, ecothiopate eye-drops, neostigmine, thiotepa	Potentiation
	Digoxin	Arrhythmias

Appendix 2: Intravenous Additives

Addition of medication to infusion fluids

Drugs may be added to a container of infusion fluid and given by slow intravenous infusion, by intermittent infusion, or via the drip tubing.

INTRAVENOUS ADDITIVE POLICIES. A local policy on the addition of drugs to intravenous fluids should be drawn up by a multi-disciplinary team in each Health District and issued as a document to the members of staff concerned.

Centralised additive services are provided in a number of hospital pharmacy departments and should be used when available in preference to making additions in hospital wards.

The information in the following section should be read in conjunction with any appropriate local policy documents.

Direct addition of medication to infusion containers

Basic guidelines

1. Drugs should only be added to infusion containers when constant plasma concentrations are needed or when the administration of a more concentrated solution would be harmful.
2. In general, only one drug should be added to any infusion container and the components should be of known compatibility (see Table). Ready-prepared solutions should be used whenever possible. Drugs should not normally be added to blood products, mannitol, or sodium bicarbonate. Only specially formulated additives should be used with fat emulsions or amino-acid solutions (see section 9.3).
3. Solutions should be thoroughly mixed by shaking and checked for absence of particulate matter before use.
4. Strict asepsis should be maintained throughout and in general the giving set should not be used for more than 24 hours.
5. The infusion container should be labelled with the patient's name, the name and quantity of additives, and the date and time of addition (and the new expiry date or time). Such additional labelling should not interfere with information on the manufacturer's label that is still valid. When possible, containers should be retained for a period after use in case they are needed for investigation.
6. It is good practice to examine intravenous infusions from time to time while they are running. If cloudiness, crystallisation, change of colour, or any other sign of interaction or contamination is observed the infusion should be discontinued.

Problems involving additives

MICROBIAL CONTAMINATION. The accidental entry and subsequent growth of micro-organisms converts the infusion fluid pathway into a potential vehicle for infection with micro-organisms, particularly species of *Candida, Enterobacter,* and *Klebsiella*. Ready-prepared infusions containing the additional drugs, or infusions prepared by an additive service (when available) should therefore be used in preference to making extemporaneous additions to infusion containers on wards etc. However, when this is necessary strict aseptic procedure should be followed.

INCOMPATIBILITY. Physical and chemical incompatibilities may occur with loss of potency, increase in toxicity, or other adverse effect. The solutions may become opalescent or precipitation may occur, but in many instances there is no visual indication of incompatibility. Interaction may take place at any point in the infusion fluid pathway, and the potential for incompatibility is increased when more than one substance is added to the infusion fluid. Information on compatibility is given in the accompanying Table. The suitability of additions may also be checked by reference to manufacturer's literature and additional information is usually available in hospital pharmacies.

Common incompatibilities. Precipitation reactions are numerous and varied and may occur as a result of pH, concentration changes, 'salting-out' effects, complexation or other chemical changes. Precipitation or other particle formation must be avoided since, apart from lack of control of dosage on administration, it may initiate or exacerbate adverse effects. This is particularly important in the case of drugs which have been implicated in either thrombophlebitis (e.g. diazepam) or in skin sloughing or necrosis caused by extravasation (e.g. sodium bicarbonate, thiopentone sodium and certain cytotoxic drugs). It is also especially important to effect solution of colloidal drugs and to prevent their subsequent precipitation in order to avoid a pyrogenic reaction (e.g. amphotericin).

It is considered undesirable to mix beta-lactam antibiotics, such as semi-synthetic penicillins and cephalosporins, with proteinaceous materials on the grounds that immunogenic and allergenic conjugates could be formed.

A number of preparations undergo significant loss of potency when added singly or in combination to large volume infusions. Examples include ampicillin in infusions that contain glucose or lactates, mustine hydrochloride in isotonic saline and gentamicin/carbenicillin combinations. The breakdown products of dacarbazine have been implicated in adverse effects.

Blood. Because of the large number of incompatibilities, drugs should not normally be added to blood and blood products for infusion purposes. Examples of incompatibility with blood include hypertonic mannitol solutions (irreversible crenation of red cells), dextrans (rouleaux formation and interference with cross-matching), glucose (clumping of red cells), and oxytocin (inactivated).

If the giving set is not changed after the administration of blood, but used for other infusion fluids, a fibrin clot may form which, apart from blocking the set, increases the likelihood of microbial growth.

Blood should always be taken for grouping and cross-matching before infusing dextrans.

Intravenous fat emulsions may break down with coalescence of fat globules and separation of phases when additions such as antibiotics or electrolytes are made, thus increasing the possibility of embolism. Only specially formulated items such as Vitlipid® (see section 9.3) may be added to appropriate intravenous fat emulsions.

Other infusions that frequently give rise to incompatibility include amino acids, mannitol, and sodium bicarbonate.

Bactericides such as chlorocresol 0.1% or phenylmercuric nitrate 0.001% are present in some injection solutions. The total volume of such solutions added to a container for infusion on one occasion should not exceed 15 ml.

Method of making additions to infusion solutions

Ready-prepared infusions should be used whenever available. **Potassium chloride** is usually available in concentrations of 20, 27, and 40 mmol/litre in sodium chloride intravenous infusion (0.9%), glucose intravenous infusion (5%) or sodium chloride and glucose intravenous infusion. **Lignocaine hydrochloride** is usually available in concentrations of 0.1 or 0.2% in glucose intravenous infusion (5%).

When addition is required to be made extemporaneously, any product reconstitution instructions such as those relating to concentration, vehicle, mixing, and handling precautions should be strictly followed using an aseptic technique throughout. Once the product has been reconstituted, addition to the infusion fluid should be made immediately in order to minimise accidental microbial contamination and, with certain products, to prevent degradation or other formulation change which may occur; e.g. reconstituted ampicillin injection degrades rapidly on standing, and also may form polymers which could cause sensitivity reactions.

It is also important in certain instances that an infusion fluid of specific pH be used. **Amphotericin** injection (Fungizone®) requires dilution in glucose injection of pH greater than 4.2 and **frusemide** injection (Lasix®) should be added to infusions of pH greater than 5.5.

When drug additions are made to the infusion container it is important to mix thoroughly; additions should not be made to an infusion container that has been connected to a giving set, as mixing is hampered. If the solutions are not thoroughly mixed a concentrated layer of the additive may form owing to differences in density of it and the infusion. **Potassium chloride** is particularly prone to this 'layering' effect when added without adequate mixing to infusions packed in non-rigid infusion containers, and if such a mixture is administered an insidious effect on the heart may result.

A time limit between addition of the additive to the infusion and completion of administration must be imposed for certain admixtures to guarantee satisfactory drug potency and compatibility. For admixtures in which degradation occurs without the formation of toxic substances, an acceptable limit is the time taken for 10% decomposition of the drug ($t_{10\%}$). When toxic substances are produced stricter limits may be imposed. Because of the risk of introducing micro-organisms a maximum time limit of 12 hours should be imposed for additions made elsewhere than in hospital pharmacies offering central additive service.

Certain injections must be protected from light during continuous infusion to minimise oxidation, e.g. amphotericin, dacarbazine, and sodium nitroprusside.

Dilution with a small volume of an appropriate vehicle and administration using a motorised infusion pump is advocated for preparations such as heparin where strict control over administration is required. In this case the appropriate dose may be dissolved in a convenient volume (e.g. 24 to 48 ml) of sodium chloride intravenous infusion (0.9%).

Use of additives table

The Table lists preparations given by three methods—continuous infusion, intermittent infusion, and addition via the drip tubing.

Drugs for **continuous infusion** must be diluted in a large volume infusion. Penicillins and cephalosporins are not usually given by continuous infusion because of stability problems and because adequate plasma and tissue concentrations are best obtained by intermittent infusion. Where it is necessary to administer these drugs by continuous infusion, the detailed literature should be consulted as the information is not included in the Table.

Intravenous preparations that are both compatible and clinically suitable may be given by **intermittent infusion** in a relatively small volume of infusion over a short period of time, e.g. 100 ml in 30 minutes. This method is applicable where the product is incompatible or is unstable over the normal period necessary for continuous infusion or where adequate plasma and tissue concentrations are not produced by continuous infusion. The limited stability of ampicillin or amoxycillin in large volume infusions containing glucose or lactate may be overcome using this method.

Carbenicillin, dacarbazine, and ticarcillin may be given by intermittent infusion in order to achieve satisfactory plasma and tissue concentrations. Gentamicin may be administered similarly, although it is normally given by direct intravenous bolus injection for the same reason.

An in-line burette may be used for intermittent infusion techniques in order to achieve strict control over the time and rate of administration of a bolus injection, especially for infants and children and in intensive care units. Intermittent infusion may also make use of the 'piggy-back' technique provided that no additions are made to the primary infusion. In this method the drug is added to a small secondary container connected to a Ytype injection site on the primary infusion giving set; the secondary solution is usually infused within 30 minutes.

Addition via the drip tubing is indicated for a number of cytotoxic drugs in order to minimise extravasation. The preparation is added aseptically via the rubber septum of the injection site of a fast-running infusion. In general, drug preparations intended for a bolus effect should be given directly into a separate vein where possible. Failing this, administration may be made via the drip tubing provided that the preparation is compatible with the infusion fluid when given in this manner.

The **Table** covers only the common intravenous infusion fluids, glucose 5 and 10%, sodium chloride 0.9%, Ringer's solution (compound sodium chloride), compound sodium lactate (Hartmann's solution), dextrans, and fructose. Where water for injections is used, care should be taken to avoid giving hypotonic solutions. Preparations compatible with glucose 5% and with sodium chloride 0.9% are also compatible with sodium chloride and glucose infusion. For information on compatibility with other fluids the literature should be consulted.

The proprietary forms indicated in the Table have been shown to be suitable. If other forms are used, suitability should be checked with the manufacturer.

Table of intravenous additives

Additive	Method	Intravenous infusion	Comments
Acetylcysteine *Parvolex*®	C	Glucose 5%	See Emergency Treatment of Poisoning.
Actinomycin D *Cosmegen Lyovac*®	D	Glucose 5%; Sodium chloride 0.9%	
Acyclovir sodium *Zovirax IV*®	I	Sodium chloride 0.9%; Sodium chloride and glucose; Sodium lactate, compound	Initially reconstitute to 25 mg/ml in water for injections or sodium chloride 0.9% then dilute to not more than 5 mg/ml with the infusion fluid. Minimum volume 50 ml. To be given over 1 hour.
Alfentanil hydrochloride *Rapifen*®	C,I	Glucose 5%; Sodium chloride 0.9%; Sodium lactate, compound	
Alprostadil *Prostin VR*®	C	Glucose 5%; Sodium chloride 0.9%	
Amikacin sulphate *Amikin*®	I	Glucose 5%; Sodium chloride 0.9%; Sodium lactate, compound	To be given over 30 minutes.
Aminophylline	C	Glucose 5%; Sodium chloride 0.9%; Sodium lactate, compound	
Amiodarone hydrochloride *Cordarone X*®	C,I	Glucose 5%	Suggested initial infusion volume 250 ml given over 20–120 minutes. For repeat infusions up to 1.2 g in a maximum volume of 500 ml. Incompatible with sodium chloride infusion.
Amoxycillin sodium *Amoxil*®	C¹,I	Glucose 5%; Sodium chloride 0.9%	Reconstituted solutions diluted and given without delay. Suggested volume 100 ml given over 30–60 minutes.
Amoxycillin sodium	D	Glucose 5%; Sodium chloride 0.9%; Ringer's solution; Sodium lactate, compound; Dextrans	
Amoxycillin/clavulanic acid *Augmentin*®	I	Sodium chloride 0.9%; Water for injections; see also package leaflet	Suggested volume 50–100 ml given over 30–40 minutes and completed within 2 hours of reconstitution.

C = continuous; **I** = intermittent; **D** = addition via drip tubing
C¹ = continuous infusion not usually recommended

Additive	Method	Intravenous infusion	Comments
Amphotericin sodium deoxycholate complex *Fungizone*®	C	Glucose 5%	Dissolve thoroughly at reconstitution stage; preparation must be diluted in a large volume infusion; pH of the glucose must not be below 4.2. Check each container. Protect from light. Suggested infusion time 6 hours.
Ampicillin sodium *Penbritin*®	I,C[1]	Glucose 5%; Sodium chloride 0.9%	Reconstituted solutions diluted and given without delay. Suggested volume 100 ml given over 30–60 minutes.
	D	As for Amoxycillin sodium	
Ampicillin/cloxacillin (sodium salts) *Ampiclox*®	I	Glucose 5%; Sodium chloride 0.9%	Reconstituted solutions diluted and given without delay. Suggested volume 100 ml given over 30–60 minutes.
	D	As for Amoxycillin sodium	
Ampicillin/flucloxacillin (sodium salts) *Magnapen*®	I	Glucose 5%; Sodium chloride 0.9%	Reconstituted solutions diluted and given without delay. Suggested volume 100 ml given over 30–60 minutes.
	D	As for Amoxycillin sodium	
Amsacrine *Amsidine*®	I	Glucose 5%	Reconstitute with diluent provided and dilute to suggested volume 500 ml; give over 60–90 minutes. Use glass syringes. Incompatible with sodium chloride infusion.
Ancrod *Arvin*®	C	Sodium chloride 0.9%	Suggested volume 50–500 ml given over 4–12 hours.
Aprotinin *Trasylol*®	C,D	Glucose 5%; Sodium chloride 0.9%; Ringer's solution	
Atenolol *Tenormin*®	I	Glucose 5%; Sodium chloride 0.9%	Suggested infusion time 20 minutes.
Atracurium besylate *Tracrium*®	C	Glucose 5%; Sodium chloride 0.9%; Sodium lactate, compound	Stability varies with diluent
Azathioprine *Imuran*®	D	Glucose 5%; Sodium chloride 0.9%	Reconstituted solutions should be administered without delay
Azlocillin sodium *Securopen*® (5 g)	I	Glucose 5% or 10%; Sodium chloride 0.9%; Ringer's solution; Fructose 5%	Intermittent infusion suggested for doses over 2 g. To be given over 20–30 minutes.
Aztreonam *Azactam*®	I	Glucose 5%; Sodium chloride 0.9%; Ringer's solution; Sodium lactate, compound	Dissolve initially in water for injections (1 g per 3 ml) then dilute to a concentration of less than 20 mg/ml. To be given over 20–60 minutes.
Benzylpenicillin sodium *Crystapen*®	I,C[1]	Glucose 5%; Sodium chloride 0.9%	Suggested volume 100 ml given over 30–60 minutes.
Betamethasone sodium phosphate *Betnesol*®	C,I,D	Glucose 5%; Sodium chloride 0.9%	
Bleomycin sulphate	I	Sodium chloride 0.9%	To be given slowly. Suggested volume 200 ml.

Additive	Method	Intravenous infusion	Comments
Bumetanide *Burinex*®	I	Glucose 5%; Sodium chloride 0.9%	Suggested volume 500 ml given over 30–60 minutes.
Calcium gluconate	C	Glucose 5%; Sodium chloride 0.9%	Avoid bicarbonates, phosphates, or sulphates.
Carbenicillin sodium *Pyopen*®	I	Glucose 5%; Water for injections	Suggested volume 100 ml given over 30–40 minutes.
Carboplatin *Paraplatin*®	C	Glucose 5%; Sodium chloride 0.9%	Short-term infusion. Final concentration as low as 500 micrograms/ml
Carmustine *BiCNU*®	I	Glucose 5%; Sodium chloride 0.9%	Use the diluent provided to reconstitute; give over 1–2 hours.
Cefotaxime sodium *Claforan*®	I	Glucose 5%; Sodium chloride 0.9%; Sodium lactate, compound; Water for injections	Suggested volume 40–100 ml given over 20–60 minutes.
Cefoxitin sodium *Mefoxin*®	I,D,C[1]	Glucose 5% or 10%; Sodium chloride 0.9%	
Cefsulodin sodium *Monaspor*®	I,D,C[1]	Glucose 5%; Sodium chloride 0.9%; Dextran 40	
Ceftazidime pentahydrate *Fortum*®	I,D	Glucose 5 and 10%; Sodium chloride 0.9%; Sodium lactate, compound; Dextrans; Water for injections	
Ceftizoxime sodium *Cefizox*®	C,I,D	Glucose 5 and 10%; Sodium chloride 0.9%; Ringer's solution; Sodium lactate, compound	Suggested volume 50–100 ml.
Cefuroxime sodium *Zinacef*®	I,D	Glucose 5%; Sodium chloride 0.9%; Sodium lactate, compound	Suggested volume 50–100 ml given over 30 minutes.
Cephalothin sodium *Keflin*®	I,D,C[1]	Glucose 5%; Sodium chloride 0.9%; Sodium lactate, compound	
Cephamandole nafate *Kefadol*®	I,D,C[1]	Glucose 5% or 10%; Sodium chloride 0.9%; Water for injections	
Cephazolin sodium *Kefzol*®	I,D,C[1]	Glucose 5% or 10%; Sodium chloride 0.9%; Sodium lactate, compound; Water for injections	
Cephradine *Velosef*®	C,I	Glucose 5% or 10%; Sodium chloride 0.9%; Ringer's solution; Sodium lactate, compound; Water for injections	Reconstituted solutions diluted and given without delay; max. 8 hours between addition and completion of administration.
Chloramphenicol sodium succinate *Kemicetine*®	I,D	Glucose 5%; Sodium chloride 0.9%	
Cimetidine *Tagamet*®	C,I	Glucose 5%; Sodium chloride 0.9%	For intermittent infusion. Suggested volume 250 ml given over 2 hours.

C = continuous; I = intermittent; D = addition via drip tubing
C[1] = continuous infusion not usually recommended

Additive	Method	Intravenous infusion	Comments
Cisplatin *Neoplatin*®, *Platinex*® *Platosin*®	C	Sodium chloride 0.9%; Sodium chloride and glucose	Suggested volume for *Neoplatin*® and *Platinex*®, 2 litres given over 6–8 hours; for *Platosin*®, 1 litre given over 6– 8 hours.
Clindamycin phosphate *Dalacin C*®	C,I	Glucose 5%; Sodium chloride 0.9%	
Clomipramine *Anafranil*®	I	Glucose 5%; Sodium chloride 0.9%	Suggested volume 125–500 ml given over 45–120 minutes.
Clonazepam *Rivotril*®	I	Glucose 5% or 10%; Sodium chloride 0.9%	Suggested volume 250 ml.
Cloxacillin sodium *Orbenin*®	I,C[1] D	Glucose 5%; Sodium chloride 0.9% As for Amoxycillin sodium (above)	Suggested volume 100 ml given over 30–60 minutes.
Colistin sulphomethate sodium *Colomycin*®	C,I	Glucose 5%; Sodium chloride 0.9%; Ringer's solution; Fructose 5%; Dextran 40 in sodium chloride	Max. 6 hours between addition and completion of administration.
Co-trimoxazole	C		Ampoule solution has a pH of about 10. Suggested infusion time 90 minutes.
Bactrim® for infusion		Glucose 5% or 10%; Sodium chloride 0.9%; Ringer's solution: Sodium lactate, compound; Fructose 5%; Dextrans 40 or 70	
Septrin® for infusion		Glucose 5% or 10%; Sodium chloride 0.9%; Ringer's solution; Fructose 5%; Dextrans 40 or 70	
Cyclophosphamide *Endoxana*®	I,D D	Water for injections Glucose 5%	For intermittent infusion suggested volume 50–100 ml given over 5–15 minutes. Max. 30 minutes between addition and completion of administration.
Cyclosporin *Sandimmun*®	C	Glucose 5%; Sodium chloride 0.9%	Dilute to a concentration of 50 mg in 20–100 ml. Max. 12 hours between addition and completion of administration.
Cytarabine *Alexan*®, *Cytosar*®	C,I,D	Glucose 5%; Sodium chloride 0.9%	Reconstitute *Cytosar*® with the diluent provided. Check container for haze or precipitate during administration.
Dacarbazine *DTIC–Dome*®	I	Glucose 5%; Sodium chloride 0.9%	Suggested volume 125–250 ml given over 15–30 minutes. Protect infusion from light.
Desferrioxamine mesylate *Desferal*®	C,I	Glucose 5%; Sodium chloride 0.9%	
Dexamethasone sodium phosphate *Decadron*®	C,I,D	 Glucose 5%; Sodium chloride 0.9%	

Additive	Method	Intravenous infusion	Comments
Dexamethasone (*continued*) *Oradexon*®		Glucose 5% or 10%; Sodium chloride 0.9%; Ringer's solution; Sodium lactate, compound	
Diazepam			Adsorbed to some extent by the plastics of the infusion set.
Diazemuls®	C	Glucose 5% or 10%	May be diluted to a maximum concentration of 200 mg in 500 ml. Max. 6 hours between addition and completion of administration.
	D	Glucose 5% or 10%; Sodium chloride 0.9%	
Stesolid®	C	Glucose 5%; Sodium chloride 0.9%	Dilute to a concentration not greater than 10 mg in 200 ml.
Valium®	C	Glucose 5%; Sodium chloride 0.9%	Dilute to a concentration of not more than 40 mg in 500 ml. Max. 6 hours between addition and completion of administration.
Digoxin *Lanoxin*®	C	Glucose 5%; Sodium chloride 0.9%	To be given slowly. See also section 2.1.
Digoxin-specific antibody fragments *Digibind*®	I	Sodium chloride 0.9%	Dissolve initially in water for injections (4 ml/vial) then dilute with the sodium chloride 0.9% and give through a 0.22 micron Millipore filter over 20 minutes.
Dinoprost *Prostin F2 alpha*®	C	Glucose 5%; Sodium chloride 0.9%	
Dinoprostone *Prostin E2*®	C,I	Glucose 5%; Sodium chloride 0.9%	
Disodium etidronate *Didronel IV*®	C	Sodium chloride 0.9%	Dilute in large-volume infusion, suggested minimum volume 250 ml; minimum period of infusion 2 hours
Disopyramide phosphate *Dirythmin IV*®, *Rythmodan*®	C,I	Glucose 5%; Sodium chloride 0.9%; Ringer's solution; Sodium lactate, compound	Max. rate by continuous infusion 20–30 mg/hour (or 400 micrograms/kg/hour).
Dobutamine hydrochloride *Dobutrex*® (lyophilised form)			Dissolve initially in water for injections or glucose 5% (250 mg in 10–20 ml) then as for *Dobutrex Solution*.
Dobutrex® Solution	C	Glucose 5%; Sodium chloride 0.9%	Dilute to a concentration of 0.5–1 mg/ml. Give higher concentration (max. 5 mg/ml) with infusion pump. Incompatible with bicarbonate.
Dopamine hydrochloride *Intropin*®	C	Glucose 5%; Sodium chloride 0.9%; Sodium lactate, compound	Dilute to a concentration of 1.6 mg/ml. Incompatible with bicarbonate.

C = continuous; I = intermittent; D = addition via drip tubing
C¹ = continuous infusion not usually recommended

Additive	Method	Intravenous infusion	Comments
Doxorubicin hydrochloride *Doxorubicin Rapid Dissolution* (Farmitalia)	**D**	Glucose 5%; Sodium chloride 0.9%	Reconstitute with water for injections or sodium chloride 0.9%.
Electrolytes *Addiphos*®	**C**	Glucose 5% or 10%	Suggested volume 500 ml.
Epirubicin hydrochloride *Pharmorubicin*®	**D**	Sodium chloride 0.9%	Reconstitute with water for injections (10 mg in 5 ml, 50 mg in 25 ml).
Epoprostenol *Flolan*®	**I**	Sodium chloride 0.9%	Reconstitute with the diluent provided (pH 10.5) to make a concentrate. Use this concentrate within 12 hours and store at 2°–8°C. Dilute with not more than 6 times the volume of sodium chloride 0.9% before use.
Erythromycin lactobionate *Erythrocin*®	**C,I**	Glucose 5% (neutralised with sodium bicarbonate); Sodium chloride 0.9%; Sodium lactate, compound	Dissolve initially in water for injections (1 g in 20 ml) then dilute to a concentration of 1 mg/ml for continuous infusion and 1–5 mg/ml for intermittent infusion.
Ethacrynic acid (sodium salt) *Edecrin*®	**D**	Glucose 5%; Sodium chloride 0.9%	pH of glucose infusion should be adjusted to above 5.
Ethanol	**C**	Glucose 5%; Sodium chloride 0.9%; Ringer's solution; Sodium lactate, compound	Dilute to a concentration of 5–10%
Etoposide *Vepesid*®	**I**	Sodium chloride 0.9%	Dilute to a concentration of not more than 250 micrograms/ml and give over not less than 30 minutes and not more than 6 hours. Check container for haze or precipitate during administration. May dissolve certain types of filter.
Flecainide acetate *Tambocor*®	**C,I**	Glucose 5%; Sodium chloride 0.9%; Sodium lactate, compound	Minimum volume in infusion fluids containing chlorides 500 ml.
Flucloxacillin sodium *Floxapen*®	**I,C**[1] **D**	Glucose 5%; Sodium chloride 0.9% As for Amoxycillin sodium	Suggested volume 100 ml given over 30–60 minutes.
Flumazenil *Anexate*®		Glucose 5%; Sodium chloride 0.9%	
Fluorouracil sodium	**C,D**	Glucose 5%	For continuous infusion suggested volume 500 ml given over 4 hours.
Folinic acid (calcium salt) *Calcium Leucovorin*®, *Refolinon*®	**C**	Glucose 10%; Sodium chloride 0.9%; Sodium lactate, compound	
Frusemide (sodium salt) *Dryptal*®, *Lasix*®	**C**	Sodium chloride 0.9%; Ringer's solution	Infusion pH must be above 5.5. Glucose solutions are unsuitable.

Additive	Method	Intravenous infusion	Comments
Fusidic acid (diethanolamine salt) *Fucidin*®	C	Glucose 5%; Sodium chloride 0.9%; Fructose 20%	Reconstitute with the buffer solution provided and dilute to a maximum equivalent to 1 mg sodium fusidate/ml. To be given over not less than 6 hours.
Gentamicin sulphate *Cidomycin*®	I,D	Glucose 5%; Sodium chloride 0.9%	Suggested volume for intermittent infusion 50–100 ml given over 20 minutes
Glyceryl trinitrate *Nitrocine*®, *Nitronal*®, *Tridil*®	C	Glucose 5%; Sodium chloride 0.9%	For *Tridil*® dilute to a concentration of not more than 400 micrograms/ml. For *Nitrocine*® suggested infusion concentration 100 micrograms/ml. Incompatible with polyvinyl chloride infusion containers such as Viaflex® or Steriflex®. Use glass or polyethylene containers or give via syringe pump.
Heparin sodium	C	Glucose 5%; Sodium chloride 0.9%	Administration with a motorised pump may be advisable.
Hydralazine hydrochloride *Apresoline*®	C	Sodium chloride 0.9%; Ringer's solution	Suggested infusion volume 500 ml.
Hydrocortisone sodium phosphate *Efcortesol*®	C,I,D	Glucose 5%; Sodium chloride 0.9%	
Hydrocortisone sodium succinate *Efcortelan Soluble*®, *Solu-Cortef*®	C,I,D	Glucose 5%; Sodium chloride 0.9%	
Ifosfamide *Mitoxana*®	C	Sodium chloride 0.9%; Sodium chloride and glucose	Suggested infusion volume 3 litres given over 24 hours.
	I,D	Sodium chloride 0.9%; Sodium chloride and glucose	For intermittent infusion give over 30–120 minutes.
Insulin	C	Sodium chloride 0.9%; Sodium lactate, compound	Adsorbed to some extent by plastics of infusion set. See also section 6.1.3. Ensure insulin is not injected into 'dead space' of injection port of the infusion bag.
Iron dextran *Imferon*®	I	Glucose 5%; Sodium chloride 0.9%	Suggested volume 500 ml.
Isoprenaline hydrochloride *Isuprel*®, *Saventrine IV*®	C	Glucose 5%; Sodium chloride and glucose	Dilute in a large-volume infusion. Suggested minimum volume 500 ml. pH of the infusion must be below 5.
Isosorbide dinitrate *Cedocard IV*®, *Isoket 0.1%*®	C	Glucose 5%; Sodium chloride 0.9%	Adsorbed to some extent by polyvinyl chloride infusion containers such as Viaflex® or Steriflex®. Preferably use glass or polyethylene containers or give via a syringe pump.

C = continuous; I = intermittent; D = addition via drip tubing
C¹ = continuous infusion not usually recommended

Additive	Method	Intravenous infusion	Comments
Isoxsuprine hydrochloride *Duvadilan*®	C	Glucose 5%; Sodium chloride 0.9%	Suggested infusion concentration 0.02%.
Kanamycin sulphate *Kannasyn*®	I	Glucose 5%; Sodium chloride 0.9%	To be given slowly.
Labetalol hydrochloride *Trandate*®	I	Glucose 5%; Sodium chloride and glucose	Dilute to a concentration of 1 mg/ml. Suggested volume 200 ml. Adjust rate with in-line burette.
Latamoxef disodium *Moxalactam*®	I,D	Glucose 5%; Sodium chloride 0.9%; Sodium lactate, compound; Water for injections	
Lignocaine hydrochloride *Xylocard 20%*®	C	Glucose 5%; Sodium chloride 0.9%; Ringer's solution; Dextrans	Dilute in a large-volume infusion. Suggested infusion concentration 0.2%. Use ready-prepared solution when available.
Lincomycin hydrochloride *Lincocin*®	C	Glucose 5%; Sodium chloride 0.9%	Dilute in a large-volume infusion. Suggested minimum volume 250 ml. Minimum period of infusion 1 hour.
Mecillinam *Selexidin*®	I	Glucose 5%; Sodium chloride 0.9%	Reconstituted solutions diluted and given without delay. Suggested infusion time 15–30 minutes.
Melphalan *Alkeran*®	C,D	Sodium chloride 0.9%	Reconstitute with the diluent provided. Max. 8 hours between addition and completion of administration.
Mesna *Uromitexan*®	C,D	Sodium chloride and glucose; Sodium chloride 0.9%	Max. 24 hours between addition and completion of administration.
Metaraminol tartrate *Aramine*®	C,D	Glucose 5%; Sodium chloride 0.9%; Ringer's solution; Sodium lactate, compound; Dextran 70	Suggested infusion volume 500 ml.
Methicillin sodium *Celbenin*®	I,C[1]	Glucose 5%; Sodium chloride 0.9%	Suggested volume 100 ml given over 30–60 minutes.
	D	As for Amoxycillin sodium	
Methocarbamol *Robaxin*®	I	Glucose 5%; Sodium chloride 0.9%	Dilute to a concentration of not less than 1 g in 250 ml.
Methotrexate sodium	C,D		Dilute in a large-volume infusion.
Methotrexate (Lederle)		Glucose 5%; Sodium chloride 0.9%; Sodium lactate, compound; Ringer's solution	Max. 24 hours between addition and completion of administration.
Methotrexate (Tillotts)		Glucose 5%; Sodium chloride 0.9%; Ringer's solution; Dextrans	Max. 24 hours between addition and completion of administration.
Emtexate®		Sodium chloride 0.9%	Max. 8 hours between addition and completion of administration.
Methyldopa hydrochloride *Aldomet*®	I	Glucose 5%	Suggested volume 100 ml given over 30–60 minutes.

Additive	Method	Intravenous infusion	Comments
Methylprednisolone sodium succinate *Solu-Medrone*®	C,I,D	Glucose 5%; Sodium chloride 0.9%	
Metoclopramide hydrochloride *Maxolon High Dose*®	C	Glucose 5%; Sodium chloride 0.9%; Sodium lactate, compound	Loading dose, dilute with 50–100 ml and give over 15–30 minutes; maintenance dose, dilute with 500 ml and give over 8–12 hours.
	I		Dilute with at least 50 ml and give over at least 15 minutes.
Mexiletine hydrochloride *Mexitil*®	C	Glucose 5%; Sodium chloride 0.9%	
Mezlocillin sodium *Baypen*® (5 g)	I	Glucose 5% and 10%; Sodium chloride 0.9%; Ringer's solution; Fructose 5%; Water for injections	Suggested volume 50 ml given over 15–20 minutes.
Miconazole *Daktarin*®	C,I	Glucose 5%; Sodium chloride 0.9%	Minimum period of infusion 30 minutes. For intermittent infusion suggested volume 200–500 ml.
Mithramycin *see* Plicamycin			
Mitozantrone hydrochloride *Novantrone*®	D	Glucose 5%; Sodium chloride 0.9%	Suggested volume at least 50 ml given over at least 3–5 minutes.
Mustine hydrochloride	D	Glucose 5%; Sodium chloride 0.9%	
Naftidrofuryl oxalate *Praxilene Forte*®	I	Glucose 5% or 10%; Sodium chloride 0.9%; Dextran 40; Fructose 10%	Suggested volume 250–500 ml given over 90–120 minutes.
Naloxone *Min-I-Jet Naloxone Hydrochloride*® *Narcan*®	C	Glucose 5%; Sodium chloride 0.9%	Dilute to a concentration of 4 micrograms/ml.
Netilmicin sulphate *Netillin*®	I,D	Glucose 5% or 10%; Sodium chloride 0.9%	For intermittent infusion suggested volume 50–200 ml given over 30–120 minutes.
Noradrenaline solution strong sterile *Levophed*®	C	Glucose 5%; Sodium chloride and glucose	Dilute in a large-volume infusion. pH of the infusion solution must be below 6.
Oxytocin *Syntocinon*®	C	Glucose 5%; Sodium chloride 0.9%; Ringer's solution; Fructose 20%; Dextrans 40 or 70	Dilute in a large-volume infusion.
Pentamidine isethionate	I	Glucose 5%; Sodium chloride 0.9%	Dissolve initially in water for injections (300 mg in 3–5 ml) then dilute in 50–250 ml; give over at least 60 minutes.
Phenoxybenzamine hydrochloride *Dibenyline*®	I	Sodium chloride 0.9%	To be given over not less than 60 minutes.
Phentolamine mesylate *Rogitine*®	I	Glucose 5%; Sodium chloride 0.9%	To be given over: 10 minutes (diagnostic), 180 minutes (therapy).

C = continuous; I = intermittent; D = addition via drip tubing
C¹ = continuous infusion not usually recommended

Additive	Method	Intravenous infusion	Comments
Phenylephrine hydrochloride	I	Glucose 5%; Sodium chloride 0.9%	
Piperacillin sodium *Pipril*®	I	Glucose 5%; Sodium chloride 0.9%; Sodium lactate, compound; Water for injections; Dextrans	Minimum infusion volume 50 ml given over 20–40 minutes.
Plicamycin *Mithracin*®	I	Glucose 5%	Suggested volume 1000 ml given over 4–6 hours.
Polymyxin B sulphate *Aerosporin*®	C	Glucose 5%	Suggested volume 200–500 ml given over 60–90 minutes.
Potassium canrenoate *Spiroctan-M*®	I	Glucose 5%; Sodium chloride 0.9%	Suggested volume 250 ml.
Potassium chloride	C	Glucose 5%; Sodium chloride 0.9%	Dilute in a large-volume infusion. Mix thoroughly to avoid 'layering', especially in non-rigid infusion containers. Use ready-prepared solutions when possible.
Prednisolone sodium phosphate *Codelsol*®	C,I,D	Glucose 5%; Sodium chloride 0.9%	Max. 24 hours between addition and completion of administration.
Propofol *Diprivan*®	D	Glucose 5%; Sodium chloride 0.9%	Not to be mixed with other therapeutic agents or infusion fluids; to be administered via a Y-piece close to injection site.
Quinine dihydrochloride	C	Sodium chloride 0.9%	To be given over 4 hours.
Ranitidine hydrochloride *Zantac*®	I	Glucose 5%; Sodium chloride 0.9%; Sodium lactate, compound	
Rifampicin *Rifadin*®, *Rimactane*® infusion	I	Glucose 5%; Sodium lactate, compound	To be given over 2–3 hours.
Ritodrine hydrochloride *Yutopar*®	C	Glucose 5%; Sodium chloride 0.9%	Dilute in a large-volume infusion.
Salbutamol sulphate *Ventolin*® for intravenous infusion	C	Glucose 5%; Sodium chloride 0.9%	Suggested volume 500 ml as a solution containing 10 micrograms/ml.
Sodium calciumedetate *Ledclair*®	C	Glucose 5%; Sodium chloride 0.9%	Dilute to a concentration of not more than 3%. Suggested volume 250–500 ml given over at least 1 hour.
Sodium nitroprusside *Nipride*®	C	Glucose 5%	Suggested volume 500–1000 ml. Reconstitute with diluent provided. Protect infusion from light. Max. 4 hours from addition to completion of administration.
Streptokinase *Kabikinase*®	C	Glucose 5%; Sodium chloride 0.9%	
Streptase®		Sodium chloride 0.9%	
Sulphadiazine sodium	C	Sodium chloride 0.9%	Suggested volume 500 ml. Ampoule solution has a pH of over 10.

Additive	Method	Intravenous infusion	Comments
Suxamethonium chloride *Anectine®*, *Scoline®*	C	Glucose 5%; Sodium chloride 0.9%	
Terbutaline sulphate *Bricanyl®*	C	Glucose 5%; Sodium chloride 0.9%	Suggested volume 500 ml. To be given over 8–10 hours.
Tetracosactrin *Synacthen®*	C	Glucose 5%; Sodium chloride 0.9%	Suggested volume 500 ml given over 6 hours.
Tetracycline hydrochloride *Achromycin Intravenous®*	C	Glucose 5%; Sodium chloride 0.9%; Sodium lactate, compound	Minimum volume 100 ml. To be given over not more than 12 hours.
Theophylline (solubilised with lysine) *Labophylline®*	C	Glucose 5%; Sodium chloride 0.9%	
Thiopentone sodium *Intraval®*	C,D	Sodium chloride 0.9%	Check container for haze or precipitate before administration.
Ticarcillin sodium *Ticar®*	I	Glucose 5%; Water for injections	Suggested volume 100–150 ml given over 30–40 minutes.
Ticarcillin sodium/ clavulanic acid *Timentin®*	I	Glucose 5%; Water for injections	Suggested volume glucose 5%, 50–150 ml (depending on dose) water, 25–100 ml given over 30–40 minutes.
Tinidazole *Fasigyn®*	I	Glucose 5%; Sodium chloride 0.9%	800 mg to be given over at least 30 minutes or *pro rata.*
Tobramycin sulphate *Nebcin®*	I,D	Glucose 5%; Sodium chloride 0.9%	For intermittent infusion suggested volume 100–150 ml given over 20–60 minutes.
Tocainide hydrochloride *Tonocard®*	I	Glucose 5%; Sodium chloride 0.9%	Suggested volume 50–100 ml given over 15–30 minutes.
Treosulfan *Treosulfan* (Leo)	I	Water for injections	Infusion suggested for doses above 5 g. Use diluted to a concentration of 5 g in 100 ml.
Trimetaphan camsylate *Arfonad®*	I	Glucose 5%; Sodium chloride 0.9%	Suggested infusion concentration 0.05–0.1%. Suggested volume 100–500 ml.
Trimethoprim lactate *Monotrim®*	D	As for Syraprim® (below); also Sodium chloride 0.9%; Sodium lactate, compound; Dextrans 40 or 70 in sodium chloride	
Syraprim®	I,D	Glucose 5%; Fructose 5%	
Trisodium edetate *Limclair®*	C	Glucose 5%; Sodium chloride 0.9%	Suggested volume 500 ml given over 2–3 hours.
Urea *Ureaphil®*	C	Glucose 5% or 10%	
Urokinase *Urokinase* (Leo)	C	Sodium chloride 0.9%	
Vancomycin hydrochloride *Vancocin®*	I,C¹	Glucose 5%; Sodium chloride 0.9%	Suggested volume 100–200 ml given over 60 minutes.

C = continuous; I = intermittent; D = addition via drip tubing
C¹ = continuous infusion not usually recommended

Additive	Method	Intravenous infusion	Comments
Vasopressin, synthetic *Pitressin*®	I	Glucose 5%	Suggested concentration 20 units/100 ml given over 15 minutes.
Vecuronium bromide *Norcuron*®	I	Glucose 5%; Sodium chloride 0.9%; Ringer's solution	Reconstitute with the diluent provided.
Vidarabine *Vira-A*®	C	Glucose 5%; Sodium chloride and glucose; Sodium lactate, compound	Solubility in infusion fluid is limited. It must be given diluted in a large-volume infusion and administered over 12–24 hours.
Vinblastine sulphate *Velbe*®	D	Sodium chloride 0.9%; Water for injections	Reconstitute with the diluent provided.
Vincristine sulphate *Oncovin*®	D	Sodium chloride 0.9%; Water for injections	Reconstitute with the diluent provided.
Vindesine sulphate *Eldisine*®	D	Glucose 5%; Sodium chloride 0.9%	Reconstitute with the diluent provided.
Vitamins B & C *Pabrinex*®, *Parentrovite IVHP*®	I,D	Glucose 5%; Sodium chloride 0.9%	Ampoule contents should be mixed, diluted, and administered without delay.
Vitamins, multiple			See also section 9.3.
Multibionta®	I	Glucose 5%; Sodium chloride 0.9%	Dilute 10 ml in not less than 250 ml of infusion fluid (adults).
Solivito N®	I	Glucose 5% or 10%	Suggested volume 500–1000 ml given over 2–3 hours.

C = continuous; I = intermittent; D = addition via drip tubing
C¹ = continuous infusion not usually recommended

Appendix 3: Borderline Substances

In certain conditions some foods (and toilet preparations) have characteristics of drugs and the Advisory Committee on Borderline Substances advises as to the circumstances in which such substances may be regarded as drugs. The Advisory Committee's recommendations are listed below. Prescriptions issued in accordance with the Committee's advice and endorsed 'ACBS' will normally not be investigated.

NON-PRESCRIBABLE PREPARATIONS

The following have been considered by the ACBS and may **not** be prescribed on form FP10, having been included in Schedule 3A to the NHS (General Medical and Pharmaceutical Services) Regulations 1974:

ALCOHOLIC BEVERAGES
Wines, tonic wines and similar preparations. (Where the therapeutic qualities of alcohol are required rectified spirit, suitably flavoured and diluted, should be prescribed.)

ANTI-SMOKING PREPARATIONS
Nicobrevin; Nicorette; Respaton.

DISINFECTANTS (ANTISEPTICS)
Drugs only when ordered in such quantities and with such directions as are appropriate for the treatment of patients. Not to be regarded as drugs if ordered for general hygienic purposes.

FOODS
Cantaflour; Carnation Build-up; Complan; Efamol capsules; Energen starch-reduced bran crispbread; Ensure Plus HN; Flora margarine; Forta puddings; Fortimel; Fortison low sodium; GF gluten-free maize biscuits with chocolate or hazelnuts, gluten-free thin wafer bread; Glucodin; Guar crispbread; Isomil ready-to-feed and liquid concentrate; Laevoral; Linoleic acid; Modifast; Nutritionally Complete Supplemented Fasting Formula; Osmolite HN; Rite-Diet gluten-free canned rich fruit cake, chocolate chip cookies, half-coated chocolate or sultana biscuit and soya bran, Lincoln, shortcake, custard cream biscuits; Safflower seed oil; Saxin; SMA, Gold Cap Powder, Gold Cap Ready-to-feed, and White cap powder; Sorbitol; Soyagen; Sweetex; Tritamyl gluten-free bread mix; Trufree plain flour, pasta mix, sweet biscuit and bread mix; Twocal HN; Wate-on tablets.
Note: Neither gluten-free products nor those containing linoleic acid (e.g. safflower and sunflower seed oils) should be regarded as drugs in the management of *multiple sclerosis.*

TOILET PREPARATIONS
Acnaveen Bar; Acne Aid Bar; Atrixo; Cidal; Covermark Removing Cream; Dansac Skin Lotion; Derbac Soap; Dermacolor Cleansing Cream, Cleansing Milk, and Cleansing Lotion; Emulave Bar; Gamophen; Genatosan; Ipsel

Hygienic Baby Salve; Lacto-Calamine; Lysaldin; Neutrogena Soap; Nivea; Oilatum Bar; Simple Soap; United Skin Care Programme; Woodwards Nursery Cream.

VITAMIN PREPARATIONS
Drugs only when used in the management of actual or potential vitamin deficiency.

PRESCRIBABLE PREPARATIONS

The following list indicates the clinical conditions and the products which the ACBS has approved for the management of those conditions. Details of the products are given in section 9.4 (food preparations) and chapter 13 (toilet preparations).

FOODS
Conditions for which the foods indicated may be prescribed on FP10.

Amino acid metabolic disorders and similar protein disorders: see phenylketonuria; histidinaemia; homocystinuria; maple syrup urine disease; synthetic diets; low-protein products.

Anorexia nervosa: Clinifeed; Enrich; Ensure; Ensure Plus; Ensure Powder; Flexical; Fortisip Energy-Plus, Flavoured, and Standard; Fortison Energy-Plus and Standard; Fresubin Liquid, Sip Feeds and Plus F; Isocal; Liquisorb; Liquisorbon MCT; Osmolite; Triosorbon; Vivonex.

Bowel fistulas: Clinifeed; Elemental 028 and 028 orange; Enrich; Ensure; Ensure Plus; Ensure Powder; Flexical; Forceval Protein; Fortisip Energy-Plus, Flavoured, and Standard; Fortison Energy-Plus and Standard; Fresubin Liquid, Sip Feeds and Plus F; Isocal; Liquisorb; Liquisorbon MCT; Maxipro HBV; Osmolite; Pepti-2000 LF; Peptisorb; Peptisorbon; Triosorbon; Vivonex.

Calcium intolerance: Locasol and Locasol New Formula.

Carbohydrate malabsorption: Calogen. See also synthetic diets; malabsorption states.

Disaccharide intolerance (without isomaltose intolerance): Caloreen; Maxijul LE, Liquid, and Super Soluble; Polycal; Polycose powder. See also lactose intolerance; lactose with sucrose intolerance.

Glucose and galactose intolerance: Comminuted chicken meat (Cow & Gate); Fructose; Galactomin Formula 19 (fructose formula).

Isomaltose intolerance: Glucose (dextrose).

Lactose intolerance: Comminuted chicken meat (Cow & Gate); Formula S (Cow & Gate); Fortison Soya; Galactomin Formula 17 (glucose formula full fat) and Formula 18 (glucose formula reduced fat); Isomil powder; Nutramigen; Portagen; Pregestimil; Prosobee; Wysoy.

Lactose with sucrose intolerance: Aminex; Comminuted Chicken Meat (Cow & Gate); Galactomin Formula 17 (glucose formula full fat) and Formula 18 (glucose formula reduced fat); Pregestimil.

Sucrose intolerance: Glucose (dextrose) and see also synthetic diets; malabsorption states; lactose with sucrose intolerance.

Cirrhosis of the liver and chronic liver disease: see liver disease.

Coeliac disease: see gluten-sensitive enteropathies.

Cystic fibrosis: see malabsorption states.

Disaccharide intolerance: see carbohydrate malabsorption.

Dysphagia (associated with: intrinsic disease of the oesophagus, e.g. oesophagitis; neuromuscular disorders, e.g. multiple sclerosis and motor neurone disease; major surgery and/or radiotherapy for cancer of the upper digestive tract; protracted severe inflammatory disease of the upper digestive tract, e.g. Stevens-Johnson syndrome and epidermolysis bullosa): Clinifeed; Elemental 028 and 028 orange; Enrich; Ensure; Ensure Plus; Ensure Powder; Forceval Protein; Fortisip Energy-Plus, Flavoured, and Standard; Fortison Energy-Plus and Standard; Fresubin Liquid, Sip Feeds and Plus F; Isocal; Liquisorb; Liquisorbon MCT; Maxipro HBV; Osmolite; Reabilan; Triosorbon; Vivonex; Wyeth Standard Enteral Feed.

Epilepsy (ketogenic diet in): Alembicol D; Calogen; Liquigen; Medium-Chain Triglyceride Oil (MCT).

Galactokinase deficiency and galactosaemia: Formula S (Cow & Gate); Galactomin Formula 17 (glucose formula full fat) and Formula 18 (glucose formula reduced fat); Isomil powder; Nutramigen; Pregestimil; Prosobee Liquid and Powder; Wysoy.

Gastrectomy (total): Clinifeed; Elemental 028 and 028 orange; Enrich; Ensure; Ensure Plus; Ensure Powder; Flexical; Forceval protein; Fortisip Energy-Plus, Flavoured, and Standard; Fortison Energy-Plus and Standard; Fresubin Liquid, Sip Feeds and Plus F; Isocal; Liquisorb; Liquisorbon MCT; Maxipro HBV; Osmolite; Pepti-2000 LF; Peptisorb; Peptisorb; Reabilan; Triosorbon; Vivonex.

Glucose/galactose intolerance: see carbohydrate intolerance.

Gluten-sensitive enteropathies: Aglutella gluten-free low-protein macaroni, pasta spirals, semolina, spaghetti, spaghetti rings, tagliatelle; Aproten products (anellini, biscuits, crispbread, ditalini, flour, rigatini, tagliatelle); Bi-Aglut biscuits and gluten-free toast; Ener-G brown rice bread; Gluten-free biscuits (Farley); Gluten-free crackers (GF Dietary Supplies); Glutenex (Cow & Gate); Juvela gluten-free corn mix, gluten-free loaf and high-fibre loaf (sliced and unsliced), gluten-free mix and fibre mix; Juvela low-protein loaf (sliced and unsliced) and low-protein mix; Liga gluten-free rusks (Cow & Gate); Polial gluten-free biscuits; Rite-Diet gluten-free high-fibre bread (with added soya-bran); Rite-Diet gluten-free white bread 400 g; Rite-Diet gluten-free white bread mix; Rite-Diet gluten-free brown bread mix; Rite-Diet gluten-free bread with soya bran (dispensed in tin); Rite-Diet gluten-free high-fibre crackers; Rite-Diet low-protein flour mix; Rite-Diet gluten-free flour mix; Rite-Diet gluten-free low-protein bread (dispen-

sed in tin, with or without salt); Rite-Diet low-protein white bread (with added fibre); Rite-Diet gluten-free digestive biscuits, sweet (without chocolate or sultanas) biscuits, savoury biscuits, and gluten-free crackers; Rite-Diet low-protein spaghetti (short cut), spaghetti rings, and macaroni; Tritamyl gluten-free flour; Tritamyl PK flour; Trufree special dietary flours No. 1, No. 2 with rice bran, No. 3 for Cantabread, No. 4 white, No. 5 brown, No. 6 plain, No. 7 self-raising; Verkade gluten-free biscuits.

Glycogen storage disease: Caloreen; Corn Flour or Corn Starch; Glucose (dextrose); Maxijul LE, liquid, and Super Soluble; Polycal; Polycose powder.

Histidinaemia: HF(2), and see also low-protein products; synthetic diets.

Homocystinuria: Albumaid RVHB X Methionine; Albumaid RVHB Complete X Methionine, and see also low-protein products; synthetic diets.

Hypercholesterolaemia (familial): Corn oil; Sunflower oil.

Hyperlipoproteinaemia type 1: Liquigen; Medium Chain Triglyceride Oil.

Hypoglycaemia: Caloreen; Corn Flour or Corn Starch; Maxijul LE, liquid, and Super Soluble; Polycal; Polycose powder, and see also glycogen storage disease.

Hypoproteinaemia: Casilan; Dialamine; Forceval Protein; Maxipro HBV; ProMod; Protifar.

Intestinal lymphangiectasia: see malabsorption states.

Intestinal surgery: see malabsorption states.

Isomaltose intolerance: see carbohydrate malabsorption.

Lactose intolerance: see carbohydrate malabsorption.

Liver disease (i.e. chronic liver disease, cirrhosis): Aglutella Azeta cream-filled wafers; Aglutella gluten-free low-protein macaroni, pasta spirals, semolina, spaghetti, spaghetti rings, tagliatelle; Alembicol D; Aminex; Aproten products (anellini, biscuits, crispbread, ditalini, flour, rigatini, tagliatelle); Caloreen; dp Low-Protein butterscotch-flavoured or chocolate-flavoured chip cookies; Fortical; Hepatic Aid; Hycal; Juvela low-protein loaf (sliced and unsliced) and low-protein mix; Liquigen; Maxijul LE, liquid, and Super Soluble; MCT (1) Powder; Medium Chain Triglyceride Oil; Polycal; Polycose powder; Portagen; Rite-Diet gluten-free low-protein bread (dispensed in tin with or without salt); Rite-Diet low-protein white bread (with added fibre); Rite-Diet gluten-free low-protein crackers; Rite-Diet low-protein flour mix; Rite-Diet low-protein cream-filled biscuits (chocolate flavour) and sweet biscuits; Rite-Diet low-protein macaroni, spaghetti (short cut), and spaghetti rings; Rite-Diet low-protein chocolate cream wafers and vanilla cream wafers; Tritamyl PK flour.

Low-protein products: Aglutella Azeta cream-filled wafers*; Aglutella gluten-free low protein (macaroni, pasta spirals, semolina, spaghetti, spaghetti-rings, tagliatelle; Aminex*; Aproten products (anellini, biscuits, crispbread, ditalini, flour, rigatini, tagliatelle); dp Low-Protein butterscotch-flavoured or chocolate-flavoured chip cookies*; Juvela low-protein loaf (sliced and unsliced); Juvela low-protein mix; Rite-Diet gluten-free low-protein bread (dispensed in tin, with or without salt); Rite-Diet low-protein white bread (with added fibre); Rite-Diet low-protein gluten-free crackers; Rite-Diet low-protein flour mix; Rite-Diet low-protein cream-filled biscuits (chocolate flavour)*; Rite-Diet low-protein sweet biscuits; Rite-Diet low-protein macaroni, spaghetti (short cut), and spaghetti rings; Rite-Diet low-protein chocolate cream and vanilla cream wafers*; Tritamyl PK flour.

*Not prescribable on ACBS for coeliac disease, dermatitis herpetiformis, steatorrhoea due to gluten sensitivity

Malabsorption states: (see also gluten-sensitive enteropathies; liver disease; milk protein intolerance and synthetic diets).

  (a) Protein sources: Albumaid Complete; Comminuted Chicken Meat (Cow & Gate); Forceval Protein; Maxipro HBV.
  (b) Fat: Alembicol D; Calogen; Liquigen; Medium Chain Triglyceride Oil.
  (c) Carbohydrate: Caloreen; Fortical; Hycal; Maxijul LE; liquid, and Super Soluble; Polycal; Polycose powder.
  (d) Complete Feeds: Clinifeed; Elemental 028 and 028 orange; Enrich; Ensure; Ensure Plus; Ensure Powder; Flexical; Fortisip Energy-Plus, Flavoured, and Standard; Fortison Energy-Plus and Standard; Fresubin Liquid, Sip Feeds, and Plus F; Isocal; Liquisorb; Liquisorbon MCT; MCT (1) Powder (with appropriate vitamin and mineral supplements); Nutranel; Osmolite; Pepti-2000 LF; Peptisorb; Peptisorbon; Portagen; Pregestimil; Reabilan; Triosorbon; Vivonex.
  (e) Minerals: Aminogran Mineral Mixture; Metabolic Mineral Mixture.
  (f) Vitamins: As appropriate, and see synthetic diets.

Maple syrup urine disease: MSUD Aid, and see also low-protein products; synthetic diets.

Milk protein intolerance: Comminuted Chicken Meat (Cow & Gate); Formula S (Cow & Gate); Fortison Soya; Isomil powder; Nutramigen; Pregestimil; Prosobee liquid and powder; Wysoy, and see also synthetic diets.

Nutritional support for adults (for precise conditions for which these products have ACBS approval, see details in section 9.4):

  A. (a) Nutritionally complete feeds (chemically defined diets, whole protein based), for oral, sip or tube feeding.
      (i) Gluten-Free: Clinifeed; Fortisip Energy-Plus, Flavoured, and Standard; Fortison Energy-Plus and Standard; Fresubin Liquid, Sip Feeds, and Plus F (vegetable soup flavour); Liquisorbon MCT; Peptisorb; Triosorbon.
      (ii) Lactose- and Gluten-Free: Enrich; Ensure, Ensure Plus, Ensure Powder; Isocal; MCT (1) Powder (with appropriate vitamin and mineral

supplements); Osmolite; Portagen; Reabilan.
      (b) Elemental and Low-lactose: Flexical; Nutranel; Vivonex.

  B. **Nutritional source supplements;** see synthetic diets; malabsorption states.
      (a) Carbohydrates; lactose-free and gluten-free; Caloreen*; Fortical*; Hycal*; Maxijul LE*, liquid, and Super Soluble; Polycal; Polycose powder.
          *Have low electrolyte content.
      (b) Fat:
          (i) Calogen.
          (ii) Alembicol D; MCT Oil; Liquigen.

  C. **Nitrogen sources:** Albumaid Complete (hydrolysed protein based); Casilan (whole protein based, low-sodium); Forceval Protein (whole protein based, low-sodium); Maxipro HBV (whole protein based, low-sodium); Pro-Mod (whey protein based, low-sodium).

  D. **Minerals:** Aminogran Mineral Mixture; Metabolic Mineral Mixture.

Phenylketonuria: Aglutella Azeta cream-filled wafers; Aglutella gluten-free low-protein macaroni, pasta spirals, semolina, spaghetti, spaghetti rings, tagliatelle; Albumaid XP and XP Concentrate; Aminex; Aminogran Food Supplement and Mineral Mixture; Aproten products (annellini, biscuits, crispbread, ditalini, flour, rigatini, tagliatelle); Calogen; Caloreen; dp Low-Protein butterscotch-flavoured or chocolate-flavoured chip cookies; Juvela low-protein loaf (sliced and unsliced); Juvela low-protein mix; Lofenalac; Maxamaid XP; Metabolic Mineral Mixture; Milupa PKU3; Minafen; PK Aid 1; Polycal; Polycose powder; Rite-Diet gluten-free low-protein bread (dispensed in tin, with or without salt); Rite-Diet low-protein white bread (with added fibre); Rite-Diet low-protein flour mix; Rite-Diet low-protein cream-filled biscuits (chocolate flavour), sweet biscuits and low-protein gluten-free crackers; Rite-Diet low-protein macaroni, spaghetti (short cut), and spaghetti rings; Rite-Diet low-protein chocolate cream and vanilla cream wafers; Tritamyl PK flour, and see low-protein products and synthetic diets.

Protein intolerance: see milk protein intolerance, low-protein products, synthetic diets, and amino acid metabolic disorders.

Renal failure: Aglutella Azeta cream-filled wafers; Aglutella gluten-free low-protein macaroni, pasta spirals, semolina, spaghetti, spaghetti rings, tagliatelle; Aminex; Aproten products (annellini, biscuits, crispbread, ditalini, flour, rigatini, tagliatelle; Calogen; Caloreen; Dialamine; dp Low-Protein butterscotch-flavoured or chocolate-flavoured chip cookies; Fortical; Hycal; Juvela low-protein loaf (sliced and unsliced) and low-protein mix; Maxijul LE, liquid, and Super Soluble; Polycal; Polycose powder; Rite-Diet gluten-free low-protein bread (dispensed in tin, with or without salt); Rite-Diet low-protein white bread (with added fibre); Rite-Diet low-protein gluten-free crackers; Rite-Diet low-protein flour mix; Rite-Diet low-protein cream-filled biscuits (chocolate flavour); Rite-Diet low-protein sweet biscuits; Rite-Diet low-protein macaroni, spaghetti (short cut), and spaghetti rings; Rite-Diet low-protein chocolate cream and vanilla cream wafers; Tritamyl PK flour.

Short bowel syndrome: see malabsorption states.

Sodium dietary reduction: Rite-Diet low-sodium bread.

Sucrose intolerance: see carbohydrate malabsorption.

Synthetic diets:

(a) Fat: Alembicol D; Calogen; Liquigen; Medium Chain Triglyceride Oil.

(b) Carbohydrate: Caloreen; Fortical; Hycal; Maxijul LE, liquid, and Super Soluble; Polycal; Polycose powder.

(c) Minerals; Aminogran Mineral Mixture; Metabolic Mineral Mixture.

(d) Protein sources: see malabsorption states, complete feeds.

(e) Vitamins: as appropriate and see malabsorption states, nutritional support for adults.

Vomiting in infancy: Instant Carobel; Nestargel.

TOILET PREPARATIONS

Conditions for which the toilet preparations indicated may be prescribed on FP10.

Acne: Ionax scrub.

Birthmarks: see disfiguring skin lesions.

Dermatitis (includes contact, atopic and infective dermatoses, eczema and pruritic dermatoses): Betadine Skin Cleanser and Foam; Genisol; Polytar Emollient, Liquid, and Plus; Ster-Zac Bath Concentrate; T/Gel shampoo.

Dermatitis herpetiformis: see gluten-sensitive enteropathies.

Disfiguring skin lesions (birthmarks, mutilating lesions and scars): Boots Covering Cream; Covermark products; Dermacolor Camouflage System; Keromask masking cream and finishing powder; Veil Cover cream (Cleansing Creams, Cleansing Milks, and Cleansing Lotions are excluded.)

Eczema: see dermatitis.

Photodermatoses (skin protection in): Coppertone Supershade 15 and Ultrashade 23; Piz Buin Creme, SPF No. 12; RoC Opaque Total Sunblock Cream SPF 15 A & B (Colourless and tinted); RoC Total Sunblock Cream 10 (colourless); Spectraban 4 and 15.

Pruritus: see dermatitis.

Psoriasis: see scaling of the scalp.

Scabies: Tetmosol.

Scaling of the scalp (psoriasis, dandruff, eczema): Alphosyl; Betadine; Capitol; Ceanel Concentrate; Cetavlon PC; Gelcotar; Genisol; Ionil T; Polytar Emollient, Liquid, and Plus; T/Gel shampoo.

Appendix 4: Cautionary and Advisory Labels for Dispensed Medicines

In recent years there has been a growing need for patients to be given better information on the medicines they have been prescribed so that they will be reminded to take the medicine correctly and most effectively. One aspect of this is the provision of more detailed cautionary and advisory labels than have been used in the past.

What a patient learns about a medicine will include whatever the prescriber says, what the labels on the dispensed medicines say, what any patient information leaflet may say, and whatever the pharmacist says by way of explanation and encouragement. Nevertheless, the label is what the patient will see when taking each dose. Leaflets may be discarded and verbal advice forgotten.

The BNF now shows under many preparations the numbers of any labels that pharmacists are recommended to apply to the containers of preparations when they are dispensed. The wordings chosen for the labels represent a carefully considered balance between the unintelligibly short and the inconveniently long. Since any fixed set of words cannot cover the language needs of all patients it is expected that pharmacists will counsel patients.

All counselling needs to be related to the age, experience, background, and understanding of the individual patient. The patient will then be able to obtain the maximum benefit from following the directions.

Compliance with the intentions of the prescriber should be encouraged. The pharmacist should ensure that the patient understands not only how to use the medicine but also how much and how often. Any effects of the medicine on driving or work, any foods or medicines to be avoided, and what to do if a dose is missed should also be explained. There may be other matters that are better dealt with by counselling than by a label, such as the possibility of staining of the clothes or skin by a medicine.

For some preparations there is a special need for counselling, such as an unusual method or time of administration or a potential interaction with a common food or domestic remedy, and this is indicated where necessary.

Manufacturers' instructions

Many preparations are now dispensed in unbroken original packs that bear complete instructions for the patient or provide a leaflet addressed to the patient. These labels or leaflets should not normally be obscured or removed. Where it is known that such instructions are provided with an original pack intended for the patient no label has been listed under the preparation. Label 10 may be used where appropriate. Leaflets may be available from various sources advising on the administration of preparations such as eye-drops, eye ointments, inhalers, and suppositories.

Scope of the recommended labels

No label recommendations have been made for injections (except for selected systemic corticosteroids) on the assumption that they will be administered by a health professional or a well-trained patient. The labelling is not exhaustive and pharmacists are recommended to use their professional discretion in labelling new preparations and those for which no labels are shown.

Individual labelling advice is not given on the administration of the large variety of antacids and topical corticosteroid preparations, although general guidance on labelling is given in the notes relevant to these preparations (see sections 1.1 and 13.4). In the absence of instructions from the prescriber, and if on enquiry the patient has had no verbal instructions, the directions given under 'Dose' should be used on the label.

It is recognised that there may be occasions when pharmacists will use their knowledge and professional discretion and decide to omit one or more of the recommended labels for a particular patient. In this case counselling is of the utmost importance. There may also be an occasion when a prescriber does not wish additional cautionary labels to be used, in which case the prescription should be endorsed 'NCL' (no cautionary labels). The exact wording that is required instead should then be specified on the prescription.

Pharmacists have traditionally labelled medicines with various wordings in addition to those directions specified on the prescription. Such labels include 'Shake the bottle', 'For external use only', 'Not to be taken', and 'Store in a cool place', as well as 'Discard . . . . days after opening' and 'Do not use after . . . .', which apply particularly to antibiotic mixtures, diluted liquid and topical preparations, and to eye-drops. Although not listed in the BNF these labels should continue to be used when appropriate; indeed, 'For external use only' is a legal requirement on external liquid preparations, while 'Keep out of the reach of children' is a legal requirement on all dispensed medicines.

It is the usual practice for patients to take oral solid-dose preparations with water or other liquid and for this reason no separate label has been recommended.

The label or labels for each preparation are recommended after careful consideration of the information available. However, it is recognised that in some cases this information may be either incomplete or open to a different interpretation. The Executive Editor will therefore be grateful to receive any constructive comments on the labelling suggested for any preparation.

Recommended label wordings

The wordings which can be given as separate warnings are labels 1–19 and label 29. Wordings which can be incorporated in an appropriate position in the directions for dosage or administration are labels 21–28. A label has been omitted for number 20.

If separate labels are used it is recommended that the wordings be used without modification. If changes are made to suit computer requirements, care should be taken to retain the sense of the original.

(1) Warning. May cause drowsiness

To be used on children's preparations containing antihistamines, e.g., paediatric elixirs and linctuses, or other preparations given to children where the warnings of label 2 on driving or alcohol would not be appropriate.

(2) Warning. May cause drowsiness. If affected do not drive or operate machinery. Avoid alcoholic drink

To be used on preparations that can cause drowsiness, thereby affecting the ability to drive and operate hazardous machinery. The main preparations are most antihistamines; central nervous system depressants such as anxiolytics, antipsychotics, opioid analgesics, and tricyclic antidepressants; some antihypertensives; some analgesics; some antiepileptics; some antiemetics; and some muscle relaxants. Label 2 is now seen as unhelpful in relation to hypnotics, hence a new label (label 19) has been introduced to cover hypnotics, and also anxiolytics, taken at night. *It is an offence to drive while under the influence of drink or drugs.*

Label 1 is more appropriate for children.

Some of these preparations only cause drowsiness in the first few days of treatment and the patient then becomes tolerant; some only cause drowsiness in higher doses.

In such cases the patient should be told that the advice to avoid driving, etc., applies until the effects have worn off. Many of these preparations can produce a slowing of reaction time and a loss of mental concentration that can have the same effects as drowsiness on activities that require alertness to avoid hazard.

The avoidance of alcoholic drink is recommended, since the effects of CNS depressants are enhanced by alcohol, but it must be realised that a strict prohibition could lead to certain patients not taking the medicine at all. Pharmacists should explain the risk and encourage compliance, particularly in patients who may think they already tolerate the effects of alcohol (see also label 3).

Queries from patients with epilepsy regarding fitness to drive should be referred back to the patient's doctor.

There are other side-effects unrelated to drowsiness that may affect a patient's ability to drive or operate machinery safely, for example, blurred vision, dizziness, or nausea. In general, no label has been recommended to cover these cases, but the patient should be suitably counselled.

(3) Warning. May cause drowsiness. If affected do not drive or operate machinery

To be used on monoamine-oxidase inhibitor (because alcohol is covered by label 10 and the MAOI treatment card).

Some patients given CNS depressants may have been advised how much alcohol they may drink by their doctor and in such cases label 3 may be more appropriate than label 2.

(4) Warning. Avoid alcoholic drink

To be used on preparations where a reaction such as flushing may occur if alcohol is taken, e.g. metronidazole and chlorpropamide. Alcohol may also enhance the hypoglycaemia produced by some oral antidiabetic drugs but routine application of a warning label is not considered necessary.

For most interactions with alcohol label 2 is more appropriate.

(5) Do not take indigestion remedies at the same time of day as this medicine

To be used in conjunction with label 25 on preparations coated to resist gastric acid, such as enteric-coated tablets, capsules, and granules.

The coating may be ruptured prematurely in the presence of alkalis present in antacids.

Label 5 also applies to drugs such as ciprofloxacin and ketoconazole where the absorption is significantly affected by antacids; the usual period of avoidance recommended is 2 to 4 hours

(6) Do not take iron preparations or indigestion remedies at the same time of day as this medicine

To be used on preparations of doxycycline, minocycline, and penicillamine. These drugs chelate iron and calcium ions and are less well absorbed when given with iron or calcium-containing antacids. If necessary these incompatible preparations may be given about two hours apart.

(7) Do not take milk, iron preparations or indigestion remedies at the same time of day as this medicine

To be used on preparations of tetracycline (except doxycycline and minocycline). These drugs chelate iron, calcium, and magnesium ions and are then less well absorbed. If necessary these incompatible preparations may be given about two hours apart.

(8) Do not stop taking this medicine except on your doctor's advice

To be used on beta-blockers, certain antihypertensive drugs, drugs used in the treatment and prophylaxis of asthma, antituberculous drugs and allopurinol.

This label is used to encourage compliance where the drug is to be taken over long periods without the patient necessarily perceiving any benefit. Patients should be told that this label does not override the need to consult the prescriber if side-effects occur.

For certain medicines the patient should be advised to ensure that the supply does not run out.

(9) Take at regular intervals. Complete the prescribed course unless otherwise directed

To be used on preparations where a course of treatment should be completed to reduce the incidence of relapse, the development of resistance, or failure of treatment. The preparations are antimicrobial drugs given by mouth.

Very occasionally, some of these antimicrobial agents may have severe side-effects and in such cases the patient may need to be advised of reasons for stopping treatment quickly and returning to the doctor. Examples are the development of diarrhoea in patients receiving clindamycin or lincomycin (see section 5.1.6), or sensitivity reactions with the penicillins.

(10) Warning. Follow the printed instructions you have been given with this medicine

To be used particularly on anticoagulants, monoamine-oxidase inhibitors, and oral corticosteroids. The appropriate treatment card should be given to the patient and any necessary explanations given.

This label may also be used on other preparations to remind the patient of the instructions that have been given.

(11) Avoid exposure of skin to direct sunlight or sun lamps

To be used on preparations that may cause phototoxic or photoallergic reactions if the patient is exposed to ultraviolet radiation. Many drugs other than those listed (e.g. phenothiazines and sulphonamides) may on rare occasions cause reactions in susceptible patients. Reactions have also been caused by external preparations (e.g. coal tar) and by various ingredients of perfumes and cosmetics. Exposure to high intensity ultraviolet radiation from sunray lamps and sunbeds is particularly likely to cause reactions and in advising patients this should be mentioned.

Drugs involved include amiodarone, demeclocycline, nalidixic acid, and protriptyline.

(12) Do not take remedies containing aspirin while taking this medicine

To be used on preparations containing salicylate derivatives, where it may not be known to the patient that the medicine has a similar action to aspirin, and on preparations containing the uricosuric drugs probenecid and sulphinpyrazone whose activity is reduced by aspirin.

Label 12 should not be used for anticoagulants; label 10 is more appropriate.

(13) Dissolve or mix with water before taking

To be used on preparations that are intended to be dissolved in water (e.g. soluble tablets) or mixed with water (e.g. powders, granules) before use. In a few cases the manufacturer's literature indicates that other liquids such as fruit juice or milk may be used.

(14) This medicine may colour the urine or stools

To be used on preparations that may cause the patient's urine to turn unusual colours. These include anthraquinones (alkaline urine red), phenolphthalein (alkaline urine pink), triamterene (blue under some lights), levodopa (dark reddish), and rifampicin (red). Iron preparations may colour the urine and stools black.

(15) Caution flammable: keep away from naked flames

To be applied to preparations containing sufficient alcohol, acetone, ether, or other flammable solvent to render them flammable if exposed to a naked flame. The term flammable is now used by the British Pharmacopoeia and in legislation in preference to inflammable. Since both terms are now liable to cause confusion, the pharmacist should make sure that the patient understands what is meant.

(16) Allow to dissolve under the tongue. Do not transfer from this container. Keep tightly closed. Discard eight weeks after opening

To be used on glyceryl trinitrate tablets to remind the patient not to transfer the tablets to plastic or less suitable containers. The manufacturer's original pack normally carries most of this wording and it may only be necessary to add 'Discard eight weeks after opening'.

(17) Not more than . . . . in 24 hours

To be used on preparations for the treatment of acute migraine except those containing ergotamine, for which label 18 is used.

It may also be used on preparations for which no dose has been specified by the prescriber.

(18) Not more than . . . in 24 hours or . . . in any one week

To be used on preparations of ergotamine tartrate.

(19) Warning. Causes drowsiness which may persist the next day. If affected do not drive or operate machinery. Avoid alcoholic drink

To be used on those preparations (e.g. nitrazepam) which are classified as hypnotics in the BNF when they are prescribed to be taken at night. On the rare occasions (e.g. nitrazepam in epilepsy) when hypnotics are prescribed for daytime administration this label would clearly not be appropriate. Also to be used as an alternative to the label 2 wording (the choice being at the discretion of the pharmacist) for anxiolytics (e.g. diazepam) prescribed to be taken at night. It is hoped that this wording will convey adequately the problem of residual morning sedation after taking 'sleeping tablets'.

(21) . . . with or after food

To be used on preparations that are liable to cause gastric irritation with nausea and vomiting, or those that are better absorbed with food.

The incidence of gastric irritation may be reduced when some preparations are given during or immediately after a meal. The presence of food in the upper gastro-intestinal tract may reduce the rate of absorption of certain drugs. Nausea and vomiting are liable to decrease compliance and possibly lead to loss of the drug from vomiting.

Patients may on occasions be advised to take their medicine with or after food in the interest of compliance when normally it should be taken before meals. There is a wide variation in the instructions given for iron salts and their preparations. They are usually best absorbed when given on an empty stomach but may then cause irritation. They are therefore often taken with a meal.

The prescriber's instructions should be followed.

A small number of preparations are better absorbed when given with food.

The word 'food' is used in preference to 'meal' on the label. Patients differ in their interpretation of the words and may decide not to take a dose if it has to be taken with a meal that they normally omit.

Patients should be advised when to take their doses, according to their particular circumstances, and that a small amount of food is sufficient.

(22) . . . half to one hour before food

To be used on some anticholinergic or antacid preparations; some pancreatin and other enzyme preparations; most appetite suppressants; and certain other drugs whose absorption or local effect is thereby improved.

(23) . . . an hour before food or on an empty stomach

To be used on some oral antibiotics whose absorption may be reduced by the presence of food and acid in the stomach.

Many of the antibiotics introduced in recent years are less affected by acid and/or food in the stomach and may be given at any time relative to meals.

(24) . . . sucked or chewed

To be used on preparations that may be sucked or chewed. Certain preparations must be chewed before swallowing to improve their absorption or because of their size; others have been specially formulated to be chewed. All pastilles and lozenges should be sucked slowly to aid their local effect on the oropharynx. The pharmacist should use discretion as to which of these words is appropriate.

(25) . . . swallowed whole, not chewed

To be used on preparations designed for sustained release; on certain preparations that are very unpleasant or may damage the mouth or oesophagus if not swallowed whole; and with label 5 for enteric-coated preparations. Most sustained-release preparations rely on the coating of pellets, granules, tablets, or capsules or compression in a matrix material to achieve their effect. Chewing can cause premature release of active ingredient.

(26) . . . dissolved under the tongue

To be used on preparations intended for sublingual use. Several drugs are absorbed into the circulation more effectively from the mucosa of the mouth, thereby avoiding the portal circulation into the liver. Patients should be advised to hold the tablet still under the tongue and avoid swallowing until the tablet is dissolved. The buccal mucosa between the gum and cheek is occasionally specified by the prescriber and specific directions should then be used.

(27) . . . with plenty of water

To be used on preparations that should be well diluted (e.g. chloral hydrate), where a high fluid intake is required (e.g. sulphonamides), or where water is required to aid the action of the preparation (e.g. methylcellulose). The patient should be advised that 'plenty' means at least 150 ml (about a tumblerful). In most cases a beverage such as fruit juice, tea, or coffee could be used. There have been reports of solid-dose preparations sticking in the oesophagus, particularly in the elderly, and all patients should be reminded of the necessity of taking capsules and tablets with water or other liquid. As much as 100 ml may be required and the patient should stand or sit while taking the dose.

(28) To be applied sparingly . . .

To be used with external corticosteroid preparations and dithranol preparations.

The application of excessive quantities to the skin can increase the incidence of local side-effects and give rise to undesirable systemic effects.

(29) Do not take more than 2 at any one time. Do not take more than 8 in 24 hours

To be used on containers of dispensed solid dose preparations containing paracetamol for adults[1]. This label has been introduced because of the serious consequences of overdosage with paracetamol.

1. **Important.** The amounts specified here are applicable to adults.

Products and their labels

Products introduced or amended since publication of BNF No. 15 (1988) are in bold.
Proprietary names are in italic.
C = counselling advised; see BNF = consult product entry in BNF.

Acebutolol, 8
Acetazolamide, 3
Acetazolamide s/r, 3, 25
Acetylcysteine gran, 13
Achromycin, 7, 9, 23
Achromycin V, 7, 9, 23
Acipimox, 21
Acrosoxacin, 2, 23
Actidil, 2
Actifed, 2
Actifed Compound, 2
Actifed Expectorant, 2
Acupan, 14
Acyclovir susp and tabs, 9
Adalat caps, 21, C, see BNF
Adalat Retard, 21, 25
Agarol, 14
Akineton, 2
Alcopar, 13
Aldomet, 3, 8
Allegron, 2
Allopurinol, 8, 21, 27
Almazine, 2 or 19
Almodan, 9
Alophen, 14 (alkaline urine pink)
Aloral, 8, 21, 27
Aloxiprin, 12, 21
Alprazolam, 2
Alrheumat, 21
Aluline, 8, 21, 27
Alunex, 2
Alupram, 2 or 19
Ambaxin, 9
Amfipen, 9, 23
Aminophylline s/r, 25
Aminophylline tabs, 21
Amiodarone, 11
Amitriptyline, 2
Amitriptyline s/r, 2, 25
Ammonium chloride mixt, 13
Amoxil, 9
Amoxil dispersible tabs and sachets,
  9, 13
Amoxil paed susp, 9, C, use of pipette
Amoxycillin, 9
Amphotericin loz, 9, 24, C, after food
Amphotericin mixt (g.i.), 9, C, use of
  pipette
Amphotericin mixt (mouth), 9, C, use
  of pipette, hold in mouth, after food
Amphotericin tabs, 9
Ampicillin, 9, 23
Ampiclox Neonatal, 9, C, use of
  pipette
Amylobarbitone, 19
Amytal, 19
Anaflex loz, 9, 24, C, after food
Anafranil, 2
Anafranil s/r, 2, 25
Ananase Forte, 5, 25
Androcur, 2, 21
Angilol, 8
Anquil, 2
Antabuse, see BNF dosage statements
Antacids, see BNF dosage statements
Antepar tabs, 24
Antepsin, 5, C, before food, see BNF
Anthranol preps, 28
Anticoagulants, oral, 10 anticoagu-
  lant card
Antihistamines   (see   individual
  preparations)
Antoin, 13, 21
Antraderm preps, 28
Anturan, 12, 21
Anxon, 2 or 19
Apisate, 25, C, impaired reactions
APP pdr, 13
Apsifen, 21
Apsin VK, 9, 23
Apsolol, 8
Apsolox, 8
Arelix, 21

Arpimycin, 9
Artane, C, before or after food, see
  BNF
Artane Sustets, 25, C, before or after
  food, see BNF
Artracin, 21
Asacol, 25
Ascorbic acid, effervescent, 13
Asmapax, 21
Aspav, 13, 21
Aspergum, 21
Aspirin and papaveretum dispersible
  tabs, 13, 21
Aspirin dispersible tabs, 13, 21
Aspirin e/c, 5, 25
Aspirin s/r, 21
Aspirin tabs, 21
**Aspirin, paracetamol, and codeine
  tabs, 21, 29**
Astemizole, 23
Atarax, 2
Atenolol, 8
Atensine, 2 or 19
Ativan, 2 or 19
Atromid-S, 21
Augmentin, 9
Augmentin dispersible tabs, 9, 13
Auranofin, 21
Aureomycin, 7, 9, 23
Aventyl, 2
Avloclor, 5
Avomine, 2
Azapropazone, 21, C, see BNF
Azatadine, 2

Bacampicillin, 9
Baclofen, 2, 8
Bactrim, 9
Bactrim dispersible tabs, 9, 13
Banocide, 9
Baratol, 2
Baxan, 9
Becloforte, 8, 10 steroid card, C, dose
Beclomethasone dipropionate inha-
  lations, 8, 10 steroid card (high-
  dose preparations only), C, dose
Becodisks, 8, C, dose
Becotide preps, 8, C, dose
Bendogen, 21
Benemid, 12, 21, 27
Benoral susp and tabs, 21, C, avoid
  aspirin, paracetamol
Benoral gran, 13, 21, C, avoid aspirin,
  paracetamol
Benorylate, 21, C, avoid aspirin,
  paracetamol
Benorylate gran, 13, 21, C, avoid
  aspirin, paracetamol
Benperidol, 2
Bentex, C, before or after food, see
  BNF
Benylin Decongestant, 2
Benylin Expectorant, 2
Benylin Paediatric, 1
Benylin with Codeine, 2
Benzathine penicillin, 9
Benzhexol, C, before or after food, see
  BNF
Benzhexol s/r 25, C, before or after
  food, see BNF
Benzoin tincture, cpd, 15
Benztropine, 2
Bephenium, 13
Berkfurin, 9, 14, 21
Berkmycen, 7, 9, 23
Berkolol, 8
Beta-Cardone, 8
Betadren, 8
Betahistine, 21
Betaloc, 8
Betaloc-SA, 8, 25
Betamethasone, 10 steroid card

Betamethasone valerate inhalations,
  8, C, dose
Betaxolol, 8
Bethanechol, 22
Bethanidine, 21
Betim, 8
Betnelan, 10 steroid card
Betnesol injection, 10 steroid card
Betnesol tabs, 10 steroid card, 13
Bextasol, 8, C, dose
Bezafibrate, 21
Bezalip, 21
Bezalip-Mono, 21, 25
Biogastrone, 21
Biophylline, 21
Biperiden, 2
Bisacodyl tabs, 5, 25
Bisoprolol, 8
Blocadren, 8
Bolvidon, 2, 25
Bradilan, 5, 25
Bricanyl SA, 25
Brocadopa, 14, 21
Broflex, C, before or after food, see
  BNF
Bromazepam, 2
Bromelains e/c, 5, 25
Bromocriptine, 21, C, hypotensive
  reactions, see BNF
Brompheniramine, 2
Broxil, 9, 23
Brufen, 21
Buccastem, 2, C, administration, see
  BNF
Budesonide inhalations, 8, 10 steroid
  card (high-dose preparations only),
  C, dose
Buprenorphine, 2, 26
Burinex K, 25, 27, C, posture, see BNF
Buspar, C, reactions, see BNF
Butacote, 5, 21, 25
Butazolidin, 21
Butazone, 21
Butobarbitone, 19
Butriptyline, 2

Cafadol, 29
Cafergot, 18, C, dosage
Calcisorb, 13, 21, C, may be sprinkled
  on food
Calcium Resonium, 13
Calcium carbonate pdr, cpd, 13
Calcium gluconate effervescent tabs,
  13
Calcium gluconate tabs, 24
**Calcium with vitamin D tabs, C, crush
  before taking or chew**
Calthor, 9
Camcolit 250 tabs, C, fluid and salt
  intake
Camcolit 400 tabs, 25, C, fluid and salt
  intake
Caplenal, 8, 21, 27
Caprin, 25
Carbachol, 22
Carbenoxolone sodium, see BNF
Cardiacap, 22, 25
Carfecillin, 9
Carisoma, 2
Carisoprodol, 2
Cascara, 14
Catapres, 3, 8
Catapres Perlongets, 3, 8, 25
Caved-S, 24
Cedocard Retard, 25
Cefaclor, 9
Cefadroxil, 9
Cefuroxime, 9, 21, 25
Celevac (constip. or diarrhoea), see
  BNF
Celevac tabs (anorectic), 22, 24, 27, C,
  administration

Cellucon (laxative), see BNF
Cellucon tabs (anorectic), 22, 24, 27, C, administration
Centyl K, 25, 27, C, posture, see BNF
Cephalexin, 9
Cephradine, 9
Ceporex caps, mixts, and tabs, 9
Ceporex paed drops, 9, C, use of pipette
Cesamet, 2
Chalk pdr, aromatic, 13
Chemotrim, 9
Chloractil, 2
Chloral hydrate, 19, 27
Chloral paed elixir, 1, 27
Chloral mixt, 19, 27
Chlordiazepoxide, 2
Chlormethiazole, 19
Chlormezanone, 2 or 19
Chloroquine, 5
Chlorpheniramine, 2
Chlorpromazine mixts and supps, 2
Chlorpromazine tabs, 2
Chlorpropamide, 4
Chlortetracycline, 7, 9, 23
Cholestyramine, 13, C, avoid other drugs at same time
Choline magnesium trisalicylate, 12, 21
Choline theophyllinate s/r, 25
Chymocyclar, 7, 9, 23, 25
Chymoral, 5, 22, 25
Chymotrypsin e/c, 5, 22, 25
Ciclacillin, 9
Cimetidine chewable tab, C, administration
Cinnarizine, 2
Cinobac, 9
Cinoxacin, 9
Ciproxin tabs, 5, 9, 25
Ciprofloxacin, 5, 9, 25
Claradin, 13, 21
Clemastine, 2
Clindamycin, 9, 27, C, diarrhoea
Clinium, 21
Clinoril, 21
Clobazam, 2 or 19
Clofazimine, 8, 14, 21
Clofibrate, 21
Clomipramine, 2
Clomipramine s/r, 2, 25
Clomocycline, 7, 9, 23
Clonazepam, 2
Clonidine see Catapres
Clonidine s/r, 3, 8, 25
Clopixol, 2
Clorazepate, 2 or 19
Cloxacillin, 9, 23
Coal tar paint, 15
Co-Betaloc, 8
Co-Betaloc SA, 8, 25
Co-codamol tabs, 29
Co-codamol dispersible tabs, 13, 29
Co-codaprin dispersible tabs, 13, 21
Co-codaprin tabs, 21
Co-danthrusate, 14 (urine red)
Codeine phosphate tabs, 2
Codelsol (systemic), 10 steroid card
Co-dergocrine, 22
Codis, 13, 21
Co-dydramol, 21, 29
Cogentin, 2
Colestid, 13, C, avoid other drugs at same time
Colestipol, 13, C, avoid other drugs at same time
Collodion, flexible, 15
Colofac, 2
Cologel, see BNF
Colpermin, 5, 22, 25
Colven sachets, 13, 22
Comox paed susp and tabs, 9
Comox dispersible tabs, 9, 13
Complement Continus, 25
Concordin, 2, 11
Co-proxamol, 2, 10 patient information leaflet, 29
Cordarone X, 11
Cordgard, 8
Corgaretic, 8

Cortelan, 10 steroid card
Corticosteroid external preps, 28
Corticosteroid tabs, 10 steroid card
Corticosteroid injections (systemic), 10 steroid card
Cortisone, 10 steroid card
Cortistab (systemic), 10 steroid card
Cortisyl, 10 steroid card
Cosuric, 8, 21, 27
Cotazym, C, see BNF
Co-trimoxazole mixts and tabs, 9
Co-trimoxazole dispersible tabs, 9, 13
Creon, C, see BNF
Cyclizine, 2
Cyclobarbitone, 19
Cyclophosphamide, 27
Cycloserine caps, 2, 8
Cyproheptadine, 2
Cyprostat, 2, 21
Cyproterone, 2 or 3 (see preparation), 21

Daktarin oral gel, 9, C, hold in mouth, after food
Daktarin tabs, 9, 21
Dalacin C, 9, 27, C, diarrhoea
Dalmane, 19
Daneral SA, 2, 25
Dantrium, 2
Dantrolene, 2
Dapsone, 8
Davenol, 2
Dayovite, 13
Decadron (systemic), 10 steroid card
Decaserpyl, 3
Decaserpyl Plus, 3
Decortisyl, 10 steroid card
Deltacortril e/c, 5, 10 steroid card, 25
Delta-Phoricol, 10 steroid card
Deltastab (systemic), 10 steroid card
Demeclocycline, 7, 9, 11, 23
Demser, 2
De-Nol, C, administration, see BNF
De-Noltab, C, administration, see BNF
Depixol, 2
Depo-Medrone (systemic), 10 steroid card
Deponit, C, administration, see BNF
Deseril, 2, 21
Desipramine, 2
Destolit, 21
Deteclo, 7, 9, 11, 23
Dexamethasone, 10 steroid card
Dextromoramide, 2
Dextropropoxyphene, 2
DF 118, 2, 21
DHC Continus, 2, 25
Diabinese, 4
Diamorphine preps, 2
Diamox tabs, 3
Diamox Sustets, 3, 25
Diazepam, 2 or 19
Dichloralphenazone, 19, 27
Diclofenac e/c, 5, 25
Diclofenac s/r, 21, 25
Diconal, 2
Didronel, C, food and calcium, see BNF
Diethylcarbamazine, 9
Diethylpropion s/r, 25, C, impaired reactions
Diflunisal, 21, 25, C, avoid aluminium hydroxide
Digoxin elixir, C, use of pipette
Dihydrocodeine, 2, 21
Dihydrocodeine s/r, 2, 25
Diloxanide, 9
Dimenhydrinate, 2
Dimethicone, see paediatric prep
Dimethindene s/r, 2, 25
Dimotane, 2
Dimotane Expectorant, 2
Dimotane LA, 2, 25
Dimotane Plus, 2
Dimotane Plus, Paediatric, 1
Dimotane with Codeine, 2
Dimotane with Codeine Paediatric, 1
Dimotapp elixir, 2
Dimotapp paed elixir, 1
Dimotapp LA, 2, 25, C, gluten

Dindevan, 10 anticoagulant card, 14
Dioralyte, 13
Diphenhydramine, 2
Diphenylpyraline s/r, 2, 25
Dipyridamole, 22
Dirythmin SA, 25
Disalcid, 12, 21
Disodium etidronate, C, food and calcium, see BNF
Disopyramide s/r, 25
Distaclor, 9
Distalgesic, 2, 10 patient information leaflet, 29
Distamine, 6, 22
Distaquaine V-K, 9, 23
Distigmine, 22
Disulfiram, 2
Dithranol preps, 28
Dithrocream preps, 28
Dithrolan, 28
Diumide-K Continus, 25, 27, C, posture, see BNF
Dolmatil, 2
Dolobid, 21, 25, C, avoid aluminium hydroxide
Doloxene, 2
Doloxene Compound, 2, 21
Domical, 2
Dopamet, 3, 8
Dormonoct, 19
Dothiepin, 2
Doxepin, 2
Doxycycline caps and tabs, 6, 9, 27
Doxycycline syrup, 6, 9
Dozic, 2
Dramamine, 2
Droleptan, 2
Dromoran, 2
Droperidol, 2
Dulcolax tabs, 5, 25
Duogastrone, 22, 25
Duromine, 25
Dyazide, 14 (urine blue in some lights), 21
Dyspamet tab, C, administration
Dytac, 14 (urine blue in some lights), 21
Dytide, 14 (urine blue in some lights), 21

Ebufac, 21
Econocil VK, 9, 23
Economycin, 7, 9, 23
Edecrin, 2
Efcortelan soluble, 10 steroid card
Efcortesol, 10 steroid card
Effercitrate, 13
Elantan preps, 25
Elavil, 2
Electrolade, 13
Electrolyte pdr (see individual preparations)
Electrosol, 13
Emcor preps, 8
Emeside, 2
Endoxana, 27
Entamizole, 4, 9, 21, 25
Enzypan, 5, 21, 25
Epanutin Infatabs, 24
Epanutin with Phenobarbitone, 2
Epilim e/c tabs, 5, 25
Equagesic, 2, 21
Equanil, 2
Eradacin, 2, 23
Ergotamine, 18, C, dosage
Erycen, 5, 9, 25
Erymax, 5, 9, 25
Erythrocin, 9
Erythrolar susp, 9
Erythrolar tabs, 9
Erythromid, 5, 9, 25
Erythromid DS, 5, 9, 25
Erythromycin estolate, 9
Erythromycin ethylsuccinate, 9
Erythromycin ethylsuccinate gran, 9, 13
Erythromycin stearate tabs, 9
Erythromycin tabs, 5, 9, 25
Erythroped, 9
Erythroped A tabs, 9

Lithium citrate s/r, 25, C, fluid and salt intake
Lobak, 2, 29
Lodine, 21
Lofepramine, 2
Loprazolam, 19
Lopresor, 8
Lopresor SR, 8, 25
Lopresoretic, 8
Lorazepam, 2 or 19
Lormetazepam, 19
Lotussin, 2
Ludiomil, 2
Lugol's solution, 27
Luminal, 2
Lurselle, 21
Lymecycline, 7, 9, 23

Macrodantin, 9, 14, 21
Madopar, 14, 21, 25
Madopar dispersible tabs, 14, 21, C, administration, see BNF
Magnapen, 9, 23
Magnesium carbonate pdr, cpd, 13
Magnesium sulphate, 13, 23
Magnesium sulphate mixt, 23
Magnesium trisilicate oral pdr, cpd, 13
Magnesium trisilicate pdr, 13
Malarivon, 5
Manevac, 14, 25, 27
Maprotiline, 2
Marevan, 10 anticoagulant card
Marplan, 3, 10 MAOI card
Maxepa, 21
Maxolon paed liquid, C, use of pipette
Mazindol, C, impaired reactions
Mebeverine, 22
Mebhydrolin, 2
Medazepam, 2
Medihaler-ergotamine, 18, C, dosage
Medised susp, 1
Medised tabs, 2, 29
Medocodene, 29
Medomet, 3, 8
Medrone, 10 steroid card
Mefenamic acid caps, paed susp, and tabs, 21
Mefenamic acid dispersible tabs, 13, 21
Megaclor, 7, 9, 23
Melleril, 2
Menthol and benzoin inhalation, 15
Meprate, 2
Meprobamate, 2
Meptazinol, 2
Meptid, 2
Mequitazine, 2
Mesalazine, 25
Metamucil, 13
Metformin, 21
Methadone, 2
Methixene, 2
Methocarbamol, 2
Methotrimeprazine, 2
Methylcellulose (constip. or diarrhoea), see BNF
Methylcellulose tabs (anorectic), 22, 24, 27, C, see BNF
Methylcysteine, 5, 22, 25
Methyldopa, 3, 8
Methylphenobarbitone, 2
Methylprednisolone (systemic), 10 steroid card
Methyprylone, 19
Methysergide, 2, 21
Metirosine, 2
Metoclopramide paed liquid, C, use of pipette
Metoclopramide s/r caps, 22, 25
Metoclopramide s/r tabs, 25
Metopirone, 21
Metoprolol, 8
Metoprolol s/r, 8, 25
Metrolyl supps, 4, 9
Metrolyl tabs, 4, 9, 21, 25
Metronidazole mixt, 4, 9, 23
Metronidazole supps, 4, 9
Metronidazole tabs, 4, 9, 21, 25
Metyrapone, 21

Mexiletine s/r, 25
Mexitil PL Perlongets, 25
Mianserin, 2, 25
Miconazole oral gel, 9, C, hold in mouth, after food
Miconazole tabs, 9, 21
Mictral, 9, 11, 13
Midrid, 2, 17
Migraleve, 17
Migravess, 13, 17
Migravess Forte, 13, 17
Migril, 2, 18, C, dosage
Min-I-Mix Methylprednisolone, 10 steroid card
Minocin, 6, 9
Minocycline, 6, 9
Mintec, 5, 22, 25
Mintezol, 3, 21, 24
Miraxid tabs, 9, 21, 25, 27, C, posture, see BNF
Miraxid paed sachets, 9, 13, 21
Mobilan, 21
Moditen, 2
Moducren, 8
Mogadon, 19
Molipaxin, 2, 21
Monit, 25
Monit LS, 25
Mono-Cedocard, 25
Monocor, 8
Monosulfiram solution, 4
Monotrim, 9
Monovent SA, 25
Morphine preps, 2
Morphine s/r, 2, 25
Motipress, 2
Motival, 2
Motrin, 21
MST Continus, 2, 25
Muripsin, 2
Myambutol, 8
Mycardol, 22
Mynah, 8, 23
Myotonine Chloride, 22
Mysoline, 2
Mysteclin, 7, 9, 23

Nabilone, 2
Nabumetone, 21, 25
Nadolol, 8
Nalcrom, 22, C, administration, see BNF
Nalidixic acid, 9, 11
Naprosyn granules, 13, 21
Naprosyn tabs and susp, 21
Naproxen granules, 13, 21
Naproxen tabs and susp, 21
Nardil, 3, 10 MAOI card
Narphen, 2
Natamycin mixt, 9, C, use of pipette, hold in mouth, after food
Natulan, 4
Navidrex-K, 25, 27, C, posture, see BNF
Naxogin, 4, 21
Nedocromil sodium inhalation, 8
Nefopam, 14
Negram, 9, 11
Neo-NaClex-K, 25, 27, C, posture, BNF
Nepenthe, 2
Neulactil, 2
Neurodyne, 29
Niclosamide, 4, 24, 27, C, administration, see BNF
Nicofuranose, 5, 25
Nicotinic acid tabs, 21
Nicoumalone, 10 anticoagulant card
Nidazol, 4, 9, 21, 25
Nifedipine caps, 21, C, see BNF
Nifedipine tabs, 21, 25
Niferex elixir, C, infants, use of dropper
Nilstim, 22, 24, 27, C, administration
Nimorazole, 4, 21
Nitoman, 2
Nitrados, 19
Nitrazepam, 19
Nitrocontin Continus, 25
Nitrofurantoin tabs, 9, 14, 21
Nivaquine, 5

Nizoral, 5, 9, 21
Nobrium, 2
Noctec, 19, 27
Noludar, 19
Noctesed, 19
Noradran, 2
Nordox, 6, 9, 27
Norflex, 25
Norgesic, 29
Normacol preps, 25, 27, see BNF
Normax, 14 (urine red)
Normison, 19
Nortriptyline, 2
Norval, 2, 25
Nuelin, 21
Nuelin SA preps, 25, 27
Nu-K, 25, 27, C, see BNF
Numotac, 25
Nu-Seals Aspirin, 5, 25
Nutrizym, 5, 21, 25
Nutrizym GR, C, administration, see BNF
Nystan pastilles, 9, 24, C, after food
Nystan susp (g.i.), 9, C, use of pipette
Nystan susp (mouth), 9, C, use of pipette, hold in mouth, after food
Nystan tabs, 9
Nystatin mixt (g.i.), 9, C, use of pipette
Nystatin mixt (mouth), 9, C, use of pipette, hold in mouth, after food
Nystatin pastilles, 9, 24, C, after food
Nystatin tabs, 9
Nystatin-Dome (g.i.), 9, C, use of 1-ml spoon
Nystatin-Dome (mouth), 9, C, use of 1-ml spoon, hold in mouth, after food

Ocusert Pilo, C, method of use
Oestriol, 25
Olbetam, 21
Opilon, 2
Opium tincture, 2
Optimax tabs, 2
Optimax pdr, 2, 13
Optimax WV, 2
Optimine, 2
Oradexon (systemic), 10 steroid card
Oramorph, 2
Orap, 2
Orbenin, 9, 23
Orovite-7 gran, 13
Orphenadrine citrate s/r, 25
Orudis caps, 21
Oruvail, 21, 25
Ovestin, 25
Oxanid, 2
Oxatomide, 2
Oxazepam, 2
Oxerutins, 21
Oxpentifylline s/r, 21, 25
Oxprenolol, 8
Oxprenolol s/r, 8, 25
Oxymycin, 7, 9, 23
Oxypertine, 2
Oxytetracycline, 7, 9, 23

Pacitron, 2
Palaprin Forte, 12, 21
Paludrine, 21
Pameton, 29
Panadeine, 29
Panadeine Forte, 2, 29
Panadeine Soluble, 13, 29
Panadol, 29
Panadol Soluble, 13, 29
Panasorb, 29
Pancrease caps, C, administration, see BNF
Pancreatin, see BNF
Pancrex gran, 25, C, dose, see BNF
Pancrex V Forte tabs, 5, 25, C, dose, see BNF
Pancrex V caps, 125 caps and pdr, C, administration, see BNF
Pancrex V tabs, 5, 25, C, dose, see BNF
Paracetamol tabs, 29
Paracetamol tabs, soluble, 13, 29
Paracodol, 13, 29

Parahypon, 29
Parake, 29
Paramax sachets, 13, 17
Paramax tabs, 17
Paramol, 21, 29
Pardale, 29
Paritane, 8
Parlodel, 21, C, hypotensive reactions, see BNF
Parlodel Starter Pack, 10, 21, C, hypotensive reactions, dosage schedule, see BNF
Parnate, 3, 10 MAOI card
Paroven, 21
Parstelin, 3, 10 MAOI card
Paxalgesic, 2, 29
Paxane, 19
Paxidal, 2
Paynocil, 21, 24
Penbritin caps and syrup, 9, 23
Penbritin paed syrup, 9, 23, C, use of pipette
Pendramine, 6, 22
Penicillamine, 6, 22
Penidural paed drops, 9, C, use of pipette
Penidural susp, 9
Pentaerythritol tetranitrate, 22
Pentaerythritol tetranitrate s/r, 22, 25
Pentazocine caps and tabs, 2, 21
Pentazocine supps, 2
Pentobarbitone, 19
Peppermint oil caps, 5, 22, 25
Peptard, 25
Percutol, C, administration, see BNF
Periactin, 2
Pericyazine, 2
Perphenazine, 2
Persantin, 22
Pertofran, 2
Pethidine, 2
Phanodorm, 19
Pharmidone, 2, 29
Phasal, 25, C, fluid and salt intake
Phenazocine, 2
Phenelzine, 3, 10 MAOI card
Phenergan, 2
Phenethicillin, 9, 23
Phenindamine, 2
Phenindione, 10 anticoagulant card, 14
Pheniramine s/r, 2, 25
Phenobarbitone elixir and tabs, 2
Phenolphthalein, 14 **(alkaline urine pink)**
Phenoxymethylpenicillin, 9, 23
Phensedyl, 2
Phentermine s/r, 25
Phenylbutazone, 21
Phenytoin chewable tabs, 24
Pholtex, 2
Phosphate-Sandoz, 13
Phyldrox, 21
Phyldrox e/c, 5, 25
Phyllocontin Continus, 25
Physeptone, 2
Phytomenadione, 24
Picolax, 13, C, see BNF
Pimafucin oral susp, 9, C, use of pipette, hold in mouth, after food
Pimozide, 2
Pindolol, 8
Piperazine tabs, 24
Pirenzepine, 22
Piretanide, 21
Piriton, 2
Piriton Spandets, 2, 25
Piroxicam caps, 21
Piroxicam dispersible tabs, 13, 21
Pivampicillin sachets, 5, 9, 13
Pivampicillin susp and tabs, 5, 9
Pivmecillinam susp, 9, 21
Pivmecillinam tabs, 9, 21, 27, C, posture, see BNF
Pizotifen, 2
Plaquenil, 5
Podophyllin paint cpd, 15, C, application, see BNF
Polynoxylin loz, 9, 24, C, after food

Ponderax Pacaps, 2, 25
Ponderax tabs, 2
Pondocillin sachets, 5, 9, 13
Pondocillin susp and tabs, 5, 9
Pondocillin Plus, 9, 21, 27, C, posture, see BNF
Ponstan, 21
Ponstan Dispersible, 13, 21
Potaba caps and tabs, 21
Potaba Envules, 13, 21
Potassium chloride s/r, see preps
Potassium citrate mixt, 27
Potassium effervescent tabs, 13, 21
Praminil, 2
Prazosin, 3, C, dose, see BNF
Precortisyl, 10 steroid card
Precortisyl Forte, 10 steroid card
Prednesol, 10 steroid card, 13
Prednisolone, 10 steroid card
Prednisone, 10 steroid card
Prefil, 22, 27, C, administration
Prestim, 8
Prestim Forte, 8
Priadel, 25, C, administration, fluid and salt intake, see BNF
Primalan, 2
Primidone, 2
Pripsen, 13
Pro-Actidil, 2, 25
Pro-Banthine, 22
Probenecid, 12, 21, 27
Probucol, 21
Procainamide Durules, 25
Procarbazine, 4
Prochlorperazine, 2
Prochlorperazine s/r, 2, 25
Prochlorperazine buccal tabs, 2, C, administration, see BNF
Prochlorperazine sachets, 2, 13
Proctofibe, C, see BNF
Progesic, 21
Proguanil, 21
Promazine, 2
Promethazine, 2
Prominal, 2
Prondol, 2
Propain, 2, 29
Propantheline, 22
Propranolol, 8
Propranolol s/r, 8, 25
Prothiaden, 2
Prothionamide, 8, 21
Protriptyline, 2, 11
Pro-Vent, 25, 27
Psoradrate, 28
Psorin, 28
Pulmicort, 8, C, dose, 10 steroid card
Pulmicort LS, 8, C, dose
Pyrazinamide, 8
Pyrogastrone liquid, 21
Pyrogastrone tabs, 21, 24

Questran, 13, C, avoid other drugs at same time
Quinalbarbitone, 19
Quinidine s/r, 25

Rabro, 21
Ranitidine dispersible tabs, 13
Redoxon effervescent, 13
Regulan, 13
Rehidrat, 13
Relifex, 21, 25
Remnos, 19
Reserpine, 3
Resonium A, 13
Restandol, 21, 25
Retcin, 5, 9, 25
Rheumacin LA, 21, 25
Rheumox, 21, C, see BNF
Rhumalgan, 5, 25
Ridaura, 21
Rifadin, 8, 14, 22, C, soft lenses
Rifampicin caps and mixt, 8, 14, 22, C, soft lenses
Rifater, 8, 14, C, soft lenses
Rifinah, 8, 14, 22, C, soft lenses
Rimactane, 8, 14, 22, C, soft lenses
Rimactazid, 8, 14, 22, C, soft lenses
Rivotril, 2

Roaccutane, 10 patient information card, 21
Robaxin, 2
Robaxisal Forte, 2, 21
Rohypnol, 19
Ronicol Timespan, 25
Rowachol, 22
Rowatinex caps, 25
Rowatinex liquid, 22, C, use of dropper
Rythmodan Retard, 25

Sabidal SR, 25
Safapryn, 5, 25
Safapryn-Co, 5, 25
Salazopyrin, 14
Salazopyrin EN-tabs, 5, 14, 25
Salbutamol s/r, 25
Salicylic acid collodion, 15
Salicylic acid lotion, 15
Salsalate, 12, 21
Sando-K, 13, 21
Sandocal, 13
Sanomigran, 2
Secadrex, 8
Seconal, 19
Sectral, 8
Securon SR, 25
Selexid susp, 9, 13, 21
Selexid tabs, 9, 21, 27, C, posture, see BNF
Senna, 14
Senokot, 14
Septrin susp and tabs, 9
Septin dispersible tabs, 9, 13
Serc, 21
Serenace, 2
Serpasil, 3
Serpasil-Esidrex, 3
Sinemet preps, 14, 21
Sinequan, 2
Sinthrome, 10 anticoagulant card
Sintisone, 10 steroid card
Slo-Indo, 21, 25
Slo-Phyllin, 25, 27 or C, administration, see BNF
Sloprolol, 8, 25
Slow Sodium, 25
Slow-Fe, 25
Slow-Fe Folic, 25
Slow-K, 25, 27, C, posture, see BNF
Slow-Pren, 8, 25
Slow-Trasicor, 8, 25
Sodium Amytal, 19
Sodium bicarbonate pdr, 13
Sodium cellulose phosphate, 13, 21, C, may be sprinkled on food
Sodium chloride s/r, 25
Sodium chloride and glucose oral pdr, cpd, 13
Sodium chloride solution-tabs, 13
Sodium cromoglycate (oral), 22, C, administration, see BNF
Sodium cromoglycate inhalations, 8
Sodium fusidate susp, 9, 21
Sodium fusidate tabs, 5, 9, 25
Sodium picosulphate pdr, 13, C, see **BNF**
Sodium salicylate mixt, 21
Sodium valproate e/c, 5, 25
Solis, 2 or 19
Solpadeine, 13, 29
Solprin, 13, 21
Solu-Cortef, 10 steroid card
Solu-Medrone, 10 steroid card
Solvazinc, 13, 21
Somnite, 19
Soneryl, 19
Soni-Slo, 25
Sorbichew, 24
Sorbid-SA, 25
Sotacor, 8
Sotalol, 8
Sotazide, 8
Sparine, 2
Stabillin V-K, 9, 23
Stafoxil, 9, 23
Staphlipen, 9, 23
Stelazine syrup and tabs, 2
Stelazine Spansule, 2, 25

Stemetil, 2
Stemetil Eff, 2, 13
Sterculia, see BNF
Stugeron, 2
Stugeron Forte, 2
Sucralfate, 5, C, before food, see BNF
Sudafed SA, 25
Sulfametopyrazine, 9, 13
Sulindac, 21
Sulphadiazine, 9, 27
Sulphadimethoxine, 9, 27
Sulphafurazole, 9, 27
Sulphamethoxypyridazine, 9, 27
Sulphasalazine e/c, 5, 14, 25
Sulphasalazine tabs, 14
Sulphathiazole, 9, 27
Sulphinpyrazone, 12, 21
Sulpiride, 2
Sulpitil, 2
Surem, 19
Surgam tabs, 21
Surgam SA caps, 21, 25
Surgam 300 sachets, 13, 21
Surgical spirit, 15
Surmontil, 2
Suscard Buccal, C, administration, see BNF
Sustac, 25
Sustamycin, 7, 9, 23, 25
Syndol, 2, 29
Synflex, 21
Syraprim, 9

Talampicillin, 9
Talpen, 9
Tavegil, 2
Tedral elixir and tabs, 21
Temazepam, 19
Temgesic, 2, 26
Tenavoid, 2
Tenoret 50, 8
Tenoretic, 8
Tenormin, 8
Tenormin LS, 8
Tensium, 2 or 19
Tenuate Dospan, 25, C, impaired reactions
Terazosin, 3, C, dose, see BNF
Terbutaline s/r, 25
Teronac, C, impaired reactions
Terramycin, 7, 9, 23
Testosterone undecanoate caps, 21, 25
Tetmosol solution, 4
Tetrabenazine, 2
Tetrabid, 7, 9, 23, 25
Tetrachel, 7, 9, 23
Tetracycline, 7, 9, 23
Tetracycline mouth-bath, see BNF
Tetralysal preps, 7, 9, 23
Tetrex, 7, 9, 23
Theodrox, 21
Theo-Dur, 25, 27
Theophylline, 21

Theophylline s/r, see preps
Thephorin, 2
Thiabendazole, 3, 21, 24
Thiethylperazine, 2
Thioridazine, 2
Thymoxamine, 21
Tiaprofenic acid gran, 13, 21
Tiaprofenic acid tabs, 21
Tiaprofenic acid s/r, 21, 25
Tiempe, 9
Tigason, 10 patient information card, 21
Tilade, 8
Timolol, 8
Tinidazole tabs, 4, 9, 21, 25
Tinset, 2, 21
Tixylix, 1 or 2
Tofranil, 2
Tolectin DS, 21
Tolerzide, 8
Tolmetin, 21
Torecan, 2
Trancopal, 2 or 19
Trandate, 8, 21
Transiderm-Nitro, C, administration, see BNF
Tranxene, 2 or 19
Tranylcypromine, 3, 10 MAOI card
Trasicor, 8
Trasidrex, 8
Trazodone, 2, 21
Tremonil, 2
Trental s/r, 21, 25
Treosulfan, 25
Triamcinolone, 10 steroid card
Triamco, 14 (urine blue in some lights), 21
Triamterene, 14 (urine blue in some lights), 21
Triazolam, 19
Triclofos sodium, 19
Trientine, 6, 22
Trifluoperazine, 2
Trifluperidol, 2
Trilisate, 12, 21
Trimeprazine, 2
Trimethoprim mixt and tabs, 9
Trimipramine, 2
Trimogal, 9
Trimopan, 9
Triominic, 2
Triperidol, 2
Tripotassium dicitratobismuthate, C, administration, see BNF
Triprolidine, 2
Triprolidine s/r, 2, 25
Triptafen, 2
Triptafen-M, 2
Tropium, 2
Tryptizol caps, 2, 25
Tryptizol mixt and tabs, 2
Tryptophan, 2
Tryptophan pdr, 2, 13
Tuinal, 19

Tylex, 2, max daily dose see BNF

Ubretid, 22
Uniflu Plus Gregovite C, 2
Unigesic, 29
Unimycin, 7, 9, 23
Uniphyllin Continus, 25, 27
Unisomnia, 19
Univer, 25
Urantoin, 9, 14, 21
Uriben, 9, 11
Urisal, 13
Uromide, 9, 14, 22
Ursodeoxycholic acid, 21
Ursofalk, 21
Uticillin, 9

Vaginyl, 4, 9, 21, 25
Valium, 2 or 19
Vallergan, 2
Valoid, 2
V-Cil-K, 9, 23
Veganin, 21, 29
Velosef, 9
Ventide, 8, C, dose
Ventolin Spandets, 25
Veractil, 2
Verapamil s/r, 25
Vertigon, 2, 25
Vibramycin caps, 6, 9, 27
Vibramycin syrup, 6, 9
Vibramycin-D, 6, 9, 13
Vidopen, 9, 23
Viloxazine, 2
Visclair, 5, 22, 25
Viskaldix, 8
Visken, 8
Vita-E Gelucaps, 24
Vivalan, 2
Volmax, 25
Voltarol tabs, 5, 25
Voltarol Retard, 21, 25

Warfarin, 10 anticoagulant card
Warfarin WBP, 10 anticoagulant card
Welldorm tabs, 19, 27

Xanax, 2

Yomesan, 4, 24, 27, C, administration, see BNF

Z Span, 25
Zaditen, 2, 8, 21
Zadstat supps, 4, 9
Zadstat tabs, 4, 9, 21, 25
Zantac dispersible tabs, 13
Zarontin, 2
Zinamide, 8
Zincomed, 21
Zinc sulphate, 21
Zinnat, 9, 21, 25
Zovirax susp and tabs, 9
Zuclopenthixol, 2
Zyloric, 8, 21, 27

Formulary

Obsolete formulae may be found in the *Compendium of Past Formulae 1933–1966* (1971) and *Supplement* (1979) issued by the National Pharmaceutical Association.

BP formulas given here relate to the BP 1980; changes in the BP 1988 have been indicated; the BP 1988 becomes official from 1st December 1988.

Dusting-powders

Chlorhexidine Dusting-powder, BP

Chlorhexidine Hydrochloride	500	mg
Sterilisable Maize Starch	99.5	g

See BP for method of preparation

Ear-drops

10 ml to be dispensed unless otherwise directed
Labelling: in the absence of instructions by the prescriber state—3 or 4 drops to be put into the affected ear

Sodium Bicarbonate Ear-drops, BP

Sodium Bicarbonate	5	g
Glycerol	30	ml
Purified Water, freshly boiled and cooled	to 100	ml

It should be recently prepared

Elixirs

PoM Chloral Elixir, Paediatric, BP

Chloral Hydrate	200	mg
Water for Preparations	0.1	ml
Black Currant Syrup	1	ml
Syrup	to 5	ml

It should be recently prepared
Diluent syrup. The diluted elixir must be freshly prepared

CD Diamorphine and Cocaine Elixir, BPC
(*Note.* See section 4.7.2)

Diamorphine Hydrochloride	5	mg
Cocaine Hydrochloride	5	mg
Alcohol (90%)	0.625	ml
Syrup	1.25	ml
Chloroform Water	to 5	ml

It must be freshly prepared
The proportion of diamorphine hydrochloride may be altered when specified by the prescriber

CD Diamorphine, Cocaine and Chlorpromazine Elixir, BPC
(*Note.* See section 4.7.2)

Diamorphine Hydrochloride	5	mg
Cocaine Hydrochloride	5	mg
Alcohol (90%)	0.625	ml
Chlorpromazine Elixir	1.25	ml
Chloroform Water	to 5	ml

It must be freshly prepared
The proportion of diamorphine hydrochloride may be altered when specified by the prescriber
5 ml contains 6.25 mg of chlorpromazine hydrochloride

PoM Isoniazid Elixir, BPC

Isoniazid	50	mg
Citric Acid Monohydrate	12.5	mg
Sodium Citrate	60	mg
Concentrated Anise Water	0.05	ml
Compound Tartrazine Solution	0.05	ml
Glycerol	1	ml
Chloroform Water, Double-strength	2	ml
Water for Preparations	to 5	ml

Diluent chloroform water. The diluted elixir must be freshly prepared

PoM Morphine and Cocaine Elixir, BPC
(*Note.* See section 4.7.2)

Morphine Hydrochloride	5	mg
Cocaine Hydrochloride	5	mg
Alcohol (90%)	0.625	ml
Syrup	1.25	ml
Chloroform Water	to 5	ml

It should be recently prepared
The proportion of morphine hydrochloride may be altered when specified by the prescriber. If above 13 mg per 5 ml the elixir becomes CD

PoM Morphine, Cocaine and Chlorpromazine Elixir, BPC
(*Note.* See section 4.7.2)

Morphine Hydrochloride	5	mg
Cocaine Hydrochloride	5	mg
Alcohol (90%)	0.625	ml
Chlorpromazine Elixir	1.25	ml
Chloroform Water	to 5	ml

It should be recently prepared
The proportion of morphine hydrochloride may be altered when specified by the prescriber. If above 13 mg per 5 ml the elixir becomes CD
5 ml contains 6.25 mg of chlorpromazine hydrochloride

Gargles

Phenol Gargle

Phenol Glycerin	5	ml
Amaranth Solution	1	ml
Water for preparations	to 100	ml

When diluted the gargle contains about 0.5% w/v of phenol
Directions for use: to be diluted with an equal quantity of warm water
300 ml to be dispensed unless otherwise directed

Inhalations

Labelling: in the absence of instructions by the prescriber, the directions for use given below the preparation should be stated

NHS Menthol and Benzoin Inhalation, BP

Menthol	2	g
Benzoin Inhalation	to 100	ml

Directions for use: add 1 teaspoonful to a pint of hot, not boiling, water and inhale the vapour.
25 ml to be dispensed unless otherwise directed

Menthol and Eucalyptus Inhalation, BP 1980[1]

Menthol	2	g
Eucalyptus Oil	10	ml
Light Magnesium Carbonate	7	g
Water for Preparations	to 100	ml

Directions for use: add 1 teaspoonful to a pint of hot, not boiling, water and inhale the vapour
25 ml to be dispensed unless otherwise directed
[1]Deleted from BP 1988

Linctuses

Codeine Linctus, Paediatric, BPC[1]
(*Note.* See section 3.9.1)

Codeine Linctus	1 ml
Syrup	to 5 ml

5 ml contains 3 mg of codeine phosphate
[1]From 1st December 1988 Paediatric Codeine Linctus BP will become official; it is the same strength as Paediatric Codeine Linctus BPC but may be prepared by diluting Codeine Linctus BP with a suitable vehicle in accordance with the manufacturer's instructions; thus a sugar-free vehicle can be chosen.

CD Diamorphine Linctus, BPC

Diamorphine Hydrochloride	3	mg
Compound Tartrazine Solution	0.06	ml
Glycerol	1.25	ml
Oxymel	1.25	ml
Syrup	to 5	ml

Diluent syrup. It must be freshly prepared

NHS Opiate Squill Linctus, BP
(Gee's Linctus)

Camphorated Opium Tincture	
Squill Oxymel	
Tolu Syrup	of each, equal parts

Diluent syrup
5 ml contains 800 micrograms of anhydrous morphine

NHS Opiate Squill Linctus, Paediatric, BP

Camphorated Opium Tincture	0.3	ml
Squill Oxymel	0.3	ml
Tolu Syrup	0.3	ml
Glycerol	1	ml
Syrup	to 5	ml

Diluent syrup
5 ml contains 150 micrograms of anhydrous morphine

Simple Linctus, BP

Citric Acid Monohydrate	125	mg
Concentrated Anise Water	0.05	ml
Amaranth Solution	0.075	ml
Chloroform Spirit	0.3	ml
Syrup	to 5	ml

Diluent syrup

Simple Linctus, Paediatric, BP

Simple Linctus	1.25	ml
Syrup	to 5	ml

Diluent syrup

Liniments

Methyl Salicylate Liniment, BP

Methyl Salicylate	25	ml
Arachis Oil	to 100	ml

It should be kept in airtight containers in a cool place
100 ml to be dispensed unless otherwise directed

Lotions

Labelling: in the absence of instructions by the prescriber, the directions for use, if any, given below the preparation should be stated

Aluminium Acetate Lotion

Aluminium Acetate Solution[2]	5	ml
Purified Water, freshly boiled and cooled	to 100	ml

It contains about 0.65% of aluminium acetate
It must be freshly prepared
To be used undiluted
500 ml to be dispensed unless otherwise directed
[2] Suppliers Macarthys, Penn, etc. on special order

Formaldehyde Lotion

Formaldehyde Solution	3	ml
Water for Preparations	to 100	ml

It must be freshly prepared
100 ml to be dispensed unless otherwise directed

Salicylic Acid Lotion, BP

Salicylic Acid	2	g
Castor Oil	1	ml
Industrial Methylated Spirit	to 100	ml

Labelling: Caution: this preparation is flammable. Do not use, or dry the hair, near a fire or naked flame
100 ml to be dispensed unless otherwise directed

Silver Nitrate Lotion

Silver Nitrate	500	mg
Purified Water, freshly boiled and cooled	to 100	ml

It must be freshly prepared, and protected from light
Directions for use: to be used undiluted
Labelling: this lotion will produce black stains on skin and clothing
50 ml to be dispensed unless otherwise directed

Sulphur Lotion, Compound, BPC

Precipitated Sulphur	4	g
Quillaia Tincture	0.5	ml
Glycerol	2	ml
Industrial Methylated Spirit	6	ml
Calcium Hydroxide Solution	to 100	ml

200 ml to be dispensed unless otherwise directed

Zinc Sulphate Lotion, BP

Zinc Sulphate	1	g
Amaranth Solution	1	ml
Water for Preparations	to 100	ml

200 ml to be dispensed unless otherwise directed

Mixtures

Labelling: mixtures, other than paediatric mixtures, and others with a dose of 5 ml, should be diluted with water before taking

Aluminium Hydroxide and Belladonna Mixture, BPC

Belladonna Tincture	0.5	ml
Chloroform Spirit	0.25	ml
Aluminium Hydroxide Mixture	to 5	ml

It must be freshly prepared

NHS Ammonia and Ipecacuanha Mixture, BP

Ammonium Bicarbonate	200	mg
Ipecacuanha Tincture	0.3	ml
Concentrated Anise Water	0.05	ml
Concentrated Camphor Water	0.1	ml
Liquorice Liquid Extract	0.5	ml
Chloroform Water, Double-strength	5	ml
Water for Preparations	to 10	ml

It should be recently prepared

Ammonium Chloride Mixture, BP

Ammonium Chloride	1	g
Aromatic Ammonia Solution	0.5	ml
Liquorice Liquid Extract	1	ml
Water for Preparations	to 10	ml

It should be recently prepared
Labelling: to be taken well diluted with water

NHS Ammonium Chloride and Morphine Mixture, BP

Ammonium Chloride	300	mg
Chloroform and Morphine Tincture	0.3	ml
Ammonium Bicarbonate	200	mg
Liquorice Liquid Extract	0.5	ml
Water for Preparations	to 10	ml

It should be recently prepared
10 ml contains 500 micrograms of anhydrous morphine

Belladonna Mixture, Paediatric, BPC

Belladonna Tincture	0.15	ml
Compound Orange Spirit	0.01	ml
Benzoic Acid Solution	0.1	ml
Glycerol	0.5	ml
Syrup	1	ml
Water for Preparations	to 5	ml

It should be recently prepared
5 ml contains 45 micrograms of belladonna alkaloids

Calcium Carbonate Mixture, Compound, Paediatric, BPC

Calcium Carbonate	50	mg
Light Magnesium Carbonate	50	mg
Sodium Bicarbonate	50	mg
Aromatic Cardamom Tincture	0.05	ml
Syrup	0.5	ml
Chloroform Water, Double-strength	2.5	ml
Water for Preparations	to 5	ml

It should be recently prepared

PoM Aromatic Chalk with Opium Mixture, BP
Chalk and Opium Mixture

Chalk	325	mg
Opium Tincture	0.5	ml
Sucrose	650	mg
Tragacanth, in powder	20	mg
Aromatic Ammonia Solution	0.5	ml
Catechu Tincture	0.5	ml
Compound Cardamom Tincture	1	ml
Chloroform Water, Double-strength	5	ml
Water for Preparations	to 10	ml

It should be recently prepared
10 ml contains 5 mg of anhydrous morphine

Chalk Mixture, Paediatric, BP
(*Note*. See Section 1.4.1)

Chalk	100	mg
Tragacanth, in powder	10	mg
Concentrated Cinnamon Water	0.02	ml
Syrup	0.5	ml
Chloroform Water, Double-strength	2.5	ml
Water for Preparations	to 5	ml

It should be recently prepared

PoM Chloral Mixture, BP

Chloral Hydrate	1	g
Syrup	2	ml
Water for Preparations	to 10	ml

It should be recently prepared
Diluent syrup 1 part with water 4 parts. The diluted mixture must be freshly prepared
Labelling: to be taken well diluted with water

Ferrous Sulphate Mixture, Paediatric, BP

Ferrous Sulphate	60	mg
Ascorbic Acid	10	mg
Orange Syrup	0.5	ml
Chloroform Water, Double-strength	2.5	ml
Water for Preparations	to 5	ml

It should be recently prepared. The use of certain types of tap water, particularly those with temporary hardness, may lead to discoloration of this mixture. Freshly boiled and cooled purified water gives a satisfactory colourless or very pale yellow product
Labelling: to be taken well diluted with water

Gentian Mixture, Acid, BPC

Concentrated Compound Gentian Infusion	1	ml
Dilute Hydrochloric Acid	0.5	ml
Chloroform Water, Double-strength	5	ml
Water for Preparations	to 10	ml

It should be recently prepared

Gentian Mixture, Alkaline, BP

Concentrated Compound Gentian Infusion	1	ml
Sodium Bicarbonate	500	mg
Chloroform Water, Double-strength	5	ml
Water for Preparations	to 10	ml

It should be recently prepared

NHS Ipecacuanha and Morphine Mixture, BP 1980[1]

Ipecacuanha Tincture	0.2	ml
Chloroform and Morphine Tincture	0.4	ml
Liquorice Liquid Extract	1	ml
Water for Preparations	to 10	ml

It should be recently prepared
10 ml contains 700 micrograms of anhydrous morphine
[1] Deleted from BP 1988

Ipecacuanha Emetic Mixture, Paediatric, BP

Ipecacuanha Liquid Extract	0.7	ml
Hydrochloric Acid	0.025	ml
Glycerol	1	ml
Syrup	to 10	ml

Available from Macarthys, Penn, etc. on special order

Kaolin and Morphine Mixture, BP

Light Kaolin, or Light Kaolin (Natural)	2	g
Sodium Bicarbonate	500	mg
Chloroform and Morphine Tincture	0.4	ml
Water for Preparations	to 10	ml

It should be recently prepared, unless the kaolin has been sterilised
10 ml contains 700 micrograms of anhydrous morphine

Kaolin Mixture, BP

Light Kaolin, or Light Kaolin (Natural)	2	g
Light Magnesium Carbonate	500	mg
Sodium Bicarbonate	500	mg
Peppermint Emulsion, Concentrated	0.25	ml
Chloroform Water, Double-strength	5	ml
Water for Preparations	to 10	ml

It should be recently prepared, unless the kaolin has been sterilised

Kaolin Mixture, Paediatric, BP 1980[1]
(*Note*. See section 1.4.1)

Light Kaolin, or Light Kaolin (Natural)	1	g
Amaranth Solution	0.05	ml
Benzoic Acid Solution	0.1	ml
Raspberry Syrup	1	ml
Chloroform Water, Double-strength	2.5	ml
Water for Preparations	to 5	ml

It should be recently prepared, unless the kaolin has been sterilised

[1]Deleted from BP 1988

Magnesium Carbonate Mixture, BPC

Light Magnesium Carbonate	500	mg
Sodium Bicarbonate	800	mg
Peppermint Emulsion, Concentrated	0.25	ml
Chloroform Water, Double-strength	5	ml
Water for Preparations	to 10	ml

It should be recently prepared

Magnesium Carbonate Mixture, Aromatic, BP

Light Magnesium Carbonate	300	mg
Sodium Bicarbonate	500	mg
Aromatic Cardamom Tincture	0.3	ml
Chloroform Water, Double-strength	5	ml
Water for Preparations	to 10	ml

It should be recently prepared

Magnesium Sulphate Mixture, BP

Magnesium Sulphate	4	g
Light Magnesium Carbonate	500	mg
Peppermint Emulsion, Concentrated	0.25	ml
Chloroform Water, Double-strength	3	ml
Water for Preparations	to 10	ml

It should be recently prepared

Magnesium Trisilicate and Belladonna Mixture, BPC

| Belladonna Tincture | 0.5 | ml |
| Magnesium Trisilicate Mixture | to 10 | ml |

It must be freshly prepared
5 ml contains 75 micrograms of belladonna alkaloids

Magnesium Trisilicate Mixture, BP

Magnesium Trisilicate	500	mg
Light Magnesium Carbonate	500	mg
Sodium Bicarbonate	500	mg
Peppermint Emulsion, Concentrated	0.25	ml
Chloroform Water, Double-strength	5	ml
Water for Preparations	to 10	ml

It should be recently prepared

CD Methadone Mixture 1 mg/ml (formerly Drug Tariff Formula)

Methadone Hydrochloride	5	mg
Green S and Tartrazine Solution	0.01	ml
Compound Tartrazine Solution	0.04	ml
Syrup, unpreserved	2.5	ml
Chloroform Water, Double-strength to	5	ml

This preparation is 2½ times the strength of Methadone Linctus and is intended only for drug dependent persons for whom treatment is normally ordered on form FP10(H.P.)(ad) or FP10(MDA)

The title includes the strength and prescriptions should be written accordingly

Note. Syrup preserved with hydroxybenzoate esters may be incompatible with methadone hydrochloride

Potassium Citrate Mixture, BP

Potassium Citrate	3	g
Citric Acid Monohydrate	500	mg
Lemon Spirit	0.05	ml
Quillaia Tincture	0.1	ml
Syrup	2.5	ml
Chloroform Water, Double-strength	3	ml
Water for Preparations	to 10	ml

It should be recently prepared
Diluent syrup
Labelling: to be taken well diluted with water

NHS Rhubarb and Soda Mixture, Ammoniated, BP

Rhubarb, in powder	250	mg
Sodium Bicarbonate	800	mg
Ammonium Bicarbonate	200	mg
Peppermint Emulsion, Concentrated	0.25	ml
Chloroform Water, Double-strength	5	ml
Water for Preparations	to 10	ml

It should be recently prepared

NHS Rhubarb Mixture, Compound, BPC[1]

Compound Rhubarb Tincture	1	ml
Light Magnesium Carbonate	500	mg
Sodium Bicarbonate	500	mg
Strong Ginger Tincture	0.3	ml
Chloroform Water, Double-strength	5	ml
Water for Preparations	to 10	ml

It should be recently prepared
[1]From 1st December 1988 Compound Rhubarb Mixture BP will become official; the formula given here should be used for extemporaneous preparation

Sodium Bicarbonate Mixture, Paediatric, BPC

Sodium Bicarbonate	50	mg
Concentrated Dill Water	0.1	ml
Ginger Syrup	0.2	ml
Syrup	1.85	ml
Chloroform Water, Double-strength	2.5	ml
Water for Preparations	to 5	ml

It should be recently prepared

Sodium Salicylate Mixture, BP

Sodium Salicylate	500	mg
Sodium Metabisulphite	10	mg
Concentrated Orange Peel Infusion	0.5	ml
Chloroform Water, Double-strength	5	ml
Water for Preparations	to 10	ml

It should be recently prepared

Sodium Salicylate Mixture, Strong, BP

Sodium Salicylate	1	g
Sodium Metabisulphite	10	mg
Peppermint Emulsion, Concentrated	0.25	ml
Chloroform Water, Double-strength	5	ml
Water for Preparations	to 10	ml

It should be recently prepared

Mouth-washes

Labelling: in the absence of instructions by the prescriber, the directions for use given under the preparation should be stated

Artificial Saliva, DPF

A suitable inert, slightly viscous, aqueous liquid; it may contain an antimicrobial preservative, normal salivary constituents, small amounts of fluoride, and colouring and flavouring agents.
If no formula is specified the following may be suitable.

Sodium Chloride	100	mg
Hypromellose '4500'	1.3	g
Benzalkonium Chloride Solution	0.02	ml
Saccharin Sodium	10	mg
Thymol	10	mg
Peppermint Oil	0.02	ml
Spearmint Oil	0.03	ml
Amaranth Solution	0.1	ml
Water for preparations	to 100	ml

Dose: up to 5 ml as required. Max. 20 ml daily.
200 ml to be dispensed unless otherwise directed
Note. For proprietary preparations, see section 12.3.4

Sodium Chloride Mouth-wash, Compound, BP

Sodium Chloride	1.5	g
Sodium Bicarbonate	1	g
Peppermint Emulsion, Concentrated	2.5	ml
Chloroform Water, Double-strength	50	ml
Water for Preparations	to 100	ml

It should be recently prepared
Directions for use: to be used with an equal quantity of warm water

Nasal Drops

Ephedrine Nasal Drops, BPC

Ephedrine Hydrochloride	500	mg
Chlorbutol	500	mg
Sodium Chloride	500	mg
Water for Preparations	to 100	ml

When Ephedrine Nasal Drops 1% is prescribed, nasal drops containing ephedrine hydrochloride 1 g/100 ml in the same vehicle is supplied

Ointments

25 g to be dispensed unless otherwise directed

Calamine and Coal Tar Ointment, BP

Calamine, finely sifted	12.5	g
Zinc Oxide, finely sifted	12.5	g
Strong Coal Tar Solution	2.5	g
Hydrous Wool Fat	25	g
White Soft Paraffin	47.5	g

Coal Tar and Salicylic Acid Ointment, BP

Coal Tar	2	g
Salicylic Acid	2	g
Emulsifying Wax	11.4	g
White Soft Paraffin	19	g
Coconut Oil	54	g
Polysorbate 80	4	g
Liquid Paraffin	7.6	g

Paraffin Ointment, BP

Hard Paraffin	3	g
White Soft Paraffin	90	g
White Beeswax	2	g
Cetostearyl Alcohol	5	g

Paints

PoM Podophyllin Paint, Compound, BP

Podophyllum Resin	15	g
Compound Benzoin Tincture	to 100	ml

Caution: This paint is very irritant to the eyes
5 ml to be dispensed unless otherwise directed

Oral Powders

Sodium Chloride and Glucose Oral Powder, Compound, BP[1]

Sodium Chloride	1	g
Sodium Bicarbonate	1.5	g
Potassium Chloride	1.5	g
Anhydrous glucose	36.4	g
or Glucose	40	g

To be dissolved in sufficient water to produce 1 litre
It should be dispensed in well-closed containers
Note: Usually in sachets of 8.8 g or 22 g to be dissolved in sufficient water to produce 200 ml or 500 ml respectively; the 8.8-g size is available as a proprietary product—see section 9.2.1.2
[1]From 1st December 1988 this will have the BP title Oral Rehydration Salts—Formula A; the title given here appears as a synonym in the BP 1988; the BP 1988 permits inclusion of suitable flow agents as well as suitable flavouring agents.
Oral Rehydration Salts—Bicarbonate (Formula B) BP 1988 specifies in 1 litre of solution: sodium chloride 3.5 g, potassium chloride 1.5 g, sodium bicarbonate 2.5 g, anhydrous glucose 20 g (*or* glucose 22 g)
Oral Rehydration Salts—Citrate (Formula C) BP 1988 specifies in 1 litre of solution: sodium chloride 3.5 g, potassium chloride 1.5 g, sodium citrate 2.9 g, anhydrous glucose 20 g
Oral Rehydration Salts Formulas B and C are recommended by the World Health Organization and the United Nations Childrens Fund

Solutions

Potassium Permanganate Solution

Potassium Permanganate	100	mg
Water for Preparations	to 100	ml

It must be freshly prepared
One part to be diluted with 7 parts of water, or as directed
The diluted solution contains potassium permanganate about 1 in 8000
500 ml to be dispensed unless otherwise directed

Water for Preparations

Potable water drawn freshly from the supply of a public water undertaking and suitable for drinking. Water obtained from the supply via a local storage tank is unsuitable for this purpose. If such a water supply is not available, or if stored water is the only source of mains water, freshly boiled and cooled purified water should be used instead. It should also be used when the potable water in a district is unsuitable for a particular preparation

Dental Practitioners' Formulary

List of Dental Preparations

The following list has been approved by the appropriate Secretaries of State, and the preparations therein may be prescribed by dental practitioners on form FP14 (GP14 in Scotland).

Acyclovir Cream, DPF
Acyclovir Suspension, DPF
Acyclovir Tablets, DPF
Amoxycillin Capsules, BP
Amoxycillin Injection, DPF
Amoxycillin Mixture, BP
Amoxycillin Oral Powder, DPF
Amoxycillin Tablets, Dispersible, DPF
Amphotericin Lozenges, BP
Amphotericin Mixture, DPF
Amphotericin Ointment, DPF
Amphotericin Tablets, DPF
Ampicillin Capsules, BP
Ampicillin Mixture, BP
Ampicillin Tablets, Paediatric, BP
Artificial Saliva, DPF
Ascorbic Acid Tablets, BP
Aspirin, Paracetamol and Codeine Tablets, DPF
Aspirin Tablets, BP
Aspirin Tablets, Dispersible, BP[1]
Aspirin Tablets, Soluble, BP[2]
Benzocaine Lozenges, DPF
Benzydamine Mouth-wash, DPF
Benzydamine Oral Spray, DPF
Benzylpenicillin Injection, BP
Carbamazepine Tablets, BP
Carmellose Gelatin Paste, DPF
Cephalexin Capsules, BP
Cephalexin Mixture, BP
Cephalexin Tablets, BP
Cephradine Capsules, BP
Cephradine Elixir, DPF
Cephradine Injection, DPF
Chlorhexidine Gluconate gels containing at least 1 per cent
Chlorhexidine Mouth-wash, DPF
Chlorpheniramine Tablets, BP
Choline Salicylate Dental Gel, BP
  (former title Choline Salicylate Dental Paste, DPF)
Clindamycin Capsules, BP
Clindamycin Injection, DPF
Clindamycin Mixture, Paediatric, DPF
Co-codamol Tablets, DPF
Co-codamol Tablets, Dispersible, DPF
Co-codaprin Tablets, Dispersible, BP
Co-dydramol Tablets, DPF
Compound Thymol Glycerin, BP
Co-trimoxazole Mixture, BP
Co-trimoxazole Mixture, Paediatric, BP
Co-trimoxazole Tablets, BP
Co-trimoxazole Tablets, Dispersible, BP
Co-trimoxazole Tablets, Double-strength, DPF
Co-trimoxazole Tablets, Double-strength, Dispersible, DPF
Co-trimoxazole Tablets, Paediatric, BP
Diazepam Capsules, BP
Diazepam Elixir, BP

Diazepam Tablets, BP
Diflunisal Tablets, BP
Dihydrocodeine Tablets, BP
Ephedrine Nasal Drops, BPC
Erythromycin Ethylsuccinate Mixture, DPF
Erythromycin Ethylsuccinate Mixture, Paediatric, DPF
Erythromycin Ethylsuccinate Oral Powder, DPF
Erythromycin Ethylsuccinate Tablets, DPF
Erythromycin Lactobionate Injection, DPF
Erythromycin Stearate Tablets, BP
Erythromycin Tablets, BP
Fusidic Acid Ointment, DPF
  (now called Sodium Fusidate Ointment, BP)
Hydrocortisone Cream, BP
Hydrocortisone Lozenges, BPC
Hydrogen Peroxide Mouth-wash, DPF
Ibuprofen Tablets, BP
Idoxuridine 5% in Dimethyl Sulphoxide, DPF
Lignocaine 5% Ointment, DPF
Lignocaine Viscous Mouth-wash, DPF
Mefenamic Acid Capsules, BP
Menthol and Eucalyptus Inhalation, BP 1980[3]
Metronidazole Mixture, DPF
Metronidazole Tablets, BP
Miconazole Oral Gel, DPF
Mouth-wash Solution-Tablets, DPF
Nitrazepam Tablets, BP
Nystatin Mixture, BP (includes sugar-free formulation)
Nystatin Ointment, BP
Nystatin Pastilles, DPF
Nystatin Tablets, BP
Oxytetracycline Capsules, BP
Oxytetracycline Tablets, BP
Paracetamol Elixir, Paediatric, BP
Paracetamol Tablets, BP
Penicillin Triple Injection, BPC
Pentazocine Tablets, BP
Pethidine Tablets, BP
Phenoxymethylpenicillin Capsules, BP
  (synonym: Penicillin VK Capsules)
Phenoxymethylpenicillin Elixir, BP
  (former title Penicillin V Elixir)
Phenoxymethylpenicillin Tablets, BP
  (synonym: Penicillin VK Tablets)
Povidone-iodine Mouth-wash, DPF
Procaine Penicillin Injection, BP
Procaine Penicillin Injection Fortified, BP
Promethazine Hydrochloride Elixir, BP
Promethazine Hydrochloride Tablets, BP
Sodium Chloride Mouth-wash, Compound, BP
Sodium Fusidate Ointment, BP
  (former title Fusidic Acid Ointment, DPF)
Sodium Perborate Mouth-wash, Buffered, DPF
Temazepam Capsules, DPF
Temazepam Elixir, DPF
Tetracycline Capsules, BP
Tetracycline Mixture, BP
Tetracycline Tablets, BP
Triamcinolone Dental Paste, BP
Vitamin B Tablets, Compound, Strong, BPC
Zinc Sulphate Mouth-wash, DPF

[1] BP 1980 title Dispersible Aspirin Tablets describes both tablets which disperse on addition of water and tablets which effervesce on addition of water; from 1st December 1988 this will only be the title for those which disperse
[2] From 1st December 1988 Soluble Aspirin Tablets BP will be title of dispersible aspirin tablets which effervesce on addition of water
[3] This preparation does not appear in BP 1988

Details of DPF preparations

Preparations on the List of Dental Preparations which are not included in the BP or BPC are described as follows in the DPF.

Although brand names have sometimes been included for identification purposes preparations on the list should be prescribed by non-proprietary name.

PoM **Acyclovir Cream,** (proprietary product: *Zovirax Cream*), acyclovir 5%

PoM **Acyclovir Suspension,** (proprietary product: *Zovirax Suspension*), acyclovir 200 mg/5 ml

PoM **Acyclovir Tablets,** (proprietary product: *Zovirax Tablets*), acyclovir 200 mg and 400 mg

PoM **Amoxycillin Injection,** (proprietary product: *Amoxil Injection*), sterile powder for reconstitution

PoM **Amoxycillin Tablets Dispersible,** (proprietary product: *Amoxil Dispersible Tablets*), amoxycillin 500 mg (as trihydrate)

PoM **Amoxycillin Oral Powder** (proprietary products: *Amoxil Sachets SF*), amoxycillin 750 mg and 3 g (as trihydrate)

PoM **Amphotericin Tablets** (proprietary product: *Fungilin Tablets*), amphotericin 100 mg

PoM **Amphotericin Mixture** (proprietary product: *Fungilin Suspension*), amphotericin 100 mg/ml

PoM **Amphotericin Ointment** (proprietary product: *Fungilin Ointment*), amphotericin 3%, in a suitable basis

Artificial Saliva, consists of a suitable inert, slightly viscous, aqueous liquid; may contain a suitable antimicrobial preservative, normal salivary constituents, small amounts of fluoride, and colouring and flavouring agents (see Formulary)

Aspirin, Paracetamol, and Codeine Tablets, aspirin 250 mg, paracetamol 250 mg, codeine phosphate 6.8 mg

Benzocaine Lozenges, benzocaine 10 mg. They are prepared by compression

Benzydamine Mouth-wash (proprietary product: *Difflam Oral Rinse*), benzydamine hydrochloride 0.15%

Benzydamine Oral Spray, (proprietary product: *Difflam Spray*), benzydamine hydrochloride 0.15%

Carmellose Gelatin Paste (proprietary product: *Orabase Paste*), gelatin, pectin, carmellose sodium, 16.58% of each in a suitable basis

PoM **Cephradine Elixir** (proprietary product: *Velosef Syrup*), cephradine 250 mg/5 ml when reconstituted with water for preparations

PoM **Cephradine Injection** (proprietary product: *Velosef Injection*), sterile powder for reconstitution

Chlorhexidine Gel (proprietary product: *Corsodyl Dental Gel*), chlorhexidine gluconate 1%

Chlorhexidine Mouth-wash (proprietary product: *Corsodyl Mouth-wash*), chlorhexidine gluconate 0.2%

PoM **Clindamycin Mixture, Paediatric** (proprietary product: *Dalacin C Paediatric Suspension*), clindamycin 75 mg (as hydrochloride palmitate)/5 ml when reconstituted with water for preparations

PoM **Clindamycin Injection** (proprietary product: *Dalacin C Phosphate Sterile Solution*), clindamycin 150 mg (as phosphate)/ml

Co-codamol Tablets, codeine phosphate 8 mg, paracetamol 500 mg

Co-codamol Tablets, Dispersible, codeine phosphate 8 mg, paracetamol 500 mg in an effervescent basis

PoM **Co-dydramol Tablets,** dihydrocodeine tartrate 10 mg, paracetamol 500 mg

PoM **Co-trimoxazole Tablets, Double-strength,** co-trimoxazole tablets BP 960 mg

PoM **Co-trimoxazole Tablets, Double-strength, Dispersible** (proprietary product: *Fectrim Forte*), co-trimoxazole tablets BP 960 mg

PoM **Erythromycin Ethylsuccinate Tablets** (proprietary product: *Erythroped A*), erythromycin ethylsuccinate 500 mg

PoM **Erythromycin Ethylsuccinate Mixture** (proprietary product: *Erythroped Suspension*), erythromycin 250 mg and 500 mg (as ethylsuccinate)/5 ml when reconstituted with water for preparations

PoM **Erythromycin Ethylsuccinate Mixture, Paediatric** (proprietary product: *Erythroped PI*), erythromycin 125 mg (as ethylsuccinate)/5 ml when reconstituted with water for preparations

PoM **Erythromycin Ethylsuccinate Oral Powder** (proprietary product: *Erythroped Sugar-free*), erythromycin 250 mg (as ethylsuccinate)/sachet

PoM **Erythromycin Lactobionate Injection** (proprietary product: *Erythrocin IV Lactobionate*), sterile powder for reconstitution

Hydrogen Peroxide Mouth-wash consists of hydrogen peroxide solution (6%), BP

PoM **Idoxuridine 5% in Dimethyl Sulphoxide,** idoxuridine 5% in dimethyl sulphoxide

Lignocaine 5% Ointment, lignocaine 5% in a suitable basis

Lignocaine Viscous Mouth-wash (proprietary product: *Xylocaine Viscous*), anhydrous lignocaine hydrochloride 20 mg/ml in a suitable basis

PoM **Metronidazole Mixture** (proprietary product: *Flagyl S*), metronidazole 200 mg (as benzoate)/5 ml

Miconazole Oral Gel (proprietary product: *Daktarin Oral Gel*), miconazole 25 mg/ml

Mouth-wash Solution-tablets, DPF, consist of tablets which may contain antimicrobial, colouring and flavouring agents in a suitable soluble effervescent basis to make a mouth-wash suitable for dental purposes

PoM **Nystatin Pastilles** (proprietary product: *Nystan Pastilles*), nystatin 100000 units

Povidone-iodine Mouth-wash (proprietary product: *Betadine Mouth-wash*), povidone-iodine 1%

Sodium Perborate Mouth-wash, Buffered (proprietary product: *Bocasan Mouth-wash*), sodium perborate 70%

PoM **Temazepam Capsules,** DPF, (soft gelatin), temazepam 10, 15, 20 and 30 mg

Note. Temazepam Capsules DPF are soft gelatin capsules; dentists have been advised to specify 'soft gelatin' to avoid inadvertent confusion with hard gelatin capsules (see section 4.1.1).

PoM **Temazepam Elixir,** temazepam 10 mg/5 ml

Zinc Sulphate Mouth-wash, consists of zinc sulphate lotion, BP (see Formulary)

Directions for use: dilute 1 part with 4 parts of warm water

Index of Manufacturers

Abbott
Abbott Laboratories Ltd,
Queenborough, Kent ME11 5EL.
Sheerness (0795) 663371

A&H
Allen & Hanburys Ltd,
Horsenden House, Oldfield Lane
North, Greenford, Middx UB6
0HB.
01-422 4225

Alcon
Alcon Laboratories (UK) Ltd,
Imperial Way, Watford WD2
4YR.
Watford (0923) 46133

Alembic Products
Alembic Products Ltd,
Oaklands House, Oaklands
Drive, Sale, Manchester M33
1NS.
061-962 4423

Allergan
Allergan Ltd,
Turnpike Rd, Cressex Industrial
Estate, High Wycombe, Bucks
HP12 3NR.
High Wycombe (0494) 444721

American Hospital Supply
Contact Du Pont.

APS
Approved Prescription Services
Ltd,
Whitcliffe House, Whitcliffe Rd,
Cleckheaton, West Yorks BD19
3BZ.
Cleckheaton (0274) 876776

Armour
Armour Pharmaceutical Co. Ltd,
St. Leonards House,
St. Leonards Rd, Eastbourne,
East Sussex BN21 3YG.
Eastbourne (0323) 21422

Arun
Arun Products Ltd,
The Square, Barnham, Bognor
Regis, West Sussex PO22 0HB.
Bognor Regis (0243) 554141

Ashe
Ashe Consumer Products Ltd,
Ashetree Works, Kingston Rd,
Leatherhead, Surrey KT22 7JZ.
Leatherhead (0372) 376151

Associated Hospital Supply,
Associated Hospital Supply,
PO Box 4, Pershore,
Worcestershire.
Pershore (0386) 554848

Astra
Astra Pharmaceuticals Ltd,
Home Park Estate,
Kings Langley,
Herts WD4 8DH.
Kings Langley (09277) 66191

Ayerst
Contact Wyeth Laboratories.

Bailey, Robert
Robert Bailey & Son PLC,
Dysart St, Great Moor,
Stockport, Cheshire
SK7 7PF.
061-483 1133

Bard
C.R. Bard International Ltd,
Pennywell Industrial Estate,
Sunderland SR4 9EW.
091-534 3131

Baxter
Baxter Healthcare Ltd,
Caxton Way, Thetford, Norfolk
IP24 3SE.
Thetford (0842) 4581

Bayer
Bayer UK Ltd,
Pharmaceutical Business Group,
Bayer House, Strawberry Hill,
Newbury, Berks RG13 1JA.
Newbury (0635) 39000

Baypharm
Contact Bayer.

Beecham
Beecham Research Laboratories,
Beecham House, Great West Rd,
Brentford, Middx TW8 9BD.
01-560 5151

Beecham Products
Contact Beecham Research
Laboratories (see above).

Bencard
Bencard,
Great West Rd, Brentford,
Middx TW8 9BD.
01-560 5151

Bengué
Bengué & Co. Ltd,
Syntex House, St. Ives Rd,
Maidenhead, Berks SL6 1RD.
Maidenhead (0628) 33191

Berk
Berk Pharmaceuticals Ltd,
St. Leonards House,
St. Leonards Rd, Eastbourne,
East Sussex BN21 3YG.
Eastbourne (0323) 641144

Bioglan
Bioglan Laboratories Ltd,
1 The Cam Centre
Wilbury Way, Hitchin,
Herts SG4 0TW.
Hitchin (0462) 38444

Bio-Medical
Bio-Medical Services Ltd.
The White House, Bishopthorpe,
York YO2 1QF.
York (0904) 702704

Biotest
Biotest (UK) Ltd,
171 Alcester Rd, Moseley,
Birmingham B13 8JR.
021-449 5267

Blake
Thomas Blake & Co,
The Byre House, Fearby, near
Masham, North Yorkshire HG4
4NF.
Ripon (0765) 89042

Boehringer Ingelheim
Boehringer Ingelheim Ltd,
Southern Industrial Estate,
Bracknell, Berks RG12 4YS.
Bracknell (0344) 424600

Boots
The Boots Co. PLC,
1 Thane Rd West, Nottingham
NG2 3AA.
Nottingham (0602) 506255

BPL
Blood Products Laboratory,
Dagger Lane, Elstree,
Borehamwood, Herts WD6 3BX.
01-953 6191

Braun
B. Braun (Medical) Ltd,
Evett Close, Stocklake,
Aylesbury, Bucks HP20 1DN.
Aylesbury (0296) 32626

Bridge
Bridge Pharmaceuticals,
Contact Smith Kline & French
Ltd.

Bristol-Myers
Bristol-Myers Pharmaceuticals,
Swakeleys House, Milton Rd,
Ickenham, Uxbridge, Middx
UB10 8NS.
Ruislip (08956) 39911

Britannia
Britannia Pharmaceuticals Ltd,
Forum House, 41–75 Brighton
Rd, Redhill, Surrey RH1 6YS.
Redhill (0737) 773741

BritCair
BritCair Laboratories Ltd,
Progress House, Albert Rd,
Aldershot GU11 1SZ.
Aldershot (0252) 333314

Brocades
Brocades (Great Britain) Ltd,
Brocades House, Pyrford Rd,
West Byfleet, Weybridge, Surrey
KT14 6RA.
Byfleet (09323) 45536

David Bull
David Bull Laboratories,
Harris Rd, Warwick CV34 5GH.
Warwick (0926) 402003

Bullen
C.S. Bullen Ltd,
7 Moss St, Liverpool L6 1EY.
051-207 6995

Burgess
Edwin Burgess Ltd,
Longwick Rd, Princes
Risborough, Aylesbury, Bucks
HP17 9RR.
Princes Risborough (08444) 6881

Cabot
Cabot Ltd,
Copyground Lane, High
Wycombe, Bucks HP12 3HE.
High Wycombe (0494) 37775

Calmic
Calmic Medical Division,
The Wellcome Foundation Ltd,
Crewe Hall, Crewe, Cheshire
CW1 1UB.
Crewe (0270) 583151

Cantassium
The Cantassium Company,
Larkhall Laboratories, 225
Putney Bridge Rd, London SW15
2PY.
01-870 0971

Care
Care Laboratories Ltd,
Lindow House, Beech Lane,
Wilmslow, Cheshire SK9 5HG.
Alderley Edge (0625) 535577

Carlton
Carlton Laboratories (UK) Ltd,
4 Manor Parade, Salvington Rd,
Durrington, Worthing, West
Sussex BN13 2JP.
Worthing (0903) 63235

Carnrick
Carnrick Laboratories,
Acres Down, Furze Hill, London
Rd, Shipston-on-Stour,
Warwickshire.
Shipston-on-Stour (0608) 61610

Ciba
CIBA Laboratories,
Wimblehurst Rd, Horsham, West
Sussex RH12 4AB.
Horsham (0403) 50101

CliniMed
CliniMed Ltd,
Cavell House, Amersham Hill,
High Wycombe, Bucks HP13
6NZ.
High Wycombe (0494) 444027

Coloplast
Coloplast Ltd,
Peterborough Business Park,
Peterborough PE2 0FX.
Peterborough (0733) 239898

Colson & Kay
Colson & Kay Ltd,
Shentonfield Rd, Manchester
M22 4RW.
061-491 1980

Concept
Concept Pharmaceuticals Ltd,
The Old Coach House,
Amersham Hill, High Wycombe,
Bucks HP13 6NQ.
High Wycombe (0494) 451938

Consolidated
Consolidated Chemicals Ltd,
The Industrial Estate, Wrexham,
Clwyd LL13 9PS.
Wrexham (0978) 661351

CooperVision
CooperVision Optics Ltd,
Permalens House, 1 Botley Rd,
Hedge End, Southampton
SO3 3HB.
Botley (04892) 5155

Cow & Gate
Cow & Gate Ltd,
Cow & Gate House, Trowbridge,
Wilts BA14 8YX.
Trowbridge (02214) 68381

Cox Pharmaceuticals
A. H. Cox & Co Ltd,
Whiddon Valley, Barnstaple,
Devon EX32 8NS.
Barnstaple (0271) 75001

CP
CP Pharmaceuticals Ltd,
Red Willow Rd, Wrexham
Industrial Estate, Clwyd LL13
9PX.
Wrexham (0978) 661261
    Also Medical Dept.
    Loughborough (0509) 611001

Crookes
Crookes Products Ltd,
PO Box 94, 1 Thane Rd West,
Nottingham NG2 3AA.
Nottingham (0602) 507431

Cupal
Cupal Ltd,
Pharmaceutical Laboratories,
Blackburn, Lancs BB2 2DX.
Blackburn (0254) 580321

Cutter
Contact Bayer.

Cuxson
Cuxson, Gerrard & Co. (IMS)
Ltd,
Oldbury, Warley,
West Midlands B69 3BB.
021-552 1355

Cyanamid
Division of Lederle Laboratories.
Contact Lederle.

Daniel
Richard Daniel & Son Ltd,
Mansfield Rd, Derby DE1 3RE.
Derby (0332) 40671

DDSA
DDSA Pharmaceuticals Ltd,
310 Old Brompton Rd, London
SW5 9JQ.
01-373 7884

De Witt
De Witt International Ltd,
Seymour Rd, London E10 7LX.
01-539 3334

Degussa
Degussa Pharmaceuticals Ltd,
The Science Park, Milton Rd,
Cambridge CB4 4FY.
Cambridge (0223) 862943

Delandale
Delandale Laboratories Ltd,
Delandale House, 37 Old Dover
Rd, Canterbury, Kent CT1 3JB.
Canterbury (0227) 766353

Dendron
Dendron Ltd,
94 Rickmansworth Rd, Watford,
Herts WD1 7JJ.
Watford (0923) 229251

Dental Health
Dental Health Promotion Ltd,
51 Greencroft Gardens, London
NW6 3II.
01-625 4389

Dermal
Dermal Laboratories Ltd,
Tatmore Place, Gosmore,
Hitchin, Herts SG4 7QR.
Hitchin (0462) 58866

Dermalex
Dermalex Co. Ltd,
Contact Labaz: Sanofi UK Ltd

DF
Duncan, Flockhart & Co. Ltd,
700 Oldfield Lane North,
Greenford, Middx UB6 0HD.
01-422 2331

Dispersa
Dispersa (United Kingdom) Ltd,
Westhead, 10 West St, Alderley
Edge, Cheshire SK9 7XP.
Alderley Edge (0625) 584788

Dista
Dista Products Ltd,
Kingsclere Rd, Basingstoke,
Hants RG21 2XA.
Basingstoke (0256) 52011

Dome/Hollister-Stier
Dome/Hollister-Stier,
Strawberry Hill, Newbury, Berks
RG13 1JA.
Newbury (0635) 39000

Dow Corning
Dow Corning Ltd, Avco House,
Castle St, Reading, Berkshire
RG1 7DZ.
Reading (0734) 596888

Downs
Contact Simcare

Du Pont
Du Pont (UK) Ltd.,
Wedgwood Way, Stevenage,
Herts SG1 4QN.
Stevenage (0438) 734549

Duphar
Duphar Laboratories Ltd,
Gaters Hill, West End,
Southampton SO3 3JD.
Southampton (0703) 472281

Dylade
Contact Fresenius Ltd.

Evans
Evans Medical Ltd,
318 High St North, Dunstable,
Beds LU6 1BE.
Dunstable (0582) 608308

Farillon
Farillon Ltd,
Ashton Rd,
Harold Hill,
Romford, Essex
RM3 8UE.
Ingrebourne (04023) 71136

Farley
Farley Health Products Ltd,
Torr Lane, Plymouth PL3 5UA.
Plymouth (0752) 24151

Farmitalia Carlo Erba
Farmitalia Carlo Erba Ltd,
Italia House, 23 Grosvenor Rd,
St. Albans, Herts AL1 3AW.
St. Albans (0727) 40041

Ferring
Ferring Pharmaceuticals Ltd,
11 Mount Road, Feltham, Middx
TW13 6JG.
01-898 8396

Fisons
Fisons plc,
Pharmaceutical Division,
12 Derby Rd, Loughborough,
Leics LE11 0BB.
Loughborough (0509) 611001

Fox
C. H. Fox Ltd,
22 Tavistock St, London WC2E
7PY
01-240 3111

FP
Family Planning Sales Ltd,
28 Kelburne Rd, Cowley, Oxford
OX4 3SZ.
Oxford (0865) 772486

Francol
Francol Surgical Ltd,
PO Box 2, High Wycombe HP14
4LJ.
Naphill (024024) 2504

Franklin
Franklin Medical Ltd,
PO Box 138, Turnpike Rd, High
Wycombe, Bucks HP12 3NB.
High Wycombe (0494) 32761

Fresenius
Fresenius Ltd,
6 Christleton Court, Stuart Rd,
Manor Park, Runcorn, Cheshire
WA7 1ST.
Runcorn (0928) 580058

Galen
Galen Ltd,
19 Lower Seagoe Industrial
Estate, Portadown, Craigavon,
Armagh BT63 5UA.
Craigavon (0762) 334974

Geigy
Geigy Pharmaceuticals,
Wimblehurst Rd, Horsham, West
Sussex RH12 4AB.
Horsham (0403) 50101

Geistlich
Geistlich Sons Ltd,
Newton Bank, Long Lane,
Chester CH2 3QZ.
Chester (0244) 47534

General Designs
General Designs Ltd,
PO Box 38E, Worcester Park,
Surrey KT4 7LX.
01-337 9366

Generics
Generics (UK) Ltd,
12 Station Close, Potters Bar,
Herts EN6 1TL.
Potters Bar (0707) 44556

GF Supplies
GF Dietary Supplies Ltd,
494 Honeypot Lane,
Stanmore, Middx HA7 1JH.
01-206 0522

Glaxo
Glaxo Laboratories Ltd,
Greenford Rd, Greenford,
Middx UB6 0HE.
01-422 3434

Glenwood
Glenwood Laboratories Ltd,
Jenkins Dale, Chatham,
Kent ME4 5RD.
0634 830535

Gold Cross
Gold Cross Pharmaceuticals,
PO Box 53, Lane End Rd, High
Wycombe, Bucks HP12 4HL.
High Wycombe (0494) 21124

Henleys
Henleys Medical Supplies Ltd,
Alexandra Works, Clarendon
Rd, London N8 0DL.
01-889 3151

Hoechst
Hoechst UK Ltd,
Pharmaceutical Division, Hoechst
House, Salisbury Rd, Hounslow,
Middx TW4 6JH.
01-570 7712

Hough
Hough, Hoseason & Co. Ltd,
22 Chapel St, Levenshulme,
Manchester M19 3PT.
061-224 3271

Hoyt
Hoyt Laboratories division of
Colgate-Palmolive Ltd,
76 Oxford St, London W1A
1EN.
01-580 2030

Hypoguard
Hypoguard Ltd,
Dock Lane, Melton,
Woodbridge, Suffolk IP12 1PE.
Woodbridge (03943) 7333

ICI
ICI Pharmaceuticals (UK),
Southbank, Alderley Park,
Macclesfield, Cheshire
SK10 4TG.
Alderley Edge (0625) 584848

Ilon
Ilon Laboratories (Hamilton)
Ltd,
Lorne St, Hamilton, Strathclyde
ML3 9AB.
Hamilton (0698) 285129

Immuno
Immuno Ltd,
Arctic House, Rye Lane, Dunton
Green, Nr Sevenoaks, Kent
TN14 5HB.
Sevenoaks (0732) 458101

IMS
International Medication Systems
(UK) Ltd,
11 Royal Oak Way South,
Daventry, Northants NN11 5PJ.
Daventry (0327) 703231

Innoxa
Innoxa (England) Ltd,
202 Terminus Rd, Eastbourne,
East Sussex BN21 3DF.
Eastbourne (0323) 639671

International Labs
International Laboratories Ltd,
Charwell House, Wilsom Rd,
Alton, Hants GU34 2TJ.
Alton (0420) 88174

J&J
Johnson & Johnson (Patient Care
Division),
Brunel Way, Slough,
Berks SL1 1XR.
Slough (0753) 31234

Jackson
Ernest Jackson & Co. Ltd,
Crediton, Devon EX17 3AP.
Crediton (03632) 2251

Janssen
Janssen Pharmaceutical Ltd,
Grove, Wantage, Oxon
OX12 0DQ.
Wantage (0235) 772966

K & K-Greeff
K & K-Greeff Ltd,
Suffolk House, George St,
Croydon CR9 3QL.
01-686 0544

K/L
K/L Pharmaceuticals Ltd,
25 Macadam Place, South
Newmoor Industrial Estate,
Irvine KA11 4HP.
Irvine (0294) 215951

KabiVitrum
KabiVitrum Ltd,
KabiVitrum House, Riverside
Way, Uxbridge, Middx UB8
2YF.
Uxbridge (0895) 51144

Kendall
The Kendall Company Ltd,
First Field Lane, Braunton,
N. Devon EX33 1ER.
Braunton (0271) 812561
Note. Contact Boots for
parenteral products.

Kerfoot
Thomas Kerfoot & Co. Ltd,
Vale of Bardsley, Ashton-under-
Lyne, Lancs OL7 9RR.
061-330 4531

Kirby-Warrick
Kirby-Warrick Pharmaceuticals
Ltd,
Mildenhall, Bury St. Edmunds,
Suffolk IP28 7AX.
Mildenhall (0638) 716321

Knoll
Knoll Ltd,
The Brow, Burgess Hill, West
Sussex RH15 9NE.
Burgess Hill (04446) 47554

LAB
Laboratories for Applied Biology
Ltd,
91 Amhurst Park, London N16
5DR.
01-800 2252

Labaz
Labaz: Sanofi UK Ltd,
Floats Rd, Wythenshawe,
Manchester M23 9NF.
061-945 4161

Lagap
Lagap Pharmaceuticals Ltd,
37 Woolmer Way, Bordon,
Hants GU35 9QE.
Bordon (04203) 8301

Lastonet
Lastonet Products Ltd,
Pool, Redruth,
Cornwall TR15 3QN.
Redruth (0209) 215151

Lederle
Lederle Laboratories,
Fareham Rd, Gosport, Hants
PO13 0AS.
Fareham (0329) 224000

Lenton
Lenton Products Ltd,
Radford Mill, Norton St,
Nottingham NG7 3HN.
Nottingham (0602) 420047

Leo
Leo Laboratories Ltd,
Longwick Rd, Princes
Risborough, Aylesbury, Bucks
HP17 9RR.
Princes Risborough (08444) 7333

Lilly
Eli Lilly & Co. Ltd,
Kingsclere Rd, Basingstoke,
Hants RG21 2XA.
Basingstoke (0256) 473241

Lipha
Lipha Pharmaceuticals Ltd,
Harrier House, High St,
Yiewsley, West Drayton, Middx
UB7 7QG.
West Drayton (0895) 449331

Lorex
Lorex Pharmaceuticals Ltd,
Old Bank House, 39 High St,
High Wycombe, Bucks HP11
2AG.
High Wycombe (0494) 26188

Loveridge
J. M. Loveridge PLC,
Southbrook Rd, Southampton
SO9 3LT.
Southampton (0703) 28411

Loxley
Loxley Medical,
Bessingby Estate, Bridlington,
North Humberside YO16 4SU.
Bridlington (0262) 75356

LRC
LRC Products Ltd,
North Circular Rd,
London E4 8QA.
01-527 2377

Lundbeck
Lundbeck Ltd,
Lundbeck House, Hastings St,
Luton LU1 5BE.
Luton (0582) 416565

3M
Contact Riker.

Macarthys
Macarthys Medical Ltd,
Chesham House, Chesham
Close, Romford RM1 4JX.
Romford (0708) 46033

Martindale
Martindale Pharmaceuticals Ltd,
Chesham House, Chesham
Close, Romford RM1 4JX.
Romford (0708) 46033

M&B
May & Baker Pharmaceuticals,
Rhone Poulenc Ltd,
Rainham Road South,
Dagenham, Essex RM10 7XS.
01-592 3060

MCP
MCP Pharmaceuticals Ltd,
Simpson Parkway, Kirkton
Campus, Livingston, West
Lothian EH54 7BH.
Livingston (0506) 412512

Medo
Medo Pharmaceuticals Ltd,
East St, Chesham, Bucks HP5
1DG.
Chesham (0494) 772071

Merck
E. Merck Ltd,
Winchester Rd, Four Marks,
Alton, Hants GU34 5HG.
Alton (0420) 64011

Merieux
Merieux UK,
Clivemont House, Clivemont Rd,
Maidenhead, Berks SL6 7BU.
Maidenhead (0628) 785291

Merrell
Merrell Dow Pharmaceuticals
Ltd,
Stana Place, Fairfield Ave,
Staines, Middx TW18 4SX.
Staines (0784) 61600

Milupa
Milupa Ltd, Milupa House,
Uxbridge Rd, Hillingdon,
Middx UB10 0NE.
01-573 9966

Molnlycke
Molnlycke Ltd, Southfields Rd,
Dunstable, Beds LU6 3EJ.
Dunstable (0582) 600211

Morson
Thomas Morson Pharmaceuticals,
Hertford Rd, Hoddesdon, Herts
EN11 9BU.
Hoddesdon (0992) 467272

MSD
Merck Sharp & Dohme Ltd,
Hertford Rd,
Hoddesdon, Herts EN11 9BU.
Hoddesdon (0992) 467272

Napp
Napp Laboratories Ltd,
Cambridge Science Park, Milton
Rd, Cambridge CB4 4GW.
Cambridge (0223) 358888

Nestlé
Nestlé Co. Ltd,
St. George's House, Croydon
CR9 1NR.
01-686 3333

Neutrogena
Neutrogena (UK) Ltd,
2 Mansfield Rd, South Croydon,
Surrey CR2 6HN.
01-680 5504

Nicholas
Nicholas Laboratories Ltd,
PO Box 17, Slough SL1 4AU.
Slough (0753) 23971

Nordic
Nordic Pharmaceuticals Ltd,
11 Mount Road, Feltham, Middx
TW13 6JG.
01-898 8665

Nordisk
Nordisk-UK,
Highview House, Tattenham
Crescent, Epsom, Surrey KT18
5QJ.
Burgh Heath (07373) 60621

Norgine
Norgine Ltd,
116 London Rd, Headington,
Oxford OX3 9BA.
Oxford (0865) 750717

Norma
Norma Chemicals Ltd,
1a Frognal, London NW3 6AN.
01-435 7627

Norton
H. N. Norton & Co. Ltd,
Patman House, George Lane,
South Woodford, London E18
2LY.
01-530 6421

Norwich Eaton
Norwich Eaton Ltd,
Hedley House, St Nicholas Ave,
Gosforth, Newcastle-Upon-Tyne
NE3 1LR.
091-279 2100

Novo
Novo Laboratories Ltd,
Ringway House, Bell Rd,
Daneshill East, Basingstoke,
Hants RG24 0QN.
Basingstoke (0256) 55055

Nycomed
Nycomed (UK) Ltd,
Nycomed House, 2111 Coventry
Rd, Sheldon, Birmingham
B26 3EA.
021-742 2444

Oral B
Oral B Laboratories Ltd,
Gatehouse Rd, Aylesbury, Bucks
HP19 3ED.
Aylesbury (0296) 32601

Organon
Organon Laboratories Ltd,
Cambridge Science Park,
Milton Rd, Cambridge,
CB4 4FL.
Cambridge (0223) 355545

Organon-Teknika
Organon-Teknika Ltd,
Cambridge Science Park,
Milton Rd, Cambridge,
CB4 4FL.
Cambridge (0223) 313650

Ortho-Cilag
Ortho-Cilag Pharmaceutical Ltd,
PO Box 79, Saunderton, High
Wycombe, Bucks HP14 4HJ.
Naphill (024024) 3541

Paines & Byrne
Paines & Byrne Ltd,
Pabyrn Laboratories, 177 Bilton
Rd, Perivale, Greenford, Middx
UB6 7HG.
01-997 1143

Panpharma
Panpharma Ltd,
Hayes Gate House, 27 Uxbridge
Rd, Hayes, Middx UB4 0JN.
01-561 8774

P-D
Parke-Davis Medical,
Mitchell House, Southampton
Rd, Eastleigh, Hants SO5 5RY.
Eastleigh (0703) 619791

Penn
Penn Pharmaceuticals Ltd,
Buckingham House, Church Rd,
Penn, High Wycombe, Bucks
HP10 8LN.
Penn (049481) 6163

Perstorp
Perstorp Pharma Ltd,
Wound-Care Division, 44 Bell
St, Henley-on-Thames, Oxon
RG9 2BA.
0491-578171

Pfizer
Pfizer Ltd,
Sandwich, Kent CT13 9NJ.
Sandwich (0304) 616161

Pharmacia
Pharmacia Ltd,
Pharmacia House, Midsummer
Boulevard, Milton Keynes MK9
3HP.
Milton Keynes (0908) 661101

Pharmax
Pharmax Ltd,
Bourne Rd, Bexley, Kent DA5
1NX.
Dartford (0322) 91321

Philip Harris
Philip Harris Medical Ltd,
Hazelwell Lane, Birmingham
B30 2PS.
021-458 2020

Phillips Yeast
Phillips Yeast Products Ltd,
Park Royal Rd, London NW10
7JX.
01-965 7533

Pickles
J. Pickles & Sons,
Beech House, 62 High St,
Knaresborough, N. Yorks HG5
0EA.
Harrogate (0423) 867314

Plough
Plough UK,
SP Consumer Products Ltd,
182-204 St. John St, London
EC1P 1DH.
01-253 2030

Porton
Porton Products Ltd,
CAMR, Porton Down,
Salisbury, Wilts SP4 0JG.
0980-610787

Procea
Procea,
Alexandra Road, Dublin 1.
Dublin (0001) 741741

Quinoderm Ltd
Quinoderm Ltd,
Manchester Rd, Oldham, Lancs
OL8 4PB.
061-624 9307

Radiol
Radiol Chemicals Ltd,
Stepfield, Witham, Essex CM8
3AG.
Witham (0376) 512538

R&C
Reckitt & Colman,
Pharmaceutical Division,
Dansom Lane, Hull HU8 7DS.
Hull (0482) 26151

Regent
Regent Laboratories Ltd,
Cunard Rd, London NW10 6PN.
01-965 3637

Rendell
W. J. Rendell Ltd,
Ickleford Manor, Hitchin,
Herts SG5 3XE.
Hitchin (0462) 32596

Richardson-Vicks
Richardson-Vicks Ltd,
Rusham Park, Whitehall Lane,
Egham, Surrey TW20 9NW.
0784-34422

Riker
Riker Laboratories,
Morley St, Loughborough, Leics
LE11 1EP.
Loughborough (0509) 268181

Robins
A. H. Robins Co. Ltd,
Sussex Manor Business Park,
Gatwick Rd, Crawley,
West Sussex RH10 2NH.
Crawley (0293) 560161

Robinsons
Robinsons of Chesterfield,
Wheat Bridge, Chesterfield,
Derbyshire S40 2AD.
Chesterfield (0246) 31101

RoC
Laboratoires RoC UK Ltd,
13 Grosvenor Crescent, London
SW1X 7EE.
01-235 9411

Roche
Roche Products Ltd,
PO Box 8, Welwyn Garden City,
Herts AL7 3AY.
Welwyn Garden (0707) 328128

Rona
Contact: Lipha Pharmaceuticals
Ltd

Rorer
Rorer Pharmaceuticals,
St Leonards House, St Leonards
Road, Eastbourne,
East Sussex BN21 3YG
Eastbourne (0323) 21422

Roterpharma
Roterpharma Ltd,
Littleton House, Littleton Rd,
Ashford, Middx.
Ashford (07842) 48279

Roussel
Roussel Laboratories Ltd,
Broadwater Park, North Orbital
Rd, Uxbridge, Middx UB9 5HP.
Uxbridge (0895) 834343

RP Drugs
RP Drugs Ltd,
RPD House, Yorkdale Industrial
Park, Braithwaite St, Leeds LS11
9XE.
Leeds (0532) 441400

Rybar
Rybar Laboratories Ltd,
30 Sycamore Rd, Amersham,
Bucks HP6 5DR.
Amersham (02403) 22741

Sallis
E. Sallis Ltd,
Vernon Works, Waterford St,
Old Basford, Nottingham
NG6 0DH.
Nottingham (0602) 787841

Salt
Salt & Son Ltd,
Saltair House, Lord St,
Nechells, Birmingham
B7 4DS.
021-359 5123

Sandoz
Sandoz Products Ltd,
Sandoz House, 98 The Centre,
Feltham, Middx TW13 4EP.
01-890 1366

Sas
Sas Pharmaceuticals Ltd,
Sas Group House, 45 Wycombe
End, Beaconsfield, Bucks HP9
1LZ.
Beaconsfield (04946) 78181

Schering
Schering Health Care Ltd,
The Brow, Burgess Hill, West
Sussex RH15 9NE.
Burgess Hill (04446) 6011

Scholl
Scholl (UK),
182 St. John St,
London EC1P 1DH.
01-253 2030

Schwarz
Schwarz Pharmaceuticals Ltd,
East St, Chesham, Bucks HP5
1DG.
Chesham (0494) 772071

Scientific Hospital Supplies
Scientific Hospital Supplies Ltd,
38 Queensland St, Liverpool L7
3JG.
051-708 8008

Searle
Searle Pharmaceuticals,
PO Box 53, Lane End Rd, High
Wycombe, Bucks HP12 4HL.
High Wycombe (0494) 21124

Serono
Serono Laboratories (UK) Ltd,
2 Tewin Court, Welwyn Garden
City, Herts AL7 1AU.
Welwyn Garden (0707) 331972

Servier
Servier Laboratories Ltd,
Fulmer Hall, Windmill Rd,
Fulmer, Slough SL3 6HH.
Fulmer (02816) 2566

Seton
Seton Products Ltd,
Tubiton House, Medlock St,
Oldham, Lancs OL1 3HS.
061-652 2222

Seton-Prebbles
As Seton

Shannon
T.J. Shannon Ltd,
59 Bradford St, Bolton BL2
1HT.
Bolton (0204) 21789

Shaw
A.H. Shaw and Partners Ltd,
Manor Rd, Ossett, West
Yorkshire WF5 0LF.
Wakefield (0924) 273474

Shire
Shire Pharmaceuticals Ltd,
13 Bridge St, Andover, Hants
SP10 1BE.
(0264) 333455

Simcare
Simcare,
Peter Rd, Lancing,
West Sussex BN15 8TJ.
Lancing (0903) 761122

Simpla
Simpla Plastics Ltd,
Phoenix Estate, Caerphilly Rd,
Cardiff CF4 4XG.
Cardiff (0222) 62100

Sinclair
Sinclair Pharmaceuticals Ltd,
Borough Rd, Godalming, Surrey
GU7 2AB.
Guildford (0483) 426644

SK&F
Smith Kline & French
Laboratories Ltd,
Welwyn Garden City, Herts AL7
1EY.
Welwyn Garden (0707) 325111

S&N
Smith & Nephew Medical Ltd,
PO Box 81, 101 Hessle Rd, Hull
HU3 2BN.
Hull (0482) 25181

S&N Pharm.
Smith & Nephew
Pharmaceuticals Ltd,
Bampton Rd, Harold Hill,
Romford, Essex RM3 8SL.
Ingrebourne (04023) 49333

Spodefell
Spodefell Ltd,
5 Inverness Mews, London W2
3QJ.
01-229 9125

Squibb
E. R. Squibb & Sons Ltd,
Squibb House, 141 Staines Rd,
Hounslow, Middx TW3 3JA.
01-572 7422

Squibb Surgicare
As Squibb

Stafford-Miller
Stafford-Miller Ltd,
Stafford-Miller House, The
Common, Hatfield, Herts AL10
0NZ.
Hatfield (07072) 61151

STD Pharmaceutical
STD Pharmaceutical Products
Ltd,
Fields Yard, Plough Lane,
Hereford HR4 0EL.
Hereford (0432) 53684

Steinhard
M. A. Steinhard Ltd,
32 Minerva Rd, London NW10
6HJ.
01-965 0194

Steriseal
Steriseal Ltd,
Thornhill Rd, Redditch,
Worcs B98 9NL.
0527-64222

Sterling Health
Sterling Health,
Sterling-Winthrop House,
Onslow St, Guildford, Surrey
GU1 4YS.
Guildford (0483) 65599

Sterling Research
Sterling Research Laboratories,
Sterling-Winthrop House,
Onslow St, Guildford, Surrey
GU1 4YS.
Guildford (0483) 505515

Stiefel
Stiefel Laboratories (UK) Ltd,
Holtspur Lane, Wooburn Green,
High Wycombe,
Bucks HP10 0AU
High Wycombe (06285) 24966

Stuart
Stuart Pharmaceuticals Ltd,
Stuart House, 50 Alderley Rd,
Wilmslow, Cheshire SK9 1RE
Wilmslow (0625) 535999

Syntex
Syntex Pharmaceuticals Ltd,
Syntex House, St. Ives Rd,
Maidenhead, Berks SL6 1RD.
Maidenhead (0628) 33191

Thackraycare
Thackraycare Ltd,
45–47 Great George St,
Leeds LS1 3BB.
Leeds (0532) 430028

Thames
Thames Laboratories Ltd,
The Old Blue School, 5 Lower
Square, Isleworth, Middx
TW7 6RL.
01-568 7071

Thornton & Ross
Thornton & Ross Ltd,
Linthwaite Laboratories,
Huddersfield HD7 5QH.
Huddersfield (0484) 842217

Tillotts
Tillotts Laboratories,
Unit 24, Henlow Trading Estate,
Henlow, Beds SG16 6DS.
Henlow Camp (0462) 813933

Torbet
Torbet Laboratories,
Boughton Lane, Maidstone,
Kent ME25 9QQ.
Maidstone (0860) 319350

Tosara
Tosara Products (UK) Ltd,
PO Box 5, 70 Picton Rd,
Liverpool L15 4NS
051-733 4432

Townendale
Townendale Pharmaceuticals,
PO Box 53, Harrogate, North
Yorks HG1 5BD.
Harrogate (0423) 62593

Travenol
Contact Baxter

Typharm
Typharm Ltd,
14 Parkstone Rd, Poole, Dorset.
Ringwood (04254) 79711

Ultra
Ultra Laboratories Ltd,
Trinity Trading Estate,
Tribune Drive, Sittingbourne,
Kent ME10 2PG.
Sittingbourne (0795) 70953

Ultrapharm
Ultrapharm Ltd,
PO Box 18, Henley-on-Thames,
Oxon RG9 2AW.
Henley-on-Thames (0491) 578016

Unigreg
Unigreg Ltd,
Spa House, 15–17 Worple Rd,
Wimbledon, London SW19 4JS.
01-946 9871

Unimed
Unimed Pharmaceuticals Ltd,
24 Steynton Ave, Bexley, Kent
DA5 3HP.
01-309 7003

United Medical
United Medical,
Staines House, 158 High St,
Staines, Middx TW18 4AZ.
(0784) 61533

Upjohn
Upjohn Ltd,
Fleming Way, Crawley, West
Sussex RH10 2NJ.
Crawley (0293) 31133

Vernon-Carus
Vernon-Carus Ltd,
Penwortham Mills, Preston,
Lancs PR1 9SN.
Preston (0772) 744493

Vestric
Vestric Ltd,
West Lane, Runcorn, Cheshire
WA7 2PE.
Runcorn (0928) 717070

Vitabiotics
Vitabiotics Ltd,
122 Mount Pleasant, Alperton,
Middx HA0 1UG.
01-903 5541

Wallace Mfg
Wallace Manufacturing Chemists
Ltd,
1a Frognal, London NW3 6AN.
01-435 7627

WBP
WB Pharmaceuticals Ltd,
Contact Boehringer Ingelheim
Ltd.

Welfare Foods
Welfare Foods (Stockport) Ltd,
63 London Rd South, Poynton,
Stockport, Cheshire SK12 1LA.
Poynton (0625) 877387

Wellcome
Wellcome Medical Division,
The Wellcome Foundation Ltd,
Crewe Hall, Crewe, Cheshire
CW1 1UB.
Crewe (0270) 583151

Windsor
Windsor Pharmaceuticals Ltd,
Ellesfield Avenue, Bracknell,
Berkshire RG12 4YS.
Bracknell (0344) 484448

Winthrop
Winthrop Laboratories,
Sterling-Winthrop House,
Onslow St, Guildford, Surrey
GU1 4YS.
Guildford (0483) 505515

W-L
Warner Lambert Health Care,
Mitchell House, Southampton
Rd, Eastleigh, Hants SO5 5RY.
Eastleigh (0703) 619791

Wyeth
Wyeth Laboratories,
Huntercombe Lane South,
Taplow, Maidenhead, Berks SL6
0PH.
Burnham (06286) 4377

Zyma
Zyma (UK) Ltd,
Westhead, 10 West St, Alderley
Edge, Cheshire SK9 7XP.
Alderley Edge (0625) 584788

Index

Clomipramine, 155, **156**
  infusion table, 450
Clomocycline, 207
Clonazepam, 180, **181**
  infusion table, 450
  interactions, 439
  status epilepticus, 183
Clonidine, 92
  hypertension, 92
  interactions, 435
  menopausal flushing, 179
  migraine, 179
  Tourette syndrome, 189
Clopamide, 75
Clopenthixol *see*
  Zuclopenthixol
Clopixol, 151, 152
Clopixol Conc, 152
Clorazepate, 141, **142**
Clorhexitulle, 401
Clotrimazole,
  anogenital, 267
  ear, 352
  skin, 387
  vaginal, 266–7
Cloxacillin, 197
  infusion table, 450
Coal tar, 375
  preparations, **376**, 477
  scalp, 383
Co-amilozide, xiii
Cobadex, 367
Cobalin-H, 296
Coban, 399
Co-Betaloc preparations, 89
Cobutolin preparations, 115
Cocaine, 161
  analgesic elixirs, 174
  eye-drops, 348
    homatropine and, 348
  local anaesthesia, 429
  poisoning by, 42
  prescribing for addicts, 9
Co-codamol tablets, 170
  dispersible, 170
Co-codaprin, tablets, 170
  dispersible, 170
Co-danthramer preparations, 64
Co-danthrusate capsules, 64
Codeine, 174
  breast-feeding, 33
  cough suppressant, 132
  diabetic diarrhoea, 241
  diarrhoea, 58, **59**
  pain, 172, **174**
  preparations, 59, **174**
    compound, 170
    linctuses, **133**, 474
  renal failure, 21
  ulcerative colitis, 60
Codelsol, **248**, 330
Co-dergocrine mesylate, 102
Codis, 170
Co-dydramol tablets, 170
Coeliac disease, ACBS, 460
Cogentin, 188
Cohepress, 399

Cohesive extensible bandages, 399
Colchicine, 333
  breast-feeding, 33
  renal failure, 21
  tablets, 333
Cold remedies, drug inter-
  actions, 435, 438
Cold sores, ACBS, 462
Colds, 317, 355
Colestid, 110
Colestipol, 110
  interactions, 433
Colifoam, 61
Colistin, 212
  bladder, 276
  eye-drops, 349
  infusion table, 450
  interactions, 444
  renal failure, 21
  skin, 385
Colitis,
  pseudomembranous, 60
  ulcerative, **60**, 245
Collodion,
  flexible, 363
  salicylic acid, 381
Collodions, 363
Colloid dressings, 401
Colofac, 53
Cologel, 63
Colomycin, 212, 385
Colostomy Plus, 70
Colpermin, 53
Coltapaste, 399
Colven, 53
  renal failure, 21
Coma
  hyperglycaemic, 240
  hyperosmolar nonketotic,
    240
  hypoglycaemic, 240
  hypothyroid, 242
  insulin, 240
  ketoacidotic, 240
Combantrin, 232
Comfeel, 70
Comfeel Ulcus, 402
Comox, 215
Complement Continus, 316
Concavit, 319
Concordin, 157
Conjugated oestrogens, 250
Conjunctivitis, 193, 341
  allergic, 343
Conjuvac preparations, 128
Conn's syndrome, 77
Conotrane, 363
Conova 30, 269
Consumer Protection Act, xi
Contact lenses, 350
  effects of drugs, 350
Containers, child-resistant, 3
Contents, vi
Contraceptives, 268–74
  oral, 268–72
    breast-feeding, 33
    combined, 268–71

Contraceptives, oral
  (*continued*)—
    elective surgery, 269
    forgotten pill, 269, 271
    interactions, 435–8,
      441–2
    liver disease, 15
    low-oestrogen, 268,
      269
    phased, 269, 270
    pregnancy, 28
    postcoital, 269
    progestogen-only, 271–2
    spermicidal, 272
Contrast media, adverse reac-
  tion reporting, 10
Controlled drugs, 7–9
  notification of addicts, 9
  prescribing, 7
  see also preparations ident-
    ified by **CD** throughout
    BNF
  travel abroad, 8
Controvlar, 253
Conversions, approximate, 6
Convulsions,
  febrile, 185
  poisoning and, 38
  see also Epilepsy
Coparvax, 287
Copholco, 134
Coppertone, preparations, 382
Co-proxamol, 170
  poisoning, 40
  tablets, 170, 172
Cordarone X, 82
Cordilox, 101
Corgard, 88
Corgaretic preparations, 89
Corlan, 357
Corn oil, 307
Corn starch, 307
Corneal ulcer, 341
Cornflour, 307
Coro-Nitro Spray, 97
Corsodyl, 359
Cortacream, 399
Cortelan, 247
Cortenema, 61
Corticosteroids, 243–9
  acne, 378
  adrenal suppression, 245
  adrenalectomy, 243
  allergic emergencies, 129
  allergy, 245
    nasal, 354
  alternate-day therapy, 246
  anaesthesia, 246, 416
  aphthous ulcers, 356, **357**
  asthma, 114, **121**
  blood disorders, 296
  breast-feeding, 33
  cautions, 245
  children, 246
  Crohn's disease, 60
  ear, 351
  epilepsy, 181
  equivalent doses, 244